The Complete Directory for People with Chronic Illness

2009/10

Ninth Edition

The Complete Directory for People with Chronic Illness

- Condition Descriptions
- Associations
- Publications
- Research Centers
- Support Groups
- Websites

A SEDGWICK PRESS Book

Grey House Publishing

PUBLISHER: Leslie Mackenzie
EDITOR: Richard Gottlieb
EDITORIAL DIRECTOR: Laura Mars-Proietti
MEDICAL EDITORS: Dr. Alan Friedman, Dr. Kristine Schmidt

PRODUCTION MANAGER: Jennifer Consolato
PRODUCTION ASSISTANTS: Jael Powell, Kristen Thatcher, Erica Schneider

MARKETING DIRECTOR: Jessica Moody

A Sedgwick Press Book
Grey House Publishing, Inc.
4919 Route 22
Amenia, NY 12501
518.789.8700
FAX 845.373.6390
www.greyhouse.com
E-MAIL: books @greyhouse.com

First edition published 1994
Ninth edition published 2009
Printed in the USA

The complete directory for people with chronic illness – 1994-2009

1053 p.; 27.5 cm
Other title: DCI
ISSN: 1080-7659

1. Chronic diseases – United States – Directories. 2. Chronic Diseases – Bibliography. 3. Chronic Disease – United States – Directories. 4. Social Support – United States – Directories. 5. Information Services – United States – Directories. 6. Rehabilitation – United States – Directories. I. Title: DCI.

RC108 .C645
616' .0025'73 96-640803

ISBN: 978-1-59237-415-1

Table of Contents

Introduction

Recent surveys report that 125 million Americans currently suffer from a chronic illness. This number is expected to reach 157 million by the year 2020. This ninth edition of *The Complete Directory for People with Chronic Illness* offers a comprehensive overview of 89 specific chronic illnesses from Addison's to Wilson's Disease, from Allergies to Cancer. Each chapter includes an easy-to-understand medical description, plus a wide range of condition-specific support services and information resources that deal with the variety of issues concerning those with a chronic illness, as well as those who support the chronic illness community.

The word "chronic" comes from the Greek word *chronos* meaning time (with Greek god Chronos often depicted as Father Time). Chronic illness, as defined by The Chronic Illness Alliance, is *. . . an illness that is permanent or lasts a long time. It may get slowly worse over time . . . or . . . go away. It may cause permanent changes to the body* (and) *will certainly affect the person's quality of life.* The National Center for Health Statistics defines chronic illness as *one lasting 3 months or more.*

However you define chronic illness, this directory will prove invaluable in dealing with the many aspects of chronic disease. It includes associations, state agencies, libraries & resource centers, research centers, magazines, newsletters, audio & video, hot lines, support groups and valuable web sites. In addition to chapters dealing with specific medical conditions, this edition includes several chapters designed to help all those in the chronic illness community, including wish foundations, death and bereavement groups and medical homes – primary care settings in the community.

The Complete Directory for People with Chronic Illness, helpful to both those dealing for the first time with the stress and crucial need-to-know issues that accompany chronic illness, as well as those already coping with chronic disease. *. . . How can I connect with others with Diabetes? . . . Which Cancer treatment is best for me? . . . What do I need to know about "protecting" my 2-year old, who was just diagnosed with a heart condition? . . . Why is my husband (or wife) angrier than our chronically ill child?* You'll find ways to answer these questions and more in the pages of this edition.

In addition to patients and their families, this directory is invaluable to hospital and medical center personnel, especially discharge planners, social service workers, and disability coordinators. *The Complete Directory for People with Chronic Illness* is full of resources crucial for people with chronic illness as they transition from diagnosis to home, work, and community life.

The Complete Directory for People with Chronic Illness provides, in one source, **comprehensive, critical, immediate information** – from national associations to children's books. It's the perfect choice for both those who find navigating the Internet overwhelming (we've done it for you) along with those who feel comfortable surfing the Net (we provide valuable, specific web sites).

New Article

Next Steps After Your Diagnosis offers information and support in five steps:

1. Take the Time you Need *2. Get the Support you Need*
3. Talk with Your Doctor *4. Seek out Information*
5. Decide on a Treatment Plan

This detailed, 21-page article, which also includes valuable phone numbers and web sites, follows the **Chronic Illness Body System** table in the front matter.

Arrangement

The 89 chronic condition chapters are arranged alphabetically by name of the disorder. Each chapter begins with a brief description of the illness, written in layman's terms with its cause, symptoms and treatment options.

Following each description are disease-specific resources. Chapters contain the following: **National Associations; State Agencies; Libraries & Resource Centers; Magazines, Newsletters, Pamphlets; Research Centers; Books for Adults; Books for Children; Support Groups & Hotlines; Audio & Video Resources; Web Sites.**

This reference work details 10,855 listings – 173 more than last edition. Thousands of listings have been verified or updated, with more data points, including web sites and additional key executives. All listings include the name of the organization or publication, address, phone, fax number (8,585), e-mail (5,518) and web site (8,631). You will find 8,633 key executives, a brief description, and other details, depending on the type of listing. Associations, for example, may include year founded and yearly dues, while Magazines may include frequency and number of pages.

In addition to the 89 chapters of chronic illnesses, *The Complete Directory for People with Chronic Illness* includes a cross reference chart of **Body Systems** in the front of the book, and several supplemental chapters in the back of the book designed to provide value to individuals with chronic illness and their families. They include: **General Resources –** information relevant to the general chronic illness community; **Wish Foundations** – organizations devoted to granting wishes of chronically and terminally ill children; **Death & Bereavement** – support services for those who find themselves or a loved one close to death or grieving a loss.

Rounding out this directory are two indexes that allow users additional access to the information: **Entry Name Index** and **Geographic Index**.

The Complete Directory for People with Chronic Illness is also available for subscription on G.O.L.D. – Grey House OnLine Database. Subscribers to G.O.L.D. can access their subscription via the Internet and do customized searches that make finding information quicker and easier. Visit http://gold.greyhouse.com for more information.

CHRONIC ILLNESS — BODY SYSTEM

The following chart lists the chronic illness and its body system(s) or disorder category. Chronic conditions not listed do not fall into a specific system(s). A cross-reference chart follows that lists the information in reverse — body system or disorder categories followed by chronic illnesses.

CHRONIC ILLNESS	BODY SYSTEM/DISORDER CATEGORY
Addison's Disease	Endocrine
Aging	Cells & Tissues
AIDS/HIV	Immune, Infectious Disease
Allergies	Immune
Alzheimer's Disease	Nervous
Amyotrophic Lateral Sclerosis	Nervous
Arthritis	Muscular, Skeletal
Asthma	Respiratory
Ataxia	Nervous
Attention Deficit Hyperactivity Disorder	Behavioral, Developmental
Autistic Spectrum Disorders	Behavioral, Developmental
Brain Tumors	Nervous
Carpal Tunnel Syndrome	Muscular, Skeletal, Nervous
Celiac Disease	Gastrointestinal
Cerebral Palsy	Nervous, Muscular
Chronic Fatigue Syndrome	Immune
Chronic Pain	Nervous
Cooley's Anemia (Thalassemia)	Blood
Congential Heart Disease	Cardiovascular
Crohn's Disease	Gastrointestinal
Cystic Fibrosis	Respiratory, Gastrointestinal
Diabetes Mellitus	Endocrine
Down Syndrome	Developmental
Eating Disorders (Anorexia Nervosa, Bulimia)	Behavioral
Endometriosis	Reproductive
Fabry Disease	Gastrointestinal
Fibromyalgia Syndrome	Muscular, Skeletal
Gastrointestinal Disorders	Gastrointestinal
Gaucher's Disease	Gastrointestinal
Growth Disorders	Developmental
Head Injuries	Nervous
Hearing Impairment	Sensory
Heart Disease	Cardiovascular
Hemophilia	Blood
Hepatitis	Infectious Disease
Hydrocephalus	Nervous
Hypertension	Cardiovascular
Impotence	Reproductive
Incontinence	Urinary
Infertility	Reproductive
Kidney Disease	Gastrointestinal

CHRONIC ILLNESS	BODY SYSTEM/DISORDER CATEGORY
Liver Disease	Gastrointestinal
Lung Disease	Respiratory
Lupus Erythematosus	Cells & Tissues
Mental Illness: General	Behavioral
Mental Illness: Depression	Behavioral
Mental Illness: Schizophrenia	Behavioral
Migraine	Cardiovascular, Nervous
Multiple Sclerosis	Nervous
Muscular Dystrophy	Nervous
Myasthenia Gravis	Nervous
Neurofibromatosis	Nervous, Dermatologic
Osteogenesis Imperfecta	Skeletal
Osteoporosis	Skeletal
Paget's Disease	Skeletal
Parkinson Disease	Nervous
Post-Polio Syndrome	Muscular, Skeletal
Prader Willi Syndrome	Endocrine
Raynaud's Disease	Cardiovascular
Sarcoidosis	Cells & Tissues, Respiratory
Scleroderma	Cells & Tissues, Dermatologic
Scoliosis	Skeletal
Seizure Disorders	Nervous
Sexually Transmitted Diseases	Reproductive, Infectious Disease
Sickle Cell Disease	Blood
Sjogren's Syndrome	Cells & Tissues
Skin Disorders	Dermatologic
Sleep Disorders	Dermatologic
Spina Bifida	Nervous, Skeletal
Spinal Cord Injuries	Nervous
Stroke	Nervous
Substance Abuse	Behavioral
Tay Sachs Disease	Nervous
Thyroid Disease	Endorcrine
Tick-Borne Disease	Infectious Disease
Tourette Syndrome	Nervous
Tuberculosis	Respiratory, Infectious Disease
Tuberous Sclerosis	Nervous, Dermatologic
Turner Syndrome	Endocrine
Ulcerative Colitis	Gastrointestinal
Visual Impairment	Sensory
War Syndromes	Nervous
Wilson's Disease	Gastrointestinal

BY BODY SYSTEM/DISORDER CATEGORY

Behavioral
Attention Deficit Disorder; Autism; Eating Disorders; Mental Illness; Substance Abuse

Blood
Cooley's Anemia; Hemophilia; Sickle Cell Disease

Cardiovascular
Heart Disease; Hypertension; Migraine; Raynaud's Disease

Cells & Tissues
Aging; Lupus Erythematosus; Scleroderma; Sjogren's Syndrome

Dermatologic
Neurofibromatosis; Scleroderma; Skin Disorders; Tuberous Sclerosis

Developmental
Attention Deficit Disorder; Autism; Down Syndrome; Growth Disorders

Endocrine
Addison's Disease; Diabetes; Turner Syndrome

Gastrointestinal
Celiac Disease; Crohn's Disease; Cystic Fibrosis; Fabry Disease; Gastrointestinal Disorders; Gaucher's Disease; Kidney Disease; Liver Disease; Ulcerative Colitis

Immune
AIDS; Allergies; Chronic Fatigue Syndrome

Infectious Disease
AIDS; Hepatitis; Sexually Transmitted Diseases; Tick-Borne Disease; Tuberculosis

Muscular
Arthritis; Carpal Tunnel Syndrome; Cerebral Palsy; Fibromyalgia Syndrome; Post-Polio Syndrome

Nervous
Agent Orange Related Injuries; Alzheimer's Disease; Amyotrophic Lateral Sclerosis; Ataxia; Brain Tumors; Carpal Tunnel Syndrome; Cerebral Palsy; Charcot-Marie-Tooth Disorder; Chronic Pain; Gulf War Syndrome; Head Injuries; Hydrocephalus; Multiple Sclerosis; Muscular Dystrophy; Myasthenia Gravis; Neurofibromatosis; Parkinson Disease; Seizure Disorders; Spina Bifida; Spinal Cord Injuries; Stroke; Tourette Syndrome; Tuberous Sclerosis

Reproductive
Endometriosis; Impotence; Infertility; Sexually Transmitted Diseases

Respiratory
Asthma; Cystic Fibrosis; Lung Disease; Tuberculosis

Skeletal
Arthritis; Carpal Tunnel Syndrome; Fibromyalgia Syndrome; Osteognesis Imperfecta; Osteoporosis; Paget's Disease; Post-Polio Syndrome; Scoliosis; Spina Bifida

Sensory
Hearing Impairment; Visual Impairment

Urinary
Incontinence

Next Steps After Your Diagnosis: Finding Information and Support

Introduction

Your doctor* gave you a diagnosis that could change your life. This article can help you take the next steps.

Every person is different, of course, and every person's disease or condition will affect them differently. But research shows that after getting a diagnosis, many people have some of the same reactions and needs.

About this Article

Next Steps After Your Diagnosis offers general advice for people with almost any disease or condition. And it has tips to help you learn more about your specific problem and how it can be treated.

The information in this article is presented in a simple way to help you scan the material and read only what you need right now. Organizations, publications, and other resources are included if you would like to know more. The on-line version www.ahrq.gov/consumer/diaginfo.htm has many additional resources and their Internet links.

Five Basic Steps

This article describes five basic steps to help you cope with your diagnosis, make decisions, and get on with your life.

Step 1: Take the time you need.
Do not rush important decisions about your health. In most cases, you will have time to carefully examine your options and decide what is best for you.

Step 2: Get the support you need.
Look for support from family and friends, people who are going through the same thing you are, and those who have "been there." They can help you cope with your situation and make informed decisions.

* Your medical care might come from a doctor, nurse, physician assistant, or another kind of clinician or health care practitioner. To keep it simple, in this article we use the term "doctor" to refer to any of these professionals with whom you might interact.

Step 3: Talk with your doctor.
Good communication with your doctor can help you feel more satisfied with the care you receive. Research shows it can even have a positive effect on things such as symptoms and pain. Getting a "second opinion" may help you feel more confident about your care.

Step 4: Seek out information.
When learning about your health problem and its treatment, look for information that is based on a careful review of the latest scientific findings published in medical journals.

Step 5: Decide on a treatment plan.
Work with your doctor to decide on a treatment plan that best meets your needs.

As you take each step, remember this: Research shows that patients who are more involved in their health care tend to get better results and be more satisfied.

Step 1:
Take the time you need.

Take time to breathe.
Don't panic, and don't
feel pressured into making
a rush decision.
Alexis, cancer survivor

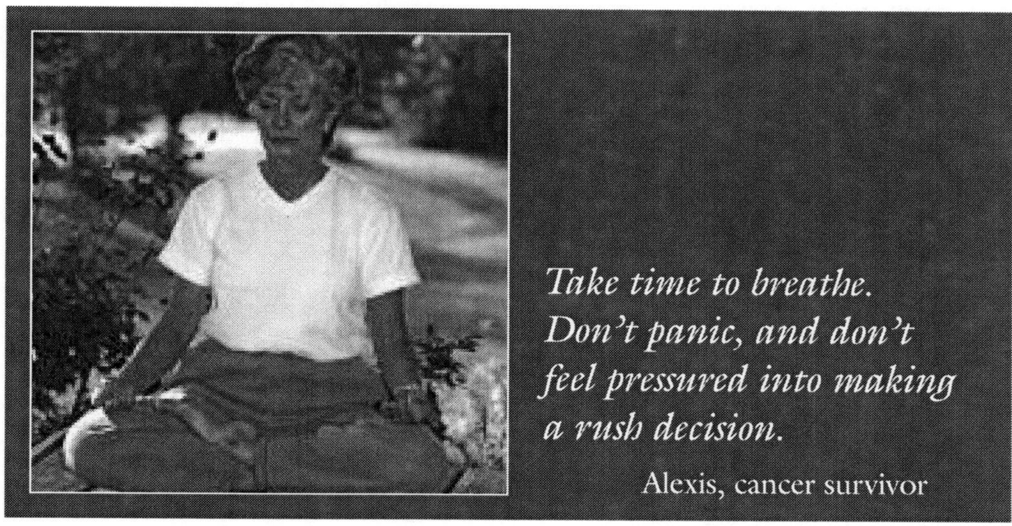

A diagnosis can change your life in an instant.

Like so many other people in your situation, you might be feeling one or more of the following emotions after getting your diagnosis:

- Afraid
- Alone
- Angry
- Anxious
- Ashamed
- Confused
- Depressed
- Helpless
- In denial
- Numb
- Overwhelmed
- Panicky
- Powerless
- Relieved (that you finally know what's wrong)
- Sad
- Shocked
- Stressed

It is perfectly normal to have these feelings. It is also normal, and very common, to have trouble taking in and understanding information after you receive the news – especially if the diagnosis was a surprise. And it can be even harder to make decisions about treating or managing your disease or condition.

Take time to make your decisions.

No matter how the news of your diagnosis has affected you, do not rush into a decision. In most cases, you do not need to take action right away. Ask your doctor how much time you can safely take.

Taking the time you need to make decisions can help you:

- Feel less anxious and stressed.
- Avoid depression.
- Cope with your condition.
- Feel more in control of your situation.
- Play a key role in decisions about your treatment.

Step 2:
Get the support you need.

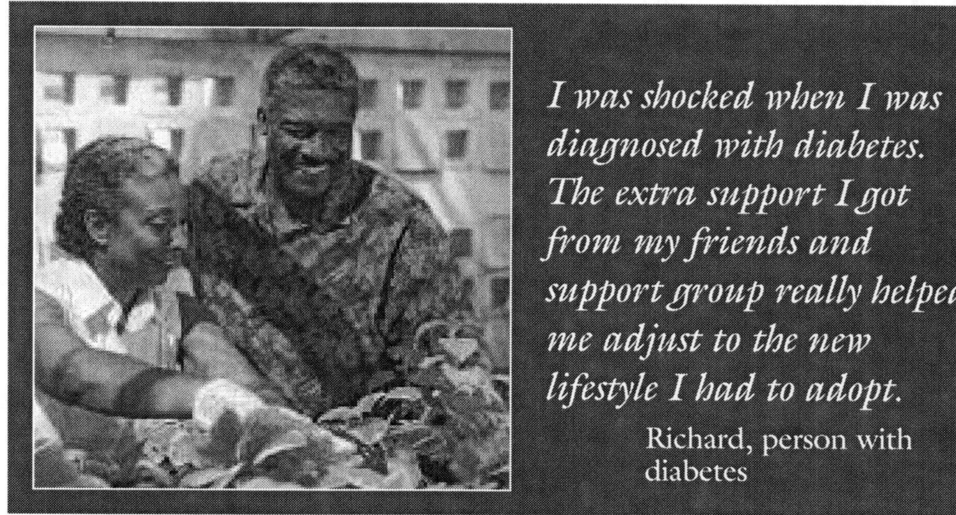

> *I was shocked when I was diagnosed with diabetes. The extra support I got from my friends and support group really helped me adjust to the new lifestyle I had to adopt.*
>
> Richard, person with diabetes

You do not have to go through it alone.

Sometimes the emotional side of illness can be just as hard to deal with as the physical side. You may have fears or concerns. You may feel overwhelmed. No matter what your situation, having other people to turn to will help you know you are not alone.

Here are the kinds of support you might want to seek:

Family and friends.

Talking to family and friends you feel close to can help you cope with your illness or condition. Just knowing that someone is there can be a comfort.

Sometimes it is hard to ask for help. And sometimes your family and friends want to help, but they do not want to intrude, or they do not know how to ask or what to offer. Think about specific ways people can help you. One idea is to ask someone to come with you to a doctor's appointment to help ask questions, take notes, and talk with you afterward.

If you do not have family or friends who can provide support, other people or groups can.

Support or self-help groups.

Support groups are made up of people with the same disease or condition who get together to share information and concerns and to help one another. Support groups may or may not be led by experts. Self-help groups are similar to support groups but usually are led by the participants. The names "support group" and "self-help group" sometimes are used to refer to either kind.

Research on support groups shows that participants feel less anxious, experience less depression, have a better quality of life, and have more success coping with their disease or condition. Similar findings have been reported for self-help groups.

On-line support or self-help groups.

The Internet has support or self-help groups for people whose concerns and situations may be similar to yours. You can also find "message boards," where you can post questions and get answers. These on-line communities can help you connect with people who can give you support and provide information.

But be careful. Not every idea or treatment you come across in these groups will be scientifically proven to be safe and effective. If you read about something interesting and new, check it out with your doctor.

Counselor or therapist.

A good counselor or therapist can help you cope with sadness, depression, and feelings of being overwhelmed. If you think this kind of help might be right for you, ask your doctor or other health care professional to recommend someone in your area.

People like you.

You might want to meet and talk with someone in your own situation. Someone who has "been there" can talk about the real-life outcomes of their treatment choices as well as how they have learned to live with their disease or condition. Some advocacy or support groups can help you make this kind of contact.

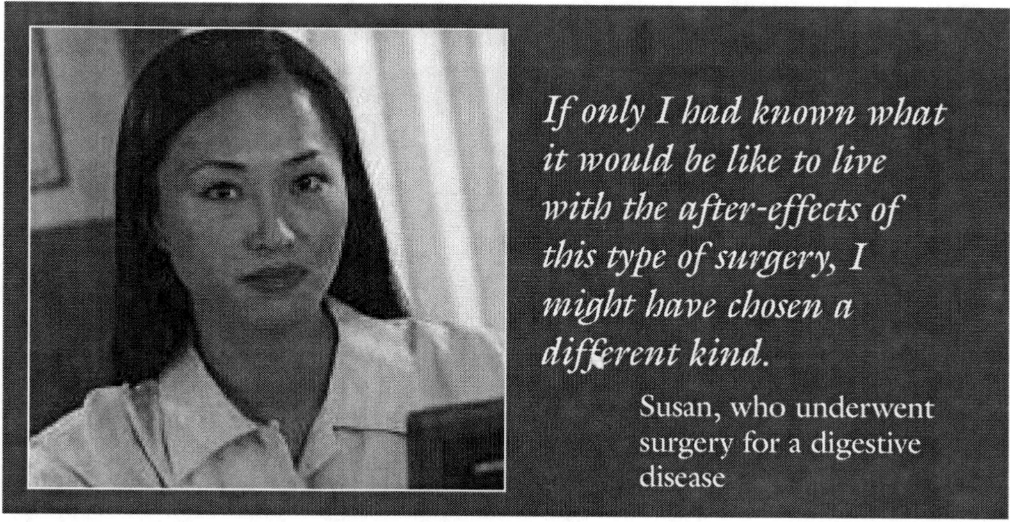

Help is available.

Take advantage of the support that is available to you. See "Where to Find More Information" on page xxx for specific places to find support. An expanded list appears in the on-line version of this article at www.ahrq.gov/consumer/diaginfo.htm.

Step 3: Talk with your doctor.

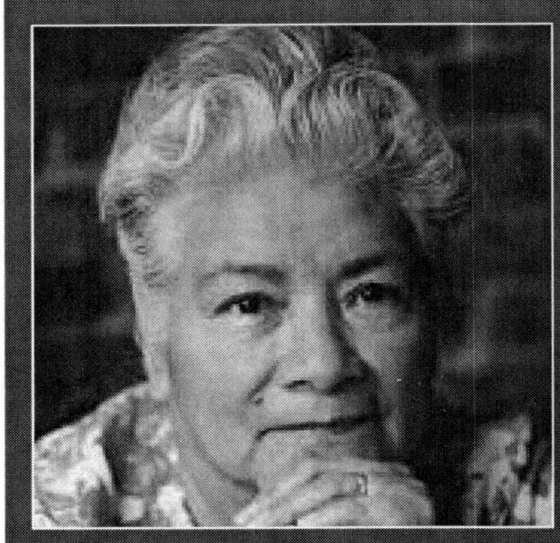

I had trouble understanding what my doctor was telling me. The words were too technical, and there was too much to absorb. I finally asked her to slow down and keep it simple. That helped a lot.

Dana, person with heart disease

Your doctor is your partner in health care.

You probably have many questions about your disease or condition. The first person to ask is your doctor.

It is fine to seek more information from other sources; in fact, it is important to do so. But consider your doctor your partner in health care—someone who can discuss your situation with you, explain your options, and help you make decisions that are right for you.

It is not always easy to feel comfortable around doctors. But research has shown that good communication with your doctor can actually be good for your health. It can help you to:

- Feel more satisfied with the care you receive.
- Have better outcomes (end results), such as reduced pain and better recovery from symptoms.

Being an active member of your health care team also helps to reduce your chances of medical mistakes, and it helps you get high-quality care.

Of course, good communication is a two-way street. Here are some ways to help make the most of the time you spend with your doctor.

Prepare for your visit.

- Think about what you want to get out of your appointment. Write down all your questions and concerns. Some suggested questions are listed on page xxiii.
- Prepare and bring to your doctor visit a list of all the medicines you take.
- Consider bringing along a trusted relative or friend. This person can help ask questions, take notes, and help you remember and understand everything once you leave the doctor's office.

Give information to your doctor.

- Do not wait to be asked.
- Tell your doctor everything he or she needs to know about your health—even the things that might make you feel embarrassed or uncomfortable.
- Tell your doctor how you are feeling—both physically and emotionally.
- Tell your doctor if you are feeling depressed or overwhelmed.

Get information from your doctor.

- Ask questions about anything that concerns you. Keep asking until you understand the answers. If you do not, your doctor may think you understand everything that is said.
- Ask your doctor to draw pictures if that will help you understand something.
- Take notes.
- Tape record your doctor visit, if that will be helpful to you. But first ask your doctor if this is okay.
- Ask your doctor to recommend resources such as Web sites, booklets, or tapes with more information about your disease or condition.

Also see "Ten Important Questions to Ask Your Doctor After a Diagnosis," on page xxiii.

Do not hesitate to seek a second opinion.

A second opinion is when another doctor examines your medical records and gives his or her views about your condition and how it should be treated. You might want a second opinion to:

- Be clear about what you have.
- Know all of your treatment choices.
- Have another doctor look at your choices with you.

It is not pushy or rude to want a second opinion. Most doctors will understand that you need more information before making important decisions about your health.

Check to see whether your health plan covers a second opinion. In some cases, health plans require second opinions.

Here are some ways to find a doctor for a second opinion:

- Ask your doctor. Request someone who does not work in the same office, because doctors who work together tend to share similar views.
- Contact your health plan or your local hospital, medical society, or medical school.
- Use the Doctor Finder on-line service of the American Medical Association at www.ama-assn.org.

Get information about next steps.

- Get the results of any tests or procedures. Discuss the meaning of these results with your doctor.
- Make sure you understand what will happen if you need surgery.
- Talk with your doctor about which hospital is best for your health care needs.

Finally, if you are not satisfied with your doctor, you can do two things: (1) talk with your doctor and try to work things out, and/or (2) switch doctors, if you are able to. It is very important to feel confident about your care.

To learn more, see "Where to Find More Information" on page xxx. The online version of this article includes additional resources.

Ten Important Questions to Ask Your Doctor After a Diagnosis

These 10 basic questions can help you understand your disease or condition, how it might be treated, and what you need to know and do before making treatment decisions.

1. What is the technical name of my disease or condition, and what does it mean in plain English?

   ____

2. What is my prognosis (outlook for the future)?

   ____

3. How soon do I need to make a decision about treatment?

   ____

4. Will I need any additional tests, and if so what kind and when?

   ____

5. What are my treatment options?

   ____

6. What are the pros and cons of my treatment options?

   ____

7. Is there a clinical trial (research study) that is right for me? (See page xxiv.)

   ____

8. Now that I have this diagnosis, what changes will I need to make in my daily life?

   ____

9. What organizations do you recommend for support and information?

   ____

10. What resources (booklets, Web sites, audiotapes, videos, DVDs, etc.) do you recommend for further information?

    ____

Step 4:
Seek out information.

I'm really glad I took the time to research my options. It stopped me from jumping into a treatment that would have been completely wrong for me.
Seth, prostate cancer survivor

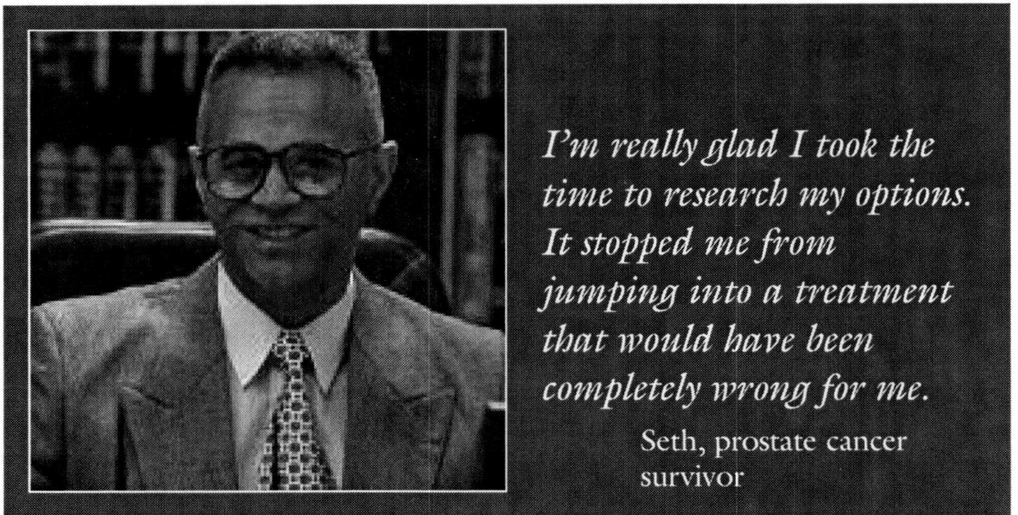

Now that you know your treatment options, you can learn which ones are backed up by the best scientific evidence. "Evidence-based" information—that is, information that is based on a careful review of the latest scientific findings in medical journals—can help you make decisions about the best possible treatments for you.

Evidence-based information comes from research on people like you.

Evidence-based information about treatments generally comes from two major types of scientific studies:

- **Clinical trials** are research studies on human volunteers to test new drugs or other treatments. Participants are randomly assigned to different treatment groups. Some get the research treatment, and others get a standard treatment or may be given a placebo (a medicine that has no effect), or no treatment. The results are compared to learn whether the new treatment is safe and effective.
- **Outcomes research** looks at the impact of treatments and other health care on health outcomes (end results) for patients and populations. End results include effects that people care about, such as changes in their quality of life.

Take advantage of the evidence-based information that is available.

Health information is everywhere—in books, newspapers, and magazines, and on the Internet, television, and radio. However, not all information is good information. Your best bets for sources of evidence-based information include the Federal Government, national nonprofit organizations, medical specialty groups, medical schools, and university medical centers.

Some resources are listed below, grouped by type of information. See "Where to Find More Information" on page xxx for additional ideas. The online version of Next Steps After Your Diagnosis lists many more, and includes links to Internet sites.

Information.

Information about your disease or condition and its treatment is available from many sources. Here are some of the most reliable:

- **healthfinder®:** www.healthfinder.gov/organizations/OrgListing.asp
  The healthfinder® site—sponsored by the U.S. Department of Health and Human Services—offers carefully selected health information Web sites from government agencies, clearinghouses, nonprofit groups, and universities.
- **Health Information Resource Database:**
  www.health.gov/nhic/#Referrals
  Sponsored by the National Health Information Center, this database includes 1,400 organizations and government offices that provide health information upon request. Information is also available over the telephone at 800-336-4797.
- **MEDLINEplus®:** www.nlm.nih.gov/medlineplus
  MedlinePlus® has extensive information from the National Institutes of Health and other trusted sources on over 650 diseases and conditions. The site includes many additional features.
- **National nonprofit groups** such as the American Heart Association, American Cancer Society, and American Diabetes Association can be valuable sources of reliable information. Many have chapters nationwide. Check your phone book for a local chapter in your community. The Health Information Resource Database (www.health.gov/nhic/#Referrals) can help you find national offices of nonprofit groups.

- **Health or medical libraries** run by government, hospitals, professional groups, and other reliable organizations often welcome consumers. For a list of libraries in your area, go to the MedlinePlus® "Find a Library" page at http://www.nlm.nih.gov/medlineplus/libraries.html.

Current medical research.

You can find the latest medical research in medical journals at your local health or medical library, and in some cases, on the Internet. Here are two major online sources of medical articles:

- **MEDLINE/PubMed®:** http://www.ncbi.nlm.nih.gov/entrez/query.fcgi
  PubMed® is the National Library of Medicine's database of references to more than 14 million articles published in 4,800 medical and scientific journals. All of the listings have information to help you find the articles at a health or medical library. Many listings also have short summaries of the article (abstracts), and some have links to the full article. The article might be free, or it might require a fee charged by the publisher.
- **PubMed Central:** http://www.pubmedcentral.nih.gov/
  PubMed Central is the National Library of Medicine's database of journal articles that are available free of charge to users.

Clinical trials.

Perhaps you wonder whether there is a clinical trial that is right for you. Or you may want to learn about results from previous clinical trials that might be relevant to your situation. Here are two reliable resources:

- **ClinicalTrials.gov:** http://clinicaltrials.gov/ct/g
  ClinicalTrials.gov provides regularly updated information about federally and privately supported clinical research on people who volunteer to participate. The site has information about a trial's purpose, who may participate, locations, and phone numbers for more details. The site also describes the clinical trial process and includes news about recent clinical trial results.
- **Cochrane Collaboration:** www.cochrane.org
  The Cochrane Collaboration writes summaries ("reviews") about evidence from clinical trials to help people make informed decisions. You can search and read the review abstracts free of charge at http://www.cochrane.org/

reviews/index.htm. Or you can read plain-English consumer summaries of the reviews at www.informedhealthonline.org.

The full Cochrane reviews are available only by subscription. Check with your local medical or health library (see page xxxii) [link back to library section in on-line version] to see whether you can access the full reviews there.

Outcomes research.

Outcomes research provides research about benefits, risks, and outcomes (end results) of treatments so that patients and their doctors can make better informed decisions. The U.S. Agency for Healthcare Research and Quality (AHRQ) supports improvements in health outcomes through research, and sponsors products that result from research such as:

- **National Guideline Clearinghouse™:** www.guideline.gov
  The National Guideline Clearinghouse™ is a database of evidence-based clinical practice guidelines and related documents. Clinical practice guidelines are documents designed to help doctors and patients make decisions about appropriate health care for specific diseases or conditions. The clearinghouse was originally created by AHRQ in partnership with the American Medical Association and America's Health Insurance Plans.

Steer clear of deceptive ads and information.

While searching for information either on or off the Internet, beware of "miracle" treatments and cures. They can cost you money and your health, especially if you delay or refuse proper treatment. Here are some tip-offs that a product truly is too good to be true:

- Phrases such as "scientific breakthrough," "miraculous cure," "exclusive product," "secret formula," or "ancient ingredient."
- Claims that the product treats a wide range of ailments.
- Use of impressive-sounding medical terms. These often cover up a lack of good science behind the product.
- Case histories from consumers claiming "amazing" results.
- Claims that the product is available from only one source, and for a limited time only.

- Claims of a "money-back guarantee."
- Claims that others are trying to keep the product off the market.
- Ads that fail to list the company's name, address, or other contact information.

To learn more about finding evidence-based information, see "Where to Find More Information," page xxx. The on-line edition of this article has many additional resources.

Step 5:
Decide on a treatment plan.

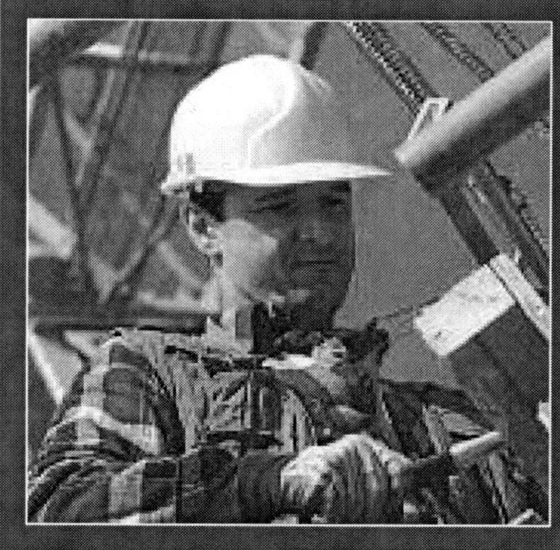

My doctor told me I had done one of the hardest but most important things a patient has to do: Face up to the diagnosis and make decisions. It feels good to be where I am now.

Bob, person with a neurological disorder

At this point, you have learned about your disease or condition and how it can be treated or managed. Your information may have come from the following sources:

- Your doctor.
- Second opinions from one or more other doctors.
- Other people who are or were in the same situation as you.
- Information sources such as Web sites, health or medical libraries, and nonprofit groups.

Work with your doctor to make decisions.

When you are ready to make treatment decisions, you and your doctor can discuss:

- Which treatments have been found to work well, or not work well, for your particular condition.
- The pros and cons of each treatment option.

Make sure that your doctor knows your preferences and feelings about the different treatments – for example, whether you prefer medicine over surgery.

Once you and your doctor decide on one or more treatments that are right for you, you can work together to develop a treatment plan. This plan will include everything that will be done to treat or manage your disease or condition—including what you need to do to make the plan work.

Remember, being an active member of your health care team helps to reduce your chances of medical mistakes, and it helps you get high-quality care.

Take another deep breath.

You have taken important steps to cope with your diagnosis, make decisions, and get on with your life. Remember two things:

- Call on others for support as you need it.
- Make use of evidence-based information for any future health decisions.

Where to Find More Information

Get the support you need.

American Self-Help Group Clearinghouse
http://mentalhelp.net/selfhelp/

National Board for Certified Counselors (NBCC)
3 Terrace Way, Suite D
Greensboro, NC 27403-3660
336-547-0607.
www.nbcc.org

National Institute of Mental Health
Public Information and Communications Branch
6001 Executive Boulevard, Room 8184, MSC 9663
Bethesda, MD 20892-9663
Phone: 866-615-6464 (toll-free)
TTY: 301-443-8431
http://www.nimh.nih.gov/HealthInformation/GettingHelp.cfm

Talk to your doctor.

Be an Active Member of Your Health Care Team. Food and Drug Administration. 2004. http://www.fda.gov/cder/consumerinfo/active_member.htm. Phone: 888-INFO-FDA (888-463-6332).

Be Informed: Questions to Ask Your Doctor Before You Have Surgery. Agency for Healthcare Quality and Research. 1995. http://www.ahrq.gov/consumer/surgery.htm. Phone: 800-358-9295.

Five Steps to Safer Health Care. Agency for Healthcare Research and Quality. 2003. http://www.ahrq.gov/consumer/5steps.htm. Phone: 800-358-9295.

Getting a Second Opinion Before Surgery. Centers for Medicare & Medicaid Services. 2004. www.medicare.gov/Publications/Pubs/pdf/02173.pdf. Phone: 800-MEDICARE (800-633-4227).

How to Get a Second Opinion. National Women's Health Information Center. 2003. http://www.4woman.gov/pub/secondopinion.htm. Phone: 1-800-994-WOMAN.

Quick Tips – When Planning for Surgery. Agency for Healthcare Research and Quality. 2002. http://www.ahrq.gov/consumer/quicktips/tipsurgery.htm. Phone: 800-358-9295.

Quick Tips – When Talking with Your Doctor. Agency for Healthcare Research and Quality. 2002. http://www.ahrq.gov/consumer/quicktips/doctalk.htm. Phone: 800-358-9295.

Talking with Your Doctor: A Guide for Older People. National Institute on Aging. 2002. www.niapublications.org/pubs/talking/index.asp. Phone: 800-222-2225. |

Seek out information.

2005 Toll-Free Numbers for Health Information. National Health Information Center. www.health.gov/nhic/pubs/tollfree.htm. Phone: 800-336-4797.

AARP Health Guide. AARP. 2004. www.aarp.org/health/healthguide. Phone: 888-OUR-AARP (888-687-2277).

HON Code of Conduct (HONcode) for Medical and Health Web Sites Health on the Net Foundation. http://www.hon.ch/HONcode/

How to Evaluate Health Information on the Internet: Questions and Answers. National Cancer Institute. 2003. http://cis.nci.nih.gov/fact/2_10.htm. Phone: 800-4-CANCER (800-422-6237).

How to Find Medical Information. National Institute of Arthritis and Musculoskeletal and Skin Diseases. 2001. http://www.niams.nih.gov/hi/topics/howto/howto.htm. Phone: 877-22-NIAMS (877-226-4267) (toll-free).

JAMA Patient Page: Health Information on the Internet. The Medem Network. http://www.medem.com/medlb/article_detaillb.cfm?article_ID=ZZZLJLLLTMC&sub_cat=603

National Guideline Clearinghouse™. Agency for Healthcare Research and Quality. http://www.guideline.gov/

NOAH: New York Online Access to Health. http://www.noah-health.org/

A User's Guide to Finding and Evaluating Health Information on the Web. Medical Library Association. 2003. http://www.mlanet.org/resources/userguide.html#1

Virtual Treatments Can Be Real-World Deceptions. Federal Trade Commission. 2001. http://www.ftc.gov/bcp/conline/pubs/alerts/mrclalrt.htm

Your Guide to Choosing Quality Health Care. Agency for Healthcare Research and Quality. 2002. http://www.ahrq.gov/consumer/qntool.htm. Phone: 800-358-9295.

AHRQ consumer publications:

20 Tips to Help Prevent Medical Errors—Practical tips and questions to ask. (AHRQ 00-P038)

20 Tips to Help Prevent Medical Errors in Children (AHRQ 02-P034)

Five Steps to Safer Health Care—Shorter version of 20 Tips. (AHRQ 03-M007)

Ways You Can Help Your Family Prevent Medical Errors!—Easy-to-read version, with drawings. (AHRQ 01-0017)

Your Guide to Choosing Quality Health Care—Based on research about the information people want and need when choosing health plans, doctors, treatments, hospitals, and long-term care. (AHRQ 99-012)

Improving Health Care Quality: A Guide for Patients and Their Families—Short version of *Your Guide to Choosing Quality Health Care.* (AHRQ 01-0004)

Quick Checks for Quality—Checklist to use when choosing health plans, doctors, treatments, hospitals, and long-term care. (AHRQ 99-R027)

Quick Tips:

- ***When Getting Medical Tests*** (AHRQ 01-0040b)
- ***When Getting a Prescription*** (AHRQ 01-0040c)
- ***When Planning for Surgery*** (AHRQ 01-0040d)
- ***When Talking with Your Doctor*** (AHRQ 01-0040a)

To order AHRQ publications:

For electronic copies of these publications, go to the AHRQ Web site at www.ahrq.gov/consumer

For print copies, contact the AHRQ Publications Clearinghouse at 800-358-9295.

Description

1 **Addison's Disease**

Addison's disease is a rare disorder that stems from the malfunction of the adrenal glands located on top of the kidneys. In this disease, there is a deficiency of hormones produced by the adrenal cortex, the gland's firm outer layer. Most often, Addison's disease results from destruction of the adrenal gland. This glandular destruction may result from unusual infections, malignant tumors, an autoimmune process or other rare disorders. At least half of all cases of Addison's disease result from patient's developing antibodies against their own adrenal tissue (autoimmune process).

There can be increased water excretion in the urine and lowered blood pressure, which can lead to severe dehydration and other major complications. The symptoms of Addison's disease increase with the progression of the disease. Early signs may include fatigue, loss of appetite, low blood pressure (hypotension), weakness and significant loss from the kidneys of water and minerals. Other symptoms may include darkened scars and skin folds, as well as dark freckles on the head and shoulders. In the later stages, nausea may develop, as well as dizziness, further dehydration, low blood sugar (hypoglycemia) and mental changes including confusion.

Patients who are treated early have an excellent prognosis, but it is imperative that treatment be instituted immediately and vigorously. In order to counteract the hormonal loss, physicians prescribe steroid hormone replacement therapy. Certain doses ofhormones need to be increased during times of illness and surgery. Treatment should never be stopped, even for a day, without the advice of a physician. Persons on treatment should wear an alert bracelet to let emergency medical providers know of their diagnosis.

National Agencies & Associations

2 **Endocrine Society**
8401 Connecticut Avenue 301-941-0200
Chevy Chase, MD 20815 888-363-6274
Fax: 301-941-0259
e-mail: societyservices@endo-society.org
www.endo-society.org
Source of state-of-the-art research and clinical advancements in endocrinology and metabolism. Dedicated to promoting excellence in research education and clinical practice in the field of endocrinology. Prime advocate and integrative force for clinicians.
Robert M Carey MD, President
Lisa H Fish MD, VP Physician in Practice

3 **National Adrenal Diseases Foundation**
505 Northern Boulevard 516-487-4992
Great Neck, NY 11021 Fax: 516-829-5710
e-mail: nadfmail@aol.com
www.nadf.us
Nonprofit organization dedicated to offer support information and research for individuals having diseases of the adrenal glands. Goals of the organization include assisting patients through informational and educational activities as well as support programs.
Paul Marguli MD, Medical Director
Melanie G Wong, Executive Director

4 **National Institute of Diabetes & Digestive & Kidney Diseases**
National Institutes of Health
31 Center Drive, MSC 2560 301-496-4000
Bethesda, MD 20892-2560 e-mail: NIHInfo@OD.NIH.GOV
www.diabetes.niddk.nih.gov
Conducts and supports research on many of the most serious diseases affecting public health. The Institute supports much of the clinical research on the diseases of internal medicine and related subspecialty fields as well as many basic science disiplines.
Dr. Griffin Rodgers, Acting Director

Support Groups & Hotlines

5 **National Health Information Center**
PO Box 1133 310-565-4167
Washington, DC 20013 800-336-4797
Fax: 301-984-4256
e-mail: info@nhic.org
www.health.gov/nhic
Offers a nationwide information referral service, produces directories and resource guides.

Magazines

6 **Endocrine News**
Endocrine Society
8401 Connecticut Avenue 301-941-0200
Chevy Chase, MD 20815 888-363-6274
Fax: 301-941-0259
e-mail: societyservices@endo-society.org
www.endo-society.org
Endocrine News is the source of trends and insights for members of the endocrine community.
Monthly
Leonard Wartofsky MD, MPH, President
Carolyn Becker, MD, VP Physician in Practice

Newsletters

7 **Addison News**
6142 Territorial
Pleasant Lake, MI 49272 www2.dmci.net/users/hoffmanrj

8 **NADF News**
505 Northern Boulevard 516-487-4992
Great Neck, NY 11021 Fax: 516-829-5710
e-mail: nadfmail@aol.com
www.nadf.us
Official newsletter of the National Adrenal Diseases Foundation. Contains information on the latest research, question and answer column by an endocrinologist and helpful hints for those with Addison's Disease.
Monthly
Erin A Foley-Moundry, President/Director
Paul Margulies MD, Editor

Web Sites

9 **Healing Well**
www.healingwell.com
An online health resource guide to medical news, chat, information and articles, newsgroups and message boards, books, disease-related web sites, medical directories, and more for patients, friends, and family coping with disabling diseases, disorders, or chronic illnesses. Includes free e-mail, free homepages, and a monthly newsletter.

10 **Health Finder**
www.healthfinder.gov
Searchable, carefully developed web site offering information on over 1000 topics. Developed by the US Department of Health and Human Services, the site can be used in both English and Spanish.

11 **Health Link USA**
www.healthlinkusa.com

Health information concerning treatment, cures, prevention, diagnosis, risk factors, research, support groups, email lists, personal stories and much more. Updated regularly.

12 **Helios Health**

www.helioshealth.com

Online resource for your health information. Detailed information about specific health topics, access to expert advice from our Medical Advisory Board, and up-to-date health news.

13 **Hormone Foundation**

www.hormone.org

Helpful database of endocrinologists by state and information on many conditions covered by the affiliate, Endocrine Society.

14 **MedicineNet**

www.medicinenet.com

An online resource for consumers providing easy-to-read, authoritative medical and health information.

15 **Medscape**

www.mywebmd.com

Search engine providing links to websites with information on illnesses, diseases and disorders.

16 **National Adrenal Disease Foundation**

www.medhelp.org

Information and links for those affected by Addison's, Cushing's, Congenital Adrenal Hyperplasia, Hyper and Hypoaldosteronism and adrenal tumors.

17 **WebMD**

www.webmd.com

Information on Addison's disease, including an overview of the disease, symptoms and home treatment.

Description

18 **Aging**

The elderly population in the United States is growing faster than any other segment of the population, and has done so since 1900. It is estimated that this trend will continue at least through the year 2050. According to the 2000 US Census, 13 percent of the population is older than 65. One in eight persons is over 85 years, classified as "old old." By 2040, it is anticipated that one person in five will exceed 65 years of age, and the number of people over 85 will increase to four times their number today, representing the aging of the baby boomers.

Aging is not a disease, but part of the normal life cycle, and many seniors retain good health and live independently for long past the traditional age of retirement. In time, however, most will develop one or more chronic conditions; for those over 75 years of age, the most common conditions are hypertension, heart disease, hearing loss, arthritis, and cataracts. By the year 2030, 150 million Americans are expected to have a chronic condition, and 42 million will be limited in their ability to work or live independently. Treating this population will require many medical and nonmedical services, integrated to provide a comprehensive continuum of care. See also *Alzheimer's Disease.*

National Agencies & Associations

19 **American Association of Homes and Services for the Aging**
2519 Connecticut Avenue NW
Washington, DC 20008-1520
202-783-2242
Fax: 202-783-2255
e-mail: info@aahsa.org
www.aahsa.org
National association of more than 4 000 nonprofit nursing homes continuing care retirement communities independent living centers and community service providers serving more than 60,000 older Americans each year.
William L Minnix Jr, President and CEO
Katrinka Smi Sloan, COO and SVP Member Services

20 **American Association of Retired Persons**
601 E Street NW
Washington, DC 20049
888-687-2277
e-mail: member@aarp.org
www.aarp.org
AARP is the nation's leading organization for people age 50 and older. It serves their needs and interests through information and education, advocacy and community services provided by a network of local chapters and experienced volunteers.
William D Novelli, CEO
Jennie Chin Hansen, President

21 **Commission on Accreditation of Rehabilitation Services**
CARF International
4891 East Grant Road
Tucson, AZ 85712
520-325-1044
888-281-6531
Fax: 520-318-1129
e-mail: fturtz@carf.org
www.carf.org
CARF reviews and grants accreditation services nationally and internationally at the request of a facility or program. Their standards are rigorous, so those services that meet them are among the best available.
Amanda Birch, Adminstrator of Operations
Brian Boon, Ph.D., President/Chief Executive Officer

22 **Gerontological Society of America**
1220 L Street NW
Washington, DC 20005
202-842-1275
Fax: 202-842-1150
e-mail: geron@geron.org
www.geron.org
Nonprofit professional organization with more than 5000 members in the field of aging. Provides researchers, educators, practitioners and policy makers with opportunities to understand, advance, integrate and use basic and applied research on aging populations.
James Appleby, Executive Director
Linda Krogh Harootyan, Deputy Executive Director

23 **Institute for Life Course and Aging**
222 College Street
Toronto, Ontario, M5T-3J1
416-978-0377
Fax: 416-978-4771
www.aging.utoronto.ca
The Institute is a research centre under the auspices of the School of Graduate Studies at the University of Toronto.
Prof Lynn McDonald, Director
Susan Murphy, Administration

24 **International Federation on Ageing**
4398 Boul. Saint-Laurent
Montreal, Quebec, H2W-1Z5
514-396-3358
e-mail: jbarratt@ifa-fiv.org
www.ifa-fiv.org
To inform, educate and promote policies and practice to improve the quality of life of older persons around the world.
Dr Jane Barratt, Secretary General
Greg Shaw, Director, International Relations

25 **National Council on Aging**
1901 L Street NW
Washington, DC 20036
202-479-1200
Fax: 202-479-0735
TTY: 202-479-6674
TDD: 202-479-6674
e-mail: info@ncoa.org
www.ncoa.org
The nation's first charitable organization dedicated to promoting the dignity, independence, well-being and contributions of older Americans. NCOA serves as a national voice and powerful advocate on behalf of older Americans.
James P Firman EdD, President/CEO
Howard Bedlin, VP Public Policy and Advocacy

26 **Problems of the Elderly Committee**
740 15th Street NW
Washington, DC 20005-1009
202-662-1500
Fax: 202-662-1501
e-mail: crimjustice@abanet.org
www.abanet.org/crimjust
This Committee examines the issues that affect the elderly as victims of street crime, identity theft, financial exploitation and other crimes of which they are targets. The committee looks at issues arising from the aging prisons populations and the elders as perpetrators of crime, also.
Lori G Levin, Co-Chair
Benjamin F Overton, Co-Chair

27 **Senior Resource**
4521 Campus Drive
Irvine, CA 92612
858-793-7901
877-793-7901
Fax: 858-792-9080
e-mail: questions@seniorresource.com
www.seniorresource.com
An agency that helps seniors to understand aging and gives different resources consisting of sociologic changes; metabolic changes; positive aging; and physical changes.
Bryan D Hatchell, Chair

28 **US Administration on Aging**
1 Massachusetts Avenue
Washington, DC 20201
202-619-0724
Fax: 202-357-3555
e-mail: aoainfo@aoa.hhs.gov
www.aoa.gov
The Administration on Aging an agency in the US Department of Health and Human Services is one of the nation's largest providers of home and community-based care for older persons and their caregivers.
Edwin L Walker, Acting Assistant Secretary
Carol Crecy, Director Office of Communications

State Agencies & Associations

Alaska

29 **AARP Alaska State Office**
3601 C Street
Anchorage, AK 99503
866-227-7447
Fax: 907-341-2270
e-mail: ak@aarp.org
www.aarp.org/states/ak

AARP is a nonprofit nonpartisan membership organization for people age 50 and over. AARP is dedicated to enhancing the quality of life as one ages, in addition to facilitating social change and delivering value to members through information and advocacy.

Fred Jenkins, Development Director
George Hieronymus, AARP Alaska State President

Arizona

30 **AARP Arizona: Phoenix Collier Center**
Collier Center
201 E Washington Street
Phoenix, AZ 85004-2428
866-389-5649
Fax: 602-256-2928
e-mail: azaarp@aarp.org
www.aarp.org/states/az

AARP is a nonprofit nonpartisan membership organization for people age 50 and over. AARP is dedicated to enhancing the quality of life as one ages, in addition to facilitating social change and delivering value to members through information and advocacy.

Leonard J Kirschner PhD, Arizona AARP State President
David Mitchell, Arizona AARP State Director

Arkansas

31 **AARP Arkansas State Office: Little Rock**
1701 Centerview Drive
Little Rock, AR 72211
866-544-5379
Fax: 501-227-7710
e-mail: araarp@aarp.org
www.aarp.org/states/ar

AARP is a nonprofit nonpartisan membership organization for people age 50 and over. AARP is dedicated to enhancing the quality of life as one ages, in addition to facilitating social change and delivering value to members through information and advocacy.

Mary Dillard, Arkansas AARP State President
Pat Jones, Arkansas AARP State Media Relations

California

32 **AARP California State Office: Pasadena**
200 S Los Robles Avenue
Pasadena, CA 91101-2422
866-448-3615
Fax: 626-583-8500
e-mail: calosangeles@aarp.org
www.aarp.org/states/ca

AARP is a nonprofit nonpartisan membership organization for people age 50 and over. AARP is dedicated to enhancing the quality of life as one ages, in addition to facilitating social change and delivering value to members through information and advocacy.

Helen Russ, California AARP State President
Thomas A Porter, California AARP State Director

33 **AARP California State Office: Sacramento**
1415 L Street
Sacramento, CA 95814
866-448-3614
Fax: 916-446-2223
e-mail: casacramento@aarp.org
www.aarp.org/states/ca

AARP is a nonprofit nonpartisan membership organization for people age 50 and over. AARP is dedicated to enhancing the quality of life as one ages, in addition to facilitating social change and delivering value to members through information and advocacy.

Helen Russ, California State AARP President
Thomas A Porter, California State AARP Director

Colorado

34 **AARP Colorado State Office: Denver**
303 E 17th Avenue
Denver, CO 80203-5012
866-554-5376
Fax: 303-764-5999
e-mail: coaarp@aarp.org
www.aarp.org/states/co

AARP is a nonprofit nonpartisan membership organization for people age 50 and over. AARP is dedicated to enhancing the quality of life as one ages, in addition to facilitating social change and delivering value to members through information and advocacy.

Robert Martinez, Colorado AARP State President
Jon Looney, Colorado AARP State Director

Florida

35 **AARP Florida State Office: St. Petersburg**
400 Carillon Parkway
Saint Petersburg, FL 33716
866-595-7678
Fax: 727-571-2278
TTY: 727-561-9544
e-mail: flaarp@aarp.org
www.aarp.org/states/fl

AARP is a nonprofit nonpartisan membership organization for people age 50 and over. AARP is dedicated to enhancing the quality of life as one ages, in addition to facilitating social change and delivering value to members through information and advocacy.

Kathy Marma, Florida AARP State Media Relations
Thomas Thame MD, Florida AARP State Board of Directors

36 **Goodwill Industries-Suncoast**
Goodwill Industries-Suncoast
10596 Gandy Boulevard
St. Petersburg, FL 33702
727-523-1512
888-279-1988
Fax: 727-563-9300
TDD: 727-579-1068
e-mail: chris.ward@goodwill-suncoast.com
www.goodwill-suncoast.org/

A nonprofit community based organization whose purpose is to improve the quality of life for people who are disabled, disadvantaged and/or aged. This mission is accomplished through a staff of over 1,200 employees providing independent living skills, affordable housing, career assessment/planning, job skills, training, placement, and job retention assistance. Goodwill Industries-Suncoast services Citrus, Hernando, Highlands, Hillsborough, Levy, Marion, Pasco, Pinellas, Polk and Sumter Counties.

R Lee Waits, President/Chief Executive Officer
Chris Ward, Marketing and Media Relations Manager

Georgia

37 **AARP Georgia: Atlanta**
999 Peachtree Street NE
Atlanta, GA 30309-4421
866-295-7281
Fax: 404-881-6997
e-mail: gaaarp@aarp.org
www.aarp.org/states/ga

AARP is a nonprofit nonpartisan membership organization for people age 50 and over. AARP is dedicated to enhancing the quality of life as one ages, in addition to facilitating social change and delivering value to members through information and advocacy.

Matthew McWilliams, Georgia AARP State Media Relations
Will Phillips, AARP Georgia Associate State Director

Hawaii

38 **AARP Hawaii State Office: Honolulu**
1132 Bishop Street
Honolulu, HI 96813
808-843-1906
866-295-7282
Fax: 808-843-1908
e-mail: oahuaarp@hawaii.rr.com
www.aarp.org/states/hi

AARP is a nonprofit nonpartisan membership organization for people age 50 and over. AARP is dedicated to enhancing the qual-

ity of life as one ages, in addition to facilitating social change and delivering value to members through information and advocacy.
Stuart TK Ho, AARP Hawaii Interim State President
Barbara Kim Stanton, Hawaii AARP State Director

Idaho

39 **AARP Idaho State Office: Meridian**
3830 E Gentry Way
Meridian, ID 83642
866-295-7284
Fax: 208-288-4424
e-mail: aarpid@aarp.org
www.aarp.org/states/id
AARP is a nonprofit nonpartisan membership organization for people age 50 and over. AARP is dedicated to enhancing the quality of life as one ages, in addition to facilitating social change and delivering value to members through information and advocacy.
Cheryl Tussey, Idaho AARP State Media Relations
Jim Wordelman, AARP Idaho State Director

Illinois

40 **AARP Illinois State Office: Chicago**
222 N LaSalle Street
Chicago, IL 60601-1033
866-448-3613
Fax: 312-372-2204
e-mail: aarpil@aarp.org
www.aarp.org/states/il
AARP is a nonprofit nonpartisan membership organization for people age 50 and over. AARP is dedicated to enhancing the quality of life as one ages, in addition to facilitating social change and delivering value to members through information and advocacy.
Evelyn Gooden, Illinois AARP State President
Gerardo Cardenas, Illinois AARP State Media Relations

Indiana

41 **AARP Indiana State Office: Indianapolis**
One N Capitol Avenue
Indianapolis, IN 46204-2025
866-448-3618
Fax: 317-423-2211
e-mail: inaarp@aarp.org
www.aarp.org/states/in
AARP is a nonprofit nonpartisan membership organization for people age 50 and over. AARP is dedicated to enhancing the quality of life as one ages, in addition to facilitating social change and delivering value to members through information and advocacy.
Martin DeAgostino, Indiana AARP State Media Relations
June Lyle, AARP Indiana State Director

Iowa

42 **AARP Iowa State Office: Des Moines**
600 E Court Avenue
Des Moines, IA 50309
866-554-5378
Fax: 515-244-7767
e-mail: iaaarp@aarp.org
www.aarp.org/states/ia
AARP is a nonprofit nonpartisan membership organization for people age 50 and over. AARP is dedicated to enhancing the quality of life as one ages, in addition to facilitating social change and delivering value to members through information and advocacy.
Ann Black, Iowa AARP State Media Relations
Bruce Koeppl, Iowa AARP State Director

Kansas

43 **AARP Kansas State Office: Topeka**
555 S Kansas
Topeka, KS 66603
866-448-3619
Fax: 785-232-8259
e-mail: ksaarp@aarp.org
www.aarp.org/states/ks
AARP is a nonprofit nonpartisan membership organization for people age 50 and over. AARP is dedicated to enhancing the quality of life as one ages, in addition to facilitating social change and delivering value to members through information and advocacy.
Mary Tritsch, Kansas AARP State Media Relations
Maren Turner, Kansas AARP State Director

Kentucky

44 **AARP Kentucky State Office: Louisville**
10401 Linn Station Road
Louisville, KY 40223
866-295-7275
Fax: 502-394-9918
e-mail: kyaarp@aarp.org
www.aarp.org/states/ky
AARP is a nonprofit nonpartisan membership organization for people age 50 and over. AARP is dedicated to enhancing the quality of life as one ages, in addition to facilitating social change and delivering value to members through information and advocacy.
Bill Harned, AARP Kentucky State President
Fred Smith, Executive Council Community Service

Louisiana

45 **AARP Louisiana State Office: Baton Rouge**
301 Main Street
Baton Rouge, LA 70825
866-448-3620
Fax: 225-387-3400
e-mail: la@aarp.org
www.aarp.org/states/la
AARP is a nonprofit nonpartisan membership organization for people age 50 and over. AARP is dedicated to enhancing the quality of life as one ages, in addition to facilitating social change and delivering value to members through information and advocacy.
Earl A White, AARP Louisiana State President
Julia Kenny, AARP Louisiana State Director

Maine

46 **AARP Maine State Office: Portland**
1685 Congress Street
Portland, ME 04102
866-554-5380
Fax: 207-775-5727
e-mail: me@aarp.org
www.aarp.org/states/me
AARP is a nonprofit nonpartisan membership organization for people age 50 and over. AARP is dedicated to enhancing the quality of life as one ages, in addition to facilitating social change and delivering value to members through information and advocacy.
Bruce Kinney, Maine AARP State Advocacy Coordinator
Phyllis Cohn, Maine AARP State Media Relations

Massachusetts

47 **AARP Massachusetts State Office: Boston**
1 Beacon Street
Boston, MA 02108
866-448-3621
Fax: 617-723-4224
e-mail: ma@aarp.org
www.aarp.org/states/ma
AARP is a nonprofit nonpartisan membership organization for people age 50 and over. AARP is dedicated to enhancing the quality of life as one ages, in addition to facilitating social change and delivering value to members through information and advocacy.
Charlie Desmond, AARP Massachusetts State President
Claire Redmond, Executive Council Member

Michigan

48 **AARP Michigan State Office: Lansing**
309 N Washington Square
Lansing, MI 48933
866-227-7448
Fax: 517-482-2794
TTY: 877-434-7598
e-mail: miaarp@aarp.org
www.aarp.org/states/mi
AARP is a nonprofit nonpartisan membership organization for people age 50 and over. AARP is dedicated to enhancing the quality of life as one ages, in addition to facilitating social change and delivering value to members through information and advocacy.
Steve Gools, AARP Michigan State Director
Stepheni Schlinker, Michigan AARP State Media Relations

Minnesota

49 **AARP Minnesota State Office: Saint Paul**
30 E Seventh Street
Saint Paul, MN 55101
866-554-5381
Fax: 651-221-2636
e-mail: aarpmn@aarp.org
www.aarp.org/states/mn

AARP is a nonprofit nonpartisan membership organization for people age 50 and over. AARP is dedicated to enhancing the quality of life as one ages, in addition to facilitating social change and delivering value to members through information and advocacy.
Michele Kimball, AARP Minnesota State Director
Amy Gromer McDonough, AARP Minnesota State Media Relations

Missouri

50 **AARP Missouri State Office: Kansas City**
700 W 47th Street
Kansas City, MO 64112-1805
866-389-5627
Fax: 816-561-3107
e-mail: moaarp@aarp.org
www.aarp.org/states/mo

AARP is a nonprofit nonpartisan membership organization for people age 50 and over. AARP is dedicated to enhancing the quality of life as one ages, in addition to facilitating social change and delivering value to members through information and advocacy.
John McDonald, AARP Missouri State Director
Anita K Parran, AARP Missouri State Media Relations

Montana

51 **AARP Montana State Office: Helena**
30 W 14th Street
Helena, MT 59601
866-295-7278
Fax: 406-441-2230
e-mail: mtaarp@aarp.org
www.aarp.org/states/mt

AARP is a nonprofit nonpartisan membership organization for people age 50 and over. AARP is dedicated to enhancing the quality of life as one ages, in addition to facilitating social change and delivering value to members through information and advocacy.
Max Logan, AARP Montana Volunteer State President
Bob Bartholomew, AARP Montana State Director

Nebraska

52 **AARP Nebraska State Office: Lincoln**
301 S 13th Street
Lincoln, NE 68508
866-389-5651
Fax: 402-323-6908
e-mail: neaarp@aarp.org
www.aarp.org/states/ne

AARP is a nonprofit nonpartisan membership organization for people age 50 and over. AARP is dedicated to enhancing the quality of life as one ages, in addition to facilitating social change and delivering value to members through information and advocacy.
Sunny Andrews, AARP Nebraska State President
Devorah Lanner, AARP Nebraska State Media Relations

Nevada

53 **AARP Nevada State Office: Las Vegas**
5820 S Eastern Avenue
Las Vegas, NV 89119
866-389-5652
Fax: 702-938-3225
e-mail: nvaarp@aarp.org
www.aarp.org/states/nv

AARP is a nonprofit nonpartisan membership organization for people age 50 and over. AARP is dedicated to enhancing the quality of life as one ages, in addition to facilitating social change and delivering value to members through information and advocacy.
Deborah Moore, AARP Nevada Spokeswoman
Nancy Andersen, AARP Nevada State Volunteer Coordinator

New Hampshire

54 **AARP New Hampshire State Office-Manchester**
900 Elm Street
Manchester, NH 03101
866-542-8168
Fax: 603-629-0066
e-mail: nh@aarp.org
www.aarp.org/states/nh

AARP is a nonprofit nonpartisan membership organization for people age 50 and over. AARP is dedicated to enhancing the quality of life as one ages, in addition to facilitating social change and delivering value to members through information and advocacy.
Kelly Clark, AARP New Hampshire State Director
Jamie Bulen, AARP New Hampshire State Media Relations

New Jersey

55 **AARP New Jersey State Office: Princeton**
101 Rockingham Row
Princeton, NJ 08540
866-542-8165
Fax: 609-987-4634
e-mail: njaarp@aarp.org
www.aarp.org/states/nj

AARP is a nonprofit nonpartisan membership organization for people age 50 and over. AARP is dedicated to enhancing the quality of life as one ages, in addition to facilitating social change and delivering value to members through information and advocacy.
Sy Larson, AARP New Jersey State President
Jane Margesson, AARP New Jersey State Media Relations

New Mexico

56 **AARP New Mexico State Office: Sante Fe**
535 Cerrillos Road
Santa Fe, NM 87501
866-389-5636
Fax: 505-820-2889
e-mail: nmaarp@aarp.org
www.aarp.org/states/nm

AARP is a nonprofit nonpartisan membership organization for people age 50 and over. AARP is dedicated to enhancing the quality of life as one ages, in addition to facilitating social change and delivering value to members through information and advocacy.
Louis Sarabia, AARP New Mexico State President
Stan Cooper, AARP New Mexico State Director

New York

57 **AARP New York State Office: Albany**
1 Commerce Plaza
Albany, NY 12260
866-227-7442
Fax: 518-434-6949
e-mail: nyaarp@aarp.org
www.aarp.org

AARP is a nonprofit nonpartisan membership organization for people age 50 and over. AARP is dedicated to enhancing the quality of life as one ages, in addition to facilitating social change and delivering value to members through information and advocacy.
Lois Aronstein, AARP New York State Director
Madeleine Moore, AARP New York State President

58 **AARP New York State Office: New York City**
780 3rd Avenue
New York, NY 10017
866-227-7442
Fax: 212-644-6390
e-mail: nyaarp@aarp.org
www.aarp.org/states/ny

AARP is a nonprofit nonpartisan membership organization for people age 50 and over. AARP is dedicated to enhancing the quality of life as one ages, in addition to facilitating social change and delivering value to members through information and advocacy.
Lois Aronstein, AARP New York State Director
Madeleine Moore, AARP New York State President

North Carolina

59 **AARP North Carolina State Office: Raleigh**
1511 Sunday Drive
Raleigh, NC 27607
866-389-5650
Fax: 919-755-9684
TTY: 919-508-0290
e-mail: ncaarp@aarp.org
www.aarp.org/states/nc

AARP is a nonprofit nonpartisan membership organization for people age 50 and over. AARP is dedicated to enhancing the quality of life as one ages, in addition to facilitating social change and delivering value to members through information and advocacy.

Diana D Hatch, AARP North Carolina State President
Bob Garner, Communications Director

North Dakota

60 **AARP North Dakota State Office: Bismarck**
107 W Main Avenue
Bismarck, ND 58501
866-554-5383
Fax: 701-255-2242
e-mail: ndaarp@aarp.org
www.aarp.org/states/nd

AARP is a nonprofit nonpartisan membership organization for people age 50 and over. AARP is dedicated to enhancing the quality of life as one ages, in addition to facilitating social change and delivering value to members through information and advocacy.

Betty Keegan, AARP North Dakota State President
Lyle Halvorson, AARP North Dakota State Media Relations

Ohio

61 **AARP Ohio State Office: Columbus**
17 S High Street
Columbus, OH 43215-3467
866-389-5653
Fax: 614-224-9801
e-mail: ohaarp@aarp.org
www.aarp.org/states/oh

AARP is a nonprofit nonpartisan membership organization for people age 50 and over. AARP is dedicated to enhancing the quality of life as one ages, in addition to facilitating social change and delivering value to members through information and advocacy.

Kathy Keller, AARP Ohio State Media Relations
Joanne Limbach, AARP Ohio State President

Oklahoma

62 **AARP Oklahoma State Office: Edmond**
126 N Bryant Avenue
Edmond, OK 73034
866-295-7277
Fax: 405-844-7772
e-mail: ok@aarp.org
www.aarp.org/states/ok

AARP is a nonprofit nonpartisan membership organization for people age 50 and over. AARP is dedicated to enhancing the quality of life as one ages, in addition to facilitating social change and delivering value to members through information and advocacy.

Robert Bristow, AARP Oklahoma State President
Marjorie Lyons, Executive Council Member

Oregon

63 **AARP Oregon State Office: Clackamas**
9200 SE Sunnybrook Boulevard
Clackamas, OR 97015-5762
866-554-5360
Fax: 503-652-9933
e-mail: oraarp@aarp.org
www.aarp.org/states/or

AARP is a nonprofit nonpartisan membership organization for people age 50 and over. AARP is dedicated to enhancing the quality of life as one ages, in addition to facilitating social change and delivering value to members through information and advocacy.

Ray Miao, AARP Oregon State President
Don Bruland, Director

Pennsylvania

64 **AARP Pennsylvania State Office: Harrisburg**
30 N 3rd Street
Harrisburg, PA 17101
866-389-5654
Fax: 717-236-4078
e-mail: sgardner@aarp.org
www.aarp.org/states/pa

AARP is a nonprofit nonpartisan membership organization for people age 50 and over. AARP is dedicated to enhancing the quality of life as one ages, in addition to facilitating social change and delivering value to members through information and advocacy.

J Shane Creamer, AARP Pennsylvania State President
Steve Gardner, AARP Pennsylvania State Media Relations

South Carolina

65 **AARP South Carolina Office: Columbia**
1201 Main Street
Columbia, SC 29201
866-389-5655
Fax: 803-251-4374
e-mail: scaarp@aarp.org
www.aarp.org/states/sc

AARP is a nonprofit nonpartisan membership organization for people age 50 and over. AARP is dedicated to enhancing the quality of life as one ages, in addition to facilitating social change and delivering value to members through information and advocacy.

Charles A Johnson, AARP SC State President
Patrick Cobb, AARP SC State Media Relations

Tennessee

66 **AARP Tennessee State Office: Nashville**
150 4th Avenue N
Nashville, TN 37219
866-295-7274
Fax: 615-313-8414
e-mail: tnaarp@aarp.org
www.aarp.org/states/tn

AARP is a nonprofit nonpartisan membership organization for people age 50 and over. AARP is dedicated to enhancing the quality of life as one ages, in addition to facilitating social change and delivering value to members through information and advocacy.

Margot Seay, AARP Tennessee State President
Rebecca Kelly, AARP Tennessee State Director

Texas

67 **AARP Texas State Office: Austin**
98 San Jacinto Boulevard
Austin, TX 78701
866-227-7443
Fax: 512-480-9799
e-mail: rayuso@aarp.org
www.aarp.org/states/tx

AARP is a nonprofit nonpartisan membership organization for people age 50 and over. AARP is dedicated to enhancing the quality of life as one ages, in addition to facilitating social change and delivering value to members through information and advocacy.

Rafael Ayuso, AARP Texas State Media Relations
Bob Jackson, AARP Texas State Director

Utah

68 **AARP Utah State Office: Midvale**
6975 Union Park Center
Midvale, UT 84047
866-448-3616
Fax: 801-561-2209
e-mail: utaarp@aarp.org
www.aarp.org/states/ut

AARP is a nonprofit nonpartisan membership organization for people age 50 and over. AARP is dedicated to enhancing the quality of life as one ages, in addition to facilitating social change and delivering value to members through information and advocacy.

Pat Gamble Hovey, Volunteer State President of AARP Utah
Ruby Hammel, Executive Council Advocacy Coordinator

Vermont

69 **AARP Vermont State Office: Montpelier**
199 Main Street
Burlington, VT 05401
866-227-7451
Fax: 802-651-9805
e-mail: vtaarp@aarp.org
www.aarp.org/states/vt

AARP is a nonprofit nonpartisan membership organization for people age 50 and over. AARP is dedicated to enhancing the quality of life as one ages, in addition to facilitating social change and delivering value to members through information and advocacy.
Nancy C Lang, AARP Vermont State President
Dave Reville, AARP Vermont State Media Relations

Virginia

70 **AARP Virginia State Office: Richmond**
707 E Main Street
Richmond, VA 23219
866-542-8164
Fax: 804-819-1923
e-mail: vaaarp@aarp.org
www.aarp.org/states/va

AARP is a nonprofit nonpartisan membership organization for people age 50 and over. AARP is dedicated to enhancing the quality of life as one ages, in addition to facilitating social change and delivering value to members through information and advocacy.
Bill Kallio, AARP Virginia State Director
Tony Hylton, AARP Virginia State Media Relations

Washington

71 **AARP Washington State Office: Seattle**
9750 3rd Avenue NE
Seattle, WA 98115
866-227-7457
Fax: 206-517-9350
e-mail: waaarp@aarp.org
www.aarp.org/states/wa

AARP is a nonprofit nonpartisan membership organization for people age 50 and over. AARP is dedicated to enhancing the quality of life as one ages, in addition to facilitating social change and delivering value to members through information and advocacy.
John Barnett, AARP Washington State President
Doug Shadel, AARP Washington State Director

West Virginia

72 **AARP West Virginia Office: Charleston**
300 Summers Street
Charleston, WV 25301
866-227-7458
Fax: 304-344-4633
e-mail: wvaarp@aarp.org
www.aarp.org/states/wv

AARP is a nonprofit nonpartisan membership organization for people age 50 and over. AARP is dedicated to enhancing the quality of life as one ages, in addition to facilitating social change and delivering value to members through information and advocacy.
Ruth Wagner, AARP West Virginia State President
Ginger Thomp McDaniel, AARP West Virginia State Media Relations

Wisconsin

73 **AARP Wisconsin State Office: Madison**
222 W Washington Avenue
Madison, WI 53703
866-448-3611
Fax: 608-251-7612
e-mail: wistate@aarp.org
www.aarp.org/states/wi

AARP is a nonprofit nonpartisan membership organization for people age 50 and over. AARP is dedicated to enhancing the quality of life as one ages, in addition to facilitating social change and delivering value to members through information and advocacy.
Ethel Percy Andrus, Founder
Albert W Majkrzak, AARP Wisconsin State President

Wyoming

74 **AARP Wyoming State Office: Cheyenne**
2020 Carey Avenue
Cheyenne, WY 82009
866-663-3290
Fax: 307-634-3808
e-mail: wy@aarp.org
www.aarp.org/states/wy

AARP is a nonprofit nonpartisan membership organization for people age 50 and over. AARP is dedicated to enhancing the quality of life as one ages, in addition to facilitating social change and delivering value to members through information and advocacy.
Les Engelter, AARP Wyoming State President
Joanne Bowlby, AARP Wyoming State Media Relations

International

75 **AARP Virgin Islands State Office: St Croix**
93B Estate Diamond
Christiansted, St. Croix, VI 00820
866-389-5633
Fax: 340-692-2544
e-mail: viaarp@aarp.org
www.aarp.org/states/vi/

AARP is a nonprofit, nonpartisan membership organization for people age 50 and over. AARP is dedicated to enhancing the quality of life as one ages in addition to facilitating social change and delivering value to members through information, advocacy and service.
Hugo Dennis, Jr., AARP Virgin Islands State President

Libraries & Resource Centers

76 **Aging In America/Morningside House Nursing Home**
1000 Pelham Parkway South
718-409-8244
Bronx, NY 10461
Fax: 718-824-4242
e-mail: chirschberg@aiamsh.org
http://www.aginginamerica.org

Aging in America is a community-based, social service agency. Morningside House is a provider of specialized medical, nursing and rehabilitative services.

Research Centers

77 **Case Western Reserve University: Center on Aging and Health**
10900 Euclid Avenue
216-368-2000
Cleveland, OH 44106
Fax: 216-368-6389
e-mail: info@case.edu
fpb.case.edu/Centers/UCAH

Research organization conducting supporting and facilitating research into the chronically ill aged person.
Diana L Morris, Executive Director
Evelyn Duffy, Associate Director

78 **Center for the Study of Aging**
706 Madison Avenue
518-465-6927
Albany, NY 12208-3604
Fax: 518-462-1339
e-mail: iapaas@aol.com
www.centerforthestudyofaging.org

Not-for-profit educational and research center for social and medical research on aging health exercise lifelong health and fitness and programs to improve the health and quality of life for older men and women.
Sara Harris, Executive Director
Debra Treadgold, President

79 **Columbia University Center for Geriatrics Gerontology**
College of Physicians and Surgeons
630 West 168th Street
212-305-3806
New York, NY 10032
Fax: 212-305-1343
e-mail: psadmissions@columbia.edu
www.cumc.columbia.edu/dept/ps

Clinical research in geriatric/gerontology and long-term care.
Barry Gurland MD, Director

80 **Creighton University Center for Healthy Aging**
601 N 30th Street 402-280-4561
Omaha, NE 68131 Fax: 402-280-4623
e-mail: caad@creighton.edu
medicine.creighton.edu/CAAD

Focuses on human development, aging and health care for the elderly.
Patricio F Reyes, Director
David Robertson, Staff

81 **Institute for Human Development Life Course and Aging**
222 College Street 416-978-0377
Toronto, Ontario, M5T-3J1 Fax: 416-978-4771
www.aging.utoronto.ca

82 **Landon Center on Aging University of Kansas Medical Center**
University of Kansas Medical Center
3901 Rainbow Boulevard 913-588-1203
Kansas City, KS 66160 800-766-3777
Fax: 913-588-1201
e-mail: rnudo@kumc.edu
www2.kumc.edu/coa

Provides support for interdisciplinary research on the issue of age and aging.
Randolph Nudo, Director
Joan McDowd, Associate Director

83 **Purdue University: Center for Research on Aging**
Ernest C Young Hall 765-494-9692
W Lafayette, IN 47907-2108 Fax: 765-494-2180
e-mail: calc@purdue.edu
www.purdue.edu/aging

Social science research on aging health and health care delivery.
Kenneth F Ferraro, Director
Gerald C Hyner, Associate Director

84 **Roy M and Phyllis Gough Huffington Center on Aging**
Huffington Center on Aging
Baylor College of Medicine 713-798-5804
Houston, TX 77030 Fax: 713-798-6688
e-mail: Gretchen@bcm.tmc.edu
www.hcoa.org

Internal unit of Baylor College representing research into the biology of aging.
Gretchen Darlington, Director
Adam Antebi, Associate Professor

85 **University of Pennsylvania Institute on Aging**
3615 Chestnut Street 215-898-3163
Philadelphia, PA 19104-2676 Fax: 215-573-5566
e-mail: aging@mail.med.upenn.edu
www.med.upenn.edu/aging

The mission of the IOA is to improve the health of the elderly by increasing the quality and quantity of clinical and basic research as well as educational programs focusing on normal aging and age-related diseases at the UPSM and across the entire Penn campus.
John Q Trojanowski, Acting Director
Steven E Arnold, Associate Director

Support Groups & Hotlines

86 **Aging Support Group**
Consultants for Aging Families
649 Remington Street 970-498-0730
Fort Collins, CO 80524 Fax: 970-416-6567
e-mail: info@fortnet.org
www.fortnet.org/CAF

Offers help with asking for the services available for the elderly and their families and give you the ability to take advantage of expert help and support.
Dave Colliton, Executive Director
Nancy McCamridge, Director

87 **Children of Aging Parents**
PO Box 167 215-355-6611
Richboro, PA 18954 800-227-7294
Fax: 215-355-6824
e-mail: info@caps4caregivers.org
www.caps4caregivers.org/about.htm

A national clearinghouse for information catering to caregivers of the elderly. Provides information and emotional support on day-to-day caregiver issues. Publishes a quarterly newsletter and supports a small network of caregiver support groups.
Lenore Sherman, Executive Director
Karen Rosenberg, Director Senior Services

88 **National Health Information Center**
PO Box 1133 310-565-4167
Washington, DC 20013 800-336-4797
Fax: 301-984-4256
e-mail: info@nhic.org
www.health.gov/nhic

Offers a nationwide information referral service, produces directories and resource guides.

Books

89 **Activities for the Disabled, Elderly and Adults**
Haworth Press
10 Alice Street 607-722-5857
Binghamton, NY 13904-1580 800-429-6784
Fax: 607-722-0012
www.haworthpress.com

Learn how to effectively plan and deliver activities for a growing number of older people with developmental disabilities. It aims to stimulate interest and continued support for recreation program development and implementation among developmental disability and aging service systems.
136 pages Hardcover
ISBN: 1-560240-92-X

90 **Adult Children and Aging Parents**
American Counseling Association
5999 Stevenson Avenue 703-823-9800
Alexandria, VA 22304-3302 800-347-6647
Fax: 703-823-0252
www.counseling.org

Provides effective intervention strategies and suggestions for counselors who work with older persons, individually and with the family. Offers information on many vital topics such as Alzheimer's Disease, retirement, elder abuse and suicide.
216 pages
ISBN: 0-840354-48-7

91 **Aging and Family Therapy**
Haworth Press
10 Alice Street 607-722-5857
Binghamton, NY 13904-1580 800-429-6784
Fax: 607-722-0012
www.haworthpress.com

Here are creative strategies for use in therapy with older adults and their families. This book provides practitioners with information, insight, reference tools, and other sources that will contribute to more effective intervention with the elderly and their families.
244 pages Hardcover
ISBN: 0-866567-78-3

92 **Aging and Our Families**
Human Sciences Press
233 Spring Street 212-620-8000
New York, NY 10013-1522 800-221-9369
Handbook for family caregivers.
132 pages Paperback
ISBN: 0-898854-41-5

93 **Caregivers' Roller Coaster**
Loyola University Press
3441 N Ashland Avenue 773-281-1818
Chicago, IL 60657-1355 800-621-1008
www.loyolapress.com

A simply written self-help guide for caregivers of the frail elderly. Offers support for men and women, not trained professionals, who find themselves caring for aging family members in their own homes. Offers practical advice and information on Alzheimer's, Medicare, insurance and community services for the elderly.
150 pages
ISBN: 0-829407-45-6

94 **Caring for Those You Love: A Guide to Compassionate Care for the Aged**
Bethany Chaffin, author
Horizon Publishers & Distributors, Inc.
191 N 650 East 801-295-9451
Bountiful, UT 84010-3628 866-818-6277
Fax: 801-298-1305
e-mail: service@horizonpublishers.biz
www.horizonpublishers.biz
This book is a practical guide to coping with special problems of the aged and infirmed, and examines the many challenges of caring for the elderly on a personal and family level.
108 pages
ISBN: 0-882902-70-9
Duane S Crowther, Owner/CEO
Jean D Crowther, Owner/CEO

95 **Continuing Care Retirement Community Directory**
American Assoc. of Homes & Services for the Aging
901 E Street NW
Washington, DC 20004-2037 800-508-9442
Fax: 301-206-9789
A national consumer's directory of continuing care retirement communities. This directory is a vital tool for individuals searching and evaluating a community for themselves or a loved one.

96 **Court-Related Needs of the Elderly and Persons with Disabilities**
Commission on the Mentally Disabled
1800 M Street NW
Washington, DC 20036-5802 202-331-2240
www.statejustice.org/
Report of the National Conference, examines the barriers of the judicial system impeding access for the elderly and persons with disabilities.

97 **Creative Movements for Older Adults**
Human Sciences Press
233 Spring Street 212-620-8000
New York, NY 10013-1522 800-221-9369
Exercises for the elderly.
172 pages Cloth
ISBN: 0-898854-14-8

98 **Diagnosis and Treatment of Old Age**
S Karger Publishers
26 W Avon Road 860-675-7834
Farmington, CT 06085-1162 800-828-5479
Fax: 860-675-7302
www.karger.ch/company/karger.htm#10
These papers furnish a concise update on the diagnosis and treatment of Alzheimer's disease.
112 pages Hardcover
ISBN: 3-805548-44-3

99 **Elder Care**
Center For Public Representation
PO Box 260049 608-251-4008
Madison, WI 53726-0049 800-369-0388
Fax: 608-251-1263
www.law.wisc.edu/pal
A compendium of alternatives for providing and financing long-term care. This practical guide provides the most comprehensive and comforting information to help navigate a number of consumer minefields.
224 pages
ISBN: 0-873371-13-5

100 **Elderly in Modern Society**
Vance Bibliographier
PO Box 229 217-762-3831
Monticello, IL 61856-0229
A bibliography of laws and human rights for the elderly.
15 pages
ISBN: 0-792001-10-9

101 **Falling in Old Age**
Springer Publishing Company
536 Broadway 212-431-4370
New York, NY 10012-3955 877-687-7476
Fax: 212-941-7842
e-mail: marketing@springerpub.com
www.springerpub.com
Presented are practical techniques for the prevention of falls and for determining and correcting the causes.
1996 408 pages Hardcover
ISBN: 0-826152-91-0
Annette Imperati, Marketing Director

102 **Family Carebook**
CAREsource Program Development
505 Seattle Tower 206-625-9080
0eattle, WA 98101-3021
Guide to aging, the special needs of older adults, and the demands of providing care and support. Experts explain potential conflicts, planning opportunities and strategies for success.
475 pages Paperback
ISBN: 1-878866-12-5

103 **Focus on Geriatric Care and Rehabilitation**
Aspen Publishers
7201 McKinney Circle 301-251-8500
Frederick, MD 21704-8356-mail: customer.service@aspenpubl.com
www.aspenpub.com
Written for nurses, occupational therapists and administrators in geriatric settings.
Michael Brown, Publisher

104 **From Theory to Therapy: The Development of Drugs for Alzheimer's Disease**
Alzheimer's Association
225 N Michigan Avenue
Chicago, IL 60611-1696 800-272-3900
Fax: 866-699-1246
TDD: 312-335-8700
e-mail: media@alz.org
www.alz.org
Provides a layman's explanation of how experimental drugs are being developed and tested for Alzheimer's disease, and information about patient participation in clinical drug trials.

105 **Geriatric Rehabilitation Preview**
RTC on Aging
7601 E Imperial Highway
Downey, CA 90242-4155 310-940-7402
www.usc.edu/dept/gero/RRTConAging
Covers research, training activities, and other issues pertaining to the rehabilitation of elderly persons with disabilities.

106 **Health Care of the Aged**
Abraham Monk, PhD, author
Haworth Press
10 Alice Street 607-722-5857
Binghamton, NY 13904-1580 800-429-6784
Fax: 607-722-0012
www.haworthpress.com
Focusing on the need for developing new service delivery models for the aged, this book examines fiscal, political, and social criteria influencing this challenge of the 1990s. The aged are caught in the sweeping changes currently occurring in the financing, organizing and delivery of human health care services.
183 pages Hardcover
ISBN: 1-560240-65-5

107 **Healthy Aging: Good Investment & Together We Care: Helping Caregivers Find Supp.**
National Council on Aging
1901 L Street NW 202-479-1200
Washington, DC 20036 Fax: 202-479-0735
TDD: 202-479-6674
e-mail: info@ncoa.org
www.ncoa.org
Describes seven model programs that could be used in community-based organizations serving older adults.
2 Book Set
James P Firman, EdD, President/CEO

108 International Health Guide for Senior Citizen Travelers
Pilot Books
103 Cooper Street 516-422-2225
Babylon, NY 11702-2368 Fax: 516-669-4173
Covers essential pre-departure health planning such as advice on specific health concerns, disease prevention, specific travel problems, medical preparedness and assistance.
70 pages Paperback
ISBN: 0-875761-39-9
Anne Small, President

109 Living Well in a Nursing Home
Lynn Dickinson, Xenia Vosen, author
Hunter House Publishing
PO Box 2194 510-865-5282
Alameda, CA 94501 800-266-5592
Fax: 510-865-4295
e-mail: ordering@hunterhouse.com
www.hunterhouse.com
Positive aspects of nursing homes. How to recognize signs that a family member needs extra support. How to identify and select the best facility.
2005 288 pages Paperback
Cristina Sverdrup, Customer Service Manager

110 Mentally Impaired Elderly
Ellen D Taira, author
Haworth Press
10 Alice Street 607-722-5857
Binghamton, NY 13904-1580 800-429-6784
Fax: 607-722-0012
www.haworthpress.com
Provides effective support and sensitive care for the most vulnerable segment of the elderly population, those with mental impairment.
191 171 pages
ISBN: 1-560241-68-1

111 Mirrored Lives
Greenwood Publishing Group, Inc/Praeger Publishers
PO Box 6926
Portsmouth, NH 03802-6926 800-225-5800
Fax: 877-231-6980
e-mail: service@greenwood.com
www.greenwood.com
Discusses geriatric decline connected to nonterminal illness in old age. Koch takes a sensitive but thorough look at the declining years of his father.
240 pages
ISBN: 0-275936-71-6

112 Nursing Home Information Services
925 15th Street NW 202-347-8800
Washington, DC 20005-2301
Lists acceptable nursing homes across the nation and provides information about their costs, admission requirements, standards and programs.

113 Nursing Home and You: Partners in Caring
American Assn. of Homes & Services for the Aging
901 E Street NW
Washington, DC 20004-2037 800-508-9442
Fax: 301-206-9789
Offers information to nursing home staff and family members about caring for persons with Alzheimer's Disease.

114 Older Americans Information Directory
Grey House Publishing
4919 Route 22 518-789-8700
Amenia, NY 12501 800-562-2139
Fax: 518-789-0545
e-mail: books@greyhouse.com
www.greyhouse.com
Comprehensive guide to thousands of resources for and about older Aamericans, national and state organizations, government agencies, health research centers, libraries and information centers, legal resorces, discount travel information and continuing education programs. Published annually
1100 pages
ISBN: 1-930956-65-7
Leslie Mackenzie, Publisher

115 On Your Behalf
CAREsource Program Development
505 Seattle Tower 206-625-9080
Seattle, WA 98101
This book takes the mystery out of very important sets of legal options. It gives lay people as well as advisors, service providers, and caregivers the information they need to understand their options and the importance of individual choice.
16 pages Books & Video
ISBN: 1-878866-14-1

116 Physical Activity and the Aging
Human Kinetic Publishers
PO Box 5076
Champaign, IL 61825-5076 800-747-4457
Fax: 217-351-1549
www.humankinetics.com
North America's leading scholars examine the effects of aging on motor function, cardiovascular function, balance, the nervous system, changes in activity level, and possible reasons for activity level changes.
208 pages
ISBN: 0-873222-20-2

117 Planning for Long-Term Care
National Council on Aging
1901 L Street NW 202-479-1200
Washington, DC 20036 Fax: 202-479-0735
TDD: 202-479-6674
e-mail: info@ncoa.org
www.ncoa.org
Identify the various long-term care resources within your family and in your community using this thorough and readable guide.
160 pages
James P Firman, EdD, President/CEO

118 Read Easy
CAREsource Program Development
505 Seattle Tower 206-625-9080
Seattle, WA 98101
If books, audio tapes and computers can spark the imagination of the young adult and the middle aged, why not seniors as well? All it takes is commitment to make quality library resources and programs accessible and user-friendly to older readers. Read Easy is an invaluable planning and operations guide, explaining senior needs to library professionals and librarianship principles to senior care professionals.
95 pages
ISBN: 1-878866-13-3

119 Resources for Elders with Disabilities
Resources for Rehabilitation
22 Bonad Road 781-368-9094
Winchester, MA 01890 Fax: 781-368-9096
e-mail: info@rfr.org
www.rfr.org
A large print resource directory that helps elders function independently, with information on hearing loss, arthritis, osteoporoses, diabetes, vision loss, and stroke.
174 pages
ISBN: 0-929718-31-3

120 Senior Center Self: Assessment & National Accreditation Manual
National Council on Aging
1901 L Street NW 202-479-1200
Washington, DC 20036 Fax: 202-479-0735
TDD: 2024796674
e-mail: info@ncoa.org
www.ncoa.org
Based upon compliance with standards (best practices) developed by the National Institutes of Senior Centers. This program was de-

veloped under the auspices of NCOA's National Institute of Senior Centers (NISC).
Book & CD Set
James P Firman, EdD, President/CEO

121 **Senior Citizens and the Law**
Center for Public Representation
PO Box 260049 608-251-4008
Madison, WI 53726-0049 800-369-0388
Fax: 608-251-1263
An introduction to legal problems facing the elderly in Wisconsin. This edition discusses legal problems associated with Social Security, Medicare, SSI, guardianship and its alternatives, community-based services, probate, taxes, private health insurance and consumer protection.
176 pages
ISBN: 0-932622-29-1

122 **Successful Models of Community Long Term Care Services for the Elderly**
Haworth Press
10 Alice Street 607-722-5857
Binghamton, NY 13904-1580 800-429-6784
Fax: 607-722-0012
www.haworthpress.com
Experienced practitioners provide examples of successful community-based long term care service programs for the elderly.
174 pages
ISBN: 0-866569-87-9

123 **Unloving Care**
Harper Collins Publishers/Basic Books
10 E 53rd Street 212-207-7000
New York, NY 10022-5299 800-242-7737
Fax: 212-207-7203
www.harpercollins.com
A leading public health expert gives his account of the negative aspects of nursing homes.
305 pages
ISBN: 0-465088-81-3

Magazines

124 **AARP Magazine**
American Association of Retired Persons
601 East Street NW
Washington, DC 20049 888-687-2277
www.aarp.org
Serves the needs and interests of people 50 and over. With membership.
Bill Novelli, AARP CEO

125 **Abstracts in Social Gerontology**
National Council on Aging
1901 L Street NW 202-479-1200
Washington, DC 20036 Fax: 202-479-0735
TDD: 202-479-6674
e-mail: info@ncoa.org
www.ncoa.org
Detailed abstracts are provided for recent major journal articles, books, reports and other materials on many facets of aging, including adult education, demography, family relations, institutional care and work attitudes.
Quarterly
James P Firman, EdD, President/CEO

126 **Innovations**
National Council on Aging
1901 L Street NW 202-479-1200
Washington, DC 20036 Fax: 202-479-0735
TDD: 2024796674
e-mail: info@ncoa.org
www.ncoa.org
Explores significant developments in the field of aging through opinion articles, profiles and research summaries. Features articles on social trends, articles on specific aging programs and information on NCOA's activities. Members are free.
Quarterly
James P Firman, EdD, President/CEO

127 **International Journal of Technology and Aging**
Human Sciences Press
233 Spring Street 212-620-8000
New York, NY 10013-1522 800-221-9369
Fax: 212-463-0742
Designed to serve health-care professionals, researchers, academicians and industries concerned with the convergence of two recent trends, the dramatic advances in technology and the rapidly growing elderly population.

128 **Modern Maturity**
AARP
601 E Street NW
Washington, DC 20049-0003 800-424-3410
e-mail: member@aarp.org
www.aarp.org
Offers news and information of concern to those 50 and older. Features articles on current events, health, recreation, housing, family life, legislation and other issues.
6x Year

Newsletters

129 **AARP Bulletin**
American Association of Retired Persons
601 East Street NW
Washington, DC 20049 888-687-2277
www.aarp.org
Get daily news about the issues that matter to you.
Bill Novelli, AARP CEO

130 **Best Practices**
American Assoc. of Homes & Services for the Aging
2519 Connecticut Avenue NW 202-783-2242
Washington, DC 20008-1520 Fax: 202-783-2255
e-mail: info@aahsa.org
www.aahsa.org
Keeps nonprofit aging service providers informed of new trends and developments in quality of care for older persons.

131 **Bulletin**
AARP
601 E Street NW
Washington, DC 20049 800-424-3410
e-mail: member@aarp.org
www.aarp.org
11x Year

132 **CAPSule**
Children of Aging Parents
PO Box 167 215-355-6611
Richboro, PA 18954-0167 800-227-7294
Fax: 215-355-6824
e-mail: info@caps4caregivers.org
www.caps4caregivers.org
Newsletter devoted to assisting caregivers of the elderly.
12 pages Quarterly
Lenore Sherman, Executive Director
Karen Rosenberg, Director Senior Services

133 **Capital Advantage**
Capital Advantage Publishing
2731-A Prosperity Avenue 703-289-4670
Fairfax, VA 22031 Fax: 703-289-4678
e-mail: sales@capitaladvantage.com
www.capitaladvantage.com
Publishes articles on all aspects of aging including legislation, innovative programs and services.
Monthly

134 **Center for the Study of Aging Newsletter**
University of Pennsylvania Center for Aging Study
3615 Chestnut Street 215-898-3163
Philadelphia, PA 19104-4205 Fax: 215-573-8684
e-mail: www.med.upenn.edu/aging
ageweb@mail.med.upenn.edu
News and information concerning the University and Center aging activities, programs and seminars.

135 **Elderly Health Services Letter**
American Business Publishing
3100 Highway 138 732-681-1133
Wall Township, NJ 0771
Information on trends and developments in the expanding field of health services for the elderly.
Monthly
Robert Jenkins, Publisher

136 **Geriatric Care News**
DRS Geriatric Publishing Company
7435 SE 71st Street 206-232-9689
Mercer Island, WA 98040-5314
Newsletter for the elderly and their families.
Monthly
Denise Schramke, Publisher

137 **Geriatrics**
7500 Old Oak Boulevard 440-243-8100
Cleveland, OH 44130-3343
Articles for physicians and laypersons relating to care of middle-aged and elderly persons.
Monthly

138 **Gerontology News**
Gerontological Society of America
1030 15th Street NW 202-842-1275
Washington, DC 20005 Fax: 202-842-1150
e-mail: geron@geron.org
www.geron.org
It reports on policy issues, legislative actions, Society events, research results, and recently released major reports on aging. Regular features include Washington Updates; Research Highlights; Grants Available; New Resources and Reports; Data Updates; and Calls for Papers, Nominations, and Manuscripts.
Carol Ann Schutz, Executive Director

139 **Health After 50: Johns Hopkins Medical Letter**
Johns Hopkins Medical Institutions
550 Broadway 410-955-3182
Baltimore, MD 21205-2011 800-829-9170
e-mail: www.medjhu.edu
Health newsletter for people over 50.
10 pages Monthly
ISBN: 1-042188-2 -
Rodney Friedman, Publisher

140 **Lifelong Health and Fitness**
Center for the Study of Aging
706 Madison Avenue 518-465-4927
Albany, NY 12208-3604 Fax: 518-462-1339
e-mail: iapaas@aol.com
www.centerforthestudyofaging-albany.org
A quarterly newsletter published by the Center for the Study of Aging.
8 pages Quarterly
Sara Harris, Executive Director

141 **NCOA Week**
National Council on Aging
1901 L Street NW 202-479-1200
Washington, DC 20036 Fax: 202-479-0735
TDD: 202-479-6674
e-mail: info@ncoa.org
www.ncoa.org
Breaking news of NCOA initiatives, crucial legislative and policy issues, research studies, developments in work and volunteering for older adults, benefits for seniors, trends in aging, grant opportunities, and more. Members only.
Weekly
James P Firman, EdD, President/CEO

142 **Senior Focus**
National Council on Aging
1901 L Street NW 202-479-1200
Washington, DC 20036 Fax: 202-479-0735
TDD: 202-479-6674
e-mail: info@ncoa.org
www.ncoa.org
Timely, objective, and practical information on health and wellness, lifestyle, and financial issues for seniors and people who work with them.
Bi-Monthly
James P Firman, EdD, President/CEO

143 **Vital Aging Report**
National Council on Aging
1901 L Street NW 202-479-1200
Baltimore, MD Fax: 202-479-0735
TDD: 202-479-6674
e-mail: info@ncoa.org
www.ncoa.org
Packed with news about health and financial matters as well as United Senior's Health Council's innovative programs and research. The USHC is a program of the National Council on the Aging. Member price $17.50.
Quarterly
James P Firman, EdD, President/CEO

Pamphlets

144 **American Perceptions of Aging in the 21st Century**
National Council on Aging
1901 L Street NW 202-479-1200
Washington, DC 20036 Fax: 202-479-0735
TDD: 2024796674
e-mail: info@ncoa.org
www.ncoa.org
There are many interesting and important findings related to aging in America as reported by over 3000 respondents. This chartbook is intended as a handy reference for scholars, the press and advocates.
James P Firman, EdD, President/CEO

145 **Care of the Elderly in America**
Vance Bibliographies
PO Box 229 217-762-3831
Monticello, IL 61856-0229
A bibliography of aged care in America.
11 pages
ISBN: 1-555905-59-5

146 **Exploring Care Options for a Relative with Alzheimer's Disease**
American Assoc. of Homes & Services for the Aging
2519 Connecticut Avenue NW 202-783-2242
Washington, DC 20008-1520 800-508-9442
Fax: 202-783-2255
e-mail: www.aahsa.org
pub@aahsa.org

147 **Medicare Health Plan Choices: Consumer Update**
National Council on Aging
1901 L Street NW 202-479-1200
Washington, DC 20036 Fax: 202-479-0735
TDD: 202-479-6744
e-mail: info@ncoa.org
www.ncoa.org
Annually updated report contains important information about options that are available to Medicare beneficiaries. Medicare is changing, Medigap premiums are going up, and many Medicare HMOs are dropping service to seniors. Pamphlets available in single copies or packs of 50.
James P Firman, EdD, President/CEO

148 **Nonprofit Housing and Care Options for Older People**
American Assoc. of Homes & Services for the Aging
901 E Street NW
Washington, DC 20004-2037 800-508-9442
Fax: 301-206-9789
Offers information on continuing care facilities, retirement communities and more for the elderly and relatives caring for Alzheimer's patients.

149 **Time Out!**
Alzheimer's Association

225 N Michigan Avenue
Chicago, IL 60611-1696 800-272-3900
Fax: 866-669-1246
TDD: 312-335-8700
e-mail: media@alz.org
www.alz.org

Details the Association's position supporting a national respite care policy and recommends actions for federal and state policy makers.
1991 14 pages

Audio & Video

150 **Aphasia: Struggling for Understanding**
Filmakers Library
124 E 40th Street 212-808-4980
New York, NY 10016-1798 Fax: 212-808-4983
e-mail: info@filmakers.com
www.filmakers.com

What if your ability to speak or understand speech was taken away without warning, and you struggled to find words that just won't come? This film is about two people faced with the daunting task of learning to speak again,of regaining their humanity. DVD or VHS, Classroom Rental VHS also available for $65. 14 minutes in length.
DVD or VHS
Sue Oscar, Co-President

Web Sites

151 **Alliance for Aging Research**
www.agingresearch.org

Improving the health and independence of Americans as they age. Promotes medical and behavioral research into the aging process.

152 **American Association of Retired Persons**
www.aarp.org

AARP is the nation's leading organization for people age 50 and older. Information and education, advocacy, and community services provided by a network of local chapters and experienced volunteers throughout the country.

153 **American Society on Aging**
www.asaging.org

An association of diverse individuals bound together by a common goal: to support the commitment and enhance the knowledge and skills of those who seek to improve the quality of life of older adults and their families.

154 **Gerontological Society of America**
www.geron.org

Nonprofit professional organization with more than 5000 members in the field of aging. Provides researchers, educators, practitioners and policy makers with opportunities to understand, advance, integrate and use basic and applied research on aging to improve the quality of life as one ages.

155 **Healing Well**
www.healingwell.com

An online health resource guide to medical news, chat, information and articles, newsgroups and message boards, books, disease-related web sites, medical directories, and more for patients, friends, and family coping with disabling diseases, disorders, or chronic illnesses.

156 **Health Finder**
www.healthfinder.gov

Searchable, carefully developed web site offering information on over 1000 topics. Developed by the US Department of Health and Human Services, the site can be used in both English and Spanish.

157 **Healthlink USA**
www.healthlinkusa.com

Health information concerning treatment, cures, prevention, diagnosis, risk factors, research, support groups, email lists, personal stories and much more. Updated regularly.

158 **Helios Health**
www.helioshealth.com

Online resource for your health information. Detailed information about specific health topics, access to expert advice from our Medical Advisory Board, and up-to-date health news.

159 **MedicineNet**
www.medicinenet.com

An online resource for consumers providing easy-to-read, authoritative medical and health information.

160 **Medscape**
www.mywebmd.com

Medscape offers specialists, primary care physicians, and other health professionals the Web's most robust and integrated medical information and educational tools.

161 **National Council on Aging**
www.ncoa.org

Seniors Corner includes many resources and health related information on older Americans and their caregivers.

162 **National Institute of Aging**
www.nia.nih.gov

Conducts research on aging, behavioral and social research, neuroscience and neuropsychology, geriatrics, and clinical gerontology.

163 **Research Center**
www.resarch.aarp.org

Online center offering information on consumer issues, demographics, independent living and other items of interest to senior citizens.

164 **US Administration on Aging**
www.aoa.gov

An agency in the US Department of Health and Human Services, is one of the nation's largest providers of home and community-based care for older persons and their caregivers.

165 **WebMD**
www.webmd.com

WebMD provides valuable health information, tools for managing your health, and support to those who seek information.

Description

166 **AIDS/HIV**

AIDS, Acquired Immune Deficiency Syndrome, is an infectious disorder that suppresses the normal function of the human body's immune system. AIDS is a result of HIV (Human Immunodeficiency Virus) infection, which destroys the body's ability to fight infections. Specifically, the virus infects and later destroys T-cells, which are a part of the body's immune system that responds to invading organisms. This destructive process is slow and silent, which means that HIV can be contracted years before any symptoms appear. When enough T-cells have been destroyed, the body is invaded by organisms that wouldn't ordinarily be able to cause serious disease. An early symptom of HIV infection is usually an increasing number of infections. Weight loss, fever and night sweats are common. Certain cancers, especially lymphoma and Kaposi's sarcoma, also take advantage of the body's lowered resistance.

HIV transmission requires contact with body fluids and is usually spread from an infected person to a noninfected person by unprotected sexual intercourse, or by sharing needles. Mothers can give HIV infection to their children before and during childbirth and while breastfeeding.

Prevention of HIV infection is the best way to stop the AIDS epidemic. Unfortunately, progress on a vaccine has been disappointing, so avoiding contact with the virus is the primary method of prevention. Avoiding the riskier types of sexual intercourse will reduce one's risk, as will the use of a condom duringal and anal sex. Injecting drug users should not share needles. The use of needle exchange programs has decreased the spread of HIV infection. Women with HIV are encouraged to avoid pregnancy. If pregnant, HIV positive women should stay on medicine directed against HIV and should not breastfeed. Today, infants born to HIV women are treated with medication immediately after birth and this has greatly reduced the incidence of vertical transmission of the infection from mother to child. Until anti-HIV drugs became available, infected persons usually had a rapid downhill course. Today, combination drug treatment can offer most infected persons a long period of relatively good health. However, the treatment regimen is often complex and expensive, involving three or four drugs which must be taken several times a day. Since skipping doses encourages growth of virus that is resistant to the drugs, it is very important to take the drugs exactly as directed.

National Agencies & Associations

167 **AIDS Action**
1730 M Street NW
Washington, DC 20036
202-530-8030
Fax: 202-530-8031
www.aidsaction.org
National organization dedicated to the development analysis cultivation and encouragement of sound policies and programs in response to the HIV epidemic. We do this through the dissemination of information and the building and use of advocacy.
Donna Crews, Director Government Affairs
Rebecca Haag, Executive Director

168 **AIDS Coalition of Cape Breton**
150 Bentinck Street
Sydney, Nova Scotia, B1P-6H1
902-567-1766
Fax: 902-567-1766
e-mail: christineporter@accb.ns.ca
www.accb.ns.ca
Provides support and advocacy services for PLW HIV/AIDS (people living with HIV/AIDS). Services provided deal with social, legal, ethical and spiritual issues.
Christine Porter, Executive Director
Jo-Anne Rolls, PHA Program Coordinator

169 **AIDS Committee of Durham**
401-222 King Street W
Oshawa, Ontario, L1J-2K4
905-576-1445
Fax: 905-576-4610
e-mail: info@aidsdurham.com
www.aidsdurham.com
To provide HIV/AIDS related services to the infected or affected and the general community in the region of Durham.

170 **AIDS Committee of London**
388 Dundas Street
London, Ontario, N6B-1V7
519-434-1601
Fax: 519-434-1843
e-mail: info@aidslondon.com
www.aidslondon.com
Is a community-based, charitable organization providing HIV-related services to people living with and concerned about HIV/AIDS in London and area.
Peter Hayes, Executive Director
Elizabeth Lam, Office Manager

171 **AIDS Committee of Ottawa**
251 Bank Street
Ottawa, Ontario K2P 1X3,
613-238-5014
Fax: 613-238-3425
e-mail: connect@aco-cso.ca
www.aco-cso.ca
Works to empower people living with HIV/AIDS and the PLWHA (persons living with HIV/AID) community in Ottawa through promoting the well being and quality of life of those living with, or close affected by HIV/AIDS.
Kathleen Cummings, Executive Director

172 **AIDS Committee of Toronto**
399 Church Street
Toronto, Ontario, M5B-2J6
416-340-2437
Fax: 416-340-8224
www.actoronto.org
Delivers responsive, effective, and valued community-based HIV support services and education, prevention, outreach and fundraising programs that promote health, well-being, worth and rights of individuals and communities living with, affected by and at risk for HIV/AIDS, and increase awareness of HIV/AIDS.
Adrienne Giroux, Special Event Manager
Lori Lucier, Executive Director

173 **AIDS Committee of York Region**
194 Eagle Street E
Newmarket, Ontario, L3Y-1J6
905-953-0248
800-243-7717
Fax: 905-953-1372
e-mail: edacyr@bellnet.ca
www.acyr.org
The AIDS Committee of York Region envisions an informed and compassionate society, which is supportive of people living with HIV/AIDS who are striving to overcome social and service challenges, working with them towards a healthy and empowered lifestyle.
Radha Bhardwaj, Acting Executive Director

174 **AIDS Network**
600 Williamson Street
Madison, WI 53703
608-252-6540
Fax: 608-252-6559
e-mail: info@aidsnetwork.org
www.aidsnetwork.org

Provides critical AIDS care and prevention services. Sustained in these efforts by the resources expertise and passion of hundreds of volunteers and donors.
Bob Power, Executive Director
Ellen Berz, President

175 **AIDS New Brunswick**
65 Brunswick Street 506-459-7518
Fredericton, NB, E3B-1G5 800-561-4009
Fax: 506-459-5782
e-mail: sidaids@nbnet.nb.ca
www.aidsnb.com
A provincial organization committed to facilitating community-based responses to the issues of HIV/AIDS. The aim is to promote and support the health and well-being of persons living with and affected by HIV/AIDS and to reduce the spread of HIV/AIDS in New Brunswick.
Joannah Lang, Executive Director

176 **AIDS Niagara**
Normandy Resource Center 905-984-8684
St. Catharines, Ontario, L2R-3C9 800-773-9843
Fax: 905-988-1921
e-mail: info@aidsniagara.com
www.aidsniagara.com
AIDS Niagara is dedicated to improving the quality of life for those infected and/or affected by HIV/AIDS.
Steve Byers, Executive Director
Jody Yurchak, Education & Support Coordinator

177 **AIDS PEI**
144 Prince Street 902-566-2437
Charlottetown, PE, C1A-3R6 Fax: 902-626-3400
www.aidspei.com
To create a supportive environment for Persons Living with AIDS/HIV, to increase public understanding of the impact of HIV/AIDS, and to reduce the incidence of HIV/AIDS in Prince Edward Island.
Angela McKinnon, Program Coordinator

178 **AIDS Thunder Bay**
574 Memorial Avenue 807-345-1516
Thunder Bay, Ontario, P7B-3Z2 800-488-5840
Fax: 807-345-2505
e-mail: info@aidsthunderbay.org
www.aidsthunderbay.org
Provide quality, compassionate support, education and advocacy around HIV and AIDS, and related issues.
Michael Sobota, Executive Director
Kate Doornwaard, ODCC Coordinator

179 **AIDS Treatment Data Network**
611 Broadway 212-260-8868
New York, NY 10012 800-734-7104
e-mail: network@atdn.org
www.atdn.org
The Network is a national independent community-based not-for-profit organization that provides treatment access and advocacy, case management, supportive counseling and English and Spanish language information services to men women and children with HIV.

180 **AIDS.ORG**
7985 Santa Monica Blvd
W Hollywood, CA 90046 323-656-6036
www.aids.org
The mission of AIDS.ORG is to help prevent HIV infections and to improve the lives of those affected by HIV and AIDS by providing education and facilitating the free and open exchange of knowledge at any easy-to-find centralized website.
Alain Berrebi, Executive Director
Peter Dobson, Director

181 **AIDSinfo**
PO Box 6303 301-519-0459
Rockville, MD 20849-6303 800-448-0440
Fax: 301-519-6616
TTY: 888-480-3739
e-mail: contactus@aidsinfo.nih.gov
www.aidsinfo.nih.gov
AIDSinfo is a U.S. Department of Health and Human Services (DHHS) project that offers the latest federally approved information on HIV/AIDS clinical research, treatment and prevention, and medical practice guidelines for people living with HIV/AIDS, their families and friends, health care providers, scientists, and researchers.

182 **ANKORS: Kootenay AIDS Services**
101 Baker Street 250-505-5506
Nelson, BC, V1L-4H1 Fax: 250-505-5507
e-mail: info@ankors.bc.ca
www.ankors.bc.ca
ANKORS' mission is to respond to the evolving needs of those living with and affected by HIV and AIDS.
Cheryl Dowden, Executive Director
Gary Dalton, Community Care Team

183 **Access AIDS Network**
111 Elm Street 705-688-0500
Sudbury, Ontario, P3C-1T3 800-465-2437
Fax: 705-688-0423
e-mail: access@cyberbeach.net
www.accessaidsnetwork.com
A non-profit, community-based charitable organization, committed to promoting wellness, education, harm and risk reduction.
Richard Rainville, Executive Director
Christine Coutu, Clerical Intake Worker

184 **Alberta Reappraising AIDS Society**
Box 61037 403-220-0129
Calgary, Alberta, T2N-4S6 Fax: 403-289-6658
e-mail: aras@aras.ab.ca
www.aras.ab.ca
Promote critical discussion of the HIV/AIDS dogma.
David Crowe, President
Katherine Newell, Treasurer

185 **American Autoimmune Related Diseases Association**
22100 Gratiot Avenue 586-776-3900
Eastpointe, MI 48021 800-598-4668
Fax: 586-776-3903
e-mail: aarda@aarda.org
www.aarda.org
Awareness, education, referrals for patients with any type of autoimmune disease.
Virginia T. Ladd, President/Executive Director

186 **American Civil Liberties Union AIDS Project**
125 Broad Street
New York, NY 10004 www.aclu.org/HIVAIDS/HIVAIDSMain.cfm
Offers legislative and employment information public awareness materials and support for persons with HIV/AIDS and their families.
Anthony D Romero, Executive Director
Dorothy M Ehrlich, Deputy Executive Director

187 **American Federation of Teachers HIV/AIDS Education Project**
555 New Jersey Avenue NW
Washington, DC 20001-2029 202-879-4400
www.aft.org
A group of education professionals with the main purpose of their work being the education and public awareness of HIV and AIDS.
Randi Weingarten, President

188 **American Foundation for AIDS Research**
120 Wall Street 212-806-1600
New York, NY 10005-3908 800-342-2437
Fax: 212-806-1601
TTY: 800-243-7889
e-mail: kevin.frost@amfar.org
www.amfar.org
Supports research in basic clinical prevention and public policy and publishes the HIV/AIDS Treatment Directory.
Kevin Robert Frost, CEO
Bradley Jensen, Chief Financial Officer

189 **Asian & Pacific Islander Wellness Center Community HIV/AIDS Services**
730 Polk Street 415-292-3400
San Francisco, CA 94109 Fax: 415-292-3404
TTY: 415-292-3410
www.apiwellness.org
HIV Care Services is the only integrated HIV services program targeting A&PIs in Northern California. Integrates primary care with psychiatric mental health HIV treatment psychosocial support and, in response to evolving needs, targeted HIV prevention.
Lance Toma LCSW, Executive Director
AJ Carvajal, Human Resources Administrator

190 **Asian and Pacific Island Wellness Center**
730 Polk Street 415-292-3400
San Francisco, CA 94109 Fax: 415-292-3404
TTY: 415-292-3410
e-mail: info@apiwellness.org
www.apiwellness.org
Our mission is to educate support empower and advocate for Asian and Pacific Islander communities - particularly A&PIs living with or at-risk for HIV/AIDS.
Lance Toma LCSW, Executive Director
AJ Carvajal, Human Resources Administrator

191 **Better Existence with HIV**
1740 Ridge 847-475-2115
Evanston, IL 60201 Fax: 847-475-2820
www.behiv.org
Private not-for-profit AIDS service organization. Only comprehensive AIDS service provider in all northern Cook County. Effectively combines direct service and prevention programs.
Eric Nelson, Executive Director
Christine Gryszkiewi, Business Manager

192 **Black Coalition for AIDS Prevention**
110 Spadina Avenue 416-977-9955
Toronto, Ontario, M5V-2K4 Fax: 416-977-7725
e-mail: blackcap@black-cap.com
www.black-cap.com
A volunteer-driven, charitable, not-for-profit, community-based organization. We work in partnership with organizations and individuals who support in principle and practice our mission, philosophy and activities.
Davine Burton RN BA, Member

193 **British Columbia Persons with AIDS Society**
1107 Seymour Street 604-893-2200
Vancouver, BC, V6B-5S8 800-994-2437
Fax: 604-893-2251
e-mail: info@bcpwa.org
www.bcpwa.org
Exists to enable persons living with AIDS and HIV disease to empower themselves through mutual support and collective action.
Ross Harvey, Executive Director
Paul Lewand, Chair

194 **CDC National Prevention Information Network (NPIN)**
PO Box 6003 919-361-4892
Rockville, MD 20849-6003 800-458-5231
Fax: 888-282-7681
TTY: 800-243-7012
e-mail: info@cdcnpin.org
www.cdcnpin.org
The CDC National Prevention Information Network (NPIN) is the U.S. reference, referral, and distribution service for information o HIV/AIDS, sexually transmitted diseases (STD's), and tuberculosis (TB). NPIN produces, collects, catalogs, processes, stocks, and disseminates materials and information on HIV/AIDS, STD's, and TB to organizations and people working in those disease fields in international, national, state, and local settings.

195 **Canadian Foundation for AIDS Research**
165 University Avenue 416-361-6281
Toronto, Ontario, M5H-3B8 800-563-2873
Fax: 416-361-5736
www.canfar.ca
A national charitable foundation whose goal is to raise awareness in order to generate funds for research into all aspects of HIV infection and AIDS.
Elissa Beckett, Executive Director
Dana Nielsen, National Programs Manager

196 **Central Alberta AIDS Network Society**
4611-50th Avenue 403-346-8858
Red Deer Alberta, T4N 3-3Z9 877-346-8858
Fax: 403-346-2352
e-mail: receptionist@cirsoninc.ca
www.caans.org
Central Alberta AIDS Network Society is a local charity and a Turning Point agency that offers support to individuals who are infected or affected by HIV/AIDS and provides prevention and education throughout Central Alberta.
Jennifer Vanderschae, Executive Director
Mel Lewis, Health Promotion Coordinator

197 **Children Affected by AIDS Foundation**
6033 W Century Boulevard 310-258-0850
Los Angeles, CA 90045 Fax: 310-258-0851
e-mail: caaf@caaf4kids.org
www.caaf4kids.org
The mission of the Children Affected by AIDS Foundation (CAAF) is to make a positive difference in the lives of children infected with HIV and affected by AIDS. CAAF accomplishes this by helping meet their diverse, special needs, advocating and educating.
Catherine A Brown, President
Pat Crawford, Office Manager

198 **Children's AIDS Fund**
PO Box 16433 703-433-1560
Washington, DC 20041 866-829-1560
Fax: 800-557-8529
e-mail: info@childrensaidsfund.org
www.childrensaidsfund.org
The Children's AIDS Fund works to limit suffering of children and their families caused by HIV disease by providing care services resourced referrals and education.
Anita Smith, President

199 **Clinical Focus on Primary Immune Deficiency Diseases**
40 W Chesapeake Avenue 410-321-6647
Towson, MD 21204 800-296-4433
Fax: 410-321-9165
e-mail: idf@primaryimmune.org
www.primaryimmune.org
Educational monograph is designed specifically for health care professionals and focuses on topics relevant to primary immune deficiency diseases.
Marcia Boyle, President & Founder

200 **Committee of Ten Thousand**
236 Massachusetts Avenue NE 202-543-0988
Washington, DC 20002 800-488-2688
Fax: 202-543-6720
e-mail: cott-dc@earthlink.net
www.cott1.org
Represents people with hemophilia who contracted HIV/AIDS and Hepatitis C from tainted factor concentrates in the 1970s and 1980s. The only national advocacy and support agency for this seriously disabled community.
Corey S Dubin, President
Mary Lou Murphy, Co-Vice President

201 **Continuum**
255 Golden Gate Avenue 415-437-2900
San Francisco, CA 94102 Fax: 415-437-2550
TTY: 415-861-1399
e-mail: anne@continuumhiv.org
web.mac.com/tenderloinhealth
Empower and dignify the lives of underserved people with HIV and AIDS providing innovative health and human services that establish community, and reduce the rate of HIV infection.
Colm Hegarty, Director Development & Public Relations
Chiquita T Tuttle, Interim Executive Director

202 Deaf AIDS Project Family Service Foundation
Family Service Foundation
5301 76th Avenue 301-459-2121
Landover Hills, MD 20784 866-935-4658
Fax: 301-459-0675
TTY: 301-731-2116
e-mail: ssoulier@fsfinc.org
www.deafnonprofit.net/dap
The AIDS Administration established in 1987 as a division of the Maryland Department of Health and Mental Hygiene leads public health initiatives regarding HIV (Human Immunodeficiency Virus), the virus that causes AIDS.

203 Elizabeth Glaser Pediatric AIDS Foundation
1140 Connecticut Avenue NW 202-296-9165
Washington, DC 20036 888-499-4673
Fax: 202-296-9185
e-mail: info@pedaids.org
www.pedaids.org
Creates a future of hope for children and families worldwide by eradicating pediatric AIDS providing care and treatment to people with HIV/AIDS and accelerating the discovery of new treatments for other serious and life-threatening pediatric illnesses.
Pamela W Barnes, President/CEO

204 Farha Foundation
576, Sainte-Catherine Street E 514-270-4900
Montreal, QC, H2L-2E1 Fax: 514-270-5363
e-mail: farha@farha.qc.ca
www.farha.qc.ca
A fundraising organization, committed to help men, women and children living with HIV/AIDS.

205 Foundation for Children with AIDS
1800 Columbus Avenue 617-442-7442
Roxbury, MA 02119 Fax: 617-442-1705
www.hivpositive.com
A national nonprofit organization founded to improve the quality of life for drug-effected and HIV-infected children and their families. The foundation raises funds for family and community-based services for children and their families affected by HIV.
Robert Maynard, President

206 HIV West Yellowhead Services
Box 2427 780-852-5274
Jasper, Alberta, T0E-1E0 Fax: 780-852-5274
e-mail: director@hivwestyellowhead.com
www.hivwestyellowhead.com
Encourage a positive, healthy lifestyle and provide accurate information to the people living and working in the region.

207 HIV/Hepatitis C in Prison (HIP) Committee
California Prison Focus 510-665-1935
San Francisco, CA 94103 e-mail: contact@prisons.org
www.prisons.org/hivin.htm
The HIV/HCV in Prison Committee of California Prison Focus works on behalf of prisoners to fight for consistent access to quality medical care including access to all new HIV and hepatitis C medications, diagnostic testing and combination therapies.
Michelle Foy, Contact
Judy Greenspan, Contact

208 Health Information Network
PO Box 30762 206-784-5655
Seattle, WA 98113 Fax: 206-784-3240
www.healthinfonetwork.org
Offers information public awareness and support for women with HIV/AIDS and the public in general.
Kathi Knowles, Executive Director

209 Health Information Network for Women and AIDS
Positive Women's Network
2817 Rockefeller Avenue 425-259-9899
Everett, WA 98201 888-651-8931
Fax: 425-259-9880
www.pwnetwork.org
A partnership of women living with and affected by HIV/AIDS supports women in making informed choices about HIV/AIDS and health.
Kerri Mallams, Executive Director
Joanne Maurice, President

210 Heart Touch™ Project
3400 Airport Avenue 310-391-2558
Santa Monica, CA 90405 Fax: 310-391-2168
e-mail: executive@hearttouch.org
www.hearttouch.org
Non-profit educational and service organization devoted to the delivery of compassionate and healing touch to home or hospital-bound men women and children.
Jennifer Noguera, Coordinator Children's Program
Patrick Callahan, Executive Director

211 Immune Deficiency Foundation
40 W Chesapeake Avenue 410-321-6647
Towson, MD 21204-4841 800-296-4433
Fax: 410-321-9165
e-mail: idf@primaryimmune.org
www.primaryimmune.org
The only national charitable organization aimed at fighting the primary immune deficiency diseases. The founders included parents of children with primary immune deficiency immunologists who treat immune deficient patients and other individuals with an immune deficiency.
John Seymour, Vice Chair
Marcia Boyle, Chair President & Founder

212 International Council of AIDS Service Orga nization
65 Wellesley Street E 416-921-0018
Toronto Ontario, M4Y 1-1G7 Fax: 416-921-9979
e-mail: icaso@icaso.org
www.icaso.org
A global network of non-governmental and community-based organizations.
Kieran Daly, Executive Director
Sumita Banerjee, Senior Program Manager

213 Life Force: Women Fighting AIDS
175 Remsen Street 718-797-0937
Brooklyn, NY 11201-4300 Fax: 718-797-4011
e-mail: info@lifeforceinc.org
www.lifeforceinc.org
A support network offering prevention education awareness risk reduction workshops and support for woman with HIV/AIDS.
Sayida Self, Interim Executive Director
Sherlina Nageer, Chair

214 Living Positive
#50, 9912-106 Street 780-488-5768
Edmonton, Alberta, T5K-1C5 800-210-9561
Fax: 780-702-8211
www.edmlivingpositive.ca
Dedicated to providing emotional, spiritual and psychological support to all those living with HIV.
Lance Hansen, Director
Deborah Norris, Chairperson

215 Medical Library Association
65 E Wacker Place 312-419-9094
Chicago, IL 60601-7246 Fax: 312-419-8950
e-mail: info@mlahq.org
www.mlahq.org
Non-profit educational organization of more than 1,100 institutions and 3,600 individual members in the health sciences information field, committed to educating health information professionals, supporting health information research and promoting access to information.
Mary L Ryan AHIP FMLA, President
Carla J Funk, Executive Director

216 Multifaith Works
115 16th Avenue 206-324-1520
Seattle, WA 98122 Fax: 206-324-2041
e-mail: info@multifaith.org
www.multifaith.org

Non-profit non-denominational organization that provides housing and supportive services to people living with AIDS or other life-threatening illness and community education on issues of human diversity.
Arthur Padilla, Executive Director
Randy Lazenby, President

217 **NAMES Project Foundation AIDS Memorial Quilt**
AIDS Memorial Quilt
637 Hoke Street NW 404-688-5500
Atlanta, GA 30318 Fax: 404-688-5552
e-mail: info@aidsquilt.org
www.aidsquilt.org
International non-governmental non-profit organization that is the custodian of the AIDS Memorial Quilt a poignant memorial and powerful tool for use in preventing new HIV infections.
Julie Rhoad, Executive Director
Roddy Williams, Director of Operations

218 **National AIDS Fund**
729 15th Street NW 202-408-4848
Washington, DC 20005-1511 888-234-AIDS
Fax: 202-408-1818
www.aidsfund.org
The National AIDS Fund is one of America's largest philanthropic organizations dedicated to eliminating HIV/AIDS as a major health and social problem. The Fund's primary purpose is channeling critical resources to community-based organizations to fight HIV.
Kandy Ferree, President & CEO
Matthew Kessler, Director of Operations

219 **National AIDS Treatment Advocacy Project**
580 Broadway 212-219-0106
New York, NY 10012 888-26N-ATAP
Fax: 212-219-8473
e-mail: info@natap.org
www.natap.org
Educate by sending out literature e-mail lists and give forums on how to prevent HIV or how to live with it.
Jules Levin, Executive Director

220 **National Coalition on Immune System Disorders**
1090 Vermont Avenue NW 202-371-8090
Washington, DC 20005-4953 800-438-2996
Fax: 202-371-1945
Professional and lay organizations with a primary interest in the immune system and its diseases.
Robert R Humphreys, Executive Director

221 **National Hospice & Palliative Care Organization (NHPCO)**
1700 Diagonal Road 703-837-1500
Alexandria, VA 22314 800-658-8898
Fax: 703-837-1233
e-mail: nhpcoinfo@nhpco.org
www.nhpco.org
The nation's only advocate for terminally ill patients and their families. Founded in 1978, the NHPCO is the only organization devoted to hospice in the United States. Support is included from state hospice organizations, patients, families, communities, provider program members and professional/volunteer members. Represents hospice care interests to Congress, regulatory agencies, courts, voluntary organizations and the public.
Donald Schumacher, PsyD, President/CEO

222 **National Minority AIDS Education Training Center**
Howard University
1840 7th Street NW 202-865-8146
Washington, DC 20001-3029 Fax: 202-667-1382
e-mail: gdowner@howard.edu
www.nmaetc.org
Located at Howard University as a HIV/AIDS training and technical resource for providers of minority HIV-infected patients throughout the country. The NMAETC receives 100% of its funding through the MAI Initiative.
Goulda Downe PhD RD, Principal Investigator
David Luckett, Deputy Director

223 **National Native American AIDS Prevention Center**
720 S Colorado Boulevard 720-382-2244
Denver, CO 80246 Fax: 720-382-2248
e-mail: information@nnaapc.org
www.nnaapc.org
To address the impact of HIV/AIDS on American Indians Alaska Natives and Native Hawaiians through culturally appropriate advocacy research education and policy development in support of healthy Indigenous people.
Geoffrey Roth, President
Dana Pierce-Hedge, Executive Director

224 **National Prevention Information Network CDC NPIN**
CDC NPIN
PO Box 6003 404-679-3860
Rockville, MD 20849-6003 800-458-5231
Fax: 888-282-7681
TTY: 888-232-6348
e-mail: info@cdcnpin.org
www.cdcnpin.org
The CDC National Prevention Information Network (NPIN) is the U.S. reference referral and distribution service for information on HIV/AIDS, sexually transmitted diseases (STDs) and tuberculosis (TB).
Jay Laudato, Executive Director

225 **National Prison Project/ACLU AIDS in Prison Project**
915 15th Street NW 202-393-4930
Washington, DC 20005-5737 Fax: 202-393-4931
www.aclu.org
National Prison Project seeks to create constitutional conditions of confinement and strengthen prisoners' rights through class action litigation and public education. Our policy priorities include reducing prison overcrowding and improving prisoner medical care.

226 **New England AIDS Education and Training Center**
23 Miner Street 617-262-5657
Boston, MA 02215-3318 Fax: 617-262-5667
e-mail: aidsed@neaetc.org
www.neaetc.org
Our goal is to increase the number of health care providers effectively trained to counsel diagnose treat and manage the care of individuals with HIV infection and to assist in the prevention of high risk behavior which may lead to infection.
Donna M Gallagher RNC MS AN, Project Director
Calvin Cohen MD MS, Co-Research Director

227 **North Bay Aids Committee**
269 Main Street W 705-497-3560
North Bay, Ontario, P1B-2T8 Fax: 705-497-7850
e-mail: acnba@efni.com
www.aidsnorthbay.com
To assist and support all persons infected or affected by HIV/AIDS and to limit the spread of the virus through education and outreach strategies.
Jennifer Furtney, Executive Director
Steve Lamb, Support Services Coordinator

228 **Ontario HIV Treatment Network**
1300 Young Street 416-642-6486
877-743-6486
Fax: 416-640-4245
e-mail: info@ohtn.on.ca
www.ohtn.on.ca
To optimize the quality of life of people living with HIV in Ontario and to promote excellence and innovation in treatment, research, education and prevention through a collaborative network of excellence representing consumers, providers, researchers and other stakeholders.
Bill Flanagan, President
Jonathan Angel, VP

229 **Pediatric AIDS Foundation**
11150 Santa Monica Boulevard 310-314-1459
Los Angeles, CA 90025-3092 Fax: 310-314-1469
e-mail: info@pedaids.org
www.pedaids.org
A national nonprofit organization confronting medical problems unique to children infected with HIV/AIDS. The foundation funds

critically needed pediatric AIDS research and provides help to hospitals that serve the needs of children with HIV/AIDS.
Pamela W Barnes, President/CEO

230 **Peel HIV/AIDS Network**
160 Traders Boulevard
Mississauga Ontario, L4Z 3-4K1
905-361-0523
Fax: 905-361-1004
e-mail: ed@phan.ca
www.phan.ca
Committed to serving people living with and affected by HIV/AIDS and to limit the spread of the virus through support education advocacy and volunteerism.
Ketih Wong, Executive Director
Savi Sinanan, Coordinator Volunteer Services

231 **Project Inform**
1375 Mission Street
San Francisco, CA 94103
415-558-8669
800-822-7422
Fax: 415-558-0684
e-mail: web@projectinform.org
www.projectinform.org
Inform people living with HIV Advocate to facilitate research towards a cure and appropriate policies and Inspire people to make informed choices take effective action in the fight against HIV and choose hope over despair.
Dana Van Gorder, Executive Director
Michael Allerton, President

232 **Resources and Services Database Centers for Disease Control**
Centers for Disease Control
PO Box 6003
Rockville, MD 20849
877-242-9760
Fax: 301-562-1050
TTY: 240-514-2780
e-mail: info@hivatwork.org
www.brta-lrta.org
Describes more than 16 000 organizations that provide HIV and AIDS prevention education and social services. These include public health departments community and social service organizations hospitals and clinics.

233 **The AIDS Network**
140 King Street East
Hamilton, ON L8N 1B2,
905-528-0854
866-563-0563
Fax: 905-528-6311
e-mail: info@aidsnetwork.ca
Hours of operation: Monday-Friday, 9am-12pm and 1pm-5pm.
Betty Anne Thomas, Executive Director

234 **Toronto People with AIDS Foundation**
399 Church Street
Toronto, Ontario, M5B-2J6
416-506-1400
Fax: 416-506-1404
e-mail: info@pwatoronto.org
www.pwatoronto.org
The Toronto People with AIDS Foundation exists to promote the health and well-being of all people living with HIV/AIDS by providing accessible, direct, and practical support services.
Murray Jose, Executive Director
Suzanne Paddock, Director, Programs & Services

235 **UNICEF USA**
125 Maiden Lane
New York, NY 10038
212-686-5522
800-486-4233
Fax: 212-779-1679
e-mail: information@unicefusa.org
www.unicefusa.org
Supports child survival protection and development worldwide through education advocacy and fundraising for AIDS and other conditions.
Caryl M Stern, President and CEO
Edward G Lloyd, Executive Vice President and CFO

236 **Well Project**
112 Krog Street NE
Atlanta, GA 30307
404-474-3152
e-mail: info@thewellproject.org
www.thewellproject.org
The Well Project is a not for profit corporation and an initiative conceived developed and administered by HIV+ women and those who are affected by this disease. Our Founder Dawn Averitt Bridge was diagnosed with HIV in 1988.
Dawn Averitt Bridge, Founder & Board President
Richard Averitt, COO

237 **Women Alive**
1566 Burnside Avenue
Los Angeles, CA 90019
323-965-1564
800-554-4876
Fax: 323-965-9886
e-mail: info@women-alive.org
www.women-alive.org
Coalition of, by and for women living with HIV/AIDS. Created ways to help women connect with each other, bring others out of isolation, exchange information about HIV treatments and take charge of their lives.
Carrie Broadus, Executive Director
Alicia K Avalos, Associate Director

238 **Women's AIDS Network Women and Children's Service Program**
Women and Children's Service Program
10 United Nations Plaza
San Francisco, CA 94101
415-864-4376

State Agencies & Associations

Alabama

239 **Alabama Department of Public Health**
201 Monroe Street
Montgomery, AL 36104-3000
334-206-5364
800-228-0469
Fax: 334-206-2092
www.adph.org/aids
Offers health education and risk education activities including compiling a state community resource directory.
Danna Cargill, Office Manager
Jane B Cheeks, Division Director

Alaska

240 **Alaska Department of Health and Social Services: AIDS/STD Program**
3601 C Street
Anchorage, AK 99503-0249
907-269-8000
800-478-0084
Fax: 907-562-7802
e-mail: mollie_cross@health.state.ak.us
www.epi.hss.state.ak.us/hivstd
The HIV/STD Program addresses public health issues and activities with the goal of preventing sexually transmitted diseases (STDs) and HIV infection in Alaska as well as their impact on health. AIDS program offers education to providers and organizations.
John Middaug PhD, Chief Dept of Public Health/Epidemiology
Mollie Cross, Prevention Community Planning Group

Arizona

241 **Arizona Department of Health Services**
150 N 18th Avenue
Phoenix, AZ 85007
602-542-1000
800-334-1540
Fax: 602-542-0883
www.azdhs.gov
Provides HIV and AIDS seropositive surveillance case investigation and analysis and AIDS health education and training for the public.
Margery Sheridan, Division Chief
Will Humble, Interim Director

242 **Tucson Interfaith HIV/AIDS Network (TIHAN)**
1011 N Craycroft Road
Tucson, AZ 85711
520-299-6647
Fax: 520-784-0620
e-mail: friends@tihan.org
www.tihan.org
Serving interfaith communities of Tucson through compassionate care education training and spiritual support so that we can make more people aware of the health crisis which affects all of us. Also provide non-medical in-home help.
Scott Blades, Executive Director
Jess Knutson, Director Education/Community Relations

Arkansas

243 **Arkansas Department of Health AIDS Prevention Program**
AIDS Prevention Program
5800 W 10th Street
Little Rock, AR 72204
501-280-4950
Fax: 501-280-4999
www.healthyarkansas.com
Provides educational materials such as pamphlets and films conducts HIV and AIDS research and operates a speakers bureau.
Robin Thomas, Regional Director

California

244 **Aids, Medicine and Miracles**
3288 21st Street
San Francisco, CA 94110-2423
415-252-7111
Fax: 415-252-7117
e-mail: amm@aidsmedicineandmiracles.org
www.aidsmedicineandmiracles.org
Provides culturally sensitive counseling and education to stop the spread of HIV infection, and to help people face the emotional, psychological and social changes of living with HIV disease.
Gregg Cassin, Chair
Mary Ellen Roche, Secretary

245 **California Collaborative Treatment Group CCTG Data Center**
CCTG Data Center
3900 Fifth Avenue
San Diego, CA 92103-1910
619-543-5006
Fax: 619-298-1359
e-mail: rhaubrich@ucsd.edu
www.cctg.ucsd.edu
The CCTG is a multi-center clinical trials organization founded by Dr. Allen McCutchan in 1986. The primary mission of the CCTG is to improve the scientific basis for HIV patient care and HIV prevention. CCTG develops treatment protocols and drug therapies.
Richard Haub MD, Investigator/Professor of Medicine
Allen McCutc MD, Investigator/Professor of Medicine

246 **California Department of Health Services Office of Aids**
Office of Aids
1616 Capitol Avenue
Sacramento, CA 95814
916-449-5900
800-458-5231
Fax: 916-449-5909
www.dhs.ca.gov/aids
Works to develop strategies and implement programs for education and prevention testing and counseling supportive care and treatment and research to control the spread of HIV infection.
Michelle Roland, Section Chief

247 **Los Angeles County Department of Health Services**
AIDS Programs
600 S Commonwealth Avenue
Los Angeles, CA 90005
213-351-8000
800-243-7889
Fax: 213-738-0825
e-mail: aids@ph.lacounty.org
www.lapublichealth.org
Responsible for planning coordinating and implementing county wide HIV/AIDS efforts.
Charles L Henry, Director
Raymond H Johnson, Chief of Staff

248 **San Francisco AIDS Foundation (SFAF)**
995 Market Street
San Francisco, CA 94103
415-487-3000
800-367-AIDS
Fax: 415-487-3009
TTY: 415-487-3012
TDD: 415-487-8099
e-mail: feedback@sfaf.org
www.sfaf.org
SFAF provides confidential array of services-including financial benefits counseling client advocacy housing assistance HIV prevention efforts and needle exchange.
Peter Taback, Director of Communications
Sergio Cano, Volunteer Programs Coordinator

249 **San Francisco Area AIDS Education and Trai ning Center**
UCSF Box 1365
1001 Potrero Avenue
San Francisco, CA 94143-1365
415-206-8730
Fax: 415-476-3454
e-mail: sfaetc@ucsf.edu
www.ucsf.edu/sfaetc
Helps to improve the care of people living with HIV and AIDS by supporting state-of-the-art clinical consultation education and training for health care professionals and organizations in Sa Francisco San Mateo and Marin counties.
Jacqueline Tulsky, Medical Director
Ronald H Goldschmidt, Director

Colorado

250 **Colorado Center for AIDS Research: Univers ity Colorado Health Sciences Center/CFAR**
Division of Infectious Diseases
4200 E 9th Avenue
Denver, CO 80262
303-315-7233
Fax: 303-315-8681
e-mail: colorado.cfar@uchsc.edu
www.uchsc.edu/ccfar
Describes forms and patterns of use of complimentary and alternative medicine (CAM) for the treatment of HIV/AIDS.
Edward N Janoff MD, CFAR Director
Kristin Jones, CFAR Administrator

Connecticut

251 **Connecticut Department of Health Services AIDS Programs**
AIDS Programs
410 Capitol Avenue
Hartford, CT 06134
860-509-7801
800-842-0038
Fax: 860-509-7853
e-mail: webmaster.dph@ct.gov
www.dph.state.ct.us
Operates a speakers bureau provides training workshops seminars and counseling services conducts meetings and offers information and referral services.
Rosa M Biaggi, Director
William Gerrish, Communications

252 **Northwestern Connecticut AIDS Project**
100 Migeon Avenue
Torrington, CT 06790-0985
860-482-1596
800-381-2437
Fax: 860-482-3606
e-mail: general@nwctaids.org
www.freewebs.com/nwctaidsproject
A nonprofit organization offering support and a variety of services to people with AIDS and their loved ones. Provides education to all segments of the public about AIDS prevention and treatment.
Patricia Lafayette, Executive Director
Demetria McMilliAn, Program Director Client Services

Delaware

253 **Delaware Department of Health and Social Services**
Division of Public Health, HIV/STD Program
417 Federal Street
Dover, DE 19901
302-744-4700
888-459-2943
Fax: 302-739-6659
e-mail: dhssinfo@state.de.us
www.dhss.delaware.gov/dhss/dph/index.htm
Provides HIV counseling and testing prevention education and AIDS surveillance and studies.
Jamie Rivera, Director

District of Columbia

254 **Washington DC Department of Health HIV/AIDS Administration**
HIV/AIDS Administration
825 N Capitol Street NE
Washington, DC 20002
202-442-5955
www.doh.dc.gov
Mission is to reduce the incidence of HIV/AIDS and number of deaths related to HIV/AIDS in the District of Columbia by the application of sound public health practices and initiatives through HIV disease surveillance tracking, monitoring, and intervention.
Dr Pierre Vigilance, Director

Florida

255 Body Positive HIV and AIDS Research and Re source Center
1144 E McDowell Road 602-307-5330
Phoenix, AZ 85006 Fax: 602-307-5021
e-mail: cweiner@phoenixbodypositive.org
www.phoenixbodypositive.org

Body Positive is a non-profit organization created by and for people infected and affected by HIV, that provides the community with the knowledge, resources and collective strength necessary for individuals to live long and well with HIV and to prevent the spread of the disease.

Carol A Poore MBA, President and CEO
Andy Myers MD, Medical Director

256 Florida Department of Health Bureau of HIV/AIDS
Bureau of HIV/AIDS
4052 Bald Cypress Way 850- 24- 433
Tallahassee, FL 32399-1715 Fax: 850- 9-2 42
e-mail: DiseaseControl@doh.state.fl.us
www.doh.state.fl.us

Making voluntary HIV testing a routine part of medical care implementing new models for diagnosing HIV infections outside medical settings preventing new infections by working with persons diagnosed with HIV and their partners.

Tom Liberti, Bureau Chief
Janell Clemons, Administrative Assistant

257 Positive Voices
3841 NE 2 Avenue 305-891-2066
Miami, FL 33138 888-POS-CONN
Fax: 786-623-0701
e-mail: email@positiveconnections.org
www.positiveconnections.org

The Center for Positive Connections is a non-profit community based organization that is run for those infected our community. Our mission is to provide educational emotional holistic and social support at all individuals living with HIV/AIDS.

258 TBAN
7402 N 56th Street
Tampa, FL 33674-8333 813-769-5180
www.queertampa.com/tan.html

TBAN formerly The Tampa AIDS Network (TAN) is a community organization which provides prevention education emotional and physical support services and advocacy on behalf of all persons affected by HIV disease.

Vivian Candelaria, Director

Georgia

259 Georgia Department of Human Resources: Division of Public Health
AIDS Section
2 Peachtree Street 404-656-4937
Atlanta, GA 30303 800-551-2728
Fax: 404-657-3100
e-mail: gdphinfo@dhr.ga.us
http://health.state.ga.us

Provides technical support and assistance to the Public Health Districts to prevent STD and HIV infection ensuring the availability of quality STD/HIV prevention and treatment by improving quality assurance guidelines and methods by providing appropriate training.

Stewart Brown, Director

Hawaii

260 Hawaii Department of Health: Communicable Disease Division
AIDS/Sexually Transmitted Diseases Control Branch
3627 Kilauea Avenue 808-733-9010
Honolulu, HI 96816-2317 Fax: 808-733-9015
e-mail: janice.okubo@doh.hawaii.gov
www.hawaii.gov/health/about/admin

Offers research education surveillance and testing components. AIDS information and guidelines about the placement of infants children and adolescents who test positive for HIV in nursery or school settings are also available.

Chiyome Fuki MD, Director
Susan Jackson, Deputy Director

Idaho

261 Idaho Department of Health and Welfare The STD/AIDS Program
The STD/AIDS Program
450 W State Street 1st Floor 208-334-6527
Boise, ID 83720-0036 Fax: 208-332-7346
e-mail: apsportal@dhw.idaho.gov
www.healthandwelfare.idaho.gov

Program receives federal funding to support testing treatment and prevention services for Idaho's reportable sexually transmitted infections.

Richard Armstrong, Director
Tom Shananan, Public Information Manager

Illinois

262 AIDS Legal Council of Chicago
180 N Michigan Avenue 312-427-8990
Chicago, IL 60601 866-506-3038
Fax: 312-427-8419
e-mail: info@aidslegal.com
www.aidslegal.com

Legal advice and services for persons who are HIV positive or have AIDS and their companions families etc.

Ann Hilton Fisher, Executive Director
Ericka Sanchez, Administrative Staff

263 Chicago Department of Health
333 S State Street 312-747-9865
Chicago, IL 60604 Fax: 312-747-9765
TTY: 312-747-2374
e-mail: publichealth@cdph.org
egov.cityofchicago.org

Offers educational services audiovisual materials surveillance of HIV and AIDS counseling and referrals.

David Kern, Director

264 Illinois Department of Public Health: Division of Infectious Diseases
535 W Jefferson Street 217-782-4977
Springfield, IL 62761 Fax: 217-782-3987
TTY: 800-547-0466
www.idph.state.il.us

Administers the AIDS Drug Assistance Program (ADAP). Currently nearly 3 300 clients use ADAP services each month accessing 10 000 prescriptions. Client approved for ADAP must re-apply on an annual basis in order to continue to receive services.

Eric E Whitaker, Director
Randy J Dunn, State Superintendent of Education

265 Test Positive Aware Network (TPAN)
5537 N Broadway Street 773-989-9400
Chicago, IL 60640-1405 Fax: 773-989-9494
e-mail: tpan@tpan.com
www.tpan.com

Empowers people living with HIV through peer-led programming support services information dissemination and advocacy. Provides services to the broader community to increase HIV knowledge and sensitivity and to reduce the risk of infection.

Rick Bejlovec, Executive Director
Barbara Marcotte, Treatment Education Coordinator

Kansas

266 Kansas Department of Health & Environment Epidemiology & Disease Prevention: HIV
1000 SW Jackson 785-296-1500
Topeka, KS 66612-1274 Fax: 785-368-6368
e-mail: info@kdheks.gov
www.kdheks.gov

Conducts surveillance of HIV/AIDS in Kansas. Conducts Prevention Program with training for counselors and educators partial funding of counseling test sites and distribution of educational materials. Provides medications and primary care.

Kathy Donner, HIV Prevention Director
Jeni Trimble, HIV Surveillance Director

Louisiana

267 **Louisiana Department of Health & Hospitals : Office of Public Health**
Louisiana AIDS Prevention/Surveillance Program
628 N 4th Street 225-342-9500
Baton Rouge, LA 70821-0629 800-992-4379
Fax: 225-342-5568
e-mail: dhhwebadmin@la.gov
www.dhh.louisiana.gov/offices/?ID
The HIV/AIDS Program was established in 1985 to provide leadership policy development and technical assistance including HIV/AIDS education prevention and services to parish health units and community based organizations throughout the state.
William Clark, Medical Director
William Hineman, Director/Program Manager II

Maine

268 **Maine Bureau of Health: Division of Disease Control**
HIV/STD Program
286 Water Street 207-287-3747
Augusta, ME 04333 800-351-2437
Fax: 207-287-3498
TTY: 800-606-0215
e-mail: chris.zukas-lessard@maine.gov
www.maine.gov/dhhs/boh/index.htm
Provides technical assistance to state agencies and private organizations regarding AIDS education and policy development.
Chris Zukas-Lessard, Deputy Director
Dora Anne Mills, Director

Massachusetts

269 **Massachusetts Department of Health HIV/AIDS Bureau**
HIV/AIDS Bureau
250 Washington Street 617-624-6000
Boston, MA 02108 800-235-2331
Fax: 617-624-5399
TTY: 617-437-1672
www.mass.gov/dph
Assisting in preventing the spread of the HIV epidemic and the development of appropriate cost-effective health and support services which will maintain patients in the least restrictive setting.
Kevin Cranston, Director
John Auerbach, Commissioner Department of Public Health

270 **New England AIDS Education & Training Cent er (NEHEC)**
23 Miner Street 617-262-5657
Boston, MA 02215-3318 Fax: 617-262-5667
e-mail: aidsed@neaetc.org
www.neaetc.org
The New England HIV Education Consortium (NEHEC), a HRSA minority AIDS initiative program, is a training and education program serving all six states in the New England region. The principal goal of NEHEC is to address the HIV-related training, educational, and support needs of the full, spectrum of providers as they provide state-of-the-art, quality and compassionate care to individuals living with HIV/AIDS.
Donna M Gallagher RNC/MS/ANP, Principal Investigator/Project Director
Barry Sandberg MS/MPA, Assistant Director/Administrator

Michigan

271 **Michigan Department of Community Health HIV/AIDS Prevention & Intervention Secti**
HIV/AIDS Prevention & Intervention Section
109 Michigan Avenue 517-241-5900
Lansing, MI 48913 888-826-6565
Fax: 517-241-5911
www.michigan.gov/mdch
Gives general public and high-risk education grants supporting educational materials programs and a hotline.
Loretta Davis-Satter, Director Division HIV/AIDS-STD
Chris Hanson, Dental Program Coordinator

Minnesota

272 **Minnesota Department of Health: AIDS/STD Prevention Service**
Office of Infectious Diseases
717 Delaware Street SE 612-676-5414
Minneapolis, MN 55440-9272 877-925-4189
Fax: 612-623-5743
e-mail: indepcweb@health.state.mn.us
www.health.state.mn.us
This division is to prevent death and disability from HIV and other sexually transmitted diseases by providing statewide leadership regarding the prevention of transmission and the availability of health and supportive services for infected persons.
Harry Hull, Director

Mississippi

273 **Mississippi Department of Public Health: STD/HIV Prevention Program**
570 E Woodrow Wilson Drive 601-576-7400
Jackson, MS 39216 866-458-4948
Fax: 601-576-7909
www.msdh.state.ms.us
Funds two statewide hotlines one for the general public and one for the gay community. Both offer health education and risk reduction activities of the Program include baseline evaluation of public knowledge about AIDS through surveys.
Joy Sennett, Director Communicable Disease Office

Missouri

274 **Missouri Department of Health: Bureau of AIDS Prevention**
Po Box 570 573-751-6400
Jefferson City, MO 65102-0570 866-628-9891
Fax: 573-751-6010
e-mail: info@dhss.mo.gov
www.dhss.mo.gov
Human Immunodeficiency Virus (HIV) disease and infection and Acquired Immunodeficiency Syndrome (AIDS) surveillance monitors and analyzes data on the number of people infected with HIV and/or AIDS and identifies and tracks trends in disease incidence.
Margaret T Donnelly, Director
Bret Fischer, Director

Montana

275 **Montana Deptartment of Health And Human Services**
STD & HIV Prevention Program
1400 Broadway 406-444-4540
Helena, MT 59620 800-233-6668
Fax: 406-444-1861
www.dphhs.state.mt.us
This program receives a Federal grant through the Centers for Disease Control to carry out a health education/risk reduction program to detect and prevent the spread of HIV infection through a number of services.
Jane Smilie, Acting Administrator
Anna Whiting Sorrell, Director

Nevada

276 **Nevada Department of Human Resources: Heal th Program Section**
4126 Technology Way 775-684-4000
Carson City, NV 89706-2009 Fax: 775-684-4010
e-mail: nvdhr@dhhs.nv.gov
www.dhhs.nv.gov
Provides HIV counseling and testing a speakers bureau information and referrals resource materials including AIDS video recordings and education.
Harold Cook, Administrator
Martha Framsted, Public Information Officer

New Hampshire

277 **New Hampshire Department of Health and Human Services**
Division of Public Health Services

29 Hazen Drive
Concord, NH 03301-4604
603-271-4502
800-852-3345
Fax: 603-271-4934
TTY: 800-735-2964
TDD: 8007352964
www.dhhs.state.nh.us

HIV/AIDS Program receives both state and Federal funding pertaining to AIDS education risk reduction testing and surveillance.
Joyce J Welch, Program Coordinator
James Fredyma, Director

New Jersey

278 **New Jersey Department of Health: Division of AIDS Prevention & Control**
Division of HIV/AIDS Service (DHAS)
Po Box 360
Trenton, NJ 08625-0360
609-292-7837
800-367-6543
www.state.nj.us/health

Serves to coordinate and direct primary HIV activities within the Department networking with other divisions and agencies to provide information and care programs to populations in need.
Laurence E Ganges, Assistant Commissioner
Carl Peck, Director

279 **New Jersey Woman AIDS Network**
103 Bayard Street
New Brunswick, NJ 08901
732-846-4462
Fax: 732-846-2674
e-mail: office@njwan.org
www.njwan.org

A leader in identifying issues facing women with HIV/AIDS educating service providers advocating for appropriate policies and building a multicultural women and HIV/AIDS movement.
Monique Howard, Executive Director
Fiordaliza Gomez, Program Coordinator

New Mexico

280 **New Mexico Health Department: Public Health Division**
HIV/AIDS/STD Prevention & Services Bureau
1190 S Saint Francis Drive
Santa Fe, NM 87502-4182
505-827-2613
800-545-2437
Fax: 505-827-2530
www.health.state.nm.us

Provides training programs and HIV education to the general public and professionals risk reduction information AIDS school curriculums classroom presentation information and an AIDS hotline.
Don Maestas, Director

New York

281 **New York Department of Health, Office of Public Health: AIDS Institute**
AIDS Institute
Empire State Plaza
Albany, NY 12237-0001
518-474-9866
Fax: 518-473-8814
e-mail: hivpubs@health.state.ny.us
www.health.state.ny.us

Awards grants and maintains relationships with regional AIDS service groups, crisis intervention, psychosocial counseling and legal, financial and housing assistance. The Institute also offers preventive education, risk reduction education, HIV counseling and testing and patient care.
Wendy V. Gould, Coordinator Educational Materials

North Carolina

282 **North Carolina Department of Health & Natural Resources**
HIV/STD Prevention & Care
1931 Mail Service Center
Raleigh, NC 27699-1902
919-707-5000
Fax: 919-870-4829
e-mail: hivstdprevention@ncmail.net
www.ncpublichealth.com

Oversee the AIDS surveillance program HIV counseling testing partner notification health education risk reduction and public information efforts in North Carolina.
Rebecca King, Chief
Paul Buescher, Director

Ohio

283 **Ohio Department of Health: Division of Pre ventive Medicine**
HIV/AIDS Surveillance Division
246 N High Street
Columbus, OH 43215-0118
614-466-1388
800-777-4775
Fax: 614-644-1909
TTY: 800-332-AIDS
e-mail: Surveillance@odh.ohio.gov
www.odh.ohio.gov

Consists of AIDS surveillance seroprevalence programs, health care worker education, health education and risk reduction projects.
Alvin D Jackson MD, Director of Health
Anne Harnish, Assistant Director

Oklahoma

284 **Oklahoma Department of Health: AIDS Division**
1000 NE 10th
Oklahoma City, OK 73117-1207
405-271-5600
800-522-0203
Fax: 405-271-5149
www.health.state.ok.us

Provides prevention-related services and funding to the network of AIDS service delivery organizations, both public and private in Oklahoma. The Division provides services and training and certification of AIDS educators, surveillance, and seroprevalence staff.
Rocky D McElvany, Interim Commissioner of Health
Ken Feagins, Director

Oregon

285 **Oregon Department of Human Resources Health Division HIV Program**
Health Division, HIV Program
800 NE Oregon Street
Portland, OR 97232
971-673-1222
800-777-2437
Fax: 971-673-1299
TTY: 971-673-0372
e-mail: health.webmaster@state.or.us
www.oregon.gov/DHS/ph

HIV Program includes training workshops for AIDS trainers curriculum development or revision and an AIDS hotline through Cascade AIDS Project.
Veda Latin, HST Program Manager
Mitch Zahn, HIV Prevention Manager

Pennsylvania

286 **Pennsylvania Department of Health: Bureau of HIV/AIDS**
Division of HIV/AIDS
Room 933
Harrisburg, PA 17108
717-783-4677
800-662-6080
Fax: 717-772-6975
e-mail: c-hivepi@state.pa.us
www.dsf.health.state.pa.us

The purpose of the Division of HIV/AIDS is to develop and implement a multi-dimensional coordinated strategy to prevent disease and change high-risk behaviors as well as provide resources and direction for sustaining preventive behavior and avoiding infection.
Janice P Kopelman MSW LSW, Director

287 **Philadelphia Department of Public Health: AIDS Program**
AIDS Activities Coordinating Office (AACO)
1101 Market Street
Philadelphia, PA 19107
215-685-5600
800-985-AIDS
Fax: 215-685-5293
www.phila.gov/health

Administers federal state and city funded HIV/AIDS programs in Philadelphia through collaborative service contracts with community-based organizations.
Marla Gold MD, Program Coordinator
Nan Feyler, Chief of Staff

Rhode Island

288 **Rhode Island Department of Health: Division of Disease Prevention & Control**
Office of AIDS/HIV

3 Capitol Hill
Providence, RI 02908
401-222-2320
800-381-AIDS
Fax: 401-222-2488
www.health.state.ri.us

Provides health education and risk reduction activities through its AIDS program. Services include professional conferences, providing assistance for in-service programs, presentation of two courses and organization of an AIDS minority program. Also, provides public health services in HIV/AIDS and Viral Hepatitis. The office develops policies, funds community programs and conducts surveillances.

Paul G. Loberti, Chief Administrator
Lucille Minuto, Assistant Administrator

South Carolina

289 **South Carolina Department of Health & Environmental Control**
Bureau of Preventive Health Services
2600 Bull Street
Columbia, SC 29201
803-898-3432
www.scdhec.net

Provides services to prevent the spread of sexually transmitted diseases (STD's) and HIV infection to reduce associated illness and death and to provide care and support resources for persons with HIV disease.

Jeff Jones MD, Director

Tennessee

290 **Tennessee Department of Health: AIDS Program**
Cordell Hull Building, 4th Floor
425 Fifth Avenue N
Nashville, TN 37243
615-741-3111
Fax: 615-741-2491
e-mail: tn.health@tn.gov
health.state.tn.us

Provides HIV/STD education and information, as well as collecting monitoring and distributing data. Provides assistance to individuals, and intervention and treatment services.

Laurel Wood, Program Coordinator

Texas

291 **AIDS Outreach Center (AOC)**
801 W Cannon Street
Fort Worth, TX 76104
817-335-1994
Fax: 817-335-3617
e-mail: info@aoc.org
www.aoc.org

The staff and volunteers of the AIDS Outreach Center (AOC) provide a wide range of social services, outreach activities, testing and counseling, prevention education programs and public policy advocacy for men, women and children living with HIV, and their loved ones.

Allan Gould Jr, Executive Director
Michael Toole, President/Board of Directors

292 **Houston Department of Health and Human Services: Bureau of HIV Prevention**
8000 N Stadium Drive
Houston, TX 77054-1823
713-794-9020
Fax: 713-798-0830
TTY: 713-794-9092
www.houstontx.gov/health

Coordinates sexually transmitted disease surveillance, seroprevalence, contract tracing partner notification, public information, minority initiatives and health evaluation/risk reduction.

Stephen L Williams, Director

293 **Texas Department of Health: Bureau of HIV and STD Prevention**
HIV/STD Division
1100 W 49th Street
Austin, TX 78756-3199
512-458-7111
888-963-7111
TTY: 800-735-2989
TDD: 512-458-7708
www.dshs.state.tx.us

Mission is to prevent, treat, and/or control the spread of HIV, STD, and other communicable diseases to protect the health of the citizens of Texas.

David Lakey, Commissioner

Utah

294 **Utah Department of Health: Bureau of Communicable Disease Control**
Division of Epidemiology & Laboratory Services
288 N 1460 W
Salt Lake City, UT 84114-2105
801-538-6191
800-537-1046
Fax: 801-538-9923
e-mail: rrolfs@utah.gov
www.health.utah.gov/cdc

Secures and distributes funds for AIDS prevention services, provides educational programs and counseling to the general public, AIDS service organizations, health workers and groups at risk.

Robert Rolfs, Director, Bureau/State Epidemiologist
Melissa Stevens-Dimo, Manager, Communicable Diseases

Vermont

295 **Vermont Department of Health: Health Surveillance HIV/AIDS/STD/TB Program**
108 Cherry Street
Burlington, VT 05402-0070
802-863-7200
800-464-4343
Fax: 802-865-7754
TTY: 802-863-7235
www.healthvermont.gov

Provides health education and risk reduction activities nurses and other professional training, AIDS presentations, educational and media campaigns and counseling and referrals.

Rod Copeland PhD, Director HIV/AIDS Program

Virginia

296 **Virginia Department of Health: Division of HIV, STD, and Pharmacy Services**
109 Governor Street
Richmond, VA 23218
804-786-6267
800-533-4148
Fax: 804-786-7528
e-mail: hiv-stdhotline@vdh.virginia.gov.
www.vdh.virginia.gov

Supports local health departments and community-based organizations in the prevention, surveillance and treatment of HIV and other STD's, including their complications, through provision of education, information, and health care services.

Casey Riley, Director
Craig Parrish, Pharmacist

Washington

297 **Northwest AIDS Education and Training Cent er (AETC)**
901 Boren Avenue
Seattle, WA 98104
206-685-6844
Fax: 206-221-4945
e-mail: lalonde@u.washington.edu
http://depts.washington.edu/nwaetc/

Located at the University of Washington, offering HIV treatment education, clinical consultation, capacity building and technical assistance to health care professionals and agencies in Washington, Alaska, Montana, Idaho, and Oregon.

Bernadette Lalonde Ph.D, Principal Investigator/Program Director
Laurie Conratt MBA, State Programs Manager

298 **Washington Department of Health: Division of HIV/AIDS Prevention Services**
HIV Client Services
PO Box 47840
Olympia, WA 98504-7840
360-236-3434
877-376-9316
Fax: 360-236-3400
e-mail: brown.mcdonald@doh.wa.gov
www.doh.wa.gov/cfh/HIV_AIDS/Prev_Edu

Provides information and referrals to local, state and national resources relating to HIV/AIDS provides informational and educational materials to individuals, agencies and organizations and actively works with print and broadcast media to promote HIV/AIDS awareness.

Paul Brown, HIV Data Manager
Brown McDonald, HIV Prevention Services Manager

West Virginia

299 **West Virginia Department of Health & Human Resources**
HIV/AIDS & STD Program
State Capitol Complex 304-558-0684
Charleston, WV 25305-3715 800-352-6513
Fax: 304-558-1130
e-mail: wvdhhrsecretary@wvdhhr.org
www.wvdhhr.org

Provides the AIDS-related services in 15 public health HIV-counseling and testing centers which offer by appointment confidential or anonymous testing.
Martha Yeage Walker, Secretary

Wisconsin

300 **Wisconsin Department of Health and Social Services: Division of Health**
HIV/AIDS/Hepatitis Program
PO Box 2659 608-266-1251
Madison, WI 53701 800-438-1282
Fax: 608-267-2832
TTY: 888-701-1253
e-mail: DHSwebmaster@wisconsin.gov
www.dhs.wisconsin.gov

Coordinates counseling and testing sites activities and services to HIV-infected persons, produces a report that contains information and recommendations for health care workers, emergency medical technicians and food service workers.
Seth Foldy, Administrator and State Health Officer
Thomas Sieger, Deputy Administrator

Wyoming

301 **Wyoming Department of Health HIV/AIDS/Hepatitis Program**
HIV/AIDS/Hepatitis Program
401 Hathaway Building 307-777-7656
Cheyenne, WY 82002-0001 866-571-0944
Fax: 307-777-7439
wdh.state.wy.us

100 percent federally funded and responsible for the solicitation development and implementation of community AIDS prevention initiatives.
Brent D Sherard, Director and State Health Officer
Ginny Mahoney, Chief of Staff

Foundations

302 **National Hemophilia Foundation**
116 West 32nd Street 212-328-3700
New York, NY 10001 800-42H-ANDI
Fax: 212-328-3777
e-mail: handi@hemophilia.org
www.hemophilia.org

The National Hemophilia Foundation is dedicated to finding better treatments and cures for bleeding and clotting disorders and to preventing the complications of these disorders through education, advocacy and research.
Alan Kinniburgh, PhD, Chief Executive Officer

Libraries & Resource Centers

303 **AIDS Library of Philadelphia**
1233 Locust Street 215-985-4851
Philadelphia, PA 19107 Fax: 215-985-4492
e-mail: library@aidslibrary.org
www.aidslibrary.org

Improving access to health and support services, preventing HIV transmission, and raising the public awareness of HIV/AIDS related issues.

304 **National Library of Medicine**
8600 Rockville Pike 301-594-5983
Bethesda, MD 20894 888-346-3656
Fax: 301-402-1384
e-mail: custserv@nlm.nih.gov
www.nlm.nih.gov/

The National Library of Medicine (NLM), on the campus of the National Institutes of Health in Bethesda, Maryland, is the world's largest medical library. The Library collects materials in all areas of biomedicine and health care, as well as works on biomedical aspects of technology, the humanities, and the physical, life, and social sciences.
Dr Donald Lindberg, Director
Betsy L Humphreys, Deputy Director

Research Centers

305 **CDC National Prevention Information Network (NPIN)**
PO Box 6003
Rockville, MD 20849-6003 800-458-5231
Fax: 888-282-7681
TTY: 800-243-7012
e-mail: info@cdcnpin.org
www.cdcnpin.org

The CDC National Prevention Information Network (NPIN) is the U.S. reference, referral, and distribution service for information o HIV/AIDS, sexually transmitted diseases (STD's), and tuberculosis (TB). NPIN produces, collects, catalogs, processes, stocks, and disseminates materials and information on HIV/AIDS, STD's, and TB to organizations and people working in those disease fields in international, national, state, and local settings.

306 **CDC National Prevention Information Networ k**
PO Box 6003 404-679-3860
Rockville, MD 20849 800-458-5231
Fax: 888-282-7681
TTY: 800-243-7012
e-mail: info@cdcnpin.org
www.cdcnpin.org

The CDC National Prevention Information Network (NPIN) is the U.S. reference referral and distribution service for information o HIV/AIDS sexually transmitted diseases (STD's) and tuberculosis (TB). NPIN produces collects catalogs processes stocks and disseminates materials and information on HIV/AIDS STD's and TB to organizations and people working in those disease fields in international national state and local settings.

Alabama

307 **Centers for AIDS Research: University of Alabama at Birmingham**
BBRB 256
Birmingham, AL 35294-2170 205-934-2437
www.uabcfar.uab.edu

Provides expertise, resources, and services not otherwise readily obtained through traditional funding mechanisms.
Michael S. Saag, Director

308 **General Clinical Research Center: UAB**
Room 907 Medical Education Building 205-934-4852
Birmingham, AL 35294 e-mail: ccts@uab.edu
www.gcrc.uab.edu

AIDS and genetics research.
Lisa Guay-Woodford, Director
Catarina Kiefe, Co-Principal Investigator

309 **University of Alabama at Birmingham: National Cooperative Drug/AIDS**
UAB Center for AIDS Research
BBRB 256
Birmingham, AL 35294-2170 205-934-2437
www.uabcfar.uab.edu

Dr. Richard Whitley, Principal Investigator

California

310 **AIDS Clinical Trials Unit CARES Clinic**
CARES Clinic
2nd Floor Research Office 916-914-6322
Sacramento, CA 95814 Fax: 916-325-1955
e-mail: actu@ucdavis.edu
www.ucdmc.ucdavis.edu/actu

The ACTU at Davis Medical Center is dedicated to offering the latest in research clinical trials to HIV/AIDS patients throughout Northern Central California.
Nancy L Fitch, Director
Richard B Pollard, Principal Investigator

311 **Adult Research Opportunities**
150 W Washington Street 619-543-8080
San Diego, CA 92103 Fax: 619-298-0117
www.avrctrials.org
A university-based nonprofit clinical trials unit. Conduct's patient-oriented research and educational programs on HIV and other chronic infections. Studies have pioneered the development of treatments that continue to change the course of the HIV epidemic.
Kim Schafer, Chief Operating Officer AEDIRP
Kumiko Koelkebeck, Finance Assistant

312 **Center for AIDS Prevention Studies AIDS Research Institute University of C**
AIDS Research Institute, University of California
50 Beale Street 415-597-9100
San Francisco, CA 94105 Fax: 415-597-9213
e-mail: CAPS.Web@ucsf.edu
www.caps.ucsf.edu
The mission of the Center for AIDS Prevention Studies is to conduct domestic and international research to prevent the acquisition of HIV and to optimize health outcomes among HIV-infected individuals.
Stephen F Morin, Director
Susan Kegeles, Co-Director

313 **Center for Interdisciplinary Research in Immunology and Diseases at UCLA**
UCLA School of Medicine
405 Hilgard Avenue 310-825-6373
Los Angeles, CA 90095 e-mail: jlfahey@mednet.ucla.edu
dgsom.healthsciences.ucla.edu
Research into immunology and blood disorders with special focus on AIDS and HIV infections.
John L Fahey MD, Director

314 **Centers for AIDS Research: North-Central California**
UC Davis, Division of Infectious Diseases
4150 V Street 916-734-8033
Sacramento, CA 95817 Fax: 916-734-7766
e-mail: nccfar@ucdavis.edu
www.ucdmc.ucdavis.edu/nccfar
Provides expertise resources and services not otherwise readily obtained through more traditional funding mechanisms.
Richard B Pollard, Division Chief
Krystin E Cheung, Director

315 **Centers for AIDS Research: USCD Center for AIDS Research**
Center for AIDS Research
University of California San Diego 858-534-5545
La Jolla, CA 92093-0716 Fax: 858-822-5840
e-mail: cfar@ucsd.edu
cfar.ucsd.edu
Provides expertise resources and services and services not otherwise readily obtained through traditional funding mechanisms.
Douglas Richman, Director
Kim Schafer, Administrative Director

316 **Centers for AIDS Research: University of California, Los Angeles**
UCLA AIDS Institute
60-054 Center for Health Sciences 310-825-4750
Los Angeles, CA 90095-1678 Fax: 310-794-7682
e-mail: ebayrd@mednet.ucla.edu
www.uclaaidsinstitute.org
Provides expertise, resources, and services not otherwise readily obtained through traditional funding mechanisms.
Irvin S.Y. Chen, Director

317 **City of Hope National Medical Center Drug Discover/AIDS Group**
City of Hope
1500 E Duarte Road
Duarte, CA 91010 626-256-4673
www.cityofhope.org
Developmental research into the treatment of AIDS.
John A Zaia, Principal Investigator

318 **Kaiser Foundation Research Institute**
3505 Broadway
Oakland, CA 94611 510-891-3400
www.dor.kaiser.org
Paul Lairson MD, Director

319 **Stanford University General Clinical Research Center**
GCRC Administration
300 Pasteur Drive 650-724-0921
Stanford, CA 94305-5251 Fax: 650-725-6698
e-mail: gcrcstanford@stanford.edu
www.med.stanford.edu/gcrc
The Stanford General Clinical Research Center (GCRC) is the major clinical research facility for Stanford University School of Medicine. With patient care units in Stanford University Hospital and Lucile Packard Children's Hospital the center plays a crucial role in the school's bench-to-bedside research mission.
David Stevenson, Associate Program Director
Branimir I Sikic, Program Director

320 **Stanford University National Cooperative Drug Discovery/AIDS Group**
School of Medicine
300 Pasteur Drive
Stanford, CA 94305 650-723-4000
www.med.stanford.edu
Ellen Jo Baron, Director

321 **UCLA AIDS Clinical Research Center**
1399 S Roxbury Drive 310-557-2273
Los Angeles, CA 90095-3075 Fax: 310-206-3311
www.uclacarecenter.org
Ronald T Mitsuyana, Director
Judith Currier, Associate Director

322 **UCSD Antiviral Research Center**
150 W Washington Street 619-543-8080
San Diego, CA 92103 Fax: 619-298-0117
www.avrctrials.org
Develops treatment protocols and drug therapies and recruits research volunteers for AIDS studies and HIV related disorders.
Jack Degnan, Outreach Manager
Michael Giancola, Community Health Program Representative

323 **USC Internal Medicine**
1520 San Pablo Street
Los Angeles, CA 90033-1034 800-872-2273
Fax: 213-224-6687
www.usc.edu/health/internal
Research into internal medicine with specialties in cardiovascular endocrinology and diabetes gastrointestinal and liver disease geriatric medicine hematology infectious diseases nephrology oncology pulmonary and critical care and rheumatology and immunology.
Alexandra Levine, Head

324 **University of California San Francisco Center for AIDS Prevention**
Center for AIDS Prevention Studies (CAPS)
50 Beale Street 415-597-9100
San Francisco, CA 94105-3411 Fax: 415-597-9213
e-mail: CAPS.web@ucsf.edu
www.caps.ucsf.edu
The mission of the Center for AIDS Prevention Studies is to conduct domestic and international research to prevent the acquisition of HIV and to optimize health outcomes among HIV- infected individuals.
Stephen F Morin, Director
Susan Kegeles, Co-Director

325 **University of California: Institute of Health Policy Studies**
3333 California Street 415-476-4921
San Francisco, CA 94118 Fax: 415-476-0705
e-mail: claire.brindis@ucsf.edu
www.ihps.medschool.ucsf.edu
Health policy and AIDS research.
Claire Brindis, Interim Director
Daniel Dohan, Associate Director of Training

Colorado

326 Centers for AIDS Research: University of Colorado Health Sciences Center
Colorado Center for AIDS Research
4200 East 9th Avenue 303-315-7233
Denver, CO 80262 Fax: 303-315-8681
e-mail: colorado.cfar@uchsc.edu
www.uchsc.edu/ccfar
Describes forms and patterns of use of complimentary and alternative medicine (CAM) for the treatment of HIV/AIDS.
Robert T. Schooley, Director

District of Columbia

327 George Washington National Cooperative: Drug Discovery/AIDS Treatment
Department of Pharmacology & Physiology
2300 Eye Street NW 202-994-3541
Washington, DC 20037-2336 Fax: 202-994-2870
e-mail: phmsmc@gwumc.edu
www.gwumc.edu/pharm
Studies and researches natural products and synthetic anti-AIDS agents.
Susan Ceryak, Associate Research Professor
Jian-Zhong Guo, Associate Research Professor

328 Whitman Walker Clinic AIDS/Medical Services Programs
1701 14th Street NW 202-745-7000
Washington, DC 20009-3840 Fax: 202-745-0238
e-mail: info@wwc.org
www.wwc.org
A non-profit community-based health organization serving the Washington D.C. metropolitan region. Established by and for the gay and lesbian community our clinic is comprised of diverse volunteers and staff who provide or facilitate the delivery of high quality comprehensive accessible health care and community services. Especially committed to ending the suffering of all those infected and affected by HIV/AIDS.
Roberto Geidner, Director
Peter Miller, Assistant Director

Florida

329 Department of Epidemiology and Health Policy Research: University of Florida
1329 SW 16th Street 352-265-8035
Gainesville, FL 32608 Fax: 352-265-8047
e-mail: rdarbelles.ichp.ufl.edu
www.ehpr.ufl.edu
Studies into child and adolescent health financing and organization of health care delivery systems community health chronic conditions transition from pediatric to adult health care access to health care for vulnerable populations quality of life and outcomes research.
Carlos Batist, Business Manager
Kathy Clinefelter, Assistant Director of Research

330 Tampa Bay Research Institute
10900 Roosevelt Boulevard N 727-576-6675
Saint Petersburg, FL 33716-2308 Fax: 727-577-9862
e-mail: development@tampabayresearch.org
www.tampabayresearch.org
TBRI is the first independent biomedical research organization of its kind in Florida. Our scientists dedicate their lives work to conquering chronic and infectious diseases while gaining a better understanding of the immune system.
Akiko Tanaka, Co-Founder

331 University of South Florida Center for HIV Education and Research
13301 Bruce B Downs Boulevard 813-974-4430
Tampa, FL 33612-3807 Fax: 813-974-8451
e-mail: Contact@FCAETC.org
www.usfcenter.org
Serves health care professionals throughout Florida by providing education and information on the transmission control treatment and prevention of HIV and AIDS and by conducting related research and community outreach.
Michael Knox PhD, Director
Martha Fried PhD, Associate Director

Georgia

332 AIDS School Health Education Database Centers for Disease Control
Centers for Disease Control
1600 Clifton Road 404-639-3534
Atlanta, GA 30333 800-232-4636
TTY: 888-232-6348
e-mail: cdcinfo@cdc.gov
www.cdc.gov
An information awareness resource produced by the Division of Adolescent and School Health. The database offers descriptions of various educational resources for professionals relevant to the education of children and youth about HIV infection and AIDS.
Richard E Besser MD, Acting Director
Tanja Popovic, Chief Science Officer

333 Center for AIDS Research: Emory University Rollins School of Public Health
1518 Clifton Road NE 404-727-2924
Atlanta, GA 30322-4201 Fax: 404-727-9853
e-mail: cfar@emory.edu
www.cfar.emory.edu
Provides expertise resources and services not otherwise readily obtained through more traditional funding mechanisms.
James W Curran, Director
Carlos del Rio, Co-Director for Clinical Science

334 Educational Materials Database Centers for Disease Control
Centers for Disease Control
1600 Clifton Road 404-679-3860
Atlanta, GA 30333 800-458-5231
TTY: 888-232-6348
e-mail: info@cdcnpin.org
www.cdc.gov
A collection of bibliographic descriptions about hard-to-find AIDS and HIV information and educational materials.

335 Emory University: National Cooperative Drug Discovery for AIDS Treatment
Emory Healthcare Pediatrics Department
2015 Uppergate Drive
Atlanta, GA 30322 404-727-5740
www.pediatrics.emory.edu
Dr Raymond F Schanzi, Principal Investor

336 Funding Database Centers for Disease Control
Centers for Disease Control
1600 Clifton Road 404-639-3534
Atlanta, GA 30333 800-232-4636
TTY: 888-232-6348
www.cdc.gov
A listing of HIV and AIDS related funding opportunities for community-based and HIV and AIDS service organizations.

Illinois

337 Clinical Research Center Northwestern Center for Clinical Researc
Northwestern Center for Clinical Research
750 N Lake Shore Drive 312-503-1709
Chicago, IL 60611 e-mail: nucats@northwestern.edu
www.nucats.northwestern.edu
Gary L Robertson MD, Professor Emeritus
Philip Greenland, Director

Indiana

338 Purdue University Center for AIDS Research
School of Pharmacy and Pharmaceutical Sciences

575 Stadium Mall Drive
W Lafayette, IN 47907-2091
765-494-1361
Fax: 765-494-7880
e-mail: oss@pharmacy.purdue.edu
www.pharmacy.purdue.edu

Steve Byrn, Department Head
Stanley L Hem, Associate Department Head

Maryland

339 **Center for AIDS Research: Johns Hopkins University School of Medicine**
720 Rutland Avenue
Baltimore, MD 21205
www.hopkinsmedicine.org/aidsresearch
Provides expertise resources and services not otherwise readily obtained through more traditional funding mechanisms.
John G Bartlett, Director
Johns Hopkins, Associate Director

340 **Johns Hopkins University: Center for Communication Programs**
Johns Hopkins Bloomberg School of Public Health
111 Market Place
Baltimore, MD 21202
410-659-6300
Fax: 410-659-6266
e-mail: webmaster@jhuccp.org
www.jhuccp.org
Health communications family planning and AIDS prevention research.
Jane Bertrand, Director
Alice Payne Merritt, Associate Director

341 **University of Maryland Center for Research, Grants & Contracts**
Family Studies Depatrment
1204 Marie Mount Hall
College Park, MD 20742
301-405-3672
Fax: 301-314-9161
e-mail: fmst@umd.edu
www.hhp.umd.edu/FMST
Dr. R Narker Bausell, Director

342 **University of Maryland Center for Studies Family Studies Depatrment**
1204 Marie Mount Hall
College Park, MD 20742
301-405-3672
Fax: 301-314-9161
e-mail: fmsc@umd.edu
www.sph.umd.edu/fmsc
Dr R Narker Bausell, Director

343 **University of Maryland: Medical Biotechnology Center**
725 W Lombard Street
Baltimore, MD 21201-1513
410-706-8181
Fax: 410-706-8184
e-mail: lederer@umbi.umd.edu
www.umbi.umd.edu
Offers research into AIDS and HIV infection including vaccine development.
W Jonathan Lederer, Director
Kadir Aslan, Assistant Professor

Massachusetts

344 **Center for AIDS Research: Harvard Medical School, Division of AIDS**
The Landmark Buiding
401 Park Drive
Boston, MA 02215
617-384-9035
Fax: 617-384-9037
e-mail: aids@hms.harvard.edu
aids.med.harvard.edu/cfar.htm
Provides expertise resources and services not otherwise readily obtained through traditional funding mechanisms.
Bruce Walker, Director

345 **Center for Blood Research Harvard Medical School/CBR**
Harvard Medical School/CBR
200 Longwood Avenue
Boston, MA 02115
617-278-3140
Fax: 617-278-3131
e-mail: kirchhausen@crystal.harvard.edu
www.cbrinstitute.org/labs/kirchhausen
Offers research into blood disorders including multidisciplinary studies on AIDS and hemophilia cancer and diabetes research as well.
Tomas Kirchhausen, Principal Investigator
Warner Boll, Lab Member

346 **Centers for AIDS Research: University of Massachusetts Medical School**
55 Lake Avenue N
Worcester, MA 01655
508-856-8989
e-mail: publicaffairs@umassmed.edu
www.umassmed.edu/cfar
Provides expertise, resources, and services not otherwise readily obtained through traditional funding mechanisms.
Mario Stevenson, Director

347 **Dana Farber Cancer Institute National Drug Discovery Group for AIDS Treatment**
Dana-Farber Cancer Institute
44 Binney Street
Boston, MA 02115
617-632-3000
TTY: 617-632-5330
TDD: 617-632-5330
e-mail: dana-farbercontactus@dfci.harvard.edu
www.dana-farber.org
Edward Benz, President and CEO
Janet E Porter, Executive Vice President and COO

348 **Developmental Medicine Center Children's Hospital Boston**
Children's Hospital Boston
300 Longwood Avenue
Boston, MA 02115
617-355-7025
Fax: 617-730-0633
www.childrenshospital.org
Studies developmental effects of infants at risk and development effects of congenital HIV infection.
Allen C Crocker MD, Senior Associate in Medicine
Lisa H Albers Prock, Assistant in Medicine

Michigan

349 **University of Michigan: National Cooperative Drug/AIDS Group**
School of Dentistry
1011 N University Avenue
Ann Arbor, MI 48109-1078
734-763-5280
Fax: 734-763-3453
e-mail: paulk@umich.edu
www.dent.umich.edu
Focuses on the design of new drugs to fight AIDS.
John C Drach PhD, Director
Paul H Krebsbach, Department Chair

350 **Wayne State University Center for Health Research**
College of Nursing
Center for Health Research
Detroit, MI 48202
313-577-4135
Fax: 313-577-5777
e-mail: n.artinian@wayne.edu
www.nursing.wayne.edu/CHR
Facilitates interdisciplinary health research across diverse settings where nursing is practiced and healthcare is provided.
Nancy T Artinian, Director
Barbara K Redman, Dean

New York

351 **Aaron Diamond AIDS Research Center**
455 First Avenue
New York, NY 10016
212-448-5000
Fax: 212-725-1126
e-mail: webinfo@adarc.org
www.adarc.org
Committed to finding solutions to end the AIDS epidemic. In the decade and a half since HIV was identified researchers have learned more about this virus than about any other in history.
David Ho, Director & CEO
Melissa Haber, Associate Director of Development

352 **Centers for AIDS Research: Albert Einstein College of Medicine**
Albert Einstein College of Medicine
Jack and Pearl Resnick Campus
Bronx, NY 10461
718-430-2156
Fax: 718-430-2374
e-mail: cfaradm@aecom.yu.edu
www.aecom.yu.edu/cfar
Provides consultation and support to the medical and research community in the scientific evaluation of CAM therapies.
Harris Goldstein, Program Director

353 **Centers for AIDS Research: Columbia University College of Physicians**
Center for AIDS Research

617 W 168th Street 212-305-1296
New York, NY 10032 e-mail: jka8@columbia.edu
www.cumc.columbia.edu

Provides a comprehensive framework for training educational programs and research which addresses health promotion disease prevention symptom management and quality of life for individuals with HIV. The goal of the Center is to create innovative research and service approaches for the prevention and management of HIV. This objective is fulfilled through research program development and program evaluations.

Joyce K Anastasi, Director
Miriam Belleca, Study Coordinator

354 **Centers for AIDS Research: NYU School of Medicine**
550 First Avenue 212-263-8527
New York, NY 10016 e-mail: zinszh01@med.nyu.edu
www.hivinfosource.org/hivis/cfar

Provides expertise resources and services not otherwise readily obtained through traditional funding mechanisms.

Fred Valentine, Director

355 **General Clinical Research Center Mount Sinai School of Medicine**
Mount Sinai School of Medicine
1184 5th Avenue 212-241-6045
New York, NY 10029 Fax: 212-348-5811
e-mail: hugh.sampson@mssm.edu
www.mssm.edu/gcrc

Focuses on AIDS education and prevention.

Hugh Sampson, Program Director
Scott Sicherer, Associate Program Director

356 **HIV Center for Clinical and Behavioral Studies**
1051 Riverside Drive 212-543-5969
New York, NY 10032 Fax: 212-543-6003
e-mail: whiteme@pi.cpmc.comlumbia.edu
www.hivcenternyc.org

Interdisciplinary research center that investigates the behavioral causes and consequences of HIV/AIDS. Focusing on the intersections of HIV infection gender and sexuality; treatment strategies for infected populations; and innovative dissemination of scientific findings.

Anke A Ehrhardt, Director
Heino F L Meyer-Bahlbur, Associate Director

357 **Institute for Clinical Research Weill Cornell Medical College**
Weill Cornell Medical College
1300 York Avenue 212-746-3774
New York, NY 10021 Fax: 212-746-8970
e-mail: cto@med.cornell.edu
www.med.cornell.edu

The mission of the ICR is to support, advance and promote clinical and translational research enterprises at WCMC. As part of Research and Sponsored Programs (RASP) the ICR streamlines the clinical research process and offers a wide range of services, resources and training.

Marion Schwa MSW LCSW, Director
Alicia Destr MA CCRP, Senior Clinical Trials Administrator

358 **SUNY at Buffalo National Cooperative Drug Discovery Group for AIDS Treatment**
Department of Biochemistry
140 Farber Hall 716-829-2727
Buffalo, NY 14214-3000 Fax: 716-829-2725
e-mail: jluck@buffalo.edu
www.buffalo.edu

Kenneth M Blumenthal, Professor and Chairman
Elizabeth O'Brocta, Assistant to the Chairman

359 **Spellman Center for HIV Related Disease The Spellman Center**
The Spellman Center
415 W Fifty-First Street
New York, NY 10019 212-459-8130
www.stclaresny.org

David Kaufman, Director

360 **State University of New York: SUNY Stony HIV Treatment Development Center**
Center for Infectious Diseases
5120 State University of New York 631-444-1659
Stony Brook, NY 11794-5120 Fax: 631-444-2493
e-mail: rsteigbigel@notes.cc.sunysb.edu
www.stonybrookmedicalcenter.org

Human immunodeficiency virus research.

Roy T Steigbigel MD, Director
Sandra Brown RN CCRC, Study Coordinator

North Carolina

361 **Centers for AIDS Research: Univeristy of North Carolina at Chapel Hill**
UNC Center For AIDS Research
Lineberger Cancer Center 919-966-8645
Chapel Hill, NC 27599 e-mail: cfar@med.unc.edu
cfar.med.unc.edu

Administrative and shared research support to synergistically enhance and coordinate high quality AIDS research projects.

Ronald Swanstrom, Director
Myron S Cohen, Associate Director

Ohio

362 **Centers for AIDS Research: Case Western University**
Department of Medicine
Division of Infectious Diseases 216-844-8766
Cleveland, OH 44106-5029 e-mail: mxl6@case.edu
www.clevelandactu.org

Provides administrative and shared research support to enhance and coordinate high quality AIDS research projects.

Michael M Lederman, Co-Director
Jonathan Karn, Associate Director

Pennsylvania

363 **Centers for AIDS Research: University of Pennsylvania**
Penn Center for AIDS Research
353 Biomedical Research Building II 215-573-7354
Philadelphia, PA 19104-6140 Fax: 215-573-7356
e-mail: oliviere@mail.med.upenn.edu
www.med.upenn.edu/aids

Also the Children's Hospital and the Wistar Institute provides important services and research for high quality projects.

James A Hoxie, Director
Ronald G Collman, Co-Director

364 **Temple University Clinical Research Center Office of Clinical Research**
Office of Clinical Research
Parkinson Pavilion 215-204-7579
Philadelphia, PA 19140 Fax: 215-201-2684
e-mail: henry.parkman@temple.edu
www.temple.edu/medicine

CRC Unit provides space to perform clinical research on 4 West of Temple University Hospital. The CRC Unit has the potential for three rooms for inpatient/outpatient studies and an additional room for outpatient studies.

Henry Parkman, Acting Director

365 **Thomas Jefferson University: Center for Research in Medical Education**
Jefferson Medical College
1015 Walnut Street 215-955-6969
Philadelphia, PA 19107 Fax: 215-923-7583
e-mail: Joseph.Gonnella@jefferson.edu
www.jefferson.edu/jmc

Joseph Gonne MD, Director
Daniel Z Louis, Managing Director

Rhode Island

366 **Centers for AIDS Research: Brown University**
The Miriam Hospital
CFAR/RISE Building 401-793-4068
Providence, RI 02906 Fax: 401-793-4704
e-mail: vgodleski@lifespan.org
www.lifespan.org/cfar

Provides expertise resources and services not otherwise readily obtained through traditional funding mechanisms.
Charles C J Carpenter, Director
Susan Cu-Uvin, HIV and Women Core Co-Director

South Carolina

367 **Medical University of South Carolina Health Services Administration**
Medical University of South Carolina
171 Ashley Avenue 843-792-2300
Charleston, SC 29425 Fax: 843-923-27
www.musc.edu
Devoted to public health policy and health care management including AIDS research.
Kit Simpson, Director

Tennessee

368 **Centers for AIDS Research: Vanderbilt University Medical Center**
Division of Infectious Disease
1161 21st Avenue S 615-322-8972
Nashville, TN 37232-2582 e-mail: richard.daquila@vanderbilt.edu
www.mc.vanderbilt.edu/cfar
Provides expertise resources and services not otherwise readily obtained through more traditional funding mechanisms.
Richard D' Aquila, Director
Vladimir Berthaud, Associate Director

Texas

369 **Centers for AIDS Research: Baylor College of Medicine**
Department of Molecular Virology & Microbiology
One Baylor Plaza 713-798-3006
Houston, TX 77030 Fax: 713-798-5019
e-mail: jbutel@bcm.edu
www.bcm.edu/cfar
A research center that is a branch of the Centers for AIDS Research.
Janet S Butel, Director
William T Shearer, Co-Director

Vermont

370 **University of Vermont: Office of Health Promotion Research**
1 S Prospect Street 802-656-4187
Burlington, VT 05401 Fax: 802-656-8826
e-mail: ohpr@uvm.edu
www.uvm.edu/~ohpr
Research done into public policy and human health including AIDS information and evaluation.
Anne L Dorwaldt, Assistant Director
Claire Bove, Research Project Assistant

Washington

371 **Centers for AIDS Research: University of Washington, Harborview Medical Center**
Center For AIDS & STDs
325 Ninth Avenue 206-744-4239
Seattle, WA 98104-2499 Fax: 206-744-3693
e-mail: worthy@u.washington.edu
www.depts.washington.edu/cfas
Provides administrative and shared research support to synergistically enhance and coordinate high quality AIDS research projects. CFARs accomplish this through core facilities that provide expertise resource and services not otherwise readily obtained through more traditional funding mechanisms.
King K Holmes, Director
Mary Fielder, Assistant to the Director

372 **HIV Prevention Trials Unit University of Washington/Seattle HPTU Si**
University of Washington/Seattle HPTU Site
Cabrini Medical Tower 901 Boren Av 206-520-3800
Seattle, WA 98104 Fax: 206-520-3801
e-mail: hptu@u.washington.edu
www.depts.washington.edu/hptu
A worldwide collaborative clinical trials network established by the National Institutes of Health (NIH) to evaluate the safety and efficacy of non-vaccine prevention interventions alone or in combination using HIV incidence as the primary endpoint.
Connie Celum, Principal Investigator

Support Groups & Hotlines

373 **AEGIS AIDS Education Global Information Sy stem**
AEGIS
32234 Paseo Adelanto Suite B 949-248-5843
San Juan Capistrano, CA 92675 Fax: 949-248-2839
e-mail: help@aegis.org
www.aegis.org
A free 24-hour information bulletin board system and on-line database.
Sister Mary Elizabeth, Assistant Operations Director
Vanessa Robison, Assistant Director

374 **AIDS Alabama**
205-324-9822
800-592-2437
Fax: 205-324-9311
www.aidsalabama.org
Devotes its energy and resources statewide to helping people with HIV/AIDS live healthy, independent lives, and works to prevent the spread of HIV.
Kathie Hiers, Chief Executive Officer
John Cosper, Executive Director

375 **AIDS Clinical Trials Information Service**
PO Box6303 301-496-8210
Rockville, MD 20849 800-448-0440
Fax: 301-519-6616
TTY: 800-243-7012
e-mail: contactus@AIDSINFO.nif.gov
www.AIDSINFO.nih.gov
A call-in service where trained staff will tell the caller all about studies for persons who have the AIDS virus.
Ryan White, Researcher

376 **AIDS Hotline of Central New York**
AIDS Community Resources
627 W Genesee Street 315-475-2430
Syracuse, NY 13204-2347 800-343-2437
Fax: 315-472-6515
e-mail: info@aidscommunityresources
www.aidscommunityresources.com
Michael Crinnin, Executive Director
Dana Zalerino, Deputy Executive Director

377 **AIDS Support Group of Cape Cod**
508-487-9445
800-905-1170
Fax: 508-487-0565
e-mail: info@asgcc.org
www.asgcc.org
Provides services to persons living with HIV and AIDS within Cape Cod communities that maintain and enhance their quality of life, and provide health education, prevention and harm reduction outreach.
Laura Thorton, Interim Director
Madeline Miller, Administrative Director

378 **Alaskan Statewide AIDS Helpline**
907-263-2050
800-478-AIDS
Fax: 907-263-2051
www.alaskanaids.org
Not-for-profit aIDS service organization. Provides one-on-one case management, housing assistance and other supportive services to people living with HIV/AIDS as well as HIV prevention case management and outreach, and public HIV education.
Trevor Storrs, Executive Director

379 **BABES Network-YWCA**
1118 Fifth Ave
Seattle, WA 98101
206-720-5566
888-292-1912
Fax: 206-720-5901
e-mail: the_staff@babesnetwork.org
www.babesnetwork.org

A peer-based program, a sisterhood of women facing HIV together. Reduces isolation, promotes self-empowerment, enhances quality of life and serves the needs of women facing HIV and their families through peer support, advocacy, education and outreach
Kelly Hill, Outreach Coordinator/Peer Counselor
Sarah Kent, Program Manager

380 **COMPASS Program**
c/o Institute for Urban Family Health
16 East 16th Street
New York, NY 10003
212-924-7744
Fax: 212-691-4610
e-mail: info@institute2000.org
www.institute2000.org/health/rwp.htm

Medical services include HIV testing and specialized HIV medical care for adults in addition to women's health services including gynecology, PAP tests, family planning and birth control methods. Mental health services includes individual, couples, and family counseling and psychiatric evaluations and monitoring.
Neil Calman MD/ABFP/FAAFP, President/Chief Executive Officer
Weston Willett, Chief Information Officer

381 **Cascade AIDS Project Hotline**
620 SW Fifth Avenue
Portland, OR 97204
503-223-2437
Fax: 503-223-7087
e-mail: info@cascadeaids.org
www.cascadeaids.org

Provides HIV prevention and services information by phone and internet to youth and adults across Orgeon and the Northwest.
Joseph Sedillo, Hotline Coordinator

382 **Dunshee House**
303-17th Avenue East
Seattle, WA 98112
206-322-2437
Fax: 206-322-1779
www.sasg.org

A non-profit organization, builds community and cultivates powerful, healthy lives by providing emotional support and personal development services to those affected by HIV/AIDS.
Deborah Witmer, Executive Director
Kim Holstein, Resource Manager

383 **HEAL**
Sidney Hillman Family Pracitce
16 E 16th Street
New York, NY 10003-3105
212-924-7744
e-mail: healweb@thorup.com
www.thorup.com/HEAL

The Health Education AIDS Liaison provides alternative and holistic support groups and resources for people with HIV.

384 **HIV/AIDS Prevention Program**
CDC National Center for HIV, STD, & TB Prevention
1600 Clifton Road NE
404-639-3286
800-232-4636
Fax: 404-639-7394
TTY: 888-232-6348
e-mail: cdcinfo@cdc.gov
www.cdc.gov/hiv/

As a part of its overall public health mission, CDC provides leadership in helping control the HIV/AIDS epidemic by working with community, state, national, and international partners in surveillance, research, and prevention and evaluation activities. CDC's programs also work to improve treatment, care, and support for persons living with HIV/AIDS and to build capacity and infrastructure to address the HIV/AIDS epidemic in the United States and around the world.
Julie Louise Gerberding MD/MPH, CDC Director
William H Gimson, Chief Operating Officer

385 **Immunization Division Centers for Disease Control**
1600 Tullie Circle NE
Atlanta, GA 30329-2303
404-639-1880
800-311-3435
Fax: 404-639-5258
www.cdc.gov

Robert Janssen, Director

386 **King County Crisis Clinic**
206-461-3210
866-427-4747
Fax: 206-461-8368
TDD: 206-461-3219
e-mail: info@crisisclinic.org
www.crisisclinic.org

Offers a comprehensive arrray of telephone and support services that are available to every community member in King County. Communicates with callers in 155 languages through the interpretation assistance of the Teleinterpreter service and with persons with hearing impairments through our TDD.

387 **Minnesota AIDS Project AIDSLine**
612-341-2060
800-248-2437
Fax: 612-341-4057
TTY: 888-820-2437
e-mail: info@mnaidsproject.org
www.mnaidsproject.org

Hotline

388 **National Health Information Center**
PO Box 1133
Washington, DC 20013
310-565-4167
800-336-4797
Fax: 301-984-4256
e-mail: info@nhic.org
www.health.gov/nhic

Offers a nationwide information referral service, produces directories and resource guides.

389 **Project Inform Hotline**
205 13th Street
San Francisco, CA 94103-2461
415-558-8669
800-822-7422
Fax: 415-558-0684
e-mail: web@projectinform.org
www.projectinform.org

AIDS Hotline.
Skip Emerson, Executive Assistant

390 **STI Resource Center Hotline**
919-361-8488
800-227-8922
www.ashastd.org

Provides information, materials and referrals to anyone concerned about sexually transmitted infections.
Lynn Barclay, President/CEO
Deborah Arrindell, VP Health Policy

Books

391 **ABC of AIDS**
Michael W. Adler, author
BMJ Publishing Group
PO Box 281
Annapolis, MD 20701-0281
800-2FO-NBMJ
Fax: 800-2FA-XBMJ
e-mail: bmjpg@pmds.com
ww.bmjpg.com

118 pages Paperback
ISBN: 0-727915-03-7

392 **AIDS & HIV Related Diseases**
Harper Collins Publishers
10 East 53rd Street
New York, NY 10022
212-207-7000
www.harpercollins.com

An education guide for professionals and the public which covers such topics as: Understanding HIV and its effect on the immune system; HIV transmission; The history of AIDS and HIV; HIV testing; The natural course of an HIV infection; Medical treatment and those who administer them; The people who have AIDS; AIDS education.
1996 246 pages
ISBN: 0-306450-85-2

393 **AIDS & Other Manifestations of HIV Infection**
Gary Wormser, author
Academic Press (Elsevier)

1183 Westline Industrial Drive
St Louis, MO 63146 800-545-2522
Fax: 800-535-9935
e-mail: usbkinfo@elsevier.com
www.elsevier.com

Provides a timely and comprehensive update on AIDS and other HIV infections. More than 40 chapters present information on the biological properties of the etiologic viral agent and the practical day-to-day management of HIV-infected patients.
2004-4th Edi 1000 pages
ISBN: 0-127640-51-7

394 AIDS Alert
American Health Consultants
3525 Piedmnt Road 404-262-7436
Atlanta, GA 30305 800-688-2421
Fax: 800-284-3291
e-mail: customerservice@ahcpubs.com
www.ahcpub.com

Covers risks, hazards, costs and prevention of AIDS and related conditions.

Leslie Norins, Publisher

395 AIDS and HIV Related Diseases
Josh Powell, author
Plenum Publishing Corporation
233 Spring Street 212-620-8000
New York, NY 10013 800-221-9369
Fax: 212-463-0742
e-mail: books@plenum.com

An education guide for professionals and the public which covers such topics as: Understanding HIV and its effect on the immune system; HIV transmission; The history of AIDS and HIV; HIV testing; The natural course of an HIV infection; Medical treatment and those who administer them; The people who have AIDS; AIDS education.
1996 243 pages
ISBN: 0-306450-85-2

396 AIDS and Persons with Developmental Disabilities
Commission on the Mentally Disabled
1800 M Street NW 202-331-2240
Washington, DC 20036

A discussion of federal and state laws that defines the rights and responsibilities of individuals with disabilities and service providers with respect to HIV infection.

397 AIDS in the Twenty-First Century: Disease and Globalization
Tony Barnett, Alan Whiteside, author
Palgrave Macmillan
175 Fifth Avenue 212-982-3900
New York, NY 10010 800-221-7945
Fax: 212-777-6359
www.palgrave.com

2nd Edition
432 pages
ISBN: 1-403900-06-X

398 AIDS, Revised Edition
Alan E. Nourse, M.D., author
Franklin Watts c/o Grolier
90 Old Sherman Tpke 203-797-3500
Danbury, CT 06816 800-621-1115
Fax: 203-797-3197
www.grolier.com

This bestselling book has been updated with the latest findings and research into the AIDS epidemic. Includes new statistical information and findings on HIV and AIDS.
144 pages
ISBN: 0-531106-62-4

399 AIDS: A Communication Perspective
Lawrence Erlbaum Associates Publishers
10 Industrial Avenue 201-236-9500
Mahwah, NJ 07430-2262 Fax: 201-236-6396
www.erlbaum.com

ISBN: 0-805809-98-8

400 AIDS: Distinguishing Between Fact and Opinion
Teresa Opheim, author
Greenhaven Press
PO Box 9187
Farmington Hills, MI 48333-9187 800-877-GALE
Fax: 800-414-5043
e-mail: gale.galeord@thomson.com (E-Mail Orders)
www.galegroup.com/greenhaven

For beginning debaters, reports and classroom use this book offers three debates: Can AIDS be spread by casual contact? Should the Food and Drug Administration make AIDS drugs more available? Is AIDS a moral issue?.
36 pages
ISBN: 0-899086-33-0

401 AIDS: How it Works in the Body
Lorna Greenberg, author
Franklin Watts
96 Leonard Street
London EC2A 4XD, www.wattspub.co.uk
For readers ages 9-12
64 pages School Binding

402 AIDS: Trading Fears for Facts: A Guide for Young People
Karen Hein, Theresa Foy Digernimo, author
Consumer Reports Books
101 Truman Avenue
Yonkers, NY 10703-1057 www.consumerreports.org
Listed for young adult readers.
232 pages Paperback
ISBN: 0-890437-21-1

403 Amfar AIDS Handbook: The Complete Guide to Understanding HIV and AIDS
Darrell Ward, author
W.W. Norton & Company, Inc.
500 Fifth Avenue 212-354-5500
New York, NY 10110 Fax: 212-869-0856
www.norton.com

Gives a greater understanding of HIV/Aids. The causes and effects, what new treatment options are being developed.
360 pages
ISBN: 0-393316-36-X

404 Black Death: AIDS in Africa
Susan Hunter, author
Palgrave Macmillan
175 Fifth Avenue 212-982-3900
New York, NY 10010 800-221-7945
Fax: 212-777-6359
www.palgrave.com

256 pages
ISBN: 1-403962-44-8

405 Children and the AIDS Virus: A Book for Children, Parents, and Teachers
Rosmarie Hausherr, author
Clarion Books
For readers ages 4-8.
48 pages Library Binding
ISBN: 0-899198-34-1

406 Community Service Delivery for Children with HIV Infection and Families
Geneva, Woodruff & Christopher Hanson, author
South Shore Mental Health Center
6 Fort Street 617-847-1950
Quincy, MA 02169 e-mail: contactus@ssmh.org
www.ssmh.org

A manual providing guidelines for developing community-based, family-centered services for children with HIV infection and their families. Describes how services can be planned and delivered using guiding principles and practices of transagency case management.

407 **Coping When You or a Friend is HIV-Positive**
Pat Kelly, author
Hazelden Publishing & Educational Services
15251 Pleasant Valley Road 651-257-4010
Center City, MN 55012-0176 800-328-9000
Fax: 651-213-4577
e-mail: customersupport@hazeldon.org
www.hazelden.org
Provides compassionate counsel for teens who have been diagnosed with the virus.
136 pages Paperback
ISBN: 1-568381-77-8

408 **Dancing Against the Darkness: A Journey Through America in the Age of AIDS**
Steven Petrow, author
Rowman & Littlefield Publishing Group
4501 Forbes Blvd. 717-794-3800
Lanham, MD 20706 800-462-6420
Fax: 717-794-3803
e-mail: custserv@rowman.com
www.lexingtonbooks.com
218 pages Hardcover
ISBN: 0-669243-09-4

409 **Everything You Need to Know About AIDS**
Katherine White, author
Rosen Publishing Group
29 E 21st Street 212-777-3017
New York, NY 10010 800-237-9932
Fax: 888-436-4643
e-mail: customerservice@rosenpub.com
www.rosenpublishing.com
Without proper information, our teens remain at risk for AIDS. This volume presents balanced information on the disease and on safer sex precautions, in a language that readers can understand.
64 pages Library Binding
ISBN: 0-823933-14-8
Barbara Taylor, Author

410 **Everything You Need to Know About Being HIV Positive**
Amy Shire, author
Rosen Publishing Group
29 E 21st Street 212-777-3017
New York, NY 10010 800-237-9932
Fax: 888-436-4643
e-mail: customerservice@rosenpub.com
www.rosenpublishing.com
To teens who need to understand what thier options are when living with HIV on a day-to-day basis. This book explains the facts about HIV.
Hardcover
ISBN: 0-823926-14-1
Amy Shire, Author

411 **Everything You Need to Know When a Parent has AIDS**
Barbara Hermie Draimin, author
Rosen Publishing Group
29 E 21st Street 212-777-3017
New York, NY 10010 800-237-9932
Fax: 888-436-4643
e-mail: customerservice@rosenpub.com
www.rosenpublishing.com
More and more teens have a parent who has AIDS. Teens must learn where they can turn for help in dealing with this difficult situation. By presenting stories of teens in the same situation, this book helps readers deal with their anger and grief.
64 pages Library Binding
ISBN: 0-823916-90-1
Barbara Hermie Draimin DSW, Author

412 **Global AIDS: Myths and Facts, Tools for Fighting the AIDS Pandemic**
Alexander Irwin, Joyce Millen, author
South End Press
7 Brookline Street #1 617-547-4002
Cambridge, MA 02139-4146 Fax: 617-547-1333
www.southendpress.org
304 pages
ISBN: 0-896086-73-9

413 **Guide to Living With HIV Infection**
John G. Md. Bartlett, Ann K. Finkbeiner, author
John's Hopkins University Press
2715 N Charles Street 410-516-6900
Baltimore, MD 21218-4363 800-537-5487
Fax: 410-516-6968
www.press.jhu.edu
This guidebook includes detailed discussions of new drugs; special considerations of the stages of infection; facts about opportunistic infection and new information on prevention.
1996 428 pages Paperback
ISBN: 0-801867-44-4

414 **Invisible People: How the U.S. Has Slept Through the Global AIDS Pandemic**
Greg Behrman, author
Free Press Publishing Co.
1010 W CASS St 813-254-5888
Tampa, FL 33606-1307
368 pages
ISBN: 0-743257-55-3

415 **Living Well With HIV and AIDS 3rd Edition**
Allen L Gifford, author
Bull Publishing Company
PO Box 1377
Boulder, CO 80306 800-676-2855
Fax: 303-545-6354
www.bullpub.com
Helps people overcome the day-to-day physical and emotional problems caused the HIV disease, and encourages them to work with their medical team to make themselves as strong and healthy as possible.
2005 328 pages Papberback
ISBN: 0-923521-86-0
Kate Lorig, Author
Diana Laurent, Author

416 **Living on the Edge**
Michael Kelly, author
HarperCollins Canada Limited/Order Department
1995 Markham Road
Ontario, Canada M1 B 5M8, 800-387-0117
Fax: 800-668-5788
A gritty, honest, biographical account of one young man's experience from the original diagnosis via the development of the illness, how Michael has learned to live with his illness and how it has affected him and all his friends who support him.
160 pages
ISBN: 0-551027-49-5

417 **Local AIDS Sercices: The National Directory**
US Conference of Mayors
1620 I Street NW 202-293-7330
Washington, DC 20006 Fax: 202-293-2352
e-mail: info@usmayors.org
www.usmayors.org
2,500 organizations that provide various information and services for AIDS coordinates and other health-related professionals.

418 **Lynda Madaras Talks to Teens About AIDS**
Lynda Madaras, author
Waterfront Books
98 Brookes Avenue 802-658-7477
Burlington, VT 05401 800-639-6063
e-mail: helpkids@waterfrontbooks.com
www.waterfrontbooks.com
An informative book about the HIV virus and AIDS.
128 pages

419 **Night Kites**
M.E. Kerr, author
HarperCollins Children's Books
1350 Avenue of the Americas
New York, NY 10019 212-261-6500
www.harperchildrens.com
For young adults.
224 pages Paperback
ISBN: 0-064470-35-0

420 **No Longer Immune: A Counselor's Guide to AIDS**
American Counseling Association
5999 Stevenson Avenue 703-823-9800
Alexandria, VA 22304 800-347-6647
Fax: 703-823-0252
www.counseling.org
Covers a broad range of issues such as working with specific populations, handling pre- and posttesting situations, coping with fear, grief and survivor guilt, preventing caregiver burnout and dealing with countertransference.
295 pages Paperback
ISBN: 1-556200-64-1

421 **Parent Education Program-HIV/AIDS: A Challenge to Us All**
Pediatric AIDS Foundation
2950 31st Street 310-314-1459
Santa Monica, CA 90405-3092 800-499-4673
Fax: 310-314-1469
e-mail: info@pedcids.org
www.pedaids.org
This parent meeting kit with a guide book and two videos will help any adult set up a parent meeting on the subject of AIDS. This kit provides accurate information to parents about HIV/AIDS, allows parents to voice concerns and fears, gives examples of appropriate answers to your child's questions about HIV/AIDS and replaces fear with knowledge and compassion.

422 **Predicting AIDS and Other Epidemics**
Christopher Lampton, author
Franklin Watts
96 Leonard Street
London EC2A 4XD, www.wattspub.co.uk
144 pages S & L Binding

423 **Scarlet Letters**
AIDS Project Los Angeles
The David Geffen Center
Los Angeles, CA 90005 213-201-1600
www.apla.org
A bilingual (Spanidh/English) journal targeted at HIV prevention providers in the U.S. The Scarlet Letters features opinion pieces and research-based essays by invited HIV/STD prevention experts.
2 year

424 **Teen Guide to AIDS Prevention**
Alan E. Nourse, author
Franklin Watts
96 Leonard Street
London EC2A 4XD, www.wattspub.co.uk
For young adult readers.
61 pages S & L Binding

425 **We Have AIDS**
Elaine Landau, author
Franklin Watts
96 Leonard Street
London EC2A 4XD, www.wattspub.co.uk
For young adult readers.
S & L Binding

426 **What Is AIDS?**
Anna Forbes, author
The Rosen Publishing Group
PowerKids Press 212-777-3017
New York, NY 10010 800-237-9932
Fax: 888-436-4643
www.powerkidspress.com
For reader levels ages 4-8.
1st Edition 24 pages Hardcover

427 **Women & AIDS**
Diane Richardson, author
Methuen
11-12 Buckingham Gate
London SW1E 6LB, www.methuen.co.uk
The first sourcebook to provide the information women need by identifying the most accurate sources and providing valuable statistical data.
183 pages Paperback
ISBN: 0-416017-51-7

428 **Women and AIDS: A Practical Guide for Those Who Help Others**
Continuum Publishing Corporation
370 Lexington Avenue 212-532-3650
New York, NY 10017-6503
Tailored to women, this book grapples with attitudes and realities of AIDS.

429 **Women and Aids: Coping and Caring**
Plenum Publishing Corporation
233 Spring Street 212-620-8000
New York, NY 10013-1522 800-221-9369
Fax: 212-463-0742
e-mail: info@plenum.com
1996 263 pages
ISBN: 0-306452-58-8
Ann O'Leary, Editor

430 **You Have HIV: A Day at a Time**
Lynn S. Baker, author
W.B. Saunders Company
www.elsevierhealth.com
258 pages paperback
ISBN: 0-721636-06-3

Children's Books

431 **AIDS Overview Series**
Lucent Books
Thomson Gale
Farmington Hills, MI 48333-9187 800-877-4253
Fax: 800-414-5043
e-mail: gale.customerservice@thomson.com
www.gale.com/lucent
A straightforward account that teaches young adults all about the growing problem of AIDS.
1998 112 pages
ISBN: 1-560061-93-6

432 **AIDS Awareness Library**
Rosen Publishing Group
29 E 21st Street 212-777-3017
New York, NY 10010 800-237-9932
Fax: 888-436-4643
e-mail: customerservice@rosepub.com
www.rosenpublishing.com
This series of eight 24 page books, for grades K-4, speaks to children in nonthreatening langauge that provides vital information without graphic detail. This series is meant to be a gentle introduction to this frightening epidemic. Each book can also be purchased seperately for $13.95 (Set includes: Where did AIDS Come From; Myths and Facts; Living in a World with AIDS; What is AIDS; When Someone You Know Has AIDS; What You Can Do About AIDS; Heroes Against AIDS; Kids with AIDS.).
1996
ISBN: 0-823974-06-8

433 **AIDS To the Point: Confronting Youth Issues**
Diana L. Hynson, author
Abingdon Press
201 8th Avenue S 615-749-6347
Nashville, TN 37202-0801 800-251-3320
Fax: 615-749-6577
www.abingdonpress.com

A resource that offers a practical means of talking with teens, individually or in a group, about AIDS. This volume offers teaching articles, ready-to-go programs for teens, leader's guides, worship resources, facts and figures, where to go for help and a section exclusively in Spanish. This is a volume in the To The Point: Confronting Youth Issues series of books.
96 pages Paperback
ISBN: 0-687782-20-1

434 **AIDS: How it Works in the Body**
Franklin Watts Grolier
90 Old Sherman Turnpike 203-797-3500
Danbury, CT 06816-0001 Fax: 203-797-3197
www.grolier.com
Focuses on the physiological effects AIDS has on the body, explains the causes of the disease, how the immune system works to defend the body and how the HIV virus affects the immune system.
64 pages Grades 5-7
ISBN: 0-531200-74-4

435 **AIDS: Trading Fears for Facts a Guide for Teens**
Consumer Reports Books
9180 La Saint Drive 914-378-2567
Fairfield, OH 45014 Fax: 914-378-2907
Written specifically for teenage readers and filled with illustrations, this book includes the current facts about AIDS, discusses how the virus is transmitted and precautions that should be taken.

436 **AIDS: Trading Fears for Facts: A Guide for Young People**
Consumer Reports Books
9180 La Saint Drive 914-378-2567
Fairfield, OH 45014 Fax: 914-378-2907
www.consumerreports.com
1993
ISBN: 0-890432-62-4

437 **Dancing Against the Darkness: A Journey Through America in the Age of AIDS**
Heath Publishing
125 Spring Street 617-822-6650
Lexington, MA 02421-7801
A professional in the field, this author has chosen people across the nation to interview and use as examples for how the AIDS epidemic has struck America and what kind of lives it has affected.
Grades 7-12

438 **Everything You Need to Know When a Parent Has AIDS**
Barbara Hermie Draimin, DSW, author
Rosen Publishing Group
29 E. 21st Street 212-777-3017
New York, NY 10010 800-237-9932
Fax: 888-436-4643
e-mail: rosenpub@tribeca.ios.com
More and more teens have a parent who has AIDS. Teens must learn where they can turn up for health in dealing with this difficult situation. By presenting stories of teens in the same situation, this book helps readers deal with their anger and grief.

ISBN: 0-823916-90-1

439 **Impact of AIDS**
Franklin Watts Grolier
90 Old Sherman Turnpike 203-797-3500
Danbury, CT 06816-0001 800-621-1115
Fax: 203-797-3197
www.grolier.com
Examines the effects of the HIV infection and discusses the efforts in finding a cure for AIDS.
64 pages Grades 5-7
ISBN: 0-531172-25-2

440 **Night Kites**
Harper Collins
55 Avenue Road
Hazelton, Toronto, M5R3L2, 416-975-9334
www.harpercollins.com
This book focuses on two brothers, one of whom is homosexual and how they interact in the face of AIDS and the intolerance of homosexuality among the many people they know.
Grades 8-12

441 **Our Immune System**
40 W Chesapeake Avenue 410-321-6647
Towson, MD 21204-4841 800-296-4433
Fax: 410-321-9165
e-mail: idf@primaryimmune.org
www.primaryimmune.org
This booklet educates children on the immune system through a series of illustrations and animated characters, including T cells, B cells, and phagocytes. Available in many languages, including Spanish.
G. Richard Barr, Chairman
Marcia Boyle, Founder, Chairperson

442 **Predicting AIDS and Other Epidemics**
Franklin Watts Grolier
90 Old Sherman Turnpike 203-797-3500
Danbury, CT 06816-0001 800-621-1115
Fax: 203-797-3197
www.grolier.com
Surveys the efforts of scientists and researchers to predict the spread of epidemic diseases, including AIDS.
128 pages Grades 7-12
ISBN: 0-531107-85-0

443 **Problem of AIDS**
Franklin Watts Grolier
90 Old Sherman Turnpike 203-797-3500
Danbury, CT 06816-0001 800-621-1115
Fax: 203-797-3197
www.grolier.com
Part of the Let's Talk About series, this book addresses the questions and answers children and young adults have about AIDS.
32 pages Grades 3-5
ISBN: 0-531171-91-4

444 **Teen Guide to AIDS Prevention**
Franklin Watts Grolier
90 Old Sherman Turnpike 203-797-3500
Danbury, CT 06816-0001 800-621-1115
Fax: 203-797-3197
www.grolier.com
Directly addresses the questions and fears of teenagers by explaining clearly and simply what AIDS is, how it is spread, and the preventive measures young persons should take.
64 pages Grades 9-12
ISBN: 0-531109-66-6

445 **We Have AIDS**
Franklin Watts Grolier
90 Old Sherman Turnpike 203-797-3500
Danbury, CT 06816-0001 800-621-1115
Fax: 203-797-3197
www.grolier.com
This book goes beyond statistics and facts and focuses on the personal side of the disease. Offers source notes, a bibliography and an index.
128 pages
ISBN: 0-531108-98-8

446 **What's a Virus, Anyway? The Kid's Book About AIDS**
Waterfront Books
98 Brookes Avenue 802-658-7477
Burlington, VT 05401-3326
A simple introduction to help adults talk with children about the subject of AIDS.
67 pages

Magazines

447 **AIDS Alert**
American Health Consultants
Po Box 740056
Atlanta, GA 30374 800-688-2421
Fax: 800-284-3291
www.ahcpub.com

448 **AIDS Clinical Care**
New England Journal of Medicine

860 Winter Street
Waltham, MA 02451-1413
781-893-3800
800-843-6356
Fax: 781-893-0413
e-mail: nejcust@mms.org
www.massmed.org

Up to date information specifically targeted at physicians with AIDS patients.
Monthly

449 **AIDS: A Year In Review**
Lippincott Williams & Wilkins
Po Box 1620
Hagerstown, MD 21741
301-223-2300
800-638-3030
www.lww.com

450 **AIDS: International Monthly Journal**
Lippincott Williams & Wilkins
Po Box 1620
Hagerstown, MD 21741
301-223-2300
800-638-3030
www.lww.com

451 **AIDS: The Disease State Management Resource**
American Health Consultants
Po Box 740056
Atlanta, GA 30374
800-688-2421
Fax: 800-284-3291
www.ahcpub.com

452 **Critical Path AIDS Project**
2062 Lombard Street
Philadelphia, PA 19146-1315
215-545-2212
www.critpath.org

Articles and reprints on experimental treatments and alternative therapies, and a listing of Philadelphia-area resources.
Monthly

453 **Institute on Health Care for the Poor and Underserved at Meharry Medical College**
Sage Publications
1005 DB Todd Boulevard
Nashville, TN 37208
615-327-6819
800-669-1269
Fax: 615-327-6362
e-mail: vbrennan@mmc.edu

Offers health care and public health policy research focusing on poor and underserved populations.
100pages 4x a year
Dr. Amy Cato, Director
Dr. Virginia Brennan, Editor

454 **Journal of Acquired Immune Deficiency Syndrome**
Lippincott Williams & Wilkins
Po Box 1620
Hagerstown, MD 21741-2601
301-223-2300
800-638-3030
www.lww.com

An interdisciplinary journal providing a synthesis of AIDS-related information from all relevant clinical and basic sciences.
Monthly
ISBN: 0-894925-5 -
William A Hazeltine, Editor

455 **Journal of the Medical Library Association**
Medical Library Association
65 East Wacker Place
Chicago, IL 60601-7246
312-419-9094
Fax: 312-419-8950
e-mail: info@mlahq.org
www.mlahq.org

Is an international, peer-reviewed journal published quarterly that aims to advance the practice and research knowledgebase of health sciences librarianship.
Quarterly
Jean P Shipman, President

456 **POZ Magazine**
POZ Publishing
500 Fifth Avenue
New York, NY 10110-0303
212-242-2163
Fax: 212-675-8505
e-mail: poz-editor@poz.com
www.poz.com

National magazine for anyone affected by HIV/AIDS. Includes treatment options, inspiring profiles and provocative commentary.
60 pages BiMonthly

457 **Risky Business**
San Francisco AIDS Foundation Materials Dept.
333 Valencia Street
San Francisco, CA 94103-3547
415-861-3397

A comic book style magazine providing accurate information about AIDS using humor and real-life situations. Contains stories that stress the importance of knowing how AIDS is transmitted and prevented.

458 **Straight Talk: A Magazine for Teens About AIDS**
Custom Publishing Division of Rodale Press
33 E Minor Street
Emmaus, PA 18098-0001
610-967-5171

A lively magazine that includes articles about teens with AIDS, teens involved in peer education and teens at risk for getting infected. Good information is presented in an interesting format for young adults.

459 **Washington Update**
Committee of Ten Thousand
500 Belmont Street
Brockton, MA 02301
508-587-2512
e-mail: cott-dc@earthlink.net
www.cott1.org

Is a primer on government related issues of importance to COTT's constituency. From health care legislation, to regulatory affairs to Administration policy for chronic diseases. A hands-on journal for grass roots health care advocacy in our Nation's capital.
Bi-Monthly
John Rider, Contact

Newsletters

460 **AIDS Alert**
American Health Consultants
3525 Piedmont Road
Atlanta, GA 30305
e-mail: customerservice@ahcpub.com
www.ahcpub.com

AIDS Alert is the definitive source of AIDS news and advice for health care professionals. It covers up-to-the-minute developments and guidance on the entire spectrum of AIDS challenges, including treatment, education, precaustions, screening, and diagnosis.
12 year

461 **AIDS Link**
University of Cincinnati-Medical Center Info.
231 Bethesda Avenue
Cincinnati, OH 45267-0001
513-558-5661
Fax: 513-558-3136
medcenter.uc.edu/

Aimed at healthcare professionals working with HIV/AIDS inflicted patients.
Rebecca Atterrin, Editor

462 **AIDS News**
Northern California Chapter of the NHF
7700 Edgewater Drive
Oakland, CA 94621-3023
510-568-6243

Provides current information for people who need to cope mentally and physically with the issues of virus infection and transmission. Provides answers to questions about AIDS, ARC, HIV infection and transmission prevention.
BiMonthly

463 **AIDS Policy and Law**
LRP Publications
747 Dresher Road
Horsham, PA 19044-0980
www.lrp.com

A report on AIDS policy and law developments from the courts, NIH, federal and state AIDS agencies and advocacy organizations.
24 year

464 **AIDS Treatment Data Network**
611 Broadway
New York, NY 10012
212-260-8868
800-734-7104
Fax: 212-260-8869
www.atdn.org

Information bulletins covering new treatments, clinical trials, and more.

465 **AIDS Treatment News**
ATN Publications
PO Box 411256
San Francisco, CA 94141-1256 800-873-2812
www.atnonline.org
Reports on the developments in treatments for HIV disease and related infections. Also covers issues relating to research.
BiMonthly

466 **AIDS Update**
Dallas Gay Alliance
PO Box 190812 214-528-4233
Dallas, TX 75219-0812 Fax: 214-521-6424
e-mail: info@dgla.org
www.divanet.com/dgla/
Includes general information on AIDS issues and treatments.

467 **AIDS Weekly Plus**
Charles Henderson
Po Box 5528
Atlanta, GA 31107-0528 e-mail: info@hendersonnet.atl.ga.us
All aspects of AIDS epidemic coverage, including research, treatments, vaccine development, political and public policy.
46 year

468 **AIDS/STD News Report**
CD Publications
8204 Fenton Street 301-588-6380
Silver Spring, MD 0910 800-666-6380
Fax: 301-588-6385
e-mail: info@cdpublications.com
www.cdpublications.com
Formerly AIDS News Alert, provides grant listings from federal, private, and corporate sources; proposal writing tips; updates on successful programs, and the latest news on AIDS/STD federal/state legislation, research, and successful programs.
24 year

469 **APICHA News**
Asian & Pacific Islander Coalition on HIV/AIDS
275 7th Avenue 212-334-7940
New York, NY 10001-3715 866-274-2429
Fax: 212-334-7956
e-mail: APICHA@apicha.org
www.apicha.org
Provides information on prevention education, client services and advocacy for Asians and Pacific Islanders.
Quarterly

470 **APLA Update**
AIDS Project Los Angeles
3550 Wilshire Boulevard
Los Angeles, CA 90010 213-201-1600
www.apla.org
Presents news about AIDS and programs of AIDS Project Los Angeles to people affected by the disease.
20 pages

471 **BETA**
San Francisco AIDS Foundation
995 Market Street 200 415-487-3000
San Francisco, CA 94103 e-mail: feedback@sfaf.org
www.sfaf.org
Medical information.
Quarterly

472 **Being Alive**
Being Alive People with HIV/AIDS Action Coalition
621 N San Vincente Boulevard 310-289-2551
West Hollywood, CA 90069 Fax: 310-289-9866
e-mail: info@beingalivela.org
www.beingalivela.org
Medical updates, plus information on AIDS advocacy, a calendar of local events and listings of AIDS support groups.

473 **Being Alive Newsletter**
Being Alive People with HIV/AIDS Action Coalition
621 N San Vicente Blvd 310-289-2551
West Hollywood, CA 90069 Fax: 310-289-9866
e-mail: info@beingalivela.org
www.beingalivela.org
Non-profit membership organization created and operated by and for people living with HIV/AIDS that engages a sense of independence and self-determination in its members and builds a healthier and more powerful community of HIV positive people.

474 **CORPUS**
AIDS Project Los Angeles
The David Geffen Center
Los Angeles, CA 90005 213-201-1600
www.apla.org
Uses art, cultural criticism, poetry, short stories and humor to reveal challenges of HIV prevention in gay and bisexual communities.
2 year

475 **COTT News**
Committee on Ten Thousand
500 Belmont Street
Brockton, MA 02301 508-587-2512
www.cott1.org
A range of information, reportage and viewpoints regarding issues and events of importance to grass roots health care advocacy and support.
John Rider, Contact

476 **Center for AIDS Prevention Studies**
AIDS Research Institute
74 New Montgomery 415-597-9100
San Francisco, CA 94105 Fax: 415-597-9213
e-mail: capsweb@psg.ucsf.edu
www.caps.ucsf.edu
Local, national, and international interdisciplinary research.

477 **Community Health Funding Report**
CD Publications
8204 Fenton Street 301-588-6380
Silver Spring, MD 20910-4571 800-666-6380
Fax: 301-588-6385
e-mail: chf@cdpublications.com
www.cdpublications.com
Covers grants for AIDS and sexually transmitted disease related programs from federal and private sources. Includes news on national and local issues affecting AIDS and STD's and case studies of successful fundraising programs. This biweekly newsletter describes changes in funding streams for community based health programs, including AIDS programs. It lists available federal and private grant opportunities, along with Washington News Medicare/Medicaid.
18 pages BiMonthly
Mike Gerecht, Publisher
Amy Bernstein, Editor

478 **Cott Washington Update**
Committee of Ten Thousand
236 Massachusetts Avenue NE 202-543-0988
Washington, DC 20002-4971 800-488-2688
Fax: 202-543-6720
www.cott1.org
Offers legislative updates, information on clinical trials, therapies, book reviews, business and politics, a readers forum and resources pertaining to HIV/AIDS.
10 pages Monthly
Corey Dubin, President
Dave Cavenaugh, Government Relations

479 **FOCUS**
AIDS Health Project
1855 Folsom Street
San Francisco, CA 94103 415-476-3902
www.ucsf-ahp.org
A guide to AIDS research and counseling. Premier mental health newsletter.
10 year

480 **Gay Men's Health Crisis**
119 West 24th Street
New York, NY 10011 212-367-1000
www.gmhc.org
Not-for-profit, voluteer-supported and community-based organization committed to national leadership in the fight against AIDS.

481 **HIV Frontline**
Center for AIDS Prevention Studies
University of California 415-552-6356
San Francisco, CA 94114 Fax: 415-597-9213
e-mail: CAPSweb@psg.ucsf.edu
www.caps.ucsf.edu
Monthly newsletter aimed at mental health and healthcare professionals who counsel people living with HIV/AIDS.
Monthly
Dr. Leon McKusick

482 **IDF Advocate**
Immune Deficiency Foundation
40 W Chesapeake Avenue 410-321-6647
Towson, MD 21204 800-296-4433
Fax: 410-321-9165
e-mail: idf@primaryimmune.org
www.primaryimmune.org
The National Newsletter of the Immune Deficiency Foundation.
3x/year
Marcia Boyle, Founder/Chair
Christine M Belsar, Editor

483 **Immune Deficiency Foundation Newsletter**
Immune Deficiency Foundation
40 W Chesapeake Avenue 410-321-6647
Towson, MD 21204-4841 800-296-4433
Fax: 410-321-9165
e-mail: idf@primaryimmune.org
www.primaryimmune.org
Offers medical updates and technology news on the latest services, products and treatments for persons with immune diseases.
Tamara Brown, Medical Programs Manager

484 **In Focus**
Project Inform
205 13th Street 415-558-8669
San Francisco, CA 94103-2461 800-822-7422
Fax: 415-558-0684
e-mail: web@projectinform.org
www.projectinform.org
The organizational newsletter of Project Inform.
20+ pages 3x/year
Skip Emerson, Executive Assistant

485 **Just Kids**
3 Corners
5th Avenue 212-634-4879
New York, NY 10014
Covers medical and social issues faced by HIV-positive children, teens and their parents.
Annual

486 **MLA News**
Medical Library Association
65 East Wacker Place 312-419-9094
Chicago, IL 60601-7246 Fax: 312-419-8950
e-mail: info@mlahq.org
www.mlahq.org
Keeps you at the forefront of association matters and the profession as a whole. Regular departments include calendar, continuing education, employment opportunities, international news, Internet resources, personals, professional development, and technology. Columns include consumer health, expert searching, hospital librarianship, leadership and management, and new members. Members only.
Jean P Shipman, President

487 **NMAC Update**
National Minority AIDS Council
300 I Street NE
Washington, DC 20002-4389 202-544-1076
www.nmac.org
A newsletter reporting on public policy issues and information on subjects in organizational management.
BiMonthly

488 **OUTReach**
The San Francisco AID Foundation
995 Market Street 415-487-8000
San Francisco, CA 94103 Fax: 415-487-8009
TDD: 415-487-8099
www.sfaf.org
Features concise articles on a wide range of HIV/AIDS topics.

489 **PAACNOTES**
101 W Grand Avenue 312-222-1326
Chicago, IL 60610-4272 800-243-3059
A news journal of the Physicians Coalition for AIDS Care featuring articles on clinical management, scientific research and a diverse range of legal, ethical and economic issues directly affecting the care of persons with HIV disease.

490 **PERSPECTIVES**
AIDS Health Project
1855 Folsom Street
San Francisco, CA 94103 415-476-3902
www.ucsf-ahp.org
Educational resource for HIV test counselors and other health professionals.
4 year

491 **PWA Rag**
Prisoners With AIDS Rights Advocacy Group
1626 Wilcox Avenue 770-946-9346
Loa Angeles, CA 90028 e-mail: RAGNEWS@aol.com
www.hometown.aol.com
Contains articles, treatment updates, and resources for prisoners.

492 **Posistive Voice Update**
National Association of People with AIDS (NAPWA)
8401 Colesville Road 240-247-0880
Silverspring, MD 20910 Fax: 240-247-0574
e-mail: info@napwa.org
www.napwa.org

493 **Positive Living**
APLA
3550 Wilshire Boulevard 213-201-1600
Los Angeles, CA 90010 800-922-2438
Monthly

494 **Positive Outlook**
2655 Swann Avenue 813-877-5696
Tampa, FL 33609
Focuses on local people and issues in West Central Florida.
Quarterly

495 **Positive Social Support Newsletter**
Lambda Center
4228 Wisconsin Avenue NW 202-965-8434
Washington, DC 20016 877-252-6232
e-mail: contact@lambcenter.com
www.thelambdacenter.com
Sponsored by and for people with HIV.

496 **Positive Woman**
PO Box 34372 202-898-0372
Washington, DC 20043-4372
Provides medical information, including alternative and holistic therapies for HIV-positive women.
BiMonthly

497 **Positively Aware**
Test Positive Aware Network
1340 W Irving Park Road
Chicago, IL 60613-1900 773-404-8726
www.tpan.com
Chicago area HIV related services directory, that includes HIV news items, events and clinical trials in the Chicago area.
Monthly

498 **Rural Prevention Report Newsletter**
Rural Center for AIDS/STD Prevention
Indiana University 812-855-3936
Bloomington, IN 47405-3085 800-566-8644
Fax: 812-855-3936
e-mail: aids@indiana.edu
www.indiana.edu/~aids/

499 **STEP Perspective**
Seattle Treatment Exchange Project
1123 E John Street 206-329-4857
Seattle, WA 98102-5711 800-869-7837
e-mail: info@stepproject.org
www.thebody.com
Updates on treatments for HIV and related diseases condensed from journals, conferences and databases by the scientific review committee.

500 **Seasons**
National Native American AIDS Prevention Center
436 14th Street 510-444-2051
Oakland, CA 94612-2011 Fax: 510-444-1593
e-mail: information@nnaapc.org
www.nnaapc.org
Features articles and artwork by Native Americans impacted by HIV/AIDS.
Quarterly

501 **Treatment Issues**
Department of Medical Information 212-337-1950
New York, NY 10011-3601
The gay men's health crisis newsletter of experimental AIDS therapies.
10x Year

502 **Up Front Drug Information**
5701 Biscayne Boulevard 305-757-2566
Miami, FL 33137-2601
Provides information on drugs and drug referrals.

503 **Walk Talk**
AIDS Coalition Silicon Valley
Walk For AIDS Silicon Valley 408-451-WALK
San Jose, CA 95154 Fax: 408-248-7423
e-mail: info@walkforaids.org
The AIDS Coalition Silicon Valley Newsletter highlighting Walk for AIDS Silicon Valley fundraising events, issues and articles about HIV/AIDS service providers in the County.

504 **Wisconsin AIDS Update**
Wisconsin AIDS/HIV Program, Department of Health
PO Box 309 608-267-5287
Madison, WI 53701-0309 e-mail: webmaildph@dhfs.state.wi.us
www.dhfs.state.wi.us
Includes epidemiological and clinical care articles, selections from the most important current abstracts in ATIN and a statewide list of events and resources.
Quarterly

505 **World/Mundo**
PO Box 11535 415-658-6930
Oakland, CA 94611-0535
Contains letters, advice, events calendar, and information on support groups in Northern California.

Pamphlets

506 **AIDS Medicines in Development**
Pharmaceutical Research & Manufacturers of America
950 F Street NW 202-835-3400
Washington, DC 20004 Fax: 202-835-3414
www.phrma.org
An annual chart of antivirals, as well as information on diagnostics and vaccines.

507 **AIDS and Hemophilia: Protecting Yourself and Others**
Hemophilia Council of California: Bay Area Office
7700 Edgewater Drive 510-568-7074
Oakland, CA 94621 Fax: 510-568-2048
e-mail: hccoak@aol.com
Lori Drake, Mental Health Counselor/Health Educator

508 **AIDS, the Law & You**
AIDS Action Committee
131 Clarendon Street 617-536-7733
Boston, MA 02116-5145 800-424-2634
Fax: 617-437-6445
e-mail: webmaster@aac.org
www.aac.org
Discusses legal protection against AIDS-related discrimination, HIV testing and the law.

509 **Americans with Disabilities Act: What it Means for People with AIDS**
American Civil Liberties Union AIDS Project
132 W 43rd Street
New York, NY 10036-6503 212-944-9800
www.aclu.org

510 **Basics of HIV Disease: Questions and Answers**
National Hemophilia Foundation
116 W 32nd Street 888-463-6643
New York, NY 10001-3212 800-424-2634
Fax: 212-328-3777
www.hemophilia.org
This publication contains basic information about hemophilia and HIV disease.
1992 28 pages
Alan Kinniburgh, PhD, CEO

511 **Be Smart About HIV**
American Red Cross
1616 Fort Myer Drive 703-312-8724
Arlington, VA 22209-3100 Fax: 703-312-8738
www.redcross.org
This brochure offers very simple and informative information on the HIV virus, in both English and Spanish.
1996
Sandra L Mertz, Product Manager

512 **Children with AIDS: Guidelines for Parents and Caregivers**
AIDS Task Force of Central New York
627 W Genesee Street 315-415-2430
Syracuse, NY 13204-2347
Offers general information on AIDS, diet and feeding, household chores, and coping with the illness.

513 **Clinical Focus**
Immune Deficiency Foundation
40 W Chesapeake Avenue 410-321-6647
Towson, MD 21204-4841 800-296-4433
Fax: 410-321-9165
e-mail: idf@primaryimmune.org
www.primaryimmune.org
Biannual publication for medical professionals covering current issues and information regarding clinical approaches to primary immune deficiencies.
BiAnnual
Marcia Boyle, Founder/Chair

514 **Clinical Focus on Primary Immune Deficiency Diseases**
Immune Deficiency Foundation
40 W Chesapeake Avenue 410-321-6647
Towson, MD 21204-4841 800-296-4433
Fax: 410-321-9165
e-mail: idf@primaryimmune.org
www.primaryimmune.org
educational mongraph is designed specifically for health care professionals and focuses on topics relevant to primary immune deficiency diseases.
Marcia Boyle, Founder/Chair

515 **Clinical Presentation of the Primary Immunodeficiency Diseases**
Immune Deficiency Foundation
40 W Chesapeake Avenue 410-321-6647
Towson, MD 21204-4841 800-296-4433
Fax: 410-321-9165
e-mail: idf@primaryimmune.org
www.primaryimmune.org
A primer for physicians.
Tamara Brown, Medical Programs Manager

516 **Clinical Trials: Talking it Over**
NIAID, Office of Communications

Building 31 301-496-5717
Bethesda, MD 20892-0001
Educational pamphlet pertaining to clinical trials.

517 **Condoms and Sexually Transmitted Diseases, Especially AIDS**
Department of Health and Human Services
National Institutes of Health 202-673-7700
Bethesda, MD 20892-0001
Offers information on condoms and how various forms of protection can be used to prevent sexually transmitted diseases, especially HIV/AIDS.

518 **Eating Defensively: Food Safety Advice for Persons with AIDS**
AIDSinfo
PO Box 6303 301-519-0459
Rockville, MD 20849-6303 800-448-0440
Fax: 301-519-6616
TTY: 888-480-3739
e-mail: ContactUs@aidsinfo.nih.gov
www.aidsinfo.nih.gov
The food safety advice in this brochure is intended to help persons with HIV infection to reduce the risk of food poisoning, thereby avoiding an illness that could worsen their condition or even cause death.
1992

519 **HIV Infection and AIDS**
NAID Office of Communications
31 Center Drive 301-496-5717
Bethesda, MD 20892-0001
Offers information on transmission, treatment, early symptoms, diagnosis, prevention and research.

520 **HIV and AIDS During Pregnancy**
March of Dimes
233 Park Avenue South 212-353-8353
New York, NY 10003 Fax: 212-254-3518
e-mail: NY639@marchofdimes.com
www.marchdofdimes.com

521 **HIV/AIDS in the Workplace**
New York Business Group on Health
386 Park Avenue S 212-252-7440
New York, NY 10016-8804 e-mail: nybgh@nybgh.org
www.nybgh.org
Offers information on federal law and state law regarding HIV/AIDS in the workplace, universal risks, health insurance and other business costs.

522 **Hope for Children with AIDS**
Pediatric AIDS Foundation
2950 31st Street 310-394-1459
Santa Monica, CA 90405-3092 888-499-4673
Fax: 310-394-1469
e-mail: info@pedaids.org
www.pedaids.org
A brochure offering information on the latest research and advances in the area of pediatric AIDS.

523 **How to Keep an Infusion Log**
Immune Deficiency Foundation
40 W Chesapeake Avenue 410-321-6647
Towson, MD 21204-4841 800-296-4433
Fax: 410-321-9165
e-mail: idf@primaryimmune.org
www.primaryimmune.org
This brochure highlights the importance of keeping an infusion log to track the dates, product lot numbers, and adverse events of IGIV infusions. IDF supplies infusion log books for both adult and pediatric patients.
Marci Boyle, Founder/Chair

524 **IDF Patient and Family Handbook**
Immune Deficiency Foundation
40 W Chesapeake Avenue 410-321-6647
Towson, MD 21204-4841 800-296-4433
Fax: 410-321-9165
e-mail: idf@primaryimmune.org
www.primaryimmune.org
Tamara Brown, Medical Programs Manager

525 **Immune Deficiency Foundation**
40 W. Chesapeake Avenue
Towson, MD 21204 800-296-4433
e-mail: idf@primaryimmune.org
www.primaryimmune.org
Your partner for living with primary immune deficiency diseases. This brochure describes the IDF and its activities and services.

526 **Infections Linked to AIDS**
NAID Office of Communications
31 Center Drive 301-496-5717
Bethesda, MD 20892-0001
Offers information on infections related to HIV/AIDS and referral numbers of where to receive help.

527 **Our Immune System**
Immune Deficiency Foundation
40 W Chesapeake Avenue 410-321-6647
Towson, MD 21204-4841 800-296-4433
Fax: 410-321-9165
e-mail: idf@primaryimmune.org
www.primaryimmune.org
A booklet, in comic book form offering information and descriptions on the body's immune system.
22 pages
Tamara Brown, Medical Programs Manager

528 **Primary Immune Deficiency Diseases: A Guide for Nurses**
Immune Deficiency Foundation
40 W Chesapeake Avenue 410-321-6647
Towson, MD 21204-4841 800-296-4433
Fax: 410-321-9165
e-mail: idf@primaryimmune.org
www.primaryimmune.org
Offers information on primary immune deficiency diseases to nurses working with patients suffering from these illnesses.
Tamara Brown, Medical Programs Manager

529 **Taking the HIV (AIDS) Test: How to Help Yourself**
NAID Office of Communications
31 Center Drive 301-496-5717
Bethesda, MD 20892-0001
Offers information on the AIDS test, how it works, how it can help and should it be taken.

530 **Teeens, Sexually Transmitted Diseases & HIV/AIDS**
4 Brighton Road
West Sussex, RH13 5BA UK, e-mail: info@avert.org
www.avert.org
Designed for teens, and contains information on what STD's are, how to avoid becoming infected, safer sex, how to spot symptoms of STD's, STD treatment, information about HIV/AIDS, information about testing and treatment, and advice helplines.

531 **Testing Positive for HIV**
NAID Office of Communications
31 Center Drive 301-496-5717
Bethesda, MD 20892-0001
Information on what a positive HIV test means, how not to spread the disease to others, and various health and dieting tips.

532 **Testing for HIV Infection**
American Red Cross
1616 Fort Myer Drive 703-312-8724
Arlington, VA 22209-3100 Fax: 703-312-8738
1996
Sandra L Mertz, Product Manager

533 **Women, Sex, and HIV**
American Red Cross
1616 Fort Myer Drive 703-312-8724
Arlington, VA 22209-3100 Fax: 703-312-8738
1992
Sandra L Mertz, Product Manager

534 **Your Job and HIV: Are There Risks?**
American Red Cross
1616 Fort Myer Drive 703-312-8724
Arlington, VA 22209-3100 Fax: 703-312-8738
1992
Sandra L Mertz, Product Manager

Audio & Video

535 **AIDS Work: Six Healthcare Workers Face the AIDS Crisis**

Fanlight Productions
4196 Washington Street 617-469-4999
Boston, MA 02131-1731 800-937-4113
Fax: 617-469-3379
e-mail: fanlight@fanlight.com
www.fanlight.com

Two physicians and four nurses reflect on several decades of combined experience in caring for patients with HIV/AIDS.

VHS
ISBN: 1-572952-20-2
Nicole Johnson, Publicity Coordinator

536 **Does Anyone Die of AIDS Anymore?**

Louise Hogarth, author

Fanlight Productions
4196 Washington Street 617-469-4999
Boston, MA 02131 800-937-4113
Fax: 617-469-3379
e-mail: fanlight@fanlight.com
www.fanlight.com

Despire the much-hyped advances in treatment which, for some patients, have transformed HIV from a death sentence to a chronic illness, tens of thousands of people are still dying of AIDS in the United States.

2002 26 Minutes
ISBN: 1-572953-62-4
Nicole Johnson, Publicity Coordinator

537 **Roger's Story: For Cori**

Howard Shepps, author

Fanlight Productions
4196 Washington Street 617-469-4999
Boston, MA 02131-1731 800-937-4113
Fax: 617-469-3379
e-mail: fanlight@fanlight.com
www.fanlight.com

Forty-four year-old Roger shares the harrowing story of his 20-year struggle against heroin, and his recent diagnosis with AIDS.

1989 28 Minutes
ISBN: 1-572950-47-1

538 **Too Little, Too Late**

Micki Dickoff, author

Fanlight Productions
4196 Washington Street 617-469-4999
Boston, MA 02131-1731 800-937-4113
Fax: 617-469-3379
e-mail: fanlight@fanlight.com
www.fanlight.com

In this moving video, family members of people with AIDS share their pain and frustration, as well as the solace they have derived from having been able to help their loved one to a peaceful death.

1987 49 Minutes
ISBN: 1-572950-27-7

539 **Undetectable: The New Face of AIDS**

Jay Corcoran, author

Fanlight Productions
4196 Washington Street 617-469-4999
Boston, MA 02131 800-937-4113
Fax: 617-469-3379
e-mail: fanlight@fanlight.com
www.fanlight.com

Follows the stories of six individuals from diverse backgrounds as they deal with the physical and psychological implication of new HIV drug therapies.

2001 56 Minutes
ISBN: 1-572953-34-9
Nicole Johnson, Publicity Coordinator

Web Sites

540 **AIDS Action**

www.aidsaction.org

National organization dedicated to the development, analysis, cultivation, and encouragement of sound policies and programs in response to the HIV epidemic. We do this through the dissemination of information and the building and use of advocacy on behalf of all those living with and affected by HIV. Our goal is simple. Until It's Over-until no one aquires HIV, until those living with HIV have the care and services they need, and until a cure is found.

541 **AIDS.ORG**

www.aids.org

The mission of AIDS.ORG is to help prevent HIV infections and to improve the lives of those affected by HIV and AIDS by providing education and facilitating the free and open exchange of knowledge at any easy-to-find centralized website.

542 **Children Affected by AIDS Foundation**

www.caaf4kids.org

Mission is to make a positive difference in the lives of children infected with HIV and affected by AIDS.

543 **Committee of Ten Thousand**

www.cott1.org

Represents presons with hemophilia that contracted HIV/AIDS and Hepatitis C from tainted factor concentrates during the 1970s and 1980s.

544 **HIV/Hepatitis C in Prison (HIP) Committee**

www.prisons.org/hivin.htm

Fighting for consistent access to quality medical care including access to all new HIV and Hepatitis C medications, diagnostic testing and combination therapies.

545 **Healing Well**

www.healingwell.com

An online health resource guide to medical news, chat, information and articles, newsgroups and message boards, books, disease-related web sites, medical directories, and more for patients, friends, and family coping with disabling diseases, disorders, or chronic illnesses.

546 **Health Finder**

www.healthfinder.gov

Searchable, carefully developed web site offering information on over 1000 topics. Developed by the US Department of Health and Human Services, the site can be used in both English and Spanish.

547 **Healthlink USA**

www.healthlinkusa.com

Health information concerning treatment, cures, prevention, diagnosis, risk factors, research, support groups, email lists, personal stories and much more. Updated regularly.

548 **Helios Health**

www.helioshealth.com

Online resource for your health information. Detailed information about specific health topics, access to expert advice from our Medical Advisory Board, and up-to-date health news.

549 **Immune Deficiency Foundation**

www.primaryimmune.org

Offers information and referral services to immune deficient patients and their families.

550 **MedicineNet**

www.medicinenet.com

An online resource for consumers providing easy-to-read, authoritative medical and health information.

551 **Medscape**

www.mywebmd.com

Medscape offers specialists, primary care physicians, and other health professionals the Web's most robust and integrated medical information and educational tools.

552 **National AIDS Information Clearinghouse**

www.cdcnac.org

Provides information and materials for employers on national, state and local resources related to HIV/AIDS in the workplace.

553 **National Minotirty AIDS Education Training**

www.nmaetc.org

Located at Howard University, as a HIV/AIDS training and technical resource for providers of minority HIV-infected patients throughout the country. THe NMAETC receives 100% of its funding through the MAI Initiative. THe NMAETC in collaboration with ither HRSA funded programs seeks to influence health care professionals who treat minority HIV-infected patients.

554 **New England AIDS Education & Training Ctr.**

www.neaetc.org

One of eleven regional education centers funded by the Ryan White CARE Act and sponsored regionally by the Office of Community Programs at the University of Massachusetts Medical Center. The AETC Program is administered by Health Resources and Services Administration (HRSA) HIV/AIDS bureau.

555 **People with AIDS Health Group**

www.Aidsinfonyc.org

PWA is a non-profit buyers club organized to assist people with AIDS in obtaining medications — as well as provide support groups committed to the self-empowerment of people living with AIDS. They offer three programs: Treatment Education and Support, Advocacy and Public Policy, and Early Treatment Access.

556 **San Francisco Area AIDS Education Center**

www.ucsf.edu/sfaetc

Helps to improve the care of people living with HIV and AIDS by supporting state-of-the-art clinical consultation, education, and training for health care professionals and organizations in Sa Francisco, San Mateo, and Marin counties.

557 **Smart & Strong**

www.smartstrong.com

A healthcare education company that supports providers and empowers HIV positive patients through publications, seminars and innovative educational programs.

558 **WebMD**

www.webmd.com

Information on AIDS related diseases, including articles and resources.

559 **Well Project**

www.projectinform.org

Not For Profit Corporation, is an initiative conceived, developed, and administered by HIV+ women and those who are affected by this disease.

Description

560 **Allergies**

Allergy means altered reactivity. Allergies are usually characterized by a hypersensitivity to substances, such as pollens, pet dander, certain foods, some medications and molds. Such substances (allergens) can trigger an allergic response in susceptible individuals. Symptoms of allergies may present in a wide spectrum ranging from the mild sneezing, runny nose and congestion of hayfever to life-threatening reactions, known as anaphylaxis. Additional allergic reactions include itchy, watery eyes, skin rashes and asthma. More severe symptoms may include a tingling sensation in the mouth, swelling of the tongue and throat, difficulty breathing, hives, vomiting abdominal cramps, diarrhea, drop in blood pressure, loss of consciousness, and cardiovascular collapse leading to death. Allergic sypmtoms typically appear within minutes to two hours after the person has been exposed to the allergen.

Approximately 35 million people suffer from allergies in the United States. The cause of allergies is unclear, although there may be a genetic link in some people.

Treatment for allergies depends upon the specific substance, beginning with avoidance. Strict avoidance of the allergy-causing food is the only way to avoid a food allergy reaction. There are no medications that cure food allergies. Most people outgrow their food allergies, although peanuts, nuts, fish and shellfish are often considered life-long allegies.

For non-food allergies, medications such as antihistamines and inhaled bronchodilators, as well as allergy shots to reduce the allergic response, may be prescribed by doctors. Epinephrine, also called adrenaline, is the medication of choice for controlling a severe reaction. Individuals at risk of an anaphylactic reaction should have a bracelet or necklace with that information. Those who are allergic to insect stings should carry and use a pre-filled syringe of epinephrine (epipen) for prompt self-treatment.

National Agencies & Associations

561 **Allergy & Asthma Network Mothers of Asthmatics**
2751 Prosperity Avenue 703-641-9595
Fairfax, VA 22031 800-878-4403
Fax: 703-573-7794
e-mail: info@aanma.org
www.breatherville.org
Leading nonprofit membership organization dedicated to eliminating suffering and death due to asthma, allergies and related conditions through education, advocacy, community outreach and research.
Nancy Sander, Founder/President

562 **Allergy Asthma Information Association**
1-111 Zenway Boulevard
Vaughan, Ontario, L4H-3H9 905-265-3322
www.aaia.ca
To develop societal awareness of the seriousness of allergic disease, including asthma, and to enable allergic individuals, their families and caregivers, to increase control over allergy symptoms by providing leadership in information, education, advocacy, in partnership with health care professionals, business, industry and government.

563 **American Academy of Allergy, Asthma & Immunology**
555 East Wells Street 414-272-6071
Milwaukee, WI 53202-3823 800-822-2762
Fax: 414-272-6070
e-mail: info@aaaai.org
www.aaaai.org
Strives to serve the public through information on asthma and allergies, as well as referrals to allergists. Also offers pollen and mold statistics from the Committee on Pollen & Molds.
John Gardner, Media Relations Manager
Katie Tetzlaff, Communications Coordinator

564 **American Academy of Environmental Medicine**
6505 E Central Avenue 316-684-5000
Wichita, KS 67206 Fax: 316-684-5709
e-mail: administrator@aaemonline.org
www.aaem.com
Offers names of Clinical Ecologists and Allergy Specialists in the United States.
Jennifer Arm MD FAAEM, President
James F Coy MD, Secretary

565 **American College of Allergy, Asthma & Immunology**
85 West Algonquin Road 847-427-1200
Arlington Heights, IL 60005 Fax: 847-427-1294
e-mail: mail@acaai.org
www.acaai.org
This association focuses its attention on research and public awareness of allergies. Distributes informational brochures and pamphlets, offers referrals and counseling services, as well as patient care.
Daniel Ein, MD, President

566 **American Dietetic Association**
120 South Riverside Plaza 312-899-0040
Chicago, IL 60606-6995 800-877-1600
Fax: 312-899-1979
e-mail: media@eatright.org
www.eatright.org
Offers information and support to allergy sufferers. Serves the public through the promotion of optimal nutrition, health, and well-being.
Lori Ferme, Media Contact
Susan H Laramee, President

567 **Association of Birth Defect Children Birth Defect Research for Children**
930 Woodcock Road 407-245-7035
Orlando, FL 32803 e-mail: staff@birthdefects.org
www.birthdefects.org
Offers informational packets on childhood asthma and prevention.
Betty Mekdeci, Contact

568 **Asthma and Allergy Foundation of America**
1233 20th Street NW 202-466-7643
Washington, DC 20036 800-727-8462
Fax: 202-466-8940
e-mail: info@aafa.org
www.aafa.org
Nonprofit patient organization dedicated to improving the quality of life for people with asthma and allergies and their caregivers, through education, advocacy and research.
Mary Brasler, EdD, MSN, Director of Programs and Services

569 **Canadian Society of Allergy and Clinical I mmunology**
774 Echo Drive 613-730-6272
Ottawa, Ontario, K1S-5N8 Fax: 613-730-1116
e-mail: csaci@rcpsc.edu
www.csaci.medical.org
Is the advancement of the knowledge and practice of allergy, clinical immunology, and asthma for optimal patient care.
Dr Charles Frankish, President

570 **Eczema Association for Science and Education**
6600 SW 92nd Avenue 503-244-7404
Portland, OR 97223-7195 800-818-7546
Fax: 503-245-0626
e-mail: getinfo@psoriasis.org
www.nationaleczema.org
Offers resources and information for allergy patients.
Irene Crosby
Philip S Crosby

571 **Food Allergy and Anaphylaxis Network**
11781 Lee Jackson Highway
Fairfax, VA 22033-3309 800-929-4040
Fax: 703-691-2713
e-mail: faan@foodallergy.org
www.foodallergy.org
Increases public awareness about food allergies and anaphylaxis advances research and provides education, emotional support and coping strategies to patients; serves as the communication link between the food industry, the government and the airline industry.
Anne Munoz-Furlong, Founder
Jennifer Love, Marketing and Media Communications

572 **Immune Deficiency Foundation**
40 W Chesapeake Avenue 410-321-6647
Towson, MD 21204-4841 800-296-4433
Fax: 410-321-9165
e-mail: idf@primaryimmune.org
www.primaryimmune.org
The national patient organization dedicated to improving the diagnosis treatment and quality of life of persons with primary immunodeficiency diseases through advocacy education and research.
Marcia Boyle, President & Founder
John Seymour PhD LMFT, Vice Chair

573 **National Institute of Allergy and Infectious Diseases**
NIAID Office of Communications and Public Liason
6610 Rockledge Drive 301-496-5717
Bethesda, MD 20892-6612 Fax: 301-402-3573
e-mail: clane@niaid.nih.gov
www.niaid.nih.gov
Conducts and supports research on allergies; focused on understanding what happens to the body during the allergic process. Educates patients and health care workers in controlling allergic disease; offers various research centers that conduct and evaluate educational programs focused on methods to control allergic diseases.
Anthony S Fauci, MD, Director

State Agencies & Associations

California

574 **Asthma and Allergy Foundation of America: Southern California Chapter**
5900 Wilshire Boulevard 323-937-7859
Los Angeles, CA 90036 800-624-0044
Fax: 323-937-7815
e-mail: aafasocal@aol.com
www.aafasocal.com
Dedicated to controlling and curing asthma and allergic diseases through education, a network of support groups, the support of research and specialized training, increasing public awareness and providing medication and treatment to the under served. Program highlights include the Breathmobile, asthma camps and air power games for children.
Francene Lifson, Executive Director

Colorado

575 **Mountain-Plains AIDS Education and Training Center (MPAETC)**
12631 E 17th Avenue 303-724-0867
Aurora, CO 80045 Fax: 303-724-0875
e-mail: info@mpaetc.org
www.mpaetc.org
One of 12 regional AETCs funded nationwide by a grant from the U.S. Health Resources and Services Administration through the Ryan White Comprehensive AIDS Resources Emergency (CARE) Act. Provides educational programs about HIV infection for healthcare providers.
Beth Mullin Rotach, Director
Lucy Bradley-Springe, Principal Investigator

Florida

576 **Asthma and Allergy Foundation of America: Florida Chapter**
200 Orangewood Drive 727-738-1146
Dunedin, FL 34698 Fax: 727-736-4484
e-mail: cherylsmall@aafaflorida.org
www.aafa.org
Works to serve its community through programs, advocacy, education, research and national involvement.
John Little, Executive Director

Maryland

577 **Asthma and Allergy Foundation of America: Maryland/Greater Washington, DC**
1777 Reistertown Road 410-653-2880
Baltimore, MD 21208 800-727-9333
Fax: 410-653-9611
e-mail: aafamd@mail.bcpl.net
Serves the state of Maryland, District of Columbia and Northern Virginia areas. Dedicated to helping asthma and allergy sufferers successfully manage and control their disease through the education, referrals and research. Major activities include accredited child care provider course, school liaison, ashtma camp, patient assistance, collge scholarships for high school seniors and professional education courses. Breathmobile, Mobile Asthma Clinic, visiting schools in the city of Baltimore.
Linda R Boyer, Executive Director

Massachusetts

578 **Asthma and Allergy Foundation of America: New England Chapter**
220 Boylston Street 617-965-7771
Chestnut Hill, MA 02467 877-227-8462
Fax: 617-965-8886
TTY: 877-227-8462
e-mail: info@asthmaandallergies.org
www.asthmaandallergies.org
Serves Massachusetts, Rhode Island, Connecticut, Maine, New Hampshire and Vermont. Program highlights include speakers and exhibits, telephone information and referrals, tobacco control program, scholarship essay contest for high school juniors, advocacy for safer environments and training programs for school, daycare and health professionals.
Patricia Goldman, Executive Director
Sharon Schumack, Health Education Coordinator

Michigan

579 **Asthma and Allergy Foundation of America: Michigan Chapter**
17520 W 12 Mile Road 248-557-8050
Southfield, MI 40876-8768 888-444-0333
Fax: 248-557-8768
e-mail: aafamich@aol.com
Serves the state of Michigan through public forums, work place educational programs, patient advocacy, Asthma Camp and telephone referrals and information.
Karen Katz, Executive Director
Dr. Rola Bokhari-Panza, President

Missouri

580 **Asthma and Allergy Foundation of America: St. Louis Chapter**
1500 S Big Bend 314-645-2422
St. Louis, MO 63117 Fax: 314-692-2022
e-mail: aafa@aafastl.org
www.aafastl.org
This chapter has provided children who suffer from asthma and allergies with life saving medications, equipment and educational and emotional support. The founders of the St. Louis chapter identified the apparent need in their community to help children effec-

tively manage their asthma through the provision of medical resources, equipment and education.
Patricia Williams, Executive Director

Oregon

581 Asthma and Allergy Foundation of America: Oregon Chapter
14530 SW 144th Avenue 503-524-2232
Tigard, OR 97224-1445 Fax: 208-474-6839
e-mail: hensches@teleport.com
Serving the state of Oregon.
Sandra L Henschel, Executive Director

Pennsylvania

582 Asthma and Allergy Foundation of America: Southern Pennsylvania Chapter
PO Box 115 856-224-9547
Gibbstown, NJ 08027 Fax: 856-224-5893
e-mail: aafasepa@prodigy.net
In the process of establishing a vital, new program that will aid children with chronic asthma. Many parents, some who are without medical insurance, are unaware of the availability of a medical support system that can help their children. The Children at Risk program will enable parents to have their children evaluated and also receive a free one month supply of medication. Parents will also receive information regarding available options for follow up care and prescription coverage.
Debi Maines, Executive Director

Texas

583 Asthma and Allergy Foundation of America: North Texas Chapter
500 Nuffield Lane 817-297-3132
Ft. Worth, TX 76036 888-932-2232
Fax: 817-297-6564
e-mail: aafantx1@hotmail.com
Offers many educational programs and services that touch patients, caregivers, physicians and allied health professionals, including: child care provider education programs, school nurse and respiratory therapist education programs, worksite allergy education programs, spacer and peak flow meter distribution to those in need, a toll free hotline, prescription assistance information, free educational materials in English and Spanish, an electronic newsletter, professional education, etc.
Joan Hart, Executive Director

Washington

584 Asthma and Allergy Foundation of America: Washington State Chapter
108 S Jackson Street 206-368-2866
Seattle, WA 98104 800-778-2232
Fax: 206-368-2941
e-mail: aafawa@aafawa.org
www.aafawa.org
Program highlights include trainings for health care professionals on asthma and allergy management, working collaboratively with other local and regional agencies to improve the quality of life for those affected by asthma and allergies, organizing health fairs and other public events and providing educational materials and products.
Penny Nelson, Executive Director

Research Centers

585 Columbus Children's Research Institute
700 Children's Drive 614-722-2700
Columbus, OH 43205 Fax: 614-722-2716
e-mail: John.Barnard@NationwideChildrens.org
www.nationwidechildrens.org
Research institute dedicated to enhancing the health of children by engaging in the high quality cutting-edge research according to the highest scientific and ethical standards.
John A Barnard, President
Grant Morrow III, Medical Director

586 Creighton University Allergic Disease Center
601 N 30th Street 402-280-5975
Omaha, NE 68131-0001 Fax: 402-280-5961
e-mail: casalej@creighton.edu
medicine.creighton.edu/allergy/homepage.
Robert G Townley, Investigator
Thomas B Casale, Chief

587 Mayo Clinic and Foundation: Division of Allergic Diseases
Department of Immunology
200 First Street SW 507-284-2511
Rochester, MN 55905 Fax: 507-284-0161
TTY: 507-284-9786
e-mail: lee.theresa@mayo.edu
www.mayoclinic.org
Provides a focus for research into the causes prevention and management of allergic diseases.
Gerald J Gleich MD, Director

588 National Jewish Center for Immunology
Goodman Building Room 611 303-398-1287
Denver, CO 80206 800-621-0505
Fax: 303-398-1806
e-mail: martinr@njhealth.org
www.nationaljewish.org
Basic and clinical research into the causes and treatments of asthmatic disorders.
Richard J Martin, Chairman

589 National Jewish Center for Immunology and Respiratory Medicine
Goodman Buiilding Room 611 303-398-1287
Denver, CO 80206 Fax: 303-398-1806
www.nationaljewish.org
Basic and clinical research into the causes and treatments of asthmatic disorders.
Richard Martin, Chairman

590 Research Institute of Palo Alto Medical Foundation
795 El Camino Real
Palo Alto, CA 94301-2302 650-326-8120
www.pamf.org/research
Clinical and general medical sciences research including allergy and immunology disorders.
Harold S Luft, Director
Marcus Krupp, Director Emeritus

591 Scripps Research Institute
10550 N Torrey Pines Road
La Jolla, CA 92037 858-784-1000
www.scripps.edu
Richard Lern MD, President
Douglas A Bingham, Executive Vice President and Chief Opera

592 Texas Children's Allergy and Immunology Clinic
Clinical Care Center
6701 Fannin Street 832-824-1319
Houston, TX 77030 Fax: 832-825-3072
e-mail: pediai@texaschildrenshospital.org
www.texaschildrenshospital.org
William T Shearer, Chief of Service
Celine Hanson, Clinic Chief

593 University of Florida: General Clinical Research Center
University of Florida
1600 SW Archer Road 352-265-8909
Gainesville, FL 32610-0322 Fax: 352-265-8910
e-mail: stacpool@gcrc.ufl.edu
www.gcrc.ufl.edu
Studies on allergies and immunology.
Peter W Stacpoole MD, Program Director

594 University of Kansas Allergy and Immunology Clinic
University of Kansas Medical Center
3901 Rainbow Boulevard 913-588-6008
Kansas City, KS 66160 TTY: 913-588-7963
TDD: 913-588-7963
e-mail: dstechsc@kumc.edu
www.kumc.edu

This service provides complete evaluation of patients with allergic diseases such as rhinitis and asthma immunological deficiencies food and drug intolerances and autoimmune dysfunctions.
Daniel J Stechschulte Sr, Director
Kottarappat Dileepan, Professor

595 **University of Michigan Montgomery: John M. Sheldon Allergy Society**
Alllergy & Clinical Immunology
24 Frank Lloyd Wright Drive 734-647-6573
Ann Arbor, MI 48106-0380 Fax: 734-647-6263
e-mail: echoreed@med.umich.edu
www.med.umich.edu/sheldonsociety
Johannes Postma, Division Administrator
Echo Reed, Senior Administrative Assistant

596 **University of Texas Southwestern Medical Center at Dallas**
University of Texas Southwestern Medical Center
5323 Harry Hines Boulevard 214-648-3111
Dallas, TX 75390 Fax: 214-648-9119
www3.utsouthwestern.edu
Immunodermatology department researching allergies and immune disorders.
Paul R Bergstresser MD, Program Director

597 **Warren Grant Magnuson Clinical Center**
National Institute of Health
9000 Rockville Pike
Bethesda, MD 20892 800-411-1222
Fax: 301-480-9793
TTY: 866-411-1010
e-mail: prpl@mail.cc.nih.gov
www.clinicalcenter.nih.gov
Established in 1953 as the research hospital of the National Institutes of Health. Designed so that patient care facilities are close to research laboratories so new findings of basic and clinical scientists can be quickly applied to the treatment of patients. Upon referral by physicians, patients are admitted to NIH clinical studies.
John Gallin, Director
David Henderson, Deputy Director for Clinical Care

Support Groups & Hotlines

598 **ASTHMA Hotline**
American Academy of Allergy, Asthma and Immunology
555 E Wells Street 414-272-6071
Milwaukee, WI 53202 800-822-2762
Fax: 414-272-6070
www.aaai.org
Referral line offering information on allergy and asthma treatments, referrals to an allergy/immunology specialist, lay organization or support groups across the country.

599 **National Health Information Center**
PO Box 1133 310-565-4167
Washington, DC 20013 800-336-4797
Fax: 301-984-4256
e-mail: info@nhic.org
www.health.gov/nhic
Offers a nationwide information referral service, produces directories and resource guides.

Books

600 **Allergies A to Z**
Facts on File
132 W 31st Street 212-967-8800
New York, NY 10001 800-322-8755
Fax: 800-678-3633
e-mail: custserv@factsonfile.com
www.factsonfile.com
This vital resource for the one in five Americans who suffer from alleries provides reliable, up-to-date information on every aspect of this condition.
Paperback

601 **Allergy Alerts from Living with Allergies**
American Allergy Association
PO Box 7273 650-322-1663
Menlo Park, CA 94026-7273
These alerts cover a wide range of areas from dyes in medications to medication interactions, food additives like sulfites, spelt, situations that could trigger asthma, problems with collagen and even fabric softeners.

602 **Allergy Plants that Cause Sneezing and Wheezing**
Asthma and Allergy Foundation of America
1233 20th Street NW 202-466-7643
Washington, DC 20036-2330 800-727-8462
Fax: 202-466-8940
www.aafa.org
Destined to be displayed on coffee tables, the spectacular photographs in this book actually show allergy sufferers what causes their sneezing and wheezing.
64 pages Paperback

603 **Complete Book of Children's Allergies**
Allergy Central Products
96 Danbury Road 203-438-9580
Ridgefield, CT 06877-4053 800-422-3878
Fax: 203-431-8963
www.allergycontrol.com
Major childhood allergies, recommendations for treatment.
Softcover

604 **Cooking for the Allergic Child**
Allergy Central Products
96 Danbury Road 203-438-9580
Ridgefield, CT 06877-4053 800-442-3878
Fax: 203-431-8963
www.allergycontrol.com
More than 300 recipes with nutrients analysis.
Softcover

605 **Diets to Help Gluten and Wheat Allergy**
HarperCollins Canada Limited/Order Department
1995 Markham Road
Scarborough, M1B 5M8, 800-387-0117
Fax: 800-668-5788
This book offers sound and practical advice on gluten allergy wheat sensitivity and Celiac disease.
96 pages
ISBN: 0-722529-10-4

606 **Food Allergy: A Primer for People**
Asthma and Allergy Foundation of America
1233 20th Street NW 202-466-7643
Washington, DC 20036-2330 800-727-8462
Fax: 202-466-8940
www.aafa.org
Food allergies demystified.
66 pages Hardcover

607 **Human Exposure Assessment for Airborne Pollutants: Advances & Opportunity**
National Academy Press
500 5th Street NW 202-334-3313
Washington, DC 20055 888-624-8373
Fax: 202-334-2793
e-mail: zjones@nas.edu
This book explores the need for strategies to address indoor and outdoor exposures and examines the methods and tools available for finding out when significant exposures occur.

608 **Indoor Allergens: Assessing & Controlling Adverse Health Effects**
National Academy Press
500 5th Street NW 202-334-3313
Washington, DC 20055 888-624-8373
Fax: 202-334-2793
e-mail: zjones@nas.edu
This unique volume summarizes what is known about indoor allergens and how they affect human health and how they can be controlled.
320 pages Hardcover

609 **Infant Formulas for Allergic Infants and Dietetic Concerns for Toddlers**
American Allergy Association

PO Box 7273 650-322-1663
Menlo Park, CA 94026-7273
Offers information on reliable food labels, evaluations of infant formulas, FDA labeling requirements under the new law and more.

610 New Food Labels
American Allergy Association
PO Box 7273 650-322-1663
Menlo Park, CA 94026-7273
Offers clear-cut and precise information on new label word definitions.

611 Pollen Times: By State, By Month
American Allergy Association
PO Box 7273 650-322-1663
Menlo Park, CA 94026-7273
A comprehensive guide offering information on how to plan vacations while avoiding pollen problems.

612 Traveling with Allergies: Prepare and Avoid Problems
American Allergy Association
PO Box 7273 650-322-1663
Menlo Park, CA 94026-7273
Prepare for travel, recognize and minimize the risk, sidestep smoke, food allergies, pollen, mold, dander, weather and emergencies.

Children's Books

613 All About Allergies
Dutton Children's Books
375 Hudson Street 212-366-2000
New York, NY 10014-3658 Fax: 212-366-2262
www.pengiunputnam.com

1993 64 pages
ISBN: 0-525674-10-1

614 Allergies
Franklin Watts Grolier
90 Old Sherman Turnpike 203-797-3500
Danbury, CT 06816-0001 800-621-1115
Fax: 203-797-3197
www.grolier.com
Covers the major types of allergies, including those of the respiratory and gastrointestinal tracts.
112 pages Grades 7-12
ISBN: 0-531125-16-5

615 Living with Allergies
Franklin Watts Grolier
90 Old Sherman Turnpike 203-797-3500
Danbury, CT 06816-0001 800-621-1115
Fax: 203-797-3197
www.grolier.com
Shows how people with allergies are able to overcome their handicap to lead full and productive lives.
32 pages Grades 5-7
ISBN: 0-531108-57-0

Magazines

616 Allergy & Asthma Today
Allergy and Asthma Network/Mothers of Asthmatics
2751 Prosperity Avenue 703-641-9595
Fairfax, VA 22031 800-878-4403
Fax: 703-573-7794
e-mail: info@aanma.org
www.breatherville.org
Allergy & Asthma Today helps patients creat a healthier tomorrow with timely, practical and medically accurate strategies to overcome, not just cope with, asthma and allergies. The cost is part of AANMA membership.
40 pages Quarterly
Mary McGowan, Executive Director
Dawn Merritt, Managing Editor

Newsletters

617 Advice From Your Allergist
American College of Allergy & Immunology
85 W Algonguin Road
Alrlington Heights, IL 60005 847-359-2800
www.allergy.mcg.edu
Offers information on the effects, triggers and causes of allergies including house dust, pets, hay fever, hives and exercise.

618 Food Allergy News
Food Allergy and Anaphylaxis Network
10400 Eaton Place 703-691-3179
Fairfax, VA 22030-2208 800-929-4040
Fax: 703-691-2713
e-mail: faan@foodallergy.org
www.foodallergy.org
Contains allergy free recipes, practical tips such as birthday party, trick-or-treating and travel tips, a dietitian's column, medical information and product information.
12 pages BiMonthly
Anne Munoz-Furlong, Founder

619 MA Report
Allergy and Asthma Network/Mothers of Asthmatics
2751 Prosperity Avenue 703-641-9595
Fairfax, VA 22031 800-878-4403
Fax: 703-573-7794
e-mail: editor@aanma.org
www.breatherville.org
Provides up-to-date medical news, emotional support and practical strategies for overcoming asthma and allergies.
8 pages 8x Year
Mary McGowan, Executive Director
Nancy Sander, Editor-in-Chief

Pamphlets

620 Allergic Diseases
National Institute of Allergy & Infectious Disease
31 Center Drive
Bethesda, MD 20892-2520 301-496-5717
www.niaid.nih.gov/default.htm
Offers information on allergies, who gets them, diagnosis and treatments for various types of allergic diseases.

621 Allergies and You
American Lung Association
1740 Broadway 212-315-8700
New York, NY 10019-4315
Answers basic questions about allergy, particularly as it relates to asthma.

622 Eating Without Packet
American Allergy Association
PO Box 7273 650-322-1663
Menlo Park, CA 94026-7273
Twelve information sheets describing the most common food allergens, specific problems with common foods and supplements, and the facts on milk ingredient labeling, milk allergies, and milk sensitivity. Included in the packet is a 16-page handbook, Understanding Calcium and Osteoporosis.

623 FAAN Flashbacks
Food Allergy and Anaphylaxis Network
10400 Eaton Place 703-691-3179
Fairfax, VA 22030-2208 800-929-4040
Fax: 703-691-2713
e-mail: faan@foodallergy.org
www.foodallergy.org
Series of reprints on specific topics of Food Allergy News. Specific pamphlets offer information on wheat, milk, soy, egg, fish, peanuts, managing food allergy in schools and anaphylaxis.
Anne Munoz-Furlong, Founder

624 Food Allergy and Atopic Dermatitis
Food Allergy and Anaphylaxis Network

10400 Eaton Place 703-691-3179
Fairfax, VA 22030-2208 800-929-4040
Fax: 703-691-2713
e-mail: faan@foodallergy.org
www.foodallergy.org

The purpose of this booklet is to provide tips and other sources of information to help parents raise a child who is afflicted with atopic dermatitis.

12 pages

Anne Munoz-Furlong, Founder

625 **Guide to Gluten-Free Diets**
American Allergy Association
PO Box 7273 650-322-1663
Menlo Park, CA 94026-7273

Offers information on safe substitutes for baking and cooking. Differentiates celiac disease from wheat allergy. Sources of gluten in diet with warnings on when to check with the manufacturer.

626 **Helpful Hints for the Allergic Patient**
American Academy of Allergy, Asthma and Immunology
611 E Wells Street 414-272-6071
Milwaukee, WI 53202-3889 800-822-2762
Fax: 414-272-6070
www.aaaai.org

An informational brochure good for someone who has just been diagnosed with allergies.

8 pages

627 **Just One Little Bite Can Hurt! Important Facts About Anaphylaxis**
Food Allergy and Anaphylaxis Network
10400 Eaton Place 703-691-3179
Fairfax, VA 22030-2208 800-929-4040
Fax: 703-691-2713
e-mail: faan@foodallergy.org
www.foodallergy.org

Offers information on what anaphylaxis is, what the patient should do if they have a reaction and important medical safety tips regarding the illness.

8 pages Booklet

Anne Munoz-Furlong, Founder

628 **Nutrition Guide to Food Allergies**
Food Allergy and Anaphylaxis Network
10400 Eaton Place 703-691-3179
Fairfax, VA 22030-2208 800-929-4040
Fax: 703-691-2713
e-mail: faan@foodallergy.org
www.foodallergy.org

Offers answers to the most commonly asked questions about food allergies, common allergy causing foods and resources for the patient.

24 pages

Anne Munoz-Furlong, Founder

629 **Something in the Air: Airborne Allergens**
National Institute of Allergy & Infectious Disease
9000 Rockville Pike 301-496-5717
Bethesda, MD 20892-0001

Offers information on the symptoms to airborne substances, pollen, mold, dust, animal, chemical allergies and treatments for them.

Audio & Video

630 **Alexander, the Elephant Who Couldn't Eat Peanuts**
Food Allergy and Anaphylaxis Network
10400 Eaton Place 703-691-3179
Fairfax, VA 22030-2208 800-929-4040
Fax: 703-691-2713
e-mail: faan@foodallergy.org
www.foodallergy.org

Video combines the animated story of a peanut allergic elephant with interviews of children who have food allergies. Designed to show children they are not alone.

Anne Munoz-Furlong, Founder

631 **Allergic Rhinitis**
American Academy of Allergy, Asthma and Immunology
611 E Wells Street 414-272-6071
Milwaukee, WI 53202-3889 800-822-2762
Fax: 414-272-6070
www.aaaai.org

Allergic rhinitis, often called hay fever, affects the quality of life of millions of Americans. This video covers the causes and symptoms of seasonal and chronic allergic rhinitis, as well as environmental controls and treatments.

10-13 minutes

632 **Allergic Rhinitis: Nothing to Sneeze At!**
Asthma and Allergy Foundation of America
1233 20th Street NW 202-466-7643
Washington, DC 20036-2330 800-727-8462
Fax: 202-466-8940
www.aafa.org

The basics of allergic rhinitis, with a touch of humor. Common allergens, environmental control, skin testing and immunotherapy medications.

Videotape

633 **Allergic Skin Reactions**
American Academy of Allergy, Asthma and Immunology
611 E Wells Street 414-272-6071
Milwaukee, WI 53202-3889 800-822-2762
Fax: 414-272-6070
www.aaaai.org

In some people, allergy symptoms include itching redness, rashes, or hives. This video describes the symptoms, triggers, and treatment for common skin reactions such as dermatitis, hives and angioedema.

10-13 minutes

634 **An Overview of Allergy**
American College of Allergy & Immunology
800 E NW Highway 847-359-2800
Palatine, IL 60067-6580

Strengthen relationships with patients by providing them with the essential information they need.

635 **Sinusitis and Sinus Surgery**
Milner-Fenwick
2125 Greenspring Drive 410-252-1700
Timonium, MD 21093-3100 800-432-8433
Fax: 410-252-6316
e-mail: sales@milnerfenwick.com
www.milner-fenwick.com

Discusses sinusitis symptoms, causes, evaluation and treatments. Animation depicts how sinuses function and how irritants, allergies, colds or structural abnormalities cause sinus blockages. Also explains the role of medical therapy and irrigation in managing acute sinusitis.

14 minutes

Dolores McKee, Advertising Director

Web Sites

636 **American College of Allergy, Asthma**
www.acaai.org

The ACAAI is a professional association of 4900 allergists/immunologists. Established in 1942, the ACAA is dedicated to improving the quality of patient care in allergy and immunology through research, advocacy and professional and public education.

637 **American Lung Association**
www.lungusa.org

638 **Association of Birth Defect Children**
www.birthdefects.org

Offers a list of books on different kinds of allergy treatments.

639 **Asthma and Allergy Foundation of America**
www.aafa.org

Voluntary health organization dedicated to improving the quality of life for people with asthma and allergies and their caregivers through education, research and advocacy. The network of affiliated chapters and educational support groups.

640 **Food Allergy and Anaphylaxis Network**

www.foodallergy.org

Information to help families living with food allergies, and to increase public awareness about food allergies and anaphylaxis.

641 **Healing Well**

www.healingwell.com

An online health resource guide to medical news, chat, information and articles, newsgroups and message boards, books, disease-related web sites, medical directories, and more for patients, friends, and family coping with disabling diseases, disorders, or chronic illnesses.

642 **Health Finder**

www.healthfinder.gov

Searchable, carefully developed web site offering information on over 1000 topics. Developed by the US Department of Health and Human Services, the site can be used in both English and Spanish.

643 **Healthlink USA**

www.healthlinkusa.com

Health information concerning treatment, cures, prevention, diagnosis, risk factors, research, support groups, email lists, personal stories and much more. Updated regularly.

644 **Helios Health**

www.helioshealth.com

Online resource for your health information. Detailed information about specific health topics, access to expert advice from our Medical Advisory Board, and up-to-date health news.

645 **Immune Deficiency Foundation**

www.primaryimmune.org

Offers information and referral services to immune deficient patients and their families.

646 **MedicineNet**

www.medicinenet.com

An online resource for consumers providing easy-to-read, authoritative medical and health information.

647 **Medscape**

www.mywebmd.com

Medscape offers specialists, primary care physicians, and other health professionals the Web's most robust and integrated medical information and educational tools.

648 **WebMD**

www.webmd.com

Information on allergies, including articles and resources.

Description

649 **Alzheimer's Disease**

Alzheimer's disease is a degenerative neurologic disease that attacks the brain and impairs memory, thinking faculties and behavior. As the most common form of dementing illness, it afflicts 4 million adults and is twice as common in women as in men. It primarily affects older people.

In spite of diligent research, the cause of Alzheimer's disease is unknown. The disease runs in families in about 15 to 20 percent of cases, although the remainder may have some genetic component. There are multiple symptoms of Alzheimer's disease, the most pronounced being gradual memory loss. Other symptoms include the inability to perform routine tasks, loss of language skills, disorientation and personality changes. The diagnosis is largely based on an interview with the patient and family members and an examination of the patient, although brain imaging tests and blood tests may add helpful information.

The brain's cells communicate with each other through various chemicals called neurotransmitters. In Alzheimer's disease, levels of the neurotransmitter acetylcholine are decreased. Recently-released drugs which enhance the transmission of acetylcholine can cause at least limited improvement in memory during the early stages of Alzheimer's disease. A new drug, memantine, has been developed to slow the progression of advanced disease.

An extract of Ginkgo biloba may also slow memory loss and other symptoms. Some research suggests that certain activities that involve using the brain, such as reading and doing crossword puzzles, seem to reduce the risk. Because Alzheimer's disease severely affects both the patient and the family, proper planning, as well as medical and social programs tailored to the individual and to family members are essential. A well-structured and safe living environment is the best way to preserve the welfare and dignity of the person with Alzheimer's disease. See also *Aging*.

National Agencies & Associations

650 **Alzheimer Society of Canada**
20 Eglinton Avenue W 416-488-8772
Toronto, Ontario, M4R-1K8 800-618-8816
Fax: 416-488-3778
e-mail: info@alzheimer.ca
www.alzheimer.ca

Identified, develops and facilitates national priorities that enable its members to effectively alleviate the personal and social consequences of Alzheimer's disease and related disorders, promotes research and leads the search for a cure.

651 **Alzheimer's Disease Education and Referral Center**
PO Box 8250 301-495-3311
Silver Spring, MD 20907-8250 800-438-4380
Fax: 301-495-3334
e-mail: adear@alzheimers.org
www.nia.nih.gov/alzheimers

A service of the National Institute on Aging the center distributes information on Alzheimer's disease on current research activities and on services available to patients and family members. Offers a free list of publications available upon request.

652 **Alzheimer's Disease and Related Disorders Association**
International Conference on Alzheimer's Disease
225 N Michigan Avenue 312-335-5790
Chicago, IL 60601-7633 800-272-3900
Fax: 866-699-1246
TTY: 312-335-5886
e-mail: icad@alz.org
www.alz.org

Dedicated to research for the prevention cure and treatment of Alzheimer's disease and related disorders and to providing support and assistance to the afflicted patients and their families.
Harry Johns, President and CEO
Angela Geiger, Chief Strategy Officer

653 **Benjamin B Greenfield National Alzheimer's Center**
225 N Michigan Avenue 312-335-9602
Chicago, IL 60601-7633 800-272-3900
Fax: 866-699-1238
TTY: 312-335-8700
TDD: 312-335-8700
e-mail: greenfield@alz.org
www.alz.org

Located at the national Alzheimer's Association in Chicago this library offers a sizable collection of videos on a variety of subjects that may interest the Alzheimer's patient family members and caregivers.
Paul Attea, Chair
Harry Johns, President and CEO

654 **Interior Alzheimer Society**
#217, 1889 Springfield Road 250-762-3312
Kelowna, BC, V1Y-5V5 Fax: 250-762-3312
e-mail: ias@silk.net
www.alzheimer-society.ca

A registered, independent, charitable non-profit society that was founded in 1981. Mission is to support, educate, and advocate for all those affected by Alzheimer disease in the Central Okanagan area of British Columbia: the patients, caregivers, patients' families and the community.

655 **John Douglas French Alzheimer's Foundation**
11620 Wilshire Boulevard 310-445-4650
Los Angeles, CA 90025-1781 800-477-2243
Fax: 310-479-0516
e-mail: jdfaf@earthlink.net
www.jdfaf.org

Provides seed money for promising research including the cause cure and prevention of Alzheimer's disease. Also gives funding to scientists who might not otherwise be funded.
Michael M Minchin Jr, President
David Werthe, Director of Operations

State Agencies & Associations

Alabama

656 **Alzheimer's Association: North Alabama Chapter**
117A Longwood Drive SE 256-880-1575
Huntsville, AL 35801-4872 800-272-3900
Fax: 256-880-8596
e-mail: karen.motz@alz.org
www.alz.org/altn

Al Wiggins, Chair
Carolyn Rice, Vice Chair

657 **Alzheimer's Association: Southeast Alabama Chapter**
PO Box 609 334-677-6799
Dothan, AL 36302 800-272-3900
Fax: 334-671-3715
www.alz.org

Kay Jones, Executive Director

658 **Alzheimer's Association: Southwest Alabama Chapter**
PO Box 9272 334-660-5661
Mobile, AL 36691 800-272-3900
Fax: 334-660-5667
www.alz.org
Bunnie Sutton, Executive Director

Alaska

659 **Alzheimer's Disease Resource Agency of Alaska**
1750 Abbott Road 907-561-3313
Anchorage, AK 99507 800-478-1080
Fax: 907-561-3315
e-mail: dnobre@alzalaska.org
www.alzalaska.org
Dulce Nobre, Executive Director
Dawnia Clements, President

Arizona

660 **Alzheimer's Association: Desert Southwest Chapter**
1028 E McDowell Road 602-528-0545
Phoenix, AZ 85006-2622 800-272-3900
Fax: 602-528-0546
e-mail: deborah.schaus@alz.org
www.alzdsw.org
Serving the state of Arizona and Southern Nevada offices in Phoenix, Tucson, Sun City, Prescott and Las Vegas.
Deborah Schaus, Executive Director
Dawn Boeck, Development Assistant

661 **Alzheimer's Association: Northern Arizona**
225 Grove Avenue 928-771-9257
Prescott, AZ 86301-2911 800-272-3900
Fax: 520-771-9297
e-mail: donald.connell@alz.org
www.alz.org
Don Connell, Regional Director

662 **Alzheimer's Association: Northern Nevada**
225 Grove Avenue 928-771-9257
Prescott, AZ 86301 Fax: 520-771-9297
e-mail: meg.fenzi@alz.org
www.alz.org/dsw
Meg Fenzi, Regional Director
Gail Schimberg, Office Manager

663 **Alzheimer's Association: Southern Arizona**
5132 East Pima Street 520-322-6601
Tucson, AZ 85712 800-272-3900
Fax: 520-322-6739
e-mail: tormay.newman@alz.org
www.alzdsw.org
Tormay Newman, Director

664 **Alzheimer's Association: Southern Tier**
3003 S Country Club Road 520-322-6601
Tucson, AZ 85713 Fax: 520-322-6739
e-mail: felipe.jacome@alz.org
www.alz.org/dsw
Felipe Jacome, Regional Director
Debra Anderson, Programs Manager

Arkansas

665 **Alzheimer's Arkansas Programs and Services**
10411 W Markham 501-224-0021
Little Rock, AR 72205 800-689-6090
Fax: 501-227-6303
e-mail: phyllis.watkins@alzark.org
www.alzark.org
Phyllis Watkins, Executive Director
Priscilla Pittman, Program Coordinator

666 **Alzheimer's Association: Western Arkansas Chapter**
320 N Greenwood Avenue 479-783-2022
Fort Smith, AR 72901-3454 800-272-3900
Fax: 479-782-3185
e-mail: ark@alzokar.org
www.alzokar.org
Rebecca Freeman, Executive Director

California

667 **Alzheimer's Association: California Central Chapter: Ventura County Office**
1339 Del Norte Road 805-485-5597
Camarillo, CA 93010 800-272-3900
Fax: 805-485-4767
e-mail: nfeatherston@centralcoastalz.org
www.alz.org/cacentralcoast
The local chapter of the National Alzheimer's Association. The chapter stands by people with Alzheimer's disease, their families and professional caregivers through the following programs and services: a telephone helpline, support groups, respite grants.
Norma Featherston, Area Director
Carol Swinney, Office Manager

668 **Alzheimer's Association: Greater Sacramento**
530 Berant Drive 916-930-9080
Sacramento, CA 95814 800-272-3900
Fax: 916-930-9085
e-mail: webmaster@alznorcal.org
www.alznorcal.org
Mary Gillon MPA, Regional Director

669 **Alzheimer's Association: Greater North Valley Chapter**
2105 Forest Avenue 530-895-9661
Chico, CA 95928-3148 800-272-3900
Fax: 530-872-7470
e-mail: info@alznorcal.org
www.alz.org/norcal
Herb Williams, President
Eduardo Salaz, Vice President

670 **Alzheimer's Association: Los Angeles Chapter**
133 N Sunol Drive 323-881-0574
Los Angeles, CA 90063-5017 800-272-3900
Fax: 323-938-1036
www.alz.org/californiasouthland
Earl Greinetz, President
Gary L Ferrell, Secretary/Treasurer

671 **Alzheimer's Association: Monterey County Chapter**
182 El Dorado Street 831-647-9890
Monterey, CA 93940-5337 800-272-3900
Fax: 831-655-9241
e-mail: info@alznorcal.org
www.alz.org/norcal
Herb Williams, President
Eduardo Salaz, Vice President

672 **Alzheimer's Association: North Bay Chapter**
4340 Redwood Highway 415-472-4340
San Rafael, CA 94903 800-272-3900
Fax: 415-472-4350
e-mail: info@alznorcal.org
www.alz.org/norcal
Provides a continuum of services for Alzheimer's families, education and referral in Marin, Sonoma and Napa counties. To provide leadership and to eliminate Alzheimer's disease through the advancement of research while enhancing care and support services.
Herb Williams, President
Eduardo Salaz, Vice President

673 **Alzheimer's Association: Orange County Chapter**
17771 Cowan 949-955-9000
Irvine, CA 92614 800-272-3900
Fax: 949-757-3700
e-mail: helpoc@alz.org
www.alz.org/oc
Dedicated to providing services, education and advocacy for individuals, families and the community affected by Alzheimer's disease and related memory disorders. Services include: 24/7

helpline, support groups, family orientation program and care managers.
Norma Castellano, Program Specialist
Bobbie Babbage, Family Services Coordinator

674 **Alzheimer's Association: Riverside/San Bernardino Counties Chapter**
5900 Wilshire Boulevard 323-938-3379
Los Angeles, CA 90036 800-272-3900
Fax: 323-938-1036
e-mail: la.webmaster@alz.org
www.alz.org/californiasouthland
Helpline, support groups, information and education for caregivers and community.
400 Members
Earl Greinetz, President
Gary L Ferrell, Secretary/Treasurer

675 **Alzheimer's Association: San Diego Chapter**
4950 Murphy Canyon Road 858-492-4400
San Diego, CA 92123 800-272-3900
Fax: 858-492-4406
e-mail: lisa.bruner@sanalz.org
adrdsd.convio.net
Lisa Bruner, Executive Director
Anna King, Director of Programs

676 **Alzheimer's Association: San Francisco Bay Area Chapter**
1060 La Avenida 650-962-8111
Mountain View, CA 94043 800-272-3900
Fax: 650-962-9644
e-mail: info@alznorcal.org
www.alz.org/norcal
Herb Williams, President
Eduardo Salaz, Vice President

677 **Alzheimer's Association: Santa Barbara Cen tral Coast Chapter**
1528 Chapala Street 805-892-4259
Santa Barbara, CA 93101-8820 800-272-3900
Fax: 805-892-4250
e-mail: rspiegel@centralcoastalz.org
www.alz.org/cacentralcoast
The Alzheimer's Association California Central Coast Chapter serves families caring for people with Alzheimer's disease and related dementia throughout San Luis Obispo, Santa Barbara and Ventura Counties, offering a variety of educational and supportive programs.
Rhonda Spiegel, Executive Director
Carrie Wanek, Director of Finance and Operations

678 **Alzheimer's Association: Santa Cruz County Chapter**
1777-A Capitola Road 831-464-9982
Santa Cruz, CA 95062 800-272-3900
Fax: 831-464-8930
e-mail: info@alznorcal.org
www.alz.org/norcal
Herb Williams, President
Eduardo Salaz, Vice President

Colorado

679 **Alzheimer's Association: Greater Grand Junction Area Chapter**
2232 N 7th Street 970-256-1274
Grand Junction, CO 81501 800-272-3900
Fax: 970-256-0569
www.alz.org/co
Linda Mitchell, President/CEO
Laurie Frasier, Regional Director

680 **Alzheimer's Association: Rocky Mountain Chapter**
455 Sherman Street 303-813-1669
Denver, CO 80203 800-272-3900
Fax: 303-813-1670
www.alz.org/co
Linda Mitchell, President/CEO
Inge Holmes, Vice President of Administration

681 **American Homes for the Aging: Western**
5010 Aspen Drive 303-795-5465
Littleton, CO 80123 Fax: 303-794-0487
Part of the national association representing retirement communities, nursing homes and community services for the elderly.

Connecticut

682 **Alzheimer's Association: Connecticut Chapter**
96 Oak Street 860-956-9560
Hartford, CT 06106 800-356-5502
Fax: 860-956-9590
www.alzct.org
Works with all individuals and family members affected by Alzheimer's disease and related disorders; ensures humane systems of care and support and promotes research efforts to treat and cure Alzheimer's disease.
Christopher Rupp, Chairman
Daniel P Finke, Treasurer

683 **Alzheimer's Association: South Central Connecticut Chapter**
2911 Dixwell Avenue 203-230-1777
Hamden, CT 06518 800-356-5502
Fax: 203-230-1712
www.alz.org

Delaware

684 **Alzheimer's Association: Delaware Chapter**
240 N James Street 302-633-4420
Newport, DE 19804 800-272-3900
Fax: 302-633-4494
e-mail: Wendy.Campbell@alz.org
www.alz.org/desjsepa
Wendy L Campbell, President
Theresa Haenn, Vice President Development

Florida

685 **Alzheimer's Association: Broward County Chapter**
201 E Sample Road 800-861-7826
Deerfield Beach, FL 33407 800-272-3900
Fax: 954-786-1538
e-mail: barbara.grasch@alz.org
www.alz.org/seflorida
Barbara Grasch, Director of Program Services
Ellen Brown, CEO

686 **Alzheimer's Association: East Central Florida Chapter**
1250 South Harbor City Boulevard 407-729-8536
Melbourne, FL 32901 Fax: 407-729-8044
www.alz.org

687 **Alzheimer's Association: Florida Gulf Coast Chapter**
9365 US Highway 19 N 727-578-2558
Pinellas Park, FL 33782 800-772-8672
Fax: 727-578-2286
e-mail: milnel@alzflgulf.org
www.alz.org/FLGulfCoast
Provides information and services to families and professionals dealing with memory related disorders.
Gloria JT Smith, President/CEO
Paul Anderson, Vice President Finance

688 **Alzheimer's Association: Greater Miami Chapter**
1100 NW 95th Street 305-891-6228
Miami, FL 33150 800-861-7826
Fax: 305-835-2449
e-mail: reni.rizzo@alz.org
www.alz.org/seflorida
Reni Rizzo, Community Education Coordinator
Ellen Brown, CEO

689 **Alzheimer's Association: Greater Orlando Area Chapter**
988 Woodcock Road 407-228-4299
Orlando, FL 32803 800-272-3900
Fax: 407-228-4201
e-mail: info@alzflorida.org
www.alz.org/cnfl
Stu Gaines, Chair
Tish Sheesley, CEO

690 **Alzheimer's Association: Greater Palm Beach Area Chapter**
600 N Congress Avenue 561-478-3120
Delray Beach, FL 33445 800-861-7826
Fax: 561-278-4910
www.alz.org

691 **Alzheimer's Association: Northeast Florida**
2123 Mango Place 904-398-5193
Jacksonville, FL 32207 800-272-3900
Fax: 904-398-2892
www.alzorlando.org

692 **Alzheimer's Association: Northern Central Florida Chapter**
2411 NW 41st Street 352-372-6266
Gainesville, FL 32606 800-272-3900
Fax: 352-372-2038
e-mail: info@alzflorida.org
www.alz.org/cnfl

Stu Gaines, Chair
Tish Sheesley, CEO

693 **Alzheimer's Association: Northwest Florida Chapter**
119 Hollywood Boulevard 850-302-0581
Ft. Walton Beach, FL 32548 800-302-0581
Fax: 850-302-0583
www.alz.org

694 **Alzheimer's Association: Southwest Florida Chapter**
22107 Elmira Boulevard 941-235-7470
Port Charlotte, FL 33949 800-772-8672
Fax: 941-235-7473
www.alz.org

695 **Alzheimer's Association: Tampa Bay Chapter**
9365 US Highway 19 N 727-578-2558
Pinellas Park, FL 33782 800-772-8672
Fax: 941-380-5701
e-mail: milnel@alzflgulf.org
www.alz.org/FLGulfCoast

Gloria JT Smith, President/CEO
Paul Anderson, Vice President Finance

696 **Alzheimer's Association: Volusia/Flagler Branch**
111 N Frederick Avenue 386-238-0066
Daytona Beach, FL 32114-5126 Fax: 386-238-8293
www.alz.org

697 **Alzheimer's Association: West Central Florida Chapter**
PO Box 2070 813-848-8888
New Port Richey, FL 34656-2070 800-841-6669
Fax: 813-849-6124
www.alz.org

Georgia

698 **Alzheimer's Association: Atlanta Chapter**
1925 Century Boulevard 404-728-1181
Atlanta, GA 30345-4021 800-272-3900
Fax: 404-636-9768
e-mail: kim.franklin@alz.org
www.alz.org/georgia

Bennett Watts, Chair
Bruce Flechter, Treasurer

699 **Alzheimer's Association: Augusta Chapter**
1899 Central Avenue 706-731-9060
Augusta, GA 30904-5755 800-272-3900
Fax: 706-731-9099
e-mail: kim.franklin@alz.org
www.alz.org/georgia

Bennett Watts, Chair
Bruce Flechter, Treasurer

700 **Alzheimer's Association: Central Georgia Chapter**
277 Martin Luther King Jr Boulevard 478-746-7050
Macon, GA 31201-3498 800-272-3900
Fax: 478-746-6679
e-mail: kim.franklin@alz.org
www.alz.org/georgia

Bennett Watts, Chair
Bruce Flechter, Treasurer

701 **Alzheimer's Association: Greater Columbus Chapter**
5900 River Road 706-327-6838
Columbus, GA 31904-0185 800-272-3900
Fax: 706-494-0533
e-mail: kim.franklin@alz.org
www.alz.org/georgia

Bennett Watts, Chair
Bruce Flechter, Treasurer

702 **Alzheimer's Association: Greater Georgia Chapter**
1925 Century Boulevard 404-728-1181
Atlanta, GA 30345-4021 800-272-3900
Fax: 404-636-9768
e-mail: kim.franklin@alz.org
www.alz.org/georgia

Bennett Watts, Chair
Bruce Flechter, Treasurer

703 **Alzheimer's Association: Southeast Georgia Chapter**
201 Television Circle 912-920-2231
Savannah, GA 31412 800-272-3900
Fax: 912-921-7960
www.alzga.org

704 **Alzheimer's Association: Southwest Georgia Chapter**
1512-1 Gillionville Road 229-888-7676
Albany, GA 31707 Fax: 229-888-2620
www.alzga.org

Maggie Keenan, Office Volunteer
Jenny House, Director Programs and Development

Hawaii

705 **Alzheimer's Association: Honolulu Chapter**
1050 Ala Moana Boulevard 808-591-2771
Honolulu, HI 96814 800-272-3900
Fax: 808-591-9071
e-mail: info@alzhi.org
www.alz.org/hawaii

Elizabeth Stevenson, Executive Director/CEO
Chris Shirai, Chairman

706 **Alzheimer's Association: West Hawaii Chapter**
PO Box 390247 808-322-4141
Kailua Kona, HI 96739-0247 Fax: 808-322-0008
www.alz.org

Idaho

707 **Alzheimer's Association: Greater Idaho Chapter**
1111 S Orchard 208-384-1788
Boise, ID 83705-2878 800-272-3900
Fax: 208-385-7191
e-mail: suzette.albers-tunnell@alz.org
www.alz.org/idaho

Suzette Albers-Tunne, Executive Director

708 **Alzheimer's Association: Northern Idaho Chapter**
2003 Lincoln Way 208-666-2996
Coeur D Alene, ID 83814 800-272-3900
Fax: 509-473-3389
e-mail: pjchristo@alz.org
www.alz.org/inlandnorthwest

PJ Christo, Outreach Coordinator
Joel Loiacono, Executive Director

Illinois

709 **Alzheimer's Association: Central Illinois Chapter**
606 W Glen Avenue 309-681-1100
Peoria, IL 61614-4831 800-272-3900
Fax: 309-681-1101
e-mail: nikki.vulgaris@alz.org
www.alz.org/illinoiscentral

Nikki Vulgaris, Executive Director
Brett Tilly, President

710 **Alzheimer's Association: East Central Illinois Chapter**
307 West University Avenue 217-351-1726
Champaign, IL 61820-7337 888-686-1726
Fax: 217-351-2161
www.alz.org
Provides information, support, and referral services to families and individuals facing Alzheimer's disease. Includes newsletter, support groups, and education.

711 **Alzheimer's Association: Four Rivers Chapter**
401 N Wall Street 815-936-0464
Kankakee, IL 60901 800-332-4495
Fax: 815-936-9363
www.alz.org

712 **Alzheimer's Association: Greater Illinois Chapter**
4709 Golf Road 847-933-2413
Skokie, IL 60076-1260 800-272-3900
Fax: 847-933-2417
e-mail: info@alz.org
www.alzchi.org

713 **Alzheimer's Association: Greater Illinois Chapter: Carbondale Office**
402 E Plaza Drive 618-985-1095
Carterville, IL 62918-1429 800-272-3900
Fax: 618-457-7830
e-mail: GI.Chapter@alz.org
www.alz.org/illinois
Jill Schoenborn, Coordinator Outreach & Development

714 **Alzheimer's Association: Land of Lincoln Chapter**
2921 Greenbriar Drive 217-726-5184
Springfield, IL 62704-4833 800-272-3900
Fax: 217-726-5185
e-mail: GI.Chapter@alz.org
www.alz.org/illinois
Jane Field, Office Manager
James Dearing, Senior Program Manager

715 **American Homes for the Aging: Midwest Regional Office**
911 N Elm Street 630-323-6755
Hinsdale, IL 60521-3641 Fax: 630-325-0749
Regional office of the AAHA, a national professional association of nonprofit nursing homes, retirement communities and homes for the aging.

Indiana

716 **Alzheimer's Association: Central Indiana**
9135 N Meridian Street 317-575-9620
Indianapolis, IN 46260-1816 800-272-3900
Fax: 317-582-0669
e-mail: Heather.Hershberger@alz.org
www.alzindiana.org
Heather Allen Hershberger, Executive Director
Wanda Lew, Director Finance and Operations

717 **Alzheimer's Association: Central Indiana Chapter-Columbus Office**
50 E 91st Street 317-575-9620
Indianapolis, IN 46240-0547 800-272-3900
Fax: 812-376-0541
e-mail: Heather.Hershberger@alz.org
www.alz.org/indiana
Helpline, support groups, caregiver education, family care planning, safe return.
newsletter
Heather Alle Hershberger, Executive Director
Sarah Ferguson, Director of Development

718 **Alzheimer's Association: Central Virginia**
50 E 91st Street 317-575-9620
Indianapolis, IN 46240 Fax: 317-582-0669
e-mail: Heather.Hershberger@alz.org
www.alz.org/indiana
Heather Alle Hershberger, Executive Director
Wanda Lew, Director Finance and Operations

719 **Alzheimer's Association: Northern Indiana Chapter**
922 E Colfax Avenue 219-232-4121
S Bend, IN 46617-3112 888-303-0180
Fax: 219-232-4235
e-mail: AlzServicesNI@sbcglobal.net
www.alz-nic.org

Iowa

720 **Alzheimer's Association: Big Sioux Chapter**
420 Chambers Street 712-279-5802
Sioux City, IA 51101-3716 800-272-3900
Fax: 712-277-8076
e-mail: kim.mccormick@alz.org
www.alz.org/siouxland
Kim McCormick, Executive Director
Darla Vander Plaats, Vice President of Finance/Operations

721 **Alzheimer's Association: East Central Iowa Chapter**
1570 42nd Street NE 319-294-9699
Cedar Rapids, IA 52402 800-272-3900
Fax: 319-294-0068
e-mail: kelly.hauer@alz.org
www.alz.org/eci
Kelly Hauer, Executive Director
Tracey Robertson, Program Education & Outreach Coordinator

722 **Alzheimer's Association: Greater Iowa Chapter**
1730 28th Street 515-440-2722
W Des Moines, IA 50266 800-272-3900
Fax: 515-440-6385
e-mail: Carol.Sipfle@alz.org
www.alz.org/greateriowa
Carol Sipfle, Executive Director
Holly Bradford, Finance Director

723 **Alzheimer's Association: Heart of Iowa Chapter**
118 Hayward Avenue 515-292-4109
Ames, IA 50014-7259 800-407-5840
Fax: 515-292-0125
www.alz.org

724 **Greater Iowa Chapter Alzheimer's Association Quadcity Office**
736 Federal Street 563-324-1022
Davenport, IA 52803-5750 800-272-3900
Fax: 563-324-6267
e-mail: Jerry.Schroeder@alz.org
www.alz.org/greateriowa
Jerry Schroeder, Program Specialist
Julie Seier, Community Relations Coordinator

Kansas

725 **Alzheimer's Association: Heart of America Chapter**
3846 W 75th Street 913-831-3888
Prairie Village, KS 66208-4126 800-272-3900
Fax: 913-831-1916
e-mail: kerry.mees@alz.org
www.alz.org/kansascity
Debra R Brook, Executive Director
Michelle Niedens, Education Director

726 **Alzheimer's Association: Sunflower Chapter**
347 S Laura 316-267-7333
Wichita, KS 67211-4109 800-272-3900
Fax: 316-267-6369
e-mail: marsha.hills@alz.org
www.alz.org/centralandwesternkansas
Marsha Hills, Executive Director
Kathy Sikes, Program Director

727 **Alzheimer's Association: Topeka Regional Office, Heart of America Chapter**
4125 SW Gage Center Drive 785-271-1844
Topeka, KS 66604-1427 800-272-3900
Fax: 785-271-1804
e-mail: cindy.miller@alz.org
www.alz.org/kansascity
Part of the national Alzheimer's Association, serving 16 counties in northeast Kansas representing approximately 10 500 Alzhei-

mer's families. Basic services include family and professional support groups, information and referral, and caregiver's relief programs.
Debra R Brook, Executive Director
Cindy Miller, Outreach Coordinator

Kentucky

728 Alzheimer's Association: Lexington/ Bluegrass Chapter
465 E High Street 859-266-5283
Lexington, KY 40507 800-272-3900
Fax: 859-268-4764
e-mail: infoky-in@alz.org
www.alz.org/kyin
Debbie Lacy Goodman, VP Awareness & Community Relations
Tonya Cox, VP Programs & Education

729 Alzheimer's Association: Louisville Chapter
6100 Dutchmans Lane 502-451-4266
Louisville, KY 40205 Fax: 502-456-2701
e-mail: infoky-in@alz.org
www.alz.org/kyin
Teri Shirk, Chapter President & CEO
Ellen Kershaw, VP Public Policy

Louisiana

730 Alzheimer's Association: Northeast/Central Louisiana Chapter
2407 Ferrand Street 318-322-2828
Monroe, LA 71201 800-272-3900
Fax: 318-998-7360
www.alz.org

731 Alzheimer's Association: Greater New Orleans Chapter
DePaul Hospital
1040 Calhoun Street 504-895-6223
New Orleans, LA 70118-5999 800-272-3900
Fax: 504-895-0493

732 Alzheimer's Services of the Capital Area
3772 N Boulevard 225-334-7494
Baton Rouge, LA 70806 800-548-1211
Fax: 225-387-3664
e-mail: info@alzbr.org
www.alzbr.org
The mission of Alzheimer's Services of the Capital Area is to provide education and support services to memory impaired individuals as well as caregivers and professionals; and to enhance community awareness of Alzheimer's disease and related disorders.

Maine

733 Alzheimer's Association: Maine Chapter
170 US Route 1 207-772-0115
Falmouth, ME 04105-2419 800-272-3900
Fax: 207-781-3312
e-mail: laurie.trenholm@alz.org
www.alz.org/maine
Joy Heptner, Executive Director
Liz Weaver, Program Director

734 Maine Alzheimer's Care Center
154 Dresden Avenue 207-626-1770
Gardiner, ME 04345

Maryland

735 Alzheimer's Association: Central Maryland Chapter
1850 York Road 410-561-9099
Timonium, MD 21093-5122 800-272-3900
Fax: 410-561-3433
e-mail: info.maryland@alz.org
www.alz.org/maryland
Cass Naugle, Executive Director
Teri Bennett, Helpline Coordinator

736 Alzheimer's Association: Eastern Shore Chapter
209C Milford Street 410-543-1163
Salisbury, MD 21804 800-272-3900
Fax: 410-546-0184
e-mail: info.maryland@alz.org
www.alz.org/maryland
Cass Naugle, Executive Director
Elizabeth Marshall, Services Coordinator

737 Alzheimer's Association: Greater Washington DC Chapter
2524 Pensylvania Avenue Southeast 202-483-4258
Washington, DC 20020 Fax: 202-483-4164
www.alzheimersdc-md.org
Helpline-telephone referral support groups, cargiver education, respite services. We have three offices serving DC and surrounding Maryland counties.

738 Alzheimer's Association: Western Maryland Chapter
108 Byte Drive 301-696-0315
Frederick, MD 21702 800-272-3900
Fax: 301-696-9061
e-mail: info.maryland@alz.org
www.alz.org/maryland
To eliminate Alzheimer's disease through the advancement of research and to enhance care and support for individuals their families and caregivers.
Cathy Hanson, Program Coordinator
Deborah Bauer, Education Coordinator

Massachusetts

739 Alzheimer's Association: Massachusetts Chapter
311 Arsenal Street 617-868-6718
Watertown, MA 02472 800-272-3900
Fax: 617-868-6720
www.alz.org/manh
Nonprofit, national, voluntary health organization dedicated to Alzheimer research and care. Provides 24 hour helpline, support groups, a wanderers prevention program early stage patient programs, family educators, professional training, and advocacy.
James Wessle MBA, President & CEO
Betsy Fitzgerald-Cam, Vice President Communications

740 Alzheimer's Association: Western Regional Office: Massachusetts Chapter
264 Cottage Street 413-787-1113
Springfield, MA 01104 800-272-3900
Fax: 413-787-1109
www.alz.org/manh
Nonprofit organization serving family and professional caregivers in seven counties in southwest Michigan. Provides information on Alzheimer's and other diseases, educational programs, resource libraries. Train-the-trainer agency referral, autopsy liaison, and other services.
Marcia McKen Med, Manager
Annie Clattenburg, Coordinator Administrative Services

741 Alzheimer's Services of Cape Cod and the Islands
473 S Street W 508-880-0055
Raynham, MA 02767 800-272-3900
Fax: 508-880-0056
www.alz.org/manh
Pam McCormack, Manager

Michigan

742 Alzheimer's Association: East Central Michigan Chapter
G-3287 Beecher Road 810-720-2791
Flint, MI 48503 800-337-3827
Fax: 810-720-3040
www.alzgmc.org

743 Alzheimer's Association: Greater Michigan Chapter
20300 Civic Center Drive 248-351-0280
Southfield, MI 48037 Fax: 248-351-0417
www.alzgmc.org
A national network of chapters, is the largest national voluntary health organization committed to finding a cure for Alzheimer's and helping those affected by the disease. Provides a wide range of

services and programs for Alzheimers and other dementia patients for their families and for the general public.

744 **Alzheimer's Association: Greater Michigan Chapter: Upper Peninsula Region**
710 Chippewa Square
Marquette, MI 49855-4521
906-228-3910
800-272-3900
Fax: 906-228-2455
TTY: 877-204-6924
www.alz.org/gmc
Pamela Parkkila, Director

745 **Alzheimer's Association: Michigan Great Lakes Chapter: West Shore Region**
549 Seminole Road
Muskegon, MI 49444-5546
231-780-1922
800-272-3900
Fax: 231-780-1494
e-mail: Barb.Betts@alz.org
www.alz.org/mglc
Providing caregiver support groups a helpline informational materials community education and a quarterly newsletter.
Barb Betts, Program Coordinator
Valerie Hanson, Regional Coordinator

746 **Alzheimer's Association: Mid-Michigan Chapter**
4604 N Saginaw Road
Midland, MI 48640
989-839-9910
800-272-3900
Fax: 989-839-5910
TTY: 877-204-6924
www.alz.org/gmc
Dawn Spicer, Director

747 **Alzheimer's Association: Northeast Michigan Chapter**
100 Woods Circle Drive
Alpena, MI 49707
989-356-4087
800-272-3900
Fax: 989-354-0855
www.alzgmc.org

748 **Alzheimer's Association: Northwest Michigan Chapter**
1040 Walnut Street
Traverse City, MI 49686
231-929-3804
800-272-3900
Fax: 231-929-2766
www.alz.nwmi.org

Minnesota

749 **Alzheimer's Association: Minnesota/Dakotas**
4550 W 77th Street
Minneapolis, MN 55435
952-830-0512
800-272-3900
Fax: 952-830-0513
e-mail: mary.birchard@alz.org
www.alz.org/mnnd
Mary Birchard, Executive Director
Michelle Barclay, Vice President Program Services

Mississippi

750 **Alzheimer's Association: Mississippi Chapter**
1900 Dunbarton Drive
Jackson, MS 39216
601-987-0020
800-272-3900
Fax: 601-987-9020
e-mail: info@msalz.org
www.alz.org/ms
Barb Dobrosky, Program Director
Patty Dunn, Director of Administration

751 **Alzheimer's Foundation of the South: Mississippi Division**
PO Box 2394
Gulfport, MS 39503
228-867-6251
800-950-6251
Fax: 228-864-8843
e-mail: alzms@cs.com
www.alzfoundation.com
Rosemary Hudgins, Executive Director

Missouri

752 **Alzheimer's Association: Mid-Missouri Chapter**
2400 Bluff Creek Drive
Columbia, MO 65201
573-443-8665
800-272-3900
Fax: 573-499-9701
e-mail: midmoinfo@alz.org
www.alz.org/mid-missouri
Linda Newkirk, Executive Director
Joetta Coen, Director of Programs

753 **Alzheimer's Association: Northwest Missouri-Chapter**
PO Box 1241
St. Joseph, MO 64502-1241
816-364-4467
800-272-3900
Fax: 816-271-7068
www.alz-heartofamerica.org

754 **Alzheimer's Association: Southwest Missouri Chapter**
1500 S Glenstone
Springfield, MO 65804
417-886-2199
800-272-3900
Fax: 417-886-0337
e-mail: rebecca.argilagos@alz.org
www.alz-swmo.org
Rebecca Argilagos, President/CEO
Annette West, Development Director

755 **Alzheimer's Association: St. Louis Chapter**
9370 Olive Boulevard
Saint Louis, MO 63132-3214
314-432-3422
800-272-3900
Fax: 314-432-3824
e-mail: elpline@alzstl.org
www.alz.org/stl
Joan D'Ambrose, President
Jan Kraemer, Chair

Montana

756 **Alzheimer's Association: Greater Billings Area Chapter**
3010 11th Avenue N
Billings, MT 59101
406-252-3053
800-272-3900
Fax: 406-252-2933
e-mail: alzbelser@bresnan.net
www.alz.org/montana
Kelly Donovan, President
Cindy Stevick, Vice President

Nebraska

757 **Alzheimer's Association: Lincoln/Greater Nebraska Chapter**
5601 S 27th Street
Lincoln, NE 68512
402-420-2540
800-272-3900
Fax: 402-420-2541
e-mail: karen.noel@alz.org
alz.org/greatplains
Karen Noel, President/CEO
Gail McNair, Development Director

758 **Alzheimer's Association: Omaha/Eastern Nebraska Chapter**
1941 S 42nd Street
Omaha, NE 68105-2167
402-502-4301
800-272-3900
Fax: 402-502-7001
www.alz.org/midlands
Duane Gross, President and CEO
Clayton Freeman, Program Director

Nevada

759 **Alzheimer's Association: Northern Nevada Chapter**
1301 Cordone Avenue
Reno, NV 89502-6362
775-786-8061
800-272-3900
Fax: 775-786-1920
e-mail: info@alznorcal.org
www.alz.org/norcal
Herb Williams, President
Eduardo Salaz, Vice President

760 **Alzheimer's Association: Southern Nevada Chapter**
5190 S Valley View Boulevard 702-248-2770
Las Vegas, NV 89118-6062 800-272-3900
Fax: 702-248-2771
e-mail: luis.carrillo@alz.org
www.alz.org/dsw

Luis Carrillo, Regional Director
Christine Terry, Program Manager

New Hampshire

761 **Alzheimer's Association of Vermont and New Hampshire**
10 Ferry Street 603-226-5868
Concord, NH 03301-5004 800-536-8864
Fax: 603-225-8126
www.alzvtnh.org

New Jersey

762 **Alzheimer's Association: Greater New Jersey Chapter**
400 Morris Avenue 973-586-4308
Denville, NJ 07854 800-883-1180
Fax: 973-586-4342
www.alznj.org

Provides programs and services to individuals with Alzheimer's disease, thier families and caregivers, including education and training, support groups, a toll free telephone helpline and respite assistance.

763 **Alzheimer's Association: South Jersey Chapter**
3 Eves Drive 856-797-1212
Marlton, NJ 08053 800-272-3900
Fax: 609-784-8486
e-mail: Wendy.Campbell@alz.org
www.alz.org/desjsepa

Wendy L Campbell, President & CEO
Theresa Haenn, Vice President Development

New Mexico

764 **Alzheimer's Association: New Mexico Chapter**
9500 Montgomery Boulevard NE 505-266-4473
Albuquerque, NM 87111 800-272-3900
Fax: 505-266-0108
www.alz.org/newmexico

Greg Gillogly, President
John Attwood, Vice President

New York

765 **Alzheimer's Association: Sullivan/Delaware Chapter**
PO Box 911
Monticello, NY 12701 941-794-3774
www.alz.org

766 **Alzheimer's Association: Central New York Chapter**
441 W Kirkpatrick Street 315-472-4201
Syracuse, NY 13204-1361 800-272-3900
Fax: 315-472-4206
e-mail: alzcny@alzcny.org
www.alz.org/centralnewyork

Larry Malfitano, President
Christina Hasemann, Vice President

767 **Alzheimer's Association: Hudson Valley/ Rockland/Westchester NY Chapter**
2 Jefferson Plaza 845-471-2655
Poughkeepsie, NY 12601-4027 800-872-0994
Fax: 845-471-8960
e-mail: info@alzhudsonvalley.org
www.alz.org/hudsonvalley

Elaine Sproat, President & CEO
Meg Boyce, Director of Programs & Services

768 **Alzheimer's Association: Long Island Chapter**
3281 Veterans Memorial Highway 631-580-5100
Ronkonkoma, NY 11779-3521 800-272-3900
Fax: 631-580-3100
e-mail: Info@alzheimersli.org
alz.org/longisland

Voluntary health agency that provides care and consultation, information and referral, education, national safe return program and support groups to individuals with Alzheimer's, their families and/or caregivers.
Mary Ann Malack-Ragona, Executive Director/CEO
Linda Cody, Director of Development

769 **Alzheimer's Association: New York City Chapter**
360 Lexington Avenue 646-744-2900
New York, NY 10017 800-272-3900
Fax: 212-490-6037
e-mail: helpline@alznyc.org
www.alznyc.org

Lou-Ellen Barkan, President/CEO
Jed A Levine, Executive Vice President

770 **Alzheimer's Association: Northeastern New York Chapter**
Washington Avenue Extension 518-867-4999
Albany, NY 12205-2083 800-272-3900
Fax: 518-438-2219
e-mail: infoneny@alz.org
www.alz.org/northeasternny

Regional affiliate of national association. Works to educate and support families, while raising funds in support of research.
Paul A Wajda, Chair
Warren E Garling, Vice Chair

771 **Alzheimer's Association: Putnam County Chapter**
Robin Hill Corporate Park
15 Mount Ebo Road S
Brewster, NY 10509-2164 845-278-0343
www.alz.org/hudsonvalley

Stuart Greif, Program Development Specialist

772 **Alzheimer's Association: Rochester Chapter**
435 E Henrietta Road 585-760-5400
Rochester, NY 14620 800-272-3900
Fax: 585-760-5401
www.alz.org/rochesterny

Teresa A Galbier, President/CEO
Stewart C Putnam, Chair

773 **Alzheimer's Association: Southern Tier Chapter**
401 Hayes Avenue 607-785-7852
Endicott, NY 13760-5421 800-272-3900
Fax: 607-785-4004
e-mail: alzcny@alzcny.org
www.alz.org/centralnewyork

L Jane Hudreck, Regional Director

774 **Alzheimer's Association: Western New York Chapter**
2805 Wehrle Drive 716-626-0600
Williamsville, NY 14421 800-272-3900
Fax: 717-626-2255
www.alz.org/wny

David Cascio, President
Linda Sabo, Executive Director

775 **Alzheimer's Foundation of Staten Island**
789 Post Avenue 718-667-7110
Staten Island, NY 10310-6427 877-574-7068
Fax: 718-667-8431
e-mail: info@sialzheimers.org
www.sialzheimers.org

Not-for-profit health and human services organization, serving people with Alzheimer's disease and related dementias.
Gladys Schweiger, Executive Director
Nicholas Lettiere, President

North Carolina

776 **Alzheimer's Association: Eastern North Carolina Chapter**
400 Oberlin Road 919-832-3732
Raleigh, NC 27605-1351 800-228-8738
Fax: 919-832-7989
e-mail: awatkins@alznc.org
www.alznc.org

Dedicated to providing program services education for patients, families and professional caregivers, advocacy and research.
Alice Watkins, Executive Director
Rita Bhan, Developmental Director

777 **Alzheimer's Association: Western Carolina Chapter**
3800 Shamrock Drive 704-532-7392
Charlotte, NC 28215 800-272-3900
Fax: 704-532-5421
e-mail: infonc@alz.org
alz.org/northcarolina
A nonprofit voluntary organization dedicated to improving the quality of life for those with Alzheimer's and their families through a broad range of programs, including patient and family services, education, advocacy and support of research through national programs.
Beth Croom MA, Director of Programs/Education
Teresa Hoover, Program Associate/Helpline Coordinator

778 **Alzheimer's Association: Western North Carolina Chapter**
31 College Place 828-254-7363
Asheville, NC 28801-1066 800-272-3900
Fax: 828-255-0948
e-mail: infonc@alz.org
www.alz.org/northcarolina
Larry Reeves, Area Program Manager
Heidi Kimsey, Program Associate

North Dakota

779 **Alzheimer's Association: Fargo/Moorhead Regional Center**
4357 13th Avenue SW 701-277-9757
Fargo, ND 58103 800-272-3900
Fax: 701-277-9785
e-mail: gretchen.dobervich@alz.org
www.alz.org/mnnd
Gretchen Dobervich, Regional Center Director
Paulette Orth, Administrative Assistant

Ohio

780 **Alzheimer's Association: Canton Chapter**
4815 Munson Street NW 330-966-7343
Canton, OH 44718 800-272-3900
Fax: 330-996-7757
e-mail: geoachl@alz.org
www.alz.org/akroncantonyoungt
Pam Schuellerman, Executive Director
Andy Junn, Development Director

781 **Alzheimer's Association: Central Ohio Chapter**
3380 Tremont Road 614-457-6003
Columbus, OH 43221-2112 800-272-3900
Fax: 614-457-6634
e-mail: helplinecentralohio@alz.org
www.alz.org/centralohio
Michelle Chippas, Executive Director
Gregory Winslow, Director of Development

782 **Alzheimer's Association: Clark/Champaign, Miami Valley Chapter**
3797 Summit Glen Drive 937-291-3332
Dayton, OH 45449-2620 800-272-3900
Fax: 937-323-9259
e-mail: judy.turner@alz.org
www.alz.org/dayton
Judy Turner, Executive Director
Teresa Thomas, Development Director

783 **Alzheimer's Association: Cleveland Area Chapter**
23215 Commerce Park Drive 216-721-8457
Beachwood, OH 44122-1013 800-272-3900
Fax: 216-831-8585
e-mail: helpline@alzclv.org
www.alz.org/cleveland
Nancy B Udelson, Executive Director
Christine B Stevens, President

784 **Alzheimer's Association: Greater Cincinnati Chapter**
644 Linn Street 513-721-4284
Cincinnati, OH 45203-1742 800-272-3900
Fax: 513-345-8446
e-mail: sue.wilke@alz.org
www.alz.org/grtrcinc
Committed to support education, advocacy and research on behalf of those affected by Alzheimer's disease.
Sue Wilke, Executive Director
Clarissa Rentz, MSN, APRN, Program Director

785 **Alzheimer's Association: Greater East Ohio Chapter: Greater Youngstown Office**
3736 Boardman Canfield Road 330-533-3300
Canfield, OH 44406-0321 800-272-3900
Fax: 330-533-3307
www.alz.org

786 **Alzheimer's Association: Miami Valley Chapter**
3797 Summit Glen Drive 937-291-3332
Dayton, OH 45449-3661 800-272-3900
Fax: 937-291-0463
e-mail: judy.turner@alz.org
www.alz.org/dayton
Judy Turner, Executive Director
Teresa Thomas, Director of Development

787 **Alzheimer's Association: Northwest Ohio Chapter**
780 Park Avenue W 419-522-5050
Mansfield, OH 44906-7906 800-272-3900
Fax: 419-522-5318
e-mail: Alzheimers@nwoalz.org
www.alz.org/nwohio
Voluntary health organization committed to finding a cure for Alzheimer's and helping those affected by the disease.
Salli Bollin, Executive Director
Barbara Stager, Finance and Operations Director

788 **Alzheimer's Association: West Central Ohio Chapter**
892A S Cable Road 419-227-9700
Lima, OH 45805-3468 800-272-3900
Fax: 419-222-6212
e-mail: Alzheimers@nwoalz.org
www.alz.org/nwohio
A voluntary health agency providing information Alzheimer's disease and related dementias, serving 7 counties: Allen, Auglaize, Hancock, Hardin, Mercer, Putnam and Van Wert. Offers support group meetings in each county and provides a toll-free helpline.
Bob Mackowiak, Director Development and Communications
Melissa Strite, Development Coordinator

Oklahoma

789 **Alzheimer's Association: Oklahoma Chapter**
6465 S Yale 918-481-7741
Tulsa, OK 74136-7804 800-272-3900
Fax: 918-481-7745
TTY: 800-493-1411
e-mail: admin@alzokar.org
www.alz.org/alzokar
Dedicated to serving Alzheimer's patients, their families, and caregivers through education, outreach, programs, support services and public advocacy.
Judi A Ver Hoef, President/CEO
Mark Fried, Executive Vice President

Oregon

790 **Alzheimer's Association: Columbia-Willamet Chapter**
1311 NW 21st Avenue 503-413-7115
Portland, OR 97209-1610 800-272-3900
Fax: 503-413-6909
e-mail: judy.mckellar@alz.org
www.alzheimers-oregon.org
Judy McKellar, Executive Director
Dave Rianda, President

791 **Alzheimer's Association: Cascade/Coast Chapter**
1238 Lincoln Street 541-345-8392
Eugene, OR 97401 800-272-3900
Fax: 541-345-5797
e-mail: infoalzoregon@alz.org
www.alz.org/oregon
Elizabeth Eckstrom, Vice President
Mark Donham, President

792 **Alzheimer's Association: Mary's Peak Chapter**
1925 NW Circle Boulevard 541-752-1012
Corvallis, OR 97330-1312 Fax: 541-757-1395
www.alz.org

793 **Alzheimer's Association: Mid-Willamette Chapter**
PO Box 12768 503-371-7728
Salem, OR 97309-0768 Fax: 503-571-9842
e-mail: midwillamatte@alz.org
www.alz.org

Pennsylvania

794 **Alzheimer's Association: Delaware Valley Chapter**
399 Market Street 215-561-2919
Philadelphia, PA 19106 800-272-3900
Fax: 215-561-4663
e-mail: Wendy.Campbell@alz.org
www.alz.org/desjsepa
Wendy L Campbell, President
Theresa Haenn, Vice President Development

795 **Alzheimer's Association: Greater Pennsylvania Chapter: SW Regional Office**
Landmarks Building, 100 Station 412-261-5040
Pittsburgh, PA 15219 800-272-3900
Fax: 412-471-2722
www.alzpa.org
Education training, information, support groups, free newsletter, telephone support, services to caregivers and diagnosed individuals, as well as professionals.
Diane Balcom, President/CEO
Erica Hood, Director Of Programs

796 **Alzheimer's Association: Greater Mid-Ohio**
1100 Liberty Avenue 412-261-5040
Pittsburgh, PA 15222 Fax: 412-471-2722
e-mail: bob.leroy@alz.org
www.alz.org/pa
Education training information support groups free newsletter telephone support services to caregivers and diagnosed individuals as well as professionals.
Bob LeRoy, President/CEO
Erica Hood, Vice President of Programs and Services

797 **Alzheimer's Association: Laurel Mountains Chapter**
1011 Old Salem Road
Greensburg, PA 15601-1095 800-652-3370
Fax: 724-837-4567
www.alz.org

798 **Alzheimer's Association: Northeast Pennsylvania Chapter**
63 North Franklin Street 717-822-4278
Wilkes Barre, PA 18701 800-272-3900
Fax: 717-822-9915
www.alzpa.org

799 **Alzheimer's Association: Northwest Pennsylvania Chapter**
1128 State Street 814-456-9200
Erie, PA 16501 800-272-3900
Fax: 814-454-0414
e-mail: bob.leroy@alz.org
www.alz.org/pa
Bob LeRoy, President/CEO
Erica Hood, Vice President of Programs and Services

800 **Alzheimer's Association: South Central Pennsylvania Chapter**
3544 North Progress Avenue 717-651-5020
Harrisburg, PA 17110 800-272-3900
Fax: 717-651-5066
Lori Hoffmaster, Regional Director
Erin Auth, Family Services Coordinator

Rhode Island

801 **Alzheimer's Association: Rhode Island Chapter**
245 Waterman Avenue 401-421-0008
Providence, RI 02906 800-272-3900
Fax: 401-941-8988
e-mail: Elizabeth.Morancy@alz.org
www.alz.org/ri
Elizabeth Morancy, Executive Director
Rita St Pierre, Program Director

South Carolina

802 **Alzheimer's Association: Low Country Chapter**
2090 Executive Hall Road 843-571-2641
Charleston, SC 29407 800-860-1444
Fax: 843-571-6020
www.alz.org/sc
Ashton Baker, VP of Development & Communications
Fran Emerson, Program Director

803 **Alzheimer's Association: Mid-State South Carolina Chapter**
2999 Sunset Boulevard 803-791-3430
W Columbia, SC 29169-7044 800-636-3346
Fax: 803-791-8388
www.alz.org/sc
Adelle Stanley, Program Director
Elizabeth Brown, Director of Development

804 **Alzheimer's Association: Upstate South Carolina Chapter**
4124 Clemson Boulevard 864-224-3045
Anderson, SC 29621-5528 800-273-2555
Fax: 864-225-1387
e-mail: cindy.alewine@alz.org
www.alz.org/sc
Cindy Alewine, President/CEO
Velma Haggan, VP of Finance & Operations

Tennessee

805 **Alzheimer's Association: Eastern Tennessee Chapter**
2200 Sutherland Avenue 865-544-6288
Knoxville, TN 37919 800-272-3900
Fax: 865-544-6249
e-mail: janice.wade@alz.org
www.alz.org/tn
Janice Wade-Whitehea, Executive Director
Carolyn Jensen, Development Director

806 **Alzheimer's Association: Highland Rim Chapter**
201 W Lincoln Street 931-455-3345
Tullahoma, TN 37388-1004 800-272-3900
Fax: 931-455-5396
e-mail: tiffany.maicke@alz.org
www.alz.org/altn
Jaine Colley, Board Director

807 **Alzheimer's Association: Memphis Area Office**
326 Ellsworth 901-565-0011
Memphis, TN 38111 800-272-3900
Fax: 901-565-9550
e-mail: tammy.deniro@alz.org
www.alz.org/altn
Kenneth Sakauye, Board Director

808 **Alzheimer's Association: Middle Tennessee Chapter**
4205 Hillsboro Pike 615-292-4938
Nashville, TN 37215-2859 800-272-3900
Fax: 615-386-9768
e-mail: diane.gramann@alz.org
www.alz.org/altn
Mike Brent, Secretary/Treasurer

809 **Alzheimer's Association: Northeast Tennessee Chapter**
207 North Boone Street 423-928-4080
Johnson City, TN 37604 800-272-3900
Fax: 423-928-1152
e-mail: tracey.kendall@alz.org
www.myalz.org

Provide support, education, advocacy and research to those affected by Alzheimers disease and their families.
Luanne Weller, Helpline Coordinator
Tracey Kendall, Regional Director

810 **Alzheimer's Association: Southeast Tennessee Chapter**
735 Broad Street 423-265-3600
Chattanooga, TN 37402 800-272-3900
Fax: 423-265-3611
www.myalz.org
Sandy Matheson, Executive Director
Ann Lindsey, Assistant Director

Texas

811 **Alzheimer's Alliance: Texarkana Area**
1105 College Drive 903-223-8021
Texarkana, TX 75503-7812 877-312-8536
Fax: 903-792-1792
e-mail: mphillipsalz@earthlink.net
www.alztexark.org
Melba Phillips, Executive Director
Mike Stuart, President

812 **Alzheimer's Association: Capital of Texas Chapter**
3429 Executive Center Drive 512-241-0420
Austin, TX 78731 800-367-2132
Fax: 512-241-0430
e-mail: TxChapterInfo@alz.org
www.alz.org/texascapital
The Alzheimer Association Greater Austin Chapter is dedicated to providing leadership to enhance care and support services for individuals and their families while promoting the advancement of research eliminate Alzheimer's disease.
Debbie Hanna, President
Christian Wells, Program Team Leader

813 **Alzheimer's Association: El Paso Chapter**
4687 N Mesa 915-544-1799
El Paso, TX 79912-1147 800-272-3900
Fax: 915-544-8746
e-mail: Luciana.murillo@alz.org
www.alz-austin.org
Cynthia Annis, Program Specialist
Linda Gravatti, Support Team Grant Supervisor

814 **Alzheimer's Association: Greater Beaumont Area Chapter**
700 N Street 409-833-1613
Beaumont, TX 77701 800-272-3900
Fax: 409-833-1902
e-mail: richard.elbein@alz.org
www.alz.org/texas
Richard Elbein, Chief Executive Officer
Janie Lewis, Program Officer

815 **Alzheimer's Association: Greater Dallas Chapter**
4144 N Central Expressway 214-827-0062
Dallas, TX 75204-4228 800-272-3900
Fax: 214-827-2064
e-mail: Helpline@alzdallas.org
www.alz.org/greaterdallas
Provides support and assistance to persons affected by Alzheimer's disease and related dementias and their families and caregivers. Serving Collin, Cooke, Dallas, Deaton, Ellis, Fanning, Grayson, Hunt, Kaufmau, Navarro and Rockwall counties.
John R Gilchrist Jr, Executive Director
Karen Shodeke, Office Manager

816 **Alzheimer's Association: Greater East Texas Chapter**
PO Box 630636 936-569-1325
Nacogdoches, TX 75963 800-272-3900
Fax: 936-569-0514
www.alz.org/texas
Phil King, Chief Financial Officer
Ana Guerrero, Development Officer

817 **Alzheimer's Association: Greater Wichita Falls Chapter**
901 Indiana 940-767-8800
Wichita Falls, TX 76301-3206 800-272-3900
Fax: 940-322-6259
e-mail: patty.taylor@alz.org
www.alz.org/northcentraltexas
Patty Taylor, Director
Lyn Downing, Director of Development

818 **Alzheimer's Association: Houston and Southeast Texas Chapter**
2242 W Holcombe Boulevard 713-266-6400
Houston, TX 77030 800-272-3900
Fax: 713-266-6487
www.alz.org/texas
Katie Olson, Community Education/Outreach Coordinator
Noga Tobias, Corporate Outreach Coordinator

819 **Alzheimer's Association: Northeast Texas Chapter**
211 Winchester 903-509-8323
Tyler, TX 75701-8732 800-789-0508
Fax: 903-509-8373
e-mail: jana@alzalliance.org
www.alzalliance.org
Jana Humphrey, Executive Director
Sherlon Spurling, Client Services Coordinator

820 **Alzheimer's Association: Rio Grande Valley Region**
222 E Van Buren 956-440-0636
Harlingen, TX 78550 800-272-3900
Fax: 956-440-9290
www.alztexas.org
A nonprofit organization designed to educate and support individuals with Alzheimer's, their families and caregivers.

821 **Alzheimer's Association: STAR Chapter, Midland Region**
4400 N Big Spring 432-570-9191
Midland, TX 79705 800-272-3900
Fax: 432-683-2345
e-mail: debbie.erdwurm@alz.org
www.alz.org/txstar
Matt W Spahn, Chair
Eddie Garc¡a, Secretary

822 **Alzheimer's Association: South Central Texas**
7400 Louis Pasteur Drive 210-822-6449
San Antonio, TX 78229 800-272-3900
Fax: 210-824-8069
e-mail: anna.bridgman@alz.org
www.alz.org/txstar
Matt W Spahn, Chair
Eddie Garc¡a, Secretary

823 **Alzheimer's Association: Tarrant County Chapter**
101 Summit Avenue 817-336-4949
Fort Worth, TX 76102 800-272-3900
Fax: 817-336-4966
e-mail: theresa.hocker@alz.org
www.alz.org/northcentraltexas
Offers support to those afflicted with Alzheimer's disease and their families through education, support groups, case management, telephone helpline and referral to services (i.e. long term care, adult daycare, medical assistance, legal assistance etc.).
Theresa Hocker, Executive Director
Susanna Luk-Jones, Director of Program Services

Utah

824 **Alzheimer's Association: Utah Chapter**
855 E 4800 S 801-265-1944
Salt Lake City, UT 84107 800-272-3900
Fax: 801-269-1226
e-mail: utah.chapter@alz.org
www.alz.org/utah
Jack Jenks, Executive Director
Janet Wood, President

Vermont

825 **Alzheimer's Association: Vermont Chapter**
172 N Main Street 802-477-7000
Barre, VT 05641-1139 800-272-3900
Fax: 802-229-5231
e-mail: jeff.maker@alz.org
www.alz.org/vermont
Jeffery M Maker, Senior Executive Director
Laura Corrow, Program Director

Virginia

826 **Alzheimer's Association: Central Virginia Chapter**
674 Hillsdale Drive 434-973-6122
Charlottesville, VA 22901 800-272-3900
Fax: 434-973-4224
e-mail: victoria.fahrenkrog@alz.org
www.alz.org/cwva
Ron Feinman, Chair
Susan B Friedman, President & CEO

827 **Alzheimer's Association: Greater Richmond Chapter**
4600 Cox Road 804-967-2580
Glen Allen, VA 23060 800-272-3900
Fax: 804-967-2588
e-mail: sherry.peterson@alz.org
www.alz.org/grva
Alzheimer's Association provides support and services to those with Alzheimer's and their families services include: helpline, support groups, educational programs for family and professional caregivers, monthly newsletter, lending library, and a speakers
Sherry Peter MSW, CEO
Alyssa McBride, Development Director

828 **Alzheimer's Association: National Capital Area Chapter**
11240 Waples Mill Road 703-359-4440
Fairfax, VA 22030 800-272-3900
Fax: 703-359-4441
e-mail: webmaster@alz-nova.org
www.alz.org/nca
Provides support and services to those diagnosed with Alzheimer's disease and related disorders and their families. Services include information on the disease, care options, caregiving techniques and research, support groups, education and training, and advocacy.
Matthew B Aaron, Chair
Robert Comeau, Vice Chair Operations

829 **Alzheimer's Association: Piedmont-Valley Area Chapter**
674 Hillsdale Drive 434-973-6122
Charlottesville, VA 22901-4634 800-272-3900
Fax: 434-973-4224
e-mail: victoria.fahrenkrog@alz.org
www.alz.org/cwva
Ron Feinman, Chair
Susan B Friedman, President & CEO

830 **Alzheimer's Association: Roanoke Salem Chapter**
2728 Colonial Avenue 540-345-7600
Roanoke, VA 24015-0014 800-272-3900
Fax: 540-345-7900
e-mail: annette.clark@alz.org
www.alz.org/cwva
William Stokes, Vice Chair
Robert D Gilges, Treasurer

831 **Alzheimer's Association: Southeastern Virginia Chapter**
6350 Center Drive 757-459-2405
Norfolk, VA 23502 800-272-3900
Fax: 757-461-7902
e-mail: gino.colombara@alz.org
www.alz.org/seva
Provides support to people with Alzheimer's disease or related dementia and their families; educates professionals and the public about Alzheimer's disease and related dementia; supports research into causes, improved diagnosis, therapies and cures.
Gino V Colombara, Executive Director
Patricia Far Lacey, Director of Education & Family Services

832 **Alzheimer's Association: Southside Virginia Chapter**
120 S Hill Avenue 434-447-3963
S Hill, VA 23970-0310 800-272-3900
Fax: 434-447-9024
e-mail: gino.colombara@alz.org
www.alz.org/seva
Gino V Colombara, Executive Director
June Rainey, Education & Family Services Coordinator

Washington

833 **Alzheimer's Association: Inland Northwest Chapter**
601 W 5th Avenue 509-473-3390
Spokane, WA 99204 800-272-3900
Fax: 509-473-3389
e-mail: joel.loiacono@alz.org
www.alz.org/inlandnorthwest
Joel Loiacono, Executive Director
Sandra Druffel, Development Director

834 **Alzheimer's Association: Western & Central Washington Chapter**
12721 30th Avenue NE 206-363-5500
Seattle, WA 98125 800-848-7097
Fax: 206-363-5700
e-mail: nancy.dapper@alz.org
www.alz.org/alzwa
Nancy Dapper, Executive Director
Ellia Ryan, Development Director

West Virginia

835 **Alzheimer's Association: Greater Mid-Ohio Valley Chapter**
1218 Market Street 304-865-6775
Parkersburg, WV 26101 800-491-2717
e-mail: jane.marks@alz.org
www.alz.org/wv
Jane Marks, Executive Director
Laurel Kirksey, Development Director

836 **Alzheimer's Association: N Central West Virginia Chapter**
1299 Pineview Drive 304-599-1159
Morgantown, WV 26505-4543 800-491-2717
Fax: 304-291-2577
e-mail: jane.marks@alz.org
www.alz.org/wv
Jane Marks, Executive Director
Elizabeth Kreutz, Regional Coordinator

837 **Alzheimer's Association: South West Virginia Chapter**
1111 Lee Street E 304-343-2717
Charleston, WV 25301 800-491-2717
Fax: 304-343-2723
e-mail: jane.marks@alz.org
www.alz.org/wv
Jane Marks, Executive Director
Melissa Gandee, Program Director

Wisconsin

838 **Alzheimer's Association: Indianhead Chapter**
1227B Menomonie Street 715-835-7050
Eau Claire, WI 54703-5996 800-272-3900
Fax: 715-835-0597
e-mail: Mary.Bouche@alz.org
www.alz.org/gwwi
Mary B Bouche, Executive Director
Michael Furgiuele, Finance/Technical Director

839 **Alzheimer's Association: Lake Superior Chapter**
400 Chapple Avenue 715-682-3974
Ashland, WI 54806-1652 800-272-3900
Fax: 715-682-6561
e-mail: Mary.Bouche@alz.org
www.alz.org/gwwi
Mary B Bouche, Executive Director
Michael Furgiuele, Finance/Technical Director

840 Alzheimer's Association: Midstate Wisconsin Chapter
1000 N Oak Avenue
Marshfield, WI 54449
715-389-3200
Fax: 715-387-5727
www.alz.org

841 Alzheimer's Association: North Central Wisconsin Chapter
203 Schiek Plaza
Rhinelander, WI 54501
715-362-7779
800-200-1221
Fax: 715-362-1879
www.alz.org

842 Alzheimer's Association: Northeast Wisconsin Chapter
2900 Curry Lane
Green Bay, WI 54311
920-498-2110
800-360-2110
Fax: 920-498-2203
www.alz.org

843 Alzheimer's Association: Riverland Chapter
1022 Caledonia Street
La Crosse, WI 54603
608-784-5011
800-797-1656
Fax: 608-784-4428
www.alz.org

844 Alzheimer's Association: South Central Wisconsin Chapter
517 N Segoe Road
Madison, WI 53705-3172
608-232-3400
800-272-3900
Fax: 608-232-3407
e-mail: scwisc.support@alz.org
www.alz.org/scwisc

Provides support and assistance to the families of those impacted by Alzheimer's and related dementias, including educational programs, support groups, information and referral and advocacy.
150 Members
Paul Rusk, Executive Director
Danielle Luethje, Education Coordinator

845 Alzheimer's Association: Southeast Wisconsin Chapter
6130 W National Avenue
Milwaukee, WI 53214
414-479-8800
800-922-2413
Fax: 414-479-8819
TTY: 414-479-8466
e-mail: info@alzheimers.sswi.org
www.alz.org/sewi

To eliminate Alzheimer's disease through advancement of research and to enhance care and support for individuals, their families and caregivers. Individual consultation over the phone or in person. Extensive library of educational materials for loan or purchase.
Tom Hlavacek, Executive Director
Krista Scheel, Program Director

Wyoming

846 Alzheimer's Association: Wyoming Chapter
5601 S 27th Street
Lincoln, NE 68512-4331
307-421-7321
800-272-3900
e-mail: bobbie.turner@alz.org
www.alz.org/greatplains

The Alzheimer's Association of the Great Plains is dedicated to supporting those with Alzheimer's disease and their families and friends through specialized programs and services, educating families, communities, and health professionals about Alzheimer's disease.
Kevin Kirsner, Community Outreach/Development
Karen Noel, President and CEO

847 Alzheimer's Wyoming
900 Werner Court
Casper, WY 82602
307-265-7960
Fax: 307-265-7960
e-mail: alzawy@tribcsp.com
www.alzheimerswyoming.org

Alzheimer's Affiliation of Wyoming is an independent organization that makes presentations about Alzheimer's Disease; assists Alzheimer support groups; provides funds for respite care; maintains a lending library; refers patients and their families to services.
Mary Hein, Executive Director

Foundations

848 Long Island Alzheimers Foundation
5 Channel Drive
Port Washington, NY 11050
516-767-6856
Fax: 516-767-6864
e-mail: info@liaf.org
www.liaf.org

Provides information and referral services, materials, adult daycare program, support groups and caregiver conferences.
Pattie Gallatin, Executive Director

Research Centers

849 Aging and Alzheimer's Disease Center Oregon Health Sciences University
Oregon Health Sciences University
3181 SW Sam Jackson Park Road - CR1
Portland, OR 97239-3098
503-494-6976
Fax: 503-494-7499
e-mail: kaye@ohsu.edu
www.ohsu.edu/research/alzheimers

Researches causes and consequences of Alzheimer's disease and ways of clinical services. Publishes a newsletter twice a year.
Jeffrey Kaye, Director
Joan Benedict, Administrative Coordinator

850 Alzheimer's Disease Center Emory University/VA Medical Center
Wesley Woods Health Center 3rd Flo
Atlanta, GA 30329
404-728-6950
Fax: 404-286-55
e-mail: emoryadrc@emory.edu
www.med.emory.edu/ADRC

Researchers work to translate advances into improved care and diagnosis for Alzheimer's patients.
Allan Levey, Director
Stuart Zola, Co-Director

851 Alzheimer's Disease Center Kentucky University
Sanders-Brown Center on Aging
101 Sanders-Brown Building
Lexington, KY 40536-9824
859-257-1412
Fax: 859-323-2866
e-mail: rdavi3@email.uky.edu
www.mc.uky.edu/coa/clinicalcore/alzheime

Researchers work to translate advances into improved care and diagnosis for Alzheimer's patients.
William R Markesbery, Director
Mary Fern Waechter, Financial Officer

852 Alzheimer's Disease Center Mayo Clinic Mayo Medical School
Mayo Medical School
4111 Highway 52 N
Rochester, MN 55901
507-284-1324
Fax: 507-538-0878
e-mail: mayoADC@mayo.edu
www.mayoresearch.mayo.edu

Researchers work to translate advances into improved care and diagnosis for Alzheimer's patients.
Ronald Petersen, Director
Neill R Graff-Radford, Associate Director

853 Alzheimer's Disease Center Pennsylvania University School of Medicine
Ralston House
3615 Chestnut Street
Philadelphia, PA 19104
215-662-7810
e-mail: jason.karlawish@uphs.upenn.edu
www.uphs.upenn.edu/ADC

Researchers work to translate advances into improved care and diagnosis for Alzheimer's patients.
John Q Trojanowski, Director

854 Alzheimer's Disease Center: Boston University
Boston University School of Medicine
72 E Concord Street
Boston, MA 02118
617-638-5426
888-458-2823
Fax: 617-414-1197
e-mail: pfau@bu.edu
www.bu.edu/alzresearch

Researchers work to translate advances into improved care and diagnosis for Alzheimer's patients.
Neil W Kowall, Director
Richard Fine, Associate Director

855 **Alzheimer's Disease Center: Johns Hopkins University School of Medicine**
Johns Hopkins University Department of Pathology
720 Rutland Avenue 410-502-5164
Baltimore, MD 21205 Fax: 410-955-9777
e-mail: edelman1@jhmi.edu
www.alzresearch.org
Researchers work to translate advances into improved care and diagnosis for Alzheimer's patients.
Donald L Price, Director
Juan Troncoso, Co-Director

856 **Alzheimer's Disease Center: University of California, Davis**
4860 Y Street 916-734-5496
Sacramento, CA 95817 e-mail: wjjagust@lbl.gov
alzheimer.ucdavis.edu/
Researchers work to translate advances into improved care and diagnosis for Alzheimer's patients.
William J Jagust, Principal Investigator

857 **Alzheimer's Disease Center: University of Alabama at Birmingham**
1720 7th Avenue S 205-934-3847
Birmingham, AL 35294-0017 Fax: 205-975-7365
e-mail: adbrain@uab.edu
www.main.uab.edu/adc
Researchers work to translate advances into improved care and diagnosis for Alzheimer's patients.
Daniel C Marson, Director
J Michael Wyss, Associate Director

858 **Alzheimer's Disease Center: Washington University**
1660 S Columbian Way 206-277-3281
Seattle, WA 98108 800-317-5382
Fax: 206-768-5456
e-mail: wamble@u.washington.edu
www.depts.washington.edu/adrcweb
Researchers work to translate advances into improved care and diagnosis for Alzheimer's patients.
Murray A Raskind, Director
Elaine Peskind, Associate Director

859 **Alzheimer's Disease Research Center Washington University School of Medicine**
Washington University School of Medicine
4488 Forest Park Avenue 314-286-2683
St Louis, MO 63108 Fax: 314-286-2763
e-mail: morrisj@abraxas.wustl.edu
www.adrc.wustl.edu
Researchers work to translate advances into improved care diagnosis and treatment for Alzheimer's patients.
John Morris, Director
Virginia D Buckles, Executive Director

860 **Alzheimer's Disease Research Center Duke University**
Bryan ADRC
2200 W Main Street Suite A200 919-668-0820
Durham, NC 27705 866-444-2372
e-mail: kwe@duke.edu
adrc.mc.duke.edu/adrc.HTM
Researchers work to translate advances into improved care and diagnosis for Alzheimer's patients.
Kathleen A Welsh-Bohmer, Director
James Robert Burke, Associate Director

861 **Cognitive Neurology and Alzheimer's Disease Center**
CNADC
320 E Superior Street 312-908-9339
Chicago, IL 60611 Fax: 312-908-8789
e-mail: CNADC-Admin@northwestern.edu
www.brain.northwestern.edu
Researchers work to translate advances into improved care and diagnosis for Alzheimer's patients.
M -Marsel Mesulam, Director
Eileen H Bigio, Director of the Neuropathology Core

862 **Cornell University: Winifred Masterson Burke Medical Research-Dementia**
425 E 61st Street 212-821-0560
New York, NY 10021 Fax: 212-821-0576
e-mail: publicaffairs@med.cornell.edu
www.med.cornell.edu
Clinical and basic studies in metabolic aspects of the nervous system especially Alzheimer's disease.
John P Blass, Director
Sanford I Weill, Chairman

863 **Duke University Center for the Study of Aging and Human Development**
duke Duke University
Box 3003 919-660-7502
Durham, NC 27710 Fax: 919-848-8569
e-mail: webmaster@geri.duke.edu
www.geri.duke.edu
Basic and clinical research into geriatrics and gerontology focusing on a number of chronic diseases in the elderly including osteoporosis cancer heart disease infectious diseases Alzheimer's disease and other disorders leading to dysmobility.
Harvey Jay Cohen MD, Director
Linda K George, Associate Director

864 **Duke University Clinical Research Institute**
Headquarters
2400 Pratt Street
Durham, NC 27705 919-668-8700
www.dcri.duke.edu
Multidisciplinary clinical research into the cause and prevention of human diseases such as Alzheimer's.
Robert A Harrington, Director
Miriam Donohue, Chief Operating Officer

865 **Indiana University Center for Aging Research**
The Center for Aging Research
410 W 10th Street 317-423-5600
Indianapolis, IN 46202-2872 Fax: 317-423-5695
e-mail: nnienaber@regenstrief.org
iucar.iu.edu
Researchers work to translate advances into improved care and diagnosis for Alzheimer's patients.
Christopher Callahan, Director
Douglas K Miller, Associate Director

866 **Indiana University: Human Genetics Center of Medical & Molecular Genetics**
School of Medicine
975 W Walnut Street 317-274-2241
Indianapolis, IN 46202-5251 e-mail: kcornett@iupui.edu
www.medicine.iu.edu
Comprised of a core group of scientists with primary appointments in the Department and a group of molecular biologists from other departments who hold joint appointments in Medical and Molecular Genetics.
Kenneth Corn MD, Division Director/Professor
Stephen R Dlouhy PhD, Associate Director & Scientist

867 **Institute for Basic Research in Developmental Disabilities**
1050 Forest Hill Road 718-494-0600
Staten Island, NY 10314-6330 Fax: 718-494-0833
www.omr.state.ny.us
W. Ted Brown MD, PhD, Director

868 **Long Island Alzheimers Foundation**
5 Channel Drive 516-767-6856
Port Washington, NY 11050 Fax: 516-767-6864
e-mail: info@liaf.org
www.liaf.org
Researchers work to translate advances into improved care and diagnosis for Alzheimer's patients.
Fred Jenny, Executive Director
Anna Maria Warmuz, Executive Assistant

869 **Massachusetts Alzheimers Disease Research Center**
Massachusetts ADRC
Massachusetts General Hospital 617-726-3987
Boston, MA 02114 Fax: 617-726-4101
www.madrc.org

Multi-institutional consortium of Harvard affiliated facilities encompasses five Core units: an Administrative Core a Clinical Core a Database Management and Statistics Core a Neuropathology Core and an Education and Information Transfer Core. The ADRC also supports four specific research projects funded for 3-5 years and annually designates three or four pilot research projects that are funded for 1 year.
John H Growdon, Clinic Director
Catherine A Crosby, Research Associates

870 **Medical College of Georgia Alzheimers Research Center**
1120 15th Street 706-721-6900
Augusta, GA 30912 Fax: 706-721-7063
e-mail: jbuccafu@mcg.edu
www.mcg.edu/centers/alz
Clinical and basic research of Alzheimer's disease.
Jerry Buccaf MD, Director
J Warren Beach, Member

871 **Michigan Alzheimer's Disease Research Center**
University of Michigan
1500 E Medical Center Drive 734-936-4000
Ann Arbor, MI 48109-0316 e-mail: sgilman@umich.edu
www.med.umich.edu/alzheimers
Researchers work to translate advances into improved care and diagnosis for Alzheimer's patients.
Sid Gilman MD, Director
Edna Andrews-Rose, Clinical Nurse Consultant

872 **Mount Sinai School of Medicine: Alzheimers Disease Research Center**
Alzheimer's Disease Research Center
One Gustave L Levy Place 212-241-8329
New York, NY 10029 Fax: 212-369-2344
e-mail: mary.sano@mssm.edu
www.mssm.edu/psychiatry/adrc
Focuses on Alzheimer's disease research.
Mary Sano, Director
Samuel Gandy, Associate Director

873 **Neurosciences Institute of the Neurosciences Research Program**
The Neurosciences Institute
10640 John Jay Hopkins Drive 858-626-2000
San Diego, CA 92121 Fax: 858-626-2099
e-mail: info@nsi.edu
www.nsi.edu
Nonprofit organization focusing on Alzheimer's and related disorders.
Gerald M Edelman, Director

874 **Ohio State University Neuroscience Program**
1835 Neil Avenue 614-292-8185
Columbus, OH 43210 Fax: 614-921-44
www.psy.ohio-state.edu
Specializes in brain disorders such as Alzheimer's disease.
Richard Petty, Chair
Tatiana Tramel, Behavioral Neurosciences Area Assistant

875 **Taub Institute For Research On Alzheimer's Disease and the Aging Brain**
630 W 168th Street 212-305-1818
New York, NY 10032 Fax: 212-342-2849
e-mail: taubinstitute@columbia.edu.
www.cumc.columbia.edu/dept/taub
Studies Alzheimer's patients.
Michael L Shelanski MD, Director
Rafael A Lantigua MD, Deputy Director

876 **Taub Institute for Research on Alzheimers Disease and the Aging Brain**
630 West 168th Street 212-305-1818
New York, NY 10032 Fax: 212-422-49
e-mail: taubinstitute@columbia.edu
www.alzheimercenter.org
Researchers work to translate advances into improved care and diagnosis for Alzheimer's patients.
Michael L Shelanski, Co-Director
Richard Mayeux MD, Co-Director

877 **The Alzheimer's Disease & Memory Disorders Center**
ADMDC
6550 Fannin 713-798-4734
Houston, TX 77030 Fax: 713-798-5326
e-mail: rdoody@bcm.tmc.edu
www.bcm.edu/neurology/admdc
Researchers work to translate advances into improved care and diagnosis for Alzheimer's Disease and other memory disorders.
Fay M Sagullo, Administrative Assistant
Rachelle S Doody, Director

878 **The Sam and Rose Stein Institute for Research on the Aging**
University of California San Diego
9500 Gilman Drive 858-534-6299
La Jolla, CA 92093-0664 Fax: 858-534-5475
e-mail: steininstitute@ucsd.edu
www.sira.ucsd.edu
Research on aging and Alzheimer's disease.
Dilip V Jeste MD, Director
Maureen Halp MS, Executive Director

879 **University Alzheimer Center University of Alabama at Birmingham**
University of Alabama at Birmingham
1720 7th Avenue S 205-934-3847
Birmingham, AL 35294-17 800-333-6543
Fax: 205-975-7365
e-mail: adbrain@uab.edu
main.uab.edu
Researchers work to translate advances into improved care and diagnosis for Alzheimer's patients.
Daniel C Marson, Director
J Michael Wyss, Associate Director

880 **University Alzheimer Center UHC: Case Western Reserve University**
12200 Fairhill Road 216-844-6400
Cleveland, OH 44120 Fax: 216-844-6446
e-mail: Nancy.Catalani@Case.Edu
www.ohioalzcenter.org
Researchers work to translate advances into improved care and diagnosis for Alzheimer's patients.
Alan Lerner, Co-Director
Kathleen A Smyth, Administrator

881 **University of Chicago Dept of Neurology University of Chicago Hospital**
University of Chicago Hospital
5841 S Maryland Avenue 773-702-6390
Chicago, IL 60637-1470 Fax: 773-702-9076
e-mail: cgomez@neurology.bsd.uchicago.edu
neurology.uchicago.edu
Covers Translational Neuroscience Research and research programs in neuroimmunology neuromuscular disease and neurovirology provided the initial foundation and brought national recognition.
Christopher MD PhD, Professor/Chairman
Maria Del Fatima Barros, Senior Research Technician

882 **University of Illinois Health Services Research**
University of Illinois College of Medicine
1601 Parkview Avenue 815-395-0600
Rockford, IL 61107 Fax: 815-395-5887
e-mail: prrockford@uic.edu
www.uirockford.com
A unit of the University of Illinois College of Medicine at Rockford serves faculty students health care providers human services agencies and other community organizations throughout Illinois with demographic health social and economic data. The skills data and resources available to faculty and students at the college are also available to individuals and organizations needing assistance.
Joann Glacken, Research Support Services

883 **University of Maryland: Division of Infectious Diseases**
UM Baltimore Department of Medicine
725 W Lombard Street 410-706-7560
Baltimore, MD 21201 Fax: 410-706-4619
e-mail: kvardjan@ihv.umaryland.edu
medschool.umaryland.edu/infectiousdiseas

Focuses research on elderly studies including drug use treatments and infectious diseases of the aged.
Robert R Redfield, Head

884 **University of Miami: Center on Aging Center on Aging**
Center on Aging
1695 NW 9th Avenue 305-355-9080
Miami, FL 33136 Fax: 305-355-9076
e-mail: ajaret@med.miami.edu
www.centeronaging.med.miami.edu
Focuses on aged disorders such as Alzheimer's research.
Sara J Czaja, Co-Director
Carl Eisdorfer, Director

885 **Yeshiva University: Resnick Gerontology Center**
Albert Einstein College of Medicine
111 E 210 Street 718-920-6722
Bronx, NY 10467 866-633-8255
Fax: 718-655-9672
e-mail: ljacobs@aecom.yu.edu
www.aecom.yu.edu
Alzheimer's disease and other dementia studies.
Laurie G Jacobs, Division Chief
Amy R Ehrlich, Geriatrics Fellowship Program Director

Support Groups & Hotlines

886 **Alzheimer's Association Autopsy Assistance Network**
Alzheimer s Association
Western/Central Washington Chapter 206-363-5500
Seattle, WA 98125 800-848-7097
Fax: 206-363-5700
e-mail: rowena.rye@alz.org
http://alzwa.org/resources6.htm
The primary purposes of the Autopsy Assistance Network are: to provide families with information regarding autopsy; to assist in obtaining a confirmed diagnosis; provide tissue for Alzheimer's disease research; and establish diagnosis for purpose of clinical and epidemiological studies.
Nancy Dapper, Executive Director
Rowena Rye, Community Resources

887 **Alzheimer's Support Group**
Columbus Health Rehabilitation Center
2100 Midway Street 812-372-8447
Columbus, IN 47201 Fax: 812-375-5117
www.columbushrc.com/
The skilled Nursing Center includes a separate unit dedicated to the care of residents with Alzheimer's disease and other forms of dementia. The Alzheimer's program is designed to celebrate the spirit of their residents, striving to offer a comfortable and compassionate environment that emphasizes positive life experiences and active involvement in a daily routine.
Mike Spencer, Executive Director

888 **National Health Information Center**
PO Box 1133 310-565-4167
Washington, DC 20013 800-336-4797
Fax: 301-984-4256
e-mail: info@nhic.org
www.health.gov/nhic
Offers a nationwide information referral service, produces directories and resource guides.

Books

889 **36-Hour Day**
Hachette Book Group USA
3 Center Plaza
Boston, MA 02108 800-759-0190
Fax: 800-331-1664
e-mail: webmaster@hbgusa.com
www.hachettebookgroup.com
A family guide to caring for persons with Alzheimer's disease, related dementing illnesses, and memory loss later in life.
1999
ISBN: 0-446618-76-2

890 **Alzheimer Early Stages**
Daniel Kuhn MSW, author
Hunter House Publishers
1515 1/2 Park Street 510-865-5282
Alameda, CA 94501 800-266-5592
e-mail: ordering@hunterhouse.com
www.hunterhouse.com
First steps in caring and treatments. This book is for family members and friends of those recently diagnosed with Alzheimer's Disase.
288 pages Paperback
ISBN: 0-897933-97-4

891 **Alzheimer's Disease**
Springer Publishing Company
536 Broadway 212-431-4370
New York, NY 10012-3955 877-687-7476
Fax: 212-941-7842
e-mail: marketing@springerpub.com
www.springerpub.com
This volume presents the latest research and findings on Alzheimer's disease.
1996 224 pages Softcover
ISBN: 0-826196-22-5
Annette Imperati, Marketing Director

892 **Alzheimer's Disease Orientation Kit**
Alzheimer's Association
225 North Michigan Avenue
Chicago, IL 60611-1696 800-272-3900
Fax: 866-699-1246
TDD: 312-335-8700
e-mail: media@alz.org
www.alz.org
A collection of materials developed to familiarize the audience with Alzheimer's disease and its effects on the patient and family. Includes the Orientation to Alzheimer's Disease videotape, Learning Guide and Caregiver Packet.

893 **Alzheimer's Disease: A Guide to Federal Programs**
Alzheimer's Disease Education & Referral Center
PO Box 8250
Silver Spring, MD 20907-8250 800-438-4380
Fax: 301-495-3334
www.alzheimers.org
Directory of Alzheimer's disease programs sponsored by federal agencies. Lists agency by agency, it provides locations and telephone numbers for multisite activities and demonstration programs and lists information resources.

894 **Alzheimer's Disease: Activity-Focused Care**
Butterworth-Heinemann
225 Wildwood Avenue
Woburn, MA 01801 800-366-2665
Fax: 800-446-6520
www.bh.com
Information for professional and family caregivers on activity-focused care for Alzheimer's patients.
436 pages
ISBN: 0-750699-08-6

895 **Alzheimer's Disease: Advances in Neurology**
Raven Press
1185 Avenue of the Americas 212-930-9500
New York, NY 10036-2601 800-777-2295
304 pages
ISBN: 0-781700-81-7

896 **Alzheimer's Disease: Questions and Answers**
Merit Publishing International
5840 Corporate Way 561-697-1116
West Palm Beach, FL 33407 Fax: 561-477-4961
e-mail: meritpi@aol.com
www.meritpublishing.com
Answers questions about Alzheimer's, explains what it is, how it is diagnosed, causes, and how if affects functions of the brain.
1999
ISBN: 1-873413-52-1
Gene Evans, President
Martin Garrido, VP

897 **Alzheimer's Disease: Thesaurus**
Alzheimer's Disease Education & Referral Center
PO Box 8250
Silver Spring, MD 20907-8250 800-438-4380
Fax: 301-495-3334
www.alzheimers.org
To help librarians and others to save time and money when searing online for books, journal articles, videos and other materials related to Alzheimer's disease.
140 pages

898 **Alzheimer's Disease: Treatment and Family Stress: Directions for Research**
Superintendent of Documents
PO Box 371954 202-512-2250
Pittsburgh, PA 15250-7954
Presents a collection of papers giving current information on research investigations that increase the understanding of the nature and consequences of family caregiving.
486 pages

899 **Alzheimer's, Stroke and 29 Other Neurological Disorders Sourcebook**
Omnigraphics
615 Griswold Street 313-961-1340
Detroit, MI 48226-3993 800-234-1340
Fax: 800-875-1340
e-mail: customerservice@omnigraphics.com
www.omnigraphics.com
Provides vital information for the nontechnical reader focusing on Alzheimer's disease, stroke and various neurological disorders. Answers thousands of questions related to afflications of the central nervous system with each chapter reviwing a particular disorder and offers in-depth discussions.

ISBN: 0-780806-66-2
Georgiann Lauginiger, Customer Service Manager

900 **Care That Works: A Relationship Approach to Persons with Dementia**
John's Hopkins University Press
2715 N Charles Street 410-516-6900
Baltimore, MD 21218-4319 800-537-5487
Fax: 410-516-6998
www.press.jhu.edu
Focuses on building and improving the relationship between the caregiver and the person with Alzheimer's.
272 pages
ISBN: 0-801860-26-1

901 **Care of Alzheimer's Patients: A Manual for Nursing Home Staff**
Lisa P Gwyther, author
Alzheimer's Association
225 North Michigan Avenue
Chicago, IL 60611-1696 800-272-3900
Fax: 866-699-1246
TDD: 312-335-8700
e-mail: media@alz.org
www.alz.org
A care guide for nursing home staff. A useful resource for any caregiver or professional.
122 pages

902 **Caregiver Helpbook**
Legacy Health System
1015 NW 22nd Avenue 503-413-6778
Portland, OR 97210 Fax: 503-413-6911
e-mail: kshannon@lhs.org
www.legacyhealth.org
A helpful guide with useful self care tools for family caregivers of frail or ill older adults.
300 pages Paperback
ISBN: 0-937915-54-6
Kathy Shannon, Manager/Caregiver

903 **Caring for Alzheimer's Patients: A Guide for Family & Healthcare Providers**
Plenum Publishing Corporation
233 Spring Street 212-620-8460
New York, NY 10013-1522 800-221-9369
Fax: 212-463-0742
e-mail: books@plenum.com
Consists of five organizations that furnish information and resources concerning Alzheimer's Disease support groups and hospitals.
308 pages
ISBN: 0-306431-99-8

904 **Complete Guide to Alzheimer's Proofing Your Home**
Purdue University Press
509 Harrison Street 765-494-2038
West Lafayette, IN 47907-2025 800-247-6553
Fax: 765-496-2442
e-mail: pupress@purdue.edu
www.thepress.purdue.edu
Guide on how to modify homes of Alzheimer's patients to facilitate caregiving.
496 pages Paperback
ISBN: 1-557532-02-8

905 **Confronting Alzheimer's Disease**
American Assoc. of Homes and Services for Aging
2519 Connecticut Avenue NW 202-783-2242
Washington, DC 20008-2008 Fax: 202-783-2255
www.aahsa.org
A resource for administrators, professional caregivers and families dealing with Alzheimer's disease and related disorders.
225 pages

906 **Court-Related Needs of the Elderly and Persons with Disabilities**
Commission on the Mentally Disabled
1800 M Street NW 202-331-2240
Washington, DC 20036
Report of the National Conference, examines the barriers of the judicial system impeding access for the elderly and persons with disabilities.

907 **Developing Support Groups for Individuals with Early-Stage Alzheimer's Disease**
Robyn Yale, author
Health Professions Press
PO Box 10624 410-337-9585
Baltimore, MD 21285-0624 888-337-8808
Fax: 410-337-8539
www.healthpropress.com
This one-of-a-kind, step-by-step guidebook has been used as a national and international model to meet the needs of people just diagnosed with Alzheimer's disease. Clinical and administrative issues include selecting group participants, training facilitators and managing unique group topics, interactions and dynamics.
256 pages Paperback
ISBN: 1-878812-62-2

908 **Directory of Alzheimer's Disease Treatment Facilities & Home Health Care**
Oryx Press
4041 N Central Avenue 602-265-2651
Phoenix, AZ 85012-3397 800-279-4663
www.oryxpress.com
A compilation of 1,500 specialized facilities with day care, residential care, diagnosis and treatment facilities.

909 **Ginny: A Love Remembered**
Iowa State Press
2121 State Street 515-292-0155
Ames, IA 50014 800-862-6657
Fax: 515-292-3348
e-mail: orders@iowastatepress.com
iowastatepress.com
This book tells the story of midwest cartoonist Bob Artley's life with his beloved wife and their 10 year battle together against Alzheimer's disease, which finally claimed her.
278 pages Hardcover
ISBN: 0-813821-04-5
Brad Nobiling, Credit Manager

910 **Hospice Alternative**
Harper Collins Publishers/Basic Books

10 E 53rd Street 212-207-7057
New York, NY 10022-5299 800-242-7737
Fax: 212-207-7203

An account of the hospice experience. An innovative and humane way of caring for the terminally ill.
256 pages
ISBN: 0-465030-61-0

911 **Hospice Care for Patients with Advanced Progressive Dementia**
Springer Publishing Company
536 Broadway 212-431-4370
New York, NY 10012 877-687-7476
Fax: 212-941-7842
e-mail: marketing@springerpub.com
www.springerpub.com

Discusses adpating hospice care for terminally ill patients with dementia. Topics include infections, eating difficulties, and providing palliative care.
320 pages Hardcover
ISBN: 0-826111-62-9
Annette Imperati, Marketing Director

912 **I'm Just Not Myself Anymore: A Family Guide to Alzheimer's Disease**
Northwestern University Press
625 Colfax Street 847-491-5313
Evanston, IL 60208-4210 Fax: 847-491-8150
e-mail: nupress@nwu.edu
www.northwestern.edu

1993 283 pages Paperback
ISBN: 1-880416-72-7

913 **Interventions for Alzheimer's Disease: A Caregiver's Complete Reference**
Ruth M Tappen, author
Health Professions Press
PO Box 10624 410-337-9585
Baltimore, MD 21285-0624 888-337-8808
Fax: 410-337-8539
www.healthpropress.com

For professionals who plan, administer or provide services to Alzheimer's patients.
256 pages Paperback
ISBN: 1-878812-39-4

914 **Key Elements of Dementia Care**
Alzheimer's Association
225 North Michigan Avenue
Chicago, IL 60611-1696 800-272-3900
Fax: 866-699-1246
TDD: 312-355-8700
e-mail: media@alz.org
www.alz.org

Defines, describes, and illustrates dementia-capable care throughout the range of residential care settings.
1997 90 pages

915 **Nursing Home and You: Partners in Caring for a Relative with Alzheimer's Disease**
American Assn. of Homes & Services for the Aging
901 E Street NW 202-783-2242
Washington, DC 20004-2037 800-508-9442
Fax: 202-783-2255

Offers suggestions for families of nursing home residents on how to work with staff to foster smooth transitions.
32 pages

916 **Occupational Therapy Practice Guidelines for Adults with Alzheimer's Disease**
American Occupational Therapy Association
4720 Montgomery Lane 301-652-2682
Bethesda, MD 20824-1220 Fax: 301-652-7711
TDD: 800-377-8555
www.aota.org

21 pages
ISBN: 1-569001-46-4

917 **Positive Interactions Program of Activities for People with Alzheimer's**
Sylvia Nissenboim, author
Health Professions Press
PO Box 10624 410-337-9585
Baltimore, MD 21285-0624 888-337-8808
Fax: 410-337-8539
www.healthpropress.com

All interactions focus on preventing individual dignity and providing opportunities to experience meaningful involvement and satisfaction. Works in a variety of settings and promotes the OBRA quality of care guidelines.
176 pages 1997
ISBN: 1-878812-40-8
Christine Vroman, Editor

918 **Rethinking Alzheimer's Care**
Sam Fazio, Dorothy Seman, author
Health Professions Press
PO Box 10624 410-337-9585
Baltimore, MD 21285-0624 888-337-8808
Fax: 410-337-8539
www.healthpropress.com

Appropriate for all settings providing long-term care, adult day services, or assisted living, this fresh and humanistic approach to Alzheimer's care will encourage caregivers to rethink the disease experience and explore its possibilities, instead of its limitations.
200 pages Paperback
ISBN: 1-878812-62-9
Jane Stansell, Editor

919 **Speaking Our Minds: Personal Reflections from Individuals with Alzheimer's**
WH Freeman and Company
41 Madison Avenue 212-576-9400
New York, NY 10010 888-330-8477
Fax: 212-689-2383
www.whfreeman.com/generalreaders

Personal reflections of people with Alzheimer's disease.
161 pages Hardcover
ISBN: 0-716732-24-6

920 **The Comfort of Home for Alheimer's Disease A Guide for Caregivers**
M. Meyer, M. Mittelman, P. Derr, C. Epstein, author
CareTrust Publications LLC
PO Box 10283
Portland, OR 97296-0283 800-565-1533
Fax: 415-673-2005
e-mail: sales@comfortofhome.com
www.comfortofhome.com

Walks readers through all Alzheimer's stages and cover the basics from undertanding the difference between AD and normal aging, to coping with the behavioral symptoms that come with the diminishing reasoning skills. Additionaly, Comfort talks about how to provide safe physical care around other medical conditions the Alzheimer's sufferer may have, due to normal aging. Not the least of all, Comfort provides self-care tips for the caregivers to remain emotionally and mentally healthy.
2008 288 pages
ISBN: 0-978790-30-8

921 **Therapeutic Interventions in Alzheimer's**
Aspen Publishers
7201 McKinney Circle 301-698-7100
Frederick, MD 21705-0990 800-638-8437
Fax: 301-695-7931
e-mail: customerservice@aspenpub.com
www.aspenpub.com

A program of functional skills for activities of daily living.
197 pages

922 **Time for Alzheimer's: A True Story**
Emerald Ink Publishing
7141 Office City Drive
Houston, TX 77087-3722 800-324-5663
www.emeraldink.com

Based on the author's personal experience in caring for her mother.
139 pages
ISBN: 1-885373-13-3

923 **Understanding Alzheimer's Disease**
University Press of Mississippi
3825 Ridgewood Road 601-432-6205
Jackson, MS 39211-6492 Fax: 601-432-6217
e-mail: press@ihl.state.ms.us
www.upress.state.ms.us
Aimed at people with Alzheimer's, family members, caregivers, health care and human service professionals. Describes Alzheimer's from early to advanced stages. Discusses the care of AD patients, ideas to help families care for the AD patient at home, reviews treatements for the psychiatric, behavioral and cognitive effects of AD and describes research efforts to better understand AD and develop effective therapies. Price $28 Hardcover, $12 Paperback.
1996 150 pages
ISBN: 0-878059-11-3
Kathy Burgess, Advertising/Marketing Services Manager

924 **When We Become the Parent to Our Parents**
MEA Productions
55 Binks Hill Road 603-536-2641
Plymouth, NH 03264 Fax: 603-536-4851
e-mail: me.allen@juno.com
www.maryemmallen.blogspot.com
Experiences of a woman who cared for her mother and aunt, both Alzheimer's patients.
62 pages
ISBN: 0-965167-51-8
Mary Emma Allen, Author

Children's Books

925 **Grandpa Doesn't Know It's Me**
Donna Guthrie, author
Alzheimer's Association
225 North Michigan Avenue
Chicago, IL 60611-1696 800-272-3900
Fax: 866-699-1246
TDD: 312-335-8700
e-mail: media@alz.org
www.alz.org
Geared to the concerns of a young child who has a relative with Alzheimer's disease.
26 pages

926 **Grandpa's Music: A Story About Alzheimer's**
Alison Acheson, author
Albert Whitman & Company
6340 Oakton Street 847-581-0033
Morton Grove, IL 60053-2723 800-255-7675
Fax: 847-581-0039
e-mail: mail@whitmanco.com
www.albertwhitman.com
Children's book using text and illustrations to show the effects of Alzheimer's disease.

ISBN: 0-807530-52-8
Pat McPartland, Sales
Joe Campbell, Customer Service

927 **Just for Children: Helping You Understand Alzheimer's Disease**
Alzheimer's Association
225 North Michigan Avenue
Chicago, IL 60611-1676 800-272-3900
Fax: 866-699-1246
TDD: 312-335-8700
e-mail: media@alz.org
www.alz.org
Information about Alzheimer's disease written especially for children.
1997 2 pages Pack of 100

928 **Let's Talk About When Someone You Love Has Alzheimer's Disease**
Rosen Publishing Group's PowerKids Press
29 E 21st Street 212-777-3017
New York, NY 10010 800-237-9932
Fax: 888-436-4643
e-mail: customerservice@rosenpub.com
www.rosenpublishing.com
This book sensitively helps children cope with this unsettling disease.

ISBN: 0-823923-06-1
Elizabeth Weitzman, Author

929 **Through Tara's Eyes: Helping Children Cope with Alzheimer's Disease**
American Health Assistance Foundation
15825 Shady Grove Road 301-948-3244
Rockville, MD 20850 800-437-2423
Fax: 301-258-9454
www.ahaf.org
Told from the perspective of Tara who has a grandmother with Alzheimer's disease but does not know anything is wrong with her grandmother.
36 pages

930 **What's Wrong with Grandma? A Family Experience with Alzheimer's**
Margaret Shawver, author
Prometheus Books
59 John Glenn Drive 716-691-0133
Amherst, NY 14228-2197 800-421-0351
Fax: 716-691-0137
e-mail: marketing@prometheusbooks.com
www.prometheusbooks.com
The story of a family's struggle with Alzheimer's disease as told by the youngest child.
62 pages Paperback
ISBN: 1-159011-74-2
Lisa Risio, Marketing Production Manager

931 **Window of Time**
Associated Publishers Group
1501 Country Hospital Road 615-254-2450
Nashville, TN 37218 800-327-5113
Fax: 615-254-2405
e-mail: vlill@apgbooks.com
www.apgbooks.com
Illustrated book about the relationship between a grandfather with Alzheimer's and his grandson.
28 pages
ISBN: 0-963633-51-1

Magazines

932 **Alzheimer Disease and Associated Disorders: An International Journal**
Raven Press
1185 Avenue of the Americas 212-930-9500
New York, NY 10036-2601 800-777-2295
A leading international forum for reports of new research findings and new approaches to diagnosis and treatments. Contributions are offered from all scientific and medical fields.
Quarterly
ISBN: 0-89303H- -
Peter J Whitehouse

933 **Mature Health**
Haymarket Group, Ltd.
45 W 34th Street 212-239-0855
New York, NY 10001-3073
Magazine featuring articles on health aspects of aging, as well as articles on recreation and leisure.

934 **Research & Practice**
Alzheimer's Association

225 North Michigan Avenue
Chicago, IL 60611-1696 800-272-3900
Fax: 866-699-1246
TDD: 312-335-8700
e-mail: media@alz.org
www.alz.org

Provides practical information for healthcare professionals on the current status of prominent areas of Alzheimer research.
Quarterly
ISBN: 2-909342-84-0

Newsletters

935 **Advances: Progress in Alzheimer Research and Care**
Alzheimer's Association
225 North Michigan Avenue
Chicago, IL 60611-1696 800-272-3900
Fax: 866-699-1246
TDD: 312-335-8700
e-mail: media@alz.org
www.alz.org

Provides information related to research and caregiving.
Quarterly

936 **Aging and Alzheimer's Disease Center Newsletter**
Oregon Health Sciences University
3181 SW Sam Jackson Park Road 503-494-6976
Portland, OR 97201-3098 Fax: 503-494-7499
e-mail: kaye@ohsu.edu
www.ohsu.edu/som-alzheimers

Researches causes and consequences of Alzheimer's disease and ways of clinical services.
2x Year
Jeffrey Kaye, Director

937 **Alzheimer Disease and Associated Disorders**
Lippincott Williams & Wilkins
PO Box 1600
Hagerstown, MD 21741-1600 800-638-3030
Fax: 301-223-2400
e-mail: orders@lww.com
www.lww.com

A leading international forum for reports of new research findings and new approaches to diagnosis and treatment.
Quarterly Journal

938 **Alzheimer's Association: Tarrant County Chapter**
101 Summit Avenue 817-336-4949
Fort Worth, TX 76102 800-471-4422
Fax: 817-336-4966
www.alz.org/northcentraltexas

Newsletter for those afflicted with Alzheimer's disease. Includes education, support groups, case management, telephone helpline and referral to services (i.e. long term care, adult daycare, medical assistance, legal assistance, etc.).
8 pages
Theresa Hocker, Executive Director
Susanna Luk-Jones, Director Services

939 **LIAFLine Newsletter**
Long Island Alzheimers Foundation
5 Channel Drive 516-767-6856
Port Washington, NY Fax: 516-767-6864
e-mail: info@liaf.org
www.liaf.org

It is intended for caregivers, service providers and anyone interested in Alzheimer's Disease or the Foundation.
Pattie Gallatin, Executive Director

Pamphlets

940 **10 Warning Signs of Alzheimer's Disease**
Alzheimer's Association
225 North Michigan Avenue
Chicago, IL 60611-1696 800-272-3900
Fax: 866-699-1246
TDD: 312-335-8700
e-mail: media@alz.org
www.alz.org

Contains a list of symptoms and answers to the most frequently asked questions.
Pack of 100

941 **10 Ways to Help a Family Living with Alzheimer's**
Alzheimer's Association
225 North Michigan Avenue
Chicago, IL 60611-1696 800-272-3900
Fax: 866-669-1246
TDD: 312-335-8700
e-mail: media@alz.org
www.alz.org

Information specifically for friends, explaining how Alzheimer's disease affects the entire family and suggesting practical ways to assist.
1995 Pack of 100

942 **Activities at Home: Planning the Day for the Person with Dementia**
Alzheimer's Association
225 North Michigan Avenue
Chicago, IL 60611-1696 800-272-3900
Fax: 866-669-1246
TDD: 312-335-8700
e-mail: media@alz.org
www.alz.org

Guides the caregiver in planning meaningful activities for the person with dementia.
Pack of 100

943 **Alzheimer's Advocates Guide**
Alzheimer's Association
225 North Michigan Avenue
Chicago, IL 60611-1696 800-272-3900
Fax: 866-699-1246
TDD: 312-335-8700
e-mail: media@alz.org
www.alz.org

Guide for the individual advocate, offering tips in letter writing, meeting with public officials and getting results.
1993-present

944 **Alzheimer's Association National Brochure**
Alzheimer's Association
225 North Michigan Avenue
Chicago, IL 60611-1696 800-272-3900
Fax: 866-699-1246
TDD: 312-335-8700
e-mail: media@alz.org
www.alz.org

Describes the Alzheimer's Association and its services.
Pack of 100

945 **Alzheimer's Disease**
National Institutes of Health
5600 Fishers Lane
Rockville, MD 20857-0001 301-468-2600
www.nih.gov

Contains information on the diagnosis and treatment of Alzheimer's and on research that offers hope for the future. Included is a list of sources of help for both the patient and the family.

946 **Alzheimer's Disease: An Overview**
Alzheimer's Association
225 North Michigan Avenue
Chicago, IL 60611-1696 800-272-3900
Fax: 866-699-1246
TDD: 312-335-8700
e-mail: media@alz.org
www.alz.org

Basic facts on Alzheimer's disease.

947 **Alzheimer's Disease: Services You May Need**
Alzheimer's Association

225 North Michigan Avenue
Chicago, IL 60611-1696
800-272-3900
Fax: 866-699-1246
TDD: 312-335-8700
e-mail: media@alz.org
www.alz.org

Guide to services available to Alzheimer's disease caregivers.
Pack of 100

948 **Alzheimer's Disease: Statistics**
Alzheimer's Association
225 North Michigan Avenue
Chicago, IL 60611-1696
800-272-3900
Fax: 866-699-1246
TDD: 312-335-8700
e-mail: media@alz.org
www.alz.org

Indicates basic information on incidence, prevalence, cost of care, etc.
Pack of 100

949 **Caregiver Stress**
Alzheimer's Association
225 North Michigan Avenue
Chicago, IL 60611-1696
800-272-3900
Fax: 866-699-1246
TDD: 312-335-8700
e-mail: media@alz.org
www.alz.org

Learn to recognize the warning signs and discover techniques for reducing stress.
Pack of 100

950 **Caring for Alzheimer's Patients**
Human Sciences Press
233 Spring Street
New York, NY 10013-1522
212-620-8000
800-221-9369

This handbook is designed for families, friends, and health-care professionals coping with the myriad of problems encountered by those afflicted with Alzheimer's disease.
308 pages Cloth

951 **Ethical Considerations: Issues in Diagnostic Disclosure**
Alzheimer's Association
225 North Michigan Avenue
Chicago, IL 60611-1696
800-272-3900
Fax: 866-699-1246
TDD: 312-335-8700
e-mail: media@alz.org
www.alz.org

Discusses the individual's right to know the Alzheimer's diagnosis. Provides tips on disclosing the diagnosis and communicating with family members.
Pack of 100

952 **Family Guide for Alzheimer's Care in Residential Settings**
Alzheimer's Association
225 North Michigan Avenue
Chicago, IL 60611-1696
800-272-3900
Fax: 866-699-1246
TDD: 312-335-8700
e-mail: media@alz.org
www.alz.org

This guide for families corresponds to Guidelines for Dignity which can be used as a companion resource. It provides 50 checkpoints for families to consider as they plan for long-term residential care for their Alzheimer/dementia patient. A checklist to use in evaluating residential settings is included.
1992 40 pages

953 **Guidelines for Dignity**
Alzheimer's Association
225 North Michigan Avenue
Chicago, IL 60611-1696
800-272-3900
Fax: 866-699-1246
TDD: 312-335-8700
e-mail: media@alz.org
www.alz.org

A resource for providers who are offerring Alzheimer/dementia care in residential settings. Eight goals target specific issues to be addressed and present practical ideas and advice. This resource for facility professionals corresponds tp the Family Guide fpr Alzheimer Care in Residential Settings, whichi can be used as a companion resource.
1992

954 **Helping Children and Teens Understand Alzheimer's Disease: A Guide for Parents**
Alzheimer's Association
225 North Michigan Avenue
Chicago, IL 60611-1696
800-272-3900
Fax: 866-699-1246
TDD: 312-335-8700
e-mail: media@alz.org
www.alz.org

Provides parents with ways to help children and teens cope when someone close to them is diagnosed with Alzheimer's disease.
Pack of 100

955 **Home Safety for the Alzheimer's Patient**
Alzheimer's Disease Education & Referral Center
PO Box 8250
Silver Spring, MD 20908-8250
800-438-4380
Fax: 301-495-3334
e-mail: adear@alzheimers.org
www.alzheimers.org

Practical guide for those who provide in-home care to people with Alzheimer's disease or related disorders. Designed to improve home safety and identify problems and solutions to prevent accidents. Increases the patient's security and freedom.
32 pages

956 **If You Have Alzheimer's Disease: What You Should Know, What You Should Do**
Alzheimer's Association
225 North Michigan Avenue
Chicago, IL 60611-1696
800-272-3900
Fax: 866-699-1246
TDD: 312-335-8700
e-mail: media@alz.org
www.alz.org

Guide for the person with Alzheimer's disease. Includes suggestions of things to do that will help the person cope.
1994 Pack of 100

957 **Just for Teens: Helping You Understand Alzheimer's Disease**
Alzheimer's Association
225 North Michigan Avenue
Chicago, IL 60611-1696
800-272-3900
Fax: 866-699-1246
TDD: 312-335-8700
e-mail: media@alz.org
www.alz.org

Information about Alzheimer's disease aimed at teenagers.
Pack of 100

958 **Late Stage Care**
Alzheimer's Association
225 North Michigan Avenue
Chicago, IL 60611-1696
800-272-3900
Fax: 866-699-1246
TDD: 312-335-8700
e-mail: media@alz.org
www.alz.org

Suggestions for coping with caregiving problems that commonly occur late in the progression of Alzheimer's disease.
Pack of 100

959 **National Public Policy Program to Conquer Alzheimer's Disease**
Alzheimer's Association
225 North Michigan Avenue
Chicago, IL 60611-1676
800-272-3900
Fax: 866-699-1246
TDD: 312-335-8700
e-mail: media@alz.org
www.alz.org

Summary of the Association's public policy goals, objectives and policies.
1997-Present 12 pages

960 **Nutrition Screening Initiative**
Nutrition Screening Initiative
2626 Pennsylvania Avenue NW 202-625-1662
Washington, DC 20037-1618 e-mail: nsi@gmmb.com
www.cafp.org
Offers information on nutrition pertaining to older Americans and illnesses such as Alzheimer's disease.

961 **Report of the Panel on Alzheimer's Disease**
National Clearinghouse for Alcohol and Drug Abuse
PO Box 2345
Rockville, MD 20857 800-729-6686
www.health.org
52 pages

962 **Respite Care Guide: How to Find What's Right for You**
Alzheimer's Association
225 North Michigan Avenue
Chicago, IL 60611-1696 800-272-3900
Fax: 866-699-1246
TDD: 312-335-8700
e-mail: media@alz.org
www.alz.org
Designed to help caregivers and persons with dementia recognize the benefits of respite care as well as identify which respite care services will best meet their needs.
1995 18 pages

963 **Safe Return Brochure**
Alzheimer's Association
225 North Michigan Avevnue
Chicago, IL 60611-1696 800-272-3900
Fax: 866-699-1246
TDD: 312-335-8700
e-mail: media@alz.org
www.alz.org
General information on the Safe Return program. Includes the registration form.
Pack of 100

964 **Steps to Diagnosis**
Alzheimer's Association
225 North Michigan Avenue
Chicago, IL 60611-1696 800-272-3900
Fax: 866-699-1246
TDD: 312-335-8700
e-mail: media@alz.org
www.alz.org
Educates individuals and their families on the importance of seeking a diagnosis, and the various test completed to obtain an accurate diagnosis.

965 **Steps to Enhancing Communication**
Alzheimer's Association
225 North Michigan Avenue
Chicago, IL 60611-1696 800-272-3900
Fax: 866-699-1246
TDD: 312-335-8700
e-mail: media@alz.org
www.alz.org
Offers caregivers techniques for improving their approach to listening to and communication with the individual with Alzheimer's disease.
1996 Pack of 100

966 **Taxes and Alzheimer's Disease**
Alzheimer's Association
225 North Michigan Avenue
Chicago, IL 60611-1696 800-272-3900
Fax: 866-669-1246
TDD: 312-335-8700
e-mail: media@alz.org
www.alz.org
A series of three consumer education brochures about tax issues that may affect people with Alzheimer's and their families. Address the household and dependent care credit, federal employment taxes, and the itemized deduction for medical expenses. Also includes a preliminary explanation of the medical deduction for long-term care expenses clarified by the Kassebaum-Kennedy health insurance law.
1997

967 **Terms & Tips: An Alzheimer Care Handbook**
Marjorie Brandenburg, author
Alzheimer's Association
225 North Michigan Avenue
Chicago, IL 60611-1696 800-272-3900
Fax: 866-699-1246
TDD: 312-335-8700
e-mail: media@alz.org
www.alz.org
Offers an explanation for over 250 terms and offers practical caregiver ideas and tips. Primarily for people with dementia and their caregivers, family members, and all providers of hands-on assistance.
1995 84 pages

968 **Useful Information on Alzheimer's Disease**
National Clearinghouse for Alcohol and Drug Abuse
PO Box 2345
Rockville, MD 20857-0001 800-729-6686
e-mail: www.webmaster@health.org
www.health.org
24 pages

969 **You Are One of Us: Clergy/Church Connections to Alzheimer Families**
Alzheimer's Disease Education & Referral Center
PO Box 8250 301-495-3311
Silver Spring, MD 20907-8250 800-438-4380
Fax: 301-495-3334
www.alzheimers.org
Describes how clergy and church members can help families by including patients and their relatives in church activities, visiting patients and developing church programs that support family caregivers.

Audio & Video

970 **Alzheimer's Association Caregiver Resource s**
Alzheimer's Association
Western/Central Washington Chapter 206-363-5500
Seattle, WA 98125 800-848-7097
Fax: 206-363-5700
e-mail: rowena.rye@alz.org
http://alzwa.org/resources6.htm
A variety of numerous resources, materials and publications providing information for assisting those with Alzheimer's Disease including a documentation guide, informational fact sheets on topics such as bathing, dressing, eating and dealing with grief, in addition resources on long term care options and a newsletter.
Nancy Dapper, Executive Director
Rowena Rye, Community Resources

971 **Alzheimer's Association Dementia Care Conf erence**
Alzheimer's Association
225 North Michigan Avenue 312-335-5790
Chicago, IL 60601-7633 800-272-3900
Fax: 866-699-1246
TDD: 312-335-8700
e-mail: careconference@alz.org
www.alz.org/careconference/
Selected sessions from the conference discussing topics such as assisted living preconference, sexuality, intimacy and lifestyle changes, and activity intensive changing approaches to Alzheimer care.
Marisol Sukhu, Hotel/Events Information
Sheryl Trotz, Continuing Education & Presentations

972 **Alzheimer's Association Safe Return Police Training Video**
Alzheimer's Association Massachusetts Chapter
311 Arsenal Street 617-868-6718
Watertown, MA 02472 800-548-2111
Fax: 617-868-6720
e-mail: communications@alzmass.org
www.alzmass.org/

An educational package designed to help police officers recognize and respond appropriately to Alzheimer patients who may need assistance. Kit includes 1 videotape and 3 print pieces.
James Wessler, President/Chief Executive Officer
Betsy Fitzgerald, Director of Communications

973 **Alzheimer's Association: Waves of Stone Vi deo and Documentary**
Alzheimer's Association Rhode Island Chapter
245 Waterman Street 401-421-3900
Providence, RI 02906 800-272-3900
Fax: 401-421-0115
e-mail: info@alz.org
http://www.alz-ri.org/Videoshtm.htm
PBS documentary on Alzheimer's disease that discusses both scientific research and caregiver issues.
1994 57 minutes
Elizabeth Morancy, Executive Director
Rita St Pierre, Program Director

974 **Another Home for Mom**
Lori Hope, author
Fanlight Productions
4196 Washington Street 617-469-4999
Boston, MA 02131-1731 800-937-4113
Fax: 617-469-3379
e-mail: fanlight@fanlight.com
www.fanlight.com
A gentle documentary following one couple as they confront the decision of whether to place the husbands mother, who has Alzheimer's disease, in a nursing home.
1989 27 Minutes
ISBN: 1-572950-77-3

975 **Caring...Sharing: The Alzheimer's Caregiver**
Fanflight Productions
47 Halifax Street 617-469-4949
Boston, MA 02130 800-937-4113
Fax: 617-469-3379
e-mail: fanlight@fanflight.com
www.fanlight.com
Examines what it means to be a caregiver. This program will be invaluable for any person or group involved in the care of the elderly.
38 minutes
ISBN: 1-572951-22-2

976 **For Those Who Take Care: An Alzheimer's Disease Training Program for Nurses**
Alzheimer's Disease Education & Referral Center
PO Box 8250 301-495-3311
Silver Spring, MD 20907-8250 800-438-4380
Fax: 301-495-3334
www.alzheimers.org
Guide for training nursing assistants and nurses' aides in long term care facilities, adult day care and private homes. Manual, text and student handouts. Produced by the University of Kentucky.

Web Sites

977 **Alzheimer Research Forum**
www.alzforum.org
Founded as an independent, non-profit organization to create an online scientific community dedicated to developing treatments and preventions for Alzheimer's disease.

978 **Alzheimer Support**
www.alzheimersupport.com
Serves Alzheimer's sufferers and their loved ones by reporting the latest news in research and treatment, making hard-to-find, recommended nutritional supplements available at manufacturer-direct low prices, and, most importantly, donating profits from each purchase to fund Alzheimer's medical research.

979 **Alzheimer's Disease International**
www.alz.co.uk/adi
Trying to improve the quality of life for people with dimentia and their families. Facilitating the sharing of expertise and resources that exist within the membership community.

980 **Caring for Persons with Alzheimer's**
www.alz.org
Provides guidance and support for caregivers of those with Alzheimer's.

981 **Healing Well**
www.healingwell.com
An online health resource guide to medical news, chat, information and articles, newsgroups and message boards, books, disease-related web sites, medical directories, and more for patients, friends, and family coping with disabling diseases, disorders, or chronic illnesses.

982 **Health Finder**
www.healthfinder.gov
Searchable, carefully developed web site offering information on over 1000 topics. Developed by the US Department of Health and Human Services, the site can be used in both English and Spanish.

983 **Healthlink USA**
www.healthlinkusa.com
Health information concerning treatment, cures, prevention, diagnosis, risk factors, research, support groups, email lists, personal stories and much more. Updated regularly.

984 **Helios Health**
www.helioshealth.com
Online resource for your health information. Detailed information about specific health topics, access to expert advice from our Medical Advisory Board, and up-to-date health news.

985 **MEDLINEplus Health Information**
www.nlm.nih.gov/medlineplus
MedlinePlus has extensive information from the National Institutes of Health and other trusted sources on over 700 diseases and conditions.

986 **MedicineNet**
www.medicinenet.com
An online resource for consumers providing easy-to-read, authoritative medical and health information.

987 **Medscape**
www.mywebmd.com
Medscape offers specialists, primary care physicians, and other health professionals the Web's most robust and integrated medical information and educational tools.

988 **Neurology Channel**
www.neurologychannel.com
Find clearly explained, medically accurate information regarding conditions, including an overview, symptoms, causes, diagnostic procedures and treatment options. On this site it is possible to ask questions and get information from a neurologist and connect to people who have similar health interests.

989 **WebMD**
www.webmd.com
Information on Alzheimer's disease, including articles and resources.

Description

990 **Amyotrophic Lateral Sclerosis**

Amyotrophic Lateral Sclerosis, ALS, also called Lou Gehrig's disease, is a neurological disorder that affects the motor nerves in the brain and spinal cord. The cause of ALS is unknown. It is marked by progressive muscle weakness.

Initial symptoms may be subtle, but early signs of ALS can include twitching and cramping of muscles (particularly in the hands and feet), as well as difficulty in swallowing. As the disorder progresses, use of legs and arms, breathing, speaking, and swallowing become increasingly difficult.

Although the physical symptoms of ALS are most debilitating, the disease does not seem to impair intellectual functioning, although recent research indicates a significant number of people with ALS who have cognitive defects. Voluntary eye movement (blinking) and the senses also remain unaffected.

Currently, there is no cure for ALS. A regime of physical therapy and psychological support can help patients and their families.

National Agencies & Associations

991 **ALS Association National Office**
27001 Agoura Road 818-880-9007
Calabasas Hills, CA 91301-5104 800-782-4747
Fax: 818-880-9006
e-mail: alsinfo@alsa-national.org
www.alsa.org
National nonprofit voluntary health organization dedicated solely to the fight against amytrophic lateral sclerosis. Its mission: to find a cure for and improve living with ALS. The four fronts of battle are: encouraging identifying funding and monitori
Jane H Gilbert, President/CEO
Lucie Bruijn PhD, SVPresident of Research and Development

State Agencies & Associations

Arizona

992 **Arizona Chapter of the ALS Association**
4643 E Thomas Road 602-297-3800
Phoenix, AZ 85018 866-350-2572
Fax: 602-297-3804
e-mail: ken@alsaz.org
webaz.alsa.org
This chapter provides newsletters and other information to help patients and their families find sources of supplie, referrals or counseling as needed. Provides monthly support meetings, public awareness information and fundraising.
Ken Brissa, President
Elayne Achilles, President Elect/Executive Director

California

993 **ALS Association: Bay Area Chapter**
565 Commercial Street 415-904-2572
San Francisco, CA 94111 800-209-0433
Fax: 415-904-2573
e-mail: fightALS@alsabayarea.org
webaz.alsa.org
ALS Association chapters are multifaceted grass roots organizations that carry out ALSA's mission and strategic goals at the community level. The chapter, with supporting services from the national office, actively pursues the association's goals.
Fred Fisher, Executive Director
Madelon M Thomson, Director Patient/Family Services

994 **ALS Association: Greater Los Angeles Chapter**
28720 Roadside Drive 818-865-8067
Agoura Hills, CA 91301 866-750-2572
Fax: 818-865-8066
e-mail: info@alsala.org
www.alsala.org
ALS Association chapters are multifaceted grass-roots organizations that carry out ALSA's mission and strategic goals at the community level. The chapter — with supporting services from the National Office — actively pursues the Association's goals.
Fred Fisher, President and Chief Executive Officer
Lance Keene, Vice President of Development

995 **ALS Association: Greater Sacramento Chapter**
2717 Cottage Way 916-979-9265
Sacramento, CA 95825 Fax: 916-979-9271
e-mail: lou@alssac.org
www.alssac.org
ALS Association chapters are multifaceted grass roots organizations that carry out ALSA's mission and strategic goals at the community level. The chapter, with supporting services from the national office, actively pursues the association's goals.
Sandie Fredericks, President
Sean South, Vice President

996 **ALS Association: Greater San Diego CIO**
7920 Silverton 858-271-5547
San Diego, CA 92126-6350 Fax: 858-271-5687
e-mail: info@alsasd.com
www.alsasd.com
ALS Association chapters are multifaceted grass-roots organizations that carry out ALSA's mission and strategic goals at the community level. The chapter — with supporting services from the National Office — actively pursues the Association's goals.
Don Casey, Chairman
Jane Mitchell, Vice Chairman

997 **Orange County Chapter of the ALS Association**
1232 Village Way 714-285-1088
Santa Ana, CA 92705-2334 Fax: 714-285-0305
e-mail: information@alsaoc.org
weboc.alsa.org
Provides information to ALS patients families and caregivers; offers support groups, information and referrals, a loan closet and public awareness information.
Mark Hershey, President
Chad Kessler, Vice President

Colorado

998 **ALS Association: Rocky Mountain Chapter**
1201 E Colfax Avenue 303-832-2322
Denver, CO 80218 866-ALS-3211
Fax: 303-832-3365
e-mail: info@alsaco.org
www.alscolorado.org
The ALS Association chapters are multifaceted grass-roots organizations that carry out ALSA's mission and strategic goals at the community level. The chapter — with supporting services from the National Office — actively pursues the Association's goals.
Pam Rush-Negri, Executive Director
Leslie Ryan, Patient Services Director

Connecticut

999 **Connecticut Chapter of the ALS Association**
4 Oxford Road 203-874-5050
Milford, CT 06460 877-257-2281
Fax: 203-874-7070
e-mail: als.assoc@snet.net
www.alsact.org
The central source in Connecticut for services and education of ALS patients, families and caregivers. Provides ALS patients with information concerning medical care and facilities, support groups, daily living aids and other services.

District of Columbia

1000 **ALS Association: National Capital Area Chapter**
7507 Standish Place 301-978-9855
Rockville, MD 20855 Fax: 301-978-9854
e-mail: info@ALSinfo.org
www.alsinfo.org

Offers patient referrals, informational newsletters and brochures, patient support groups and meetings and fund raising for research into finding cures and treatments for ALS.
Colette Pond, Development Associate
Cathy Easter, Regional Director

Florida

1001 **ALS Association: Florida Chapter**
3242 Parkside Center Circle 813-637-9000
Tampa, FL 33619 888-257-1717
Fax: 813-637-9010
e-mail: cbright@als-florida.org
webfl.alsa.org

ALS Association chapters are multifaceted grass-roots organizations that carry out ALSA's mission and strategic goals at the community level. The chapter — with supporting services from the National Office — actively pursues the Association's goals.
Dara Alexander, President
Christine Br MSW, Care Coordinator - Southwest Florida

1002 **ALS Association: Florida Chapter East Coast Regional Office**
5005 W Laurel Street 813-637-9000
Tampa, FL 33607 888-257-1717
Fax: 813-637-9010
e-mail: office@als-florida.org
webfl.alsa.org

ALS Association chapters are multifaceted grass-roots organizations that carry out ALSA's mission and strategic goals at the community level. The chapter — with supporting services from the National Office — actively pursues the Association's goals.
Dara Alexander, President
Christine Br MSW, Care Coordinator - Southwest Florida

Georgia

1003 **ALS Association of Georgia**
1955 Cliff Valley Way 404-636-9909
Atlanta, GA 30329 888-636-9940
Fax: 404-636-9949
e-mail: info@alsaga.org
www.alsaga.org

Offers meetings, local support groups, patient support equipment loan and research for persons suffering from ALS.
Candace Wood, Executive Director
Liz Bohling, Patient Services Provider

Illinois

1004 **Lois Insolia ALS Center at Northwestern Me morial Hospital**
5550 West Touhyu 847-679-3311
Skokie, IL 60077 888-ALS-1107
Fax: 847-679-9109
e-mail: info@lesturnerals.org
www.lesturnerals.org

Utilizes a multidisciplinary approach in treating ALS. Trained specialists provide diagnostic, rehabilitative and supportive services that focus on assessment, care planning and education. Patients and loved ones are encouraged to attend the support groups offered. Provides in-home visits by ALS nurse consultants and social worker, support groups, a lending bank of equipment, and grant programs for financial aid.
Teepu Siddique MD, Director

Indiana

1005 **ALS Association: Indiana Chapter**
6525 E 82nd Street 317-915-9888
Indianapolis, IN 46250 888-508-3232
Fax: 317-573-9889
e-mail: jlewellen@alsaindiana.org
webin.alsa.org

ALS Association chapters are multifaceted grass-roots organizations that carry out ALSA's mission and strategic goals at the community level. The chapter — with supporting services from the National Office — actively pursues the Association's goals.
Jennifer Lewellen, Executive Director
Suzanne Cox, Director of Patient Services

Kansas

1006 **ALS Association: Keith Worthington Chapter**
8340 Mission Road 913-648-2062
Prairie Village, KS 66206 800-878-2062
Fax: 913-642-2431
e-mail: bcooper@alsa-midwest.org
www.alsa-midwest.org

ALS Association chapters are multifaceted grass-roots organizations that carry out ALSA's mission and strategic goals at the community level. The chapter — with supporting services from the National Office — actively pursues the Association's goals.
Beckie Cooper, Executive Director

1007 **ALS Association: Keith Worthington Chapter Central/Western Kansas Branch**
526 South Market 316-612-0188
Wichita, KS 67202 800-878-2062
Fax: 316-612-8768
e-mail: kwille@alsa-midwest.org
www.alsa-midwest.org

ALS Association chapters are multifaceted grass-roots organizations that carry out ALSA's mission and strategic goals at the community level. The chapter — with supporting services from the National Office — actively pursues the Association's goals.
Kathleen Willie, Awareness and Development

Kentucky

1008 **ALS Association: Kentucky CIO**
2375 Fortune Drive 859-294-0223
Lexington, KY 40555 800-406-7702
Fax: 859-294-0591
e-mail: alskyjenny@yahoo.com
webky.alsa.org

ALS Association chapters are multifaceted grass-roots organizations that carry out ALSA's mission and strategic goals at the community level. The chapter — with supporting services from the National Office — actively pursues the Association's goals.
Jenny Allen, Director Development & Administration
Jean Hale, Services Staff

Massachusetts

1009 **ALS Association: Massachusetts Chapter, Wakefield Office**
7 Lincoln Street 781-245-2133
Wakefield, MA 01880-3021 800-258-3323
Fax: 781-245-5414
e-mail: info@als-ma.org
www.als-ma.org

Offers informational brochures and newsletters to promote public awareness, support groups and meetings for patients and their families, and referral information for members in the Massachusetts area.
Rick J Arrowood

Michigan

1010 **ALS Association: Michigan Chapter**
24359 Northwestern Highway 648-354-6100
Southfield, MI 48075 800-882-5764
Fax: 248-354-6440
e-mail: sueb@alsofmi.org
www.alsofmichigan.org

ALS Association chapters are multi-faceted grass-roots organizations that carry out ALSA's mission. and strategic goals at the community level. The chapter — with supporting services from the National Office — actively pursues the Association's goals.
Sue Burstein-Kahn, Executive Director
Lisa Alteri, President

1011 ALS Association: West Michigan Chapter
678 Front Street 616-459-1900
Grand Rapids, MI 49504 800-387-7121
Fax: 616-459-4522
e-mail: stacey@alsa-michigan.org
webmi.alsa.org

ALS Association chapters are multi-faceted grass-roots organizations that carry out ALSA's mission. and strategic goals at the community level. The chapter — with supporting services from the National Office — actively pursues the Association's goals.
Stacey Orsted, Executive Director
Katee Stahl, Administrative Assistant

Minnesota

1012 ALS Association: Minnesota Chapter
333 N Washington Avenue 612-672-0484
Minneapolis, MN 55401 888-672-0484
Fax: 612-672-9110
e-mail: info@alsmn.org
webmi.alsa.org

ALS Association chapters are multifaceted grass-roots organizations that carry out ALSA's mission and strategic goals at the community level. The chapter — with supporting services from the National Office — actively pursues the Association's goals.
Rebecca Ayaz, Development Director
Sandy Judge, Development Director

Missouri

1013 ALS Association: Keith Worthington Chapter Central Missouri Branch Office
1721 West Elfindale 417-886-5003
Springfield, MO 65807 888-386-1200
Fax: 417-886-5003
e-mail: pblackwell@alsa-midwest.org
www.alsa-midwest.org

ALS Association chapters are multifaceted grass-roots organizations that carry out ALSA's mission and strategic goals at the community level. The chapter — with supporting services from the National Office — actively pursues the Association's goals.
Paul Blackwell, Services Staff
Valerie Gustin, Awareness and Development

1014 ALS Association: St. Louis Regional Chapter
2258 Weldon Parkway 314-432-7257
Saint Louis, MO 63146 888-873-8539
Fax: 314-432-2991
e-mail: bwessels@alsastl.org
webstl.alsa.org

A chapter serving the Eastern Missouri and Southern Illinois regions dedicated solely to finding the cause and cure of ALS through research, patient support, information and referrals and public awareness.
Robert Wessels, President
Sharon Gacki MA, Public/Professional Education

Nebraska

1015 ALS Association: Keith Worthington Chapter Nebraska Branch Office
10730 Pacific at Shaker Place 402-991-8788
Omaha, NE 68114 866-762-6361
Fax: 402-991-3690
e-mail: info@alsa-midwest.org
www.alsa-midwest.org

ALS Association chapters are multifaceted grass-roots organizations that carry out ALSA's mission and strategic goals at the community level. The chapter — with supporting services from the National Office — actively pursues the Association's goals.
Shannon Todd, Services Staff
Sherrie Hanneman, Awareness and Development

New Mexico

1016 ALS Association: New Mexico CIO
PO Box 16495 505-323-6348
Albuquerque, NM 87191-6495 e-mail: als@alsanm.org
www.alsa-nm.org

ALS Association chapters are multifaceted grass-roots organizations that carry out ALSA's mission and strategic goals at the community level. The chapter — with supporting services from the National Office — actively pursues the Association's goals.
Chuck Borgman, President
Terie Baker, Executive Director

New York

1017 ALS Association: Greater New York Chapter
42 Broadway 212-619-1400
New York, NY 10004 800-672-8857
Fax: 212-619-7409
e-mail: als@als-ny.org
www.als-ny.org

ALS Association chapters are multifaceted grass-roots organizations that carry out ALSA's mission and strategic goals at the community level. The chapter — with supporting services from the National Office — actively pursues the Association's goals.
Dorine Gordon, President
Jaqueline Reinhard, Executive Director

1018 ALS Association: Upstate New York CIO
890 7th N Street 315-413-0121
Liverpool, NY 13088 866-499-7257
Fax: 315-413-0508
e-mail: info@alsaupstateny.org
webuny.alsa.org

ALS Association chapters are multifaceted grass-roots organizations that carry out ALSA's mission and strategic goals at the community level. The chapter — with supporting services from the National Office — actively pursues the Association's goals.
Katharine Loomis, Executive Director
Shiann Atuegbu, Patient Services Coordinator

Ohio

1019 ALS Association: Northeast Ohio Chapter
2500 E 22nd Street 216-592-2572
Cleveland, OH 44115 888-592-2572
Fax: 216-592-2575
e-mail: alsa@alsaohio.org
webnoh.alsa.org

Offers telephone consultation services, support groups, caregivers support groups, equipment loan bank and a 24 hour telephone answering service for persons with ALS.
Brad Sussman, Executive Director
Fred M DeGrandis, President

1020 ALS Association: Western Ohio Chapter
1170 Old Henderson Road 614-273-2572
Columbus, OH 43220 866-273-2572
Fax: 614-273-2573
e-mail: alsohio@alsohio.org
webcsoh.alsa.org

Offers telephone consultation services, support groups, caregivers support groups, equipment loan bank and a 24 hour telephone answering service for persons with ALS.
Marlin Seymour, Executive Director
Pinky Dressm LSW, Patient Services Coordinator

Oregon

1021 ALS Association: Oregon & SW Washington CIO
310 SW Fourth Avenue 503-238-5559
Portland, OR 97204 800-681-9851
Fax: 503-296-5590
e-mail: info@alsa-or.org
webor.alsa.org

The ALS Association chapters are multifaceted grass-roots organizations that carry out ALSA's mission and strategic goals at the community level. The chapter — with supporting services from the National Office — actively pursues the Association's goals.
Cindy Burdell, Director
Lance Christ MSW, Services Director

Pennsylvania

1022 ALS Association: Greater Philadelphia Chapter
321 Norristown Road
Ambler, PA 19002
215-643-5434
877-434-7441
Fax: 215-643-9307
e-mail: alsassoc@alsphiladelphia.org
www.alsphiladelphia.org

Offers medical management of ALS at the ALS Clinical Services Center located at Hahnemann University, monthly support meetings, international programs on research, in-home evaluations, equipment loan closet and more for the ALS patient, families and caregivers.

Danielle Beaton, Development Assistant
Joan Borowsky, Development Coordinator

1023 ALS Association: Western Pennsylvania Chapter
416 Lincoln Avenue
Pittsburgh, PA 15209
412-821-3254
800-967-9296
Fax: 412-821-3549
e-mail: mbernarding@alswp.org
webwpawv.alsa.org

The mission of this chapter is to provide services and education to ALS patients, families and caregivers through medical information, support groups, assisting health care providers and providing communication devices.

Michael Bernarding, Executive Director
Marie Folino, Patient Services Director

South Carolina

1024 ALS Association: Jim (Catfish) Hunter Chapter
120-101 Penmarc Drive
Raleigh, NC 27603
919-755-9001
877-568-4347
Fax: 919-755-0910
e-mail: jerry@catfishchapter.org
www.catfishchapter.org

ALS association chapters are multifaceted grass roots organizations that carry out ALSA's mission and strategic goals at the community level. The chapter, with supporting services from the national office, actively pursues the association's goals.

Jerry Dawson RN BSN, President & CEO
Megan Gardner, Executive Director

Tennessee

1025 ALS Association: Middle Tennessee Chapter
522 E Iris Drive
Nashville, TN 37204
615-279-5551
877-216-5551
Fax: 615-279-5445
e-mail: cheri.sanders@alstn.org
webtn.alsa.org

ALS Association chapters are multifaceted grass-roots organizations that carry out ALSA's mission and strategic goals at the community level. The chapter — with supporting services from the National Office — actively pursues the Association's goals.

Cheri Sanders, Executive Director
Patty Lane, Patient Services Coordinator

Texas

1026 ALS Association: Greater Houston CIO
PO Box 271561
Houston, TX 77277-1561
713-942-2572
866-788-2572
Fax: 218-497-2572
e-mail: linda.richardson@alsa-houston.org
www.alsa-houston.org

ALS Association chapters are multi-faceted grass roots organizations that carry out ALSA's mission and stategic goals at the community level. he chapter — with supporting services from the National Office — actively pursues the Association's goals.

Linda Richardson, President
Georgia Mclain, Patient Services

1027 ALS Association: North Texas Chapter
1231 Greenway Drive
Irving, TX 75038
972-714-0088
877-714-0088
Fax: 972-714-0066
e-mail: hope@alsanorthtexas.org
webntx.alsa.org

ALS Association chapters are multi-faceted grass roots organizations that carry out ALSA's mission and strategic goals at the community level. he chapter — with supporting services from the National Office — actively pursues the Association's goals.

Kristen Stubbs, Executive Director
Leigh Craig, Development Director

1028 ALS Association: South Texas Chapter
8600 Wurzbach
San Antonio, TX 78240
210-733-5204
877-257-4673
Fax: 210-733-5206
e-mail: Information@alsasotx.org
www.alsasotx.org

ALS Association chapters are multi-faceted grass roots organizations that carry out ALSA's mission and strategic goals at the community level. he chapter — with supporting services from the National Office — actively pursues the Association's goals.

Patrick Callihan, Executive Director
Julia Dyer, Development Associate

Vermont

1029 ALS Association: Northern New England Chapter
The Champlain Mill
10 Ferry Street
Concord, NH 03301
603-226-8855
866-257-6663
Fax: 603-226-8890
e-mail: executive.director@alsanne.org
www.alsanne.org

ALS Association chapters are multifaceted grass-roots organizations that carry out ALSA's mission and strategic goals at the community level. The chapter — with supporting services from the National Office — actively pursues the Association's goals.

Kathleen L Phillips, Executive Director
Christine Richards, Patient Services Director

Washington

1030 ALS Association: Evergreen Chapter
19110 66th Avenue
Kent, WA 98032
425-656-1650
866-786-7257
Fax: 425-656-1649
e-mail: BeckyMooreED@alsa-ec.org
webwa.alsa.org

The ALS Association chapters are multifaceted grass-roots organizations that carry out ALSA's mission and strategic goals at the community level. The chapter — with supporting services from the National Office — actively pursues the Association's goals.

Rebecca Moore, Executive Director
Sonja Zimmer, Patient Services Director

1031 ALS Association: Oregon & SW Washington CIO
310 SW Fourth Avenue
Portland, OR 97204
503-238-5559
800-681-9851
Fax: 503-296-5590
e-mail: info@alsa-or.org
webor.alsa.org

The ALS Association chapters are multifaceted grass-roots organizations that carry out ALSA's mission and strategic goals at the community level. The chapter — with supporting services from the National Office — actively pursues the Association's goals.

Cindy Burdell, Director
Lance Christ MSW, Services Director

Wisconsin

1032 ALS Association: Southeast Wisconsin Chapter
2505 N 124th Street
Brookfield, WI 53005
262-784-5257
Fax: 262-784-5260
e-mail: info@alsawi.org
webwi.alsa.org

Begun in 1987 as a support group this chapter is managed by a Board of Directors from all walks of life and disciplines. All members share a dedication to carry out the mission of Hope Through Research and Support Through Caring. The goal is to help ALS

Melanie Roach-Bekos, Executive Director
Linda Lehmann, Office Manager

Research Centers

1033 ALS Center at UCSF
350 Parnassus Avenue 415-353-2108
San Francisco, CA 94117 Fax: 415-353-2524
e-mail: alscenter@ucsf.edu
www.ucsf.edu/brain/als
Research serves as a cornerstone for our patient programs allowing us to translate the most recent advancement in therapies drug development and clinical management into care for our patients.
Catherine Lomen-Hoer, Director
Carolyn Rodriguez, Clinical Coordinator

1034 ALS Clinic at Penn Neurological Institute ALS Association Greater Philadelphia Cha
ALS Association Greater Philadelphia Chapter
321 Norristown Road 215-643-5434
Ambler, PA 19002 Fax: 215-643-9307
e-mail: brenda@alsphiladelphia.org
www.pennhealth.com/als
A multidisciplinary center for the evaluation and treatment of amyotrophic lateral sclerosis (ALS) and related disorders.
Brenda Edelm LCSW BCD, Director of Patient Services
Lauren Elman, Associate Medical Director

1035 ALS Clinical Department of Neurology College of Medicine of the University of
College of Medicine of the University of Vermont
89 Beaumont Avenue 802-656-2156
Burlington, VT 05405-3456 Fax: 802-656-8577
e-mail: Rup.Tandan@uvm.edu
www.med.uvm.edu
Clinical care facility for ALS patients.
Rup Tandan MD, Vice Chairman
Robert W Hamill, Chair

1036 Center for ALS and Related Diorders The Cleveland Clinic DepartmentOf Neurol
The Cleveland Clinic DepartmentOf Neurology
9500 Euclid Avenue 216-444-5538
Cleveland, OH 44195-5227 800-223-2273
Fax: 216-445-4653
TTY: 216-444-0261
e-mail: andrewd@ccf.org
my.clevelandclinic.org
Clinical care and research facility for ALS patients.
Erik P Pioro, Director
Kathleen M Kelly, ALS Clinical Coordinator

1037 Les Turner Research Laboratory Northwestern University Medical School
Northwestern University Medical School
5550 W Touhy Avenue 847-679-3311
Skokie, IL 60077 888-ALS-1107
Fax: 847-679-9109
e-mail: info@lesturnerals.org
www.lesturnerals.org
Scientists and researchers dedicate their time to discover what causes ALS and find a cure for the disease. The international team of scientists at the Laboratory are internationally recognized for their accomplishments in the field of ALS research.
Teetu Siddique, Head
Wendy Abrams, Executive Director

1038 Mayo Clinic: Department of Neurology
200 First Street SW
Rochester, MN 55905 507-284-2511
www.mayo.edu
Ongoing reserach and treatment for ALS.
Eric J Sorenson MD, Director

1039 Motor Neuron Disease Clinic University of Connecticut Health Center
University of Connecticut Health Center
263 Farmington Avenue 860-679-4888
Farmington, CT 06030 Fax: 860-679-1454
TTY: 860-679-2242
www.uchc.edu
Kevin Felice, Director

1040 Motor Neuron Disease Program University of Michigan Health System
University of Michigan Health System
1500 E Medical Center Drive 734-936-9010
Ann Arbor, MI 48109-316 Fax: 734-153-53
www.med.umich.edu
Regional clinic that is dedicated to the diagnosis of Amyotrophic Lateral Sclerosis and improving the well-being of patients who have this disease.
Eva Feldman MD PhD, Director
Kirsten L Gruis, Co-Director

1041 Neuromuscular and ALS Center The Clinical Academic Building
The Clinical Academic Building
125 Patterson Street 732-235-7331
New Brunswick, NJ 08901 Fax: 732-235-7344
e-mail: nmalsweb@umdnj.edu
www2.umdnj.edu/nmalsweb
A multidisciplinary program for the diagnosis evaluation and long-term management of a host of neuromuscular diseases found in adults.
Jerry Belsh MD, Director
Annmarie Coyne-West, Patient Care Coordinator

1042 New England Medical Center: ALS Laboratory
800 Washington Street 617-636-5364
Boston, MA 02111-1533 Fax: 617-636-8568
www.tuftsmedicalcenter.org
Specializes in Amyotrophic Lateral Sclerosis research.
Su Wu, Director
Susan Blanchard, Vice President

1043 Solomon Park Research Institute
12815 NE 124th Street 425-650-2020
Kirkland, WA 98034 800-470-1817
Fax: 425-650-2028
e-mail: pclapshaw@soloman.org
www.solomon.org
Amyotrophic lateral sclerosis research.
Patric Clapshaw, Director
Sheila Dunagan, Office Manager

1044 Stem Cell Research Program University of Wisconsin-Madison
University of Wisconsin-Madison
1500 Highland Avenue 608-265-8668
Madison, WI 53705-2280 Fax: 608- 26- 526
e-mail: gilbert@waisman.wisc.edu
www.waisman.wisc.edu/scrp
The mission of this program is to understand the molecular mechanisms responsible for the proliferation and differentiation of stem cells and assess their safety and efficacy following transplantation into various disease models.
Jacalyn McHugh, Research Program Manager
Sue Gilbert, Administrative Assistant

1045 Virginia Mason Medical Center Neuroscience Institute
Virginia Mason Medical Center
1100 9th Avenue
Seattle, WA 98101 206-341-1900
www.virginiamason.org
Clinical care and research.
Michael Elliott, Medical Director

Support Groups & Hotlines

1046 ALS Association Free Standing Support Groups
ALS Association National Office
27001 Agoura Road 818-880-9007
Calabasas Hills, CA 91301-5104 800-782-4747
Fax: 818-880-9006
e-mail: alsinfo@alsa-national.org
www.alsa.org
We know of support groups in Alabama, California, Florida, Illinois, New York, Oklahoma, Oregon, Puerto Rico, Utah and Virginia.

1047 American Society of Human Genetics
9650 Rockville Pike 301-634-7000
Bethesda, MD 20814-3998 Fax: 301-634-7079
e-mail: estrass@genetics.faseb.org
www.faseb.org
This society will locate a genetic counselor in various areas across the United States for persons with ALS.

1048 Amyotrophic Lateral Sclerosis Toll Free Hotline
ALS Association
27001 Agoura Road 818-880-9007
Calabasas Hills, CA 91301-5104 800-782-4747
Fax: 818-880-9006
e-mail: alsinfo@alsanational.org
www.alsa.org
Informs individuals with ALS and their families of services available through the ALS Association.
Gary Leo, President
Sondi Scheck, VP Operations/Administration

1049 Les Turner Amyotrophic Lateral Sclerosis Foundation
5550 West Touhy 847-679-3311
Skokie, IL 60077 888-257-1107
Fax: 847-679-9109
e-mail: info@lesturnerals.org
www.lesturnerals.org
Support groups offer patients and family members a chance to not feel alone and frustrated in coping with ALS and offers them the support of professionals as well as others who are experiencing similar problems.
Claire Owen, Director Patient Services

1050 National Health Information Center
PO Box 1133 310-565-4167
Washington, DC 20013 800-336-4797
Fax: 301-984-4256
e-mail: info@nhic.org
www.health.gov/nhic
Offers a nationwide information referral service, produces directories and resource guides.

Books

1051 Amyotrophic Lateral Sclerosis: Guide for Patients and Families
Demos Medical Publishing
386 Park Avenue S
New York, NY 10016 800-532-8663
Fax: 212-683-0118
www.demosmedpub.com
This second edition book offers an overview and practical advice.
2001
ISBN: 1-888799-28-5

1052 Complete Bedside Companion: No Nonsense Advice on Caring for the Seriously Ill
Simon & Shuster
1230 Avenue of the Americas
New York, NY 10020 800-323-7445
Fax: 800-943-9831
www.simonsays.com
Practical counsel and methods.
1998
ISBN: 0-684843-19-6

1053 Easy-to-Swallow, Easy-to-Chew Cookbook
Wiley Publishers
10475 Crosspoint Boulevard
Indianapolis, IN 46256 877-762-2974
Fax: 800-597-3299
e-mail: customer@wiley.com
www.wiley.com
Offers over 150 tasty and nutritious recipies with simple instruction for tailoring food textures from very easy-to-chew to soft and smooth. All recipes contain nutritional information per serving.

ISBN: 0-471200-74-3

1054 Journeys with ALS
DLRC Press
PO Box 61661 757-473-1130
Virginia Beach, VA 23466 800-776-0560
e-mail: mary@davidlawrence.com
Compiled by an ALS patient, this book contains 33 first person journeys with ALS. Some are hopeful, some are sad, a few are angry. All are powerful, real-life examples of people doing their best to cope, often with humor and high spirits.
1998
ISBN: 1-880731-58-4

1055 Learning to Fall: the Blessings of an Imperfect Life
Bantam Dell Publishing Group
1540 Broadway 212-782-9186
New York, NY 10036 800-733-3000
Fax: 212-782-8890
www.bantamdell.com
The author was diagnosed with ALS in 1993. An associate professor of English at Lake Forest College in Illinois, he was just 35. In his quest to help other and himself, Simmons turned his experience with ALS into this book.
2001
ISBN: 0-553802-66-6

1056 Life on Wheels: for the Active Wheelchair User
O'Rielly & Associates
1230 Heil Quaker Boulevard
LaVegne, TN 37086 800-998-9938
Fax: 707-829-0104
www.oreilly.com
Offers practical ways to adapt and optimize the quality of your life. It covers subjects such as skin care, bowel and bladder care, sexuality, home access, maintaining a wheelchair and dealing with insurance problems.
1999
ISBN: 1-565922-53-0

1057 Non Chew Cookbook
Wilson Publishing Company
5708 Nicollet Avenue S
Minneapolis, MN 55419 800-843-2409
e-mail: nonchew@excite.com
www.nonchewcookbook.com
Soft food recipes good for the whole family.

1058 Realities in Coping with Progressive Neuromuscular Diseases
Charles Press Publishers
PO Box 15715 215-561-2786
Philadelphia, PA 19103-0715 Fax: 215-561-0191
e-mail: mailbox@charlespresspub.com
www.charlespresspub.com
This book brings together 51 eminent authorities on ALS focusing on a variety of different coping strategies for patients and families, as well as health professionals.
248 pages Hardcover only
ISBN: 0-914783-20-3

Newsletters

1059 ALS Today
Les Turner ALS Foundation
5550 West Touhy 847-679-3311
Skokie, IL 60077 888-257-1107
Fax: 847-679-9109
e-mail: info@lesturnerals.org
www.lesturnerals.org
Offers information on clinical trials, medical updates, recipes, resources and support groups available from the foundation.
3 per year

1060 LINK
ALS Association
27001 Agoura Road 818-880-9007
Calabasas Hills, CA 91301-5104 800-782-4747
Fax: 818-880-9006
e-mail: alsinfo@alsa-national.org
www.alsa.org
Offers information on a national level to all patients and chapter members of the ALS Association. Medical updates, loan equip-

ment, resources, hotlines, support groups and news of charity and fundraising events are included as well.

1061 **Massachusetts Chapter of the ALS Association Newsletter**
Massachusetts Chapter of the ALS Association
7 Lincoln Street 781-245-2133
Wakefield, MA 01880-3021 800-258-3323
Offers information on activities, events, charity and fundraising activities, resources and more for members.
BiMonthly
Ginny DelVecchio, President

1062 **Peach Lines**
ALS Association of Georgia
3795 Manor House Drive 770-642-7962
Marietta, GA 30062-5147
Chapter newsletter offering information on support groups, meetings, hotlines, resources and reviews the newest technology and daily living aids for persons with ALS in the Georgia area.
BiMonthly

1063 **Reaching Out**
Orange County Chapter of the ALS Association
16787 Beach Boulevard 949-587-9700
Huntington Beach, CA 92647-4848
Offers information on support groups, meetings, charity events, fundraising activities and more for ALS members in the Orange County area.
BiMonthly

1064 **South Texas Chapter of the ALS Association Newsletter**
2389 W Military Highway 210-493-1311
San Antonio, TX 78231
Offers chapter information on events, charities, memorials, tributes and resources for persons with ALS and their families.
BiMonthly

1065 **ALS News & Views**
Western Pennsylvania Chapter-ALS Association
1323 Forbes Avenue 412-261-5940
Pittsburgh, PA 15219-4725
Offers information on resources, medical articles, events, charities, fundraising activities and more for patients with ALS, families and caregivers in the western Pennsylvania region.
8 pages BiMonthly
Rita Patchan, Editor

Pamphlets

1066 **Basic Home Care for ALS Patients**
ALS Association
27001 Agoura Road 818-880-9007
Calabasas Hills, CA 91301-5104 800-782-4747
Fax: 818-880-9006
e-mail: alsinfo@alsa-national.org
www.alsa.org
Offers a brief overview of the disease, diet and nutrition information, elimination of swallowing problems, hygiene, equipment, communication aids, patient services and suggested readings for the ALS patient.

1067 **Maintaining Good Nutrition with ALS**
ALS Association
27001 Agoura Road 818-880-9007
Calabasas Hills, CA 91301-5104 800-782-4747
Fax: 818-880-9006
e-mail: alsinfo@alsa-national.org
www.alsa.org
Guide for patients, families and friends on nutrition for persons with ALS and other swallowing disorders.

Audio & Video

1068 **Driving Force: A Story of Life**
Production House
811 St. John's 847-433-3172
Highland Park, IL 60035 Fax: 847-433-9383
Inspiring video featuring Dr. Frank de Leon Jones, a pychiatrist and ALS patient. Despite his disease and the need for continuous medical ventilation, Dr. de Leon Jones continues his challenging medical practice and physical education responsibilities. This is a film of courage, persistence and love of life. It offers poignant messages for ALS patients, family and caregivers as well as healthcare providers. Available in VHS or DVD.
Howie Samuelson, Executive Director

1069 **Living with ALS: Adapting to Breathing Changes/Use of Non Invasive Ventilation**
ALS Association National Office
27001 Agoura Road 818-880-9007
Calabasas Hills, CA 91301-5104 800-782-4747
Fax: 818-880-9006
e-mail: alsinfo@alsa-national.org
www.alsa.org
One of a series of four videotapes distrubuted by the ALS Association.
2003

1070 **Living with ALS: Adjusting to Swallowing Difficulties & Good Nutrition**
ALS Association National Office
27001 Agoura Road 818-880-9007
Calabasas Hills, CA 91301-5104 800-782-4747
Fax: 818-880-9006
e-mail: alsinfo@alsa-national.org
www.alsa.org
One of a series of four videotapes distrubuted by the ALS Association.
2003

1071 **Living with ALS: Communication Solutions & Symptom Management**
ALS Association National Office
27001 Agoura Road 818-880-9007
Calabasas Hills, CA 91301-5104 800-782-4747
Fax: 818-880-9006
e-mail: alsinfo@alsa-national.org
www.alsa.org
One of a series of four videotapes distrubuted by the ALS Association.
2003

1072 **Living with ALS: Mobility, Activities of Daily Living, Home Adaptions**
ALS Association National Office
27001 Agoura Road 818-880-9007
Calabasas Hills, CA 91301-5104 800-782-4747
Fax: 818-880-9006
e-mail: alsinfo@alsa-national.org
www.alsa.org
One of a series of four videotapes distrubuted by the ALS Association.
2003

1073 **Ventilation: Decision Making Process**
Les Turner ALS Foundation
5550 West Touhy 847-679-3311
Skokie, IL 60077 888-257-1107
Fax: 847-679-9109
e-mail: info@lesturnerals.org
www.lesturnerals.org
Designed for ALS patients, their family members and health professionals. Includes interviews with three ventilator dependent ALS patients, family members and the medical staff from Lois Insolia ALS Center at Northwestern University Medical School. Available for loan to ALS patients.
20 Minutes

Web Sites

1074 **Healing Well**
www.healingwell.com
An online health resource guide to medical news, chat, information and articles, newsgroups and message boards, books, disease-related web sites, medical directories, and more for patients, friends,

and family coping with disabling diseases, disorders, or chronic illnesses.

1075 **Health Finder**

www.healthfinder.gov

Searchable, carefully developed web site offering information on over 1000 topics. Developed by the US Department of Health and Human Services, the site can be used in both English and Spanish.

1076 **Healthlink USA**

www.healthlinkusa.com

Health information concerning treatment, cures, prevention, diagnosis, risk factors, research, support groups, email lists, personal stories and much more. Updated regularly.

1077 **Helios Health**

www.helioshealth.com

Online resource for your health information. Detailed information about specific health topics, access to expert advice from our Medical Advisory Board, and up-to-date health news.

1078 **MedWebPlus**

www.medwebplus.com

Provides links to Amyotropic Laternal Sclerosis information, such as associations, support, and treatment centers.

1079 **MedicineNet**

www.medicinenet.com

An online resource for consumers providing easy-to-read, authoritative medical and health information.

1080 **Medscape**

www.mywebmd.com

Medscape offers specialists, primary care physicians, and other health professionals the Web's most robust and integrated medical information and educational tools.

1081 **Neurology Channel**

www.neurologychannel.com

Find clearly explained, medically accurate information regarding conditions, including an overview, symptoms, causes, diagnostic procedures and treatment options. On this site it is possible to ask questions and get information from a neurologist and connect to people who have similar health interests.

1082 **WebMD**

www.webmd.com

Information on Amyotrophic Lateral Sclerosis, including articles and resources.

Description

1083 **Arthritis**

Arthritis is a nonspecific term meaning inflammation of one or more joints. There are over 100 kinds of arthritis, many of them associated with illnesses of other body systems, such as the skin, gut, or liver. Most cases of arthritis are chronic and involve multiple joints. The three most common are rheumatoid arthritis (RA), osteoarthritis (OA), sometimes called degenerative joint disease, and gouty arthritis, or gout.Juvenile Rheumatoid Arthritis (JRA) affects children.

Rheumatoid arthritis may strike either sex at any age, but typically affects women in the early adult years. It is marked by considerable inflammation, commonly of the hands and feet. RA may also involve the knee, elbow, shoulder, ankle and neck, as well as other body systems in addition to the joints. Osteoarthritis tends to occur later in life, related to repeated wear and tear most commonly on weight-bearing joints, such as the hip and knee. Osteoarthritis often occurs earlier in people who have injured their joints in sports. Gout, which typically affects men in midlife, reflects a disorder in the body's metabolism of uric acid. Its most common feature is excruciating pain in the big toe.

Joints affected by arthritis are typically painful, stiff, and swollen. Nonspecific treatment may be used for arthritis of any sort. This includes the nonsteroidal anti-inflammatory drugs (NSAIDs) and aspirin. Steroids can be injected into the knee in OA and be indicated in an oral form for RA. Severe cases of rheumatoid arthritis are generally treated with more specific drugs that attempt to alter the body's immune system. Gouty arthritis responds to drugs that alter the production and metabolism of uric acid. For any kind of arthritis, local application of heat and cold, as well as physical therapy, are often helpful. In certain cases, joint surgery is recommended.

National Agencies & Associations

1084 **American Juvenile Arthritis Organization Arthritis Foundation**
Arthritis Foundation
PO Box 7669 — 404-872-7100
Atlanta, GA 30357-0669 — 800-283-7800
Fax: 404-872-9559
e-mail: help@arthritis.org
www.arthritis.org
A council established by the Arthritis Foundation which serves the special needs of young people with arthritis and their families. Provides information, inspiration and advocacy by identifying the needs of children with arthritis and speaks out on their behalf.
Cecile Perich, Chair
John H Klippel MD, President & CEO

1085 **Arthritis & Autoimmunity Research Centre (AARC) Foundation**
190 Elizabeth Street — 416-340-3388
Toronto, Ontario, M5G — Fax: 416-340-4896
e-mail: aarc.foundation@aarcf-uhn.ca
uhn.info@uhn.on.ca
Increase awareness of this large family of diseases, which affects over four million Canadians.
Gerri Grant, Executive Director
Pippa Shaddick, Development Manager

1086 **Arthritis Foundation**
1330 West Peachtree Street — 404-872-7100
Atlanta, GA 30309 — 800-283-7800
Fax: 404-872-0457
e-mail: help@arthritis.org
www.arthritis.org
A nonprofit organization that depends on volunteers to provide services to help people with arthritis. Supports research to find ways to cure and prevent arthritis and provides services to improve the quality of life for those affected by arthritis. Provides help through information, referrals, speakers bureaus, forums, self-help courses, and various support groups and programs nationwide.
Christina Lennon, VP

1087 **Arthritis Society**
393 University Avenue — 416-979-7228
Toronto Ontario, M5G 1-1E6 — 800-321-1433
Fax: 416-979-8366
e-mail: info@on.arthritis.ca
www.arthritis.ca
Promoting evaluating and funding research in the areas of causes prevention treatment and cures of arthritis.
Steven McNair, CEO/President
Sinead Canavan, Communications/Marketing Manager

1088 **Myositis Association**
1233 20th Street NW — 202-887-0088
Washington, DC 20036 — 800-821-7356
Fax: 202-466-8940
e-mail: tma@myositis.org
www.myositis.org
Involves swelling of the muscles. It is an inflammatory myopathies that is a disease of the muscle where there is swelling and loss of muscle.
Bob Goldberg, Executive Director
Theresa R Curry, Communications Manager

1089 **National Arthritis and Musculoskeletal & Skin Diseases Information Clearinghouse**
National Institutes of Health
31 Center Drive - MSC 2350 — 301-496-8190
Bethesda, MD 20892-2350 — Fax: 301-480-2814
e-mail: niamsinfo@mail.nih.gov
www.niams.nih.gov
Our mission is to support research into the causes treatment and prevention of arthritis and musculoskeletal and skin diseases, the training of basic and clinical scientists to carry out this research and the dissemination of information on research programs.
Stephen I Katz MD PhD, Director
Robert H Carter, Deputy Director

1090 **National Institute of Arthritis and Musculoskeletal and Skin Disease (NIAMS)**
1 AMS Circle — 301-495-4484
Bethesda, MD 20892 — 877-226-4267
Fax: 301-718-6366
TTY: 301-565-2966
e-mail: niamsinfo@mail.nih.gov
www.niams.nih.gov
The NIAMS Information Clearinghouse provides information about various forms of arthritis and rheumatic disease and bone, muscle, and skin diseases. It distributes patient and professional education materials and refers people to other sources of information.
Stephen I Katz MD, PhD, Director

State Agencies & Associations

Alabama

1091 **Alabama Chapter of the Arthritis Foundation**
2700 Hwy 280 E — 205-979-5700
Birmingham, AL 35223-3775 — 800-879-7896
Fax: 205-979-4172
e-mail: info.al@arthritis.org
www.arthritis.org
Founded in 1948 this chapter affects thousands of lives through programs services information and referrals public and profes-

sional education and more for residents of Alabama. Research is a great priority of the chapter which supports the advancemen
Lisa Hemphill, Development Director
Mandy Moulin, Community Development Director

Arizona

1092 **Arthritis Foundation: Central Arizona Chapter**
777 E Missouri Avenue 602-264-7679
Phoenix, AZ 85014 800-477-7679
Fax: 602-264-0563
e-mail: info.caz@arthritis.org
www.arthritis.org
A nonprofit health agency serving the needs of Arizona residents with arthritis. This chapter provides arthritis self-help courses, aquatic programs, foundation clubs, a juvenile arthritis parent group, exercise programs and informational brochures.
Angela McTee, Director - New Mexico
Angie Castillo, Finance Coordinator

1093 **Arthritis Foundation: Greater Southwest Chapter**
1313 E Osborn Road 602-264-7679
Phoenix, AZ 85014 800-477-7679
Fax: 602-264-0563
e-mail: info.caz@arthritis.org
www.arthritis.org
A nonprofit health agency serving the needs of Arizona, New Mexico, El Paso residents with arthritis. This chapter provides self management workshops, aquatic programs, a juvenile arthritis parent and peer group, exercise programs and informational brochures.
Vikki Scarafiotti, President
Melissa Brauer, Events Manager

Arkansas

1094 **Arthritis Foundation: Arkansas Chapter**
6213 Father Tribou Street 501-664-7242
Little Rock, AR 72205-3002 800-482-8858
Fax: 501-664-6588
e-mail: info.ar@arthritis.org
www.arthritis.org
Carla Davis, Secretary
Diane Denham, VP Finance/Administration

California

1095 **Arthritis Foundation: Northern California Chapter**
657 Mission Street 415-356-1230
San Francisco, CA 94105-4120 800-464-6240
Fax: 415-356-1240
e-mail: info.nca@arthritis.org
www.arthritis.org
Offers research into the causes of arthritis and more effective treatments; serves people in California with arthritis through information and referral services, exercise programs, self-help courses, education and other activities.
Mary Arnold, Assistant to the President
PJ Handeland, President

1096 **Arthritis Foundation: San Diego Area Chapter**
9089 Clairemont Mesa Boulevard 858-492-1090
San Diego, CA 92123-1288 800-422-8885
Fax: 858-492-9248
e-mail: info.sd@arthritis.org
www.arthritis.org
Offers various programs and services including professional seminars, a speakers bureau, public forums, exercise classes, patient and family support groups, arthritis self-help courses and medical research to the residents of the San Diego area living with arthritis.
Veronica Braun, President
Sandra Hayhurst, Director Health Promotion

1097 **Arthritis Foundation: Southern California Chapter**
800 W 6th Street 323-954-5750
Los Angeles, CA 90017-3775 800-954-2873
Fax: 323-954-5790
e-mail: info.sac@arthritis.org
www.arthritis.org
Cynthia Callihan, Administrative Assistant
Christeen Amloian, Assistant Controller

Colorado

1098 **Arthritis Foundation: Rocky Mountain Chapter**
2280 S Albion Street 303-756-8622
Denver, CO 80222-4906 800-475-6447
Fax: 303-759-4349
e-mail: info.rm@arthritis.org
www.arthritis.org
Serves Colorado, Montana, and Wyoming and is dedicated to finding solutions to over 100 forms of arthritis which affect 43 millions of people nationwide.
Isabelle Stohler, Program Manager
Laura Rosseisen, VP Development

Connecticut

1099 **Arthritis Foundation: Southern New England Chapter**
35 Cold Spring Road 860-563-1177
Rocky Hill, CT 06067 800-541-8350
Fax: 860-563-6018
e-mail: info.snc@arthritis.org
www.arthritis.org
A resource center for persons in Southern New England, Connecticut, Maine and Vermont with arthritis. Offers self-help courses, exercise programs, aquatic programs, Dial-A-Doctor helpline, and physician referrals.
Ann Louise Richman, Development Assistant
Debra McCaig, Executive Assistant

District of Columbia

1100 **Arthritis Foundation: Metropolitan Washington Chapter**
2011 Pennsylvania Avenue NW 202-537-6800
Washington, DC 20006 Fax: 202-537-6859
e-mail: info.mwa@arthritis.org
www.arthritis.org
The mission of the Arthritis Foundation is to improve lives through leadership in the prevention control and cure of arthritis and related conditions.
Calaneet Balas, President/CEO
Jacquelyn Hair, Director of Operations

Florida

1101 **Arthritis Foundation: Florida Chapter, Gulf Coast Branch**
3816 W Linebaugh Avenue 813-968-7000
Tampa, FL 33618 800-850-9455
Fax: 941-795-0348
e-mail: info.fl.b4@arthritis.org
www.arthritis.org
Dedicated to improving the quality of life for those in the seven county area of Pinellas, Pasco, Citrus, Levy, Hillsborough, Hernando and Polk, who have one or more of over 100 conditions that comprise the disease known as arthritis. Provides patient education and referal services.
Alexa Simpkins, Events Coordinator
Alvi McConahay, Regional Executive Director

Georgia

1102 **Arthritis Foundation: Georgia Chapter**
2790 Peachtree Road 404-237-8771
Atlanta, GA 30305 800-933-7023
Fax: 404-237-8153
e-mail: info.ga@arthritis.org
www.arthritis.org
A statewide health organization dedicated to reducing the devastating effects of arthritis by offering programs for people with ar-

thritis and their families, information and educational services for people with arthritis, medical professionals and the general public.
Andrea Collins, Vice President Mission Delivery
Christina Lennon, VP Resource Development

Illinois

1103 **Arthritis Foundation: Greater Chicago Chapter**
29 E Madison 312-372-2080
Chicago, IL 60602 800-795-0096
Fax: 312-372-2081
e-mail: info.gc@arthritis.org
www.arthritis.org
Offers self-help courses, wellness workshops, educational seminars, aquatic programs, brochures and publications for persons with arthritis in the state of Illinois.
Roxanne Bartol, Information Systems Coordinator
Tom Fite, President

1104 **Arthritis Foundation: Greater Illinois Chapter**
2621 N Knoxville Avenue 309-682-6600
Peoria, IL 61604-3623 800-795-9115
Fax: 309-682-6732
e-mail: greaterillinois@arthritis.org
www.arthritis.org
Audrey LeGrande, Branch Director
Craig Rogers, President Greater Illinois Chapter

Indiana

1105 **Arthritis Foundation: Indiana Chapter**
615 N Alabama 317-879-0321
Indianapolis, IN 46204 800-783-2342
Fax: 317-876-5608
e-mail: info.in@arthritis.org
www.arthritis.org
Offers programs and services for the arthritis community of Indiana.
Jenny Conder, Director of Health Promotion
Pam Chambers, Bookkeeper

Iowa

1106 **Arthritis Foundation: Iowa Chapter**
2600 72nd Street 515-278-0636
Des Moines, IA 50322-4724 866-378-0636
Fax: 515-278-2603
e-mail: info.ia@arthritis.org
www.arthritis.org
Melissa Marchant, Senior Development Director
Doyle Monsma CFRE, President/CEO

Kansas

1107 **Arthritis Foundation: Kansas Chapter**
1999 N Amidon Avenue 316-263-0116
Wichita, KS 67203-2122 800-362-1108
Fax: 316-263-3260
e-mail: info.ks@arthritis.org
www.arthritis.org
Serves 103 counties and is governed by the Volunteer Board of Directors elected from throughout the state. Services offered include water exercise classes, arthritis support groups, children's summer camp, loan closet of hospital equipment and self-help programs.
Audry Goldsmith, Financial Administrator
Betsy Gwin, Director Development

Kentucky

1108 **Arthritis Foundation: Kentucky Chapter**
2908 Brownsboro Road 502-585-1866
Louisville, KY 40206 800-633-5335
Fax: 502-585-1657
e-mail: myoung@arthritis.org
www.arthritis.org
Serves residents of 117 counties in Kentucky and the counties of Floyd and Clark in Indiana. This chapter is a resource center for funding research education programs for health professionals, community education and support services for people with arthritis.
Barbara Perez, President/CEO
Annette Beach, Annual Giving Coordinator

Maryland

1109 **Arthritis Foundation: Maryland Chapter**
9505 Reisterstown Road 410-654-6570
Owings Mills, MD 21117 800-365-3811
Fax: 410-654-9270
e-mail: info.md@arthritis.org
www.arthritis.org
This chapter supports research both locally and nationally to help find causes better treatments and ways to prevent the many forms of arthritis. Offers various educational booklets and brochures, a referral service for physician referrals, and other support services.
Ayana Charleston, Director
Bethany Farrall, Development Coordinator

Massachusetts

1110 **Arthritis Foundation: Massachusetts Chapter**
29 Crafts Street 617-244-1800
Newton, MA 02458-1287 800-766-9449
Fax: 617-558-7686
e-mail: info.ma@arthritis.org
www.arthritis.org
Offers essential information research programs and services for the close to one million Massachusetts residents with arthritis.
Suha Bekdash, Administrative Assistant
Carmen Quinonez, Finance Manager

Michigan

1111 **Arthritis Foundation: Michigan Chapter Chapter and Metro Detroit**
Chapter and Metro Detroit
1050 Wilshire Drive 248-649-2891
Troy, MI 48084-1564 800-968-3030
Fax: 248-649-2895
e-mail: info.mi@arthritis.org
www.arthritis.org
Supports research to prevent, control, and cure arthritis and related diseases. The Foundation also helps improve the lives of people with arthritis and their families by offering self-help classes, exercise programs, support groups, information and referrals.
Heather Luka, Development Manager
Jackie Appleton, Administrative Assistant

Minnesota

1112 **Arthritis Foundation: North Central Chapter**
1902 Minnehaha Avenue W 651-644-4108
Saint Paul, MN 55104 800-333-1380
Fax: 651-644-4219
e-mail: info.mn@arthritis.org
www.arthritis.org
A nonprofit organization providing programs and services to anyone affected by arthritis in the Minnesota area. Offers aquatic programs support groups juvenile arthritis support groups, research, grants program and information and referrals.
Chris Davis, Community Development Coordinator
Deb Cassidy, Assistant to the President

Mississippi

1113 **Arthritis Foundation: Mississippi Chapter**
1060 E County Line Road 601-853-7556
Ridgeland, MS 39157 800-844-8400
Fax: 601-206-8868
e-mail: infoms@arthritis.org
www.arthritis.org
Many Mississippians volunteer their services to help the chapter with fund raising and program support. Programs include land and water based exercise classes, and support groups, direct assistance

to needy individuals to purchase arthritis medications and services.
Anne Weather Robertson, Development Specialist
Barry McBride, Office Manager/Special Events

Missouri

1114 **Arthritis Foundation: Eastern Missouri Chapter**
9433 Olive Boulevard
Saint Louis, MO 63132
314-991-9333
800-406-2491
Fax: 314-991-4020
e-mail: info.emo@arthritis.org
www.arthritis.org
Denise Heidger, Community Development Specialist
Ann Mangelsdorf, Director Services

1115 **Arthritis Foundation: Western Missouri, Greater Kansas City**
1900 W 75th Street
Prairie Village, KS 66208
913-262-2233
888-719-5670
Fax: 816-753-2227
e-mail: info.wmo@arthritis.org
www.arthritis.org
The only organization in the area representing the National Office in support of its international research program and in providing services throughout the bi-state area. Offers a wide range of services and programs to deal with the needs of persons with arthritis.
Sherri Hayes, Director of Operations
Alyson Watkins, Special Events Coordinator

Nebraska

1116 **Arthritis Foundation: Nebraska Chapter**
600 N 93rd Street
Omaha, NE 68114
402-330-6130
800-642-5292
Fax: 402-330-6167
e-mail: mpuccioni@arthritis.org
www.arthritis.org
For close to 40 years the Arthritis Foundation has been the source for help and hope to the 263 000 Nebraskans and residents of Pottawattamie County Iowa with arthritis. Provides a wide variety of services designed to help people better cope with arthritis.
Cindy Doerr, Program Director/Editor
Marzia Pucci Shields, Executive Director

New Jersey

1117 **Arthritis Foundation: New Jersey Chapter**
200 Middlesex Turnpike
Iselin, NJ 08830
732-283-4300
888-467-3112
Fax: 732-283-4633
e-mail: info.nj@arthritis.org
www.arthritis.org
Offers various programs for the residents of New Jersey including support groups, self-help courses, water exercise and arthritis fitness classes and informational public forums.
Linda Gruskiewicz, President & CEO
Tanya Barbarics, Director

New Mexico

1118 **Arthritis Foundation: New Mexico Chapter**
1313 E Osborn Road
Phoenix, AZ 85014
602-264-7679
800-477-7679
Fax: 602-264-0563
e-mail: info.caz@arthritis.org
www.arthritis.org
Offers public education information, referrals, educational materials, chapter lending library, professional education resources and support groups for the residents of New Mexico.
Vikki Scarafiotti, President
Angela McTee, Director - New Mexico

New York

1119 **Arthritis Foundation: Central New York Chapter**
3300 Monroe Avenue
Rochester, NY 14618
585-264-1480
Fax: 585-264-1517
e-mail: info@uny@arthritis.org
www.arthritis.org
Nicole L Mau, Executive Director
Lynn Doescher, Marathon and Events Manager

1120 **Arthritis Foundation: Long Island Chapter**
501 Walt Whitman Road
Melville, NY 11747-2189
631-427-8272
Fax: 631-427-3546
e-mail: into.li@arthritis.org
www.arthritis.org
The mission of the Arthritis Foundation is to fund research to find the cause and cures for arthritis and to improve the quality of life for those affected. There is a wide range of programs available for patients.
Patrick T McAsey, President
Roshane Gillespie, Program Secretary

1121 **Arthritis Foundation: New York Chapter**
122 E 42nd Street
New York, NY 10168-1898
212-984-8700
Fax: 212-878-5960
e-mail: nfo.ny@arthritis.org
www.arthritis.org
Offers land exercise programs warm water resources and programs, self-help groups and courses, events and activities video clinics, peer support and a lending library to arthritis sufferers in the New York area.
Cathy Hogstrom, Community Outreach Coordinator
Michael Friedman, President

1122 **Arthritis Foundation: Rockland/Orange Unit**
Helen Hayes Hospital
Route 9W
W Haverstraw, NY 10993
845-947-3000
Fax: 845-429-9602
e-mail: ameyerowitz@arthritis.org
www.arthritis.org
Aviva Meyerowitz, Community Outreach Coordinator
Beatrice Jasanya, Community Outreach Coordinator

North Carolina

1123 **Arthritis Foundation: Carolinas Chapter**
4530 Park Road
Charlotte, NC 28209
704-529-5166
800-883-8806
Fax: 704-529-0626
e-mail: info.car@arthritis.org
www.arthritis.org
Stephani Roark, Community Development Director
Candy Fuller, Community Development Coordinator

Ohio

1124 **Arthritis Foundation: Central Ohio Chapter**
3740 Ridge Mill Drive
Hilliard, OH 43026
614-876-8200
Fax: 614-876-8363
e-mail: info.coh@arthritis.org
www.arthritis.org
Offers information and referral services, self-help courses, aquatics program equipment loans, clinics, home assessment and continuing education to help more than 350,000 people in Central Ohio, including over 5,000 children affected with the 100 types of arthritis
Stephanie Houck, Director of Special Events
David Painter, Director of Outreach

1125 **Arthritis Foundation: Northeastern Ohio Chapter**
4630 Richmond Road
Cleveland, OH 44128-5525
216-831-7000
800-245-2275
Fax: 216-831-1764
e-mail: info.neoh@arthritis.org
www.arthritis.org
Barb Cvelbar, Director of Health Promotion
Cheryl Carter, Director of Development

1126 **Arthritis Foundation: Northwestern Ohio Chapter**
29 E Madison
Chicago, IL 60602
419-537-0888
800-735-0096
Fax: 419-537-6553
e-mail: info.gc@arthritis.org
www.arthritis.org

Cherie Chatreau-Grif, Executive Director
Dawn Dayton, President

1127 **Arthritis Foundation: Ohio River Valley Chapter**
7124 Miami Avenue
Cincinnati, OH 45243
513-271-4545
800-383-6843
Fax: 513-271-4703
e-mail: info.orv@arthritis.org
www.arthritis.org

Barbara Perez, President/CEO
Annette Beach, Annual Giving Coordinator

Oklahoma

1128 **Arthritis Foundation: Oklahoma Chapter**
1200 NW 63rd Street
Oklahoma City, OK 73116
405-936-3366
800-627-5486
Fax: 405-936-0617
e-mail: info.ok@arthritis.org
www.arthritis.org

Sherri O'Neil, Executive Director
Sherri Harris, Director Special Events

Pennsylvania

1129 **Arthritis Foundation: Central Pennsylvania Chapter**
3544 North Progress Avenue
Harrisburg, PA 17110
717-763-0900
800-776-0746
Fax: 717-763-0903
e-mail: info.cpa@arthritis.org
www.arthritis.org

Serves 28 counties in the central Pennsylvania area. More than 441,233 persons in the chapter area are affected with one of the forms of arthritis seriously enough to require medical care. The chapter offers research services, professional education and training, parent and community services and public health education.

Berneta Smith, Receptionist
Carol VanRaay, Volunteer Project Director

Rhode Island

1130 **Arthritis Foundation: Southern New England Chapter**
35 Cold Spring Road
Rocky Hill, CT 06067
860-563-1177
800-541-8350
Fax: 860-563-6018
e-mail: info.sne@arthritis.org
www.arthritis.org

Offers programs and services for persons in the Rhode Island area who are living with arthritis.

Anne Louise Richman, Development Assistant
Karin O'Keefe, Executive Assistant to the President

Tennessee

1131 **Arthritis Foundation: Tennessee Chapter**
421 Great Circle Road
Nashville, TN 37228
615-254-6795
800-454-4662
Fax: 615-254-8316
e-mail: info.tn@arthritis.org
www.arthritis.org

This chapter serves the residents of Tennessee by offering research and fellowship grants, self-help courses, aquatics program, educational programs, pharmacy services, loan closet, information and referrals, public forums and seminars and support groups.

Tori Foster, Manager of Accounting/IT
Deborah German, Chairman of the Board

Texas

1132 **Arthritis Foundation: North Texas Chapter**
4300 Macarthur
Dallas, TX 75209-6524
214-826-4361
800-442-6653
Fax: 214-824-5842
e-mail: info.ntx@arthritis.org
www.arthritis.org

With over 1.5 million people in the North Texas Chapter area with arthritis, the chapter's mission is to improve lives through leadership in the prevention, control and cure of arthritis and related diseases.

Carla Brandt, CFO/COO
Jane Hynes, Director Administration/Info Systems

Utah

1133 **Arthritis Foundation: Utah/Idaho Chapter**
448 E 400 S
Salt Lake City, UT 84111
801-536-0990
800-444-4993
Fax: 801-536-0991
e-mail: info.utid@arthritis.org
www.arthritis.org

A nonprofit organization serving individuals with arthritis and their families in Utah and Idaho by providing invaluable services, programs and activities.

Lisa B Fall, President
Leslie Nelson, Program Director

Vermont

1134 **Arthritis Foundation: Northern New England Chapter**
6 Chenell Drive
Concord, NH 03301
603-224-9322
800-639-2113
Fax: 603-224-3778
e-mail: info.sne@arthritis.org
www.arthritis.org

Janet Bourne, Vice President Development
Margaret Duffy, Regional Program Director

Virginia

1135 **Arthritis Foundation: Virginia Chapter**
3805 Cutshaw Avenue
Richmond, VA 23230
804-359-1700
800-456-4687
Fax: 804-359-4900
e-mail: info.va@arthritis.org
www.arthritis.org

Founded in 1954 this chapter is a nonprofit voluntary health organization dedicated to finding the cause prevention and cure for the entire group of diseases called arthritis. Offered classes books and information to better manage arthritis.

Angela Courtney, Vice President Community Development
C Annie Magnant, President

Washington

1136 **Arthritis Foundation: Washington/Alaska Chapter**
3876 Bridge Way N
Seattle, WA 98103
206-547-2707
800-746-1821
Fax: 206-547-2707
e-mail: tzuehl@arthritis.org
www.arthritis.org

Offers arthritis helplines and information lines for residents of Washington state. Provides self-help courses arthritis aquatic programs and resources for persons living with various forms of arthritis.

Barbara Osen, North Puget Sound Branch Director
Kim Mellen, Campaign Coordinator

Wisconsin

1137 **Arthritis Foundation: Wisconsin Chapter Foundation**
1650 S 108th Street
W Allis, WI 53214-4021
414-321-3933
800-242-9945
Fax: 414-321-0365
e-mail: info@wi@arthritis.org
www.arthritis.org

Statewide programs offered. Including aquatics exercise programs, support groups, self-help courses, professional education, public education seminars, advocacy counsel, juvenile arthritis support programs and children's camp information and referral help.

Libraries & Resource Centers

1138 **New York Chapter of the Arthritis Foundation**
122 East 42nd Street 212-984-8700
New York, NY 10168-1898 Fax: 212-878-5960
e-mail: info.ny@arthritis.org
www.arthritis.org
Offers people with arthritis, their families and all those with an interest in the rheumatic diseases, information on how to live every day to its fullest, even when affected by a chronic disease.

Research Centers

1139 **Affiliated Children's Arthritis Centers of New England**
New England Medical Center
750 Washington Street 617-636-7285
Boston, MA 02111-1533 Fax: 617-350-8388
Research organization comprised of a network of 15 territory pediatric centers throughout New England and based at the Floating Hospital of New England Medical Center.
Jane G Schaller MD, Coordinator

1140 **Arthritis and Musculoskeletal Center: UAB Shelby Interdisciplinary Biomedical Rese**
Shelby Interdisciplinary Biomedical Research Bldg
1825 University Boulevard 205-934-5306
Birmingham, AL 35294-2182 Fax: 205-934-1564
www.main.uab.edu/amc
Arthritis and related rheumatic disorders are studied.
Robert Kimbe MD, Director
Jennifer A Croker, Executive Administrator

1141 **Boston University Arthritis Center**
720 Harrison Avenue 617-638-4310
Boston, MA 02118 Fax: 617-638-5226
e-mail: mikyork@bu.edu
www.bumc.bu.edu
The research efforts of the Rheumatology Section relate to basic biologic mechanisms in the pathogenesis of scleroderma vasculitis amyloidosis osteoarthritis and systemic lupus erythematosus. There are concordant research efforts in clinical investigation of these disorders including testing of novel therapies.
Eugene Kissin, Clinical Director
Paul Monach, Associate Fellowship Program Director

1142 **Boston University Medical Campus General Clinical Research Center**
715 Albany Street 617-638-4542
Boston, MA 02118 Fax: 617-638-8890
e-mail: mfholick@bu.edu
dcc2.bumc.bu.edu/gcrcweb/GCRCcampus.htm
Integral unit of the University Hospital specializing in arthritis and connective tissue studies.
Michael F Holick, Program Director
Janice Kopp, Administrative Director

1143 **Brigham and Women's Orthopedica and Arthritis Center**
Brigham and Women's Hospital
75 Francis Street 617-732-5322
Boston, MA 02115 800-BWH-9999
www.brighamandwomens.org
Research studies into arthritis and rheumatic diseases.
Matthew Lian MD, Director

1144 **Central Missouri Regional Arthritis Center Stephen's College Campus**
Stephen's College Campus
1507 E Broadway 573-882-8097
Columbia, MO 65215 Fax: 573-884-5509
e-mail: phelpsam@missouri.edu
marrtc.missouri.edu
Research into arthritis and rheumatic diseases.
Amber Phelps, Health Program Specialist

1145 **Department of Pediatrics, Division of Rheumatology**
Duke University School of Medicine
T909 Children's Health Center 919-684-6575
Durham, NC 27710-1 Fax: 919-684-6616
www.rheum.pediatrics.duke.edu
Clinical and laboratory pediatric rheumatoid studies.
Laura Schanberg MD, Cochairman
Egla Rabinovich MD, Co-Chairman

1146 **Hahnemann University Hospital, Orthopedic Wellness Center**
Hahnemann University Hospital
Broad and Vine 215-762-7000
Philadelphia, PA 19107-1511 Fax: 215-762-8109
www.hahnemannhospital.com
Research activity at Hahnemann University into the areas of arthritis.
Dr. Arnold Berman, Director

1147 **Medical University of South Carolina**
96 Jonathan Lucas Street 843-792-1991
Charleston, SC 29425 800-424-MUSC
Fax: 843-792-7121
clinicaldepartments.musc.edu/medicine/di
Offers basic and clinical research on various types of arthritis.
Richard M Silver, Division Director/Professor
Gary S Gilkeson, Vice Chairman Research

1148 **Medical University of South Carolina: Division of Rheumatology & Immunology**
96 Jonathan Lucas Street Suite 912 843-792-1991
Charleston, SC 29425 Fax: 843-792-7121
www.musc.edu
Offers basic and clinical research on various types of arthritis.
Richard M Silver, Division Director/Professor

1149 **Multipurpose Arthritis and Musculoskeletal Disease Center**
School of Medicine Rheumatology Division
1110 W Michigan Street 317-274-7177
Indianapolis, IN 46202 Fax: 317-274-7792
medicine.iupui.edu
The mission of this center is to pursue major biomedical research interests relevant to the rheumatic diseases. Current areas of emphasis include articular cartiliage biology pathogenesis and treatment of various forms of amyloidosis the pathogenesis of dermatomyositis and immunologic and biochemical markers of cartilage breakdown and repair.
Raffeal Grau, Division Director
Deborah Jenkins, Office Manager and Fellowship Coordinato

1150 **Oklahoma Medical Research Foundation**
825 NE 13th Street 405-271-6673
Oklahoma City, OK 73104-5005 800-522-0211
Fax: 405-271-OMRF
www.omrf.ouhsc.edu
Focuses on arthritis and muscoloskeletal disease research.
Gary Gorbsky PhD, Member/Program Head
Philip M Silverman PhD, Member

1151 **Rehabilitation Institute of Chicago**
345 E Superior Street 312-238-1000
Chicago, IL 60611 800-354-7342
TTY: 312-238-1059
www.ric.org
Expertise in treating a range of conditions from the most complex conditions including cerebral palsy spinal cord injury stroke and traumatic brain injury to the more common such as arthritis chronic pain and sports injuries.
Edward B Case, Executive Vice President and Chief Finan
Joanne C Smith, President and Chief Executive Officer

1152 **Rosalind Russell Medical Research Center for Arthritis at UCSF**
350 Parnassus Avenue 415-476-1141
San Francisco, CA 94117 Fax: 415-476-3526
e-mail: rrac@medicine.ucsf.edu
www.rosalindrussellcenter.ucsf.edu

Arthritis research and its probable causes.
Ephraim P Engelman MD, Director
David Wofsy, Associate Director

1153 University of Michigan: Orthopaedic Research Laboratories
University of Michigan Mott Hospital
400 N Ingalls Building 734-936-7417
Ann Arbor, MI 48109 Fax: 734-647-0003
Develops and studies the causes and treatments for arthritis including new devices and assistive aids.
Dr SA Goldstein, Director

1154 Warren Grant Magnuson Clinical Center
National Institute of Health
9000 Rockville Pike
Bethesda, MD 20892 800-411-1222
Fax: 301-480-9793
TTY: 866-411-1010
e-mail: prpl@mail.cc.nih.gov
www.clinicalcenter.nih.gov
Established in 1953 as the research hospital of the National Institutes of Health. Designed so that patient care facilities are close to research laboratories so new findings of basic and clinical scientists can be quickly applied to the treatment of patients. Upon referral by physicians, patients are admitted to NIH clinical studies.
John Gallin, Director
David Henderson, Deputy Director for Clinical Care

Support Groups & Hotlines

1155 Arthritis Foundation Information Hotline
PO Box 7669
Atlanta, GA 30357-0669 800-283-7800
e-mail: contactus@arthritis.org
www.arthritis.org
Offers information and referrals, counseling, physicians information and more to persons living with arthritis.
John H Klippel, President/CEO

1156 Kids on the Block Arthritis Programs
Arthritis Foundation
PO Box 19000 404-872-7100
Atlanta, GA 31126-1000 800-283-7800
Fax: 404-872-0457
State and local programs that use puppetry to help children understand what it is like for children and adults who have arthritis.

1157 National Health Information Center
PO Box 1133 310-565-4167
Washington, DC 20013 800-336-4797
Fax: 301-984-4256
e-mail: info@nhic.org
www.health.gov/nhic
Offers a nationwide information referral service, produces directories and resource guides.

Books

1158 250 Tips for Making Life with Arthritis Easier
Arthritis Foundation Distribution Center
PO Box 6996
Alpharetta, GA 30023-6996 800-207-8633
Fax: 770-442-9742
www.arthritis.com
What do aerosol cooking spray and snow-shoveling have in common? Learn the answer to this question, and other clever and handy tips to make your life with or without arthritis easier. Plus learn about helpful serviced you didn't know were available through you bank, post office, phone company, grocery store, and other businesses you frequent.
88 pages

1159 Arthritis 101: Questions You Have, Answers You Need
Arthritis Foundation Distribution Center
PO Box 6996
Alpharetta, GA 30009-6996 800-207-8633
Fax: 770-442-9742
www.arthritis.com
Expert reviewers answer questions about basic arthritis facts, treatments, research, surgery and more. Also, specific information about six common conditions: rheumatoid arthritis, osteoarthritis, osteoporosis, fibromyalgia, lupus and gout.
144 pages

1160 Arthritis Helpbook: A Tested Self-Management Program for Coping
Kate Lorig and James Fries, author
Da Capo Press
Order Department
Jackson, TN 38301 800-343-4499
Fax: 800-351-5073
www.perseusbooksgroup.com/dacapo
This book teaches people proven techniques to reduce pain and increase dexterity, build a calcium-rich diet and maintain a healthy weight, design an exercise program that matches their needs, find tips and gadgets that solve common problems, overcome fatigue, depression, and other troubling feelings associated with these health issues, and learn about all available arthritis medications and surgeries.
2006 288 pages 6th Edition
ISBN: 0-201409-63-1

1161 Arthritis Self-Help Products
Aids for Arthritis
35 Wakefield Drive
Medford, NJ 08055-3204 609-654-6918
www.aidsforarthritis.com
Offers lists of arthritis self-help devices.

1162 Arthritis Self-Management
RA Rapaport Publishing
150 W 22nd Street 212-989-0200
New York, NY 10011-2421 800-234-0923
Fax: 212-989-4786
e-mail: editor@arthritis-self-mgmt.com
Publishes practical, how to information, focusing on the day-to-day and long term aspects of arthritis in a positive and upbeat style. Gives subscribers up-to-date news, facts and advice to help them mai tain their wellness and make informed decisions regarding their health.
48+ pages Bi-Monthly
Christine Martin Grove, Editor
Ingrid Strauch, Executive

1163 Arthritis: What Exercises Work
St. Martin's Press
175 5th Avenue 212-674-5151
New York, NY 10010-7848 800-221-7945
Fax: 212-420-9314
1993 160 pages
ISBN: 0-312097-43-3

1164 Arthritis: Your Complete Exercise Guide
Human Kinetics Press
PO Box 5076 217-351-5076
Champaign, IL 61825-5076 800-747-4457
Fax: 217-351-2674
www.humankinetics.com
1993 152 pages Paperback
ISBN: 0-873223-92-6
Steve Ruhlig, Marketing Director

1165 Bone Up on Arthritis
Arthritis Foundation
PO Box 6996
Alpharetta, GA 30009-6996 800-207-8633
Fax: 770-442-9742
www.arthritis.com
A self-help education packet designed for home-study use, this program can improve your pain and function levels by teaching proven self-help techniques.
w/Audio Tapes

1166 Clinical Care in the Rheumatic Disease
Arthritis Foundation Distribution Center

PO Box 6996
Alpharetta, GA 30023-6996 800-207-8633
Fax: 770-442-9742
www.arthritis.com

This book was written for all health professionals caring for people with rheumatic diseases and for students in these disciplines.
224 pages

1167 **Educational Rights for Children with Arthritis: A Parents Manual**
AJAO
1314 Spring Street NW
Atlanta, GA 30309-2810 404-872-7100
www.arthritis.org/

A self-instructional manual helping parents to identify and obtain school services needed by their child with arthritis. Covers laws and special services, explores strategies for working with school personnel and stresses good communication and advocacy techniques.

1168 **Exercise Beats Arthritis**
Bull Publishing Company
PO Box 1377
Boulder, CO 80306 800-676-2855
Fax: 303-545-6354
www.bullpub.com

Easy-to-follow program will help arthritis sufferers of all ages manage the problems of living with this condition. In depth look at minimizing the pain and limitations of arthritis, keep their joints mobile, increase muscle strength, strengthen bones and ligaments, perform daily tasks more easily.
1998 144 pages
ISBN: 0-923521-45-3

1169 **Help Yourself Cookbook**
Arthritis Foundation
PO Box 6996
Alpharetta, GA 30023-6996 800-207-8633
Fax: 770-442-9742
www.arthritis.com

158 pages

1170 **Living With Rheumatoid Arthritis**
John's Hopkins University Press
2715 N Charles Street 410-516-6900
Baltimore, MD 21218-4319 800-537-5487
Fax: 410-516-6998
www.press.jhu.edu

This book offers practical and usable answers to the questions of everyday life. The authors provide clear explanations of the causes, diagnosis and treatment of the disease and why medication, joint protection, physical activity and good nutrition are essential components of care.
1993 312 pages Paperback
ISBN: 0-801871-47-6

1171 **Personal Guide to Living Well with Fibromyalgia**
Arthritis Foundation Distribution Center
PO Box 6996
Alpharetta, GA 30023-6996 800-207-8633
Fax: 770-442-9742
www.arthritis.com

With this guide you'll learn the latest information about fibromyalgia, what researchers have uncovered about its causes, and an overview of the best treatment options available. Helpful worksheets and tables allow you to manage your condition and document your progress.
224 pages

1172 **Primer on the Rheumatic Diseases**
Arthritis Foundation
PO Box 6996
Alpharetta, GA 30023-6996 800-207-8633
www.arthritis.com

Written to educate medical students and family physicians, this is the authoritative guide on the rheumatic diseases.
513 pages

1173 **Toward Healthy Living: A Wellness Journal**
Arthritis Foundation Distribution Center
PO Box 6996
Alpharetta, GA 30023-6996 800-207-8633
Fax: 770-442-9742
www.arthritis.com

This spiral-bound journal has ample pages where you can record your thoughts, plus scales to monitor your mood and pain. Throughout the book you will also find wisdom from a variety of famous and ordinary people - those who live with chronic ilness, and those whose life lessons can help you gain a more positive outlook on daily living.
144 pages

1174 **Understanding Juvenile Rheumatoid Arthritis**
American Juvenile Arthritis Organization
PO Box 19000
Atlanta, GA 31126-1000 800-283-7800

A manual for health professionals to use in teaching children with JRA and their families about disease management and self-care.
372 pages

1175 **We Can: A Guide for Parents of Children with Arthritis**
AJAO
1330 W Peachtree Street NW
Atlanta, GA 30309-2904 404-872-7100
www.arthritis.org/

Offers parents tips for daily living and practical points for helping their child toward independent adulthood.

Children's Books

1176 **Arthritis**
Franklin Watts Grolier
90 Old Sherman Turnpike 203-797-3500
Danbury, CT 06816-0001 800-621-1115
Fax: 203-797-3197
www.grolier.com

This book offers a clear explanation of the various forms and effects of the disease of arthritis and what treatments are available.
96 pages Grades 7-12
ISBN: 0-531108-01-5

1177 **JRA and Me**
American Juvenile Arthritis Organization
PO Box 19000
Atlanta, GA 31126-1000 800-283-7800

A workbook for school-aged children who have juvenile arthritis. This book offers a variety of educational games, puzzles and worksheets to teach children about their illness and how to take care of themselves.
57 pages

1178 **Living with Arthritis**
Franklin Watts Grolier
90 Old Sherman Turnpike 203-797-3500
Danbury, CT 06816-0001 800-621-1115
Fax: 203-797-3197
www.grolier.com

Shows how people with arthritis can overcome their pain and lead productive, full lives.
32 pages Grades 5-7

1179 **Yard Sale Coloring Book**
American Juvenile Arthritis Organization
PO Box 19000
Atlanta, GA 31126-1000 800-283-7800

A coloring/activity book based on a Kids on the Block script, written for third and fourth grade students. It can be used with Kids on the Block performances, as a stand-alone piece or with a free lesson plan packet.

Magazines

1180 **Arthritis Today**
Arthritis Foundation
1330 W Peachtree Street NW 404-872-7100
Atlanta, GA 30309-2922 800-933-0032
Fax: 404-872-9559

The authoritative and respected source of information for persons with arthritis, their families and health professionals who manage their care. As the official magazine of the Arthritis Foundation, it is backed by the Foundation's experience of 44 years and leadership in the fight against arthritis. This magazine gives its readers the advice, information and inspiration they need to live better with arthritis.
Monthly

Newsletters

1181 **AJAO Newsletter**
American Juvenile Arthritis Organization
1330 W Peachtree Street NW
Atlanta, GA 31126-2904 404-872-7100
www.arthritis.org/answers
Offers information and updates about the organization's activities and events. Legislative information, medical updates, camp information and more for children living with arthritis.
Quarterly
Janet Austin MEd, Editor

1182 **Arthritis Accent**
Arthritis Foundation Southern N.E. Chapter
35 Cold Spring Road 860-563-1177
Rocky Hill, CT 06067-3166 800-541-8350
Fax: 860-563-6018
Information on chapter events and activities.
Quarterly

1183 **Arthritis Foundation of Illinois**
Greater Chicago Chapter
29 East Madison 312-372-2080
Chicago, IL 60602 800-735-0096
Fax: 312-372-2081
e-mail: info.gc@arthritis.org
www.arthritis.org
Marilynn J Cason, Chairman

1184 **Arthritis Foundation: Newsletter of Nebraska Chapter**
10846 Old Mill Road 402-330-6130
Omaha, NE 68154 800-642-5292
Fax: 402-330-6167
e-mail: mpuccioni@arthritis.org
www.arthritis.org
Contains information on research, medication, different types of arthritis and features on oustanding volunteers.
3x Year
Cindy Doerr, Program Director/Editor

1185 **Arthritis Foundation: Southern Arizona Chapter**
6464 E Grant Road 520-290-9090
Tucson, AZ 85715 800-444-5426
Offers updated information and news on chapter activities and events for persons with arthritis.
Monthly
Richard M Brown EdD, CFRE, President

1186 **Arthritis News**
Arthritis Foundation - WI Chapter
1650 S 108th Street 414-321-3933
West Allis, WI 53214 800-242-9945
Fax: 414-321-0365
e-mail: info.wi@arthritis.org
www.arthritis.org
Offers information on activities, events, medical research, information and referrals to persons living in the Wisconsin area that are afflicted with arthritis.
Quarterly
Judy Haugsland, CEO

1187 **Arthritis Observer**
Rocky Mountain Chapter of the Arthritis Foundation
2280 S Albion Street 303-756-8622
Denver, CO 80222-4906 800-475-6647
Fax: 303-759-4349
e-mail: info.m@arthitis.org
www.arthritis.org
Offers chapter information and educational programs to the community as well as updates on fund-raising events, resources, publications and medical updates for the arthritis community.
Quarterly

1188 **Arthritis Reporter**
New York Chapter of the Arthritis Foundation
122 E 42nd Street 212-984-8700
New York, NY 10168-0002 Fax: 212-878-5960
e-mail: info.ny@arthritis.org
www.arthritis.org
Chapter newsletter offering information on upcoming events, activities and groups for the arthritis community.
Quarterly

1189 **Arthritis Update of Rhode Island**
Arthritis Foundation Rhode Island Office
Airport Office Park 401-739-3773
Warwick, RI 02886 Fax: 401-739-8990
e-mail: info.sne@arthritis.org
www.arthritis.org
Offers information, activities, events and updates on the chapter.
Quarterly

1190 **Arthritis Volunteer**
Tennessee Chapter of the Arthritis Foundation
1719 W End Avenue 615-320-7626
Nashville, TN 37203-5123 Fax: 615-329-3982
Keeps members up-to-date on arthritis developments and on programs, services and special events in Tennessee.
Quarterly

1191 **Factor Fax**
Arthritis Foundation: Northeast California Chapter
3040 Explorer Drive 916-368-5599
Sacramento, CA 95827 800-571-3456
Fax: 916-368-5596
e-mail: info.neca@arthritis.org
www.arthritis.org
Offers information on all of the chapter's activites, events and resources for the arthritis community of central California.
Patrick Dunlap, VP Events/Programs/Services
Edward Kelley, Motion Coordinator

1192 **Focus**
Arthritis Foundation: Central Ohio Chapter
3740 Ridge Mill Drive 614-876-8200
Hilliard, OH 43026-9231 Fax: 614-876-8363
www.arthritis.org
Offers updated information on arthritis as well as news of the services and activities of the chapter.
Quarterly
Irene Baird, President

1193 **Health Points**
TyH Publications
17007 E Colony Drive
Fountain Hills, AZ 85268 800-801-1406
e-mail: editor@e-tyh.com
National newsletter with articles on complementary therapy, latest nutrition news, disability issues and much more. Focus is on fibromyalgia, chronic fatigue, arthritis and chronic pain.
Quarterly

1194 **News Across Our Horizons**
Northern & Southern New England Chapter
35 Cold Spring Road 860-563-1177
Rocky Hill, CT 06060 800-541-8350
Fax: 860-563-6018
e-mail: info.sne@arthritis.org
www.arthritis.org
Chapter newsletter offering information on programs, activities and events of the foundation, medical and research articles and resources for persons with arthritis.

1195 **Newsletter of the Central Pennsylvania Chapter**
Central Pennsylvania Chapter/Arthritis Foundation

17 S 19th Street
Camp Hill, PA 17011-5459
717-763-0900
800-776-0746
Fax: 717-763-0903
e-mail: info.cpa@arthritis.org
www.arthritis.org

Offers information on activities and events of the Chapter.
Quarterly

1196 Spectrum
Michigan Chapter of the Arthritis Foundation
1050 Wilshire Drive
Troy, MI 48084-1564
248-649-2891
800-968-3030
Fax: 248-649-2895
e-mail: info.mi@arthritis.org
www.arthritis.org

Promotes various activities and programs and provides current information about arthritis.

1197 Volunteer Voice
Kentucky Chapter of the Arthritis Foundation
410 W Chestnut Street
Louisville, KY 40202-2368
502-893-9771
800-633-5335

Newsletter offering information and updates on chapter activities, events, camps, juvenile programs and government/legislative information.

Pamphlets

1198 Americans with Disabilities Act Resource Manual
Arthritis Foundation
PO Box 7669
Atlanta, GA 30357-0669
404-872-7100
800-283-7800
Fax: 404-872-0457

1199 Ankylosing Spondylitis
Arthritis Foundation
PO Box 7669
Atlanta, GA 30357-0669
404-872-7100
800-283-7800
Fax: 404-872-0457

1200 Arthritis Answers: Basic Information About Arthritis
Arthritis Foundation
PO Box 7669
Atlanta, GA 30357-0669
404-872-7100
800-283-7800
Fax: 404-872-0457

1201 Arthritis Foundation Services
Arthritis Foundation
PO Box 7669
Atlanta, GA 30357-0669
404-872-7100
800-283-7800
Fax: 404-872-0457

1202 Arthritis Information: Advocacy and Government Affairs
Arthritis Foundation
PO Box 7669
Atlanta, GA 30357-0669
404-872-7100
800-283-7800
Fax: 404-872-0457

1203 Arthritis Information: Children
Arthritis Foundation
PO Box 7669
Atlanta, GA 30357-0669
404-872-7100
800-283-7800
Fax: 404-872-0457

List of materials for children with arthritis, their families and the health professionals who care for them.

1204 Arthritis and Diet Information Package
NAMSIC/National Institutes of Health
1 AMS Circle
Bethesda, MD 20892-0001
301-495-4484
877-226-4267
Fax: 301-718-6366
TTY: 301-565-2966
e-mail: niamsinfo@mail.nih.gov
www.nih.gov/niams/

Offers information on nutrition and diet pertaining to the arthritis community.
16 pages

1205 Arthritis and Employment: You Can Get the Job You Want
Arthritis Foundation
PO Box 7669
Atlanta, GA 30357-0669
404-872-7100
800-283-7800
Fax: 404-872-0457

1206 Arthritis and Inflammatory Bowel Disease
Arthritis Foundation
PO Box 7669
Atlanta, GA 30357-0669
404-872-7100
800-283-7800
Fax: 404-872-0457

1207 Arthritis and Pregnancy
Arthritis Foundation
PO Box 7669
Atlanta, GA 30357-0669
404-872-7100
800-283-7800
Fax: 404-872-0457

How arthritis affects pregnancy, managing pregnancy and a new baby.

1208 Arthritis and Vocational Rehabilitation
Arthritis Foundation
2970 Peachtree Road NW
Atlanta, GA 30305
404-237-8771
800-933-7023
Fax: 404-237-8153
e-mail: info.ga@arthritis.org
www.arthritis.org

1209 Arthritis in Children Information Package
NAMSIC/National Institutes of Health
1 AMS Circle
Bethesda, MD 20892-0001
301-495-4484
877-226-4267
Fax: 301-718-6366
TTY: 301-565-2966
e-mail: niamsinfo@mail.nih.gov
www.nih.gov/niams/

1210 Arthritis in Children and La Artritis Infantojuvenil
American Juvenile Arthritis Organization
PO Box 19000
Atlanta, GA 31126-1000
800-283-7800

A medical information booklet about juvenile rheumatoid arthritis. This booklet is written for parents or other adults and includes details about different forms of JRA, medications, therapies and coping issues.

1211 Arthritis on the Job: You Can Work With It
Arthritis Foundation
PO Box 7669
Atlanta, GA 30357-0669
404-872-7100
800-283-7800
Fax: 404-872-0457

1212 Arthritis: Do You Know?
Arthritis Foundation
PO Box 7669
Atlanta, GA 30357-0669
404-872-7100
800-283-7800
Fax: 404-872-0457

A brief overview of arthritis and the services of the Arthritis Foundation.

1213 Aspirin and Other Nonsteroidal Anti-Inflamatory Drugs
Arthritis Foundation
PO Box 7669
Atlanta, GA 30357-0669
404-872-7100
800-283-7800
Fax: 404-872-0457

1214 Back Pain
Arthritis Foundation
PO Box 7669
Atlanta, GA 30357-0669
404-872-7100
800-283-7800
Fax: 404-872-0457

1215 Behcet's Disease
Arthritis Foundation
PO Box 7669
Atlanta, GA 30357-0669
404-872-7100
800-283-7800
Fax: 404-872-0457

1216 Bursitis, Tendionitis and Other Soft Tissue Rheumatic Syndromes
Arthritis Foundation
PO Box 7669
Atlanta, GA 30357-0669
404-872-7100
800-283-7800
Fax: 404-872-0457

1217 **CPPD Crystal Deposition Disease**
Arthritis Foundation
PO Box 7669 404-872-7100
Atlanta, GA 30357-0669 800-283-7800
Fax: 404-872-0457

1218 **Corticosteriod Medications**
Arthritis Foundation
PO Box 7669 404-872-7100
Atlanta, GA 30357-0669 800-283-7800
Fax: 404-872-0457

1219 **Diet and Arthritis**
Arthritis Foundation
PO Box 7669 404-872-7100
Atlanta, GA 30357-0669 800-283-7800
Fax: 404-872-0457

1220 **Ehlers-Danlos Syndrome**
Arthritis Foundation
PO Box 7669 404-872-7100
Atlanta, GA 30357-0669 800-283-7800
Fax: 404-872-0457

1221 **Exercise and Your Arthritis**
Arthritis Foundation
PO Box 7669 404-872-7100
Atlanta, GA 30357-0669 800-283-7800
Fax: 404-872-0457
Types of exercise for people with arthritis and how to do them.

1222 **Family**
Arthritis Foundation
PO Box 7669 404-872-7100
Atlanta, GA 30357-0669 800-283-7800
Fax: 404-872-0457
Effects of arthritis on family life and ways to cope.

1223 **Family: Making the Difference**
Arthritis Foundation
PO Box 7669 404-872-7100
Atlanta, GA 30357-0669 800-283-7800
Fax: 404-872-0457

1224 **Gold Treatment**
Arthritis Foundation
PO Box 7669 404-872-7100
Atlanta, GA 30357-0669 800-283-7800
Fax: 404-872-0457

1225 **Gout**
Arthritis Foundation
PO Box 7669 404-872-7100
Atlanta, GA 30357-0669 800-283-7800
Fax: 404-872-0457

1226 **Guide to Effective Volunteer Lobbying**
Arthritis Foundation
PO Box 7669 404-872-7100
Atlanta, GA 30357-0669 800-283-7800
Fax: 404-872-0457

1227 **Health, Life and Disability Insurance for People with Arthritis**
Arthritis Foundation
PO Box 7669 404-872-7100
Atlanta, GA 30357-0669 800-283-7800
Fax: 404-872-0457
Information about these three types of insurance.

1228 **Hydroxychloroquine**
Arthritis Foundation
PO Box 7669 404-872-7100
Atlanta, GA 30357-0669 800-283-7800
Fax: 404-872-0457

1229 **Individuals with Arthritis**
Mainstream
1030 5th Street NW 202-898-1400
Washington, DC 20001-2504
Mainstreaming individuals with arthritis into the workplace.
12 pages

1230 **Juvenile Dermatomyositis**
Arthritis Foundation
PO Box 7669 404-872-7100
Atlanta, GA 30357-0669 800-283-7800
Fax: 404-872-0457
www.arthritis.org

1231 **Living and Loving: Information About Sexuality and Intimacy**
Arthritis Foundation
PO Box 7669 404-872-7100
Atlanta, GA 30357-0669 800-283-7800
Fax: 404-872-0457

1232 **Managing Your Activities**
Arthritis Foundation
PO Box 7669 404-872-7100
Atlanta, GA 30357-0669 800-283-7800
Fax: 404-872-0457

1233 **Managing Your Fatigue**
Arthritis Foundation
PO Box 7669 404-872-7100
Atlanta, GA 30357-0669 800-283-7800
Fax: 404-872-0457

1234 **Managing Your Health Care**
Arthritis Foundation
PO Box 7669 404-872-7100
Atlanta, GA 30357-0669 800-283-7800
Fax: 404-872-0457

1235 **Managing Your Pain**
Arthritis Foundation
PO Box 7669 404-872-7100
Atlanta, GA 30357-0669 800-283-7800
Fax: 404-872-0457

1236 **Managing Your Stress**
Arthritis Foundation
PO Box 7669 404-872-7100
Atlanta, GA 30357-0669 800-283-7800
Fax: 404-872-0457

1237 **Methotrexate**
Arthritis Foundation
PO Box 7669 404-872-7100
Atlanta, GA 30357-0669 800-283-7800
Fax: 404-872-0457

1238 **Myositis**
Arthritis Foundation
PO Box 7669 404-872-7100
Atlanta, GA 30357-0669 800-283-7800
Fax: 404-872-0457

1239 **Osteoarthritis**
Arthritis Foundation
PO Box 7669 404-872-7100
Atlanta, GA 30357-0669 800-283-7800
Fax: 404-872-0457
Offers introductions, examples, explanations and research pertaining to this type of arthritis.

1240 **Osteonecrosis**
Arthritis Foundation
PO Box 7669 404-872-7100
Atlanta, GA 30357-0669 800-283-7800
Fax: 404-872-0457

1241 **Overcoming Rheumatoid Arthritis**
Michigan Chapter of the Arthritis Foundation
1050 Wilshire Drive 248-649-2891
Troy, MI 48084-1564 800-968-3030
Fax: 248-649-2895
e-mail: info.mi@arthritis.org
www.arthritis.org
Provides extensive information about the disease and treatment, with an emphasis on what you can do for yourself.

1242 **Penicillamine**
Arthritis Foundation

PO Box 7669
Atlanta, GA 30357-0669
404-872-7100
800-283-7800
Fax: 404-872-0457

1243 **Polyarteritis Nodosa and Wegener's Granulomatosis**
Arthritis Foundation
PO Box 7669
Atlanta, GA 30357-0669
404-872-7100
800-283-7800
Fax: 404-872-0457

1244 **Polymyalgia Rheumatica and Giant Cell Arthritis**
Arthritis Foundation
PO Box 7669
Atlanta, GA 30357-0669
404-872-7100
800-283-7800
Fax: 404-872-0457

1245 **Pseudoxanthoma Elasticum Fact Sheet**
Arthritis Foundation
PO Box 7669
Atlanta, GA 30357-0669
404-872-7100
800-283-7800
Fax: 404-872-0457

1246 **Psoriatic Arthritis Information Package**
NAMSIC/National Institutes of Health
1 AMS Circle
Bethesda, MD 20892-0001
301-495-4484
877-226-4267
Fax: 301-718-6366
TTY: 301-565-2966
e-mail: niamsinfo@mail.nih.gov
www.nih.gov/niams/

1247 **Q&A's About Arthritis and Rheumatic Disease**
NIH/National Institutes of Health
1 AMS Circle
Bethesda, MD 20892-0001
301-495-4484
877-226-4267
Fax: 301-718-6366
TTY: 301-565-2969
e-mail: niamsinfo@mail.nih.gov
www.nih.gov/niams

This pamphlet offers information, technical articles and research on arthritis and related disorders. Also included are referral organizations to help patients uncover more information.

1248 **Reflex Sympathetic Dystrophy Syndrome Fact Sheet**
Arthritis Foundation
PO Box 7669
Atlanta, GA 30357-0669
404-872-7100
800-283-7800
Fax: 404-872-0457

1249 **Reiter's Syndrome**
Arthritis Foundation
PO Box 7669
Atlanta, GA 30357-0669
404-872-7100
800-283-7800
Fax: 404-872-0457

1250 **Rheumatoid Arthritis Information Package**
NAMSIC/National Institutes of Health
1 AMS Circle
Bethesda, MD 20892-0001
301-495-4484
877-226-4267
Fax: 301-718-6366
TTY: 301-565-2966
e-mail: niamsinfo@mail.nih.gov
www.nih.gov/niams

Offers an introduction and definition of rheumatoid arthritis, treatments, causes, objectives, daily living, resources and medical information.

1251 **Surgery: Information to Consider**
Arthritis Foundation
PO Box 7669
Atlanta, GA 30357-0669
404-872-7100
800-283-7800
Fax: 404-872-0457

1252 **Thinking About Tomorrow: A Career Guide for Teens with Arthritis**
Arthritis Foundation
PO Box 7669
Atlanta, GA 30357-0669
404-872-7100
800-283-7800
Fax: 404-872-0457

1253 **When Your Student Has Arthritis: A Guide for Teachers**
Arthritis Foundation
PO Box 7669
Atlanta, GA 30357-0669
404-872-7100
800-283-7800
Fax: 404-872-0457

A medical information booklet written for teachers or other adults who have arthritis. The booklet describes different forms of juvenile arthritis, how arthritis might affect the child at school, and how to help the child work around these problems.

Audio & Video

1254 **FIT Video**
Arthritis Foundation
550 Pharr Road
Altlanta, GA 30023-6996
404-237-8771
800-933-7023
Fax: 404-237-8153
e-mail: info.ga@arthritis.org
www.arthritis.org

1255 **In Control**
Arthritis Foundation
1330 W Peachtree Street NW
Atlanta, GA 30309-2922
404-872-7100
800-283-7800
Fax: 404-872-0457

An excellent at-home program which includes video, audio cassettes and the Arthritis Helpbook. Provides tools to help meet the challenges of arthritis.

1256 **PACE I**
Arthritis Foundation
PO Box 6996
Alpharetta, GA 30023-6996
800-207-8633

1257 **PACE II**
Arthritis Foundation
PO Box 6996
Alpharetta, GA 30023-6996
800-207-8633
Fax: 770-442-9742
www.arthritis.com

1258 **Pathways to Better Living**
Arthritis Foundation
PO Box 6996
Alpharetta, GA 30023-6996
800-207-8633
Fax: 770-442-9742
www.arthritis.com

1259 **Pool Exercise Program**
Arthritis Foundation Distribution Center
PO Box 6996
Alpharetta, GA 30023-6996
800-207-8633
Fax: 770-442-9742
www.arthritis.com

This video features water exercises that will help you increase and maintain joint flexibility, strengthen and tone muscles, and increase endurance. All exercises are performed in water at chest level. No swimming skills are necessary.

Web Sites

1260 **American Juvenile Arthritis Organization**
www.arthritis.com

Serves the special needs of young people with arthritis and their families. Provides information, inspiration and advocacy.

1261 **Arthritis Foundation**
www.arthritis.org

Provide services to help through information, referrals, speakers bureaus, forums, self-help courses, and various support groups and programs nationwide.

1262 **Healing Well**
www.healingwell.com

An online health resource guide to medical news, chat, information and articles, newsgroups and message boards, books, disease-related web sites, medical directories, and more for patients, friends, and family coping with disabling diseases, disorders, or chronic illnesses.

1263 **Health Finder**

www.healthfinder.gov

Searchable, carefully developed web site offering information on over 1000 topics. Developed by the US Department of Health and Human Services, the site can be used in both English and Spanish.

1264 **Healthlink USA**

www.healthlinkusa.com

Health information concerning treatment, cures, prevention, diagnosis, risk factors, research, support groups, email lists, personal stories and much more. Updated regularly.

1265 **Helios Health**

www.helioshealth.com

Online resource for your health information. Detailed information about specific health topics, access to expert advice from our Medical Advisory Board, and up-to-date health news.

1266 **MedicineNet**

www.medicinenet.com

An online resource for consumers providing easy-to-read, authoritative medical and health information.

1267 **Medscape**

www.mywebmd.com

Medscape offers specialists, primary care physicians, and other health professionals the Web's most robust and integrated medical information and educational tools.

1268 **National Arthritis & Musculoskeletal & Skin Diseases Information Clearinghouse**

www.nih.gov/niams

Provides clinical and public information and research to increase understanding of the many rheumatic diseases and related disorders. Also provides lists and order forms for their resources and materials.

1269 **WebMD**

www.webmd.com

Information on arthritis, including articles and resources.

Description

1270 **Asthma**

Asthma is a respiratory disorder that causes shortness of breath, wheezing, coughing and chest tightness. About 12 million people in the U.S. have asthma, and its incidence is increasing. It is the leading cause of hospitalization for children; however, some children with asthma will outgrow the disorder by the time they are teenagers or adults. Asthma ranges from mild illness to life-threatening episodes.

Numerous environmental factors trigger an asthma attack including allergies, infections, exercise, cold weather and stress. Treatment consists of avoiding or minimizing factors that cause an asthma attack, for example pet dander and pollen.

In addition, several medications are used to relieve asthma symptoms by opening lung airways, known as bronchodilation. Many of these drugs can be inhaled so that they work directly on the lungs. Inhaled steroids may be used for long-term control. Research and new therapies are being directed at trying to find medications that will prevent asthma from occurring. See also *Lung Disease.*

National Agencies & Associations

1271 **Allergy & Asthma Network Mothers of Asthmatics**
2751 Prosperity Avenue 703-641-9595
Fairfax, VA 22031 800-878-4403
Fax: 703-573-7794
e-mail: info@aanma.org
www.breatherville.org
A national nonprofit network of families with a desire to overcome allergies and asthma by producing the most accurate timely practical and livable alternatives to suffering.
Nancy Sander, Founder/President
Hiwote Aberra, Database/Member Services Coordinator

1272 **American Academy of Allergy, Asthma & Immunology**
555 East Wells Street 414-272-6071
Milwaukee, WI 53202-3823 800-822-2762
Fax: 414-272-6070
e-mail: info@aaaai.org
www.aaaai.org
Strives to serve the public through information on asthma and allergies, as well as referrals to allergists. Also offers pollen and mold statistics from the Committee on Pollen & Molds.
John Gardner, Media Relations Manager
Katie Tetzlaff, Communications Coordinator

1273 **American Lung Association**
61 Broadway 212-315-8700
New York, NY 10006 800-LUN-GUSA
www.lungusa.org
The mission of the American Lung Association is to prevent lung disease and promote lung health. Founded in 1904 to fight tuberculosis, the American Lung Association today fights disease in all its forms, with special emphasis on asthma, tobacco control and environmental health.
James M Anderson, Secretary

1274 **Association of Birth Defect Children Birth Defect Research for Children**
800 Celebration Avenue 407-566-8304
Celebration, FL 34747 Fax: 407-566-8341
e-mail: staff@birthdefects.org
www.birthdefects.org
Non-profit organization that provides parents and expectant parents with information about birth defects and support services for their children. Sponsors the National Birth Defect Registry, a research project that studies associations between birth defects and genetics.
Betty Mekdeci, Contact

1275 **Asthma Society of Canada**
4950 Yonge Street 416-787-4050
Toronto, Ontario, M2N-6K1 866-787-4050
Fax: 416-787-5807
e-mail: info@asthma.ca
www.asthma.ca
A national registered healthcare charity, operating within a civil society business structure.
Frank Viti, CEO
Robert Peacock MA CFRE, VP Advancement

1276 **Asthma and Allergy Information Association**
1233 20th Street NW 202-466-7643
Washington, DC 20036 800-611-7011
Fax: 202-466-8940
e-mail: info@aafa.org
www.aafa.org
A not-for-profit organization, is the leading patient organization for people with asthma and allergies, and the oldest asthma and allergy patient group in the world. AAFA provides practical information, community based services and support through a national network of chapters and support groups. AAFA develops health education, organizes state and national advocacy efforts and funds research to find better treatments and cures.
William McLin, Executive Director

1277 **National Advisory Allergic and Infectious Disease Council**
6610 Rockledge Drive 301-496-5717
Bethesda, MD 20892-6612 866-284-4107
Fax: 301-402-3573
TTY: 800-877-8339
TDD: 800-877-8339
e-mail: afauci@niaid.nih.gov
www.niad.nih.gov
The National Institute of Allergy and Infectious Diseases (NIAID) conducts and supports basic and applied research to better understand treat and ultimately prevent infectious immunologic and allergic diseases.
Anthony S Fauci MD, Director
H Clifford Lane MD, Acting Deputy Director

State Agencies & Associations

Alaska

1278 **Asthma and Allergy Foundation of America: Alaska Chapter**
PO Box 201927
Anchorage, AK 99520-1927 e-mail: aafaalaska@gci.net
www.aafaalaska.com
Formed in April, 2001, the AAFA Alaska chapter is moving quickly to provide educational programs and information about asthma and allergies through classes, workshops and educational materials. Focused not only on reaching children and adults with asthma information, but also health care professionals, caregivers, childcare providers and school personnel.
Suzi Jackson, Executive Director

California

1279 **Asthma and Allergy Foundation of America: Southern California Chapter**
5900 Wilshire Boulevard 323-937-7859
Los Angeles, CA 90036 800-624-0044
Fax: 323-937-7815
e-mail: aafasocal@aol.com
www.aafasocal.com
Dedicated to controlling and curing asthma and allergic diseases through education, a network of support groups, the support of research and specialized training, increasing public awareness and providing medication and treatment to the under served. Program

highlights include the Breathmobile, asthma camps and air power games for children.
Francene Lifson, Executive Director

Massachusetts

1280 Asthma and Allergy Foundation of America: New England Chapter
220 Boylston Street 617-965-7771
Chestnut Hill, MA 02467 877-227-8462
Fax: 617-965-8886
TTY: 877-227-8462
e-mail: info@asthmaandallergies.org
www.asthmaandallergies.org
Serves Massachusetts, Rhode Island, Connecticut, Maine, New Hampshire and Vermont. Program highlights include speakers and exhibits, telephone information and referrals, tobacco control program, scholarship essay contest for high school juniors, advocacy for safer environments and training programs for school, daycare and health professionals.
Patricia Goldman, Executive Director
Sharon Schumack, Health Education Coordinator

Michigan

1281 Asthma and Allergy Foundation of America: Michigan Chapter
17520 West 12 Mile Road 248-557-8050
Southfield, MI 40876-8768 888-444-0333
Fax: 248-557-8768
e-mail: aafamich@sbcglobal.net
www.aafa.org
Serves the state of Michigan through public forums, work place educational programs, patient advocacy, Asthma Camp and telephone referrals and information.
Karen Katz, Executive Director
Dr. Rola Bokhari-Panza, President

Missouri

1282 Asthma and Allergy Foundation of America: Greater Kansas City Chapter
9140 Ward Parkway 816-333-6608
Kansas City, MO 64114 888-542-8252
Fax: 816-333-6684
e-mail: info@aafakc.org
www.aafakc.org
Provides college scholarships, Family Asthma Education Day, adult discussion groups, Superkids Asthma Day Camp for grades 1-5, professional education, ACT, health fair participation, breathing machine, peak flow meter and spacer distribution programs. They also have a quarterly newsletter, an asthma action line, emergency medication assistance, assistance to local school districts, free educational materials, seminars for worksite clinicians and daycare workers and the smoke-free dining group.
Noel Albert, Executive Director

1283 Asthma and Allergy Foundation of America: St. Louis Chapter
1500 South Big Bend 314-645-2422
St. Louis, MO 63117 Fax: 314-692-2022
e-mail: aafa@aafastl.org
www.aafastl.org/
The Asthma and Allergy Foundation of America (AAFA), St. Louis Chapter, was founded in 1981 by a group of volunteer board-certified allergists, including Dr. Phillip Korenblat of Washington University and Dr. Raymond Slavin of St. Louis University. AAFA St. Louis provides services to the community in helping children effectively manage their asthma through the provision of medical resources, equipment and education.
Robert Novelly, Executive Director
Amy Leipholtz, Development Director

New Jersey

1284 Asthma and Allergy Foundation of America: Southeast Pennsylvania Chapter
32 Caspertown Street 856-224-9547
Gibbstown, NJ 08027 Fax: 856-224-5893
e-mail: aafasepa@prodigy.net
www.aafa.org
In the process of establishing a vital, new program that will aid children with chronic asthma. Many parents, some who are without medical insurance coverage, are unaware of the availability of a medical support system that can help their children. The Children at Risk program will enable parents to have their children evaluated and also receive a free one month supply of medication. Parents will also receive information regarding available options for follow up care and prescription coverage.
Debi Maines, Executive Director

Oregon

1285 Asthma and Allergy Foundation of America
14530 SW 144th Avenue 503-579-8375
Tigard, OR 97224 Fax: 208-474-6839
e-mail: hensches@teleport.com
Serving the state of Oregon.
Sandra L Henschel, Executive Director

1286 Asthma and Allergy Foundation of America: Oregon Chapter
14530 Southwest 144th Avenue 503-579-8375
Tigard, OR 97224-1445 Fax: 208-474-6839
e-mail: hensches@teleport.com
Serving the state of Oregon.
Sandra L Henschel, Executive Director

Texas

1287 Asthma and Allergy Foundation of America
9101 Quarter Horse Lane 817-297-3132
Fort Worth, TX 76123 888-933-AAFA
Fax: 817-563-5696
e-mail: info@aafatexas.org
www.aafatexas.org
Offers many educational programs and services that touch patients, caregivers, physicians and allied health professionals, including: child care provider education programs, school nurse and respiratory therapist education programs, and worksite allergy educacation.
Joan Hart, Executive Director
Jim Rosenthal, President

1288 Asthma and Allergy Foundation of America: North Texas Chapter
155 Southwood 817-483-8131
Burleson, TX 76028 888-933-AAFA
Fax: 817-563-5696
e-mail: aafantx@hotmail.com
www.aafa.org
Offers many educational programs and services that touch patients. caregivers, physicians and allied health professionals, including: child care provider education programs, school nurse and respiratory therapist education programs, worksite allergy education programs, spacer and peak flow meter distribution to those in need, a toll free hotline, prescription assistance information, free educational materials in English and Spanish, an electronic newsletter, professional education, etc.
Joan Hart, Executive Director

Washington

1289 Ysthma and Allergy Foundation of America: Washington Chapter
1233 20th Street 206-368-2866
Washington, DC 20036 800-727-8462
Fax: 206-368-2941
e-mail: Info@aafa.org
www.aafa.org
Program highlights include trainings for health care professionals on asthma and allergy management, working collaboratively with other local and regional agencies to improve the quality of life for those affected by asthma and allergies, organizing health seminars and educations programs.
Mary Brasle, Director of Programs and Services
Amy Patterson, Director Administration/Governance

Foundations

1290 **Asthma and Allergy Foundation of America**
1233 20th Street NW
Washington, DC 20036
202-466-7643
800-727-8462
Fax: 202-668-40
e-mail: info@aafa.org
www.aafa.org
AAFA provides practical information, community based services and support through a national network of chapters and support groups. AAFA develops health education, organizes state and national advocacy efforts and funds research to find better treatments and cures
William McLin, Executive Director

Research Centers

1291 **Brigham and Women's Hospital: Rheumatology Immunology, and Allergy Division**
75 Francis Street
Boston, MA 02115
617-525-1000
Fax: 617-525-1001
www.brighamandwomens.org
Internationally renowned for excellence in clinical care clinical investigation and basic research. A faculty of 36 board certified rheumatologists and allergists provide eldtive urgent and emergency consultations as necessary.
Michael B Brenner MD, Division Chief
Jonathan S Coblyn, Clinical Director Rheumatology

1292 **Childrens Hospital Immunology Division Children's Hospital**
Children's Hospital
300 Longwood Avenue
Boston, MA 02115
617-355-6117
www.childrenshospital.org
Organizational research unit of the Children's Hospital that focuses on the causes prevention and treatments of asthma infections and allergies.
Hans Oettgen, Associate Chief
Raif S Geha, Chief

1293 **Clinical Immunology, Allergy, and Rheumatology**
Tulane Medical School
1700 Perdido Street
New Orleans, LA 70112-1210
504-988-5578
Fax: 504-988-3686
www.som.tulane.edu/medciar
Mauel Lopez MD, Director

1294 **Duke Asthma, Allergy and Airway Center**
4309 Medical Park Drive
Durham, NC 27704
919-620-7300
www.aaac.duhs.duke.edu
Raffeal Rau, President

1295 **Johns Hopkins University: Asthma and Allergy Center**
5501 Hopkins Bayview Circle
Baltimore, MD 21224-6821
410-550-2101
e-mail: jhuallergy@jhmi.edu
www.hopkinsmedicine.org/allergy
Studies of allergic diseases and individuals with allergic disease pulmonary diseases and diseases involving inflammation and immunological processes.
Bruce S Bochner, Director
Peter S Creticos, Clinical Director

1296 **National Jewish Division of Immunology National Jewish Medical and Research Cen**
National Jewish Medical and Research Center
1400 Jackson Street
Denver, CO 80206-2762
303-398-1337
800-550-6227
Fax: 303-270-2125
e-mail: harbeckr@njc.org
www.njc.org
The only medical center in the country whose research and patient care resources are dedicated to respiratory and immunologic diseases.
John Cambier, Chairman
Ronald J Harbeck, Medical Director

1297 **Northwestern University: Division of Allergy and Immunology**
The Feinberg School of Medicine
240 E Huron
Chicago, IL 60611
312-695-4000
Fax: 312-695-4141
e-mail: rpschleimer@northwestern.edu
www.medicine.northwestern.edu
A referral center of local regional and national stature.ÿ Areas of clinical excellence include asthma allergic bronchopulmonary aspergillosis idiopathic anaphylaxis drug allergy occupational immunologic lung disease and allergen immunotherapy.
Robert P Schleimer PhD, Chief
Leslie C Grammer MD, Associate Chief for Clinical Affairs

1298 **University of Virginia: General Clinical Research Center**
University of Virginia Health System
PO Box 800787
Charlottesville, VA 22908-0787
434-924-2394
Fax: 434-924-9960
e-mail: gcrc@virginia.edu
www.healthsystem.virginia.edu/internet/g
Focuses on asthmatic disorders.
Arthur Garso Jr MD MPH, Principal Investigator
Eugene J Barrett, Program Director

1299 **University of Wisconsin: Asthma, Allergy and Pulmonary Research Center**
600 Highland Avenue
Madison, WI 53792-2454
608-263-1300
Fax: 608-262-6743
www.medicine.wisc.edu
Richard Hong, Head

Support Groups & Hotlines

1300 **Allergy & Asthma Networks Hotline**
Allergy and Asthma Network/Mothers of Asthmatics
2751 Prosperity Avenue
Fairfax, VA 22031
703-641-9595
800-878-4403
Fax: 703-573-7794
www.breatherville.org
Mary McGowan, Executive Director

1301 **Asthma and Allergy Foundation of America**
1233 20th Street NW
Washington, DC 20036
202-466-7643
Fax: 202-466-8940
e-mail: info@aafa.org
www.aafa.org
The foundation was formed to alleviate suffering and loss from asthma and allergy disorders. The foundation offers a nationwide network of chapters and support groups and provides education and emotional support for persons with allergies and asthma. Also funds research for improved treatments and ultimately a cure.

1302 **National Health Information Center**
PO Box 1133
Washington, DC 20013
310-565-4167
800-336-4797
Fax: 301-984-4256
e-mail: info@nhic.org
www.health.gov/nhic
Offers a nationwide information referral service, produces directories and resource guides.

1303 **Physician Referral and Information Line**
American Academy of Allergy Asthma and Immunology
611 East Wells Street
Milwaukee, WI 53202-3889
414-272-6071
800-822-2762
Fax: 414-272-6070
www.aaaai.org
Referral line offering information on allergy and asthma, referral to an allergy/immunology specialist.

1304 **Support for Asthmatic Youth**
Asthma and Allergy Foundation of America
1080 Glen Cove Avenue
Glen Head, NY 11545-1565
516-625-5735
Fax: 516-625-2976
A network of educational/support groups for adolescents between the ages of 9 and 17. All meetings are free and feature guest speakers, informational programs, games and other fun activities.
Renee Theodorakis MA, Director Adolescent Services

Books

1305 Asthma Care Training for Kids
Asthma and Allergy Foundation of America
1233 20th Street NW 202-466-7643
Washington, DC 20036 Fax: 202-466-8940
e-mail: info@aafa.org
www.aafa.org
Designed to help children ages 7-12 and their parents take charge of their asthma. In a series of three action filled sessions, children and their parents meet separately with their peers to learn about asthma management.

1306 Asthma Organizer
Allergy and Asthma Network/Mothers of Asthmatics
2751 Prosperity Avenue 703-641-9595
Fairfax, VA 22031-4397 800-878-4403
Fax: 703-573-7794
www.mothersofasthmatics.org
Includes daily symptom diary and forms to track medications, office visits and updates to your personal management plan. Information on peak flow monitoring, managing asthma at school, understanding asthma activators, and allergy-proofing also included. Available in Spanish.
Loose Leaf
Mary McGowan, Executive Director

1307 Asthma Resources Directory
Allergy and Asthma Network/Mothers of Asthmatics
2751 Prosperity Avenue 703-641-9595
Fairfax, VA 22031-4397 800-878-4403
Fax: 703-573-7794
www.mothersofasthmatics.org
Comprehensive listings of thousands of products, services, and resources for allergy and asthma questions.
Mary McGowan, Executive Director

1308 Asthma Self-Help Book
Asthma and Allergy Foundation of America
1233 20th Street NW 202-466-7643
Washington, DC 20036 Fax: 202-466-8940
e-mail: info@aafa.org
www.aafa.org
A thorough, practical look at asthma that includes information from the National Heart, Lung and Blood Institute's 1991 Asthma Guidelines.

1309 Asthma in the School: Improving Control with Peak Flow Monitoring
Asthma and Allergy Foundation of America
1233 20th Street NW 202-466-7643
Washington, DC 20036 Fax: 202-466-8940
e-mail: info@aafa.org
www.aafa.org
Comprehensive and practical guide to help the school nurse monitor and assist students with asthma.

1310 Asthma in the Workplace
John H Dekker & Sons
2941 Clydon Street SW 616-538-5160
Grand Rapids, MI 49509 Fax: 616-538-0720
1993 664 pages
ISBN: 0-824787-99-4

1311 Asthma: The Complete Guide
Asthma and Allergy Foundation of America
1233 20th Street NW 202-466-7643
Washington, DC 20036-2330 800-727-8462
Fax: 202-466-8940
www.aafa.org
An excellent self-management guide for asthma and allergy patients and their families.
357 pages Paperback

1312 Breathing Disorders: Your Complete Exercise Guide
Human Kinetics
PO Box 5076 217-351-5076
Champaign, IL 61825-5076 800-747-4457
Fax: 217-351-2674
www.humankinetics.com
1993 144 pages Paperback
ISBN: 0-873224-26-4
Steve Ruhlig, Marketing Director

1313 Bronchial Asthma: Principles of Diagnosis and Treatment
Humana Press
999 Riverview Drive 973-256-1699
Totowa, NJ 07512 Fax: 973-256-8341
e-mail: humana@humanapr.com
www.humanapress.com
2001 496 pages
ISBN: 0-896038-61-0

1314 Children with Asthma: A Manual for Parents
Allergy Control Products
PO Box 793 203-438-9580
Ridgefield, CT 06877-0793 800-422-3878
Fax: 203-431-8963
www.allergycontrol.com
Known as the asthma bible, this second edition is sprinkled with anecdotes by patients and their parents.
296 pages Paperback

1315 Conquering Asthma
Michael Newhouse, MD, author
B.C Decker, Inc.
50 King Street E, Floor 2 PO Box620 905-522-7017
Ontario, Canada L8N 3K7, 800-568-7281
Fax: 905-522-7839
e-mail: info@bcdecker.com
www.bcdecker.com
This text shows asthmatics how to live a healthier and happier life hardly aware that they have asthma.
1998 107 pages Paperback
ISBN: 1-896998-01-1

1316 Coping with Asthma
Rosen Publishing Group
29 E 21st Street 212-777-3017
New York, NY 10010 800-237-9932
Fax: 888-436-4643
e-mail: customerservice@rosenpub.com
www.rosenpublishing.com
This book prepares students by explaining to them the dangers of asthma, a condition which, when properly treated, is completely manageable.

ISBN: 0-823929-69-8
Carolyn Simpson, Author

1317 Understanding Asthma
Phil Lieberman, MD, author
University Press of Mississippi
3825 Ridgewood Road 601-432-6205
Jackson, MS 39211-6492 Fax: 601-432-6217
e-mail: kburgess@ihl.state.ms.us
www.upress.state.ms.us
A guide to how the disease behaves and how the latest therapies work.
1999 120 pages Paperback
ISBN: 1-578061-42-3
Kathy Burgess, Advertising/Marketing Services Manager

Children's Books

1318 All About Asthma
Asthma and Allergy Foundation of America
1233 20th Street NW 202-466-7643
Washington, DC 20036-2330 800-727-8462
Fax: 202-466-8940
www.aafa.org

Written by a 10-year-old with asthma, this cleverly illustrated book explains causes and symptoms, and ways to control asthma to lead a normal life.
39 pages Paperback

1319 **Asthma**
Franklin Watts Grolier
90 Old Sherman Turnpike 203-797-3500
Danbury, CT 06816-0001 800-621-1115
Fax: 203-797-3197
www.grolier.com
This book offers vital information on causes and treatments, plus advice on how to prevent flare-ups.
96 pages Grades 7-12
ISBN: 0-531106-97-7

1320 **Asthma Challenge**
Asthma and Allergy Foundation of America
1233 20th Street NW 202-466-7643
Washington, DC 20036 Fax: 202-466-8940
e-mail: info@aafa.org
www.aafa.org
An exciting new team game for large or small groups. Custom designed, full color, stand up board and two sets of pretested question cards. Teens and adults win AAFA Bucks as they test their knowledge in categories like Sneezes and Wheezes and Asthma Nuts and Bolts.

1321 **Best of Superstuff Activity Booklet**
American Lung Association
1740 Broadway 212-315-8700
New York, NY 10019-4315
For young children with asthma featuring a series of activities designed to help youngsters cope with asthma.
32 pages Ages 6-8

1322 **Bronkie the Bronchiasaurus**
Asthma and Allergy Foundation of America
1233 20th Street NW 202-466-7643
Washington, DC 20036-2330 800-727-8462
Fax: 202-466-8940
www.aafa.org
A Super Nintendo role-playing adventure in which players manage the asthma of two dinosaurs. They must avoid triggers, maintain their peak-flow and take daily medications. Only then can they use their strongest defense - the powerful breath blast. Designed for ages 7 to 15.

1323 **Childhood Asthma: Learning to Manage**
Asthma and Allergy Foundation of America
1233 20th Street NW 202-466-7643
Washington, DC 20036-2330 800-727-8462
Fax: 202-466-8940
www.aafa.org
Self-paced, entertaining activity books for home use featuring practical guidelines for managing childhood asthma with a focus on using peak flow meters.

1324 **Clubhouse Kids Learn About Asthma**
Asthma and Allergy Foundation of America
1233 20th Street NW 202-466-7643
Washington, DC 20036-2330 800-727-8462
Fax: 202-466-8940
www.aafa.org
Interactive CD-ROM helps children ages 4-12 learn about asthma at their own pace. Sound, animation and game-like features draw players into the life of Janie, who has just been diagnosed with asthma.

1325 **I'm a Meter Reader**
Allergy and Asthma Network/Mothers of Asthmatics
2751 Prosperity Avenue 703-641-9595
Fairfax, VA 22031-4397 800-878-4403
Fax: 703-573-7794
www.mothersofasthmatics.org
Provides expert advice on how a peak flow meter can help detect when an asthma attack can occur in an easy to understand format with colorful illustrations. Available in Spanish. Companion video, I'm a Meter Reader, available as part of a set for $12.00.
Ages 4-9
Mary McGowan, Executive Director
Nancy Sander, Editor-in-Chief

1326 **Let's Talk About Having Asthma**
Rosen Publishing Group's PowerKids Press
29 E 21st Street 212-777-3017
New York, NY 10010 800-237-9932
Fax: 888-436-4643
e-mail: customerservice@rosenpub.com
www.rosenpublishing.com
This book talks about the cause and treatments for asthma as well as the precautions sufferers should take. Recommended for grades K-4.

ISBN: 0-823950-32-8

1327 **Lion Who Had Asthma**
Asthma and Allergy Foundation of America
1233 20th Street NW 202-466-7643
Washington, DC 20036-2330 800-727-8462
Fax: 202-466-8940
www.aafa.org
A beautifully illustrated book that encourages preschoolers to use their imaginations and take their asthma medications.
24 pages Hardcover

1328 **Luke Has Asthma Too!**
Allergy Control Products
PO Box 793
Ridgefield, CT 06877-0793 800-422-3878
Fax: 203-431-8963
This gentle book will make for good reading with children, whether they have asthma or not.

1329 **Scorpions**
Harper & Row
10 E 53rd Street
New York, NY 10022-5299 212-207-7000
www.harpercollins.com
This novel, while not wholly dedicated to examining the ramifications of asthma on a child's life, does incorporate the theme into a compelling narrative.
Grades 6-9

1330 **So You Have Asthma Too!**
Allergy and Asthma Network/Mothers of Asthmatics
2751 Prosperity Avenue 703-641-9595
Fairfax, VA 22031-4397 800-878-4403
Fax: 703-573-7794
www.mothersofasthmatics.org
A children's illustrated book, offering a clear description and understanding of childhood asthma. Available in Spanish. Also see companion video, SO YOU HAVE ASTHMA TOO!, available as part of a set for $12.00.
Mary McGowan, Executive Director
Nancy Sander, Editor-in-Chief

1331 **Winning Over Asthma**
Asthma and Allergy Foundation of America
1233 20th Street NW 202-466-7643
Washington, DC 20036-2330 800-727-8462
Fax: 202-466-8940
www.aafa.org
Simple coloring book explains asthma through a story about five-year-old Graham.
30 pages Paperback

Magazines

1332 **Controlling Asthma**
American Lung Association
1740 Broadway 212-315-8700
New York, NY 10019-4315

For parents of children with asthma, this newsmagazine tells how parents can help their child deal with the many problems presented by asthma.
16 pages

1333 **Starting Strong-Staying Strong: A Resource Guide for Educational Support Groups**
Asthma and Allergy Foundation of America
1233 20th Street NW 202-466-7643
Washington, DC 20036 800-727-8462
Fax: 202-466-8940
e-mail: info@aafa.org
www.aafa.org
A resource guide to help educational support groups get organized, publicize and remain successful. Great for people who want to start an asthma or allergy support group and for existing group leaders who want to strengthen their programs. Filled with stories of success and struggle from other group leaders, medical advisors and group members across the country. A companion CD-ROM provides additional tips.
Guide + CD-ROM
William McLin, Executive Director
Mike Tringale, Director Marketing/Communications

Newsletters

1334 **Advance**
Asthma and Allergy Foundation of America
1233 20th Street NW 202-466-7643
Washington, DC 20036-2330 800-727-8462
Fax: 202-466-8940
www.aafa.org
A bi-monthly , 8 page newsletter for patients and their families filled with timely and useful information about managing asthma and allergies.
BiMonthly

1335 **Allergy & Asthma ADVOCATE Newsletter**
American Academy of Allergy, Asthma and Immunology
611 E Wells Street 414-272-6071
Milwaukee, WI 53202 800-822-2762
Fax: 414-272-6070
www.aaaai.org
Offers tips and medical information on allergies and asthma via articles written by allied health and physician AAAAI members.
6 pages Quarterly

1336 **FreshAAIR**
Asthma and Allergy Foundation of America
1233 20th Street NW 202-466-7643
Washington, DC 20036 800-727-8462
Fax: 202-466-8940
e-mail: info@aafa.org
www.aafa.org
Filled with lots of information about asthma, seasonal allergies, food allergies, back-to-school tips for parents, educational materials and much more.
Teens Bi-Monthly
William McLin, Executive Director
Mike Tringale, Director Marketing/Communications

1337 **Leaders Link**
Asthma and Allergy Foundation of America
1233 20th Street NW 202-466-7643
Washington, DC 20036 800-727-8462
Fax: 202-466-8940
e-mail: info@aafa.org
www.aafa.org
Provides useful and timely insights on how to plan and lead asthma and allergy support group meetings, how to keep your support group active and strong, and useful ideas from other support groups. Each issue features a special section for food allergy support groups.
Bi-Monthly
William McLin, Executive Director
Mike Tringale, Director Marketing/Communications

1338 **MA Report**
Allergy and Asthma Network/Mothers of Asthmatics
2751 Prosperity Avenue 703-641-9595
Fairfax, VA 22031-4397 800-878-4403
Fax: 703-573-7794
www.mothersofasthmatics.org
Offers information on medical breakthroughs, patient care, public awareness, activities and events focusing on the allergy and asthma patient. This newsletter keeps a patient fully informed with medical articles written by experts in the field.
Monthly
Mary McGowan, Executive Director
Nancy Sander, Editor-in-Chief

Pamphlets

1339 **About Asthma**
American Lung Association
1740 Broadway 212-315-8700
New York, NY 10019-4315
A popular style pamphlet explaining symptoms, treatment and more for persons with asthma.
16 pages

1340 **Adverse Reactions to Foods**
American Academy of Allergy, Asthma and Immunology
611 E Wells Street 414-272-6071
Milwaukee, WI 53202-3889 800-822-2762
Fax: 414-272-6070
www.aaaai.org
A patient's guide to problem foods, food additives, diagnosis, and treatment.

1341 **Allergies and You**
American Lung Association
1740 Broadway 212-315-8700
New York, NY 10019-4315
Answers basic questions about allergy, particularly as it relates to asthma.

1342 **Allergies to Animals**
American Academy of Allergy, Asthma and Immunology
611 E Wells Street 414-272-6071
Milwaukee, WI 53202-3889 800-822-2762
Fax: 414-272-6070
www.aaaai.org

1343 **Allergy & Asthma**
American Academy of Allergy, Asthma and Immunology
611 E Wells Street 414-272-6071
Milwaukee, WI 53202-3889 800-822-2762
Fax: 414-272-6070
www.aaaai.org
An informational brochure discussing major topics of allerges and asthma.

1344 **Allergy and Asthma: An Informational Brochure**
American Academy of Allergy, Asthma and Immunology
611 E Wells Street 414-272-6071
Milwaukee, WI 53202-3889 800-822-2762
Fax: 414-272-6070
www.aaaai.org
Offers information on asthma, its symptoms, causes, diagnosis and treatments.

1345 **Anaphylaxis**
American Academy of Allergy, Asthma and Immunology
611 E Wells Street 414-272-6071
Milwaukee, WI 53202-3889 800-822-2762
Fax: 414-272-6070
www.aaaai.org

1346 **Asthma Alert**
American Lung Association
1740 Broadway 212-315-8700
New York, NY 10019-4315
Quick reference folders with information on asthma, the symptoms and what to do in an emergency.

1347 **Asthma Handbook**
American Lung Association

1740 Broadway 212-315-8700
New York, NY 10019-4315
Explains asthma, gives self-care methods for handling it and helps patients work more effectively with their doctor.
28 pages

1348 **Asthma Lifelines**
American Lung Association
1740 Broadway 212-315-8700
New York, NY 10019-4315
Promotional brochure providing descriptions of ALA asthma education materials.
12 pages

1349 **Asthma and Allergies in Seniors**
American Academy of Allergy, Asthma and Immunology
611 E Wells Street 414-272-6071
Milwaukee, WI 53202 800-822-2762
Fax: 414-272-6070
www.aaaai.org

1350 **Asthma and Pregnancy**
American Academy of Allergy, Asthma and Immunology
611 E Wells Street 414-272-6071
Milwaukee, WI 53202-3889 800-822-2762
Fax: 414-272-6070
www.aaaai.org

1351 **Asthma and the School Child**
American Academy of Allergy, Asthma and Immunology
611 E Wells Street 414-272-6071
Milwaukee, WI 53202-3889 800-822-2762
Fax: 414-272-6070
www.aaaai.org

1352 **Atopic Dermatitis**
American Academy of Allergy, Asthma and Immunology
611 E Wells Street 414-272-6071
Milwaukee, WI 53202-3889 800-822-2762
Fax: 414-272-6070
www.aaaai.org
This brochure offers information on symptoms, diagnosi, treatment, and prognosis.

1353 **Being Close**
National Jewish Center for Immunology
1400 Jackson Street 303-388-4461
Denver, CO 80206-2762
A booklet offering information to patients suffering from a respiratory disorder such as emphysema, asthma or tuberculosis, that discusses sexual problems and feelings.

1354 **Childhood Asthma**
American Academy of Allergy, Asthma and Immunology
611 E Wells Street 414-272-6071
Milwaukee, WI 53202-3889 800-822-2762
Fax: 414-272-6070
www.aaaai.org

1355 **Childhood Asthma: A Guide for Parents**
Asthma and Allergy Foundation of America
1233 20th Street NW 202-466-7643
Washington, DC 20036-2330 800-727-8462
Fax: 202-466-8940
www.aafa.org
This colorful booklet helps parents learn all about asthma in children.
32 pages

1356 **Childhood Asthma: A Matter of Control**
American Lung Association
1740 Broadway 212-315-8700
New York, NY 10019-4315
A guide for parents of children with asthma, this booklet covers topics such as identifying asthma signs and symptoms as well as controlling the condition.
28 pages

1357 **Consumer Guide to Health Care Plans**
American Academy of Allergy, Asthma and Immunology
611 E Wells Street 414-272-6071
Milwaukee, WI 53202-3889 800-822-2762
Fax: 414-272-6070
www.aaaai.org
Gives answers to some commonly asked questions on health care.

1358 **Efficacy of Asthma Education, Selected Abstracts**
American Lung Association
1740 Broadway 212-315-8700
New York, NY 10019-4315
Abstracts documenting the efficacy of asthma education programs for physicians and other health professionals.

1359 **Exercise-Induced Asthma & Bronchospasm**
American Academy of Allergy, Asthma and Immunology
611 E Wells Street 414-272-6071
Milwaukee, WI 53202-3889 800-822-2762
Fax: 414-272-6070
www.aaaai.org
This brochure covers testing, treatment, and other advice on how to deal with exercise-induced asthma.

1360 **Facts About Asthma**
American Lung Association
1740 Broadway 212-315-8700
New York, NY 10019-4315
Primary public information leaflet on asthma.
12 pages

1361 **Facts About Peak Flow Meters**
American Lung Association
1740 Broadway 212-315-8700
New York, NY 10019-4315
Discusses the use of a peak flow meter for adults and children with asthma.
8 pages

1362 **Healthy Breathing**
National Jewish Center for Immunology
1400 Jackson Street 303-388-4461
Denver, CO 80206-2762
Offers patients with lung or respiratory disorders information on exercise and healthy breathing.

1363 **Helping Others Breathe Easier**
Allergy and Asthma Network/Mothers of Asthmatics
2751 Prosperity Avenue 703-641-9595
Fairfax, VA 22031-4397 800-878-4403
Fax: 703-573-7794
www.mothersofasthmatics.org
Offers information on educational resources, support groups and the Network for persons afflicted with asthma or allergic disorders.
Mary McGowan, Executive Director
Nancy Sander, Editor-in-Chief

1364 **Home Control of Allergies and Asthma**
American Lung Association
1740 Broadway 212-315-8700
New York, NY 10019-4315
Discusses substances in the home that may trigger asthma and allergy problems and offers suggestions for controlling them.
12 pages

1365 **Immunitherapy**
American Academy of Allergy, Asthma and Immunology
611 E Wells Street 414-272-6071
Milwaukee, WI 53202-3889 800-822-2762
Fax: 414-272-6070
www.aaaai.org
This brochure offers information on administration, benefits, and potential side effects of immune therapy.

1366 **Inhaled Medications for Asthma**
American Academy of Allergy, Asthma and Immunology
611 E Wells Street 414-272-6071
Milwaukee, WI 53202-3889 800-822-2762
Fax: 414-272-6070
www.aaaai.org
This brochure gives helpful information on classes of inhaled medication, types of inhalation devices, spacers and holding chambers, how proper training is necessary.

1367 Latex Allergy
American Academy of Allergy, Asthma and Immunology
611 E Wells Street 414-272-6071
Milwaukee, WI 53202-3889 800-822-2762
Fax: 414-272-6070
www.aaaai.org

1368 Making the Most of Your Next Doctor Visit
American Academy of Allergy, Asthma and Immunology
611 E Wells Street 414-272-6071
Milwaukee, WI 53202-3889 800-822-2762
Fax: 414-272-6070
www.aaaai.org
A personal asthma management monitor. Includes personal tracking charts to help you along.
10 pages

1369 Many Faces of Asthma
American Lung Association
1740 Broadway 212-315-8700
New York, NY 10019-4315
Provides an overview of asthma as a major public health problem, describes what happens during asthma attacks and explains how asthma is treated and managed.
12 pages

1370 Nocturnal Asthma
National Jewish Center for Immunology
1400 Jackson Street 303-388-4461
Denver, CO 80206-2762
Offers information to patients about how to understand and manage asthma at night.

1371 Occupational Asthma
American Academy of Allergy, Asthma and Immunology
611 E Wells Street 414-272-6071
Milwaukee, WI 53202-3889 800-822-2762
Fax: 414-272-6070
www.aaaai.org
This brochure also contains a list of most common agents theat cause occupational asthma and who is at risk.

1372 Occupational Asthma: Lung Hazards on the Job
American Lung Association
1740 Broadway 212-315-8700
New York, NY 10019-4315
Discusses occupational asthma, a form of asthma in which airways overreact to various irritants in the workplace.

1373 Outpatient Treatment of Asthma
American Academy of Allergy, Asthma and Immunology
611 E Wells Street 414-272-6071
Milwaukee, WI 53202-3889 800-822-2762
Fax: 414-272-6070
www.aaaai.org

1374 Peak Flow Meter: A Thermometer for Asthma
American Academy of Allergy, Asthma and Immunology
611 E Wells Street 414-272-6071
Milwaukee, WI 53202-3889 800-822-2762
Fax: 414-272-6070
www.aaaai.org

1375 Pollen and Spores Around the World
American Academy of Allergy, Asthma and Immunology
611 E Wells Street 414-272-6071
Milwaukee, WI 53202-3889 800-822-2762
Fax: 414-272-6070
www.aaaai.org
Multi-paged brochure offering graphes and tables of pollen levels and different times of the year in different parts of the country.
10 pages

1376 Removing House Dust and Other Allergic Irritants From Your Home
American Academy of Allergy, Asthma and Immunology
611 E Wells Street 414-272-6071
Milwaukee, WI 53202-3889 800-822-2762
Fax: 414-272-6070
www.aaaai.org
This brochure covers some good ideas on how to reduce dust in the home.

1377 Role of the Allergist & Clinical Immunologist in Patient Care
American Academy of Allergy, Asthma and Immunology
611 E Wells Street 414-272-6071
Milwaukee, WI 53202-3889 800-822-2762
Fax: 414-272-6070
www.aaaai.org
An informational brochure containing definitions and addresses for further information.

1378 School Information Packet
Allergy and Asthma Network/Mothers of Asthmatics
2751 Prosperity Avenue 703-641-9595
Fairfax, VA 22031-4397 800-878-4403
Fax: 703-573-7794
www.mothersofasthmatics.org
Practical, medical, and legal information for school administrators and parents of students with asthma.
Mary McGowan, Executive Director
Nancy Sander, Editor-in-Chief

1379 Standards for the Diagnosis and Care of Patients with Asthma
American Lung Association
1740 Broadway 212-315-8700
New York, NY 10019-4315
Standards developed by the American Thoracic Society, the medical section of the ALA. For physicians.
24 pages

1380 Student Asthma Action Card
Asthma and Allergy Foundation of America
1233 20th Street NW 202-466-7643
Washington, DC 20036-2330 800-727-8462
Fax: 202-466-8940
www.aafa.org
Indispensable tool for familiarizing school personnel with asthma triggers, daily medications and emergency directions for each of their students with asthma.

1381 Superstuff
American Lung Association
1740 Broadway 212-315-8700
New York, NY 10019-4315
Kit specifically designed to help the elementary schoolchild with asthma to learn how to manage the condition. The kit contains teaching tools, puzzles, riddles, stories and games.

1382 Teens Talk to Teens About Asthma
Asthma and Allergy Foundation of America
1233 20th Street NW 202-466-7643
Washington, DC 20036-2330 800-727-8462
Fax: 202-466-8940
www.aafa.org
Quotes and thoughts from teens capture the essence of what it feels like to have asthma.

1383 There are Solutions for the Student with Asthma
American Lung Association
1740 Broadway 212-315-8700
New York, NY 10017
Leaflet telling how parents and school personnel can work together to make life easier for children with asthma.
4 pages

1384 Tips to Remember
American Academy of Allergy, Asthma and Immunology
611 E Wells Street 414-272-6071
Milwaukee, WI 53202-3889
A set of 23 tip sheets offering information on various topics including allergy and asthma treatments, pregnancy and asthma, animal allergies, sinusitis and more.

1385 Tips to Remember Brochures
American Academy of Allergy, Asthma and Immunology
611 E Wells Street 414-272-6071
Milwaukee, WI 53202-3889 800-822-2762
Fax: 414-272-6070
www.aaaai.org

Thirty three colorful brochures offered on numerous topics in allergy, asthma, and immunology.

1386 **Triggers of Asthma**
American Academy of Allergy, Asthma and Immunology
611 E Wells Street 414-272-6071
Milwaukee, WI 53202-3889 800-822-2762
Fax: 414-272-6070
www.aaaai.org
This brochure gives helpful information on what will cause an asthma attack.

1387 **Understanding Asthma**
National Jewish Center for Immunology
1400 Jackson Street 303-388-4461
Denver, CO 80206
Offers a brief introduction to asthma and then goes into the physiology of asthma, the triggers of asthma, and diagnosis and monitoring of asthma.
27 pages

1388 **Understanding Immunology**
National Jewish Center for Immunology
1400 Jackson Street 303-388-4461
Denver, CO 80206-2762
Offers information to patients and the public on the body's defenses. Explains how immunity develops, the basics of immunologic medicine and coping with respiratory disorders.

1389 **Understanding Your Child with Asthma**
National Jewish Center for Immunology
1400 Jackson Street 303-388-4461
Denver, CO 80206-2762 800-222-5264
Offers information on patient care, research, education and adult programs offered by the Association.

1390 **Understanding the Pollen and Mold Season**
American Academy of Allergy, Asthma and Immunology
611 E Wells Street 414-272-6071
Milwaukee, WI 53202-3889 800-822-2762
Fax: 414-272-6070
www.aaaai.org

1391 **Unproven Methods in Diagnosing and Treating Allergies**
Asthma and Allergy Foundation of America
1233 20th Street NW 202-466-7643
Washington, DC 20036-2330 800-727-8462
Fax: 202-466-8940
www.aafa.org

1392 **Use of Steroids for Asthma and Allergies**
American Academy of Allergy, Asthma and Immunology
611 E Wells Street 414-272-6071
Milwaukee, WI 53202-3889 800-822-2762
Fax: 414-272-6070
www.aaaai.org

1393 **What Every Patient Should Know About Asthma & Allergy Medications**
American Academy of Allergy, Asthma and Immunology
611 E Wells Street 414-272-6071
Milwaukee, WI 53202-3889 800-822-2762
Fax: 414-272-6070
www.aaaai.org

1394 **What is an Allergic Reaction?**
American Academy of Allergy, Asthma and Immunology
611 E Wells Street 414-272-6071
Milwaukee, WI 53202-3889 800-822-2762
Fax: 414-272-6070
www.aaaai.org
This brochure gives helpful information on what will cause an allergic reaction.

1395 **Your Child and Asthma**
National Jewish Center for Immunology
1400 Jackson Street 303-388-4461
Denver, CO 80206-2762
A booklet offerring information to parents and family about their child with asthma. Offers information on diagnosis, treatments, triggers and family concerns.

Audio & Video

1396 **Asthma Handbook Slides**
American Lung Association
1740 Broadway 212-315-8700
New York, NY 10019-4315
Slides and script based on The Asthma Handbook for asthma patients and others.
Film

1397 **Asthma Management**
American Academy of Allergy, Asthma and Immunology
611 E Wells Street 414-272-6071
Milwaukee, WI 53202-3889 800-822-2762
Fax: 414-272-6070
www.aaaai.org
Although there is currently no cure for asthma, attacks can be controlled by appropriate asthma management. This video describes what happens during an asthma attack, how your allergists diagnoses asthma, and ways your allergist can help you to manage your condition.
10-13 minutes

1398 **Asthma and the Athlete**
American Academy of Allergy, Asthma and Immunology
611 E Wells Street 414-272-6071
Milwaukee, WI 53202 800-822-2762
Fax: 414-272-6070
www.aaaai.org
In the past, people with asthma were sometimes discouraged from exercising. Today we know that everyone, including asthmatics, can benefit from physical actilvity. This video details which exercises are best for those with asthma, and how an allergist can help asthmatic athletes to properly manage and treat their disease.
10-13 minutes

1399 **Environmental Control Measures**
American Academy of Allergy, Asthma and Immunology
611 E Wells Street 414-272-6071
Milwaukee, WI 53202-3889 800-822-2762
Fax: 414-272-6070
www.aaaai.org
By conrtolling your environment, you can reduce your exposure to substances called allergens that trigger your allergic symptoms. This program depicts common outdoor and indoor allergens, methods an allergist uses to diagnose which substances you're allergic to, and how to reduce your exposure to allergic triggers.
10-13 minutes

1400 **I'm a Meter Reader**
Allergy and Asthma Network/Mothers of Asthmatics
2751 Prosperity Avenue 703-641-9595
Fairfax, VA 22031-4397 800-878-4403
Fax: 703-573-7794
www.mothersofasthmatics.org
Provides expert advice on how a peak flow meter can help detect when an asthma attack can occur in an easy to understand format. Companion book, I'm a Meter Reader, available as part of a set for $12.00.
Video
Mary McGowan, Executive Director
Nancy Sander, Editor-in-Chief

1401 **Immunotherapy**
American Academy of Allergy, Asthma and Immunology
611 E Wells Street 414-272-6071
Milwaukee, WI 53202-3889 800-822-2762
Fax: 414-272-6070
www.aaaai.org
Immunotherapy, of allergy shots, is a long-term allergy and asthma treatment program that helps control allergic symptoms and reduces the need for medications. Learn more about immunotherapy through this video, which includes information on allergy testing and how your allergist determines if immunotherapy is right for you.
10-13 minutes

1402 **Managing Asthma in School: An Action Plan**
Asthma and Allergy Foundation of America

1233 20th Street NW 202-466-7643
Washington, DC 20036-2330 800-727-8462
Fax: 202-466-8940
www.aafa.org

Gives the basics of asthma and a plan for school nurses, parents and physicians to work together.
14 minutes

1403 **Managing Childhood Asthma**
American Lung Association
Box 596-COL 212-245-8000
New York, NY 10001 800-586-4872
Fax: 312-440-9374
e-mail: webmaster@ala.org
www.ala.org

What parents need to know to manage asthma. 22 minutes.
Video

1404 **Pharmacologic Therapy of Pediatric Asthma**
American Lung Association
1740 Broadway 212-315-8700
New York, NY 10019-4315

A Learning Resource Program developed by a joint committee of the American Thoracic Society and the ALA.
Film

1405 **Regular Kid**
American Lung Association
1740 Broadway 212-315-8700
New York, NY 10019-4315

This film shows how families and children cope with asthma problems. Proven asthma management strategies are presented through the experiences of four children with asthma, ranging in age from toddler to teenager.
Film

1406 **So You Have Asthma Too!**
Allergy and Asthma Network/Mothers of Asthmatics
2751 Prosperity Avenue 703-641-9595
Fairfax, VA 22031-4397 800-878-4403
Fax: 703-573-7794
www.mothersofasthmatics.org

Offers a clear description and understanding of childhood asthma. Also see companion book, So You Have Asthma Too!, available as part of a set for $12.00.
Video
Mary McGowan, Executive Director
Nancy Sander, Editor-in-Chief

1407 **Stinging Insect Allergy**
American Academy of Allergy, Asthma and Immunology
611 E Wells Street 414-272-6071
Milwaukee, WI 53202-3889 800-822-2762
Fax: 414-272-6070
www.aaaai.org

Although many people are afraid of stinging insects such as bees, the stings of these insects actually cause some people to have serious allergic reactions. This video tells how to recognize and avoid stinging insects, what to do if you are stung and how to identify symptoms of an allergic reaction and get medical help.
10-13 minutes

1408 **Understanding Allergic Reactions**
American Academy of Allergy, Asthma and Immunology
611 E Wells Street 414-272-6071
Milwaukee, WI 53202-3889 800-822-2762
Fax: 414-272-6070
www.aaaai.org

During an allergic reaction, your body responds to a substance generally considered harmless to most people. This video portrays what happens in you body's immune system during an allergic reaction, how to avoid allergic substances, and methods your allergist uses to treat your allergies.
10-13 minutes

1409 **What School Personnel Should Know About Asthma**
American Lung Association
1740 Broadway 212-315-8700
New York, NY 10019-4315

Professionally produced videotape discussing the triggers, symptoms and management of childhood asthma.
Videotape

1410 **You're in Charge: Teens with Asthma**
Asthma and Allergy Foundation of America
1233 20th Street NW 202-466-7643
Washington, DC 20036-2330 800-727-8462
Fax: 202-466-8940
www.aafa.org

Designed for young adults dealing with the daily challenges of asthma management. Teens share their experiences and use of peak flow meters and prescribed medications.
10 minutes

Web Sites

1411 **American Academy of Allergy, Asthma**
www.aaaai.org

Largest professional medical specialty organization in the United States. Mission is the advancement of knowledge and practice of allergy, asthma and immunology for optimal patient care.

1412 **American College of Allergy, Asthma**
www.acaai.org

The ACAAI is a professional association of 4900 allergists/immunologists. Established in 1942, the ACAA is dedicated to improving the quality of patient care in allergy and immunology through research, advocacy and professional and public education.

1413 **American Lung Association**
www.lungusa.com

Mission is to prevent lung disease and to promote lung health. As the oldest voluntary health organization in the United States, achieving the goals through thousands of volunteers and staff.

1414 **Asthma and Allergy Foundation of America**
www.aafa.org

Information to alleviate suffering and loss from asthma and allergy disorders.

1415 **Gazoontite**
www.gazoontite.com

Provides links to websites involving asthma and also asthma-related products, such as books and guides.

1416 **Healingwell**
www.healingwell.com

An online health resource guide to medical news, chat, information and articles, newsgroups and message boards, books, disease-related web sites, medical directories, and more for patients, friends, and family coping with disabling diseases, disorders, or chronic illnesses.

1417 **Health Finder**
www.healthfinder.gov

Searchable, carefully developed web site offering information on over 1000 topics. Developed by the US Department of Health and Human Services, the site can be used in both English and Spanish.

1418 **Healthlink USA**
www.healthlinkusa.com

Health information concerning treatment, cures, prevention, diagnosis, risk factors, research, support groups, email lists, personal stories and much more. Updated regularly.

1419 **Helios Health**
www.helioshealth.com

Online resource for your health information. Detailed information about specific health topics, access to expert advice from our Medical Advisory Board, and up-to-date health news.

1420 **MedicineNet**
www.medicinenet.com

An online resource for consumers providing easy-to-read, authoritative medical and health information.

1421 **Medscape**
www.mywebmd.com

Medscape offers specialists, primary care physicians, and other health professionals the Web's most robust and integrated medical information and educational tools.

1422 WebMD

www.webmd.com

Provides links to over 100 articles involving asthma information.

Description

1423 **Ataxia**

Ataxia refers to a group of diseases that cause failure of muscular coordination, resulting in a staggered gait, the inability to stand or sit straight and the inability to make smooth, voluntary movements. All ataxias involve deterioration of the cerebellum and/or the brain and spinal structures that communicate with it. Conditions that are associated with ataxia may be hereditary or sporadic.

The most common hereditary ataxia is Friedreich's ataxia, which typically begins between 5 and 15 years of age. At first there is gait unsteadiness and slurred speech which progresses to weakness of the extremities. Some patients develop spinal deformity or cardiac problems. Other, less common hereditary ataxias generally begin during adult life. Sporadic cases also begin in adulthood and may be due to toxins, such as alcohol, or may be of unknown cause. Sporadic cases are often a symptom of some other disease, such as multiple sclerosis, stroke, or vitamin deficiencies. Although essentially all patients will become wheelchair-dependent at some point, the outlook for long-term survival is good.

Treatment for any of the ataxias is aimed at the underlying cause, but often supportive, with physical therapy, assistive devices, psychological support, career counseling and treatment of complications. Genetic counseling is appropriate for those with the hereditary forms and their families.

National Agencies & Associations

1424 **National Ataxia Foundation**
2600 Fernbrook Lane 763-553-0020
Minneapolis, MN 55447 Fax: 763-553-0167
e-mail: naf@ataxia.org
www.ataxia.org
The National Ataxia Foundation is dedicated to improving the lives of persons affected by ataxia through support education and research.
Michael Parent, Executive Director
Susan Hagen, Patient Services Director

Support Groups & Hotlines

1425 **National Health Information Center**
PO Box 1133 310-565-4167
Washington, DC 20013 800-336-4797
Fax: 301-984-4256
e-mail: info@nhic.org
www.health.gov/nhic
Offers a nationwide information referral service, produces directories and resource guides.

Alabama

1426 **Alabama Ambassador: National Ataxia Foundation**
123 Leigh Ann Road 256-828-4858
Hazel Green, AL 35750 e-mail: diannebw@aol.com
www.ataxia.org
Ambassadors are often in areas not served by a support group or chapter.
Dianne Blaine-Williamson, NAF Ambassador

1427 **Alabama Support Group: National Ataxia Foundation**
16 Oaks Circle 205-531-2514
Birmingham, AL 35244 e-mail: donnellyB6132@aol.com
www.ataxia.org
Becky Donnelly, Group Contact

Arizona

1428 **Phoenix Area Support Group: National Ataxi Foundation**
2322 W Sagebrush Drive 480-726-3579
Chandler, AZ 85224-2155 e-mail: rtg22@cox.net
www.ataxia.org
Rita Garcia, Director

1429 **Tucson Support Group: National Ataxia Foundation**
7665 E Placita Luna Preciosa 520-885-8326
Tucson, AZ 85710 e-mail: bbeck15@cox.net
Bart Beck, Director

California

1430 **California Ambassador: National Ataxia Foundation**
315 W Alamos 559-281-9188
Clovis, CA 93612 e-mail: mike betchel@yahoo.com
www.ataxia.org
Mike Betchel, NAF Ambassador

1431 **Los Angeles Support Group: National Ataxia Foundation**
339 W Palmer 818-246-5758
Glendale, CA 91204 e-mail: harryluther@sbcglobal.net
www.ataxia.org
Sid Luther, President

1432 **Northern California Support Group: National Ataxia Foundation**
26840 Eldridge Avenue 510-783-3190
Hayward, CA 94544 e-mail: rsisbig@aol.com
www.ataxia.com
Deborah Ominctin, Leader

1433 **Orange County Support Group: National Ataxia Foundation**
829 W Gary Ave 323-788-7751
Montebello, CA 90640 e-mail: dnavar@ucla.edu
www.ataxia.org
Daniel Navar, Group Leader

1434 **San Diego Support Group: National Ataxia Foundation**
2087 Granite Hills Drive 619-447-3753
El Cajon, CA 92019 e-mail: sdasg@cox.net
www.ataxia.org
Earl McLaughlin, Group Leader

Colorado

1435 **Denver Support Group: National Ataxia Foundation**
5902 W Maplewood Drive 303-973-8035
Littleton, CO 80123 e-mail: tom_sathre@acm.org
www.ataxia.org
Tom Sathre, Group Leader

Florida

1436 **Florida Ambassador: National Ataxia Foundation**
302 Beach Drive 850-654-2817
Destin, FL 30541 e-mail: csugars@cox.net
www.ataxia.org
Ambassadors are often in areas not served by a support group or chapter.
Christina Sugars, NAF Ambassador

1437 **Northwest Florida Support Group: National Ataxia Foundation**
54 Troon Terrace 904-273-4644
Ponte Vedra, FL 32082-3321 e-mail: jmcgranepvb@bellsouth.net
www.ataxia.org
June McGrane, Group Leader

1438 **West Central FL Support Group: National A taxia Foundation**
9753 Elm Way 813-453-1084
Tampa, FL 33635 e-mail: flataxia@yahoo.com
www.ataxia.org
Crystal Frohna, Group Leader

Georgia

1439 **Georgia Support Group: National Ataxia Foundation**
320 Peters Street 404-822-7451
Savannah, GA 30313 e-mail: rookssgj@yahoo.com
www.ataxia.org

Greg Rooks, Group Leader

Illinois

1440 **Chicago Area Support Group: National Ataxia Foundation**
410 W Mahogany Ct 847-496-7544
Palatine, IL 60067 e-mail: caasg2@aol.com
www.ataxia.org

Craig Lisack, Group Leader

1441 **Chicago Metro Support Group: National Ataxia Foundation**
5633 N Kenmore 773-334-1667
Chicago, IL 60660 e-mail: cmarsh34@ameritech.net
www.ataxia.org

Chris Marsh, Group Leader

Indiana

1442 **Southern Indiana Support Group: National Ataxia Foundation**
1102 Ridgewood Drive 812-630-4783
Huntingburg, IN 47542 e-mail: monicasfaith@insightbb.com
www.ataxia.org

Monica Smith, Group Leader

Louisiana

1443 **Louisiana Support Group: National Ataxia Foundation**
2250 Gause Blvd 985-643-0783
Slidell, LA 70431 e-mail: ataxia1@earthlink.net
www.ataxia.org

Carla Hagler, Group Leader

Maine

1444 **Maine Support Group: National Ataxia Foundation**
PO Box 113
Bowdoinham, ME 04008 e-mail: rollins@gwi.net
www.ataxia.org

Kelly Rollins, Group Leader

Maryland

1445 **Chesapeake Area Support Group: National Ataxia Foundation**
3200 Baker Circle 301-644-1836
Adamstown, MD 21710-9666 e-mail: carljlauter@erols.com
www.ataxia.org

Carl J Lauter, Group Leader

Massachusetts

1446 **New England Area Support Group: National Ataxia Foundation**
45 Juliette Street
Andover, MA 01810 978-475-8072
www.ataxia.org

Donna Gorzela, Group Leader

Michigan

1447 **Detroit Support Group: National Ataxia Foundation**
20217 Wyoming 313-736-2827
Detroit, MI 48221 e-mail: tinyt48221@yahoo.cpom
www.ataxia.org

Tanya Tunstul, Group Leader

Minnesota

1448 **Minnesota Ambassador: National Ataxia Foundation**
5179 Meadow Drive SE 504-282-7127
Rochester, MN 55904 e-mail: logoetz@gmail.com
www.ataxia.org

Lori Goetzman, NAF Ambassador

1449 **Twin Cities Area Support Group: National Ataxia Foundation**
2549 32nd Avenue S 612-724-3487
Minneapolis, MN 55406 e-mail: lschultz@bitstream.net
www.ataxia.org

Lenore Healy Schultz, Group Leader

Mississippi

1450 **Mississippi Area Support Group: National Ataxia Foundation**
PO Box 17005
Hattisburg, MS 39404 e-mail: daglio1@bellsouth.net
www.ataxia.org

Camille Daglio, Group Leader

Missouri

1451 **Kansas City Support Group: National Ataxia Foundation**
17700 E 17th Terrace Court S
Independence, MO 64057 816-257-2428
www.ataxia.org

Lois Goodman, Group Leader

1452 **Mid Missouri Support Group: National Ataxia Foundation**
1609 Cocoa Court 573-474-7232
Columbia, MO 65202 e-mail: rogercooley@localnet.com
www.ataxia.org

Roger Cooley, Contact

New York

1453 **Central NY Area Support Group: National Ataxia Foundation**
2849 Bingley Road
Cazenovia, NY 13035 e-mail: johnsons@summitsolutions.net
www.ataxia.org

Linda Johnson, President

1454 **New York Ambassador National Ataxia Foundation**
36 W Redoubt Rd 763-553-0020
Fishkill, NY 12524 e-mail: vrabsolutely@aol.com
www.ataxia.org

Valerie Ruggiero, NAF Ambassador

1455 **Tri-State Area Support Group: National Ataxia Foundation**
Northgate 6C 212-844-8711
Bronxville, NY 10708 e-mail: markmeghan@aol.com
www.ataxia.org

Mark Mitchell, Group Leader

Ohio

1456 **Central Ohio Support Group: National Ataxia Foundation**
7852 Country Court 440-255-8284
Mentor, OH 44060 e-mail: wurbanski@oh.rr.com
www.ataxia.org

Cecilia Urbanski, Group Leader

1457 **North East Ohio Support Group National Ataxia Foundation**
Box 148 440-693-4454
Mesopotamia, OH 44439 e-mail: kakah@windstream.net
www.ataxia.org

Joe Miller, President

1458 **Ohio Ambassador: National Ataxia Foundation**
1283 Westfield SW 330-499-4060
North Canton, OH 44720 e-mail: jkardos@juno.com
www.ataxia.org

James Kardos, NAF Ambassador

Oklahoma

1459 **Oklahoma Ambassador: National Ataxia Foundation**
5700 SE Hazel Road 918-331-9530
Bartlesville, OK 74006 e-mail: droopydog36@hotmail.com
www.ataxia.org

Darrell Owens, NAF Ambassador

Oregon

1460 **Willamette Valley Support Group: National Ataxia Foundation**
Albany General Hospital 541-812-4162
Albany, OR 97321 Fax: 541-812-4614
e-mail: malindam@samhealth.org
www.ataxia.org

Malinda Moore, President

Pennsylvania

1461 **South East Pennsylvania Support Group: National Ataxia Foundation**
610-272-1502
e-mail: lizout@aol.com
www.ataxia.org

Liz Nussear, Group Leader

South Carolina

1462 **Carolinas Support Group: National Ataxia National Ataxia Foundation**
1305 Cely Road 864-220-3395
Easley, SC 29642 e-mail: cecerussell@hotmail.com
www.ataxia.org

Cece Russell, Group Leader

Texas

1463 **Houston Support Group: National Ataxia Foundation**
9405 Highway 6 S 281-693-1826
Houston, TX 77083 e-mail: angelahcloud@aol.com
www.ataxia.org

Angela Cloud, Group Leader

1464 **North Texas Support Group: National Ataxia Foundation**
7 Wentworth Court
Trophy Club, TX 76262 e-mail: cheve11e@sbcglobal.net
www.ataxia.org

David Henry Jr, Group Leader

1465 **Texas Ambassador: National Ataxia Foundation**
356 Las Brisas Blvd 830-557-6050
Seguin, TX 78155-0193 e-mail: acemom@peoplepc.com
www.ataxia.org

Barbara Pluta, NAF Ambassador

Utah

1466 **Utah Support Group: National Ataxia Founda tion**
Moran Eye Clinic 801-585-2213
Salt Lake City, UT 84132 e-mail: julia.kleinschmidt@hsc.utah.edu
www.ataxia.org

Dr Julia Kleinschmidt, Group Leader

Washington

1467 **Seattle Support Group: National Ataxia Foundation**
14104 107th Avenue 425-823-6239
Kirkland, WA 98034 e-mail: ataxiaseattle@comcast.net
www.ataxia.org

Milly Lewendon, Group Leader

1468 **Washington Ambassador National Ataxia Foundation**
PO Box 19045
Spokane, WA 99219 509-482-8501
www.ataxia.org

Linda Jacoy, Ambassador

Books

1469 **Directory of National Genetic Voluntary Organizations**
Genetic Alliance
4301 Connecticut Avenue NW 202-966-5557
Washington, DC 20008-2369 800-336-4363
Fax: 202-966-8553
e-mail: info@genticalliance.org
www.genticalliance.org

Lists hundreds of organizations and associations dealing with genetic conditions.

1470 **Hereditary Ataxia: Guidebook for Managing Speech & Swallowing**
National Ataxia Foundation
2600 Fernbrook Lane N 763-553-0020
Minneapolis, MN 55447-4752 Fax: 763-553-0167
e-mail: naf@mr.net
www.ataxia.org

1471 **Living with Ataxia**
National Ataxia Foundation
2600 Fernbrook Lane N 763-553-0020
Minneapolis, MN 55447-4752 Fax: 763-553-0167
e-mail: naf@mr.net
www.ataxia.org

Compassionate resource for people who have or may be at risk of having ataxia, and for their families. This book explains the nature and causes of ataxia, the basic genetics that underlie many kinds of ataxia, discusses medical management of ataxia, provides practical advice for everyday living, points the way to many useful resources and assures that living a good life is an entirely reasonable aspiration, even with ataxia.
112 pages

1472 **Ten Years to Live**
National Ataxia Foundation
2600 Fernbrook Lane N 763-553-0020
Minneapolis, MN 55447-4752 Fax: 763-553-0167
e-mail: naf@mr.net
www.ataxia.org

Struggles of the Schut family with hereditary ataxia.

ISBN: 0-962716-63-1

Newsletters

1473 **Alert**
Alliance of Genetic Support Groups
4301 Connecticut Avenue NW 301-652-5553
Washington, DC 20008-2304 800-336-4363
e-mail: alliance@capaccess.org
www.medhelp.org/www/agsg2.htm

Functions as a vehicle of communication between the Alliance and its constituency. Provides timely and useful information on genetics research.
Monthly

1474 **GENES Information Services**
Genetic Network of the Empire State
Empire State Plaza 518-474-7148
Albany, NY 12201 Fax: 518-474-8590

1475 **Generations**
National Ataxia Foundation
2600 Fernbrook Lane N 763-553-0020
Minneapolis, MN 55447-4752 Fax: 763-553-0167
e-mail: naf@mr.net
www.ataxia.org

Provides the latest in ataxia research, information on coping, reference material, updates on chapters and support groups and personal stories on living with ataxia. With a readership of more than 25,000, this publication is distributed throughout the US and the world. This publication is for ataxia families, the medical community, ataxia researchers and interested individuals. This publication is free to NAF members.
Quarterly

1476 **Genexus**
Great Plains Genetic Service Network
The University of Iowa 319-356-2674
Iowa City, IA 52242 Fax: 319-356-3347

1477 **Great Lakes Genetic News**
Great Lakes Regional Genetics Group
1500 Highland Avenue 608-266-2907
Madison, WI 53705-2274 Fax: 608-263-3496

1478 **MARGIN**
Mid-Atlantic Regional Human Genetics Network
260 S Broad Street 215-456-7910
Philadelphia, PA 19102-5021 Fax: 215-456-7911

1479 **MSRGSN Newsletter**
Mountain States Regional Genetics Service Network
4300 Cherry Creek Drive S 303-692-2423
Denver, CO 80246 Fax: 303-782-5576
e-mail: joyce.hooker@state.co.us
www.mostgene.org

8-12 pages
Joyce Hooker, Coordinator

1480 **NERG News**
New England Regional Genetics Group
PO Box 670 207-839-5324
Mount Desert, ME 04660-0670 Fax: 207-839-8637

1481 **SERGG**
Southeast Regional Genetics Group
PO Box 1642 404-778-8551
Decatur, GA 30031-1642 Fax: 404-778-8562
e-mail: mlane@sergginc.org
sergginc.org

Pamphlets

1482 **Alliance Brochure**
Genetic Alliance
4301 Connecticut Avenue NW 202-966-5557
Washington, DC 20008-2304 Fax: 202-966-8553
e-mail: info@geneticalliance.org
www.geneticalliance.org
Explains the services and programs offered by the alliance.

1483 **Ataxia Fact Sheet**
National Ataxia Foundation
2600 Fernbrook Lane N 763-553-0020
Minneapolis, MN 55447-4752 Fax: 763-553-0167
e-mail: naf@mr.net
www.ataxia.org
Describes ataxia as a symptom and its association with other medical problems as well as the hereditary types.

1484 **Familial Spastic Paraplegia**
National Ataxia Foundation
2600 Fernbrook Lane N 763-553-0020
Minneapolis, MN 55447-4752 Fax: 763-553-0167
e-mail: naf@mr.net
www.ataxia.org
Defines this disorder and notes symptoms, causes and treatments.

1485 **Frenkel's Exercises**
National Ataxia Foundation
2600 Fernbrook Lane N 763-553-0020
Minneapolis, MN 55447-4752 Fax: 763-553-0167
e-mail: naf@mr.net
www.ataxia.org
Describes an exercise program designed for those with ataxia.

1486 **Friedrich's Ataxia**
National Ataxia Foundation
2600 Fernbrook Lane N 763-553-0020
Minneapolis, MN 55447-4752 Fax: 763-553-0167
e-mail: naf@mr.net
www.ataxia.org
Describes symptoms, diagnosis, genetics and hints on coping.

1487 **Gene Testing for Ataxia**
National Ataxia Foundation
2600 Fernbrook Lane N 763-553-0020
Minneapolis, MN 55447-4752 Fax: 763-553-0167
e-mail: naf@mr.net
www.ataxia.org
Describes the latest information about who should consider it and where to have it done.

1488 **Health Insurance**
National Ataxia Foundation
2600 Fernbrook Lane N 763-553-0020
Minneapolis, MN 55447-4752 Fax: 763-553-0167
e-mail: naf@mr.net
www.ataxia.org
Offers health insurance advice for persons with ataxia.

1489 **Hereditary Ataxia: Brochure**
National Ataxia Foundation
2600 Fernbrook Lane N 763-553-0020
Minneapolis, MN 55447-4752 Fax: 763-553-0167
e-mail: naf@mr.net
www.ataxia.org
Describes recessive and dominant ataxias, information on how hereditary ataxia is transmitted and explanations of the NAF's role in education, service and prevention.

1490 **Hereditary Ataxia: Fact Sheets**
National Ataxia Foundation
2600 Fernbrook Lane N 763-553-0020
Minneapolis, MN 55447-4752 Fax: 763-553-0167
e-mail: naf@mr.net
www.ataxia.org
Various ataxia fact sheets relating to specific forms of hereditary ataxia. Individual ataxia fact sheets include Friederich's ataxia and specific forms of spinocerebellar ataxias (SCAs).

1491 **Incorporating Consumers into Regional Genetics Networks**
Genetic Alliance
4301 Connecticut Avenue NW 202-966-5557
Washington, DC 20008-2304 Fax: 202-966-8553
e-mail: info@geneticalliance.org
www.geneticalliance.org

1492 **Informed Consent: Participation In Genetic Research Studies**
Genetic Alliance
4301 Connecticut Avenue NW 202-966-5557
Washington, DC 20008-2304 Fax: 202-966-8553
e-mail: info@genticalliance.org
www.geneticalliance.org
This booklet explains the nature of genetic research with its benefits and risks.

1493 **Pen-Pal Directory**
National Ataxia Foundation
2600 Fernbrook Lane N 763-553-0020
Minneapolis, MN 55447-4752 Fax: 763-553-0167
e-mail: naf@mr.net
www.ataxia.org
National, state and international directory of others who are affected by ataxia. Available to NAF Pen-Pal members only. Application available.

1494 **Students with Friedreich's Ataxia**
National Ataxia Foundation
2600 Fernbrook Lane N 763-553-0020
Minneapolis, MN 55447-4752 Fax: 763-553-0167
e-mail: naf@mr.net
www.ataxia.org
Worksheet for teachers, parents and others who need to understand the physical constraints of ataxia.

Audio & Video

1495 **Together...There Is Hope**
National Ataxia Foundation
2600 Fernbrook Lane N 763-553-0020
Minneapolis, MN 55447-4752 Fax: 763-553-0167
e-mail: naf@mr.net
www.ataxia.org
Video discussing ataxias genetic patterns of inheritance and the National Ataxia Foundation and its research efforts.

Web Sites

1496 **Healing Well**
www.healingwell.com
An online health resource guide to medical news, chat, information and articles, newsgroups and message boards, books, disease-re-

lated web sites, medical directories, and more for patients, friends, and family coping with disabling diseases, disorders, or chronic illnesses.

1497 Health Finder

www.healthfinder.gov

Searchable, carefully developed web site offering information on over 1000 topics. Developed by the US Department of Health and Human Services, the site can be used in both English and Spanish.

1498 Healthlink USA

www.healthlinkusa.com

Health information concerning treatment, cures, prevention, diagnosis, risk factors, research, support groups, email lists, personal stories and much more. Updated regularly.

1499 Helios Health

www.helioshealth.com

Online resource for your health information. Detailed information about specific health topics, access to expert advice from our Medical Advisory Board, and up-to-date health news.

1500 MedicineNet

www.medicinenet.com

An online resource for consumers providing easy-to-read, authoritative medical and health information.

1501 Medscape

www.mywebmd.com

Medscape offers specialists, primary care physicians, and other health professionals the Web's most robust and integrated medical information and educational tools.

1502 National Ataxia Foundation

www.ataxia.org

Information on ataxia, ataxia research, listing of chapters and support groups and related links. Researchers may download NAF's ataxia reserch application guidelines and forms. Exerpts of articles in NAF's quarterly news publication, Generations. Online registration for NAF's annual membership meetings. Caladar of events on NAF activities. This site is for ataxia familes, the medical community, ataxia reserachers and interested individuals.

1503 WebMD

www.webmd.com

Information on Ataxia, including articles and resources.

Description

1504 **Attention Deficit Hyperactivity Disorder**

Attention Deficit-Hyperactivity Disorder, ADHD, and Attention Deficit Disorder, ADD, are neurologically based disorders. ADHD primarily affects children, with 2 to 4 percent of the school-age population in the United States having some symptoms. In about 25 percent of attention deficit cases, hyperactivity is not present, and it is thus labeled ADD. ADHD's three major symptoms are distractability, impulsivity and hyperactivity. The dominant symptom of ADD is day dreaming or tuning out. ADHD is seen 10 times more frequently in boys than girls. Studies show that 90 percent have academic problems or are underachievers, although these difficulties may not begin until the middle school years.

While studies suggest that about 50 percent of children with these disorders will improve at puberty, both ADHD and ADD can exist throughout a lifetime and, in fact, may first be diagnosed in teen or adult years.

Often, an affected individual experiences difficulties that can impact learning, peer relations, family life, and self-esteem. These difficulties may manifest themselves through angry outbursts, self-imposed social isolation, blaming others, a quickness to fight, and a high sensitivity to criticism.

Treatment of ADHD and ADD include: education programs with resource or tutorial help; psychological programs to improve self-esteem and help families and individuals deal with associated stress; and medical therapy. Treatment must be individualized to address both intrinsic charateristics of the child and relevant environmental factors, and be coordinated with a variety of interventions within the school, home and community.

Many professionals agree that medication, when appropriate, combined with counseling, best controls symptoms. Stimulant medications, including the new longer active agents, are the drugs of choice. To identify children with this disorder and to develop the most appropriate treatment plan, parents will need to consult with a psychiatrist, pediatric neurologist, or pediatrician.

National Agencies & Associations

1505 **Children & Adults with Attention Deficit Disorders**
8181 Professional Place 301-306-7070
Landover, MD 20785 800-233-4050
Fax: 301-306-7090
www.chadd.org

CHADD's primary objectives are: to provide a support network for parents and caregivers; to provide a forum for continuing education; to be a community resource and disseminate accurate evidence-based information about AD/HD to parents, educators and adults.
E Clarke Ross, CEO
Ruth Hughes, Chief Program Officer Community Service

1506 **Council for Exceptional Children**
1110 N Glebe Road 703-620-3660
Arlington, VA 22201-5704 800-224-6830
Fax: 703-264-9494
TTY: 866-915-5000
e-mail: service@cec.sped.org
www.cec.sped.org

Advocates appropriate policies standards and development for individuals with special needs. Provides professional development for special educators.
Bruce Ramirez, Executive Director
Joan Melner, Assistant Executive Director

1507 **Feingold Association of the US**
554 E Main Street 631-369-9340
Riverhead, NY 11901 800-321-3287
Fax: 631-369-2988
e-mail: help@feingold.org
www.feingold.org

Helps families of children with learning and behavior problems including attention deficit disorder. Also helps chemically-sensitive and salicylate-sensitive adults. Program is based upon a diet which primarily eliminates certain synthetic food additives.

1508 **Learning Disabilities Association of America**
4156 Library Road 412-341-1515
Pittsburgh, PA 15234-1349 888-300-6710
Fax: 412-344-0224
e-mail: info@LDAAmerica.org
www.ldaamerica.org

An information and referral center for parents and professionals dealing with learning disabilities.
Barbara Lefler, Director of Affiliate Services

1509 **National Center for Learning Disabilities**
381 Park Avenue S 212-545-7510
New York, NY 10016-8806 888-575-7373
Fax: 212-545-9665
www.ncld.org

One of the foremost nonprofit organizations committed to improving the lives of the estimated one in ten children with learning disabilities raising public awareness and understanding.
James H Wendorf, Executive Director
Sheldon H Horowitz EdD, Director/Professional Services

1510 **National Dissemination Center for Children with Disabilities**
PO Box 1492 202-884-8200
Washington, DC 20013 800-695-0285
Fax: 202-884-8441
e-mail: nichcy@aed.org
www.nichcy.org

Publishes free, fact filled newsletters. Arranges workshops. Advises parents on the laws entitling children with disabilities to special education and other services.
Dr Suzanne Ripley, Contact

Libraries & Resource Centers

1511 **HEATH Resource Center**
American Council on Education
2134 G Street NW 202-973-0904
Washington, DC 20052-0001 800-544-3284
Fax: 202-994-3365
e-mail: askheath@gwu.edu
http://www.heath.gwu.edu/

The HEATH Resource Center of The George Washington University, Graduate School of Education and Human Development, is the national clearinghouse on postsecondary education for individuals with disabilities.
Dr Lynda West, Principal Investigator
Dr Joel Gomez, Co-Principal Investigator

Support Groups & Hotlines

1512 **Attention Deficit Information Network**
475 Hillside Ave 617-455-9895
Needham, MA 02194

Offers support and information to families of children with attention deficit disorder, adults with ADD and professionals through an international network of 60 parent and adult chapters.

1513 **Federation of Families for Children's Ment al Health**
9605 Medical Center Drive 240-403-1901
Rockville, MD 20850 Fax: 240-403-1909
e-mail: ffcmh@ffcmh.org
www.ffcmh.org/
Provides information, support and referrals through federation chapters throughout the country. This national parent run organization focuses on the needs of children with broad mental health problems.
Sandra Spencer, Executive Director
Pat Hunt, Director Policy & Research

1514 **National Health Information Center**
PO Box 1133 310-565-4167
Washington, DC 20013 800-336-4797
Fax: 301-984-4256
e-mail: info@nhic.org
www.health.gov/nhic
Offers a nationwide information referral service, produces directories and resource guides.

Books

1515 **ADHD Parenting Handbook: Practical Advice for Parents from Parents**
Colleen Alexander-Roberts, author
Taylor Trade Publishing
4501 Forbes Boulevard 301-459-3366
Lanham, MD 20706 Fax: 301-429-5743
e-mail: custserv@nbnbooks.com
www.rlpgtrade.com
This book is a compilation of practical advice and tips for handling day-to-day activities that would routinely become problematic for ADHD children, such as getting dressed for school, going to bed, performing chores, completeing homework, and playing with other children.
Paperback
ISBN: 0-878338-62-4

1516 **ADHD in Schools: Assessment and Intervention Strategies**
Guilford Publications
72 Spring Street 212-431-9800
New York, NY 10012-4068 800-365-7006
Fax: 212-966-6708
This landmark volume emphasizes the need for a team effort among parents, community-based professionals, and educators. Provides practical information for educators that is based on empirical findings. Chapters focus on: how to identify and assess students who might have ADHD; the relationship between ADHD and learning disabilities; how to develop and implement classroom-based programs; communication strategies to assist physicians; and the need for community-based treatments.
269 pages Hardcover
ISBN: 0-898622-45-0

1517 **ADHD: Handbook for Diagnosis & Treatment**
Western Psychological Services
12031 Wilshire Boulevard 310-478-2061
Los Angeles, CA 90025-1201 800-648-8857
Fax: 310-478-7838
www.wpspublish.com
This second edition helps clinicians diagnose and treat Attention Deficit Hyperactivity Disorder. Written by an internationally recognized authority in the field, it covers the history of ADHD, its primary symptoms, associated conditions, developmental course and outcome, and family context. A workbook companion manual is also available.
700 pages

1518 **Attention Deficit Disorder: A Different Perception**
Underwood-Miller
708 Westover Drive
Lancaster, PA 17601-1242 717-285-2255
www.vance.hw.nl/dbase/publisher
1993 180 pages Paperback
ISBN: 0-887331-56-4

1519 **Attention Deficit Disorder: Learning Disabilities**
Random House
25 Van Zant Street 410-848-1900
East Norwalk, CT 06855-1726 800-726-0600
Fax: 800-214-1438
www.randomhouse.com
Realities, myths, and controversial treatments. Section I tries to dispel the myths and discusses proven treatments for ADHD and LD. Section II explains how the scientific community evaluates new treatment methods, and Section III summarizes alternative treatments and discusses scientific evidence pertaining to its usefulness.
256 pages
ISBN: 0-385469-31-4

1520 **Attention Deficit Hyperactivity Disorder: What Every Parent Wants to Know**
Paul H Brookes Publishing Company
PO Box 10624 301-337-9580
Baltimore, MD 21285-0624 800-638-3775
Fax: 410-337-8539
e-mail: custserv@brookspublishing.com
www.brookespublishing.com
1993 320 pages Paperback
ISBN: 1-557661-41-3
Dante Washington, Customer Service Representative

1521 **Coping with ADD/ADHD**
Rosen Publishing Group
29 E 21st Street 212-777-3017
New York, NY 10010-6209 800-237-9932
Fax: 888-436-4643
e-mail: customerservice@rosenpub.com
www.rosenpublishing.com
At least 3.5 million American youngsters suffer from ADD. This book defines the syndrome and provides specific information about treatment and counseling.
150 pages Hardcover
ISBN: 0-823931-96-X

1522 **Helping Your ADD Child With or Without Hyperactivity**
John F Taylor PhD, author
Random House Inc.
Department of Library Marketing 800-733-3000
New York, NY 10017 800-726-0600
Fax: 212-940-7381
e-mail: crownpublicity@randomhouse.com
www.randomhouse.com
Inside this book you will find step-by-step tools for helping your ADD or ADHD child. From extensive screening for spotting the initial signs to the pros and cons of nutritional, psychological, and drug treatments.
2001
ISBN: 0-761527-56-7

1523 **Hyperactive Children Grown Up**
Guilford Publications
72 Spring Street 212-431-9800
New York, NY 10012-4068 800-365-7006
Fax: 212-966-6708
Long considered a standard in the field, this book explores what happens to hyperactive children when they grow into adulthood. Updated and expanded, this second edition describes new developments in ADHD, current psychological treatments of ADHD, contemporary perspectives on the use of medications, and assessment, diagnosis and treatment of ADHD adults.
473 pages Hardcover
ISBN: 0-898620-39-2

1524 **LD Child and the ADHD Child**
1406 Plaza Drive
Winston-Salem, NC 27103-1485
336-768-1374
800-222-9796
Fax: 336-768-9194
e-mail: blairpub@aol.com
www.blairpub.com

The author recommends other options that can be explored to treat LD and ADHD children without drugs.
Paperback
ISBN: 0-895871-42-4
John F Blair, Publisher

1525 **Managing Attention Deficit Hyperactivity Disorder In Children**
Sam and Michael Goldstein, author
John Wiley and Sons, Inc.
Customer Service-Consumer Accounts
Indianapolis, IN 46256
877-762-2947
Fax: 800-597-3299
e-mail: consumers@wiley.com
www.wiley.com

A proven approach to the diagnosis and management of one of the most challenging childhood disorders. In this book the authors describe a proven multidisciplinary approach to the diagnosis and treatment of childhood ADHD, developed at the prestigous Neurology, Learning and Behavior Center in Salt Lake City.
1998 896 pages
ISBN: 0-471121-58-9

1526 **Maybe You Know My Kid: A Parent's Guide to Identifying ADHD**
Birch Lane Press
120 Enterprise Avenue S
Secaucus, NJ 07094-1902
800-447-2665

The author writes about her family experiences with their son, David, who has attention deficit disorder. Contains a comprehensive review of important issues plus descriptions of some helpful management techniques.
222 pages

1527 **Medications for Attention Disorders and Related Medical Problems**
Specialty Press
300 NW 70th Avenue
Plantation, FL
954-792-8100
800-233-9273
Fax: 954-792-8545
e-mail: sales@addwarehouse.com
www.addwarehouse.com

A comprehensive handbook covering the history, characteristics, and causes of ADHD. The equal importance of appropriate academic programming, counseling, and medication are stressed throughout.
415 pages Hardcover

1528 **Parents Helping Parents: A Directory of Support Groups for ADD**
CibaGelgy, Pharmaceuticals Division
External Communications
Summit, NJ 07901
908-277-5000
Fax: 973-781-2601

1529 **Parents' Hyperactivity Handbook: Helping the Fidgety Child**
Plenum Press
233 Spring Street
New York, NY 10013-1578
212-620-8000
Fax: 212-463-0742
e-mail: info@plenum.com

1993 306 pages
ISBN: 0-306444-65-8

1530 **Rethinking Attention Deficit Disorders**
Miriam Cherkes-Julkowski, author
Brookline Books
PO Box 1209
Brookline, MA 02445
617-734-6772
800-666-2665
Fax: 617-734-3952
www.brooklinebooks.com

Gives the classroom teacher useful information that provides ideas and strategies for working with children suffering from ADD.
1997 Paperback
ISBN: 1-571290-37-0

1531 **The New ADD in Adults Workbook**
Lynn Weiss, PhD, author
Taylor Trade Publishing
4501 Forbes Boulevard
Lanham, MD 20706
301-459-3366
Fax: 301-429-5743
e-mail: custserv@nbnbooks.com
www.rlpgtrade.com

This book, now in its 3rd edition, not only touches on and dispels the most recent clinical findings, but it also emphasizes the bigger perspective, focusing on the empowerment and diversity issues facing everyone on the ADD continuum today. It persuades readers to work through their challenges with practical, prescriptive exercises and insights.
1997 Paperback
ISBN: 0-878338-50-0

1532 **You Mean I'm Not Lazy, Stupid or Crazy?**
Tyrell & Jerem Press
PO Box 20089
Cincinnati, OH 45220-0089
800-622-6611

A new self-help book is the first written by ADD adults for ADD adults. This comprehensive guide provides accurate information, practical how-tos and moral support.

1533 **Attention Deficit/Hyperactivity Disorder**
Guilford Publications
72 Spring Street
New York, NY 10012-4068
212-431-9800
800-365-7006
Fax: 212-966-6708

A second edition that is the handbook on the diagnosis and treatment of ADHD in the 1990s. A companion workbook is also available with forms that may be photocopied.
747 pages Hardcover
ISBN: 0-898624-43-6

Children's Books

1534 **Self-Control Games & Workbook**
Western Psychological Services
12031 Wilshire Boulevard
Los Angeles, CA 90025-1201
310-478-2061
800-648-8857
Fax: 310-478-7838

This game is designed to teach self-control in academic and social situations. Addresses a total of 24 impulsive, inattentive and hyperactive behaviors. The companion workbook reinforces the use of positive self-statements, and problem-solving techniques, instead of expressing anger.
Game

1535 **Shelley, the Hyperactive Turtle**
Woodbine House
6510 Bells Mill Road
Bethesda, MD 20817-1636
800-843-7323
Fax: 301-897-5838

Entertaining picture book for use with very young children. Sensitive text and colorful illustrations help children understand ADHD.
20 pages
Carol Schwartz, Illustrator

Magazines

1536 **Attention**
Children & Adults with Attention Deficit Disorder
8181 Professional Place
Landover, MD 20785-7221
301-306-7070
800-233-4050
Fax: 301-306-7090
TTY: 301-429-0641

Quarterly

Newsletters

1537 **ADHD Report**
Guilford Publications

72 Spring Street 212-431-9800
New York, NY 10012-4068 800-365-7006
Fax: 212-966-6708

Presents the most up-to-date information on the evaluation, diagnosis and management of ADHD in children, adolescents and adults. This important newsletter is an invaluable resource for all professionals interested in ADHD.
BiMonthly
ISBN: 1-065802-5 -

1538 **Chadder**
Children & Adults with Attention Deficit Disorder
8181 Professional Place 301-306-7070
Landover, MD 20785-7221 800-233-4050
Fax: 301-306-7090
TTY: 301-429-0641
Quarterly

1539 **Challenge**
Challenge
PO Box 488 978-462-0495
West Newbury, MA 01985-0688 800-233-2322
National newsletter on ADD/ADHD that carries interviews with nationally-known scientists, as well as physicians, psychologists, social workers, educators, and other practitioners in the field of ADHD.
12 pages BiMonthly
Jean C Harrison, Executive Director

1540 **Pure Facts**
Feingold Association of the US
PO Box 6550 703-768-3287
Alexandria, VA 22306-0550
Monthly newsletter with articles on nutrition and behavior and lists of approved brand-name foods.

Pamphlets

1541 **ADHD**
Learning Disabilities Association of America
4156 Library Road 412-341-1515
Pittsburgh, PA 15234-1349 888-300-6710
Fax: 412-344-0224
e-mail: info@ldaamerica.org
www.ldaamerica.org
A booklet for parents offering information on Attention Deficit Hyperactivity Disorders and learning disabilities.
Sheila Buckley, Executive Director

1542 **ADHD in the Classroom**
Guilford Publications
72 Spring Street 212-431-9800
New York, NY 10012-4068 800-365-7006
Fax: 212-966-6708
Designed specifically to help teachers with their ADHD students, thereby providing a better learning environment for the entire class.

1543 **Attention Deficit Disorders and Hyperactivity**
Council for Exceptional Children
1110 N Glebe Road 703-620-3660
Arlington, VA 22201 888-232-7733
Fax: 703-264-9494
e-mail: service@cec.sped.org
www.cec.sped.org
Published by the Council for Exceptional Children.

1544 **COGREHAB**
Life Science Associates
1 Fennimore Road 631-472-2111
Bayport, NY 11705-2115 Fax: 631-472-8146
e-mail: lifesciassoc@pipeline.com
lifesciassoc.home.pipeline.com
Divided into six groups for diagnosis and treatment of attention, memory and perceptual disorders to be used by and under the guidance of a professional.
$95 - $1,950

1545 **Fact Sheet: Attention Deficit Hyperactivity Disorder**
Learning Disabilities Association of America
4156 Library Road 412-341-1515
Pittsburgh, PA 15234-1349 888-300-6710
Fax: 412-344-0224
e-mail: info@ldaamerica.org
www.ldaamerica.org
A pamphlet offering factual information on ADHD.
Sheila Buckley, Executive Director

1546 **Helping Adolescents with ADHD and Learning Disabilities**
Learning Disabilities Association of America
4156 Library Road 412-341-1515
Pittsburgh, PA 15234-1349 888-300-6710
Fax: 412-344-0224
e-mail: info@ldaamerica.org
www.ldaamerica.org
Sheila Buckley, Executive Director

Audio & Video

1547 **ADD Stepping Out of the Dark**
ADD Videos
PO Box 622 845-255-3612
New Paltz, NY 12561-0622 Fax: 845-883-6452
A powerful, effective video, ideal for health professionals, educators and parents providing a visual montage designed to promote an understanding and awareness of attention deficit disorder. Based on actual accounts of those who have ADD, including a neurologist, an office worker, and parents of children with ADD. The video allows the viewer to feel the frustration and lack of attention that ADD brings to many.
Video
Lenae Madonna, Producer

1548 **ADHD in Adults**
Guilford Publications
72 Spring Street 212-431-9800
New York, NY 10012-4068 800-365-7006
Fax: 212-966-6708
This program integrates information on ADHD with the actual experiences of four adults who suffer from the disorder. Representing a range of professions, from a lawyer to a mother working at home, each candidly discusses the impact of ADHD on his or her daily life. These interviews are augmented by comments from family members and other clinicians who treat adults with ADHD.
Video

1549 **ADHD: What Do We Know?**
Guilford Publications
72 Spring Street 212-431-9800
New York, NY 10012-4068 800-365-7006
Fax: 212-966-6708
An introduction for teachers and special education practitioners, school psychologists and parents of ADHD children. Topics outlined in this video include the causes and prevalence of ADHD, ways children with ADHD behave, other conditions that may accompany ADHD and long-term prospects for children with ADHD.
Video

1550 **Around the Clock**
Guilford Publications
72 Spring Street 212-431-9800
New York, NY 10012-4068 800-365-7006
Fax: 212-966-6708
This videotape provides both professionals and parents a helpful look at how the difficulties facing parents of ADHD children can be handled.

1551 **Attention Deficit Disorder**
Pro-Ed, Inc.
8700 Shoal Creek Boulevard 512-451-3246
Austin, TX 78757-6897 800-897-3202
Fax: 800-397-7633
e-mail: info@proedinc.com
www.proedinc.com/

A video and book providing helpful suggestions for both home and classroom management of students with attention deficit disorder.
216 pages Paperback
ISBN: 0-890797-42-0
Krista Anderson, Technical Advisor
Matt Synatschk, Books & Materials Permissions Editor

1552 **Educating Inattentive Children**
Western Psychological Services
12031 Wilshire Boulevard
Los Angeles, CA 90025-1201
800-648-8857
Fax: 310-478-7838
An excellent resource for teachers who encounter inattention and hyperactivity in the classroom. It helps teachers distinguish deliberate misbehavior from the incompetent, nonpurposeful behavior of the inattentive child.
Video

1553 **It's Just Attention Disorder**
Western Psychological Services
12031 Wilshire Boulevard
Los Angeles, CA 90025-1201
310-478-2061
800-648-8857
Fax: 310-478-7838
This ground-breaking videotape takes the critical first steps in treating attention-deficit disorder: it enlists the inattentive or hyperactive child as an active participant in his or her treatment.
Video

1554 **Why Won't My Child Pay Attention?**
Western Psychological Services
12031 Wilshire Boulevard
Los Angeles, CA 90025-1201
310-478-2061
800-648-8857
Fax: 310-478-7838
Practical and reassuring videotape, noted child psychologist tells parents about two of the most common and complex problems of childhood: inattention and hyperactivity.
Video

Web Sites

1555 **Attention Deficit Information Network**
www.addinfonetwork.com
Offers support and information to families of children and adults with ADD and to professionals.

1556 **Healing Well**
www.healingwell.com
An online health resource guide to medical news, chat, information and articles, newsgroups and message boards, books, disease-related web sites, medical directories, and more for patients, friends, and family coping with disabling diseases, disorders, or chronic illnesses.

1557 **Health Finder**
www.healthfinder.gov
Searchable, carefully developed web site offering information on over 1000 topics. Developed by the US Department of Health and Human Services, the site can be used in both English and Spanish.

1558 **Healthlink USA**
www.healthlinkusa.com
Health information concerning treatment, cures, prevention, diagnosis, risk factors, research, support groups, email lists, personal stories and much more. Updated regularly.

1559 **Helios Health**
www.helioshealth.com
Online resource for your health information. Detailed information about specific health topics, access to expert advice from our Medical Advisory Board, and up-to-date health news.

1560 **MedicineNet**
www.medicinenet.com
An online resource for consumers providing easy-to-read, authoritative medical and health information.

1561 **Medscape**
www.mywebmd.com
Medscape offers specialists, primary care physicians, and other health professionals the Web's most robust and integrated medical information and educational tools.

1562 **WebMD**
www.webmd.com
Information on Attention Deficit Disorder, including articles and resources.

Description

1563 **Autistic Spectrum Disorders**

Autistic Spectrum Disorders, ASD, includes (from most to least severe) autism, high-functioning autism (HFA), Asperger's syndrome, and PDD-NOS (pervasive development disorder — not otherwise specified). ASD typically appear during the first three years of life. Autism involves severe impairment of social and communication development. HFA symptoms are less severe, but include delayed language development. Asperger's is similar to HFA, but with no speech delay. PPD-NOS describes autistic categories that do not fit into any of the above. ASD affects behavior, communication, social interaction and other neurological functions.

ASD has numerous symptoms, all of which reduce the child's ability to communicate and interact. Many autistic children have abnormal social relationships, impaired understanding, and uneven intellectual development with mental retardation in most cases. They may exhibit repetitive movement (i.e., rocking, spinning, and hand twisting), avoid making eye contact, and have impaired verbal skills. Occasionally, children with ASD will have decreased sensitivity to pain, and have abnormal responses to light, touch and sound. The disorder can include self-injury and bizarre behavior.

ASD is two to four times more common in boys than in girls. It is found in people of all ethnic backgrounds, and throughout the world. In 2003, one in 500 children were diagnosed with ASD, up from one in 3,500 thirty years ago.

In some cases, ASD may be linked to damage to the brain or nervous system. Studies of twins with autism point to a possible genetic link. ASD has been associated with the following risk factors: pre- and perinatal birth complications; prenatal infections with certain viruses; abnormalities of the brain detected with a CT scan or MRI (although no specific defects in the brain struture have been consistently identified). More recently, usual childhood vaccines, environmental toxins, and pollutents are being questioned to explain the sharp rise in ASD cases in recent decades, but researchers have been unable to confirm these findings.

Although there are no known cures for ASD, experts advocate early and intense behavioral, developmental and speech therapy. Medications may alleviate some of the accompanying behavior problems, but provide minimal help for the disorder itself and are generally not used. There is strong emphasis on early diagnosis, early intervention, and individualized educational programs to provide the opportunity for maximum development for the child with Autistic Spectrum Disorder.

National Agencies & Associations

1564 **ARRISE**
9238 Parklane Avenue 847-451-2740
Franklin Park, IL 60131-2836

Provides information about autism.

1565 **Autism Research Institute**
4182 Adams Avenue 619-281-7165
San Diego, CA 92116-2536 866-366-3361
Fax: 619-563-6840
www.autism.com

A clearinghouse for research on autism and related disorders of learning and behavior. Conducts and compiles research findings to provide people with the latest research available.
Stephen M Edelson PhD, Director

1566 **Autism Services Center**
929 Fourth Avenue 304-525-8014
Huntington, WV 25701-0507 Fax: 304-525-8026
www.autismservicescenter.org

Provides educational information to the public and professional communities on autism provides case management activities and referrals for persons afflicted with autism and their families.
Ruth Christ Sullivan, Founder and Executive Director

1567 **Autism Society of America**
7910 Woodmont Avenue 301-657-0881
Bethesda, MD 20814-3067 800-328-8476
Fax: 301-657-0869
e-mail: info@autism-society.org
www.autism-society.org

A national charitable organization with the mission of providing as much information as possible about autism and the various options, approaches, methods and systems available to parents of children with autism, family members and professionals.
Lee Grossman, President/CEO
Barbara Newhouse, Chief Operating Officer

1568 **Autism Treatment Center of America**
2080 S Undermountain Road 413-229-2100
Sheffield, MA 01257 877-766-7473
Fax: 413-229-3202
e-mail: correspondence@option.org
www.autismtreatmentcenter.org

Since 1983 the Autism Treatment Center of America has provided innovative training programs for parents and professionals caring for children challenged by Autism Autism Spectrum Disorders Pervasive Developmental Disorder (PDD) and other developmental disorders.
Barry Neil Kaufman, Co-Founder/Co-Creator Son-Rise Program
Bryn Hogan, Director Son-Rise Program

1569 **Autism Treatment Center of America: Son-Rise Program**
2080 South Undermountain Road 413-229-2100
Sheffield, MA 01257 877-766-7473
Fax: 413-229-3202
e-mail: correspondence@option.org
www.son-rise.org

Since 1983, the Autism Treatment Center of America has provided innovative training programs for parents and professionals caring for children challenged by Autism, Autism Spectrum Disorders, Pervasive Developmental Disorder (PDD) and other developmental difficulties. The Son-Rise Program teaches a specific yet comprehensive system of treatment and education designed to help families and caregivers enable their children to dramatically improve in all areas of learning.
Sean Fitzgerald, Assistant Director Son-Rise Program

1570 **Community Services for Autistic Adults & Children**
8615 E Village Avenue 240-912-2220
Montgomery Village, MD 20886 Fax: 301-926-9384
e-mail: csaac@csaac.org
www.csaac.org

The Community Services for Autistic Adults & Children is a non-profit organization dedicated to helping those with autism. Since 1979 CSAAC has served over 150 individuals and helped people with autism find housing, employment and other community services.
Ian Paregol, Executive Director
Peter Donaghy, Chief Financial Officer

1571 **National Institute of Neurological Disorders and Stroke**
NIH Neurological Institute
Bethesda, MD 20824
301-496-5751
800-352-9424
Fax: 301-402-2186
TTY: 301-468-5981
www.ninds.nih.gov
The mission of NINDS is to reduce the burden of neurological disease - a burden borne by every age group, by every segment of society, by people all over the world.
Story C Landis, PhD, Director
Walter J Koroshetz, Deputy Director

State Agencies & Associations

Alabama

1572 **Autism Society of Alabama**
Birmingham, AL 35243
205-951-1364
877-4AU-TISM
Fax: 205-967-8244
e-mail: info@autism-alabama.org
www.autism-alabama.org
Ryan Thomas, President
Jennifer Muller, Executive Director

1573 **Autism Society of North Alabama**
PO Box 2902
Huntsville, AL 35801-2902
256-776-0505
e-mail: sherron@northalabamaautism.org
www.northalabamaautism.org
Teresa White, President
Carol Wright, Vice President

Arizona

1574 **Autism Society of Pima County**
PO Box 44156
Tucson, AZ 85733-4156
520-770-1541
Fax: 520-319-5979
e-mail: az-pimacounty@autismsocietyofamerica.org
www.tucsonautism.org
Peter Earhart, President
Stephanie Hillÿ, Vice President

California

1575 **Autism Society of California**
PO Box 15247
Long Beach, CA 90815-0600
562-943-3335
800-700-0037
e-mail: brubin698@earthlink.net
www.autismsocietyca.org
Dean Wilson, President
Gregory Fletcher, First Vice President

Colorado

1576 **Autism Society of Colorado**
550ÿSÿWadsworth Boulevard
Lakewood, CO 80226-4169
720-214-0794
Fax: 720-274-2744
e-mail: co-colorado@autismsocietyofamerica.org
www.autismcolorado.org
Betty Lehman, Executive Director
Lorri Park, ProgramsÿDirector

Connecticut

1577 **Autism Society of Connecticut**
PO Box 1404
Guilford, CT 06437
888-453-4975
www.autismsocietyofct.org

Delaware

1578 **Autism Society of Delaware**
924 Old Harmony Road
Newark, DE 19713
302-224-6020
Fax: 302-224-6017
e-mail: delautism@delautism.org
www.delautism.org
Theda Ellis, Executive Director
Kim Siegel, Development Director

District of Columbia

1579 **Autism Society of District Columbia**
5167 7th Street NE
Washington, DC 20011-2624
202-561-5300
Fax: 202-561-8634
e-mail: dc-washington@autismsocietyofamerica.org
www.autism-society.org/chapter130
Sondra Cunningham, President
Rhoda McLees Smith

Florida

1580 **Autism Society of Greater Orlando**
4743 Hearthside Drive
Orlando, FL 32837-5445
407-855-0235
e-mail: contact@asgo.orgÿ
www.asgo.org
Donna Lorman, President
Marzena Batignani, Vice President

Georgia

1581 **Autism Society of Greater Georgia**
PO Box 3707
Suwanee, GA 30024
770-904-4474
Fax: 770-904-4476
www.asaga.com
Steve Doran, President
Cindy Pike, Executive Director

Hawaii

1582 **Autism Society of Hawaii**
PO Box 2995
Honolulu, HI 96802-2995
808-282-3676
e-mail: naomig122@hotmail.com
www.autismhawaii.org
Evelyn Akamine, President
Naomi Grossman

Idaho

1583 **Autism Society of Treasure Valley**
PO Box 44831
Boise, ID 83711-9404
208-336-5676
Fax: 202-884-5582
e-mail: Autism.asatvc@yahoo.com
www.asatvc.org

Illinois

1584 **Autism Society of Illinois**
2200 S Main Street
Lombard, IL 60148-5366
630-691-1270
888-691-1270
Fax: 630-932-5620
e-mail: info@autismillinois.org
www.autismillinois.org
Karen McDonough, Executive Director
Kym Bills, President

Indiana

1585 **Autism Society of Indiana**
4740 Kingsway Drive
Indianapolis, IN 46205-0252
317-695-0252
Fax: 317-815-0859
e-mail: info@inautism.org
www.inautism.org
Susan Pieples, President

Iowa

1586 **Autism Society of Iowa**
4549 Waterford Drive
W Des Moines, IA 50265-2059
515-327-9075
888-722-4799
Fax: 319-557-1169
e-mail: autism50ia@aol.com
www.autismia.org

Kansas

1587 **Autism Society of Kansas Autism Society of America**
Autism Society of America

PO Box 860984 913-706-0042
Shawnee, KS 66286-2325 Fax: 316-943-3292
e-mail: ks-johnsoncounty@autismsocietyofamerica.
www.autismsocietyoftheheartland.org

Bill Robinso, President
DeeDee Velasquez-Per, Board Member

Kentucky

1588 **Autism Chapter of Bluegrass Chapter**
243 Shady Lane
Lexington, KY 40503-2034 859-299-9000
www.asbg.org

Sara Spragens, President

1589 **Autism Society of Western Kentucky**
230 Second Street Suite 206 270-826-0510
Henderson, KY 42419-1647 e-mail: nboyett1956@yahoo.com
www.autism.org

Nancy Boyett, President

Louisiana

1590 **Autism Society of Louisiana**
5430 S Woodchase Court
Baton Rouge, LA 70808 800-955-3760
e-mail: pjmanco@cox.net
www.lastateautism.org

Pat Giamanco, President

Maine

1591 **Autism Society of Maine**
72B Main Street
Winthrop, ME 04364-1406 800-273-5200
Fax: 207-377-9434
e-mail: nancy@asmonline.org
www.asmonline.org

Kim Humphrey, President
Lynda Mazzola, Vice President

Maryland

1592 **Autism Society of Baltimore-Chesapeake**
PO Box 10822 410-655-7933
Parkville, MD 21234-0822 e-mail: questions@bcc-asa.org
www.bcc-asa.org

Massachusetts

1593 **Autism Society of Massachusetts**
47 Walnut Street 781-237-0272
Wellesley Hills, MA 02481-2108 Fax: 781-237-5020
e-mail: asamasschapter@hotmail.com
www.geocities.com/asamasschapter

Michigan

1594 **Autism Society of Michigan**
1213 Center Street 517-882-2800
Lansing, MI 48906-5338 800-223-6722
Fax: 517-862-2816
e-mail: mi-michigan@autismsocietyofamerica.org
www.autism-mi.org

Kathy Johnson, President
Penny Bearden, Vice President

Minnesota

1595 **Autism Society of Minnesota**
2380 Wycliff Street 651-647-1083
St Paul, MN 55114-1257 Fax: 651-642-1230
e-mail: info@ausm.org
www.ausm.org

Pam Erickson, Executive Director
Laurie Dixon, Associate Director

Mississippi

1596 **Autism Society of Gateway Chapter**
7777 Bonhomme Avenue 314-863-0077
St Louis, MO 63105 Fax: 314-863-7494
e-mail: PegiSues@aol.com
www.autism-society.org

Pegi Price, President

Nebraska

1597 **Autism Society of Nebraska**
1672 Van Dorn Street 402-472-4346
Lincoln, NE 68502 877-375-0120
e-mail: autismsociety@autismnebraska.org
www.autismnebraska.org

Shawn Neff, President
Georgann Albin, Executive Director

Nevada

1598 **Autism Society of Northern Nevada**
3490 Southampton Drive 775-786-9315
Reno, NV 89509-8911 Fax: 775-786-0984
www.autism-society.org/chapter547

Paul Deane, Vice President
Dinah Deane, President

New Hampshire

1599 **Autism Society of New Hampshire**
PO Box 68 603-679-2424
Concord, NH 03302-0068 Fax: 301-657-0869
e-mail: info@nhautism.com
www.nhautism.com

Stacey Shannon, President

New Jersey

1600 **Autism Society of Southwest New Jersey**
10 Shadow Oak Court 856-722-8518
Mount Laurel, NJ 08054-2113 e-mail: CMedo@aol.com
www.autism-society.org

New Mexico

1601 **Autism Society of New Mexico**
PO Box 30955 505-332-0306
Albuquerque, NM 87190-0955 e-mail: nmautism@nmautismsociety.org
www.nmautismsociety.org

New York

1602 **Autism Society of Albany**
PO Box 3487 518-355-2191
Schenectady, NY 12303 Fax: 518-355-2191
e-mail: info@albanyautism.org
www.albanyautism.org

Cindy Barkowski, Contact

North Carolina

1603 **Autism Society of North Carolina**
505 Oberlin Road 919-743-0204
Raleigh, NC 27605-1345 800-442-2762
Fax: 919-743-0208
e-mail: info@autismsociety-nc.org
www.autismsociety-nc.org

Scott Badesch, Chief Executive Officer
David Laxton, Director Communications

North Dakota

1604 **Autism Society of North Dakota**
628 6th Avenue 701-281-8254
Alice, ND 58031 e-mail: Jocelyn@AutismND.org
www.AutismND.org

Jocelyn Sloan, President

Ohio

1605 **Autism Society of Greater Cincinnati**
PO Box 43027
Cincinnati, OH 45243-0027
513-561-2300
Fax: 513-561-4748
e-mail: asgc@cinci.rr.com
www.autismcincy.org

Christi Carnahan, Secretary
Ken Jones, President

1606 **Autism Society of Ohio Tri-County Chapter**
1749 S Raccoon Road
Austintown, OH 44515
330-720-2066
e-mail: TriCountyAutism_ASO@Yahoo.com
www.triautism.com

Terry Chapin, President
Jack Campbell, Vice President

Oklahoma

1607 **Autism Society of Central Oklahoma**
PO Box 720103
Norman, OK 73070
405-370-3220
e-mail: ASOCO-owner@yahoogroups.com
www.asofok.org

Jeremy Rand, Contact

Oregon

1608 **Autism Society of Oregon**
PO Box 396
Marylhurst, OR 97036-0396
503-636-1676
888-288-4761
Fax: 503-636-1696
e-mail: info@oregonautism.com
www.oregonautism.com

Jenny Schoonbee, President
Genevieve Athens, Executive Director

Pennsylvania

1609 **Autism Society of Greater Harrisburg**
PO Box 101
Enola, PA 17025-0856
717-732-8400
800-277-2425
e-mail: georgia.rackley@verizon.net
www.autismharrisburg.com

Georgia Rackley, President
Sherry Christian, Vice President

Rhode Island

1610 **Autism Society of Rhode Island**
PO Box 16603
Rumford, RI 02916
401-595-3241
e-mail: LRego@asa-ri.org
www.asa-ri.org

Lisa Rego, President

South Carolina

1611 **Autism Society of South Carolina**
806 Twelfth Street
W Columbia, SC 29169
803-750-6988
800-438-4790
Fax: 703-750-8121
e-mail: scas@scautism.org
www.scautism.org

Craig Stoxen, President & CEO
Tim Conroy, Chief Operating Officer & Vice President

South Dakota

1612 **Autism Society of Black Hills**
521 7th Street
Rapid City, SD 57701-4347
605-737-0377
e-mail: sheritony@rap.midco.net
www.autismsd.com

Sandy Burns, President
Sheri Perkins

Tennessee

1613 **Autism Society of East Tennessee**
PO Box 30015
Knoxville, TN 37930
865-824-2897
Fax: 865-824-2896
e-mail: asaetc@gmail.com
www.asaetc.org

John Thomas, President
Ron Bowling, Vice President

Texas

1614 **Autism Society of Dallas**
10503 Metric Drive
Dallas, TX 75243
214-208-0792
e-mail: autismsociety_dallas@yahoo.com
www.autism-society.org

Carolyn Garver, Contact
Pamela Lane, President

Vermont

1615 **Autism Society of Vermont Autism Society of America**
Autism Society of America
PO Box 978
White River Junction, VT 05001-0978
800-559-7398
e-mail: vt-vermont@autismsocietyofamerica.org
www.autism-info.org

Virginia

1616 **Autism Society of Northern Virginia**
PO Box 1334
Vienna, VA 22183-1334
703-495-8444
Fax: 703-571-8138
e-mail: info@asanv.org
www.asanv.org

Kymberly S DeLoatche, Executive Director
Christopher Waddell, President

Washington

1617 **Autism Society of Washington**
1101 Eastside Street SE
Olympia, WA 98501
888-ASW-4YOU
Fax: 253-503-1157
e-mail: info@autismsocietyofwa.org
www.autismsocietyofwa.org

Patty Gee, President & Executive Director

West Virginia

1618 **Autism Socity of West Virginia**
PO Box 1024
Wayne, WV 25570
304-272-9834
e-mail: wv-westvirginia@autismsocietyofamerica.o
www.aswv.org

Kim Farley, President
Ginny Gattlieb, 1st VP

Wisconsin

1619 **Autism Society of Wisconsin**
1477 Kenwood Drive
Menasha, WI 54952
920-558-4602
888-428-8476
Fax: 920-553-0034
e-mail: asw@asw4autism.org
www.asw4autism.org

Nancy Alar, President
Dale Prahl, Vice President

Libraries & Resource Centers

1620 **Autism Services Center**
929 4th Avenue
Huntington, WV 25710-0507
304-525-8014
Fax: 304-258-26
http://www.autismservicescenter.org/

ASC is a nonprofit, licensed behavioral health care agency. Though specializing in autism, the agency provides comprehen-

sive, community integrated services for individuals with all developmental disabilities. throughout their lifespan.
Dr Ruth Christ Sullivan, Director

1621 Emory Autism Resource Center
Emory University 404-727-8350
Atlanta, GA 30322-0001 Fax: 404-727-3969
www.psychiatry.emory.edu/PROGRAMS/autism
The Emory Autism Resource Center is a component of the Department of Psychiatry and Behavioral Sciences of Emory University's School of Medicine. It is the only Georgia resource that provides a comprehensive continuum of services specially designed to meet the needs of children and adults with autism and their families.
Gail G McGee, PhD, Director
Michael J Morrier, MA, Assistant Dir Research Coordinator

1622 Indiana Resource Center for Autism (IRCA)
Indiana Institute on Disability & Community
2853 E 10th Street 812-855-6508
Bloomington, IN 47408-2696 Fax: 812-855-9630
www.iidc.indiana.edu/irca
The Indiana Resource Center for Autism staff conduct outreach training and consultations, engage in research, and develop and disseminate information focused on building the capacity of local communities, organizations, agencies, and families to support children and adults across the autism spectrum in typical work, school, home, and community settings.
Dr Cathy Pratt PhD, Center Director
Dr Scott Bellini PhD, Assistant Director

Research Centers

1623 Center for Neurodevelopmental Studies
5430 W Glenn Drive 623-915-0345
Glendale, AZ 85301 800-352-3792
Fax: 623-937-5425
e-mail: admin@ccnsaz.org
www.thechildrenscenteraz.org
Effective treatment methods for autism and developmental disabilities are subjects researched and studied at the Center.
Lorna Jean King, Founder

1624 Division TEACCH University of North Carolina at Chapel H
University of North Carolina at Chapel Hill
100 Renee Lynne Court 919-966-5156
Carrboro, NC 27510-6305 Fax: 919-966-4003
e-mail: teacch@unc.edu
www.teacch.com
This organization is the division for the treatment and education of Autistic and related communication handicapped children.
Catherine Jones, Office Manager/Parent Intake Coordinator
Elaine Coonrod, Clinical Director

1625 Facilitated Communication Institute at Syracuse University
University of Syracuse
370 Huntington Hall 315-443-9379
Syracuse, NY 13244-2340 Fax: 315-443-2274
e-mail: fcstaff@syr.edus
www.inclusioninstitutes.org
College offering facilitated learning research into communication with persons who have autism or severe disabilities. Offers books videos and public awareness information on the research projects.
Marilyn Chadwick
Dr Christine Ashby

1626 Institute for Basic Research in Developmental Disabilities
1050 Forest Hill Road 718-494-0600
Staten Island, NY 10314-6356 Fax: 718-494-0833
www.mor.state.ny.us/ws/ws_ibr_resources
Conducts research into neurodegenerative diseases, Alzheimer's disease, developmental disabilities, fragile X syndrome, Down's syndrome, autism, epilepsy and basic science issues underlying all developmental disabilities.

1627 National Alliance for Autism Research
2 Park Avenue 212-252-8584
New York, NY 10016 Fax: 212-252-8676
e-mail: contactus@autismspeaks.org
www.autismspeaks.org
The National Alliance for Autism Research has merged with Autism Speaks to further reach for the goal of finding the causes the best prevention and treatments and a cure for autism.
Glenn Tringali, Executive Vice President
Mark Roithmayr, President

1628 State University of New York Health Sciences Center
SUNY Downstate Medical Center
450 Clarkson Avenue 718-270-2431
Brooklyn, NY 11203-2098 Fax: 718-270-1271
e-mail: health@downstate.edu
www.hscbklyn.edu
Child psychiatry research programs.
John C Larosa, President

1629 The West Virginia Autism Training Center Marshall University
Marshall University
1 John Marshall Drive 304-696-2332
Huntington, WV 25755 800-344-5115
www.marshall.edu/coe/atc
The Autism Training Center was established through the efforts of parents of children with autism throughout West Virginia to provide education training and treatment programs for West Virginians who have Autism Pervasive Developmental Disorder (NOS) or Asperger's Disorder and have been formally registered with the Center.

Support Groups & Hotlines

1630 Autism Society of America
7910 Woodmont Avenue 301-657-0881
Bethesda, MD 20814-3065 800-328-8476
Fax: 301-657-0869
e-mail: info@autismsociety.org
www.autismsociety.org
Provides support groups nationwide for persons with autism and their families.
Lee Grossman, President

1631 Genetic Alliance
4301 Connecticut Avenue NW 202-966-5557
Washington, DC 20008-2369 800-336-4363
Fax: 202-668-8533
e-mail: info@geneticalliance.org
www.geneticalliance.org
A coalition of voluntary genetic support groups, consumers and professionals addressing the needs of individuals and families affected by genetic disorders from a national perspective.
Sharon Terry, President/Chief Executive Offficer
Karen White, Education/Information Director

1632 National Autism Hotline Autism Services Center
Autism Services Center
PO Box 507 304-525-8014
Huntington, WV 25710-507 Fax: 304-525-8026
www.autismservicescenter.org
Service agency for individuals with autism and developmental disabilities, and their families. Assists families and agencies attempting to meet the needs of individuals with autism and other developmental disabilities. Makes available technical assistance in designing treatment programs and more. The hotline provides informational packets to callers and assists via telephone when possible.
Ruth Sullivan, Director

1633 National Health Information Center
PO Box 1133 310-565-4167
Washington, DC 20013 800-336-4797
Fax: 301-984-4256
e-mail: info@nhic.org
www.health.gov/nhic
Offers a nationwide information referral service, produces directories and resource guides.

Books

1634 A Miracle to Believe In
Option Indigo Press

2080 S Undermountain Road
Sheffield, MA 01257
413-229-2100
800-714-2779
Fax: 413-229-8931
e-mail: www.optionindigo.org
indigo@bcn.net

A group of people from all walks of life come together and are transformed as they reach out, under the direction of the Kaufmans, to help a little boy the medical world had given up as hopeless. This heartwarming journey of loving a child back tolife will not only inspire you, the reader, but presents a compelling new way to deal with life's traumas and difficulties.

379 pages
ISBN: 0-440201-08-2

1635 **A Parent's Guide to Asperger's Syndrome & High-Functioning Autism**
Guilford Press
72 Spring Street
New York, NY 10012
800-365-7006
Fax: 212-966-6708
e-mail: info@guilford.com
www.guilford.com

For parents of children on the higher end of the autistic spectrum. All educators, the authors provide the basic on diagnosis, causes, and treatment.

2002 278 pages
ISBN: 1-572307-67-6

1636 **Activities for Developing Pre-Skill Concepts In Children with Autism**
Toni Flowers, author
Autism Society of North Carolina Bookstore
505 Oberlin Road
Raleigh, NC 27605-1345
919-743-0204
800-442-2762
Fax: 919-743-0208
e-mail: info@autismsociety-nc.org
www.autismsociety-nc.org

Chapters include auditory development, concept development, social development and visual-motor integration.

1637 **Asperger Syndrome or High-Functioning Autism?**
Plenum Publishing Corporation
233 Spring Street
New York, NY 10013-1522
212-741-6680
Fax: 212-463-0742

ISBN: 0-306457-46-6

1638 **Asperger's Syndrome: A Guide for Parents and Professionals**
taylor & Francis
325 Chestnut Street
Philadelphia, PA 19106
215-625-8900
www.tonyattwood.com

Offers insight into the identification and treatment of children on the higher functioning end of ASD.

201 pages
ISBN: 1-853025-77-1

1639 **Autism Society of North Carolina Bookstore**
505 Oberlin Road
Raleigh, NC 27605-1345
919-743-0204
800-442-2762
Fax: 919-743-0208
e-mail: info@autismaociety-nc.org
www.autismsociety-nc.org

Offers one of the largest selections of books about autism.

1640 **Autism Through the Lifespan: The Eden Model**
Woodbine House
6510 Bells Mill Road
Bethesda, MD 20817-1636
301-897-3570
800-843-7323
Fax: 301-897-5838

Presents Eden's comprehensive model for helping children and adults with autism, offering services that extend over their entire lifespan. An overview of what is known about autism today, discussions about Eden's approach to behavior modification, placement and treatment, curriculum from early childhood to adulthood, staffing issues, integration, decision making, and parental roles. Also contains dozens of examples and case histories that illustrate the program's successes.

1998 383 pages Paperback
ISBN: 0-933149-28-x

1641 **Autism Treatment Guide**
Elizabeth King Gerlach, author
Autism Society of North Carolina Bookstore
505 Oberlin Road
Raleigh, NC 27605-1345
919-743-0204
800-442-2762
Fax: 919-743-0208
e-mail: info@autismsociety-nc.org
www.autismsociety-nc.org

This 3rd edition offers many of the most current findings in treatments fo autism spectrum disorder. First published in 1993 and updated regularly, this concise handbook provides hundres of resource listings and suggested readings pertaining to ASD. This is a must-have reference book for parents and professionals

2003 157 pages Softcover

1642 **Autism and Asperger Syndrome Preparing for Adulthood**
Autism Society of North Carolina Bookstore
505 Oberlin Road
Raleigh, NC 27605-1345
919-743-0204
800-442-2762
Fax: 919-743-0208
e-mail: info@autismsociety-nc.org
www.autismsociety-nc.org

Chapters include topics such as what becomes of adults with ASD, interventions for ASD, problems af communication, social functioning in adulthood, sterotyped, ritualistic, and obsessional behaviors, secondary education, post-secondary education, finding and coping with employment, pyschiatric disturbances in adulthood, leagal issues, sexual relationships and marriage, and enhancing independence.

2004 388 pages Softcover

1643 **Autism in Adolescents and Adults**
Plenum Press
233 Spring Street
New York, NY 10013-1578
212-620-8000
Fax: 212-463-0742
e-mail: info@plenum.com

A survey of the needs, problems and services for autistic adolescents and adults.

456 pages
ISBN: 0-306410-57-5

1644 **Autism...Nature, Diagnosis and Treatment**
Guilford Press
72 Spring Street
New York, NY 10012
800-365-7006
Fax: 212-966-6708
e-mail: info@guilford.com
www.guilford.com

Covers perspectives, issues, neurobiological issues and new directions in diagnosis and treatment.

417 pages
ISBN: 0-898627-24-9

1645 **Autism: Explaining the Enigma**
Uta Frith, author
Blackwell Publishing
Commercer Place
Malden, MA 02148
781-388-8200
800-862-6657
Fax: 781-388-8210
www.blackwellpublishing.com

Explains the nature of autism.

2003 264 pages
ISBN: 0-631229-01-9

1646 **Autism: Identification, Education and Treatment**
Dianne Zager, author
Lawrence Earlbaum Associates
10 Industrial Avenue
Mahwah, NJ 07430
201-258-2200
800-926-6579
Fax: 201-236-0072
www.erlbaum.com

Chapters include medical treatments, early intervention and communication development in autism.

2005 608 pages
ISBN: 0-805845-79-8

1647 **Autism: The Facts**
Oxford University Press

2001 Evans Road
Cary, NC 27513-2010
212-726-6000
800-451-7556
Fax: 919-677-1303
www.oup-usa.org

1993 128 pages
ISBN: 0-192623-28-1

1648 Autistic Adults at Bittersweet Farms
Haworth Press
10 Alice Street
Binghamton, NY 13904-1580
607-722-5857
800-429-6784
Fax: 607-722-0012
www.haworthpress.com

A touching view of an inspirational residential care program for autistic adolescents and adults.
205 pages Paperback
ISBN: 1-560240-57-0

1649 Beyond Gentle Teaching
J.J McGee and F.J Menolascino, author
Springer
233 Spring Street
New York, NY 10013
212-460-1500
800-777-4643
Fax: 212-460-1575
e-mail: service-ny@springer.com
www.springer.com

A nonaversive approach to helping those in need, caregivers.
252 pages Hardcover
ISBN: 0-306438-56-1

1650 Biology of the Autistic Syndromes
Christopher Gillberg and Mary Coleman, author
Blackwell Publishing, Inc.
Commerce Place
Malden, MA 02148
781-388-8200
800-862-6657
Fax: 781-388-8210
www.blackwellpublishing.com

Autism is not a disease but a syndrome of different diseases. In this completely reworked and updated 3rd edition, the authors adress the difficulties this presents for clinical diagnosis with diagnostic aids and clear guidlines for medical evaluation. This is an essential text text for clinicians and will also be of interest to parents of autistic children.
2000 340 pages
ISBN: 1-898683-22-0

1651 Children with Autism
Woodbine House
6510 Bells Mill Road
Bethesda, MD 20817-1636
301-897-3570
800-843-7323
Fax: 301-897-5838
e-mail: info@woodbinehouse.com
www.woodbinehouse.com

Recommended as the first book parents should read, this volume offers information and a complete introduction to autism, while easing the family's fears and concerns as they adjust and cope with their child's disorder.
368 pages Paperback
ISBN: 0-933149-16-6

1652 Communication Unbound: How Facilitated Communication Is Challenging Views
Teachers College Press
1234 Amsterdam Avenue
New York, NY 10027
212-678-3929
Fax: 212-678-4149
e-mail: tcpress@tc.columbia.edu
www.teacherscollegepress.com

Addresses the ways in which we receive persons with autism in our society, our community and our lives.
1993 221 pages

1653 Diagnosis Autism: Now What? 10 Steps to Improve Treatment Outcomes
Lawrence P Kaplan, PhD, author
Autism Society of North Carolina Bookstore
505 Oberlin Road
Raleigh, NC 27605-1345
919-743-0204
800-442-2762
Fax: 919-743-0208
e-mail: info@autismsociety-nc.org
www.autismsociety-nc.org

This practical guide was written to help parents of children with autism spectrum disorder form successful pediatric partnerships with physicians and other healthcare practitioners involved in their child's diagnosis and treatment. Containing chrts and worksheets, sample questions, research resources, and numerous planning strategies, this guide will aid parents and caregivers as they strive to build collaborative relationships with their child's case management team.
2005

1654 Effective Teaching Methods for Autistic Children
Rosalind C Oppenheim, author
Charles C Thomas Publisher
2600 S 1st Street
Springfield, IL 62704-4730
217-789-8980
800-258-8980
Fax: 217-789-9130
e-mail: books@ccthomas.com
www.ccthomas.com

The Rimland School for Autistic Children in Evanston, Illinois, with a Foreward by Bernard Rimland. This enlightening monograph is seven chapters detailing the specific problems encountered in teaching autistic children. Anecdotal reports of seven such children bring to light the need for special training and provide an insight into their handling. Related research is reviewed and discussed.
1974 116 pages Paperback
ISBN: 0-398028-58-3

1655 Encounters with Autistic States
Jason Aronson
PO Box 15100
York, PA 17405-7100
800-782-0015
Fax: 201-840-7242
www.aronson.com

Hardcover
ISBN: 0-765700-62-

1656 Handbook of Autism and Pervasive Developmental Disorders
Autism Society of North Carolina Bookstore
505 Oberlin Road
Raleigh, NC 27605-1345
919-743-0204
800-442-2762
Fax: 919-743-0208
e-mail: info@autismsociety-nc.org
www.autismsociety.org

A list of contributors address such topics as characteristics of autistic syndromes and interventions.
2005 1317 pages 2 volumes

1657 Helping Children with Autism Learn: A Guide to Treatment Approaches
Oxford University Press
2001 Evans Road
Cary, NC 27513
212-726-6000
800-451-7556
Fax: 919-677-1303

Shows parents and educators what the need to do to reach autistic children.
1993 320 pages
ISBN: 0-195138-11-2

1658 Hidden Child: The Linwood Method for Reaching the Autistic Child
Woodbine House
6510 Bells Mill Road
Bethesda, MD 20817-1636
301-897-3570
800-843-7323
Fax: 301-897-5838
e-mail: info@woodbinehouse.com
www.woodbinehouse.com

Chronicle of the Linwood Children's Center's successful treatment program for autistic children.
286 pages Paperback
ISBN: 0-933149-06-9

1659 I'm Not Autistic on the Typewriter
TASH

11201 Greenwood Avenue N 206-361-8870
Seattle, WA 98133-8612
An introduction to the facilitated communication training method.

1660 Keys to Parenting the Child with Autism
Marlene Targ Brill, M.Ed, author
Barrons Educational Series, Inc.
250 Wireless Boulevard
Hauppauge, NY 11788
800-645-3476
Fax: 631-434-3723
e-mail: fbrown@barronseduc.com
www.barronseduc.com
This book explains what autism is and how it is diagnosed.
2001 224 pages
ISBN: 0-764112-92-9

1661 Let Community Employment Be the Goal for Individuals with Autism
Autism Society of North Carolina Bookstore
505 Oberlin Road 919-743-0204
Raleigh, NC 27605-1345 800-442-2762
Fax: 919-743-0208
e-mail: info@autismsociaty-nc.org
www.autismsociety-nc.org
A guide designed for people who are responsible for preparing individuals with autism to enter the work force.
1993 66 pages Booklet

1662 Let Me Hear Your Voice A Family's Triumph Over Autism
Catherine Maurice, author
Autism Society of North Carolina Bookstore
505 Oberlin Road 919-743-0204
Raleigh, NC 27605-1345 800-442-2762
Fax: 919-743-0208
e-mail: info@autismsociety-nc.org
www.autismsociety-nc.org
The Maurice family's second and third children were diagnosed with autism. This book recounts their experience with a home program using behavior therapy.
1993 371 pages Softcover
ISBN: 0-679408-63-0

1663 Management of Autistic Behavior
Pro-Ed, Inc.
8700 Shoal Creek Boulevard 512-451-3246
Austin, TX 78757-6897 800-897-3202
Fax: 800-397-7633
e-mail: info@proedinc.com
www.proedinc.com
Comprehensive and practical book that tells what works best with specific problems.
450 pages Paperback
ISBN: 0-890791-96-1
Lindy Jordaan, Marketing Coordinator

1664 Navigating the Social World: A Curriculum for Individuals with Asperger's Syndrome
Future Horizons
721 W Abram Street
Arlington, TX 76013 800-489-0727
Fax: 817-277-2270
www.futurehorizons-autism.com
Help parents to improve communications and other skills that are difficult for ASD children.
350 pages
ISBN: 1-885477-82-1

1665 Neurobiology of Autism
Johns Hopkins University Press
2715 N Charles Street 410-516-6936
Baltimore, MD 21218-4319 Fax: 410-516-6998
www.jhupbooks.com
This book discusses recent advances in scientific research that point to a neurobiological basis for autism and examines the clinical implications of this research.
272 pages
ISBN: 0-801856-80-9

1666 News from the Border: A Mother's Memoir of Her Autistic Son
Houghton Mifflin Company/Order Processing
222 Berkeley Street 617-351-5000
Boston, MA 02116 800-225-3362
www.hmco.com
A searingly honest account of the author's family experiences with autism. Raising an autistic child is the central, ongoing drama of her married life and this riveting account of acceptance and coping.
1993 384 pages Cloth

1667 Pervasive Developmental Disorders: Finding a Diagnosis and Getting Help
O'Reilly & Associates
1005 Gravenstein Highway N 707-829-0515
Sebastopol, CA 95472-3858 800-998-9938
Fax: 707-829-0104
www.oreilly.com
Published for parents and patients with PDD-NOS and atypical PDD.
Paperback
ISBN: 1-565925-30-0

1668 Please Don't Say Hello
Human Sciences Press
233 Spring Street 212-620-8000
New York, NY 10013-1522
Paul and his family moved into a new neighborhood. Paul's brother was autistic. The children thought that Eddie was retarded until they learned that there were skills that he could do better than they could.
1976 47 pages Paperback
ISBN: 0-898851-99-8

1669 Psychoeducational Profile (PEP-3): TEACCH Individualized Psychoeducational Assessm
Autism Society of North Carolina Bookstore
505 Oberlin Road 919-743-0204
Raleigh, NC 27605-1345 800-442-2762
Fax: 919-743-0208
e-mail: info@autismsociety-nc.org
www.autismsociety-nc.org
This is the revised edition of Psychoeducational Profile, a widely recognized assessment tool used to identify the learning strengths and weaknesses of children with autism spectrum disorder (ASD). Developed by Division TEACCH clinicians, this instrument has been updated in several ways, including improved psychometric properties, revised function domains, new items and sub-tests, within-group comparison data, and the addition of key documentation.
2005

1670 Raising a Child with Autism: A Guide to Applied Behavior Analysis for Parents
Taylor & Francis
325 Chestnut Street 215-625-8900
Philadelphia, PA 19106 Fax: 215-625-2940
Applied behavior analysis activities that parents can use with ASD children. Inlcuded is helpful guidance for toilet training, daily living, and increasing communication and sibling interaction.
173 pages
ISBN: 1-853029-10-6

1671 Reaching the Autistic Child: A Parent Training Program
Martin Kozloff, author
Brookline Books/Lumen Editions
PO Box 1209 617-734-6772
Brookline, MA 02445 800-666-2665
Fax: 617-734-3952
www.brooklinebooks.com
Detailed case studies of social and behavioral change in autistic children and their families show parents how to implement the principles for improved socialization and behavior.
1998 Softcover
ISBN: 1-571290-56-7

1672 Record Book for Individuals with Autism Spectrum Disorders
Marci Wheeler and Cathy Pratt, PhD, author
Autism Society of North Carolina Bookstore

505 Oberlin Road 919-743-0204
Raleigh, NC 27605-1345 800-442-2762
Fax: 919-743-0208
e-mail: info@autismsociety-nc.org
www.autismsociety-nc.org

This valuable resource provides a method for organizing and documenting information that will help parents track their child's development. This record book is divided into several categories, including: developmental and family history, sleeping and eating patterns, medical history, education history, behavior problems, skill development, and vital information. The book contains reproducible pages that will help parents keep important information up to date.

2000 44 pages Spiral Bound

1673 Record Book for Individuals with Autism Sp ectrum Disorders

Indiana Resource Center for Autism
2853 East 10th Street 812-855-6508
Bloomington, IN 47408-2696 Fax: 812-855-9630
TTY: 812-855-9396
e-mail: iidc@indiana.edu
www.iidc.indiana.edu/irca/fmain1.html

Throughout your lifetime, or that of a loved one with and autism spectrum disorder, various professionals will request information about previous approaches, assessments, treatments, illnesses, and other issues. This book was developed with input from parents, to provide a place to keep information about a child so that it is organized and easily accessible.

2000 44 pages

1674 Riddle of Autism: A Psychological Analysis

Jason Aronson
PO Box 15100
York, PA 17405-7100 800-782-0015
Fax: 201-840-7242
www.aronson.com

Dr. Victor examines the myths that cloud an understanding of this disorder and describes the meanings of its specific behavioral symptoms.

356 pages Softcover
ISBN: 1-568215-73-8

1675 Siblings of Children with Autism: A Guide. for Families

Woodbine House
6510 Bells Mill Road 301-897-3570
Bethesda, MD 20817 800-843-7323
Fax: 301-897-5838
www.woodbinehouse.com

Resource for families with autistic children and nonautistic siblings examines the perceptions, needs, compromises, and inevitable stresses that brothers and sisters face.

160 pages
ISBN: 1-890627-29-1

1676 TEACCH Transition Assessment Profile

Autism Society of North Carolina Bookstore
505 Oberlin Road 919-743-0204
Raleigh, NC 27605-1345 800-442-2762
Fax: 919-743-0208
e-mail: info@autismsociety-nc.org
www.autismsociety-nc.org

This new assessment profile is a major revision of the AAPEP. This comprehensive test was developed for older children and adolescents with autism spectrum disorder, particularly those who have transition needs. This assessment tool is structured to satisfy those provisions in the 2004 Individuals with Disabilities Education Act, which requires that adolescents be evaluated and also provided with a transition plan.

2007 Kit

1677 Targeting Autism: What We Know, Don't Know and Can Do to Help Young Children

University of California Press
1445 Lower Ferry Road 205-978-5000
Ewing, NJ 08618 800-777-4726
Fax: 800-999-1958
www.ucpress.com

Provides strong overviews of current work being done with autism and addresses the diferent life cycles of children with the condition through preschool, elementary school, and adolescence.

240 pages
ISBN: 0-520234-80-4

1678 Tasks Galore for the Real World

Laurie Eckenrode, Pat Fennell, and Kathy Hearsey, author

Autism Society of North Carolina Bookstore
505 Oberlin Road 919-743-0204
Raleigh, NC 27605-1345 800-442-2762
Fax: 919-743-0208
e-mail: info@autismsociety-nc.org
www.autismsociety-nc.org

These visually structured tasks are strategies that translate complex, everyday life skills into simpler, meaningful learning situations. The myriad of ideas in this guide will be valuable to anyone developing functional, daily living goals for a child or client.

2004

1679 Teach Me Language: A Language Manual for Children with Autism

Sabrina Freeman, PhD and Lorelei Dake, BA, author

Autism Society of North Carolina Bookstore
505 Oberlin Road 919-743-0204
Raleigh, NC 27605-1345 800-442-2762
Fax: 919-743-0208
e-mail: info@autismsociety-nc.org
www.autismsociety-nc.org

This book contains behaviorally based exercises and drills that adress common language weaknesses in children and incorporate professional speech pathology methods. These exercises were designed for children who are attentive, able to follow simple directions, have learned the basics of low-level language, and are visual learners. The activities and exercises are appropriate for children and young adults ages 5-18.

1997 410 pages Spiral Bound

1680 Teaching Children with Autism: Strategies to Enhance Communication and Socializing

Kathleen Ann Quill, author

Thomson Delmar Learning
Attn: Order Fullfillment
Florence, KY 41022 800-347-7707
Fax: 800-487-8488
www.delmarlearning.com

This book describes teaching strategies and instructional adaptations which promote communication and socialization in children with autism. It offers specific strategies that capitalize on the individual strengths and learning styles of the autistic child.

1996
ISBN: 0-827362-69-2

1681 Teaching Community Skills and Behaviors to Students with Autism or Related Problems

Indiana Resource Center for Autism
2853 East 10th Street 812-855-6508
Bloomington, IN 47408-2696 Fax: 812-855-9630
TTY: 812-855-9396
e-mail: iidc@indiana.edu
www.iidc.indiana.edu/irca/fmain1.html

Emphasizing the needs of the person with autism and the philosophy of community integration, this book cover the process of successful community-based teaching.

1988 117 pages

1682 The Autism Sourcebook

Karen Siff Exkorn, author

Autism Society of North Carolina Bookstore
505 Oberlin Road 919-743-0204
Raleigh, NC 27605-1345 800-442-2762
Fax: 919-743-0208
e-mail: www.autismsociety-nc.org
www.autismsociety-nc.org

This comprehensive handbook is for parents of newly diagnosed children who are looking for information about ASD, its diagnosis, treatment options, and practical strategies in one in-depth text.
2005

1683 The Everything Parent's Guide to Children with Autism
Adelle Jameson Tilton, author
Autism Society of North Carolina Bookstore
505 Oberlin Road 919-743-0204
Raleigh, NC 27605-1345 800-442-2762
Fax: 919-743-0208
e-mail: info@autismsociety-nc.org
www.autismsociety-nc.org
This book offers a wealth of information and reassuring advice for parents of newly diagnosed children. It is filled with hundreds of helpful tips, unique insights, and real-life situations, this is an essential guide for parents and family members.
2004 285 pages Softcover

1684 Understanding the Nature of Autism A Guide to the Autism Spectrum Disorders
Janice E Janzen, author
Autism Society of North Carolina Bookstore
505 Oberlin Road 919-743-0204
Raleigh, NC 27605-1345 800-442-2762
Fax: 919-743-0208
e-mail: info@autismsociety-nc.org
www.autismsociety-nc.org
Straightforward and comprehensive information that can be used by parents and professionals to develop curricula and programs for children with autism spectrum disorder. This important resource is a standard text used by educators, parents, and caregivers.
2003 508 pages Softcover

1685 When Snow Turns to Rain
Woodbine House
6510 Bells Mill Road 301-897-3570
Bethesda, MD 20817-1636 800-843-7323
Fax: 301-897-5838
e-mail: info@woodbinehouse.com
www.woodbinehouse.com
A gripping personal account of one family's experiences with autism. Chronicles a family's journey from parental bliss to devastation, as they learn that their son has autism. This book delves into diagnosis, treatments and attitudes toward persons with autism.
1993 250 pages Paperback
ISBN: 0-933149-63-8

1686 Autism Spectrum Disorders: The Complete Guide
Chantal Sicile-Kira, author
Autism Society of North Carolina Bookstore
505 Oberlin Road 919-743-0204
Raleigh, NC 27605-1345 800-442-2762
Fax: 919-743-0208
e-mail: info@autismsociety-nc.org
www.autismsociety-nc.org
This reference guide was written to help parents, professionals, and other members of the community learn more about autism spectrum disorder, and it presents a thorough overview of the disorder, from diagnosis through adulthood.
2004 360 pages Softcover

Children's Books

1687 Joey and Sam
Illana Katz and Edward Ritvo, MD, author
Autism Society of North Carolina Bookstore
505 Oberlin Road 919-743-0204
Raleigh, NC 27605-1345 800-442-2762
Fax: 919-743-0208
e-mail: ASNC@aol.com
A unique and invaluable tool for teaching children about others who are different. This awrd-winning and heartwarming sibling storybook examines the similarities and differences in behavior and educational experiences of two brothers, one of whom has autism.
1993 Softcover
ISBN: 1-882388-00-3

1688 Kristy and the Secret of Susan
Scholastic
800-724-6527
www.scholastic.com
This book discusses Kristy and her new baby-sitting charge, Susan. Susan can't speak but sings beautifully. Susan is autistic. Part of the Babysitters Club series.

1689 Russell is Extra Special
Charles A Amenta III. MD, author
Autism Society of North Carolina Bookstore
505 Oberlin Road 919-743-0204
Raleigh, NC 27605-1345 800-442-2762
Fax: 919-743-0208
e-mail: info@autismsociety-nc.org
www.autismsociety-nc.org
A sensitive portrayal of an autistic boy written by his father.
Hardcover

1690 Wild Boy of Aveyron
Harlan Lane, author
Harvard University Press
79 Garden Street
Cambridge, MA 02138 800-405-1619
Fax: 800-406-9145
e-mail: contact_HUP@harvard.edu
www.hup.harvard.edu
A dramatic account of a wild boy of nature and a young French doctor who shaped the modern education of retarded, deaf, and preschool children.
368 pages
ISBN: 0-674953-00-2

Newsletters

1691 Autism Research Review International
Autism Research Institute
4182 Adams Avenue 619-281-7165
San Diego, CA 92116-2536 Fax: 619-563-6840
www.autismresearchchinstitute.com
A quarterly newsletter published by the Autism Research Institute.
8 pages Quarterly
Dr. Bernard Rimland, Director

Pamphlets

1692 Avoiding Unfortunate Situations
Autism Society of North Carolina Bookstore
505 Oberlin Road 919-743-0204
Raleigh, NC 27605-1345 800-442-2762
Fax: 919-743-0208
e-mail: info@autismsociety-nc.org
www.autismsociety-nc.org
A collection of tips and information from and about people with autism and other developmental disabilities and their encounters with law enforcement agencies.

1693 Developing a Functional and Longitudinal Individual Plan
Nancy Dalrymple, author
Autism Society of North Carolina Bookstore
505 Oberlin Road 919-743-0204
Raleigh, NC 27605-1345 800-442-2762
Fax: 919-743-0208
e-mail: info@autismspectrum-nc.org
www.autismspectrum-nc.org
It is the author's view that a functional, longitudinal approach should be taken when educating persons with autism spectrum disorder, and that the developmentof an individualized plan should incorporate school, home, and community. This guide discusses the importance of defining strengths, striving for independent func-

tioning, and determining which activitiesshould recieve priority in the areas of self-care, social and leisure activities, and employment.
1989 11 pages Booklet

1694 Enabling Communication in Children with Autism
Autism Society of North Carolina Bookstore
505 Oberlin Road 919-743-0204
Raleigh, NC 27605-1345 800-442-2762
Fax: 919-743-0208
e-mail: info@autismsociety-nc.org
www.autismsociety-nc.org
Based on a 2 year research project, the goal of this book is to help teachers develop more communication-enabling enviroments for children with atuism spectrum disorder who use little or no speech. The authors illustrate many communication-enabling strategies, including the minimal speech approach, proximal communication, prompting, and multipointing.
2001 207 pages Softcover

1695 Job Seeker Involvment in Securing Employme nt
Nancy Kalina, author
Indiana Resource Center for Autism
2853 East 10th Street 812-855-6508
Bloomington, IN 47408-2696 Fax: 812-855-9630
TTY: 812-855-9396
e-mail: iidc@indiana.edu
www.iidc.indiana.edu/irca/fmain1.html
A walk through the job development process, from identifying job options and writing a resume to negotiating workplace supports with a potential employer. Each step provides opportunities for the peronal with autism, or another disability, to become actively involved in their job search process.
1997 22 pages

1696 Learning to be Independent and Responsible
Nancy Dalrymple, author
Indiana Resource Center for Autism
2853 East 10th Street 812-855-6508
Bloomington, IN 47408-2696 Fax: 812-855-9630
TTY: 812-855-9396
e-mail: iidc@indiana.edu
www.iidc.indiana.edu/irca/fmain1.html
People with autism build trust in people and environments through successful interactions. Individualized, supportive programs, utilizing positive instructional and environmental supports that lead to increased opportunities, chouse, and motivation are described in this booklet.
1989 11 pages

1697 Parents as Trainers of Legislators, Other Parents and Researchers
Autism Services Center
101 Richmond Street 304-525-8014
Huntington, WV 25702-1513 Fax: 304-525-8026
Reprint offering information on parents of autistic children that learn early in their child's life how little professionals know about autism.

1698 Sex, Sexuality, and the Autism Specrtum
Wendy Lawson, author
Autism Society of North Carolina Bookstore
505 Oberlin Road 919-743-0204
Raleigh, NC 27605-1345 800-442-2762
Fax: 919-743-0208
e-mail: info@autismsociety-nc.org
www.autismsociety-nc.org
The author, a psychologist, who has Aspergers Syndrome, presents her unique perspective on sexuality and interpersonal relationships. Filled with honest insights and positive advice, this is a valuable guide for persons with ASD and the people who live and work with them.
2005 175 pages Softcover

1699 Son-Rise Method
Option Institute
2080 S Undermountain Road 413-229-2100
Sheffield, MA 01257-9643 Fax: 413-229-8931
e-mail: sonrise@option.org
www.son-rise.org
Describes a program Barry and Samahria Kaufman developed to help heal their once-autistic son.

1700 What Is Autism
Autism Society of America
7910 Woodmont Avenue 301-657-0881
Bethesda, MD 20814-3065 800-328-8476
Fax: 301-657-0869
e-mail: info@autism-society.org
www.autism-society.org
Offers a definition and introduction to autism, produces a wide range of autism information written for various audiences. Offers a quarterly magazine, national conference, nationwide chapter network and many other resources.

Audio & Video

1701 A Sense of Belonging: Including Students w ith Autism in their School Community
Indiana Resource Center for Autism
2853 East 10th Street 812-855-6508
Bloomington, IN 47408-2696 Fax: 812-855-9630
TTY: 812-855-9396
e-mail: iidc@indiana.edu
www.iidc.indiana.edu/irca/fmain1.html
Highlights the efforts of two elementary and one middle school in Indiana in teaching students with autism in general education settings. Comments from parents, school administrators, classmates, and educators illustrate the role they each played in supporting students with autism in becoming active learners in their school community. Includes practical strategies for teaching the student with autism.
1997 20 minutes

1702 Autism: A Strange, Silent World
Filmakers Library
124 E 40th Street 212-808-4980
New York, NY 10016-1798 Fax: 212-808-4983
e-mail: info@filmakers.com
www.filmakers.com
British educators and medical personnel offer insight into autism's characteristics and treatment approaches through the cameos of three children.
Video Cassette
Sue Oscar, Co-President

1703 Autism: A World Apart
Karen Cunninghame, author
Fanlight Productions
4196 Washington Street 617-469-4999
Boston, MA 02131-1731 800-937-4113
Fax: 617-469-3379
e-mail: fanlight@fanlight.com
www.fanlight.com
In this documentary, three families show us what the textbooks and studies cannot, what it's like to live with autism day after day, raise and love children who may be withdrawn and violent and unable to make personal connections with their families.
1988 29 Minutes
ISBN: 1-572950-39-0

1704 Developing IEPs Under the New Idea Regulations
LRP Publications
747 Dresher Road
Horsham, PA 19044-2247 800-341-7874
Fax: 215-784-9639
e-mail: custserve@lrp.com
www.lrp.com
A practical, step-by-step approach makes it easy to understand the legal and educational issues surrounding IEPs.
26 minutes

1705 **Discipline Under the New Idea: Practical Methods and Procedures**
LRP Publications
747 Dresher Road
Horsham, PA 19044-2247
800-341-7874
Fax: 215-784-9639
e-mail: custserve@lrp.com
www.lrp.com
Provides practical explanation of the discipline methods and procedures school officials are permitted to use for students with disabilities.
26 minutes

1706 **Embracing Play: Teaching Your Child with Autism**
Woodbine House
6510 Bells Mill Road
Bethesda, MD 20817
301-897-3570
800-843-7323
Fax: 301-897-5838
www.woodbinehouse.com
Guide for parents who incorporate applied behavior analysis with their child.
1993 47 minutes

1707 **Functional Behavioral Assessments: How to Do Them Right!**
LRP Publications
747 Dresher Road
Horsham, PA 19044-2247
800-341-7874
Fax: 215-784-9639
e-mail: custserve@lrp.com
www.lrp.com
Assist you in understanding why a behavior problem has occured, so you can maximize the effectiveness of a planned intervention.
18 minutes

1708 **Getting Started with Facilitated Communication**
Syracuse University, Facilitated Communication Ins
370 Huntington Hall
Syracuse, NY 13244-2340
315-443-9379
Fax: 315-443-9218
e-mail: fcstaff@syr.edu
soeweb.syr.edu/thefci/
Describes in detail how to help individuals with autism and/or severe communication difficulties to get started with facilitated communication.
Videotape

1709 **Going to School with Facilitated Communication**
Syracuse University, School of Education
805 S Krouse
315-443-2693
Syracuse, NY 13244-0001
A video in which students with autism and/or severe disabilities illustrate the use of facilitated communication focusing on basic principles fostering facilitated communication.
Videotape

1710 **I Want My Little Boy Back**
Autism Treatment Center of America
2080 S Undermountain Road
Sheffield, MA 01257
413-229-2100
800-714-2779
Fax: 413-229-8931
e-mail: www.son-rise.org
information@son-rise.org
This BBC documentary follows an English family with a child with autism before, during, and after their time at the Son-Rise Program. It uniquely captures the heart of the Son-Rise Program and is extremely useful in understanding the program's techniques.
Lauren Astor, Public Relations Manager

1711 **I'm Not Autistic on the Typewriter**
Syracuse University, School of Education
805 S Krouse
315-443-2693
Syracuse, NY 13244-0001
A video introducing facilitated communication, a method by which persons with autism express themselves.
Videotape

1712 **Invisible Wall: Autism**
PRIMEDIA/Films Media Group
Films for Humanities & Sciences
Princeton, NJ 08543
800-257-5126
Fax: 609-671-0266
e-mail: custserv@filmsmediagroup.com
www.films.com/
It features interviews with Ivar Lovaas, the creator of applied behavior analysis therapy.
2001 52 minutes
Dean B Nelson, Chairman/President/CEO PRIMEMEDIA
Kevin Neary, Chief Financial Officer/PRIMEDIA

1713 **Public Schools and Students with Autism: Components of a Defensible Program**
LRP Publications
747 Dresher Road
Horsham, PA 19044-2247
800-341-7874
Fax: 215-784-9639
e-mail: custserve@lrp.com
www.lrp.com
This video assists you in understanding transition planning, documentation of student progress and proven strategies you can implement in your program.
13 minutes

1714 **Standards and Inclusion: Can We Have Both?**
LRP Publications
747 Dresher Road
Horsham, PA 19044-2247
800-341-7874
Fax: 215-784-9639
e-mail: custserve@lrp.com
www.lrp.com
Addresses the critical issues educators face when supporting students with disabilities in inclusive settings. Through dynamic, powerful presentations by two inclusion experts.
40 minutes

1715 **Understanding Autism**
Suzanne Newman, author
Fanlight Productions
4196 Washington Street
Boston, MA 02131-1731
617-469-4999
800-937-4113
Fax: 617-469-3379
e-mail: fanlight@fanlight.com
www.fanlight.com
Parents of children with autism discuss the nature and symptoms of this lifelong disability and outlines a treatment program based on behavior modification principles.
1993 19 Minutes
ISBN: 1-572951-00-1

Web Sites

1716 **Autism Research Institute**
www.autism.com/ari/
A clearinghouse for research on autism and related disorders of learning and behavior. Conducts and compiles research findings to provide people with the latest research available.

1717 **Autism Resources**
www.autism-resources.com
Provides links, frequently asked questions, and excellent bibliography of more than 700 books.
1993 47 minutes

1718 **Autism Society of America**
www.autism-society.org
Providing as much information as possible about autism and the various options, approaches, methods and systems available to parents of children with autism, family members and those professionals who work with them.

1719 **Autism Treatment Center of America**
www.autismtreatment.com
Since 1983, the Autism Treatment Center of America has provided innovative training programs for parents and professionals caring for children challenged by Autism, Autism Spectrum Disorders, Pervasive Developmental Disorder (PDD) and other developmental difficulties. The Son-Rise Program teaches a specific yet com-

prehensive system of treatment and education designed toh elp families and caregivers enable their children to dramatically improve in all areas of learning.

1720 **Community Services for Autistic Adults & Children**
www.csaac.org
Private nonprofit agency dedicated to serving persons disabled by autism. Helping these individuals to remain in their communities to live, work, and play.

1721 **Healing Well**
www.healingwell.com
An online health resource guide to medical news, chat, information and articles, newsgroups and message boards, books, disease-related web sites, medical directories, and more for patients, friends, and family coping with disabling diseases, disorders, or chronic illnesses.

1722 **Health Finder**
www.healthfinder.gov
Searchable, carefully developed web site offering information on over 1000 topics. Developed by the US Department of Health and Human Services, the site can be used in both English and Spanish.

1723 **Healthlink USA**
www.healthlinkusa.com
Health information concerning treatment, cures, prevention, diagnosis, risk factors, research, support groups, email lists, personal stories and much more. Updated regularly.

1724 **Helios Health**
www.helioshealth.com
Online resource for your health information. Detailed information about specific health topics, access to expert advice from our Medical Advisory Board, and up-to-date health news.

1725 **MedicineNet**
www.medicinenet.com
An online resource for consumers providing easy-to-read, authoritative medical and health information.

1726 **Medscape**
www.mywebmd.com
Medscape offers specialists, primary care physicians, and other health professionals the Web's most robust and integrated medical information and educational tools.

1727 **National Alliance for Autism Research**
www.naar.org
The first organization in the United States dedicated to funding and accelerating biomedical research focusing on autism spectrum disorders.

1728 **National Institute of Mental Health: Autism**
Office of Communications
6001 Executive Boulevard 301-443-4513
Bethesda, MD 20892-9663 866-615-6464
Fax: 301-443-4279
e-mail: nimhinfo@nih.gov
www.nimh.nih.gov/healthinformation/
Maintains a series of autism information links as well as downloadable booklets that provide a good instruction to the condition.
1993 47 minutes
Thomas R Insel, MD, Director

1729 **Son Rise Program**
www.son-rise.org
Describes an effective, loving and respectful method for treating children with autism. It teaches parents and healing professionals how to set up a home based program using the child's motivation to reach their special child.

1730 **WebMD**
www.webmd.com
Information on Autism, including articles and resources.

Description

1731 **Birth Defects**

Birth defects, or congenital abnormalities, occur in 3 to 4 percent of newborns and can include structural defects of the heart, major blood vessels, kidneys, urinary tract, gastrointestinal tract, skeleton and nervous system. The incidence of specific abnormalities varies with the type of defect. These defectsmay be single or several defects may occur together, often known as a syndrome.

Although in many instances the cause of the defect is unknown, genetic factors may cause many single malformations and syndromes. Some syndromes, such as Down syndrome, result from chromosomal abnormalities. Factors during the pregnancy can sometimes result in defects, such as taking certain drugs (coumadin, dilantin), maternal illness (diabetes), and various infections (German measles, Rubella).

Prior to birth, ultrasound evaluation of the fetus and testing of the amniotic fluid surrounding it can identify some defects. If a defect is identified and is serious, parents can decide how or if they wish the pregnancy to proceed. Other abnormalities may not be identified until birth. Treatment and outcome vary greatly, depending on the type and severity of the defect. Parents and other family members need honest information and emotional support when caring for a child born with congenital defects. If genetic factors are suspected, the parents should receive genetic counseling. See also *Spina Bifida and Congenital Heart Disease.*

National Agencies & Associations

1732 **Birth Defect Research for Children**
800 Celebration Avenue
Celebration, FL 34747
407-566-8304
Fax: 407-566-8341
e-mail: staff@birthdefects.org.
www.birthdefects.org
A nonprofit organization that provides information about birth defects of all kinds to parents and professionals. Offers a library of medical books and files of information on less common categories of birth defects and is involved in research to discover causes and prevention.
Betty Mekdeci, Executive Director
John Bragg, Administrative Assistant

1733 **CAPP National Parent Resource Center**
95 Berkeley Street
Boston, MA 02116
617-482-2915
800-331-0688
Fax: 617-482-2915
A parent-run resource system designed to further the needs and goals of family-centered community-based coordinated care for children with special health needs and their families. Offers written materials, training packages, workshops and presentations.

1734 **Cleft Palate Foundation**
1504 E Franklin Street
Chapel Hill, NC 27514-2820
919-933-9044
800-24C-LEFT
Fax: 919-933-9604
e-mail: info@cleftline.org
www.cleftline.org
Major services are provided through CLEFTLINE, a 24 hour toll free hotline for anyone affected by a facial birth defect. We provide free educational materials referrals to local treatment and support groups and hope.
Nancy C Smythe, Executive Director
Rafael Goldberg, Member Services Manager

1735 **Cornelia de Lange Syndrome Foundation**
302 W Main Street
Avon, CT 06001
860-676-8166
800-223-8355
Fax: 860-676-8337
e-mail: info@cdlsusa.org
www.cdlsusa.org
Provides information about birth defects caused by Cornelia de Lange Syndrome.
Liana Garcia-Fresher, Executive Director
Barbara Koontz, Information Coordinator

1736 **Easter Seals**
230 W Monroe Street
Chicago, IL 60606
312-726-6200
800-221-6827
Fax: 312-726-1494
TTY: 312-726-4258
e-mail: info@easter-seals.org
www.easter-seals.org
Provides services to children and adults with disabilities as well as support to their families.
Reenie Kavalor, VP Medical/Rehabilitation Services

1737 **Federation for Children with Special Needs**
1135 Tremont Street
Boston, MA 02120
617-236-7210
800-331-0688
Fax: 617-572-2094
e-mail: fcsninfo@fcsn.org
fcsn.org
A center for parents and parent organizations to work together on behalf of children with special needs.
Richard J Robison, Executive Director
Peter Brenna CPA, Board of Director

1738 **March of Dimes Birth Defects Foundation**
1275 Mamaroneck Avenue
White Plains, NY 10605
914-997-4488
www.marchofdimes.com
Our mission is to improve the health of babies by preventing birth defects premature birth and infant mortality. The March of Dimes carries out this mission through programs of research community services education and advocacy to save babies' lives.

1739 **National Early Childhood Technical Assistance Center**
Campus Box 8040 UNC-CH
Chapel Hill, NC 27599-8040
919-962-2001
Fax: 919-966-7463
TDD: 919-843-3269
e-mail: nectac@unc.edu
www.nectac.org
Assists states and other designated governing jurisdictions as they develop multidisciplinary, coordinated and comprehensive services for children with special needs.
Pascal Trohanis, Director
Judi Shaver, Operations Coordinator

1740 **National Foundation for Facial Reconstruction**
317 East 34th Street
New York, NY 10016
212-263-6656
Fax: 212-263-7534
e-mail: info@nffr.org
www.nffr.org
The National Foundation for Facial Reconstruction addresses the plight of children with a facial disfigurement by supporting state of the art treatment, innovative research, psychosocial support and medical training that inspires a new generation of pediatric doctors.
Whitney Burnett, Executive Director
Michele B Golombuski, MS, Associate Executive Director

1741 **Parent Professional Advocacy League**
45 Bromfield Street
Boston, MA 02108
617-542-7860
866-815-8122
Fax: 617-542-7832
e-mail: info@ppal.net
www.ppal.net
An organization of families of children with mental emotional or behavioral needs and concerned professionals. PALS support groups are run in many areas across the country.
Lisa Lambert, Executive Director

Research Centers

1742 **Boston University Center for Human Genetics**
715 Albany Street 617-638-7083
Boston, MA 02118-2394 Fax: 617-638-7092
e-mail: amilunski@bu.edu
www.bumc.bu.edu
Offers research into genetic disorders and growth disorders.
Aubrey Milun MD, Director
Jeff Milunsky, Co-Director

1743 **California Teratogen Information Service UC San Diego School of Medicine Dept of**
UC San Diego School of Medicine Dept of Pediatrics
9500 Gilman Drive 619-294-6291
La Jolla, CA 92093 800-532-3749
Fax: 619-220-0228
e-mail: ctispregnancy@ucsd.edu
www.ctispregnancy.org
Statewide service operated by the California Teratogen Information Service (CTIS) and Clinical Research Program. Our goal is to promote healthy pregnancies through education and research.
Kenneth Lyon Jones MD, Medical Director
Christina D Chambers, Program Director

1744 **Department of Reproductive Genetics: Magee Women's Hospital**
300 Halket Street 412-647-4168
Pittsburgh, PA 15213-3108 800-454-8155
Fax: 412-641-1032
e-mail: dbrucha@mail.magee.edu
www.upmc.com/HospitalsFacilities/Hospita
Obstetrical and gynecological teaching unit of the University of Pittsburgh School of Medicine. A full-service women's hospital and now has expanded to include a range of services for women and men.
W Allen Hogge, Clinical Investigator
Jie Hu, Assistant Investigator

1745 **Division Of Developmental and Behavioral Pediatrics**
Children's Hospital Medical Center of Cincinnati
3333 Burnet Avenue 513-636-4200
Cincinnati, OH 45229-3039 800-344-2462
TTY: 513-636-4900
www.cincinnatichildrens.org
The Division of Developmental and Behavioral Pediatrics provides services for infants children and adolescents from birth to age 21 who are experiencing developmental or behavioral problems.
David J Schonfeld, Director
Matthew W Zurad, Business Director

1746 **Georgetown University Child Development Center**
Box 571485 202-687-5000
Washington, DC 20057 Fax: 202-687-8899
e-mail: gucdc@georgetown.edu
www.gucchd.georgetown.edu
The mission of the GUCCHD is to bring together policy, research and clinical practice for the betterment of individuals and families, especially children youth and those with special needs including: development disabilities and special health care needs, mental health needs, young children and those in the child welfare system.
John De Gioia, President
Neal Horen, Co-Director Training and Technical Assis

1747 **Louisiana State University Genetics Section of Pediatrics**
200 Clay Avenue 504-896-9524
New Orleans, LA 70118 Fax: 504-894-3997
e-mail: ylacas@lsuhsc.edu
www.medschool.lsuhsc.edu
Yves Lacassie, Section Head
Mary Camille Fournet, Research Associate

1748 **New England Regional Genetics Group**
PO Box 920288 781-444-0126
Needham, MA 02492 Fax: 781-444-0127
e-mail: mfgnergg@verizon.net
www.nergg.org
Human genetic services and educational planning pertaining to birth defects.
Mary-Frances Garber, Executive Director
Cindy Ingham, Co-Director

1749 **Teratology OTIS**
1295 N Martin 520-626-3547
Tucson, AZ 85721 866-626-6847
e-mail: OTISPregnancy@pharmacy.arizona.edu.
www.otispregnancy.org
Teratology Information Services are comprehensive and multidisciplinary resources for medical consultation on prenatal exposures. TIS interpret information regarding known and potential reproductive risks into risk assessments that are communicated to individuals of reproductive age and health care providers.
Dee Quinn, Executive Director
Myla Moretti, President

1750 **Thomas Jefferson University: Daniel Baugh Institute**
329 Jefferson Alumni Hall
1020 Locust Street 215-503-7823
Philadelphia, PA 19107 Fax: 215-503-2636
e-mail: James.Schwaber@mail.dbi.tju.edu
www.dbi.tju.edu
Cares for both out and in-patients with complex problems involving a wide variety of infectious diseases. The Division has an active clinical research program bringing state-of-the-art treatments to patients.
James Schwaber, Director
Boris N Kholodenko, Director Computational Cell Biology

1751 **University of Illinois at Chicago Craniofacial Center**
College of Medicine
180 DENT M/C 588 312-996-7546
Chicago, IL 60612 Fax: 312-413-1157
e-mail: dreisber@uic.edu
www.uic.edu
David J Reisberg, Director

1752 **University of Iowa Birth Defects and Genetic Disorders Unit**
Iowa Registry for Congenital/Inherited Disorders
M107 Oakdale Hall 319-335-4107
Iowa City, IA 52242-5000 866-274-4237
Fax: 319-335-4030
e-mail: ircid@uiowa.edu
www.uiowa.edu
Established through the joint efforts of the University of Iowa the Iowa Department of Public Health and the Iowa Department of Human Services to monitor birth defects in the state.
Paul A Romitti, Director
Kim Keppler-Noreuil, Clinical Director for Birth Defects

1753 **University of Miami: Mailman Center for Child Development**
1601 NW 12th Avenue 305-243-6801
Miami, FL 33136-6820 Fax: 305-243-5978
TTY: 305-243-5937
TDD: 305-243-5937
peds2.med.miami.edu/mailman
Focuses on birth defects and children's illnesses.
Dr Robert Stempfel Jr, Director

1754 **Wayne State University: CS Mott Center for Human Growth and Development**
275 E Hancock Street 313-577-1485
Detroit, MI 48201 Fax: 313-577-8554
home.med.wayne.edu
Human growth and development disorders.
Dr Robert Sokol, Director

1755 **Wichita Medical Research & Education Foundation**
3306 E Central Avenue 316-686-7172
Wichita, KS 67208-3104 e-mail: info@wichitamedicalresearch.org
www.wichitamedicalresearch.org
The Wichita Medical Research Foundation promotes research for the development of new medical skills and knowledge which serve patients from Wichita and throughout Kansas.
Peggy L Johnson, Executive Director/COO
Dwight Oxley, President

Support Groups & Hotlines

1756 **CUNY: Teratogen Information Service**
People
1219 N Forest Road
Williamsville, NY 14221-3292
716-634-8132
888-773-0753
Fax: 716-634-3889
www.people-inc.org
Luther Robinson MD

1757 **Connecticut Pregnancy Exposure Information Service**
University of Connecticut Health Center
263 Farmington Avenue
Farmington, CT 6030-1
860-679-2100
800-325-5391
Fax: 860-679-4815
www.uchc.edu
Philip E Austin, President
James F Abromaitis, Commissioner

1758 **Illinois Teratogen Information Service (IT IS)**
680 North Lake Shore Drive
Chicago, IL 60611
312-252-4847
800-252-4847
Fax: 312-981-4366
e-mail: mgaudette@fetal-exposure.org
www.fetal-exposure.org/
The Illinois Teratogen Information Service (ITIS) is free statewide service that provides information regarding all types of exposures during pregnancy. This service is available to women who are pregnant or planning a pregnancy, fathers, physicians, and other healthcare providers in the State of Illinois.
Mara Gaudette MS/CGC, Genetic Counselor/Coordinator ITIS
Eugene Pergament MD/Ph.D, Medical Geneticist/ITIS Staff

1759 **Indiana Teratogen Information Service**
Indiana University Medical Center
975 W Walnut Street
Indianapolis, IN 46202
317-274-2241
medicine.iu.edu
A telephone inquiry service, available to physicians, nurses, midwives, other health professionals caring for pregnant women, women who are already pregnant, and women thinking about becoming pregnant. Also provides central, up-to-date, information from computerized sources, professional articles and expert consultantants
David D Weaver MD, Director

1760 **Missouri Teratogen Information Service**
University of Missouri Health Care
1 Hospital Drive
Columbia, MO 65212-1
573-882-7299
Fax: 573-882-1593
e-mail: umhs-muhealth@missouri.edu
www.muhealth.org/
The Missouri Teratogen Information Services (MOTIS) helps promote healthy pregnancies by providing, counseling, education and information.
James Ross, Chief Executive Officer
James C Poehling, Chief Operating Officer

1761 **National Health Information Center**
PO Box 1133
Washington, DC 20013
310-565-4167
800-336-4797
Fax: 301-984-4256
e-mail: info@nhic.org
www.health.gov/nhic
Offers a nationwide information referral service, produces directories and resource guides.

1762 **Nebraska Information Service**
University of Nebraska Medical Center
985440 Nebraska Medical Center
Omaha, NE 68198-5440
402-559-5071
Fax: 402-559-7248
Teratogen Information Project
Beth Conover APRN, MS, Genetic Counselor
Kathleen Caldwell, Project Assistant

1763 **New Jersey Pregnancy Risk Information Service**
254 Easton Avenue
New Brunswick, NJ 8901-1766
732-745-6659
DebraLynn Day Salvatore, Medical Director

1764 **PALS Support Groups**
Parent Professional Advocacy League
59 Temple Place
Boston, MA 02111
617-542-7860
866-815-7860
Fax: 617-542-7832
e-mail: info@ppal.net
www.ppal.net
Offers emotional support to parents and families of disabled children.
Donna Welles, Executive Director
Lisa Lambert, Assistant Director

1765 **Pregnancy Healthline: Pennsylvania Hospital**
8th & Spruce Streets
Philadelphia, PA 19107
215-829-3601
Betsy Schick-Boschetto MSN

1766 **Pregnancy Risk Line**
288 N 1460 W
Salt Lake City, UT 84113
801-328-2229
800-822-2229
health.utah.gov/prl
Provides valuable information to women who are pregnant, considering becoming pregnant, or breastfeeding, and to their healthcare providers.
David Sunwell MD, Executive Director

1767 **Pregnancy Safety Hotline**
Western Pennsylvania Hospital
4800 Friendship Avenue
Pittsburgh, PA 15224-1722
412-687-7233
www.wphs.org
Michael Kerr MS

1768 **Teratogen Information Services**
University of Florida Health Science Center
PO Box 100296
Gainesville, FL 32610-0296
352-392-3050
www.health.ufl.edu
Donna H Poynor MA

1769 **Teratogen and Birth Defects Information Project**
University of South Dakota
414 E Clark Street
Vermillion, SD 57069-2307
605-677-5011
877-269-6837
Fax: 605-677-6534
e-mail: urelate@usd.edu
www.usd.edu
James Abbott, University President
Rod Parry, Dean of the Medical School

1770 **University of Iowa Teratogen Information Service**
University of Iowa Teratogen
200 Hakins Drive
Iowa City, IA 52242
319-353-7877
800-777-8442
www.uihealthcare.com
Donna Katen Bahensky, Chief Executive Officer
Anne Madenrice, Chief Operations Officer

1771 **University of Nebraska Medical Center Tera Togen Project**
Genetic Medicine-Munroe-Meyer Institute
985430 Nebraska Medical Center
Omaha, NE 68198-5430
402-559-6800
800-656-3937
Fax: 402-559-6688
e-mail: gbschaef@unmc.edu
www.unmc.edu/dept/mmi/
The section of Genetic Medicine provides comprehensive services for a variety of patients and their families. Direct services include diagnosis, interpretation of risks, supportive counseling, and suggestions/referrals for further management. The department participates in clinics, inpatient consultation, and the Teratogen Information Project.
G Bradley Schaefer MD/FAAP/FACMG, Director Genetics Department

1772 **Vermont Pregnancy Risk Information Service**
Vermont Regional Genetics Center
1 Mill Street
Burlington, VT 05401-1530
800-932-4609
Alan E Guttmacher MD

Books

1773 **Bendectin Report**
930 Woodcock Road 407-245-7035
Orlando, FL 32812 800-313-2232
www.birthdefects.org
Report on research connecting the anti-nausea medication, Bendectin, with birth defects. Includes latest judicial opinion confirming $24 million judgment in a Bendectin case.
90 pages

1774 **Dursban Report**
930 Woodcock Road 407-245-7035
Orlando, FL 32812 800-313-2232
www.birthdefects.org
Report on research and latest EPA findings on Dursban and health problems, including MCS and birth defects.
90 pages

1775 **Environmental Birth Defect Digest**
930 Woodcock Road 407-245-7035
Orlando, FL 32812 800-313-2232
www.birthdefects.org
Compendium of research briefs from the world medical literature, plus original articles covering birth defects associated with medications, radiation, chemicals, toxic sites, dioxin, pesticides, lead, mercury, Bendectin, aspartame and more.
42 pages

1776 **Understanding Birth Defects**
Franklin Watts Grolier
90 Old Sherman Turnpike 203-797-3500
Danbury, CT 06816-0001 800-621-1115
Fax: 203-797-3197
www.grolier.com
What birth defects are, their genetic and environmental origins and what can be done to help, plus the problems of low birth weight are discussed.
128 pages
ISBN: 0-531109-55-0

Children's Books

1777 **Don't Feel Sorry for Paul**
JB Lippincott
530 Walnut Street 215-521-8300
Philadelphia, PA 19105 Fax: 215-521-8902
www.ilkins.com
Paul is seven and was born with deformities of both hands and feet. Paul must wear a prosthesis on both feet so that he can walk. He has a third prosthesis for his right hand. The third prosthesis has a pair of hooks Paul uses as fingers.
94 pages Hardcover
ISBN: 0-397315-88-0

1778 **God, the Universe and Hot Fudge Sundaes**
Houghton, Mifflin & Company
222 Berkeley Street
Boston, MA 02108-3107 617-351-5000
www.hmco.com

Newsletters

1779 **ABDC Newsletter**
Association of Birth Defect Children
5400 Diplomat Circle 407-629-1466
Orlando, FL 32810-5603 800-313-2232
www.birthdefects.org
Offers updated information on the association activities, events and medical updates. Back issues available.
8 pages Quarterly

1780 **NewsLine**
Federation for Children with Special Needs
95 Berkeley Street 617-482-2915
Boston, MA 02116-6230 800-331-0688
Offers information for parents and families on resources, medical updates, activities, fund-raising events and association news for their disabled children.
Quarterly

1781 **PAL News**
Parent Professional Advocacy League
95 Berkeley Street 617-482-2915
Boston, MA 02116-6264 800-331-0688
Offers information on medical and technological updates in the area of research on birth defects, support groups and family resources for persons with disabled children.
Quarterly

Pamphlets

1782 **After School...Then What? The Transition to Adulthood**
Federation for Children with Special Needs
95 Berkeley Street 617-482-2915
Boston, MA 02116-6230 800-331-0688
Preparing for the transition after high school for children with special needs.

1783 **Agent Orange and Birth Defects**
930 Woodcock Road 407-245-7035
Orlando, FL 32812 800-313-2232
www.birthdefects.org
Research booklet, including the latest findings from the National Birth Defect Registry and government research connecting Agent Orange to birth defects.
42 pages

1784 **Birth Defects & Genetics: The Genetics Revolution**
March of Dimes Birth
233 Park Avenue South 212-353-8353
New York, NY 10003 Fax: 212-254-3518
e-mail: NY639@marchofdimes.com
www.marchofdimes.com
Offers information on genetic testing and what it means to the patient and family members.

1785 **Childhood Illnesses in Pregnancy: Chicken Pox & Fifth Disease**
March of Dimes
233 Park Avenue South 212-353-8353
New York, NY 10003 Fax: 212-254-3518
e-mail: NY639@marchofdimes.com
www.marchofdimes.com
Located on the March of Dimes website.

1786 **Cleft Lip & Palate**
March of Dimes
233 Park Avenue South 212-353-8353
New York, NY 10003 Fax: 212-254-3518
e-mail: NY639@marchofdimes.com
www.marchofdimes.com
Located on March of Dimes website.

1787 **Club Foot and Other Foot Deformities**
March of Dimes
233 Park Avenue South 212-353-8353
New York, NY 10003 Fax: 212-254-3518
e-mail: NY639@marchofdimes.com
www.marchofdimes.com

1788 **Genetic Counseling**
March of Dimes
233 Park Avenue South 212-353-8353
New York, NY 10003 Fax: 212-254-3518
e-mail: NY639@marchofdimes.com
www.marchofdimes.com

1789 **Gulf War and Birth Defects**
930 Woodcock Road 407-225-7035
Orlando, FL 32812 800-313-2232
www.birthdefects.org
Information booklet on recent data from the National Birth Defect Registry and other research related to Gulf War exposures and birth defects.
30 pages

1790 **How to Find More About Your Child's Birth Defect or Disability**
Association for Birth Defect Children
5400 Diplomat Circle
Orlando, FL 32810-5603 800-922-9234
www.birthdefects.org
An informational fact sheet that encourages parents who have a child with a birth defect or disability to become the expert on the child's disability with some suggestions on how to educate themselves.

1791 **Low Birthweight**
March of Dimes
233 Park Avenue South 212-353-8353
New York, NY 10003 Fax: 212-254-3518
e-mail: NY639@marchofdimes.com
www.marchofdimes.com
Fact Sheets: one or two page review written for the general public. Also available electronically on the website: www.marchofdimes.com

1792 **PKU Quick Reference and Fact Sheet**
March of Dimes
233 Park Avenue South 212-353-8353
New York, NY 10003 Fax: 212-254-3518
e-mail: NY639@marchofdimes.com
www.marchofdimes.com
Phenylketonuria (PKU) is an inherited disorder that affects the way the body is able to process food. If left untreated, it causes mental retardation. How PKU is passed on and how it is treated are outlined. The Information Fact Sheet is located on the March of Dimes website.

1793 **Teaching Social Skills to Youngsters with Disabilities**
Federation for Children with Special Needs
95 Berkeley Street 617-482-2915
Boston, MA 02116-6230 800-331-0688
Explains the importance of instruction and training to learn appropriate social behavior.

1794 **Toxoplasmosis**
March of Dimes
233 Park Avenue South 212-353-8353
New York, NY 10003 Fax: 212-254-3518
e-mail: NY639@marchofdimes.com
www.marchofdimes.com
Fact Sheets: one or two page review written for the general public. Also available electronically at the website: www.marchofdimes.com

Audio & Video

1795 **Genetics and Inherited Traits**
March of Dimes
233 Park Avenue South 212-353-8353
New York, NY 10003 Fax: 212-254-3518
e-mail: NY639@marchofdimes.com
www.marchofdimes.com

1796 **Why My Child**
5400 Diplomat Circle 407-629-1466
Orlando, FL 32810-5603 800-313-2232
www.birthdefects.org
A 9 1/2 minute video that explores the feelings every parent has when their child is born with a birth defect. Emmy-award-winning producer, Karen Dorsett, has created a compelling video that begins with the parents' question, Why my child? and follows through to concerns about links between birth defects and environmental exposures to drugs, pesticides, dioxin, radiation, hazardous wastes, etc.

Web Sites

1797 **Association for Birth Defect Children**
www.birthdefects.org
Provides information about birth defects of all kinds to parents and professionals. Offers a library of medical books and files of information on less common categories of birth defects and is involved in research to discover possible links between environmental exposures and birth defects.

1798 **Healing Well**
www.healingwell.com
An online health resource guide to medical news, chat, information and articles, newsgroups and message boards, books, disease-related web sites, medical directories, and more for patients, friends, and family coping with disabling diseases, disorders, or chronic illnesses.

1799 **Health Finder**
www.healthfinder.gov
Searchable, carefully developed web site offering information on over 1000 topics. Developed by the US Department of Health and Human Services, the site can be used in both English and Spanish.

1800 **Healthlink USA**
www.healthlinkusa.com
Health information concerning treatment, cures, prevention, diagnosis, risk factors, research, support groups, email lists, personal stories and much more. Updated regularly.

1801 **Helios Health**
www.helioshealth.com
Online resource for your health information. Detailed information about specific health topics, access to expert advice from our Medical Advisory Board, and up-to-date health news.

1802 **March of Dimes Birth Defects Foundation**
www.modimes.org
Information on chapters situated across the countryand can be located through the web site, National Office, or telephone book. The Resource Center answers questions relating to preconception health, pregnancy, childbirth and birth defects.

1803 **MedicineNet**
www.medicinenet.com
An online resource for consumers providing easy-to-read, authoritative medical and health information.

1804 **Medscape**
www.mywebmd.com
Medscape offers specialists, primary care physicians, and other health professionals the Web's most robust and integrated medical information and educational tools.

1805 **WebMD**
www.webmd.com
Information on birth defects, including articles and resources.

Description

1806 **Brain Tumors**

Brain tumors are either primary (originate in the brain) or metastatic (travel from other cancer sites). About 29,000 people in the United States are diagnosed with primary brain tumors each year; approximately 50 percent of those are benign (noncancerous). Cancerous brain tumors originating in the brain make up roughly 2 percent of all cancers. They may occur at any age but are most common in early adult and middle life. Metastatic brain tumors (those that spread from other cancers) occur in 20 to 40 percent of all cancers.

There are many different types of brain tumors, each with a distinctive appearance under the microscope and a characteristic pattern of onset, progression, location and response to treatment. Depending on the exact site and rate of growth of the tumor, symptoms may include change in personality, moodiness, impaired vision and hearing, headaches, nausea, vomiting, seizures, lethargy and a varying degree of weakness. Some cancers have a genetic basis. In most cases, the cause of an individual's brain tumor is not known.

The treatment of brain tumors, as in many other cancers, consists of a combination of surgical removal, chemotherapy and radiation therapy. Steroids reduce swelling, and antiseizure medication is commonly given. If the disease or its treatment has caused damage to the brain's functioning, the patient may also need physical therapy, speech therapy, or general supportive care. The prognosis depends on the patient's age and on the location, extent and precise type of the tumor. See also *Head Injuries.*

National Agencies & Associations

1807 **American Brain Tumor Association**
2720 River Road 847-827-9910
Des Plaines, IL 60018-4117 800-886-2282
Fax: 847-827-9918
e-mail: info@abta.org
www.abta.org

Services includes over 40 publications which address brain tumors their treatment and coping with the disease. Materials address brain tumors in all age groups. Provide free social service consultations and a mentorship program for new brain tumor support groups.
Elizabeth M Wilson, Executive Director
Geri Jo Duda RN, Patient Services

1808 **Brain Tumor Society**
124 Watertown Street 617-924-9997
Watertown, MA 02472 800-770-8287
Fax: 617-924-9998
e-mail: info@tbts.org
www.tbts.org

Exists to find a cure for brain tumors and strives to improve the quality of life of brain tumor patients and their families. Disseminates educational information and provides access to psycho-social support and raises funds.
N Paul TonThat, Executive Director
Mark Cole, Deputy Executive Director

1809 **National Brain Tumor Foundation**
22 Battery Street 415-834-9970
San Francisco, CA 94111-5520 800-934-2873
Fax: 415-834-9980
e-mail: nbtf@braintumor.org
www.braintumor.org

Nonprofit health organization which raises funds for research and provides information and support to patients, their family members and friends and health professionals. Sponsors national and regional conferences, patient and caregiver programs.
Harriet Patt MPH, Director of Patient Services

1810 **National Institute of Neurological Disorders and Stroke**
PO Box 5801 301-496-5751
Bethesda, MD 20824 800-352-9424
Fax: 301-402-2186
TTY: 301-468-5981
www.ninds.nih.gov

Supports research on brain tumors and nervous disorders. The Information Center will send free printed materials on brain tumors.
Story C Landis, PhD, Director

Foundations

1811 **Brain Tumor Foundation for Children**
6065 Roswell Road NE 404-252-4107
Atlanta, GA 30328 Fax: 404-252-4108
e-mail: bfc@bellsouth.net
www.braintumorkids.org

Provides information and emotional support for families of children with brain tumors. They also raise funds for brain tumor research and provide a telephone network system of parents who offer emotional support.
Rick Sauers, Chairman/Co-Founder
R Hal Meeks, Jr, President

1812 **Children's Brain Tumor Foundation**
274 Madison Avenue 212-448-9494
New York, NY 10016 866-228-HOPE
Fax: 212-448-1022
e-mail: info@cbtf.org
www.cbtf.org

Children's Brain Tumor Foundation (CBTF) is a national organization whose mission is to improve the treatment, quality of life and long-term outlook for children with brain and spinal cord tumors through research, support, education, and advocacy to families and survivors. CBTF provides research and quality of life grants, offers information and support via our toll free line, written educational material, meet the unique needs of childhood brain tumor survivors.
Robert Budlow, President
Joseph B Fay, Executive Director

1813 **Pediatric Brain Tumor Foundation**
302 Ridgefield Court 828-665-6891
Asheville, NC 28806 800-253-6530
Fax: 828-655-6894
e-mail: pbtfus@pbtfus.org
www.pbtfus.org

Dedicated to finding the cause and cure of childhood brain tumors through the support of medical research. Increases public awareness, aids in early detection and treatment, supports a national database on all primary brain tumors. Helps to provide hope and emotional support for the thousands of children and families affected by this life threatening disease.
Michael Traynor, President
Glenn Wilcox, Vice President

Research Centers

1814 **Brain Research Center Children s Hospital National Medical Cen**
Children s Hospital National Medical Center

111 Michigan Avenue NW
Washington, DC 20010
202-884-2120
800-787-0021
Fax: 202-884-5226
www.dcchildrens.com

Edwin K Zechman Jr, Chief Executive Officer
Mark L Batshaw, Chief Medical Officer

1815 **Brain Research Foundation**
111 W Washington Street
Chicago, IL 60602
312-759-5150
Fax: 312-759-5151
e-mail: info@theBRF.org
www.brainresearchfdn.org

The Brain Research Foundation is a charitable foundation supporting research into causes and cures for brain-related illnesses. With help of over 100 scientists at the University of Chicago's Brain Research Institute great progress is being made to treat diseases of the brain among them brain tumors multiple sclerosis Alzheimer's disease Parkinson disease pediatric epilepsy LAS learning disorders and depression.
Gwill L Newman, Chairman
Nathan Hansen, Board Director

1816 **Brain Tissue Resource Center McLean Hospital**
McLean Hospital
115 Mill Street
Belmont, MA 02478
617-855-2000
800-272-4622
Fax: 617-855-3199
e-mail: mcleaninfo@mclean.harvard.edu
www.brainbank.mclean.org

A centralized resource for the collection and distribution of human brain specimens for brain research.
Francine M Benes, Director
Edward D Bird, Director Emeritus

1817 **Central Brain Tumor Registry of the US**
244 E Ogden avenue
Hinsdale, IL 60521
630-655-4786
Fax: 630-655-1756
e-mail: cbtrus@aol.com
www.cbtrus.org

Nonprofit resource for gathering and distributing current statistics on all primary brain tumors for the entire US. Includes data on benign borderline and malignant primary brain tumors.
Carol Kruchko, President /Administrator
Jeri Dolan, Executive Administrator

1818 **University of California, San Francisco Brain Tumor Research Center**
Department of Neurological Surgery
1855 Folsom Street
San Francisco, CA 94143-1631
415-476-3923
Fax: 415-376-3934
e-mail: garritye@neurosurg.ucsf.edu
www.neurosurgery.medschool.ucsf.edu

Continuously funded by grants from the National Institutes of Health Since 1072, the Brain Tumor Research Center at UCSF is internationally recognized as a major research and treatment center for adults and children with tumors of the brain and spinal cord. This center emphasizes translational research into the biology and behavior of brain tumors - research in which scientists and health care clinicians work in partnership to translate laboratory findings of new or improved forms of therapy.
Charles B Wilson, Director

Support Groups & Hotlines

1819 **National Health Information Center**
PO Box 1133
Washington, DC 20013
310-565-4167
800-336-4797
Fax: 301-984-4256
e-mail: info@nhic.org
www.health.gov/nhic

Offers a nationwide information referral service, produces directories and resource guides.

1820 **Parent-to-Parent Network**
Children's Brain Tumor Foundation
274 Madison Avenue
New York, NY 10016
212-448-9494
866-228-HOPE
Fax: 212-448-1022
e-mail: info@cbtf.org
www.cbtf.org

Allows families to share their experiences with those having similar concerns. Parents become better advocates for their children, and survivors become stronger advocates for themselves.
Robert Budlow, President
Joseph B Fay, Executive Director

Alabama

1821 **Pediatric Brain Tumor Support Group**
Children's Hospital
1600 7th Avenue S
Birmingham, AL 35233-1785
205-939-9090

Groups for parents and siblings of brain tumor patients. Related to Children's Hospital of Alabama. Babysitting available.
Paula Teague

Arizona

1822 **Arizona Brain Tumor Support Group**
Barrow Neurological Ins of St. Joe's Hospital
350 W Thomas Road
Phoenix, AZ 85013
623-205-6446
www.braintumorfoundation.org

Lanette Veres, Director

1823 **Southern Arizona Brain Tumor Support Group**
Arizona Cancer Cetner
1515 N Campbell Avenue
Tucson, AZ
520-694-4605
www.braintumorfoundation.org

Marsha Drozdoff, Contact

California

1824 **Bereavement Group for Children**
Corstone Center
33 Buchanan Drive
Sausalito, CA 94965-2535
415-331-6161
Fax: 415-331-4545
e-mail: info@corstone.org
www.corstone.org

Steve Leventhal, Executive Director
Richard Cuadra, MS, Program Director

1825 **Brain Tumor & Family Support Group**
100 E Valencia Mesa Drive
Fullerton, CA 92835
714-446-7182

1826 **Brain Tumor Information Line**
National Brain Tumor Foundation
22 Battery Street
San Francisco, CA 94111-5520
415-834-9970
800-934-2873
Fax: 415-834-9980
e-mail: nbtf@braintumor.org
www.braintumor.org

Quickly access brain tumor information and resources.
12 pages
Rob Tufel, Director Patient Services

1827 **Brain Tumor Support Group: Fresno**
7130 N Millbrook Avenue
Fresno, CA 93726
559-450-5528
e-mail: kkennedy@samc.com

1828 **Brain Tumor Support Group: Modesto**
1441 Florida Avenue
Modesto, CA 95350
209-523-0999

1829 **Brain Tumor Support Group: Palo Alto**
National Brain Tumor Foundation
c/o Stanford Cancer Center
Stanford, CA 94305
415-834-9970
800-934-2873
Fax: 650-736-0607
e-mail: nbtf@braintumor.org
www.braintumor.org

Time: Last Monday of each month, 7:30-9:00 PM. No meeting in December. The National Brain Tumor Foundation (NBTF) main-

tains a comprehensive list of brain tumor support groups for patients and their families. 160 support groups spread across the United States and Canada are currently listed.
Joanie Taylor RN, Support Group Coordinator (650-343-4791)
Sharon Lamb RN, Support Group Coordinator (415-661-1442)

1830 **Brain Tumor Support Group: San Francisco**
National Brain Tumor Society
22 Battery Street 415-834-9970
San Francisco, CA 94111-5520 Fax: 415-834-9980
e-mail: info@braintumor.org
www.braintumor.org
N Paul TonThat, Executive Director

1831 **Brain Tumor Support Group: Santa Barbara**
Cancer Foundation of Santa Barbara
300 W Pueblo Street 805-682-7300
Santa Barbara, CA 93105 Fax: 805-898-3608
www.ccsb.org
Cathie Nelson MSW, Facilitator

1832 **Brain Tumor Support Group: Santa Rosa**
Coast Rehab Hospital
151 Sotoyome Conference Room 415-476-2966
Santa Rosa/Petaluma, CA
Jane Rabbitt, RN

1833 **Brain Tumor Support Group: South Bay**
667 Chapman Street 650-498-7573
San Jose, CA 95126-2145
Jamie Vavroutsos, LCSW

1834 **Brain Tumor Support Group: West Los Angeles**
2716 Ocean Park Boulevard 310-314-2564
West Los Angeles, CA 90405

1835 **Children Living with Illness**
The Center for Attitudinal Healing
33 Buchanan Drive 415-331-6161
Sausalito, CA 94965 Fax: 415-331-4545
www.healingcenter.org
For children who are ill, have an ill sibling, or an ill parent. Parent group meets separately at the same time.
Lynn Scott

1836 **Inland Empire Brain Tumor Support Group**
Kaiser Fontana Neurosurgery Waiting Room
Medical Annex Building 2 909-780-7136
Fontana, CA 92334 e-mail: smelton@pacbell.net
Meets first Tuesday of each month at 6:30 p.m.
Sue Melton, Information
Sheri Kyander, Information

1837 **King Drew Brain Tumor Support Group**
12021 S Wilmington Avenue
Los Angeles, CA 90059 800-934-2873

1838 **Neuro-Oncology Information and Support Group**
Sister Mary Pia Regional Cancer Center
1800 N California Street
Stockton, CA 95204-6019 209-467-6550
www.stjosephscares.org
For patients and family members living with primary and metastatic brain tumors as well as spinal cord tumors. Free child care and refreshments are provided.
Jim Linderman

1839 **Neuroscience Institute Brain Tumor Support Group**
Hospital of the Good Samaritan
637 S Lucas Avenue 213-977-2234
Los Angeles, CA 90017-1912 866-895-7688
Fax: 213-482-2157
Support groups for caregivers, spouses, and gamma knife patients.
Cherrie Dela Cruz, Office Manager

1840 **Neuroscience Institute Brain Tumor Hotline**
Hospital of the Good Samaritan
637 Lucas Avenue
Los Angeles, CA 90017-1912 800-762-1692
e-mail: info@goodsam.org
www.goodsam.org
Diana Selover, LCSW

1841 **Peninsula Support & Education Group for Parents of Children with Brain Tumors**
Parents Helping Parents
3041 Olcott Street 408-727-5775
Santa Clara, CA 95054-3222 866-747-4040
Fax: 408-727-0182
e-mail: info@php.com
www.php.com
A comprehensive family resource center providing information, training, guidance and support to families of children with special needs and the professionals who serve them.
Mary Ellen Peterson, Chief Executive Officer

1842 **Sacramento Area Brain Tumor Support Group**
Lawrence J. Ellison Ambulatory Care Center
UC Davis medical Center 916-734-3590
Sacramento, CA 95817 Fax: 916-734-5706
e-mail: nbtf@braintumor.org
www.braintumor.org/
Educational topics presented, additional informational materials available. Monthly meetings including a speaker usually having between 20 and 30 people attending. Patients, family members and friends are all welcome. Mailing list available. Date/Time: First Thursday of each month, 6:30 - 8:30 p.m.
Karen Smith RN, Support Group Coordinator (916-734-5613)
Freda Muizelaar BSW, Support Group Coordinator (916-734-5613)

1843 **Support Group for Caregivers of Brain Tumor Patients**
UCLA Medical Center
200 UCLA Medical Plaza 310-206-6731
Los Angeles, CA 90095 e-mail: cabe@mednet.ucla.edu
Guest speakers on occasion.
Cheryl Abe LCSW, Clinical Social Worker
Pamela Hoft LCSW, Clinical Social Worker

1844 **Vital Options International**
4419 Coldwater Canyon Avenue 818-508-5657
Studio City, CA 91604-1479 800-477-7666
Fax: 818-788-5260
e-mail: info@vitaloptions.org
www.vitaloptions.org/
Vital Options International TeleSupport Cancer Network is a not-for-profit cancer communications, support and advocacy organization whose mission is to facilitate a global cancer dialogue by using communications technology to reach every person touched by cancer. Vital Options provides a variety of cancer communications projects for patients of all ages and disease types, as well as for their families, friends and healthcare providers.
Selma R Schimmel, Chief Executive Officer/Founder
Felice Bachrach, Advocacy Relations Manager

1845 **Wellness Community Cancer Support Groups**
Wellness Community
3276 Mc Nutt Avenue 925-933-0107
Walnut Creek, CA 94597 Fax: 925-330-0249
e-mail: jbouquin@twc-bayarea.org
www.twc-bayarea.org/
The mission of The Wellness Community is to help people affected by cancer enhance their health and well-being through participation in a professional program of emotional support, education, and hope. Many general support groups, workshops, classes, etc. offered. Calendar available.
James Bouquin, Executive Director
Margaret Stauffer, Program Director

1846 **Support Group for Parents of Children with Brain Tumors**
Oakland Children's Hospital
747 52nd Street 510-428-3885
Oakland, CA 800-400-PEDS
www.kidsfirst.org
Contact can be reached at extension 2161.
Trish Murphy

Colorado

1847 **Brain Tumor Resource and Vital Encouragement**
Childrens Hospital
1056 19th Avenue 303-861-8888
Denver, CO e-mail: webmaster@tchden.org
www.tchden.org
Pediatric focus. Education and support. Retreats for parents of brain tumor patients.
Joanne Pearson, Outpatient Oncology

1848 **Colorado Brain Tumor Support Group**
Swedish Medical Center
Englewood, CO 80113 303-806-7420
www.braintumorfoundation.org
Lorre Gibson, Contact

Connecticut

1849 **Connecticut Brain Tumor Support Group**
Yale New Haven Children's Hospital
20 York Street 203-785-7528
New Haven, CT 06510 Fax: 203-688-2395
www.braintumorfoundation.org
Angela Thomas LCSW, Facilitator

Delaware

1850 **Pediatric Brain Tumor Support Group**
Ronald McDonald House
PO Box 269 302-661-4077
Wilmington, DE 19899-3629 e-mail: izienberg@kidshealth.org
www.kidshealth.org
Meets first Monday of each month from 7:30 to 9:30 p.m.
Niel Izienberg, Chief Executive Officer

District of Columbia

1851 **Washington DC Metropolitan Area Support Group**
George Washington University
2150 Pennsylvania Aveneu NW 202-994-4035
Washington, DC 20037-3201
Margaret Fiore, RN

Florida

1852 **Angels in the Sun Brain Tumor Support Group**
Wellness Community
3900 Clark Road 941-921-5539
Sarasota, FL 34233
John Kleinbaum, Program Director

1853 **Brain Tumor Support Group**
Miami Children's Hospital Foundation
3000 SW 62nd Avenue 305-662-8386
Miami, FL 33155 e-mail: maria.penate@mch.com
Call for schedule.
Maria Penate RN, Facilitator
Raquel Pasaron, Facilitator

1854 **Florida Brain Tumor Association**
PO Box 770182 954-755-4307
Coral Springs, FL 33077-0182 e-mail: sshetsky@fbta.info
www.fbta.info
Provides hope, support and education to brain tumor survivors, their families and friends; conquers brain tumors by funding research into their causes and cures; and enriches the quality of life of those touched by brain tumors
Sheryl Shetsky, President
Gary L Kornfeld, VP

1855 **Florida Brain Tumor Support Group**
Healthpark Medical Ctr, Meeting Rm
Ft Meyers, FL 33919 239-433-4396
www.braintumorfoundation.org
Dona Ross, President

1856 **Hollywood Brain Tumor Support Group**
PO Box 770182 954-755-4307
Coral Springs, FL 33077-0182 e-mail: sshetsky@fbta.info
www.fbta.info
Sheryl Shetsky, President
Gary L Kornfeld, VP

1857 **Tampa Bay Area Brain Tumor Support Group**
St. Joseph's Hospital, Medical Arts Building
3001 Martin Luther King Boulevard 813-870-4327
Tampa Bay, FL
Contact is St. Joseph's Hospital. Educational materials available.

Georgia

1858 **All Ages Support Group**
Brain Tumor Foundation for Children
6065 Roswell Road NE 404-252-4107
Atlanta, GA 30328-4015 Fax: 404-252-4108
e-mail: info@braintumorkids.org
www.braintumorkids.org/
Patient Support Group Activities includes bowling, fishing, craft parties, picnics, sporting events, holiday parties, etc. These activities, social events and more are provided for children of all ages and their families.
Mary Campbell, Executive Director
R Hal Meeks Jr, President

1859 **Emory Clinic Brain Tumor Support Group**
Emory Clinic
1365 Clifton Road 404-778-5770
Atlanta, GA 30322 e-mail: terri_armstrong@emory.org
www.emoryhealthcare.org
Meet on the first Thursday of each month from 1 to 3 p.m.
Jeffrey J Olson, Director
Erwin G Van Meir, Director

1860 **Hearts and Minds**
Piedmont Hospital
1968 Peachtree Road NW 404-373-5202
Atlanta, GA Fax: 404-605-5000
www.piedmonthospital.org
Neal Kuhlhorst

1861 **SBTF Brain Tumor Support Group**
PO Box 422471 404-843-3700
Atlanta, GA 30342 e-mail: info@sbtf.org
www.sbtf.org
Improves the quality of life for brain tumor patients and their families.
Steve Andrews, President

Illinois

1862 **Brain Tumor Support Group**
Northwestern Memorial Hospital
251 E Huron 312-695-8143
Chicago, IL 60611 Fax: 312-695-4075
Meets on the third Monday of each month from 5 to 6 p.m.
Mary Ellen Maher-DeLeon, Facilitator

1863 **Parents of Children with Brain Tumors PCBT**
Children's Memorial Hospital
2400 Children's Plaza 773-880-4485
Chicago, IL 60614-2300 800-543-7362
Fax: 773-880-4036
e-mail: webfeedback@childrensmemorial.org.
www.childrensmemorial.org
Meets quarterly and publishes a monthly newsletter. Library available at meetings (at CMH). Educational speakers and family functions.
Ann Ingold, Facilitator

Indiana

1864 **Brain Tumor Support Group**
Community Hospital East
1500 North Ritter Avenue 317-355-1411
Indianapolis, IN 46219 e-mail: m.w.kemf@att.net
www.ecommunity.com/east

Meets the third Wednesday of each month from 6:30 to 7:30 p.m.
Michael Kemf, Facilitator
Marsha Cline, Facilitator

1865 Primary Brain Cancer Support Group
Women's Cancer Center at Lutheran Hospital
7950 West Jefferson Boulevard 260-435-7959
Fort Wayne, IN 46804 Fax: 260-435-7632
e-mail: women.cancer.center@lutheranhosp.com
www.lutheranhospital.com/cancer/wcc.htm
Meets on the first Tuesday of every month at 6:00 p.m.
Linda Jordan RN, Facilitator
Wendy Rowland, Oncology Nurse Specialist

Iowa

1866 Neurological Center of Iowa
Iowa Clinic
1215 Pleasant Street 515-241-5760
Des Moines, IA 50309-1418 Fax: 515-241-6090
www.iowaclinic.com/
Networks people in similar situations.
Ed Brown, Chief Executive Officer

1867 Quad Cities Brain Tumor Support Group
Genesis Medical Center
1401 W Central Park City 563-421-1905
Davenport, IA 52803 e-mail: christyp@genesishealth.com
Meetings are on the 4th Monday of each month from 6:30 to 8:00 p.m.
Pat Christy RN, Facilitator

Kentucky

1868 Brain Tumor Support Group: Kentucky
Markley Cancer Center
800 Rose Street 606-257-4310
Lexington, KY
Educational materials.
Claire Courtney

Louisiana

1869 Brain Tumor Support Group
3939 Houma Boulevard, Doctor's Row 504-835-5715
Metairie, LA 70005 e-mail: gmom224@cox.net
Meets on the third Sunday of each month at 1:30 p.m., call to confirm.
Gayle Johnson, Contact Person

Maine

1870 Brain Tumor Support Group: Maine
Maine Medical Center
22 Braunhall Street 207-871-4527
Portland, ME 04102 Fax: 207-662-6212
www.mmc.org/
Meets on the second Tuesday of each month from 7:00 to 9:00 p.m.
Nancy Fortier LCSW, Facilitator (207-662-4527)

Maryland

1871 Brain Tumor Networking Group
Wellness Communities Baltimore
901 Dulaney Valley Road 410-832-2719
Towson, MD 21204 Fax: 410-337-0937
e-mail: cancerhelp@hopewellcancersupport.org
Meets on the fourth Monday of each month from 7:00 to 8:30 p.m.
Robin Katts, Facilitator

Massachusetts

1872 Brain Tumor Support Group: Boston
Brigham & Women's Hospital/Dana Farber Cancer Inst
44 Binney Street, Dana Building 617-732-6826
Boston, MA 02115 Fax: 617-734-8342
www.partners.org
Meets the first Thursday of each month from 12:00 to 1:30 pm and Third Thursday of each month from 5:30 to 7:00 pm.
Nancy Bailey RN, Facilitator
Nancy Diferna LCSW, Facilitator

1873 Brain Tumor Support Group: Lahey
Lahey Clinic Medical Center
41 Mall Road
Burlington, MA 01805 978-538-4625
www.lahey.org
Meets on the first and third Monday each month from 7:00 to 9:00 p.m.
Michele Lucas, Facilitator

1874 Brain Tumor Support Group: Waltham
Massachusetts General West
40 2nd Avenue 617-726-1061
Waltham, MA 02451 Fax: 800-697-2593
Meets the second and fourth Tuesday of every month from 7:00 to 8:30 p.m.
Michelle Lucas, Facilitator
Jean Kracher, Facilitator

1875 Neurological Support Group of St. Luke's Hospital
101 Page Street 508-997-1515
New Bedford, MA 02740-3464
Contact can be reached at extension 2764.
Diane Robinson RN

1876 Parent Education/Support Group
Dana Farber Cancer Institute
44 Binney Street 617-632-3301
Boston, MA 2115 800-525-5068
e-mail: dana.farbercontactus@dfci.harvard.edu
www.dfci.harvard.edu
For parents of children with brain tumors. Please call for schedule.
Beverly Lavalley Run, Facilitator
Edward Benz Jr, President

Michigan

1877 Brain Tumor Networking Group
Gilda's Club Metro Detroit
3517 Rochester Road 248-577-0800
Royal Oak, MI 48073 Fax: 248-577-0898
e-mail: webmaster@gildasclubdetroit.org
www.gildasclubdetroit.org/mk3.asp
Meets on the fourth Tuesday of each month from 6:00 to 8:00 p.m.
Joe Perry, Program Director
Meg Callow, Development Director

1878 Brain Tumor Support Group for Patients & Families
University of Michigan Medical Center
1500 East Medical Center Drive 734-936-7910
Ann Arbor, MI 48109-316 Fax: 734-936-8763
www.braintumor.org/
Offers support for patients and their families. Meets the third Tuesday of each month from 7:00 to 8:30 p.m.
Mary Delisle-Berry, Support Group Coordinator
Kathy Wilson, Support Group Coordinator

1879 Brain Tumor Support Group: Ann Arbor
St Joseph Mercy Hospital Cancer Care Center
5301 East Huron River Drive
Ann Arbor, MI 734-712-3658
www.sjmh.com
Paula Nedela, Clinical Manager

1880 Brain Tumor Support Group: Spectrum
Spectrum Health East
1840 Wealthy SE 616-774-7278
Grand Rapids, MI 49506 Fax: 616-454-9004
Meets on the second Monday of each month from 7:00 to 9:00 p.m.
Nancy Rude, Facilitator

Missouri

1881 Brain Cancer Support Group MidAmerica Cancer Center
St John s Regional Health Center

1235 E Cherokee Avenue
Springfield, MO 65804-2212
417-820-2000
800-909-8326
www.stjohns.net

Primary and metastatic brain tumors; patients, families, friends welcome.
Connie Zimmerman

1882 **Brain Tumor Support Network: St. Louis**
Wellness Community of Greater St. Louis
1058 Old Des Peres Road
Saint Louis, MO 63131
314-238-2000
Fax: 314-909-9900
e-mail: info@wellnesscommunitystl.org
www.wellnesscommunitystl.org/

Alternates between speakers and support time. Provides literature, lending library of books and audiotapes, newsletters.
Amy Eilers MSW/LCSW, Program Director
Mary Luntz, Program Coordinator

1883 **Pediatric Brain Tumor Support Network**
St. Louis Children's Hospital
1 Childrens Place
Saint Louis, MO 63110
314-454-4805
www.stlouischildrens.org

New Mexico

1884 **People Living Through Cancer Support Group s**
3939 San Pedro Boulevard NE C-8
Albuquerque, NM 87110
505-242-3263
888-441-4439
Fax: 505-242-6756
e-mail: pltc@pltc.org
www.pltc.org/

People Living Through Cancer is a grassroots non-profit organization founded in 1983 in Albuquerque, New Mexico by cancer survivors. With a full-time staff and numerous volunteers, they offer support and education to cancer survivors, their families and friends.
Bernadette Lujan MPA, Executive Director
Patricia Torn, Support Services Program Manager

New York

1885 **Brain Tumor Support Group: Albany**
Albany Medical Center
Hematology/Oncology Waiting Room
Albany, NY 12208
518-282-6696
e-mail: webmaster@mail.am.edu
www.amc.edu

Facilitated by Susan Weaver, MD, and Christina Blanchard, CSW, PhD. Contact number reaches Patient Services.

1886 **Brain Tumor Support Group: Long Island**
230 Main St. Emma Clark Library
Setauket, NY
516-747-8749
Billie Wilczek

1887 **Long Island Adult Brain Tumor Support Group: Nassau Chapter**
999 Old Country Road
Plainview, NY 11803-4927
516-938-0077
e-mail: bcrescenzo@lancer-ins.com
www.virtulatrials.com/support
Billie Wilczek

1888 **People Treated for Brain Tumors and Their Caregivers**
Memorial Sloan-Kettering Cancer Center
215 E 68th Street
Manhattan, NY
212-717-3527
www.mskcc.org

The Post-Treatment Resource Program (PTRP) offers support groups, lectures, and open house meetings. Newsletter, lending library, and special counseling also available.
Melinda Friedrich CSW

1889 **Support for Parents of Children with Brain Tumors**
19 E 88th Street
Manhattan, NY 10128-0558
212-534-8877
Marcia Greenleaf MD

North Carolina

1890 **Brain Tumor Support Group: Raleigh Area**
Raleigh Community Hospital
3400 Wake Forest Road
Raleigh, NC 27609-7373
919-846-0923
www.raleighcommunity.com

Lectures, educational materials, and newsletter. Home and hospital visitation.
Louise Clark, Director

1891 **Duke Brain Tumor Support Group**
Preston Robert Tisch Brain Tumor Center at Duke
Duke University Medical Center
Durham, NC 27710
919-684-5301
Fax: 919-848-1391
e-mail: calho006@mc.duke.edu
www.cancer.duke.edu/btc/

Support groups for cancer patients and their family and friends in coping with the disease. Time: 1st Wednesday of the month, 3:00-4:00 PM.
Roberta D Calhoun-Eagan LCSW, Clinical Social Worker (919-681-1687)
Amy E Powell LCSW, Social Worker/Family Support

1892 **Duke Pediatric Brain Tumor Family Support Program**
Preston Robert Tisch Brain Tumor Center
Duke University Medical Center
Durham, NC 27710
919-668-2327
Fax: 919-668-2485
e-mail: korpi001@mc.duke.edu
www.cancer.duke.edu/btc/

Assists the families of pediatric patients with identifying strengths and supports available for coping with the emotional and social impact of the brain tumor on the family, offering information about resources in the community in addition to both individual and group supportive counseling.
Darell D. Binger, MD, PhD, Director

Ohio

1893 **Brain Tumor Support Group: Southwest Ohio**
Kettering Hospital
3535 Southern Boulevard
Dayton, OH 45429-1221
937-687-3325
www.ketthealth.com

Educational materials.
Darlene Carroll

1894 **Neuro-Oncology Support Group**
Wellness Community of Greater Cincinnati
4918 Cooper Road
Cincinnati, OH 45242
513-791-4060
Fax: 513-791-8239
e-mail: bcrawford@cancer-support.org
www.cancer-support.org

Weekly support groups for people with cancer and their loved ones. Stress management, nutrition exercise and cancer education programs. Brain tumor networking group for patients and family members available.
Bonnie Crawford MSW, Program Director

1895 **Support Group for Parents of Children with Brain Tumors**
Cincinnati Childrens Hospital Medical Center
Childrens Hospital Medical Center
Cincinnati, OH 45229-3039
513-636-4200
800-344-2462
www.cincinnatichildrens.org/default.htm
Thomas Boat, Director
Stephen Daniels, Associate Chair

Pennsylvania

1896 **Brain Tumor Support Group: Bradford**
Bradford Regional Medical Center
116 Interstate Parkway
Bradford, PA 16701-1036
814-362-8329
www.brmc.org
Michelle Elilson, Executive Officer

1897 **Brain Tumor Support Group: Lehigh Valley**
St. John's Lutheran Church
5th and Chestnut Street
Emmaus, PA
610-776-2566

24-hour phone service for patients and families affected by brain tumors.
Dolores Fioriglio

1898 Brain Tumor Support Group: Pittsburgh
Pittsburgh Cancer Institute
Monte Fiore Hospital, 7 Main Lounge 412-624-1115
Pittsburgh, PA 800-237-4724
www.upci.upmc.edu
Contact is the Cancer Info and Referral Services.

1899 Presbyterian Hospital Pittsburgh Cancer Center
University of Pittsburgh Medical Center
Desoto and O'Hara Streets
Pittsburgh, PA 15213 412-647-8762
www.upmc.com
Jeffrey Romoff, President

1900 Support Group for Parents of Children with Brain Tumors
Children's Hospital of Philadelphia
34th & Civic Center Boulevard
Philadelphia, PA 609-924-7367
www.chop.edu
Six newsletters each year, informal meetings alternate with guest speakers.
Marion Roemner

Tennessee

1901 Brain Tumor Support Group: Nashville
Southern Hills Medical Center
391 Wallace Road, Building Conf 615-781-4190
Nashville, TN 37211-4851
Elizabeth Spurgeon

Texas

1902 Brain Tumor Support Group: West Texas
Abilene Regional Medical Center
1680 Antilley Road
Abilene, TX 79606-5267 915-698-7566
www.abilene.com
Jana Boss RN

1903 Brain Tumor Support Network: Houston Area
Jessie Jones Rotary House International
1600 Holcombe Boulevard 713-792-0760
Houston, TX 77030-4012
Dialogue, sharing, and educational programs.
Wendy Nes LMSW/ACP

1904 Shirvers Cancer Center Brain Tumor Support Group
University of Texas Nursing School
1700 Red River Street
Austin, TX 78701-1412 512-469-7378
www.utexas.edu
Ann Harris
Karen Martin

1905 We've Just Begun to Live Brain Tumor Support Group
Audie Murphy VA Hospital
7400 Merton Minter Street 210-617-5300
San Antonio, TX 78284-5701
Contact can be reached at extension 4720.
Greta Ford

Utah

1906 Peer-Led Brain Tumor Support Group
University of Utah Hospital and Clinics
50 N Medical Drive
Salt Lake City, UT 84132-0001 801-581-2584
www.med.utah.edu
Karen Elliott

Washington

1907 Northwest Hospital Brain Tumor Group Support Hotline
Northwest Hospital
1550 N 115th Street 206-364-0500
Seattle, WA 98133 e-mail: neighbor2nwh@nwhsea.org
www.nwhospital.org
Steve Marshal, Director

West Virginia

1908 Brain Tumor Support Group: Southern West Virginia
First Presbyterian Church
16 Broad Street 304-744-0393
Charleston, WV 25301-2487
Jeri McDonald

Wisconsin

1909 Brain Tumor Support Group: John Sierzant Lutheran Hospital, Gunderson Clinic
1836 S Avenue 608-791-9862
LaCrosse, WI
Esther Lindeman RN

1910 LODAT: Brain Tumor Support Group
Children's Hospital of Wisconsin
Room 888
Milwaukee, WI 414-962-8984
www.braintumor.org
Living One Day At a Time is a parent support group for families of chidren with cancer. Monthly newsletter, informational meetings, social activities for families, and bereavement support.
Frances Swigart

Books

1911 Brain Tumor Resource Directory
National Brain Tumor Foundation
22 Battery Street 415-834-9970
San Francisco, CA 94111-5520 800-934-2873
Fax: 415-834-9980
e-mail: nbtf@braintumor.org
www.braintumor.org
Comprehensive reference for healthcare providers, the directory contains the names and phone numbers of various organizations that offer services and products of particular interest to brain tumor patients and their families.
Rob Tufel, Director Patient Services

1912 Death Be Not Proud: A Memoir
Harper Collins
10 E 53rd Street
New York, NY 10022 212-207-7000
www.harpercollins.com
The father of a young man diagnosed with glioblastoma multiforme wrote this 50-year-old classic.

ISBN: 0-060929-89-8

1913 Resource Guide for Parents of Children with Brain and Spinal Cord Tumors
Children's Brain Tumor Foundation
274 Madison Avenue 212-448-9494
New York, NY 10016 866-228-HOPE
Fax: 212-448-1022
e-mail: info@cbtf.org
www.cbtf.org
Contains practical information to sort out the complexities of medical procedures, interruptions in school and social life, and uncertainty about the future.
Robert Budlow, President
Joseph B Fay, Executive Director

1914 Support Group Directory
National Brain Tumor Foundation
22 Battery Street 415-834-9970
San Francisco, CA 94111-5520 800-934-2873
Fax: 415-834-9980
e-mail: nbtf@braintumor.org
www.braintumor.org
Directory listing support groups in the US and Canada, pediatric support groups, online support groups and additional resources on the North American Brain Tumor Coalition. Available online only.
Rob Tufel, Director Patient Services

1915 **That's Unacceptable: Surviving a Brain Tumor: My Personal Story**
Rebecca L Libutti, author
Krystal Publishing
PO Box 221 908-889-6038
Martinsville, NJ 08836 800-833-9327
Fax: 908-889-6038
e-mail: RLibutti@aol.com
www.krystalpublishing.com
Written by a ten-year survivor of glioblastoma multiforme, the book's title was the author's first response to the initial discouragement she received about pursuing aggressive treatment.
198 pages Paperback
RL Libutti

1916 **The Essential Guide to Brain Tumors**
National Brain Tumor Foundation
22 Battery Street 415-834-9970
San Francisco, CA 94111-5520 800-934-2873
Fax: 415-834-9980
e-mail: nbtf@braintumor.org
www.braintumor.org
Full of information concerning the brain, how it functions, what causes tumors, types of brain tumors, managing symptoms, and even surviving brain tumorrs.
80 pages
Rob Tufel, Director Patient Services

1917 **Understanding and Coping with Your Child's Brain Tumor**
National Brain Tumor Foundation
22 Battery Street 415-834-9970
San Francisco, CA 94111-5520 800-934-2873
Fax: 415-834-9980
e-mail: nbtf@braintumor.org
www.braintumor.org
Guide for families contains information for parents of children with brain tumors, including information about diagnosis, tumor types, treatment methods, social and emotional support and more. It also contains a glossary, along with listings of organizations and resources.
52 pages
Rob Tufel, Director Patient Services

Children's Books

1918 **My Name is Buddy**
Dave Bauer, author
National Brain Tumor Foundation
22 Battery Street 415-834-9970
San Francisco, CA 94111-5520 800-934-2873
Fax: 415-834-9980
e-mail: nbtf@braintumor.org
www.braintumor.org
Unique book for children with brain tumors. The reader follows Buddy, a Golden Retriever, on his journey through a brain tumor diagnosis and treatment. This true story uses photographs and narrative to describe Buddy's experiences before and after surgery and talks about his feelings and fears as a brain tumor patient.
Rob Tufel, Director Patient Services

Newsletters

1919 **Butterfly Bulletin**
Brain Tumor Foundation for Children
6065 Roswell Road NE 404-252-4107
Atlanta, GA 30328-4015 Fax: 404-252-4108
e-mail: info@braintumorkids.org
www.braintumorkids.org
Reporting on news and events of the Brain Tumor Foundation for Children.
Quarterly
Rick Sauers, Chairman/Co-Founder
R Hal Meeks, Jr, President

1920 **Caring Hand**
Pediatric Brain Tumor Foundation
302 Ridgefield Court 828-665-6891
Asheville, NC 28806 800-253-6530
Fax: 828-655-6894
e-mail: pbtfus@pbtfus.org
www.pbtfus.org
The Caring Hand is a regular newsletter, distributed free of charge to patient families, caregivers and medical/social work professionals.
Michael Traynor, President
Glenn Wilcox, Vice President

1921 **Childhood Brain Tumor Foundation Newsletter**
Childhood Brain Tumor Foundation
20312 Watkins Meadow Drive 310-515-2900
Germantown, MD 20876-4259 877-217-4166
e-mail: cbtf@childhoodbraintumor.org
www.childhoodbraintumor.org
Seeking second opinions, access to healthcare, and combating discrimination.

1922 **Helping Hand**
Pediatric Brain Tumor Foundation
302 Ridgefield Court 828-665-6891
Asheville, NC 28806 800-253-6530
Fax: 828-655-6894
e-mail: pbtfus@pbtfus.org
www.pbtfus.org
The Helping Hand is a regular newsletter, distributed free of charge to Ride for Kids®and supporters.
Michael Traynor, President
Glenn Wilcox, Vice President

1923 **Message Line Newsletter**
American Brain Tumor Association
2720 S River Road 847-827-9910
Des Plaines, IL 60018-4117 800-886-2282
Fax: 847-827-9918
e-mail: info@abta.org
www.abta.org
Describes research advances and announces updates to publications.
TriAnnual
Elizabeth Wilson, Executive Director
Geri Jo Duda, RN, Patient Services

1924 **SEARCH**
National Brain Tumor Foundation
22 Battery Street 415-834-9970
San Francisco, CA 94111-5520 800-934-2873
Fax: 415-834-9980
e-mail: nbtf@braintumor.org
www.braintumor.org
Newsletter that covers topics of current interest to brain tumor survivors and their families.
Quarterly
Rob Tufel, Director Patient Services

1925 **TLC (Tips for Living And Coping)**
American Brain Tumor Association
2720 S River Road 847-827-9910
Des Plaines, IL 60018-4117 800-886-2282
Fax: 847-827-9918
e-mail: info@abta.org
www.abta.org
E-bulletin of news, research and development finds, support and treatment information.

ISBN: 0-944093-37-X
Elizabeth Wilson, Executive Director
Geri Jo Duda, RN, Patient Services

Pamphlets

1926 **Clinical Trial Fact Sheet**
National Brain Tumor Foundation

22 Battery Street
San Francisco, CA 94111-5520
415-834-9970
800-934-2873
Fax: 415-834-9980
e-mail: nbtf@braintumor.org
www.braintumor.org

Lists of clinical trial by state, tumor type and/or treatment type.

1927 **Coping with Your Loved One's Brain Tumor**
National Brain Tumor Foundation
22 Battery Street
San Francisco, CA 94111-5520
415-834-9970
800-934-2873
Fax: 415-834-9980
e-mail: nbtf@braintumor.org
www.braintumor.org

Describes important coping stategies for caregivers and family members of a loved one with a brain tumor.
12 pages Booklet

1928 **Dictionary for Brain Tumor Patients**
American Brain Tumor Association
2720 S River Road
Des Plaines, IL 60018-4117
847-827-9910
800-886-2282
Fax: 847-827-9918
e-mail: info@abta.org
www.abta.org

Offers a dictionary of terms used in the diagnosis and everday living with brain tumors.
Paperback
ISBN: 0-944093-27-2
Elizabeth Wilson, Executive Director
Geri Jo Duda, RN, Patient Services

1929 **Ependymoma**
American Brain Tumor Association
2720 S River Road
Des Plaines, IL 60018-4117
847-827-9910
800-886-2282
Fax: 847-827-9918
e-mail: info@abta.org
www.abta.org

ISBN: 0-944093-40-X
Elizabeth Wilson, Executive Director
Geri Jo Duda, RN, Patient Services

1930 **Glioblastoma Multiforme and Anaplastic Astrocytoma**
American Brain Tumor Association
2720 S River Road
Des Plaines, IL 60018-4117
847-827-9910
800-886-2282
Fax: 847-827-9918
e-mail: info@abta.org
www.abta.org

ISBN: 0-944093-36-1
Elizabeth Wilson, Executive Director
Geri Jo Duda, RN, Patient Services

1931 **Living with A Brain Tumor**
American Brain Tumor Association
2720 S River Road
Des Plaines, IL 60018-4117
847-827-9910
800-886-2282
Fax: 847-827-9918
e-mail: info@abta.org
www.abta.org

A guide for brain tumor patients.
2004
ISBN: 0-944093-54-X
Elizabeth Wilson, Executive Director
Geri Jo Duda, RN, Patient Services

1932 **Medulloblastoma**
American Brain Tumor Association
2720 S River Road
Des Plaines, IL 60018-4117
847-827-9910
800-886-2282
Fax: 847-827-9918
e-mail: info@abta.org
www.abta.org

Paperback
ISBN: 0-944093-33-7
Elizabeth Wilson, Executive Director
Geri Jo Duda, RN, Patient Services

1933 **Meningioma**
American Brain Tumor Association
2720 S River Road
Des Plaines, IL 60018-4117
847-827-9910
800-886-2282
Fax: 847-827-9918
e-mail: info@abta.org
www.abta.org

ISBN: 0-944093-23-X
Elizabeth Wilson, Executive Director
Geri Jo Duda, RN, Patient Services

1934 **Metastatic Brain Tumors**
American Brain Tumor Association
2720 S River Road
Des Plaines, IL 60018-4117
847-827-9910
800-886-2282
Fax: 847-827-9918
e-mail: info@abta.org
www.abta.org

ISBN: 0-944093-26-4
Elizabeth Wilson, Executive Director
Geri Jo Duda, RN, Patient Services

1935 **Oligodendroglioma and Mixed Glioma**
American Brain Tumor Association
2720 S River Road
Des Plaines, IL 60018-4117
847-827-9910
800-886-2282
Fax: 847-827-9918
e-mail: info@abta.org
www.abta.org

Pamphlet
ISBN: 0-944093-43-4
Elizabeth Wilson, Executive Director
Geri Jo Duda, RN, Patient Services

1936 **Organizing a Support Group**
American Brain Tumor Association
2720 S River Road
Des Plaines, IL 60018-4117
847-827-9910
800-886-2282
Fax: 847-827-9918
e-mail: info@abta.org
www.abta.org

Elizabeth Wilson, Executive Director
Geri Jo Duda, RN, Patient Services

1937 **Pituitary Tumors**
American Brain Tumor Association
2720 S River Road
Des Plaines, IL 60018-4117
847-827-9910
800-886-2282
Fax: 847-827-9918
e-mail: info@abta.org
www.abta.org

Pamphlet
ISBN: 0-944093-44-2
Elizabeth Wilson, Executive Director
Geri Jo Duda, RN, Patient Services

1938 **Primer of Brain Tumors**
American Brain Tumor Association
2720 S River Road
Des Plaines, IL 60018-4117
847-827-9910
800-886-2282
Fax: 847-827-9918
e-mail: info@abta.org
www.abta.org

A patient's reference manual offering information on brain tumors.

ISBN: 0-944093-35-3
Elizabeth Wilson, Executive Director
Geri Jo Duda, RN, Patient Services

1939 **Radiation Therapy of Brain Tumors: A Basic Guide**
American Brain Tumor Association

2720 S River Road
Des Plaines, IL 60018-4117
847-827-9910
800-886-2282
Fax: 847-827-9918
e-mail: info@abta.org
www.abta.org

ISBN: 0-944093-28-0
Elizabeth Wilson, Executive Director
Geri Jo Duda, RN, Patient Services

1940 **Returning to Work: Strategies for Brain Tumor Patients**
National Brain Tumor Foundation
22 Battery Street
San Francisco, CA 94111-5520
415-834-9970
800-934-2873
Fax: 415-834-9980
e-mail: nbtf@braintumor.org
www.braintumor.org

Reviews brain tumor survivors rights with respect to returning to work and suggests several strategies to make it an easier transition to go back into the workplace.
16 pages Brochure
Rob Tufel, Director Patient Services

1941 **Stereotactic Radiosurgery**
American Brain Tumor Association
2720 S River Road
Des Plaines, IL 60018-4117
847-827-9910
800-886-2282
Fax: 847-827-9918
e-mail: info@abta.org
www.abta.org

ISBN: 0-944093-42-6
Elizabeth Wilson, Executive Director
Geri Jo Duda, RN, Patient Services

1942 **Understanding Brain Tumors: Glioblastoma Multiforme**
National Brain Tumor Foundation
22 Battery Street
San Francisco, CA 94111-5520
415-834-9970
800-934-2873
Fax: 415-834-9980
e-mail: nbtf@braintumor.org
www.braintumor.org

Helps patients and caregivers understand more about the diagnosis and treatment of glioblastoma multiforme.
16 pages
Rob Tufel, Director Patient Services

1943 **Using A Medical Library**
American Brain Tumor Association
2720 S River Road
Des Plaines, IL 60018-4117
847-827-9910
800-886-2282
Fax: 847-827-9918
e-mail: info@abta.org
www.abta.org

Elizabeth Wilson, Executive Director
Geri Jo Duda, RN, Patient Services

1944 **What You Need to Know About Brain Tumors**
National Cancer Institute
Building 31
Bethesda, MD 20892-0001
301-435-3848
800-422-6237
www.nci.nih.gov

Offers factual information about brain tumors, possible causes, primary and secondary tumors, symptoms, diagnosis, treatment, side effects, followup care, support and medical terms.

1945 **When Your Child Returns to School**
American Brain Tumor Association
2720 S River Road
Des Plaines, IL 60018-4117
847-827-9910
800-886-2282
Fax: 847-827-9918
e-mail: info@abta.org
www.abta.org

Guides parents and teachers through a successful return to school when a child has had a brain tumor.
Paperback
ISBN: 0-944093-21-3
Elizabeth Wilson, Executive Director
Geri Jo Duda, RN, Patient Services

Audio & Video

1946 **Conference Audiotapes**
National Brain Tumor Foundation
22 Battery Street
San Francisco, CA 94111-5520
415-834-9970
800-934-2873
Fax: 415-834-9980
e-mail: nbtf@braintumor.org
www.braintumor.org

Audiotapes of keynote addresses and conference workshops from NBTF's biennial National Brain Tumor Conferences where leading researchers, physicians and health professionals address a range of issues affecting brain tumor survivors, such as new approaches to radiation and surgery, research and coping skills for families.
Rob Tufel, Director Patient Services

1947 **Strategies for Healing**
National Brain Tumor Foundation
414 13th Street
Oakland, CA 94612
510-839-9777
800-934-2873
Fax: 510-839-9779
e-mail: nbtf@braintumor.org
www.braintumor.org

CD-Rom contains vital information about treatment options and self-care for newly diagnosed patients and their families.
Rob Tufel, Director Patient Services

Web Sites

1948 **American Brain Tumor Association**
www.abta.org

Provide free social service consultations; a mentorship program for new brain tumor support group leaders; a nationwide database of established support groups; the Connections pen-pal program; networking with organizations that provide services to patients and families; a resource listing of physicians offering investgative treatments.

1949 **Brain Tumor Society**
124 Watertown Street
Watertown, MA 02472
617-924-9997
800-770-8287
Fax: 617-924-9998
e-mail: info@tbts.org
www.tbts.org

Disseminates educational information and provides access to psycho-social support and raises funds to advance carefully selected scientific research projects, improve clinical care and find a cure.

1950 **Healing Well**
www.healingwell.com

An online health resource guide to medical news, chat, information and articles, newsgroups and message boards, books, disease-related web sites, medical directories, and more for patients, friends, and family coping with disabling diseases, disorders, or chronic illnesses.

1951 **Health Finder**
www.healthfinder.gov

Searchable, carefully developed web site offering information on over 1000 topics. Developed by the US Department of Health and Human Services, the site can be used in both English and Spanish.

1952 **Healthlink USA**
www.healthlinkusa.com

Health information concerning treatment, cures, prevention, diagnosis, risk factors, research, support groups, email lists, personal stories and much more. Updated regularly.

1953 **Helios Health**
www.helioshealth.com

Online resource for your health information. Detailed information about specific health topics, access to expert advice from our Medical Advisory Board, and up-to-date health news.

1954 **MedicineNet**
www.medicinenet.com

An online resource for consumers providing easy-to-read, authoritative medical and health information.

1955 **Medscape**

www.mywebmd.com

Medscape offers specialists, primary care physicians, and other health professionals the Web's most robust and integrated medical information and educational tools.

1956 **National Brain Tumor Foundation**

www.braintumor.org

Nonprofit health organization which raises funds for research and provides information and support to patients, their family members and friends and health professionals. Sponsors national and regional conferences, patient and caregiver programs, support groups, special patient programs including a teleconference series, a newsletter, a medical advice nurse and a wide variety of patient information about treatments, tumor types and coping. Also has a web site listing patient resources.

1957 **Pediatric Brain Tumor Foundation of the US**

www.ride4kids.org

Goal is to create an awareness about this growing disease among children and adults so that fundraising programs may continue to expand in increased laboratory research.

1958 **WebMD**

www.webmd.com

Information on Brain Tumors, including articles and resources.

Description

Cancer

Cancer is a general term for more than 100 diseases characterized by abnormal or uncontrolled growth of cells. The resulting mass, or disease, can invade and destroy surrounding normal tissue. Cancer cells from the tumor can also spread (metastasize) through the blood or lymph (plasmatic fluid) to start new cancers in other parts of the body. In 2008, about 1,437,180 new cancer cases were diagnosed, and about 565,650 Americans died from their disease. Cancer is the second leading cause of death in the U.S., exceeded only by heart disease. Although these figures seem bleak, most cancers are potentially curable if detected at an early stage.

Cancer, also called a malignancy (from Latin, meaning bad), can be either a solid tumor (carcinoma), such as lung cancer, or a disorder of blood cell formation, such as leukemia.

Cancer is caused by an interplay of internal and external factors, individually or in combination. Abnormal genes can cause multiple changes that affect cell growth. Environmental factors, such as cigarette smoke, (also called a carcinogen – causing cancer) and exposure to radiation, play a role. Many cancers can be prevented by health awareness. For example, 90 percent of the over one million skin cancers that will be diagnosed this year could be drastically reduced by protection from solar rays. Lung cancer, one of the most prevalent and hazardous cancers could be drastically reduced by eliminating tobacco use. The American Cancer Society estimates that 30 percent of all cancer deaths are related to cigarette smoking.

Cancer treatment may be curative – removes the tumor in the hope that it will not reoccur, or palliative – prolongs life and minimize discomfort when a cure is not possible. A treatment program typically includes a combination of surgery, radiation therapy, and chemotherapy. Immunotherapy is the newest form of treatment and uses agents known as biologic-response modifiers (BRM), to alter the immune system in its response to malignant growth. Brief descriptions of the more common cancers follow.

Brain Cancer

Brain cancer occurs at varying rates but overall it comprises approximately 5.6 cases per 100,000 populations each year. They are most common in early or middle adult life and incidence in the elderly population is increasing. Overall incidence is about equal in males and females.

The seriousness of brain tumors is determined by their size, location, and rate of growth. While brain cancer does not normally spread to others areas, many other cancers have the propensity of spreading throughout the nervous system and producing metastatic tumors in the brain. In adults, these tumors are most commonly from cancer of the lung, breast, or skin (melanoma). Symptoms include headaches, seizures, behavior problems, changes in eating or sleeping habits, lethargy and clumsiness. See also Brain Tumors.

Breast Cancer

Breast cancer is the most common malignant tumor in women in the western hemisphere. Approximately 182,460 new cases of breast cancer in women were diagnosed in 2008. As many as one in nine women will develop breast cancer during her lifetime. Incidence of breast cancer increases under the following conditions: age; (two-thirds of cases develop after age 55); a close relative (mother, sister) with breast cancer; a previous history of breast cancer; a previous history of breast cancer; exposure to radiation. Other risk factors include not having children, early onset of menstruation, and estrogen replacement therapy.

Early detection can be lifesaving. Many breast cancers are self-diagnosed. More than 80 percent of breast cancers occur as a painless mass. Monthly breast self-examination for women of all ages is crucial. The American Cancer Society recommends that women aged 20-39 have a clinical breast examination performed every three years. Depending on the presence of known risk factors, patients should undergo mammography either yearly or every other year between 40 and 50 years, and yearly after age 50.

Warning signs that can aid women in detecting breast cancer include lumps, swelling, skin irritation, tenderness of the nipple, and dimpling of the skin. Treatments vary, depending on when the cancer is discovered and whether it has spread. Research has shown that the traditional radical mastectomy (removal of the entire breast) canoften be replaced by lumpectomy (removal of just the tumor), coupled with radiation therapy. Chemotherapy or hormonal manipulation is also prescribed in some cases. The five year survival rate for localized (not spread) breast cancer has improved in recent years from 78 percent to 97 percent.

Colon and Rectal Cancer

In western countries, colon and rectal (colorectal) cancer account for more new cases of cancer per year than any other anatomic site except the lung. The incidence begins to rise at age 40 and peaks at age 60 to 75. Incidence of colorectal cancer increases in people who eat low-fiber diets that are high in animal protein, fat, and refined carbohydrates.

Symptoms vary, depending on the location and size of the tumor. Vague signs include weight loss, reduced appetite, and general malaise. More specific signs include rectal bleeding, blood in the stool, or a change in bowel habits.

A digital rectal examination and testing the stool for the presence of blood are important screening tests. Flexible sigmoidoscopy in which the doctor inserts a thin, flexible tube into the rectum shows tumors in 60 percent of cases. A colonoscopy is performed when a tumor is believed to be higher up the colon. These procedures are used to visualize abnormalities and take tissue samples (biopsy).

Treatment consists of surgical removal of the tumor, followed by radiotherapy and/or chemotherapy.

Leukemia

Leukemia is a disorder characterized by uncontrolled growth of abnormal and immature white or red blood cells, and is divided into acute and chronic forms. Although leukemia is often thought of as a childhood disease, it strikes 10 times as many adults as children. New treatment, especially for acute leukemia in children has resulted in dramatic improvements in the 5- year survival rates. Today, the likelihood of disease remission is greater than 95 percent, with 30 percent chance of the disease reappearing.

Warning signs of leukemia are related to the disruption of the different cells in the blood: weakness and fatigue are caused by anemia (decreased red blood cells); easy bruising and hemorrhages (e.g. nosebleeds) from reduced clotting cells (platelets); and repeated infections from abnormal white cells. Generalized symptoms include weight loss and malaise.

Treatment for leukemia includes chemotherapy with a wide variety of anticancer drugs. Transfusions restore red cells and platelets, and frequent infections are treated with antibiotics. Bone marrow transplants, in which new blood cells are provided, are one of the most recent and successful advances in the treatment of this disease.

Liver Cancer

Liver cancer comprises only about 0.6 percent of all cancers diagnosed in the United States. Risk include hepatitis B infection, hepatitis C infection, and exposure to any agent that causes liver damage, including alcohol. The remaining patients have no underlying liver disorder.

Symptoms include abdominal pain, weight loss, and a mass on the upper right side of the abdomen. The outlook for patients with liver cancer is usually grim. Surgery provides the best hope, but is suitable in only a few cases. Most experts remain wary of the benefit of liver transplantation. See also Liver Disease.

Lung Cancer

Lung cancer is one of the most prevalent cancers with an estimated 170,000 new cases each year. The frequency is increasing rapidly. Originally a disease that primarily affected men older than 60, lung cancer has become the second most common cause of cancer in women.

Cigarette smoking and exposure to industrial substances, such as asbestos, are strongly linked to lung cancer. Recent research has shown that exposure to secondhand smoke increases the risk for this disease.

Warning signs of lung cancer are persistent coughing, shortness of breath,sputum streaked with blood, chest pain, and reoccurring pneumonia or bronchitis. Early detection is difficult, as symptoms do not appear until the disease is in advanced stages. Treatment includes surgical removal of the lung if the cancer has not spread (metastasized) and/or chemotherapy and radiation therapy. Survival rates depend on tumor size, location, and whether or not the disease has spread. Because lung cancer is so difficult to treat, public health efforts are focused on prevention. See also Lung Disease.

Oral Cancer

Oral cancer represents approximately 2 percent of all newly diagnosed cancers, and 1.5 percent of cancer deaths. Incidence is more than twice as high in men as in women, and is most frequently found in men over age 40. Risk factors include cigarette, pipe, and cigar smoking, as well as the use of chewing tobacco and excessive intake of alcohol.

Oral cancer symptoms include a sore that bleeds easily, or a lump, thickening, or persistent red or white patch in the mouth. Difficulties in chewing and swallowing are symptoms of progressive disease.

Oral cancer can affect any part of the mouth, and primary care physicians and dentists often detect the disease during routine check-ups. Treatment consists of surgical removal (frequently disfiguring), radiation therapy, or a combination of both.

Ovarian Cancer

Ovarian cancer develops in 1 in 70 women and accounts for 4 percent of cancers in women. Despite its low incidence, it is the cause of more deaths in women than any other female reproductive cancer. Incidence rates are highest in the industrialized nations.

Risk factors include prior history of breast cancer and not having had children. Women who become pregnant at an early age, who have early menopause, and who use oral contraceptives are at less risk.

Ovarian cancer symptoms usually do not appear until the disease is well developed. The most common sign is an enlarging abdomen from of accumulated fluid; digestive disturbance such as discomfort, gas and distention, may also occur.

Often an abdominal mass is discovered during a routine pelvic examination in women who are symptom free. Therefore, women age 18 or older, or earlier if they are sexually active should have annual check-ups. (The Pap smear detects cervical cancer, not ovarian cancer.) Once diagnosed, 78 percent of ovarian cancer patients survive longer than one year and more than 52 percent survive longer than five years. If the disease is diagnosed before it has spread to the other parts of the body, the five-year survival rate is 95 percent.

Treatment includes surgical removal, followed by varying combinations of chemotherapy. As in all cancers, early detection is the key to effective therapy.

Pancreatic Cancer

Pancreatic cancer is one of the most dangerous cancers because it is difficult to detect and responds poorly to anticancer therapy. The incidence of this tumor has been increasing during the 20th century with nearly 30,000 cases diagnosed in 2001. Men are affected more commonly than women, and the average age of diagnoses is from 55 to 65 years.

There is an increased incidence in those who smoke, consume a fatty diet and, to a lesser extent, who are diabetics. Chronic inflammation of the pancreas, especially among alcoholics, is also a predisposing cause.

Pancreatic cancer runs a particularly silent course, with no symptoms until it has significant advanced. The overall 5- year survival rate for patients with pancreatic cancer is less than 5 percent. Surgery is the mainstay of therapy, but only is appropriate for 15 percent of patients; radiation and/or chemotherapy are often part of treatment.

Prostate Cancer

Approximately 1 in 6 men will develop prostate cancer by 85. Incidencerates are higher among blacks and increases with age.

Early prostate cancer is symptom free. Pain and difficulty urinating, are late signs of prostate cancer. More than 50 percent of patients have a nodule that can be felt by a digital examination.

The American Cancer Society recommends that beginning at age 50, the digital rectal examination and PSA (prostatespecific antigen) blood test should be performed annually to men with a life expectancy of at least 10 years, due to the slow growth of prostate cancer. African- American males, who are at a greater risk of developing prostate cancer, should start screening at age 45, as should men with a close relative (father, brother) was diagnosed with prostate cancer at a young age.

Surgery, radiation and hormones are all used to treat prostate cancer, depending on age and health of the patient and how far the disease has progressed.

Skin Cancer

There are over one million cases of skin cancer that are diagnosed each year. The vast majority of these cases, called basal cell or squamous cell cancers, appear on areas that are most exposed to the sun and are highly curable. Melanoma is the most serious skin cancer and accounts for 4 percent of cases. Diagnosis of melanomas has more than doubled since the mid-70s and is estimated now to develop in 1 of 50 Americans. Similar to the more benign skin cancers, melanoma develops as the result of excessive exposure to the sun and has a higher incidence among those who work outdoors. Persons with fair complexions are at particular risk.

The warning signs of skin cancer include a persistent skin lesion, especially those that change in the size, color or shape. Other signs include scaliness, oozing, bleeding, pain or spread of pigmentation.

Prevention plays a key role in the development of melanoma, especially avoiding the sun's ultraviolet rays between 10 a.m. and 3 p.m. Sunscreens and protective clothing should be worn by those who spend the majority of their time outside, those who easily sunburn, and all children. In addition, early detection is critical because, despite advances in treatment, including the use of biologic response modifiers, melanoma is difficult to cure.

Stomach Cancer

Stomach (or gastric) cancer is most common among those living in northern areas of the U.S., and poor African-American populations. Its incidence increases with age; more than 75 percent of patients are over 50 years of age.

Diet and infection are believed to play a role in the development of stomach cancer. It is also more common in persons with vitamin B12 deficiency (pernicious anemia). Other causes are under investigation.

Symptoms of stomach cancer are usually vague, and include indigestion, abdominal discomfort, bloating, heartburn, and weight loss.

Removal of the tumor when possible offers the only hope of cure. The prognosis is good if the tumor is limited, but most patients are not diagnosed until their disease has spread.

Testicular Cancer

Cancer of the testes accounts for approximately 1 percent of all male cancers. However, unlike most cancers, testicular cancer usually occurs in the 15 to 40 age group; with the average age at diagnosis is 32 years.

The cause of testicular cancer is uncertain, but the incidence is increased in men with cogenital crytorochidism (a failure of one or both testes to descend). Some researchers believe that getting an infection with a virus, such as mumps, may play a role.

Fortunately, testicular cancer is one of the most curable of all cancers, In order to discover it early, men must perform selfexamination at regular intervals to feel for local abnormal growths such as lumps or nodules. Pain in the scrotal sac can also occur, although more than 90 percent of patients have a painless, solid testicular swelling.

Treatment of testicular cancer may include surgical removal, radiation, and chemotherapy.

Urinary Tract Cancer

Urinary tract cancers comprise about 9 percent of new cancer cases each year in men and 4 percent in women. The two most common urinary tract cancers are of the bladder and kidney.

Overall, the incidence rate is three times greater among men than women, and usually occurs in patients who are 40-70 years of age. Smoking is the greatest risk factor, with smokers having twice the incidence of nonsmokers. African-Americans, those living in urban areas, and workers exposed to dye, rubber, or leather are also at higher risk.

Common symptoms of bladder cancer include microscopic or observable blood in the urine and painful, increased, and urgent urination. Pain the lower back may also be present. Bladder cancer may be treated by surgical removal of the tumor combined with chemotherapy.

Risk factors for kidney (renal) cancer are cigarette smoking (most important) and obesity in women. Symptoms are similar to those in bladder cancer and may also include weight loss, nausea, and vomiting.

Total removal of the cancerous kidney is the treatment of choice and is used in nearly 90 percent of cases; radiation therapy and chemotherapy are relatively ineffective. Biologic response modifiers are promising but must responses are limited in duration.

Uterine and Cervical Cancer

The overall incidence of cervical cancer has decreased over the past 40 years, due mainly to regular checkups and the use of the Pap smear test for early detection. Risk factors include intercourse at an early age, cigarette smoking, multiple sex partners, and history of a sexually transmitted disease. Infection with the virus that causes genital warts (HPV), is responsible for half of all cases of cervical cancer.

Warning signs include bleeding outside the normal menstrual cycle or after menopause. Cervical cancer in most patients is treated with surgery, radiation, or a combination of both. Due to a recently developed vaccine that is 100 percent effective against HPV, the rates of cervical cancer have sharply decreased.

The American Cancer Society recommends that all women who are, or have been, sexually annual Pap test and pelvic examination. After three or more consecutive satisfactory examinations with normal findings, the Pap test may be performed less frequently, after being discussed with your health care provider.

Uterine cancer has been increasing since the 1970s. Risk factors include obesity, diabetes, high blood pressure, late onset of menopause, and estrogen-only hormone replacement therapy. Symptoms for most women include some form of abnormal bleeding from the uterus.

Treatment for uterine and cervical cancers include surgery, radiation therapy, hormone therapy and, occasionally, chemotherapy.

National Agencies & Associations

1959 **American Bone Marrow Donor Registry**
PO Box 8841
Mandeville, LA 70470-8841
985-626-1749
800-745-2452
Fax: 985-626-7414
e-mail: jakabmdr@bellsouth.net
www.charityadvantage.com/abmdr

A registry of bone marrow donors. Provides information on donor searches and recruitment.

1960 **American Cancer Society**
1599 Clifton Road NE
Atlanta, GA 30329-4250
404-320-3333
800-ACS-2345
TTY: 800-228-4327
www.cancer.org

A nationwide community based voluntary health organization dedicated to eliminating cancer as a major health problem by preventing saving lives and diminishing suffering through research education advocacy and services. Provides free printed materials.
Stephen F Sener, President
Thomas G Burish, Chairman

1961 **American Prostate Society**
PO Box 870
Hanover, MD 21076-3117
410-859-3735
877-859-3735
Fax: 410-850-0818
e-mail: ameripros@mindspring.com
www.americanprostatesociety.com

The only organization dedicated exclusively to using existing medical capabilities to reduce death due to prostate cancer and to reduce unnecessary or ineffective prostate therapies for prostate growth.

1962 **American Society of Colon and Rectal Surgeons**
85 W Algonquin Road
Arlington Heights, IL 60005-4460
847-290-9184
Fax: 847-290-9203
e-mail: ascrs@facsrs.org
www.fascrs.org

ASCRS Represents more than 1000 board certified colon and rectal surgeons and other surgeons dedicated to advancing and promoting the science and practice of the treatment of patients with cancer and other diseases affecting the colon and related areas.
Anthony Sena MD, President
James W Fleshman MD, President Elect

1963 **Americas Association for the Care of the Children**
P.O. Box 2154
Boulder, CO 80306-2154
303-527-2742
www.aacchildren.net

Carries out a variety of programs to promote the health of children. Publishes educational materials on child health of interest to parents, educators and health professionals.
Laurene Philips, President
Douglas Johnson, Vice President

1964 **Association for Research of Childhood Cancer**
PO Box 251
Buffalo, NY 14225-0251
716-681-4433
e-mail: president@arocc.org
www.arocc.org

A nonprofit organization staffed by volunteers and formed in 1971 by parents who had lost children to pediatric cancer. Charter members raise funds by various projects in order to provide seed money to various pediatric research centers.
Anne O'Donnell, President

1965 **Association for the Cure of Cancer of the Prostate**
1250 4th Street
Santa Monica, CA 90401
310-570-4700
800-757-2873
Fax: 310-570-4701
e-mail: info@prostatecenterfoundation.org
www.capcure.org

Goal is to find better treatments and a cure for recurrent prostate cancer. Pursues the mission by reaching out to individuals corpora-

tions and others to harness society's resources - both financial and human - to fight this deadly disease.
Mike Milken, Founder/Chairman
James Blair, General Partner

1966 **Bone Marrow Foundation**
30 E End Avenue 212-838-3029
New York, NY 10128 800-365-1336
Fax: 21- 22- 008
e-mail: theBMF@BoneMarrow.org
www.bonemarrow.org
Goal is to improve the quality of life for bone marrow and stem cell transplant patients and their families by providing financial aid education and emotional support.
Christina Merrill, Founder and Executive Director, Secretary

1967 **Breast Cancer Action**
55 New Montgomery Street 415-243-9301
San Francisco, CA 94105 877-2ST-OPBC
Fax: 415-243-3996
e-mail: info@bcaction.org
www.bcaction.org
Breast Cancer Action carries the voices of people affected by breast cancer to inspire and compel the changes necessary to end the breast cancer epidemic.
Barbara Brenner, Executive Director

1968 **Breast Cancer Society of Canada**
118 Victoria Street N 519-336-0746
Sarnia, Ontario, N7T-5W9 800-567-8767
Fax: 519-336-5725
e-mail: bcsc@bcsc.ca
www.bcsc.ca
Is a registered charitable organization established in 1991 in Point Edwards Ontario. Our mandate is to fund vital Canadian research into improving the detection, prevention and treatment of breast cancer as well as to ultimately find a cure and create awareness through education.
Rany Xanthopoulo, Executive Director
Dawn Hamilton, Fundraising & Administrative Coordinator

1969 **Burger King Cancer Caring Center**
4117 Liberty Avenue 412-622-1212
Pittsburgh, PA 15224 Fax: 412-622-1216
e-mail: info@cancercaring.org
www.cancercaring.org
Provides a wide variety of support services to cancer patients their families and friends including support groups, education classes, personal counseling and telephone helpline.
Rebecca Whitlinger, Executive Director
Bonnie Shiel MSW LSW, Director Support Services

1970 **Canadian Breast Cancer Network (CBCN)**
300-331 Cooper Street 613-230-3044
Ottawa, Ontario, K2P-0G5 800-685-8820
Fax: 613-230-4424
e-mail: cbcn@cbcn.ca
www.cbcn.ca
Is a survivor-directed, national network of organizations and individuals. CBCN is a national link between all groups and individuals concerned about breast cancer, and represents the concerns of all Canadians affected by breast cancer and those at risk.
Jackie Manthorne, Executive Director
Chantale Lavoie, Program Coordinator

1971 **Canadian Cancer Society**
1639 Yonge Street 416-488-5400
Toronto, Ontario, M4T-2W6 800-268-8874
Fax: 416-488-2872
www.cancer.ca
Is a national, community-based organization of volunteers whose mission is the eradication of cancer and the enhancement of the quality of life of people living with cancer.
Stephen Roche, Chair

1972 **Cancer Care Public Information Associates**
Public Information Associates
275 7th Avenue 212-302-2400
New York, NY 10001 800-813-4673
Fax: 212-712-8495
e-mail: info@cancercare.org
www.cancercare.org
Non-profit social service agency with the goal of helping cancer patients and their families and friends cope with the impact of cancer. Treats people at all stages of illness and provides help to both patients and families.
Diane S Blum, Executive Director

1973 **Candlelighters Childhood Cancer Foundation**
10400 Connecticut Avenue 301-962-3520
Kensington, MD 20895 800-366-2223
Fax: 301-962-3521
e-mail: staff@candlelighters.org
www.candlelighters.org
Founded by parents of children with cancer. Candlelighters helps families of pediatric and adolescent cancer patients cope with the educational and emotional needs of the disease. The organization is the largest distributor of free childhood cancer books and other materials.
Ruth Hoffman MPH, Executive Director

1974 **Colon Cancer Canada**
5915 Leslie Street 416-785-0449
Toronto, On, M2H-1J8 888-571-8547
Fax: 416-785-0450
e-mail: info@coloncancercanada.ca
www.coloncancercanada.ca
Raise public awareness for this deadly disease and to raise money for vital research.

1975 **Colorectal Cancer Association of Canada**
5 Place Ville Marie 514-875-7745
Montreal, QC, H3B-2G2 Fax: 514-875-7746
e-mail: admin@ccac-accc.ca
www.ccac-accc.ca
Non-profit organization dedicated to improving the quality of life of patients and increasing awareness of the disease.
Barry D Stein, President
Heidi Watts, Program Director

1976 **ENCORE YWCA-National Board**
YWCA-National Board
726 Broadway 212-614-2827
New York, NY 10003-9502 800-953-7587
The YWCA's discussion and exercise program for women who have had breast cancer surgery. Designed to restore physical strength and emotional well-being.

1977 **Foundation for Dignity**
37 S 20th Street 215-567-2828
Philadelphia, PA 19103
Offers counseling and seminars concerning the employment rights of cancer patients and for human services workers. The society offers an extensive list of publications dealing with all aspects of cancer prevention and care.
Barbara Hoffman, Staff Attorney

1978 **International Association of Laryngectomees**
American Cancer Society
Box 691060 757-888-0324
Stockton, CA 95269-1060 866-425-3678
Fax: 209-472-0516
e-mail: ialhq@larynxlink.com
www.larynxlink.com
Consists of loacal clubs worldwide that provides services and information to patients who have undergone laryngectomies and their families. Members are given information on first aid, postoperative care, rehabilitation, esophageal speech and other speech alternatives. Directories of speech instructors and self-care supplies for the surgical site are distributed.
Jack Henslee, Executive Director

1979 **International Society for Dermatologic Surgery**
Rosenparkklinik GmbH 212-213-5439
Germany, e-mail: info@isdsworld.org
www.isdsworld.com

Goals of this organization are to promote high standards of patient care, provide continuing education and research in dermatologic surgery and encourage public interest in this field.
Antonio Picoto, Executive Director

1980 **Leukemia Society of America**
1311 Mamaroneck Avenue 914-949-5213
White Plains, NY 10605 800-955-4572
Fax: 914-949-6691
www.leukemia.org
A national voluntary health agency dedicated to curing leukemia lymphoma Hodgkin's disease and myeloma and to improving the quality of life of patients and their families.

1981 **Leukemia and Lymphoma Society**
1311 Mamaroneck Avenue 914-949-5213
White Plains, NY 10605 800-955-4572
Fax: 914-949-6691
www.lls.org
The Leukemia and Lymphoma Society is the world's largest voluntary health organization dedicated to funding blood cancer research education and patient services.
John Walter, President & CEO

1982 **Make Today Count**
1235 E Cherokee 417-885-3324
Springfield, MO 65804-2263 800-432-2273
Fax: 417-888-7426
smsu.edu/nursing/community
An organization that helps patients and their families cope with cancer and other serious diseases and improve their quality of life.
Connie Zimmerman, Director

1983 **National Alliance of Breast Cancer Organizations**
9 E 37th Street
New York, NY 10016 888-806-2226
Fax: 212-689-1213
e-mail: nabcoinfo@aol.com
www.nabco.org
A network of breast cancer organizations that provides information assistance and referral to anyone with questions about breast cancer and acts as a voice for the interests and concerns of breast cancer survivors and women at risk.

1984 **National Cancer Institute**
6116 Executive Boulevard
Bethesda, MD 20892-8322 800-422-6237
TTY: 800-332-8615
e-mail: cancergovstaff@mail.nih.gov
www.cancer.gov
One of the largest organizations dealing solely with cancer in its many forms. Offers educational information public awareness research grants and more for patients their families and health care professionals. Offers a hotline and on-line support.
Deborah Pear RN MPH, Chief Public Inquiries Office

1985 **National Cancer Institute of Canada**
10 Alcorn Avenue 416-961-7223
Toronto, Ontario, M4V-3B1 Fax: 416-961-4189
e-mail: research@cancer.ca
www.ncic.cancer.ca
Was formed through a joint initiative of the Department of National Health and Welfare and the Canadian Cancer Society.
Dr Elizabeth Eisenhauer, President

1986 **National Coalition for Cancer Survivorship**
1010 Wayne Avenue 301-650-9127
Silver Spring, MD 20910 888-622-7937
Fax: 301-565-9670
e-mail: info@canceradvocacy.org
www.canceradvocacy.org
Survivor led advocacy organization working exclusively on behalf of people with all types of cancer and their families. Dedicated to assuring quality and care for all Americans.
Ellen Storall, President/CEO

1987 **National Foundation for Cancer Research**
4600 EW Highway 301-654-1250
Bethesda, MD 20814 800-321-2873
Fax: 301-654-5824
e-mail: info@nfcr.org
www.nfcr.org
Contracts with major universities for basic science cancer research in the fields of biophysics, theoretical physics and biochemistry.
Franklin C Salisbury Jr, President
Sujuan Ba, Chief Operating Officer

1988 **National Hospice & Palliative Care Organization (NHPCO)**
1700 Diagonal Road 703-837-1500
Alexandria, VA 22314 800-658-8898
Fax: 703-837-1233
e-mail: nhpcoinfo@nhpco.org
www.nhpco.org
The nation's only advocate for terminally ill patients and their families. Founded in 1978, the NHPCO is the only organization devoted to hospice in the United States. Support is included from state hospice organizations, patients, families, communities, provider program members and professional/volunteer members. Represents hospice care interests to Congress, regulatory agencies, courts, voluntary organizations and the public.
Donald Schumacher, PsyD, President/CEO

1989 **National Hospice & Palliative Care Org.**
1731 King Street 703-837-1500
Alexandria, VA 22314 Fax: 703-837-1233
e-mail: nhpco_info@nhpco.org
www.nhpco.org
The nation's only advocate for terminally ill patients and their families. Founded in 1978, the NHPCO is the only organization devoted to hospice in the United States. Support is included from state hospice organizations, patients, families and communities.
Donald Schum PsyD, President/CEO
Galen Miller PhD, Executive Vice President

1990 **National Institute on Aging Information Center**
31 Center Drive MSC 2292 301-496-1752
Bethesda, MD 20892 800-222-2225
Fax: 301-496-1072
TTY: 800-222-4225
www.nih.gov/nia
Concerned with the health problems of older Americans. The Center offers free printed materials including fact sheets about going to the hospital and about prostate problems.
Richard J Hodes MD, Director

1991 **National Kidney and Urologic Diseases Information Clearinghouse**
31 Center Drive,MSC 2560 301-654-4415
Bethesda, MD 20892-2560 800-891-5390
Fax: 301-907-8906
e-mail: nkudic@info.niddk.nih.gov
www.niddk.nih.gov
A service of the Federal Government's National Institute for Diabetes and Digestive and Kidney Diseases. Offers free information about benign prostate enlargement and other noncancerous urinary tract problems.

1992 **National Marrow Donor Program**
3001 Broadway Street NE 612-627-5800
Minneapolis, MN 55413-1763 800-627-7692
www.marrow.org
Created to improve the effectiveness of the search for bone marrow donors so that a greater number of bone marrow transplantations can be carried out.
Jeffrey W Chell MD, CEO
Patricia A Coppo MS, COO

1993 **National Ovarian Cancer Coalition**
500 NE Spanish River Boulevard 561-393-0005
Boca Raton, FL 33431 888-OVA-RIAN
Fax: 561-393-7275
e-mail: NOCC@ovarian.org
www.ovarian.org
Our mission is to raise awareness about ovarian cancer and to promote education about this disease. By dispelling myths and misun-

derstandings the coalition is committed to improve the overall survival rate and quality of life for women with ovarian cancer.
April Donahue, President

1994 **New Brunswick Innovation Foundation**
440 King Street, Suite 602 506-452-2884
Fredericton, NB, E3B-5H8 877-554-6668
Fax: 506-452-2886
e-mail: info@nbif.ca
www.nbif.ca
An independent corporation, has the mission to contribute to building the province's innovation capacity.
Barrie Black, President/CEO

1995 **Rethink Breast Cancer**
296 Richmond Street W 416-920-0980
Toronto, Ontario, M5V-1X2 Fax: 416-920-5798
e-mail: hello@rethinkbreastcancer.com
www.rethinkbreastcancer.com
Is a charity helping young people who are concerned about and affected by breast cancer through innovative breast cancer education, research and support programs.
MJ DeCoteau MA, Executive Director

1996 **Skin Cancer Foundation**
149 Madison Avenue 212-725-5176
New York, NY 10016-8728 800-754-6490
Fax: 212-725-5751
e-mail: info@skincancer.org
www.skincancer.org
Conducts public and medical education programs to help reduce skin cancer. Major goals are to increase public awareness of the importance of taking protective measures against the damaging rays of the sun and to teach people how to recognize the early signs.
Perry Robins MD, President

1997 **Support for People with Oral and Head and Neck Cancer**
PO Box 53 516-759-5333
Locust Valley, NY 11560-0053 800-377-0928
Fax: 516-671-8794
e-mail: info@spohnc.org
www.spohnc.org
Nonprofit organization founded in 1991 to address the broad emotional physical and humanistic needs of oral and head and neck cancer patients.
Nancy E Leupold, President/Founder

1998 **Y-ME National Breast Cancer Organization**
212 W Van Buren 312-986-8338
Chicago, IL 60607 800-221-2141
e-mail: askyme@y-me.org
www.y-me.org
Provides support information and education to anyone touched by breast cancer. Support and information are available 24 hours through the National Breast Cancer Hotline which is staffed by breast cancer survivors who are trained peer counselors.
Margaret Kirk, CEO

State Agencies & Associations

Alabama

1999 **American Cancer Society: Alabama**
1100 Ireland Way 205-879-2242
Birmingham, AL 35205 Fax: 205-930-8895
e-mail: scarlet.thompson@cancer.org
www.cancer.org/docroot/com/com_0.asp
The American Cancer Society is the nationwide community-based voluntary health organization dedicated to eliminating cancer as a major health problem by preventing cancer, saving lives and diminishing suffering from cancer, through research and education.
Scarlet Thom (205-930-8889), Media/Public Relations Alabama

2000 **Leukemia Society of America: Alabama Chapter**
Leukemia Society of America
100 Chase Park S 205-989-0098
Birmingham, AL 35244 888-560-9700
Fax: 205-989-0099
www.leukemia-lymphoma.org
Dedicated to finding cures for leukemia and related cancers and to improving the quality of life for patients and their families.
Valerie Hunton, Executive Director

Alaska

2001 **American Cancer Society: Alaska**
3851 Piper Street 907-277-8696
Anchorage, AK 99508 Fax: 907-263-2073
e-mail: leslie.jones@cancer.org
www.cancer.org
The American Cancer Society is the nationwide community-based voluntary health organization dedicated to eliminating cancer as a major health problem by preventing cancer saving lives and diminishing suffering from cancer through research and education.
Leslie Jones (251-414-1303), Media/Public Relations Alaska

Arizona

2002 **American Cancer Society: Arizona**
4212 N 16th Street 602-224-0524
Phoenix, AZ 85016 800-227-2345
Fax: 602-778-7699
e-mail: meg.kondrich@cancer.org
www.cancer.org
The American Cancer Society is the nationwide community-based voluntary health organization dedicated to eliminating cancer as a major health problem by preventing cancer saving lives, and diminishing suffering from cancer through research and education.
Meg Kondrich (602-381-3092), Media/Public Relations Arizona

2003 **International Holistic Center**
PO Box 15103 928-771-2826
Phoenix, AZ 85060-5103 e-mail: ihcinc@cox.net
www.holisticresources.org
Provides information and referrals concerning holistic health care in Arizona and beyond.
Stan Kalson, Director

2004 **Leukemia Society of America: Mountain States Chapter**
Leukemia Society of America
3877 N 7th Street 602-567-7600
Phoenix, AZ 85014 800-568-1372
Fax: 602-567-7601
www.leukemia-lymphoma.org
Dedicated to finding cures for leukemia and related cancers and to improving the quality of life for patients and their families. Serves New Mexico and the Greater El Paso, TX area.
Tim Metzer, Executive Director

Arkansas

2005 **American Cancer Society: Arkansas**
901 N University 501-664-3480
Little Rock, AR 72207 Fax: 501-603-5223
e-mail: jodie.spears@cancer.org
www.cancer.org
The American Cancer Society is the nationwide community-based voluntary health organization dedicated to eliminating cancer as a major health problem by preventing cancer, saving lives, and diminishing suffering from cancer, through research and education.
Jodie Spears (501-603-5210), Media/Public Relations Arkansas

2006 **Health Resource**
933 Faulkner Street 501-329-5272
Conway, AR 72034 800-949-0090
Fax: 501-329-9489
e-mail: research@thehealthresource.com
www.thehealthresource.com
A medical information service which provides clients with an individualized, in depth research report on his or her specific health problem. Reports include latest treatment options, mainstream, experimental and alternative and top specialists.
Janice Guthrie, Director/Researcher
Shirley Effinger, Researcher

California

2007 American Cancer Society: Central Los Angel es
3333 Wilshire Boulevard 213-386-6102
Los Angeles, CA 90010 Fax: 213-480-0806
e-mail: katherine.spangle@cancer.org
www.cancer.org
The American Cancer Society is the nationwide community-based voluntary health organization dedicated to eliminating cancer as a major health problem by preventing cancer, saving lives, and diminishing suffering from cancer, through research and education.
Katie Spangl (213-736-5075), Media/Public Relations Los Angeles Area

2008 American Cancer Society: East Bay/Metropol itan Region
1700 Webster Street 510-832-7012
Oakland, CA 94612 Fax: 510-763-8826
e-mail: patty.guinto@cancer.org
www.cancer.org
The American Cancer Society is the nationwide community-based voluntary health organization dedicated to eliminating cancer as a major health problem by preventing cancer, saving lives, and diminishing suffering from cancer, through research and education.
Patty Guinto (510-452-5229), Media/Public Relations East Bay Area

2009 American Cancer Society: Fresno/Madera Cou nties
2222 W Shaw Avenue 559-451-0722
Fresno, CA 93711 Fax: 559-451-0744
e-mail: erica.jones@cancer.org
www.cancer.org
The American Cancer Society is the nationwide community-based voluntary health organization dedicated to eliminating cancer as a major health problem by preventing cancer, saving lives, and diminishing suffering from cancer, through research and education.
Erica Jones (559-451-0163), Media/Public Relations Fresno CA

2010 American Cancer Society: Inland Empire
1240 Palmyrita Avenue 951-683-6415
Riverside, CA 92507 Fax: 951-682-6804
e-mail: beckie.mooreflati@cancer.org
www.cancer.org
The American Cancer Society is the nationwide community-based voluntary health organization dedicated to eliminating cancer as a major health problem by preventing cancer, saving lives, and diminishing suffering from cancer, through research and education.
Beckie Moore Flati 714-779-8104, Media/Public Relations Riverside Region

2011 American Cancer Society: Orange County
1940 E Deere Avenue 949-261-9446
Santa Ana, CA 92705-5718 Fax: 949-261-9419
e-mail: jennifer.horspool@cancer.org
www.cancer.org
The American Cancer Society is the nationwide community-based voluntary health organization dedicated to eliminating cancer as a major health problem by preventing cancer, saving lives, and diminishing suffering from cancer, through research and education.
Jennifer Hor (949-567-0637), Media/Public Relations Orange County

2012 American Cancer Society: Sacramento County
1765 Challenge Way 916-446-7933
Sacramento, CA 95815 Fax: 916-64 -977
e-mail: maria.robinson@cancer.org
www.cancer.org
The American Cancer Society is the nationwide community-based voluntary health organization dedicated to eliminating cancer as a major health problem by preventing cancer, saving lives, and diminishing suffering from cancer, through research and education.
Maria Robins (916-446-7933), Media/Public Relations Sacramento County

2013 American Cancer Society: San Diego County
2655 Camino Del Rio N 619-299-4200
San Diego, CA 92108 800-227-2345
Fax: 619-296-0928
e-mail: robin.brown@cancer.org
www.cancer.org
The American Cancer Society is the nationwide community-based voluntary health organization dedicated to eliminating cancer as a major health problem by preventing cancer, saving lives, and diminishing suffering from cancer, through research and education.
Robin Brown (619-682-7439), Media/Public Relations San Diego CA

2014 American Cancer Society: San Francisco Cou nty
201 Mission Street 415-394-7100
San Francisco, CA 94105 Fax: 415-495-1877
e-mail: patty.guinto@cancer.org
www.cancer.org
The American Cancer Society is the nationwide community-based voluntary health organization dedicated to eliminating cancer as a major health problem by preventing cancer, saving lives and diminishing suffering from cancer, through research and education.
Patty Guinto (510-452-5229), Media/Public Relations San Francisco

2015 American Cancer Society: Santa Clara Count y/Silicon Valley/Central Coast Region
747 Camden Avenue 408-871-1062
Campbell, CA 95008 Fax: 408-871-2993
e-mail: angie.carrillo@cancer.org
www.cancer.org
The American Cancer Society is the nationwide community-based voluntary health organization dedicated to eliminating cancer as a major health problem by preventing cancer, saving lives and diminishing suffering from cancer, through research and education.
Angie Carril (408-688-0106), Media/Public Relations Silicon Valley

2016 American Cancer Society: Santa Maria Valle y
426 E Barcellus 805-922-2354
Santa Maria, CA 93454 Fax: 805-925-1424
e-mail: jeb.baird@cancer.org
www.cancer.org
The American Cancer Society is the nationwide community-based voluntary health organization dedicated to eliminating cancer as a major health problem by preventing cancer, saving lives and diminishing suffering from cancer, through research and education.
Jeb Baird (805-560-6819), Media/Public Relations Santa Maria

2017 American Cancer Society: Sonoma County
1451 Guerneville Road 707-545-6720
Santa Rosa, CA 95403 Fax: 707-545-3179
e-mail: angie.carrillo@cancer.org
www.cancer.org
The American Cancer Society is the nationwide community-based voluntary health organization dedicated to eliminating cancer as a major health problem by preventing cancer, saving lives and diminishing suffering from cancer, through research and education.
Angie Carril (408-688-0106), Media/Public Relations Central Coast

2018 Cancer Control Society and Cancer Book House
2043 N Berendo Street 213-663-7801
Los Angeles, CA 90027 Fax: 323-663-7757
www.cancercontrolsociety.com
An informational organization offering books, films, videos, clinic tours and lists of patients with cancer.
Lorraine Rosenthal, Co-Founder
Frank Cousineau, President

2019 City of Hope National Medical Center Beckman Research Institute
Beckman Research Institute
1500 E Duarte Road 626-256-4673
Duarte, CA 91010 800-826-4673
e-mail: tpogue@coh.org
www.cityofhope.org
City of Hope is an innovative biomedical research, treatment and educational institution dedicated to the prevention and cure of cancer and other life-threatening illness.
Stephen J Foreman, Chair

2020 Leukemia & Lymphoma Society: Orange, Riverside, And San Bernadino Counties
2020 E 1st Street 714-881-0610
Santa Ana, CA 92705 888-535-9300
Fax: 714-881-0616
www.leukemia-lymphoma.org
Dedicated to finding cures for leukemia and related cancers and to improving the quality of life for patients and their families.

2021 Leukemia Society of America: San Diego/Hawaii Chapter
Leukemia Society of America

8575 Gibbs Drive
San Diego, CA 92123
858-277-1800
888-535-9300
Fax: 858-277-1748
www.leukemia.org
Dedicated to finding cures for leukemia and related cancers and to improving the quality of life for patients and their families.
Keith Turner, Executive Director

2022 **Leukemia Society of America: Greater Sacramento Area Chapter**
Leukemia Society of America
4604 Roseville Road
North Highlands, CA 95660
916-348-1793
Fax: 916-348-7864
www.leukemia.org
Dedicated to finding cures for leukemia and related cancers and to improving the quality of life for patients and their families.
Tracy Latino, Executive Director

2023 **Leukemia Society of America: Greater Los Angeles Chapter**
Leukemia Society of America
6033 W Century Boulevard
Los Angeles, CA 90045
310-342-5800
Fax: 310-342-5801
www.leukemia-lymphoma.org
Dedicated to finding cures for leukemia and related cancers and to improving the quality of life for patients and their families.
Donna Lynch, Executive Director

2024 **Leukemia Society of America: Northern California Chapter**
Leukemia Society of America
1390 Market Street
San Francisco, CA 94102
415-625-1100
Fax: 415-625-1155
www.leukemia.org
Dedicated to finding cures for leukemia and related cancers and to improving the quality of life for patients and their families.

2025 **Leukemia Society of America: Tri-County Chapter**
Leukemia Society of America
2020 E 1st Street
Santa Ana, CA 92705
714-881-0610
888-535-9300
Fax: 714-881-0616
www.leukemia-lymphoma.org
Dedicated to finding cures for leukemia and related cancers and to improving the quality of life for patients and their families.
Sam Thomas, Executive Director

2026 **National Health Federation**
PO Box 688
Monrovia, CA 91017
626-357-2181
Fax: 626-303-0642
e-mail: contact-us@thenhf.com
www.thenhf.com
A nonprofit consumer-oriented organization devoted to health matters. Dedicated to preserving freedom of choice in health care issues, prevention of diseases and the promotion of wellness.
Scott Tips, President
Sylvia Provenza, Vice-President

2027 **Regional Cancer Foundation**
1200 Gough Street
San Francisco, CA 94109
415-775-9956
Fax: 415-346-8652
e-mail: mail@regionalcancerfoundation.org
www.regionalcancerfoundation.org
This foundation offers, at no charge, a second opinion consultation to individuals diagnosed with cancer. The patient and a family member or friend meet with an interdisciplinary panel of local cancer specialists with expertise in radiation therapy, chemotherapy, and cancer treatment plans.
William Gillis, CEO
Arhur J Inerfield, Chairman

Colorado

2028 **American Cancer Society: Colorado**
2255 S Oneida Street
Denver, CO 80224
303-758-2030
Fax: 303-759-1615
e-mail: lynda.solomon@cancer.org
www.cancer.org
The American Cancer Society is the nationwide community-based voluntary health organization dedicated to eliminating cancer as a major health problem by preventing cancer, saving lives and diminishing suffering from cancer, through research and education.
Lynda Solomo 720-524-5470, Media/Public Relations Colorado
Joel Quevill 719-636-5101, Media/Public Relations Colorado

Connecticut

2029 **American Cancer Society: Connecticut**
Meriden Executive Park
Meriden, CT 06450
203-379-4700
Fax: 203-379-5060
e-mail: simone.upsey@cancer.org
www.cancer.org
The American Cancer Society is the nationwide community-based voluntary health organization dedicated to eliminating cancer as a major health problem by preventing cancer, saving lives and diminishing suffering from cancer, through research and education.
Simone Upsey (203-379-4717), Media/Public Relations NH/MS/NL Counties
Christian Me (203-563-1510), Media/Public Relations LF/FF Counties

2030 **Leukemia Society of America: Connecticut Chapter**
Leukemia Society of America
300 Research Parkway
Meriden, CT 06450
203-379-0445
888-282-9465
Fax: 203-379-0451
www.leukemia.org
Founded in 1949 to help serve and educate the communities and residents who have been touched by leukemia, lymphoma, multiple myeloma and Hodgkin's disease.

2031 **Leukemia Society of America: Central Connecticut Chapter**
Leukemia Society of America
300 Research Parkway
Meriden, CT 06450
203-379-0445
888-282-9465
Fax: 203-379-0451
www.leukemia.org
Founded in 1971 to help serve the residents of the counties of New Haven, New London and parts of Middlesex and Litchfield who have been touched by leukemia, lymphoma, multiple myeloma and Hodgkin's disease.

2032 **Leukemia Society of America: Fairfield County Chapter**
Leukemia Society of America
25 Third Street
Stamford, CT 06905
203-967-8326
Fax: 203-325-8559
www.leukemia.org
Dedicated to finding cures for leukemia and related cancers and to improving the quality of life for patients and their families.

Delaware

2033 **American Cancer Society: Delaware**
92 Reads Way
New Castle, DE 19720
302-324-4427
Fax: 302-324-4233
e-mail: dawn.ward@cancer.org
www.cancer.org
The American Cancer Society is the nationwide community-based voluntary health organization dedicated to eliminating cancer as a major health problem by preventing cancer, saving lives, and diminishing suffering from cancer, through research and education.
Dawn Ward (410-933-5134), Media/Public Relations Delaware

2034 **Leukemia & Lymphoma Society Leukemia Society of America**
Leukemia Society of America
100 W 10th Street
Wilmington, DE 19801
302-661-7300
800-220-1617
Fax: 302-661-0363
www.leukemia-lymphoma.org
Our mission is to cure leukemia, lymphoma, Hodgkin's disease and myeloma and to improve the quality of life of patients and their families.

District of Columbia

2035 **American Cancer Society: District of Colum bia**
1875 Connecticut Avenue NW
Washington, DC 20009
202-483-2600
Fax: 202-483-1174
e-mail: angela.collins@cancer.org
www.cancer.org

The American Cancer Society is the nationwide community-based voluntary health organization dedicated to eliminating cancer as a major health problem by preventing cancer, saving lives, and diminishing suffering from cancer, through research and education.
Angela Colli (202-483-2600), Media/Public Relations Washington DC

2036 **American Institute for Cancer Research**
1759 R Street NW
Washington, DC 20009
202-328-7744
800-843-8114
Fax: 202-328-7226
e-mail: aicrweb@aicr.org
www.aicr.org

Not-for-profit research and educational organization. Provides grants for research into the causes, development, prevention and treatment of cancer through diet and nutrition. Offers publications, research results, conferences and various public services.

2037 **Center for Science in the Public Interest**
1875 Connecticut Avenue NW
Washington, DC 20009
202-332-9110
Fax: 202-265-4954
e-mail: cspi@cspinet.org
www.cspinet.org

The nation's leading consumer group concerned with food and nutrition issues. Focuses on diseases that result from consuming too many calories, too much fat, sodium and sugar such as cancer and heart disease.
William Corr, Board of Directors
Tom Gegax, Board of Directors

Florida

2038 **American Cancer Society: Florida**
2006 W Kennedy Boulevard
Tampa, FL 33606
813-254-3630
Fax: 813-349-4431
e-mail: cynthia.dunlap@cancer.org
www.cancer.org

The American Cancer Society is the nationwide community-based voluntary health organization dedicated to eliminating cancer as a major health problem by preventing cancer, saving lives, and diminishing suffering from cancer, through research and education.
Cynthia Dunl (941-365-2858), Media/Public Relations Tampa Region
Kristen Redd (727-546-9822), Media/Public Relations Tampa Region

2039 **Leukemia & Lymphoma Society: Suncoast Chapter**
Leukemia Society of America
3507 E Frontage Road
Tampa, FL 33607
813-963-6461
800-436-6889
Fax: 813-963-1306
www.leukemia.org

Serves patients with leukemia, lymphoma, multiple myeloma and Hodgkin's disease in Charlotte, Citrus, Collier, DeSoto, Hardee, Hernando, Hillsborough, Lee, Manatee, Pasco, Pinellas and Sarasota counties.

2040 **Leukemia Society of America: Central Florida Chapter**
Leukemia Society of America
3319 Maguire Boulevard
Orlando, FL 32803-3720
407-898-0733
Fax: 407-896-8645
www.leukemia.org

Dedicated to finding cures for leukemia and related cancers and to improving the quality of life for patients and their families.

2041 **Leukemia Society of America: Northern Florida Chapter**
Leukemia Society of America
9143 Phillips Highway
Jacksonville, FL 32256
904-538-0721
800-868-0072
Fax: 904-538-9245
www.leukemia.org

Dedicated to finding cures for leukemia and related cancers and to improving the quality of life for patients and their families.

2042 **Leukemia Society of America: Palm Beach Area Chapter**
Leukemia Society of America
4360 Northlake Boulevard
Palm Beach Gardens, FL 33410
561-775-9954
888-478-8550
Fax: 561-775-0930
www.leukemia.org

Dedicated to finding cures for leukemia and related cancers and to improving the quality of life for patients and their families.

2043 **Leukemia Society of America: Southern Florida Chapter**
Leukemia Society of America
3325 Hollywood Boulevard
Hallandale, FL 33021
954-961-3234
Fax: 954-961-7376
www.leukemia.org

Dedicated to finding cures for leukemia and related cancers and to improving the quality of life for patients and their families.

Georgia

2044 **American Cancer Society: Georgia**
50 Williams Street
Atlanta, GA 30303
404-315-1123
Fax: 404-315-9348
e-mail: elissa.mccrary@cancer.org
www.cancer.org

The American Cancer Society is the nationwide community-based voluntary health organization dedicated to eliminating cancer as a major health problem by preventing cancer, saving lives, and diminishing suffering from cancer, through research and education.
Elissa McCra (404-949-6418), Media/Public Relations Georgia

2045 **Kidscope**
2045 Peachtree Road
Atlanta, GA 30309
404-892-1437
www.kidscope.org

A nonprofit organization formed to help families and children better understand the effects from cancer in a parent. The name can also be read as Kids Cope - one of the goals being to improve the chances that a child will successfully cope with the diagnosis.
H Elizabeth King PhD, Board Member
Carol Webb PhD, Board Member

2046 **Leukemia Society of America: Georgia Chapter**
Leukemia Society of America
3715 Northside Parkway
Atlanta, GA 30327
404-720-7900
800-399-7312
Fax: 404-720-7878
e-mail: dick.brown@lls.org
www.leukemia-lymphoma.org

Dedicated to finding cures for leukemia and related cancers and to improving the quality of life for patients and their families.
Dick Brown, Executive Director
Maureen Quin Davidson, Director TNT

Hawaii

2047 **American Cancer Society: Hawaii**
2370 Nuuanu Avenue
Honolulu, HI 96817
808-595-7544
800-ACS-2345
Fax: 808-595-7545
TTY: 866-228-4327
e-mail: milton.hirata@cancer.org
www.cancer.org

The American Cancer Society is the nationwide community-based voluntary health organization dedicated to eliminating cancer as a major health problem by preventing cancer, saving lives, and diminishing suffering from cancer, through research and education.
Milton Hirata, Media Relations Contact - Hawaii

Idaho

2048 **American Cancer Society: Idaho**
2676 Vista Avenue
Boise, ID 83705
208-345-2184
800-ACS-2345
Fax: 208-343-9922
TTY: 866-228-4327
e-mail: jim.ryan@cancer.org
www.cancer.org

The American Cancer Society is the nationwide community-based voluntary health organization dedicated to eliminating cancer as a major health problem by preventing cancer, saving lives, and diminishing suffering from cancer, through research and education.
Jim Ryan, Media Relations Contact - Idaho

Illinois

2049 **American Cancer Society: Illinois**
225 N Michigan Avenue
Chicago, IL 60601
312-372-0471
800-ACS-2345
Fax: 312-372-0910
TTY: 866-228-4327
e-mail: melissa.leeb@cancer.org
www.cancer.org
The American Cancer Society is the nationwide community-based voluntary health organization dedicated to eliminating cancer as a major health problem by preventing cancer, saving lives, and diminishing suffering from cancer, through research and education.
Melissa Leeb, Media Relations Contact - Illinois

2050 **Leukemia Society of America: Illinois Chapter**
Leukemia Society of America
651 W Washington Boulevard
Chicago, IL 60661
312-651-7350
800-742-6595
Fax: 312-463-0980
e-mail: pam.swenk@lls.org
www.leukemia.org
Dedicated to finding cures for leukemia and related cancers and to improving the quality of life for patients and their families.
Pam Swenk, Executive Director
Jennifer Hufnagel, Director Donor Development

Indiana

2051 **American Cancer Society: Indiana**
5635 W 96th Street
Indianapolis, IN 46278
317-344-7800
800-ACS-2345
Fax: 317-344-7810
TTY: 866-228-4327
e-mail: leslie.smith@cancer.org
www.cancer.org
The American Cancer Society is the nationwide community-based voluntary health organization dedicated to eliminating cancer as a major health problem by preventing cancer, saving lives, and diminishing suffering from cancer, through research and education.
Leslie Smith Babione, Media Relations Contact - Indianapolis
Katie Burton (317-280-6643), Media/Public Relations Indiana

2052 **Leukemia Society of America: Indiana Chapter**
Leukemia Society of America
941 E 86th Street
Indianapolis, IN 46240
317-726-2270
800-846-7764
Fax: 317-726-2280
e-mail: amy.kwas@lls.org
www.leukemia.org
Dedicated to finding cures for leukemia and related cancers and to improving the quality of life for patients and their families.
Amy Kwas, Executive Director
Sarah Moore, Deputy Executive Director

Iowa

2053 **American Cancer Society: Iowa**
8364 Hickman Road
Des Moines, IA 50325
515-253-0147
800-ACS-2345
Fax: 515-253-0806
TTY: 866-228-4327
e-mail: chuck.reed@cancer.org
www.cancer.org
The American Cancer Society is the nationwide community-based voluntary health organization dedicated to eliminating cancer as a major health problem by preventing cancer, saving lives, and diminishing suffering from cancer, through research and education.
Chuck Reed, Media Relations Contact - Iowa
Kathy Holdefer, Media Relations Contact - Iowa

2054 **People Against Cancer**
604 E Street
Otho, IA 50569-0010
515-972-4444
800-662-2326
Fax: 515-972-4415
e-mail: info@PeopleAgainstCancer.net
www.peopleagainstcancer.com
A nonprofit grassroots organization whose mission is to find the best cancer therapy for people with cancer worldwide.
Frank Wiewel, Executive Director

Kansas

2055 **American Cancer Society: Kansas City**
6700 Antioch
Merriam, KS 66024
913-432-3277
800-ACS-2345
Fax: 913-432-1732
TTY: 866-228-4327
e-mail: christine.winter@cancer.org
www.cancer.org
The American Cancer Society is the nationwide community-based voluntary health organization dedicated to eliminating cancer as a major health problem by preventing cancer, saving lives, and diminishing suffering from cancer, through research and education.
Christine Winter, Media Relations Contact

2056 **Leukemia Society of America: Kansas Chapter**
Leukemia Society of America
300 N Main
Wichita, KS 67202
316-266-4050
800-779-2417
Fax: 316-266-4960
e-mail: gerstenk@ks.leukemia-lymphoma.org
www.leukemia.org
Dedicated to finding cures for leukemia and related cancers and to improving the quality of life for patients and their families.
Sean McParland, Divisional Director
Kelly Gerstenkorn, Managing Director

2057 **Leukemia Society of America: Mid-America Chapter**
Leukemia Society of America
6811 W 63rd Street
Shawnee Mission, KS 66202
913-262-1515
800-256-1075
Fax: 913-262-2167
e-mail: janna.lacock@lls.org
www.leukemia.org
Dedicated to finding cures for leukemia and related cancers and to improving the quality of life for patients and their families.
Janna LaCock, Executive Director
Jill Ring, Development Director

Kentucky

2058 **American Cancer Society: Kentucky**
701 W Muhammad Ali Boulevard
Louisville, KY 40203
502-584-6782
800-ACS-2345
Fax: 502-584-6767
TTY: 866-228-4327
e-mail: stephanie.schrenger@cancer.org
www.cancer.org
The American Cancer Society is the nationwide community-based voluntary health organization dedicated to eliminating cancer as a major health problem by preventing cancer, saving lives, and diminishing suffering from cancer, through research and education.
Stephanie Schrenger, Media Relations Contact - Kentucky

2059 **Leukemia Society of America: Kentucky Chapter**
Leukemia Society of America
600 E Main Street
Louisville, KY 40202-2661
502-584-8490
800-955-2566
Fax: 502-589-5316
e-mail: karyl.ferman@lls.org
www.leukemia.org
Founded in 1975 to serve Kentucky and Southern Indiana residents touched by leukemia and its related cancers. Goal is to find a cure for leukemia and its related cancers and to improve the quality of life for patients and their families.
Karyl D Ferman, Executive Director
Katie Anderson, Director Team in Training

Louisiana

2060 **American Cancer Society: Louisiana**
2605 River Road
New Orleans, LA 70121
504-469-0021
800-ACS-2345
Fax: 504-219-2290
TTY: 866-228-4327
e-mail: jewel.m.bush@cancer.org
www.cancer.org
The American Cancer Society is the nationwide community-based voluntary health organization dedicated to eliminating cancer as a

major health problem by preventing cancer, saving lives, and diminishing suffering from cancer, through research and education.
Jewel M Bush, Media Relations Contact

Maine

2061 **American Cancer Society: Maine**
1 Bowdoin Mill Island 207-373-3700
Topsham, ME 04086 800-ACS-2345
Fax: 207-725-6680
TTY: 866-228-4327
e-mail: susan.clifford@cancer.org
www.cancer.org
The American Cancer Society is the nationwide community-based voluntary health organization dedicated to eliminating cancer as a major health problem by preventing cancer, saving lives, and diminishing suffering from cancer, through research and education.
Susan Clifford, Media Relations Contact - Maine

Maryland

2062 **American Cancer Society: Maryland**
8219 Town Center Drive 410-931-6850
Baltimore, MD 21236 800-ACS-2345
Fax: 410-931-6875
TTY: 866-228-4327
e-mail: dawn.ward@cancer.org
www.cancer.org
The American Cancer Society is the nationwide community-based voluntary health organization dedicated to eliminating cancer as a major health problem by preventing cancer, saving lives, and diminishing suffering from cancer, through research and education.
Dawn Ward, Media Relations Contact - Baltimore Area

2063 **Leukemia Society of America: Maryland Chapter**
Leukemia Society of America
11350 McCormick Road 410-527-0220
Hunt Valley, MD 21031-2001 800-242-4572
Fax: 410-527-0510
e-mail: sharon.yateman@lls.org
www.leukemia.org
Dedicated to finding cures for leukemia and related cancers and to improving the quality of life for patients and their families.
Sharon E Yateman MSW LCSW, Executive Director
Allyson Yospe, Deputy Executive Director

2064 **Rose Kushner Breast Cancer Advisory Center**
PO Box 757 301-897-3445
Malaga Cove, CA 90274 Fax: 301-897-3444
e-mail: lkkushner@yahoo.com
www.rkbcac.org
Provides a mail service offering referrals to health professionals as well as information about detection, diagnosis, treatment and physical and psychological rehabilitation for patients with breast cancer.

Massachusetts

2065 **American Cancer Society: Boston**
18 Tremont Street 617-556-7400
Boston, MA 02108 800-ACS-2345
Fax: 617-263-6825
TTY: 866-228-4327
e-mail: kate.langstone@cancer.org
www.cancer.org
The American Cancer Society is the nationwide community-based voluntary health organization dedicated to eliminating cancer as a major health problem by preventing cancer, saving lives, and diminishing suffering from cancer, through research and education.
Kate Langstone, Media Relations Contact - Boston Area

2066 **American Cancer Society: Central New Engla nd Region-Weston MA**
9 Riverside Road 781-894-6633
Weston, MA 02493 800-ACS-2345
Fax: 781-314-2699
TTY: 866-228-4327
e-mail: jessica.saporetti@cancer.org
www.cancer.org
The American Cancer Society is the nationwide community-based voluntary health organization dedicated to eliminating cancer as a major health problem by preventing cancer, saving lives, and diminishing suffering from cancer, through research and education.
Jessica Saporetti, Media Relations Contact

Michigan

2067 **Leukemia Society of America: Michigan Chapter**
1421 E 12 Mile Road 248-581-3900
Madison Heights, MI 48071 800-456-5413
Fax: 248-581-3901
e-mail: peggy.shriver@lls.org
www.leukemia.org
Peggy Shriver, Executive Director
Robin R Rhea, Director Operations

Minnesota

2068 **American Cancer Society: Duluth**
130 W Superior Street 218-727-7439
Duluth, MN 55802 800-ACS-2345
Fax: 218-727-8069
TTY: 866-228-4327
e-mail: janis.rannow@cancer.org
www.cancer.org
The American Cancer Society is the nationwide community-based voluntary health organization dedicated to eliminating cancer as a major health problem by preventing cancer, saving lives, and diminishing suffering from cancer, through research and education.
Janis Rannow, Media Relations Contact

2069 **American Cancer Society: Mendota Heights Mendota Heights**
Mendota Heights
2520 Pilot Knob Road 651-255-8100
Mendota Heights, MN 55120 800-ACS-2345
Fax: 651-255-8133
TTY: 866-228-4327
e-mail: lou.harvin@cancer.org
www.cancer.org
The American Cancer Society is the nationwide community-based voluntary health organization dedicated to eliminating cancer as a major health problem by preventing cancer, saving lives, and diminishing suffering from cancer, through research and education.
Lou Harvin, Media Relations Contact
Janis Rannow, Media Relations Contact

2070 **American Cancer Society: Rochester**
2900 43 Street NW 507-287-2044
Rochester, MN 55901 800-ACS-2345
Fax: 507-287-2178
TTY: 866-228-4327
e-mail: janis.rannow@cancer.org
www.cancer.org
The American Cancer Society is the nationwide community-based voluntary health organization dedicated to eliminating cancer as a major health problem by preventing cancer, saving lives, and diminishing suffering from cancer, through research and education.
Janis Rannow, Media Relations Contact

2071 **American Cancer Society: Saint Cloud**
3721 23rd Street S 320-255-0220
Saint Cloud, MN 56301 800-239-7028
Fax: 320-255-5517
TTY: 866-228-4327
e-mail: janis.rannow@cancer.org
www.cancer.org
The American Cancer Society is the nationwide community-based voluntary health organization dedicated to eliminating cancer as a major health problem by preventing cancer, saving lives, and diminishing suffering from cancer, through research and education.
Janis Rannow, Media Relations Contact

2072 **Leukemia Society of America: Minnesota Chapter**
5217 Wayzata Boulevard
Golden Valley, MN 55426
763-852-3000
888-220-4440
Fax: 763-852-3001
e-mail: Murray.Schmidt@lls.org
www.leukemia.org

Murray Schmidt, Executive Director
Vickie Shaw, Deputy Executive Director

Mississippi

2073 **American Cancer Society: Jackson**
1380 Livingston Lane
Jackson, MS 39213
601-362-8874
800-ACS-2345
Fax: 601-362-8876
TTY: 866-228-4327
e-mail: kelly.lindsay@cancer.org
www.cancer.org

The American Cancer Society is the nationwide community-based voluntary health organization dedicated to eliminating cancer as a major health problem by preventing cancer, saving lives, and diminishing suffering from cancer, through research and education.
Kelly Lindsay, Media Relations Contact

2074 **Leukemia Society of America: Mississippi Chapter**
408 Fontaine Place
Ridgeland, MS 39157
601-956-7447
877-538-5364
Fax: 601-956-6957
e-mail: Travis.Lee@lls.org
www.leukemia.org

Travis Lee, Campaign Director Team in Training
Natalie Michael, Campaign Director Team in Training

Missouri

2075 **American Cancer Society: Saint Louis**
4207 Lindell Boulevard
Saint Louis, MO 63108
314-286-8100
800-ACS-2345
Fax: 314-286-8160
TTY: 866-228-4327
e-mail: christine.winter@cancer.org
www.cancer.org

The American Cancer Society is the nationwide community-based voluntary health organization dedicated to eliminating cancer as a major health problem by preventing cancer, saving lives, and diminishing suffering from cancer, through research and education.
Christine Winter, Media Relations Contact

Montana

2076 **American Cancer Society: Montana**
3550 Mullan Road
Missoula, MT 59808
406-542-2191
800-ACS-2345
Fax: 406-327-0146
TTY: 866-228-4327
e-mail: jim.ryan@cancer.org
www.cancer.org

The American Cancer Society is the nationwide community-based voluntary health organization dedicated to eliminating cancer as a major health problem by preventing cancer, saving lives, and diminishing suffering from cancer, through research and education.
Jim Ryan, Media Relations Contact

Nebraska

2077 **American Cancer Society: Nebraska**
9850 Nicholas Street
Omaha, NE 68114
402-393-5800
800-ACS-2345
Fax: 402-393-7790
TTY: 866-228-4327
e-mail: mike.lefler@cancer.org
www.cancer.org

The American Cancer Society is the nationwide community-based voluntary health organization dedicated to eliminating cancer as a major health problem by preventing cancer, saving lives, and diminishing suffering from cancer, through research and education.
Mike Lefler, Media Relations Contact

2078 **Leukemia Society of America: Nebraska Chapter**
10832 Old Mill Road
Omaha, NE 68154
402-344-2242
888-847-4974
Fax: 402-344-2422
e-mail: pattie.gorham@lls.org
www.leukemia.org

Pattie Gorham, Executive Director
Tonya Schroeder, Patient Services Manager - Portland Area

Nevada

2079 **American Cancer Society: Nevada**
6165 S Rainbow Boulevard
Las Vegas, NV 89118
702-798-6877
800-ACS-2345
Fax: 702-798-0530
TTY: 866-228-4327
e-mail: paulette.anderson@cancer.org
www.cancer.org

The American Cancer Society is the nationwide community-based voluntary health organization dedicated to eliminating cancer as a major health problem by preventing cancer, saving lives, and diminishing suffering from cancer, through research and education.
Paulette Anderson, Media Relations Contact

New Hampshire

2080 **American Cancer Society: New Hampshire Gail Singer Memorial Building**
Gail Singer Memorial Building
2 Commerce Drive
Bedford, NH 03110
603-472-8899
800-ACS-2345
Fax: 603-472-7093
TTY: 866-228-4327
e-mail: peter.davies@cancer.org
www.cancer.org

The American Cancer Society is the nationwide community-based voluntary health organization dedicated to eliminating cancer as a major health problem by preventing cancer, saving lives, and diminishing suffering from cancer, through research and education.
Peter Davies, Media Relations Contact

2081 **New Hampshire Cancer Pain Initiative**
125 Airport Road
Concord, NH 03301
603-225-0900
e-mail: info@nhpain.org.
www.nhpain.org

Made up of concerned people who have joined together to promote the alleviation of cancer pain through education, research and advisory activities.

New Jersey

2082 **American Cancer Society: New Jersey**
2600 US Highway 1
N Brunswick, NJ 08902
732-297-8000
800-ACS-2345
Fax: 732-297-9043
TTY: 866-228-4327
e-mail: marjorie.kaplan@cancer.org
www.cancer.org

The American Cancer Society is the nationwide community-based voluntary health organization dedicated to eliminating cancer as a major health problem by preventing cancer, saving lives, and diminishing suffering from cancer, through research and education.
Marjorie Kaplan, Media Relations Contact

2083 **Leukemia Society of America: Northern New Jersey Chapter**
Leukemia Society of America
116 South Euclid Avenue
Westfield, NJ 07090
908-654-9445
Fax: 908-654-9496
www.leukemia.org

Dedicated to finding cures for leukemia and related cancers and to improving the quality of life for patients and their families.

2084 **Leukemia Society of America: Southern New Jersey Chapter**
Leukemia Society of America
216 Haddon Avenue
Westmont, NJ 08108-2811
856-869-0200
888-920-8557
Fax: 856-869-7383
www.leukemia.org

Dedicated to finding cures for leukemia and related cancers and to improving the quality of life for patients and their families.

New Mexico

2085 American Cancer Society: New Mexico
10501 Montgomery Boulevard NE 505-260-2105
Albuquerque, NM 87111 800-ACS-2345
Fax: 505-266-9513
TTY: 866-228-4327
e-mail: john.weisgerber@cancer.org
www.cancer.org
The American Cancer Society is the nationwide community-based voluntary health organization dedicated to eliminating cancer as a major health problem by preventing cancer, saving lives, and diminishing suffering from cancer, through research and education.
John Weisgerber, Media Relations Contact

2086 Leukemia Society of America: Mountain States Chapter
Leukemia Society of America
3411 Candelaria NE 505-872-0141
Albuquerque, NM 87107 888-286-7846
Fax: 505-872-2480
www.leukemia.org
Dedicated to finding cures for leukemia and related cancers and to improving the quality of life for patients and their families. Serves New Mexico and the Greater El Paso, TX area.
Deborah Hoffman, Executive Director
Mikki Aronoff, Patient Services Manager - Portland Area

New York

2087 American Cancer Society: Central New York Region/East Syracuse
6725 Lyons Street 315-437-7025
E Syracuse, NY 13057 800-ACS-2345
Fax: 315-437-8233
TTY: 866-228-4327
e-mail: kim.mcmahon@cancer.org
www.cancer.org
The American Cancer Society is the nationwide community-based voluntary health organization dedicated to eliminating cancer as a major health problem by preventing cancer, saving lives, and diminishing suffering from cancer, through research and education.
Kim McMahon, Media Relations Contact

2088 American Cancer Society: Long Island
75 Davids Drive 631-436-7070
Hauppauge, NY 11788 800-ACS-2345
Fax: 631-436-5380
TTY: 866-228-4327
e-mail: jennifer.cucurullo@cancer.org
www.cancer.org
The American Cancer Society is the nationwide community-based voluntary health organization dedicated to eliminating cancer as a major health problem by preventing cancer, saving lives, and diminishing suffering from cancer, through research and education.
Jennifer Cucurullo, Media Relations Contact

2089 American Cancer Society: New York City
132 W 32nd Street 212-586-8700
New York, NY 10001-3983 800-ACS-2345
Fax: 212-237-3855
TTY: 866-228-4327
e-mail: jennifer.cucurullo@cancer.org
www.cancer.org
The American Cancer Society is the nationwide community-based voluntary health organization dedicated to eliminating cancer as a major health problem by preventing cancer, saving lives, and diminishing suffering from cancer, through research and education.
Jennifer Cucurullo, Media Relations Contact

2090 American Cancer Society: Queens Region/Reg o Park
97-99 Queens Boulevard 718-263-2224
Rego Park, NY 11374 800-ACS-2345
Fax: 718-261-0758
TTY: 866-228-4327
e-mail: jennifer.cucurullo@cancer.org
www.cancer.org
The American Cancer Society is the nationwide community-based voluntary health organization dedicated to eliminating cancer as a major health problem by preventing cancer, saving lives, and diminishing suffering from cancer, through research and education.
Jennifer Cucurullo, Media Relations Contact

2091 American Cancer Society: Westchester Regio n/White Plains
2 Lyon Place 914-949-4800
White Plains, NY 10601 800-ACS-2345
Fax: 914-397-8851
TTY: 866-228-4327
e-mail: jennifer.cucurullo@cancer.org
www.cancer.org
The American Cancer Society is the nationwide community-based voluntary health organization dedicated to eliminating cancer as a major health problem by preventing cancer, saving lives, and diminishing suffering from cancer, through research and education.
Jennifer Cucurullo, Media Relations Contact

2092 Foundation for Advancement in Cancer Therapy
Old Chelsea Station
New York, NY 10113 212-741-2790
www.fact-ltd.org
Distributes information on cancer prevention and nontoxic therapies for cancer.
Ruth Sackman, President/Co-founder

2093 Leukemia & Lymphoma Society Chapter: New York City
475 Park Avenue S 212-376-7100
New York, NY 10016 800-955-4572
Fax: 212-448-9214
e-mail: ossom@lls.org
www.leukemia-lymphoma.org
Dedicated to finding cures for leukemia and related cancers and to improving the quality of life for patients and their families. Educational materials, support services and financial aid available. Volunteer opportunities.
Michael Osso, Executive Director
Sara Lipsky, Deputy Executive Director

2094 Leukemia Society of America: Westchester/Hudson Valley Chapter
Leukemia Society of America
1313 Mamaroneck Avenue 914-949-0084
White Plains, NY 10605 Fax: 914-949-0391
www.leukemia.org
Dedicated to finding cures for leukemia and related cancers and to improving the quality of life for patients and their families.

2095 Leukemia Society of America: Central New York Chapter
Leukemia Society of America
401 N Salina Street 315-471-1050
Syracuse, NY 13203 800-690-8944
Fax: 315-471-6434
e-mail: chip.lockwood@lls.org
www.leukemia.org
Dedicated to finding cures for leukemia and related cancers and to improving the quality of life for patients and their families.
Chip Lockwood, Executive Director
Kristen Duggleby, Campaign Director Donor Relations

2096 Leukemia Society of America: Long Island Chapter
Leukemia Society of America
555 Broadhollow Road 631-752-8500
Melville, NY 11747 Fax: 631-752-9066
e-mail: tammy.philie@lls.org
www.leukemia.org
Established to serve Long Islanders with leukemia, lymphoma, Hodgkin's disease and myeloma, their families and friends.
Tammy Philie, Executive Director
Nicole Kowaleski, Deputy Executive Director

2097 Leukemia Society of America: Upstate New York Chapter
Leukemia Society of America
5 Computer Drive W 518-438-3583
Albany, NY 12205 866-255-3583
Fax: 518-438-6431
e-mail: Maureen.Thornton@lls.org
www.leukemia.org

Dedicated to finding cures for leukemia and related cancers and to improving the quality of life for patients and their families.
Maureen O'Brien-Thor, Executive Director
Raechel Hunt, Patient Services Manager - Portland Area

2098 **Leukemia Society of America: Western New York & Finger Lakes Chapter**
Leukemia Society of America
4053 Maple Road
Amherst, NY 14226
716-834-2578
800-784-2368
Fax: 716-837-0335
e-mail: nancy.hails@lls.org
www.leukemia.org
Dedicated to finding cures for leukemia and related cancers and to improving the quality of life for patients and their families.
Nancy Hails, Executive Director
Luann Burgio, Deputy Executive Director

North Carolina

2099 **American Cancer Society: North Carolina**
8300 Health Park
Raleigh, NC 27615
919-334-5218
800-ACS-2345
Fax: 919-841-1422
TTY: 866-228-4327
e-mail: jbright@cancer.org
www.cancer.org
The American Cancer Society is the nationwide community-based voluntary health organization dedicated to eliminating cancer as a major health problem by preventing cancer, saving lives, and diminishing suffering from cancer, through research and education.
Jeff Bright, Media Relations Contact

2100 **Leukemia Society of America: Eastern North Carolina Chapter**
Flagship Building
401 Harrison Oaks Boulevard
Cary, NC 27513
919-677-3993
800-936-9337
Fax: 919-677-3992
e-mail: tiffany.armstrong@lls.org
www.leukemia.org
Tiffany Armstrong, Executive Director
Loreal Massiah, Patient Services Manager - Portland Area

2101 **Leukemia Society of America: North Carolina Chapter**
Leukemia Society of America
5950 Fairview Road
Charlotte, NC 28210
704-998-5012
800-888-9934
Fax: 704-998-5010
www.leukemia.org
Dedicated to finding cures for leukemia and related cancers and to improving the quality of life for patients and their families.

2102 **Leukemia Society of America: North Texas Leukemia Society of America**
5950 Fairview Road
Charlotte, NC 28210
704-998-5012
Fax: 704-998-5010
e-mail: jane.weaver@lls.org
www.leukemia.org
Dedicated to finding cures for leukemia and related cancers and to improving the quality of life for patients and their families.
Jane Weaver, Executive Director
Keri Norris, Office Manager

North Dakota

2103 **American Cancer Society: North Dakota**
4646 Amber Valley Parkway
Fargo, ND 58104
701-232-1385
800-ACS-2345
Fax: 701-232-1109
TTY: 866-228-4327
e-mail: jim.ryan@cancer.org
www.cancer.org
The American Cancer Society is the nationwide community-based voluntary health organization dedicated to eliminating cancer as a major health problem by preventing cancer, saving lives, and diminishing suffering from cancer, through research and education.
Jim Ryan, Media Relations Contact

Ohio

2104 **American Cancer Society: Ohio**
870 Michigan Avenue
Columbus, OH 43215
888-227-6446
Fax: 877-227-2838
TTY: 866-228-4327
e-mail: robert.paschen@cancer.org
www.cancer.org
The American Cancer Society is the nationwide community-based voluntary health organization dedicated to eliminating cancer as a major health problem by preventing cancer, saving lives, and diminishing suffering from cancer, through research and education.
Robert Paschen, Media Relations Contact

2105 **Leukemia Society of America: Central Ohio Chapter**
Leukemia Society of America
2225 City Gate Drive
Columbus, OH 43219
614-476-7194
800-686-CURE
Fax: 614-476-7189
e-mail: phil.tanner@lls.org
www.leukemia.org
Dedicated to finding cures for leukemia and related cancers and to improving the quality of life for patients and their families.
Phil Tanner, Executive Director
Dan Swisher, Office Manager

2106 **Leukemia Society of America: Northern Ohio Chapter**
Leukemia Society of America
23297 Commerce Park
Cleveland, OH 44122
216-910-1200
800-589-5721
Fax: 216-910-1201
e-mail: frank.canning@lls.org
www.leukemia.org
Dedicated to finding cures for leukemia and related cancers and to improving the quality of life for patients and their families.
Frank Canning, Field Director
Nancy Toghill, Office Manager

2107 **Leukemia Society of America: Southern Ohio Chapter**
Leukemia Society of America
2300 Wall Street
Cincinnati, OH 45212
513-361-2100
Fax: 513-361-2109
e-mail: michelle.steed@lls.org
www.leukemia.org
Dedicated to finding cures for leukemia and related cancers and to improving the quality of life for patients and their families. This chapter serves a 22-county geographic area.
Michelle Steed, Executive Director

Oklahoma

2108 **American Cancer Society: Oklahoma**
6525 N Meridian
Oklahoma City, OK 73116
405-843-9888
800-ACS-2345
Fax: 405-848-0795
TTY: 866-228-4327
e-mail: christina.lindholm@cancer.org
www.cancer.org
The American Cancer Society is the nationwide community-based voluntary health organization dedicated to eliminating cancer as a major health problem by preventing cancer, saving lives, and diminishing suffering from cancer, through research and education.
Christina Li (816-218-7171), Media/Public Relations

2109 **Leukemia Society of America: Oklahoma Chapter**
Leukemia Society of America
500 N Broadway
Oklahoma City, OK 73102
405-943-8888
888-828-4572
Fax: 405-943-8355
e-mail: sherry.martin@lls.org
www.leukemia.org
Dedicated to finding cures for leukemia and related cancers and to improving the quality of life for patients and their families.
Sherry Marti MSW LCSW, Patient Services Manager - Portland Area
Jill Hull, Campaign Director Team in Training

Oregon

2110 **American Cancer Society: Oregon**
0330 SW Curry Street
Portland, OR 97239
503-295-6422
800-ACS-2345
Fax: 503-228-1062
TTY: 866-228-4327
e-mail: gretchen.rosenberger@cancer.org
www.cancer.org

The American Cancer Society is the nationwide community-based voluntary health organization dedicated to eliminating cancer as a major health problem by preventing cancer, saving lives, and diminishing suffering from cancer, through research and education.
Gretchen Rosenberger, Media Relations Contact

2111 **Leukemia Society of America: Oregon Chapter**
Leukemia Society of America
9320 SWBarbur Boulevard
Portland, OR 97219
503-245-9866
800-466-6572
Fax: 503-245-9865
e-mail: Sarah.Varner@lls.org
www.leukemia.org

Dedicated to finding cures for leukemia and related cancers and to improving the quality of life for patients and their families.
Sarah Varner, Executive Director
Sue Sumpter, Patient Services Manager - Portland Area

Pennsylvania

2112 **American Cancer Society: Harrisburg Capital Area Unit**
Capital Area Unit
3211 N Front Street
Harrisburg, PA 17110
215-985-5336
888-227-5445
Fax: 717-231-5784
TTY: 866-228-4327
e-mail: john.held@cancer.org
www.cancer.org

The American Cancer Society is the nationwide community-based voluntary health organization dedicated to eliminating cancer as a major health problem by preventing cancer, saving lives, and diminishing suffering from cancer, through research and education.
Colleen Fitz (215-985-5357), Media Relations Contact
John Held, Media Relations Contact

2113 **American Cancer Society: Philadelphia**
1626 Locust Street
Philadelphia, PA 19103
215-985-5336
888-227-5445
Fax: 215-985-5406
TTY: 866-228-4327
e-mail: john.held@cancer.org
www.cancer.org

The American Cancer Society is the nationwide community-based voluntary health organization dedicated to eliminating cancer as a major health problem by preventing cancer, saving lives, and diminishing suffering from cancer, through research and education.
John Held, Media Relations Contact
Colleen Fitz 215-985-5357, Media/Public Relations

2114 **American Cancer Society: Pittsburgh**
320 Bilmar Drive
Pittsburgh, PA 15205
215-985-5336
888-227-5445
Fax: 412-919-1101
TTY: 866-228-4327
e-mail: dcatena@cancer.org
www.cancer.org

The American Cancer Society is the nationwide community-based voluntary health organization dedicated to eliminating cancer as a major health problem by preventing cancer, saving lives, and diminishing suffering from cancer, through research and education.
Dan Catena, Media Relations Contact

2115 **Leukemia Society of America: Central Pennsylvania Chapter**
800 Corporate Circle
Harrisburg, PA 17110
717-652-6520
800-822-2873
Fax: 717-652-8614
e-mail: beth.mihmet@lls.org
www.leukemia.org

Elizabeth Mihmet, Executive Director
Danielle Bubnis, Patient Services Manager

2116 **Leukemia Society of America: Eastern Pennsylvania Chapter**
555 N Lane
Conshohocken, PA 19428
610-238-0360
800-482-CURE
Fax: 484-530-0833
e-mail: ursula.raczak@lls.org
www.leukemia.org

Lydia Hernandez-Vele, Executive Director
Ursula Raczak, Deputy Executive Director

2117 **Leukemia Society of America: Western Pennsylvania/West Virginia Chapter**
Leukemia Society of America
333 E Carson Street
Pittsburgh, PA 15219-1439
412-395-2873
800-726-2873
Fax: 412-395-2888
e-mail: massaric@lls.org
www.leukemia.org

Tina Massari, Executive Director
Jeanne Caliguiri, Development Director

Rhode Island

2118 **American Cancer Society: Rhode Island**
931 Jefferson Boulevard
Warwick, RI 02886
401-722-8480
800-ACS-2345
Fax: 401-421-0535
TTY: 866-228-4327
e-mail: jim.beardsworth@cancer.org
www.cancer.org

The American Cancer Society is the nationwide community-based voluntary health organization dedicated to eliminating cancer as a major health problem by preventing cancer, saving lives, and diminishing suffering from cancer, through research and education.
Jim Beardsworth, Media Relations Contact

2119 **Leukemia Society of America: Rhode Island Chapter**
1150 Pontiac Avenue
Cranston, RI 02920
401-943-8888
Fax: 401-943-1377
e-mail: koconisb@lls.org
www.leukemia.org

Bill Koconis, Executive Director
Gloria Hincapie, Patient Services Manager

South Carolina

2120 **American Cancer Society: South Carolina**
128 Stonemark Lane
Columbia, SC 29210
803-750-1693
800-ACS-2345
Fax: 803-750-4000
TTY: 866-228-4327
e-mail: mjwardle@cancer.org
www.cancer.org

The American Cancer Society is the nationwide community-based voluntary health organization dedicated to eliminating cancer as a major health problem by preventing cancer, saving lives, and diminishing suffering from cancer, through research and education.
Mary Jane Wardle, Media Relations Contact

2121 **Leukemia Society of America: South Carolina Chapter**
1247 Lake Murray Boulevard
Irmo, SC 29063
803-749-4299
Fax: 803-749-4088
www.leukemia.org

2122 **Leukemia Society of America: South/West**
107 Westpark Boulevard
Columbia, SC 29210
803-731-4060
Fax: 803-731-4066
e-mail: paul.jeter@lls.org
www.leukemia.org

Paul Jeter, Executive Director
Cassandra Wineglass, Patient Services Manager

South Dakota

2123 **American Cancer Society: South Dakota**
4904 S Technopolis Drive
Sioux Falls, SD 57106
605-361-8277
800-ACS-2345
Fax: 605-361-8537
TTY: 866-228-4327
e-mail: charlotte.hofer@cancer.org
www.cancer.org

The American Cancer Society is the nationwide community-based voluntary health organization dedicated to eliminating cancer as a major health problem by preventing cancer, saving lives, and diminishing suffering from cancer, through research and education.
Charlotte Ho (605-376-3758), Media Relations Contact

Tennessee

2124 **American Cancer Society: Tennessee**
2000 Charlotte Avenue
Nashville, TN 37203
615-327-0991
800-ACS-2345
Fax: 615-341-7335
TTY: 866-228-4327
e-mail: brian.gillespie@cancer.org
www.cancer.org
The American Cancer Society is the nationwide community-based voluntary health organization dedicated to eliminating cancer as a major health problem by preventing cancer, saving lives, and diminishing suffering from cancer, through research and education.
Brian Gillespie, Media Relations Contact

2125 **Leukemia & Lymphoma Society: Tennessee Chapter**
404 BNA Drive
Nashville, TN 37217
615-331-2980
800-332-2980
Fax: 615-331-2941
e-mail: winslowm@tn.leukemia-lymphoma.org
www.leukemia-lymphoma.org
Founded in 1982 to better serve the needs of Tennesseans. Offers contribution funded community services, family support groups, free educational materials and financial assistance for those affected by leukemia, Hodgkin's disease, myeloma and lymphomas.
Colleen Grady, Executive Director
Mary Winslow, Patient Services Manager

Texas

2126 **American Cancer Society: Texas**
2433 Ridgepoint Drive
Austin, TX 78754
512-919-1800
800-ACS-2345
Fax: 512-919-1846
TTY: 866-228-4327
e-mail: justine.hall@cancer.org
www.cancer.org
The American Cancer Society is the nationwide community-based voluntary health organization dedicated to eliminating cancer as a major health problem by preventing cancer, saving lives, and diminishing suffering from cancer, through research and education.
Justin Hall, Media Relations Contact

2127 **Leukemia Society of America: North Texas Chapter**
Leukemia Society of America
8111 LBJ Freeway
Dallas, TX 75251
972-239-0959
800-800-6702
Fax: 972-239-0892
e-mail: Tina.Garcia@lls.org
www.leukemia.org
Dedicated to finding cures for leukemia and related cancers and to improving the quality of life for patients and their families.
Tina Garcia, Executive Director
Sarah Bayley, Donor Development Director

2128 **Leukemia Society of America: South/West Texas Chapter**
Leukemia Society of America
431 Isom Road
San Antonio, TX 78216-4170
210-377-1775
800-683-2458
Fax: 210-344-3717
www.leukemia.org
Dedicated to finding cures for leukemia and related cancers and to improving the quality of life for patients and their families.
Jon Walter, President/CEO
Jimmy Nangle, CFO

2129 **Leukemia Society of America: Texas Gulf Coast Chapter**
Leukemia Society of America
5005 Mitchelldale
Houston, TX 77092
713-680-8088
Fax: 713-683-9504
e-mail: BillieSue.Parris@lls.org
www.leukemia.org
Dedicated to finding cures for leukemia and related cancers and to improving the quality of life for patients and their families.
Billie Sue Parris, Executive Director
Jane Thompson, Office Manager

Utah

2130 **American Cancer Society: Utah**
941 E 3300 S
Salt Lake City, UT 84106
801-483-1500
800-ACS-2345
Fax: 801-483-1558
TTY: 866-228-4327
e-mail: patricia.monsoor@cancer.org
www.cancer.org
The American Cancer Society is the nationwide community-based voluntary health organization dedicated to eliminating cancer as a major health problem by preventing cancer, saving lives, and diminishing suffering from cancer, through research and education.
Patricia Monsoor, Media Relations Contact

Vermont

2131 **American Cancer Society: Vermont**
121 Connor Way
Williston, VT 05495
802-872-6300
800-ACS-2345
Fax: 802-872-6399
TTY: 866-228-4327
e-mail: chris.falk@cancer.org
www.cancer.org
The American Cancer Society is the nationwide community-based voluntary health organization dedicated to eliminating cancer as a major health problem by preventing cancer, saving lives, and diminishing suffering from cancer, through research and education.
Chris Falk, Media Relations Contact

Virginia

2132 **American Cancer Society: Virginia**
4240 Park Place Court
Glen Allen, VA 23060
804-527-3700
800-ACS-2345
Fax: 804-527-3797
TTY: 866-228-4327
e-mail: domenick.casuccio@cancer.org
www.cancer.org
The American Cancer Society is the nationwide community-based voluntary health organization dedicated to eliminating cancer as a major health problem by preventing cancer, saving lives, and diminishing suffering from cancer, through research and education.
Domenick Casuccio, Media Relations Contact

2133 **Arlin J Brown Information Center**
PO Box 251
540-752-9511
Fort Belvoir, VA 22060-0251
An information clearinghouse on types of cancer health methods and nontoxic cancer therapies.

2134 **Leukemia Society of America: National Capital Area Chapter**
Leukemia Society of America
5845 Richmond Highway
Alexandria, VA 22303
703-399-2900
Fax: 703-399-2901
e-mail: donna.mckelvey@lls.org
www.leukemia.org
Serves the greater Washington DC metropolitan area including Northern Virginia Prince George's and Montgomery counties.
Donna Mckelvey, Executive Director
Beth Rather Gorman, Deputy Executive Director

Washington

2135 **American Cancer Society: Washington**
728 134th Street SW
Everett, WA 98204
425-741-8949
Fax: 425-741-9638
e-mail: liz.lamb-ferro@cancer.org
www.cancer.org
The American Cancer Society is the nationwide community-based voluntary health organization dedicated to eliminating cancer as a major health problem by preventing cancer, saving lives, and diminishing suffering from cancer, through research and education.
Liz Lamb-Ferro, Media Relations Contact

2136 CanHelp
PO Box 1678
Livingston, NJ 07039
360-297-5221
800-364-2341
Fax: 888-800-0201
e-mail: joan@canhelp.com
www.canhelp.com

Offers reports for cancer patients on orthodox and alternative therapies.
Patrick M McGrady, Founder
Joan Runfola LCSW, Director/Founder

2137 Washington Leukemia and Lymphoma Society: Alaska Chapter
Leukemia Society of America
530 Dexter Avenue N
Seattle, WA 98109
206-628-0777
888-345-4572
Fax: 206-292-9791
e-mail: wachapter@lls.org
www.leukemia-lymphoma.org

Dedicated to finding cures for leukemia and related cancers and to improving the quality of life for patients and their families.
Anne Gillingham, Executive Director
Kimberly Conn, Deputy Executive Director

West Virginia

2138 American Cancer Society: West Virginia
301 RHL Boulevard
Charleston, WV 25309
304-746-9950
800-ACS-2345
Fax: 304-746-9962
TTY: 866-228-4327
e-mail: amy.wentz@cancer.org
www.cancer.org

The American Cancer Society is the nationwide community-based voluntary health organization dedicated to eliminating cancer as a major health problem by preventing cancer, saving lives, and diminishing suffering from cancer, through research and education.
Amy Wentz Berner, Media Relations Contact

Wisconsin

2139 American Cancer Society: Wisconsin
N19 W24350 Riverwood Drive
Waukesha, WI 53188
262-523-5500
800-ACS-2345
Fax: 262-523-5533
TTY: 866-228-4327
e-mail: peter.balistrieri@cancer.org
www.cancer.org

The American Cancer Society is the nationwide community-based voluntary health organization dedicated to eliminating cancer as a major health problem by preventing cancer, saving lives, and diminishing suffering from cancer, through research and education.
Peter Balistrieri, Media Relations Contact

2140 Leukemia Society of America: Wisconsin Chapter
Leukemia Society of America
200 S Executive Drive
Brookfield, WI 53005
262-790-4701
800-261-7399
Fax: 262-790-4706
e-mail: bede.barthpotter@lls.org
www.leukemia.org

Founded in 1963 to serve Wisconsites touched by leukemia, lymphoma, Hodgkin's disease and myeloma.
Bede Barth Potter, Executive Director
Karen Ropel, Deputy Executive Director

Wyoming

2141 American Cancer Society: Wyoming
333 S Beech Street
Casper, WY 82601
307-577-4892
800-ACS-2345
Fax: 307-234-0926
TTY: 866-228-4327
e-mail: joel.quevillon@cancer.org
www.cancer.org

The American Cancer Society is the nationwide community-based voluntary health organization dedicated to eliminating cancer as a major health problem by preventing cancer, saving lives, and diminishing suffering from cancer, through research and education.
Joel Quevillon, Media Relations Contact

Foundations

2142 Chemotherapy Foundation
183 Madison Avenue
New York, NY 10016
212-213-9292
Fax: 212-133-31
www.chemotheraphyfoundation.org

The Chemotherapy Foundation is dedicated to developing more effective methods of treatment for the control and cure of cancer. They provide educational materials and provide funds for innovative chemotherapy research, and sponsor professional and public educational symposia.
Shirley Cox, Executive Director

2143 Dermatology Foundation
1560 Sherman Avenue
Evanston, IL 60201-4808
847-328-2256
Fax: 847-328-0509
e-mail: dfgen@dermatologyfoundation.org
www.dermfnd.org

The Foundation focuses on funding research that will advance patient care, and help develop and retain tomorrow's teachers and clinical leaders in the specialty.
Sandra Rahn Benz, Executive Director

2144 National Children's Cancer Society
One South Memorial Drive
Saint Louis, MO 63102
314-241-1600
800-882-6227
Fax: 314-241-1996
e-mail: pbeck@children-cancer.org
www.children-cancer.org

Our mission is to improve the quality of life for children with cancer and their families worldwide. We serve as a financial, emotional, educational, and medical resource for those in need, at every stage of their illness and recovery. The NCCS provides direct financial assistance to families for expenses not covered by insurance during their treatment; including transportation, lodging, gas money, medical assistance, health insurance premiums, and phone cards.
Mark Slocomb, Chairman
Mark Stolze, President/CEO

Libraries & Resource Centers

2145 Cancer Federation
PO Box 1298
Banning, CA 92220
951-849-4325
Fax: 951-849-0156
e-mail: info@cancerfed.org
www.cancerfed.com

The Federation is a not-for-profit organization that provides information, counseling, educational materials and meetings for the cancer patients, their families and friends.
John Steinbacher, Executive Director

2146 Cancer Information Service
National Cancer Institute
6116 Executive Boulevard
Bethesda, MD 20892-8322
301-435-3848
800-422-6237
TTY: 800-332-8615
http://cis.nci.nih.gov/

The National Cancer Institute's Cancer Information Service is a national resource for information and education about cancer. The CIS provides the latest and most accurate cancer information to patients and their families, the public, and health professionals by talking with people one-on-one through its Telephone Service, working with organizations through its Partnership Program, participating in research efforts to find the best ways to help people.

2147 Patient Advocates for Advanced Cancer Treatments (PAACT)
PO Box 141695
Grand Rapids, MI 49514-1695
616-453-1477
Fax: 616-453-1846
e-mail: paact@paactusa.org
www.paactusa.org

Provides support and advocacy for prostate cancer patients, their families, and the general public at risk. Information relative to the advancements in the detection, diagnosis, evaluation, and treatment of prostate cancer. Information, referrals, phone help, conferences, newsletter.
Richard H. Profit, Jr., President

Research Centers

2148 Purdue Cancer Center Purdue University
Purdue University
201 S University Street 765-494-9129
W Lafayette, IN 47907-2064 Fax: 765-494-9193
e-mail: pccinfo@purdue.edu
www.cancer.purdue.edu
Provide a forum for 75 of Purdue's best and brightest scientists to collaborate across campus and nationwide to prevent cancer to ease its detection and to cure it.
Timothy Ratliff, Director
Andrea Gregory-Kreps, Operations Manager

Alabama

2149 Birmingham VA Medical Center: Research and Development
700 S 19th Street 205-933-8101
Birmingham, AL 35233 866-487-4243
Fax: 205-933-4484
www.birmingham.va.gov
An acute tertiary care facility with particularly strong programs in both medicine and surgery andÿserves as the primary referral center for the state. We provide health care services to eligible veterans in the VA Southeast Network .
John Kennedy, Acting Chief of Staff
Rica Lewis-Payton, Medical Center Director

2150 Breast Cancer Resource Foundation of Alabama
PO Box 531225 205-871-4653
Birmingham, AL 35253 Fax: 205-966-2376
e-mail: Jennifer.Galbreath@ccc.uab.edu
www.bcrfa.org
Dedicated to finding a cure for breast cancer.
Dianne Mooney, President
Jennifer Galbreath, Program Director

2151 University of Alabama At Birmingham Comprehensive Cancer Center
UAB Comprehensive Cancer Center
1802 6th Avenue S 205-975-8222
Birmingham, AL 35294-3300 800-UAB-0933
e-mail: josh.till@ccc.uab.edu
www3.ccc.uab.edu
The Center provides advanced cancer care research and education based on stringent peer-reviewed data.
Edward E Partridge, Director and Associate Director for Comm
Kirby I Bland, Deputy Director

Arizona

2152 Southwest Association for Education in Biomedical Research
PO Box 210101 520-621-3931
Tucson, AZ 85721-0101 Fax: 520-621-3355
e-mail: swaebr@ahsc.arizona.edu
www.swaebr.org
The mission of the Southwest Association for Education in Biomedical Research is to develop and implement a strong proactive campaign to educate school children as well as the general public in the vital role biomedical research plays in their everyday lives.
Charles Atkinson, President

2153 University of Arizona Cancer Center
1515 N Campbell Avenue
Tucson, AZ 85724-5024 520-694-2873
www.azcc.arizona.edu
Comprehensive cancer center for diagnosis treatment and prevention.
David S Alberts, Director

California

2154 Burnham Institute Cancer Center The Burnham Institute for Medical Resear
The Burnham Institute for Medical Research
10901 N Torrey Pines Road 858-646-3100
La Jolla, CA 92037 Fax: 858-646-3199
e-mail: info@burnham.org
www.burnham.org
Known for world-class capabilities in stem cell research and drug discovery technologies. Dedicated to revealing the fundamental molecular causes of disease and devising the innovative therapies of tomorrow.
Kristiina Vu MD PhD, Director
John Reed, President and Chief Executive Officer

2155 City of Hope Comprehensive Cancer Research Center
1500 E Duarte Road 626-256-4673
Duarte, CA 91010 800-256-4673
Fax: 626-930-5394
e-mail: tkronitis@coh.org
www.cityofhope.org
Excellence in biomedical research patient-centered medical care and community outreach.
Theodore G Krontiris MD, Director
Richard Jove, Deputy Director

2156 Geraldine Brush Cancer Research Institute California Pacific Medical Center
California Pacific Medical Center
2330 Clay Street
San Francisco, CA 94115 415-600-1728
www.cpmc.org
Warren S Browner, Director

2157 Ida and Joseph Friend Cancer Resource Center
1600 Divisadero Street 415-885-3693
San Francisco, CA 94143 Fax: 415-885-3701
e-mail: cancerresource@ucsfmedctr.org
www.cancer.ucsf.edu/crc
The Cancer Resource Center supports wellness and the healing process by providing patients and their loved ones with information emotional support and community resources. The CRC maintains a multimedia library provides access to specialized health databases and offers research assistance. We host diverse support groups and classes and direct people to other community resources. All CRC programs are free.
Frank Mccorm PhD, Director

2158 Jonsson Comprehensive Cancer Center University of California At Los Angeles
University of California At Los Angeles
8-684 Factor Building 310-825-5268
Los Angeles, CA 90095-1781 888-662-8252
Fax: 310-206-5553
e-mail: jcccinfo@mednet.ucla.edu
www.cancer.mednet.ucla.edu
UCLA's Jonsson Comprehensive Cancer Center (JCCC) has established an international reputation for developing new cancer therapies providing the best in experimental treatments and expertly guiding and training the next generation of medical researchers.
Judith Gasson, Director
James Economou, Executive Director

2159 Melanoma Research Foundation
170 Township Line Road
Hillsborough, NJ 08844 800-673-1290
Fax: 908-281-0937
e-mail: info@melanoma.org
www.melanoma.org
Founded in October 1996 by melanoma patients and their families to support research which will lead to cure for melanoma. Strictly a volunteer organization - not one person will receive compensation for his or her efforts.
Randy Lomax, Chairman

2160 Northern California Cancer Center
2201 Walnut Avenue 510-608-5000
Fremont, CA 94538-2334 800-511-2300
Fax: 510-608-5095
www.nccc.org
The North California Cancer Center is dedicated to understanding the causes prevention and detection of cancer and to improving the quality of life for individuals living with cancer.
Sally Glaser, Interim Executive Director
Rebecca Chekouras, Interim Development Director

2161 **Pediatric Cancer Research Laboratory Children's Hospital of Orange County**
Children's Hospital of Orange County
455 S Main Street
Orange, CA 92868-3874 714-997-3000
www.choc.org
CHOC is the first hospital devoted exclusively to caring for children in Orange County.
Dr Mitchell Cairo, Director

2162 **Rebecca and John Moores UCSD Cancer Center**
3855 Health Sciences Drive 585-534-7600
La Jolla, CA 92093-0658 Fax: 858-534-7628
e-mail: dedavis@ucsd.edu
www.cancer.ucsd.edu
One of the just 39 centers in the US to hold a National Cancer Institute designation as a Comprehensive Cancer Center. As such it ranks among the top centers in the nation conducting basic and clinical cancer research providing advanced patient care and serving the community through outreach and education programs.
John Alksne, Professor Surgery
Michael Andre, Adjunct Professor Radiology

2163 **Salk Institute Cancer Center Salk Institute for Biological Studies**
Salk Institute for Biological Studies
PO Box 85800 858-453-4100
San Diego, CA 92186-5800 Fax: 858-453-8534
e-mail: communications@salk.edu
www.salk.edu
The Cancer Center was established in 1970. It is one of only eight basic research cancer centers in the country designated by the National Cancer Institute. The center includes 22 faculty members 150 postdoctoral researchers 45 graduate students and 80 research assistants. It comprises about half of the research at the Salk Institute.
Walter Eckhart, Professor and Laboratory Head
William R Brody, President

2164 **Salk Institute for Biological Studies**
PO Box 85800 858-453-4100
San Diego, CA 92186-5800 Fax: 858-453-8534
e-mail: communications@salk.edu
www.salk.edu
Cellular and molecular biology research focusing mainly on cancer.
William R Brody, President
Marsha A Chandler, Executive Vice President

2165 **Santa Barbara Breast Cancer Institute**
5333 Hollister Avenue 805-964-8883
Santa Barbara, CA 93111-2341
Otto Sartorius, Director

2166 **Stanford University: Beckman Center for Molecular and Genetic Medicine**
School of Medicine, Department of Biochemistry
Beckman Center B400
Stanford, CA 94305 650-723-6161
cmgm.stanford.edu
Dr Paul Berg, Emeritus Professor Biochemistry
Robert Baldwin, Emeritus Faculty Academic Council Bioc

2167 **USC/Norris Comprehensive Cancer Center**
1441 Eastlake Avenue
Los Angeles, CA 90033-1048 323-865-3000
uscnorriscancer.usc.edu
Major regional and national resource for cancer research treatment prevention and education.
Peter A Jones, Director
Robert W Haile, Associate Director for Cause & Preventio

2168 **University of California Berkeley Cancer Research Laboratory**
447 Life Science Addition 510-642-4711
Berkeley, CA 94720-2751 Fax: 510-642-5741
e-mail: crl@berkeley.edu
biology.berkeley.edu/crl
Basic research with a special emphasis on mammary cancer and tumor immunotherapy.
Astar Winoto, Director
Judith Yee, Manager

2169 **University of California: Los Angeles Bone Marrow Transplantation Program**
200 UCLA Medical Plaza
Los Angeles, CA 90024 www.healthcare.ucla.edu/transplant
Treatment of leukemia and anemia.
David W Golde MD, Director

Colorado

2170 **AMC Cancer Research Center**
1600 Pierce Street 303-233-6501
Denver, CO 80214 800-321-1557
Fax: 303-239-3400
e-mail: contactus@amc.org
www.amc.org
Offers research activities publications meetings educational activities public services testing services community-based cancer control programs and knowledge of cancer mortality rates.
Carolyn Draper, Assistant to the Executive Director
Gail Eckhardt, Clinical Science

2171 **Colorado Cancer Research Program**
2253 S Oneida Street 303-777-2663
Denver, CO 80224 888-785-6789
Fax: 303-777-2642
e-mail: ccrp@co-cancerresearch.org
www.co-cancerresearch.org
A nonprofit community-based cancer program established to provide community hospitals and physicians access to a wide range of cancer research trials in order to provide their patients with greater options for the treatment control and prevention.
Jane Hajovsky, Executive Director
Eduardo Pajon, Principal Investigator

2172 **University of Colorado Cancer Center**
13001 E 17th Place 720-848-0300
Aurora, CO 80045 800-473-2288
Fax: 720-848-0360
e-mail: CancerCenter.Webmaster@uchsc.edu
www.uccc.info
UCCC consortium is the hub for cancer research in Colorado. With eight programs 17 shared core resources and nearly 400 members from three universities and six institutions UCCC is responsible for the majority of cancer research in the Rocky Mountain region.
Tim Byers, Interim Director
Anthony Elias, Associate Director for Clinical Research

Connecticut

2173 **Yale University Comprehensive Cancer Center**
333 Cedar Street 203-785-4095
New Haven, CT 06520-8028 866-925-3226
Fax: 203-785-4116
www.yalecancercenter.org
A National Cancer Institute designated comprehensive cancer center for over 30 years Yale Cancer Center is one of only 40 Centers in the nation and the only comprehensive center in Southern New England.
Richard Edelson, Director
Jose Costa, Deputy Director

District of Columbia

2174 **Georgetown University: Vincent T Lombardi Cancer Research Center**
3800 Reservoir Road NW
Washington, DC 20057 202-444-4000
lombardi.georgetown.edu
Established in 1970 the Lombardi Comprehensive Cancer Center is named for the legendary Green Bay Packers and Washington Redskins coach Vince Lombardi who was treated for cancer at Georgetown University Hospital.
Louis M Weiner, Director
Peter G Shields, Deputy Director

2175 Howard University Cancer Center
2041 Georgia Avenue NW 202-806-7697
Washington, DC 20060-0001 Fax: 202-462-8928
e-mail: ladams-campbell@howard.edu
cancer.howard.edu
Reduce the burden of cancer through research education and service with emphasis on the unique ethnic and cultural aspects of minority and underserved populations.
Lucile Adams-Campbel, Director
Wayne A I Frederick, Interim Director

Florida

2176 Rambaugh-Goodwin Institute for Cancer Research
1850 NW 69th Avenue 954-587-9020
Plantation, FL 33313 Fax: 954-587-6378
e-mail: info@rgicr.org
www.rgicr.org
RGI is committed to rapidly developing anti-cancer therapies in conjunction with industrial and academic partners using efficient models of cancer growth and metastasis with the aim of moving novel compounds to market in the shortest time possible.
Claire Thuning-Robin, Director

2177 UM/Sylvester Comprehensive Cancer Center
1475 NW 12th Avenue 305-243-1000
Miami, FL 33136 800-545-2292
www.sylvester.org
UMHC offers an outpatient clinic a 40-bed inpatient unit a comprehensive treatment unit the Mohs surgery center/dermatology clinic the Rosenfield GI Center a cardiology lab and clinic a radiology/imaging suite an interventional radiology clinic the Spine Institute clinics on-site laboratory and pharmacy the Courtelis Center for Psychosocial Oncology the Jill Selevan Chapel a cafeteria as well as administrative offices.
W Jarrard Goodwin, Director
Jess De Jesus, Executive Director

Georgia

2178 Emory University: Georgia Center for Cancer Statistics
Rollins School of Public Health
1462 Clifton Road NE 404-727-8700
Atlanta, GA 30322 Fax: 404-727-7261
e-mail: gccs@sph.emory.edu
www.sph.emory.edu/gccs
Serves as a cancer registry for five counties of metropolitan Atlanta and ten rural counties of central Georgia.
Raymond S Greenberg MD PhD, Director

2179 Emory University: Winship Cancer Institute
1365-C Clifton Road NE 404-778-1900
Atlanta, GA 30322 888-946-7447
www.cancer.emory.edu
A clinical cancer center coordinating basic and clinical cancer research.
Brian Leyland-Jones, Director
Paul W Doetsch, Deputy Directory for Basic Research

Hawaii

2180 Pacific Health Research Institute
700 Bishop Street 808-524-4411
Honolulu, HI 96813 Fax: 808-524-5559
e-mail: info@phrihawaii.org
www.phrihawaii.org
Located in Honolulu Hawaii Pacific Health Research Institute (PHRI) is the largest independent biomedical research institute in the state. Since its founding on 1960 as an independent not for profit 501(c)(3) research institute PHRI today has become a leader in biomedical research in the Pacific. Indeed its researchers are performing complex investigations aimed at conquering some of the most debilitating and lethal diseases that afflict humankind.
Bruce R Stevenson, Executive Director/CEO
Helen Petrovitch, Chair Department of Research

2181 University of Hawaii: Cancer Research Center
1236 Lauhala Street 808-586-3010
Honolulu, HI 96813 Fax: 808-586-3052
e-mail: cvogel@crch.hawaii.edu
www.crch.org
The mission of the Cancer Research Center of Hawaii is to reduce the burden of cancer through research education and service with an emphasis on the unique ethnic culture and environmental characteristics of Hawaii and the Pacific.
Carl-Wilhelm Vogel, Professor (Researcher)
Michele Carbone, Interim Cancer Center Director

Illinois

2182 Kellogg Cancer Care Center Evanston Hospital
Evanston Hospital
2650 Ridge Avenue 847-570-2000
Evanston, IL 60201 888-364-6400
www.enh.org
Integral unit of the Evanston Hospital this center researches treatment and diagnosis of cancer including phase 1 and phase 2 studies.
Janardan D Khandekar, Chairman Department of Medicine
Ying Wu, Research Associate

2183 Leukemia Research Foundation
3520 Lake Avenue 847-424-0600
Wilmette, IL 60091-8021 888-558-5385
Fax: 847-424-0606
e-mail: info@lrfmail.org
www.leukemia-research.org
To conquer leukemia lymphoma and myelodysplastic syndromes by funding research into their causes and cures and to enrich the quality of life of those touched by these diseases.
Kevin Radelet, Executive Director
Cindy Kane, Senior Director of Development

2184 Oncology Hematology Associates of Central Illinois
8940 N Wood Sage Road 309-243-3000
Peoria, IL 61615-7828 866-662-6564
www.ohaci.com
Research into cancer treatments.
Robert Cooper, Director
Paul A S Fishkin, Hematology Internal Medicine Medical O

2185 Robert H Lurie Comprehensive Cancer Center of Northwestern University
Galter Pavilion 675 N Street Clair 312-908-5250
Chicago, IL 60611 866-587-4322
e-mail: cancer@northwestern.edu
www.lurie.northwestern.edu
Lurie Cancer Center is a founding member of the National Comprehensive Cancer Network an exclusive alliance of 21 of the nation's leading cancer centers.
Steven T Rosen, Director
Leonidas Platanias, Deputy Director

2186 University of Chicago Cancer Research Center
5841 S Maryland Avenue 773-702-6180
Chicago, IL 60637 877-824-0600
e-mail: cancerresources@uccrc.org
uccrc.uchicago.edu
The University of Chicago Cancer Research Center (UCCRC) employs a wealth of intellectual technological and financial resources to pursue a comprehensive collaborative research program involving more than 200 renowned scientists and clinicians.
Mary Ellen Connellan, Executive Director
Justin Ullman, President

2187 University of Chicago: Clinical Nutrition Research Unit
5841 S Maryland Avenue
Chicago, IL 60637-1463 773-702-1000
www.uchicago.edu
Provide superior healthcare in a compassionate manner ever mindful of each patient's dignity and individuality.
Michael D Sitrin MD, Director
James L Madara, CEO

Indiana

2188 Mary Margaret Walther Program Walther Cancer Institute
Walther Cancer Institute
9292 N Meridian Street
Indianapolis, IN 46260
317-708-6101
Fax: 317-708-6102
e-mail: info@walther.org
www.walther.org

Focuses research on all types of cancer studies.
Leonard J Betley, Chairman
James E Ruckle, President/CEO

Iowa

2189 Iowa Oncology Research Association
300 E Locust
Des Moines, IA 50314-2501
515-244-7586
888-244-6061
Fax: 515-244-3037
e-mail: sherrijr@iora.org
www.iora.org

Clinical cancer studies and research.
Sherri Rickabaugh, Administrator
Becky Berrett, Research Assistants

2190 University of Iowa: Holden Comprehensive Cancer Center
UI Hospitals and Clinics
University of Iowa
Iowa City, IA 52242
319-353-8620
800-777-8442
Fax: 319-353-8988
e-mail: cancer-center@uiowa.edu
www.uihealthcare.com/depts/cancercenter

The Holden Cancer Center promotes interactive high-quality cancer research high-quality health care related to the prevention detection and treatment of cancer and educates cancer professionals and the citizens of Iowa about cancer.
John Buatti, Deputy Director for Clinical Care
George Weiner, Director

Kansas

2191 Kansas State University: Terry C Johnson Center for Basic Cancer Research
Center for Basic Cancer Research
1 Chalmers Hall
Manhattan, KS 66506
785-532-6705
Fax: 785-532-6707
e-mail: marcia@k-state.edu
www.k-state.edu/cancer.center

The mission of the Terry C. Johnson Center for Basic Cancer Research is to further the understanding of cancers by funding basic cancer research and supporting higher education training and public outreach.
Rob Denell, Director
S Keith Chapes, Associate Director

Kentucky

2192 Henry Vogt Cancer Research Institute James Graham Brown Cancer Center
James Graham Brown Cancer Center
529 S Jackson Street
Louisville, KY 40202
502-562-4158
866-530-5516
e-mail: info@ulh.org
www.louisville.edu/hsc/centers

The overall goal of the scientists in the Henry Vogt Cancer Research Institute is to study mechanisms relevant to tumor cell biology at the basic and translational level in order to provide insights that will contribute to the ultimate prevention and cure of malignant diseases.
Donald M Miller, Director
John W Eaton, Deputy Director

2193 Kentucky Cancer Program
2365 Harrodsburg Road
Lexington, KY 40504-3381
859-219-0772
Fax: 859-219-0548
e-mail: dka@kcp.uky.edu
www.kcp.uky.edu

The KCP provides a variety of cancer programs and services to health professionals the public patients and survivors.
Debra Armstong, Director
Diane Frasure, Administrative Associate

2194 University of Kentucky: Children Cancer Study Group
Markey Cancer Center
800 Rose Street
Lexington, KY 40536
859-257-4500
866-340-4488
Fax: 859-323-2074
www.mc.uky.edu/markey

Kentucky Children's Hospital is the only children's hospital in the region. Patients range in age from infants through adolescents and have a variety of illness and injuries.
Michael Karpf, Executive Vice President for Health Affa
Frank Butler, VP for Medical Center Operations

2195 University of Kentucky: Lucille Parker Markey Cancer Center
800 Rose Street
Lexington, KY 40536
859-247-4500
866-340-4488
Fax: 859-323-2074
www.mc.uky.edu/markey

The Markey Cancer Center mission is to eliminate the morbidity and mortality of cancer through a comprehensive program of research education clinical care and community outreach.
Alfred M Cohen MD FACS, Director
Michael Karpf, Executive Vice President for Health Affa

Louisiana

2196 Baton Rouge Regional Tumor Registry Mary Bird Perkins Cancer Center
Mary Bird Perkins Cancer Center
4950 Essen Lane
Baton Rouge, LA 70809
225-767-0847
Fax: 225-215-1215
www.marybird.org

The Louisiana Tumor Registry is composed of a central office and regional registries that collect and process cancer incidence data from the state's eight established geographic regions. These eight geographic areas are based on Louisiana's historic health districts.
Lori McCallum, Center Director
Richard A Lipsey, Chairman

2197 Tulane University Pulmonary Diseases Critical Care and Enviromental Medicine
School of Medicine
1430 Tulane Avenue
New Orleans, LA 70112
504-988-8600
800-588-5300
e-mail: cesteves@tulane.edu
www.som.tulane.edu/pulmdis/facilities

Provides state-of-the-art care to patients and teaching to trainees through several areas of academic excellence that include: Interstitial Lung Diseases; Asthma; Cystic Fibrosis; Sleep Disorders; Interventional Pulmonology; Lung Cancer; Smoking Cessation; Critical Care; and Environmental Medicine.
Charlene L Esteves, Executive Secretary
Sandy Ditta, Senior Research Administrator

Maryland

2198 Frederick Cancer Research Center
PO Box B
Frederick, MD 21702-1201
301-846-1000
Fax: 301-846-1108
web.ncifcrf.gov

Direct research into the causes treatment and prevention of cancer AIDS and related diseases.
Craig W Reynolds, Associate Director
Jo Anne Barb, Secretary

2199 Johns Hopkins University: Sydney Kimmel Comprehensive Cancer Center
The Harry and Jeanette Weinberg Buidling
401 N Broadway
Baltimore, MD 21231-0005
410-955-5222
www.hopkinskimmelcancercenter.org

Johns Hopkins Kimmel Cancer Center has active programs in clinical research laboratory research education community outreach and prevention and control.
William Nelson, Director
Roger Abounader, Assistant Professor of Neurology and Onc

2200 **National Foundation for Cancer Research National Foundation for Cancer Research**
National Foundation for Cancer Research
4600 E W Highway
Bethesda, MD 20814-3206
301-654-1250
800-321-2873
Fax: 301-654-5824
e-mail: info@nfcr.org
www.nfcr.org
NFCR promotes and facilitates collaboration among scientists to accelerate the pace of discovery from bench to bedside. NFCR is committed to Research for a Cure - cures for all types of cancers.
Sujuan Ba MD, COO
Franklin C Salisbury Jr, President

2201 **Warren Grant Magnuson Clinical Center**
National Institute of Health
9000 Rockville Pike
Bethesda, MD 20892
800-411-1222
Fax: 301-480-9793
TTY: 866-411-1010
e-mail: prpl@mail.cc.nih.gov
www.clinicalcenter.nih.gov
Established in 1953 as the research hospital of the National Institutes of Health. Designed so that patient care facilities are close to research laboratories so new findings of basic and clinical scientists can be quickly applied to the treatment of patients. Upon referral by physicians, patients are admitted to NIH clinical studies.
John Gallin, Director
David Henderson, Deputy Director for Clinical Care

Massachusetts

2202 **Boston University Cancer Research Center**
820 Harrison Avenue
Boston, MA 02118
617-638-8265
Fax: 617-638-6518
e-mail: sfenness@bu.edu
www.bumc.bu.edu/clinicaltrials
The Office of Clinical Research (OCR) was established on July 1 1998 to serve as the central focus for clinical research support conduct and training at Boston University Medical Center.
Douglas V Faller, Director
Salli Fennessey, Manager

2203 **Dana-Farber Institute: Department of Biostatistics and Computational Biology**
44 Binney Street
Boston, MA 02115
617-632-3012
Fax: 617-632-2444
e-mail: biostatistics@jimmy.harvard.edu
www.dana-farber.org
Integral unit of the Institute organized into laboratories of biostatistics computing and epidemiology.
Marvin Zelen, Researcher
David P Harrington, Chairman

2204 **Massachusetts Institute of Technology Center for Cancer Research**
MIT Center for Cancer
40 Ames Street
Cambridge, MA 02142
617-253-6403
Fax: 617-252-1891
e-mail: cancer@mit.edu
web.mit.edu/ccr
The mission of MIT Cancer Center is to apply tools of basic science and technology to determine how cancer is caused progresses and responds to treatment. Through this effort they have developed an increasingly complete understanding of the nature of cancer cells which has led directly to improved treatments for the disease.
Dr Tyler Jacks, Director
Dr Jaqueline Lees, Associate Director

2205 **Massachusetts Institute of Technology: Center for Cancer Research**
40 Ames Street
Cambridge, MA 02142
617-253-6403
Fax: 617-253-1891
e-mail: cancer@mit.edu
web.mit.edu/ccr
The Koch Institute includes over 40 laboratories and more than 500 researchers located at headquarters and across the MIT campus. Koch Institute will continue the CCR's tradition of scientific excellence while also seeking to directly promote innovative ways to diagnose monitor and treat cancer through advanced technology.
Tyler Jacks, Director
Dr Jaqueline Lees, Associate Director

Michigan

2206 **Gershenson Radiation Oncology Center Barbara Ann Karmanos Cancer Institute**
Barbara Ann Karmanos Cancer Institute
4100 John Road
Detroit, MI 48201
313-745-9191
800-527-6266
Fax: 313-745-2314
e-mail: info@karmanos.org
www.karmanos.org
Radiation therapy and cancer treatment and research.
Arthur T Porter MD, President

2207 **Meyer L Prentis Comprehensive Cancer Center of Metropolitan Detroit**
Barbara Ann Karmanos Cancer Institute
110 E Warren Avenue
Detroit, MI 48201
313-833-0715
Fax: 313-831-8714
www.karmanos.org

2208 **Meyer L Prentis Comprehensive Cancer Cente Barbara Ann Karmanos Cancer Institute**
110 E Warren Avenue
Detroit, MI 48201
313-833-0715
800-527-6266
Fax: 313-831-8714
e-mail: info@karmanos.org
www.karmanos.org

2209 **University of Michigan: Cancer Center Cancer Research Committee**
Cancer Research Committee
1500 E Medical Center Drive
Ann Arbor, MI 48109-094
734-764-0039
800-865-1125
Fax: 734-936-9582
www.cancer.med.umich.edu
The U-M Comprehensive Cancer Center provides its patients diagnostic treatment and support services in a collaborative environment focused on excellence in patient care.
Irwin J Goldstein, Associate Dean for Research
Max S Wicha, Director

2210 **Wayne State University Center for Molecular Medicine and Genetics**
Wayne State University School of Medicine
3127 Scott Hall
Detroit, MI 48201
313-577-5323
Fax: 313-577-5218
e-mail: info@genetics.wayne.edu
www.genetics.wayne.edu
Research focusing on human conditions such as cancer and neuromuscular disorders.
Lawrence I Grossman, Professor/Director
Jeffrey A Loeb, Associate Director

Minnesota

2211 **Mayo Comprehensive Cancer Center**
200 First Street SW
Rochester, MN 55905-0001
507-284-2511
Fax: 507-284-0161
TTY: 507-284-9786
www.mayo.edu
Scientists and physician investigators conduct wide-ranging research to improve patient care while training the next generation of medical scholars.
Denis Cortese, President/Chief Executive Officer
Robert A Rizza, Director

2212 **University of Minnesota Masonic Cancer Center**
Division of Oncology
420 Delaware Street SE
Minneapolis, MN 55455
612-624-8484
800-226-2376
Fax: 612-626-3069
e-mail: ccinfo@umn.edu
www.cancer.umn.edu
The Masonic Cancer Center fosters this mission by creating a collaborative research environment focused on the causes prevention

detection and treatment of cancer; applying that knowledge to improve quality of life for patients and survivors; and sharing its discoveries with other scientists students professionals and the community.
Philip Mcglave, Deputy Director
John Kersey, Founding Director Emeritus

Missouri

2213 Cancer Research Center
3501 Berrywood Drive 573-875-2255
Columbia, MO 65201 Fax: 873-443-1202
www.cancerresearchcenter.org
Not only does the Cancer Research Center offer research they also offer community outreach programs to educate church groups civic clubs and other organizations about their research and cancer prevention.
Abe Eisenstark, Research Director
Marnie Clark, Director

Nebraska

2214 Lincoln Cancer Center
4600 Valley Road 402-483-2827
Lincoln, NE 68510-4844 Fax: 402-483-4184
Barb Morton, Director

2215 University of Nebraska at Omaha Eppley Institute for Research in Cancer
University of Nebraska
987878 University of Nebraska Medic 402-559-4090
Omaha, NE 68198-6805 e-mail: hmmaurer@unmc.edu
www.unmc.edu/eppley
To improve the health of Nebraska through premier educational programs innovative research the highest quality patient care and outreach to underserved populations.
Harold M Maurer, Chancellor
Thomas H Rosenquist, Vice Chancellor

New Hampshire

2216 Cancer and Leukemia Group B
230 W Monroe 773-702-9171
Chicago, IL 60606 Fax: 312-345-0117
e-mail: marciak@uchicago.edu
www.calgb.org
Integral unit of the Institute specializing in leukemia research and prevention.
Marcia Kelly, Administrative Coordinator
Kathy Karas, Director Protocol Operations

2217 Norris Cotton Cancer Center Dartmouth-Hitchcock Medical Center
Dartmouth-Hitchcock Medical Center
One Medical Center Drive 603-653-9000
Lebanon, NH 03756 800-639-6918
Fax: 603-653-9003
e-mail: cancercenter@dartmouth.edu
www.cancer.dartmouth.edu
The Cancer Center provides a positive environment for treatment cure and recovery for patients with all forms of cancer.
Mark Israel MD, Director
Burton L Eisenberg, Deputy Director

New Jersey

2218 Melanoma Research Foundation
170 Township Line Road
Hillsborough, NJ 08844 800-673-1290
Fax: 908-281-0937
e-mail: info@melanoma.org
www.melanoma.org
Founded in October 1996 by melanoma patients and their families to support research which will lead to cure for melanoma. Strictly a volunteer organization - not one person will receive compensation for his or her efforts.
Randy Lomax, Chairman

New Mexico

2219 University of New Mexico Cancer Research and Treatment Center
University of New Mexico
900 Camino de Salud NE 505-272-4946
Albuquerque, NM 87131-0001 800-432-6806
Fax: 505-272-1465
www.cancer.unm.edu
One of the nation's 60 premier National Cancer Institute (NCI)-Designated Cancer Centers and we have been named one of "America's Best Cancer Hospitals" by U.S. News & World Report. UNM Cancer Center provides cancer diagnosis and treatment to over 40% of the adults and virtually all of the children diagnosed with cancer each year in New Mexico.
Cheryl Willman, Director/CEO
John A Trotter, Deputy EVP for Health Sciences

2220 University of New Mexico: Cancer Research and Treatment Center
900 Camino de Salud NE 505-272-4946
Albuquerque, NM 87131-5001 800-432-6806
Fax: 505-272-1465
www.cancer.unm.edu
One of the nation's 60 premier National Cancer Institute (NCI)-Designated Cancer Centers and we have been named one of "America's Best Cancer Hospitals" by U.S. News & World Report. UNM Cancer Center provides cancer diagnosis and treatment to over 40% of the adults and virtually all of the children diagnosed with cancer each year in New Mexico.
Cheryl Willman, Director/CEO
John A Trotter, Deputy EVP for Health Sciences

2221 University of New Mexico: Center for Non-Invasive Diagnosis
Mind Imaging Center/University of New Mexico
1101 Yale Boulevard NE 505-272-5774
Albuquerque, NM 87131-0001 Fax: 505-272-4056
www.hsc.unm.edu
Cardiology and cancer research.

2222 University of New Mexico: Center for Non-I Mind Imaging Center/University of New Me
1101 Yale Boulevard NE 505-272-5774
Albuquerque, NM 87131 Fax: 505-272-4056
hsc.unm.edu
Cardiology and cancer research.

New York

2223 Ackerman Institute for the Family
149 E 78th Street 212-879-4900
New York, NY 10075 Fax: 212-744-0206
e-mail: ackerman@ackerman.org
www.ackerman.org
Independent nonprofit research organization specializing in family therapy teaching and clinical services.
Lois Braverman, President/CEO
Evan Imber-B PhD, Director

2224 Albany Medical College Joint Center for Cancer and Blood Disorders
43 New Scotland Avenue 518-262-3125
Albany, NY 12208 877-AMC-8008
Fax: 518-262-3165
TTY: 518-262-1180
www.amc.edu
Offers research in the fields of cancer and blood disorders focusing on radiotherapy pathology and surgery.
Herbert Abbott, General Pediatric
Mitra Abessi, Internal Medicine

2225 Albert Einstein Cancer Center Albert Einstein College of Medicine
Albert Einstein College of Medicine
1300 Morris Park Avenue 718-430-2302
Bronx, NY 10461 Fax: 718-430-2000
e-mail: aecc@aecom.yu.edu
www.aecom.yu.edu/cancer

The goal of AECC is to foster basic clinical population-based and translational research that addresses all aspects of the cancer problem.
I David Goldman MD, Director
Richard Seither, Director of Administration

2226 Association for Research of Childhood Cancer
PO Box 251 716-681-4433
Buffalo, NY 14225-0251 e-mail: president@arocc.org
www.arocc.org
The Association was chartered by New York State in that year as a not-for-profit corporation whose primary purpose was to fund the major pediatric research centers in Western New York.
Larry Lorenz, Vice President
Anne O'Donnel, President

2227 Bassett Research Institute
One Atwell Road 607-547-3456
Cooperstown, NY 13326 800-227-7388
e-mail: research.institute@bassett.org
www.bassett.org
Research institute committed to seeking new information and new strategies for preventing detecting and treating disease.
Wiliiam F Streck MD, President/CEO

2228 Cancer Institute of Brooklyn
927 49th Street 718-972-5816
Brooklyn, NY 11219-2923 Fax: 718-972-8693
Jo-Ann Hertz, Executive Director

2229 Cancer Research Institute: New York
One Exchange Plaza 55 Broadway 212-688-7515
New York, NY 10006 800-992-2623
Fax: 212-832-9376
e-mail: info@cancerresearch.org
www.cancerresearch.org
The Cancer Research Institute is the world's only non-profit organization dedicated exclusively to the support and coordination ofÿlaboratory and clinical efforts that will lead to the immunological treatment control and prevention of cancer.
Jill O'Donnel-Tormey, Executive Director
Leslie Salter, Assistant to the Executive Director

2230 Columbia University Comprehensive Cancer Center
701 W 168th Street 212-305-4186
New York, NY 10032-2704 Fax: 212-305-6889
I Bernard Weinstein, Director

2231 Medical Foundation of Buffalo Hauptman-Woodward Medical Research Insti
Hauptman-Woodward Medical Research Institute
700 Ellicott Street 716-898-8600
Buffalo, NY 14203-1102 Fax: 716-898-8660
www.hwi.buffalo.edu
Nonprofit organization devoted to cancer research.
Herbert A Hauptman PhD, President/Nobel Laureate
Eaton E Lattman, Executive Director & CEO

2232 Memorial Sloan-Kettering Cancer Center
1275 York Avenue 212-639-2000
New York, NY 10065 800-525-2225
e-mail: publicaffairs@mskcc.org
www.mskcc.org
Sloan-Kettering Institute has endeavored to lead the way in basic science research oftentimes translating those advances into clinical treatments.
Harold Varmus, Lab Head
Thomas J Kelly, Director

2233 New York University Cancer Institute New York University Medical Center
New York University Medical Center
530 First Avenue 212-263-7300
New York, NY 10016 888-769-8633
Fax: 212-263-0715
www.nyucancerinstitute.org
The mission of the NYU Cancer Institute is to decrease and eliminate cancer as a significant health problem throughout New York the national and the world by developing and maintaining excellent programs in patient care research education and prevention.
William Carroll, Director
Lauren E Hackett, Executive Director of Administration

2234 Roswell Park Cancer Institute National Cancer Institute
National Cancer Institute
Elm & Carlton Streets 716-845-2300
Buffalo, NY 14263 877-275-7724
e-mail: askrpci@roswellpark.org
www.roswellpark.org
Roswell Park Cancer Institute has made fundamental contributions to reducing the cancer burden and has successfully maintained an exemplary leadership role in setting the national standards for cancer care research and education.
David Hohn MD, President/CEO
Jonathan Ada PharmD, Assistant Vice President / Chief of Pha

2235 State University of New York Health Science Center At Brooklyn
450 Clarkson Avenue
Brooklyn, NY 11203 718-270-1000
www.downstate.edu
Downstate includes Colleges of Medicine Nursing and Health Related Professions and a School of Graduate Studies as well as its own teaching hospital an M.P.H. Program and extensive research facilities.
John C LaRosa, President
John B Clark, Interim Chancellor

2236 University of Rochester: James P Wilmot Cancer Center
601 Elmwood Avenue 585-275-0842
Rochester, NY 14642 866-494-5668
Fax: 585-276-0158
www.stronghealth.com/services/cancer
To use education science and technology to improve health transforming the patient experience with fresh ideas and approaches steeped in disciplined science and delivered by health care professionals who innovate take intelligent risks and care about the lives they touch.
Richard I Fisher MD, Director

North Carolina

2237 Cancer Center of Wake Forest University at Bowman Gray School of Medicine
Wake Forest University School Of Medicine
Medical Center Boulevard 336-716-4264
Winston-Salem, NC 27157 800-446-2255
Fax: 336-716-9593
e-mail: medadmit@wfubmc.edu
www1.wfubmc.edu/cancer
Provide a superb education as well as personal support. Beyond the academic experiences offered at our medical school we encourage the development of our students as caring physicians dedicated to providing the very best care professionally and personally to all patients.
William B Applegate M D M P, Dean

2238 Duke Comprehensive Cancer Center
2424 Erwin Road 919-684-3377
Durham, NC 27705 888-ASK-DUKE
Fax: 919-684-5653
www.cancer.duke.edu
One of only 39 centers in the country designated by the National Cancer Institute (NCI) as a 'comprehensive cancer center ' Duke combines cutting-edge research with compassionate care. Our team of nationally recognized physicians and staff treat nearly 6 000 new patients per year giving them the extensive experience that yields better results. In fact U.S. News & World Report rates Duke #7 in the nation for cancer care and best in the Southeast.
H Kim Lyerly, Director
Anthony Means, Deputy Director

2239 University of North Carolina UNC Lineberger Comprehensive Cancer Center
School of Medicine
450 W Drive 919-966-3036
Chapel Hill, NC 27599-7295 Fax: 919-966-3015
e-mail: lccc@med.unc.edu
cancer.med.unc.edu

The Center provides multidisciplinary programs for most cancers giving patients the benefit of many medical specialists in one place often in one visit.
H Shelton Earp, Director
Michael O'Malley, Associate Director

Ohio

2240 **Case Western Reserve University: Ireland Cancer Center**
University Hospitals of Cleveland
11100 Euclid Avenue 216-844-3951
Cleveland, OH 44106 800-641-2422
www.uhhospitals.org/irelandcancer

2241 **Case Western Reserve University: Ireland C University Hospitals of Cleveland**
11100 Euclid Avenue 216-844-3951
Cleveland, OH 44106 800-641-2422
www.uhhospitals.org/irelandcancer
Information and support to patients, families and the public.

2242 **Children's Hospital Research Foundation**
700 Childrens Drive 614-722-2000
Columbus, OH 43205-2696 Fax: 614-722-5995
e-mail: CommunityLink@NationwideChildrens.org
www.nationwidechildrens.org
Offers research activities into Reye's Syndrome genetics and children's cancer chemotherapy.
Grant Morrow III, Medical Director
Steve Allen, Chief Executive Officer

2243 **Medical College of Toledo: Cancer Research Division**
Department of Pathology
3000 Arlington Avenue 419-383-3470
Toledo, OH 43614-2595 Fax: 419-383-6130
e-mail: utmc.webmaster@utoledo.edu
utmc.utoledo.edu
Researches into all aspects of cancer.
Jill Zyrek-Betts, Assistant Professor

2244 **Ohio State University Comprehensive Cancer Center**
Arthur G James Cancer Hospital
320 W 10th Avenue 614-293-7521
Columbus, OH 43210-1240 e-mail: michael.caligiuri@osumc.edu
www.osuccc.osu.edu
A national and international leader in researchÿwhich translates to high-quality patient care and educational programs for residents of Ohio and beyond.
Michael A Caligiuri M D, Director
John C Byrd, Associate Director

2245 **Ohio State University General Clinical Research Center**
The Ohio State University Davis Me 614-293-8750
Columbus, OH 43210 Fax: 614-293-3796
e-mail: william.malarkey@osumc.edu
www.crc.osu.edu
Provides facilities and financial support for inpatient and outpatient cancer research.
William Malaykey, Program Director
David Phillips, Administrative Director

2246 **The Cancer Prevention Institute**
601 W Riverview Avenue 937-227-9400
Dayton, OH 45406 877-274-4543
Fax: 937-293-7652
e-mail: info@pch-dayton.org
www.cancerpreventioninstitute.org
Nonprofit organization focusing research activities primarily on cancer prevention anti-cancer drugs early diagnosis of cancer and bone marrow toxicity. previously known as the Hipple Cancer Research Center.

Oklahoma

2247 **Natalie Warren Bryant Cancer Center St. Francis Hospital**
St. Francis Hospital
6600 S Yale Avenue 918-488-6688
Tulsa, OK 74136 e-mail: webadministrator@saintfrancis.com
www.saintfrancis.com/locations/nwbcc
Jake Henry Jr, President/Chief Executive Officer
Barry Steichen, Executive Vice President/Chief Administr

2248 **Oklahoma Medical Research Foundation Immunobiolgy & Cancer Research**
Oklahoma Medical Research Foundation
825 North East 13th Street 405-271-7430
Oklahoma City, OK 73104-5005 800-522-0211
Fax: 405-271-7016
www.omrf.ouhsc.edu
Paul W Kincade Ph.D, Program Head

2249 **Oklahoma Medical Research Foundation: Oklahoma Medical Research Foundation**
825 N E 13th Street 918-488-6688
Oklahoma City, OK 73104 Fax: 405-271-7016
e-mail: OMRF-President@omrf.org
www.omrf.ouhsc.edu
Conducting basic research to benefit society and integrity in research is essential to expanding our knowledge of the basic biological processes fundamental to life.
Paul W Kincade Ph D, Program Chair
Stephen M Prescott, President

2250 **Samuel Roberts Noble Foundation Biomedical Division**
Samuel Roberts Noble Foundation
2510 Sam Noble Parkway 580-223-5810
Ardmore, OK 73401 Fax: 580-224-6217
www.noble.org
One of the largest international offshore drilling contractors in the world.
Michael A Cawley, CEO/President
Wadell Altom, Senior Vice President /Agricultural Divi

Pennsylvania

2251 **Abramson Cancer Center of the University of Pennsylvania**
3535 Market Street
Philadelphia, PA 19104-4283 800-789-PENN
Fax: 215-349-5445
e-mail: craig@mail.med.upenn.edu
www.penncancer.com
National leader in cancer research patient care and education.
Craig B Thompson MD, Director
Caryn Lerman, Deputy Director

2252 **Allegheny Singer Research Institute West Penn Allegheny Health System**
West Penn Allegheny Health System
4800 Friendship Avenue 412-359-6896
Pittsburgh, PA 15224 866-680-0004
Fax: 412-359-8610
e-mail: tchakurd@wpahs.org
www.wpahs.org
Thomas Chakurda, Vice President Communications and Marke

2253 **Fox Chase Cancer Center**
333 Cottman Avenue 215-728-6900
Philadelphia, PA 19111-2497 888-369-2427
www.fccc.edu
Franklin Hoke, Assistant Vice President for Communicati
Diana Quattrone, Associate Director of Public Affairs

2254 **Temple University FELS Institute for Cancer Research**
School of Medicine
3420 N Broad Street 215-707-7000
Philadelphia, PA 19140 Fax: 215-707-7000
www.temple.edu/medicine
Policies and programs are oriented toward research and training in cancer-related basic biological and biochemical sciences with progressive extension into the areas of molecular developmental and chemical biology to advance knowledge of the etiology and pathogenesis of cancer. A major goal of the Institute is to utilize the advances made in basic science programs to develop novel targeted therapies for the treatment of cancer.
E Premkumar Reddy PhD, Director
Judith Danie (Litvin), Associate Professor Anatomy and Cell Bi

2255 University of Pittsburgh Cancer Institute
5150 Centre Avenue 412-647-2811
Pittsburgh, PA 15232 e-mail: PCI-INFO@upmc.edu
www.upci.upmc.edu
Since 1985 the UPCI has been committed to improving the understanding of how cancer develops; to characterizing new lifesaving approaches for cancer prevention detection diagnosis and treatment; and to educating future generations of scientists and clinicians.
Nancy E Davidson MD, Committee Chair
Ronald Herberman, Director Emeritus/ Senior Advisor

Rhode Island

2256 Brown University Division of Biology and Medicine
BioMed Research Admin, Brown Medical School
97 Waterman Street 401-863-3281
Providence, RI 02912-0001 Fax: 401-863-2660
bms.brown.edu
Interdisciplinary studies in biological and medical sciences including studies in health care problems and fields of research such as cancer and diabetes.
Pierre Gallleti, VP
Edward J Wing, Medicine / Biological Sciences

2257 Roger Williams Clinical Cancer Research Center
Roger Williams General Hospital
825 Chalkstone Avenue
Providence, RI 02908 401-456-2000
www.rwmc.com

2258 Roger Williams Clinical Cancer Research Ce Roger Williams General Hospital
825 Chalkstone Avenue
Providence, RI 02908 401-456-2000
www.rwmc.com
Provides the most advanced specialty care.

South Carolina

2259 Children's Center for Cancer and Blood Disorders
University of South Carolina School of Medicine
7 Richland Medical Park
Columbia, SC 29203 803-434-3503
www.palmettohealth.org
Joint clinical and basic research of juvenile cancer and blood disorders.

2260 Children's Center for Cancer and Blood Dis University of South Carolina School of M
7 Richland Medical Park 803-434-3503
Columbia, SC 29203 800-775-2287
www.palmettohealth.org
Joint clinical and basic research of juvenile cancer and blood disorders.

Tennessee

2261 St. Jude Children's Research Hospital
262 Danny Thomas Place 901-495-3300
Memphis, TN 38105 Fax: 901-495-4011
e-mail: donors@stjude.com
www.stjude.org
One of the world's premier pediatric cancer research centers.
Harvey J Cohen, Chair
William Evan PharmD, Director/CEO

2262 University of Tennessee Memphis: Cancer Center
N327 Van Vleet Building 3 N Dunlap 901-448-5150
Memphis, TN 38163-0001 Fax: 901-528-5033
Alvin M Mauer MD, Director

Texas

2263 Baylor University Bone Marrow Transplantation Research Center
Baylor Research Institute
3434 Live Oak Street
Dallas, TX 75204 214-820-2687
www.baylorhealth/com
Offers bone marrow transplantation research in leukemia studies.

2264 Baylor University Bone Marrow Transplantat Baylor Research Institute
3434 Live Oak Street 214-820-2687
Dallas, TX 75204 Fax: 800-922-9567
www.baylorhealth.edu
Offers bone marrow transplantation research in leukemia studies.

2265 Cancer Therapy and Research Center
7979 Wurzbach Road 210-450-1000
San Antonio, TX 78229 800-340-2872
www.ctrc.net
The mission of the Cancer Therapy & Research Center is to conquer cancer through research prevention and treatment.

2266 San Antonio Cancer Institute
7703 Floyd Curl Drive 210-567-2710
San Antonio, TX 78229 Fax: 210-567-2709
www.saci.uthsca.edu
Dr Tyler J Curiel, Director

2267 Southwest Foundation for Biomedical Research
PO Box 760549
San Antonio, TX 78245-0549 210-258-9400
www.sfbr.org
Advancing the health of our global community through innovative biomedical research.
John R Hurd, Chairman
Lewis J Moorman III, Vice-Chairman

2268 University of Texas: MD Anderson Cancer Center
1515 Holcombe Boulevard 713-792-6161
Houston, TX 77030-4009 800-392-1611
www.mdanderson.org
To eliminate cancer in Texas the nation and the world through outstanding programs that integrate patient care research and prevention and through education for undergraduate and graduate students trainees professionals employees and the public.
John Mendelsohn, President -Executive Committee
Raymond DuBois, Executive Vice President

2269 University of Texas: Medical Branch at Galveston Cancer Center
301 University Boulevard 409-772-1506
Galveston, TX 77555 Fax: 409-747-1938
TTY: 409-772-4200
e-mail: public.affairs@utmb.edu
www.utmb.edu
The mission of The University of Texas Medical Branch at Galveston is to provide scholarly teaching innovative scientific investigation and state-of-the-art patient care in a learning environment to better the health of society.
B Mark Evers, Director

Utah

2270 Brigham Young University Cancer Research Center
E181 Benson Science Building 801-422-3913
Provo, UT 84602 e-mail: cancer_research@byu.edu
cancerresearch.byu.edu
Provide a rigorous research training program for students.
Daniel L Simmons, Director
Merrill J Christensen, Board Member

2271 Huntsman Cancer Institute University of Utah School of Medicine
University of Utah School of Medicine
2000 Circle of Hope 801-585-0303
Salt Lake City, UT 84112 877-585-0303
Fax: 801-585-5886
e-mail: public.affairs@hci.utah.edu
www.huntsmancancer.org
Understand cancer from its beginnings to use that knowledge in the creation and improvement of cancer treatments to relieve the suffering of cancer patients and to provide education about cancer risk prevention and care.
Mary C Beckerle, Executive Director
Wallace Akerley, Senior Director of Clinical Research

Vermont

2272 **University of Vermont Cancer Center University of Vermont**
University of Vermont
E-213 Given Buildinge 802-656-4414
Burlington, VT 05405 877-540-4673
Fax: 802-656-8788
e-mail: vcc@uvm.edu
www.vermontcancer.org
Richard Branda, Interim Director
Marianne Baggs, Assistant to the Director

Virginia

2273 **Cancer Research Foundation of America**
1600 Duke Street 703-836-4412
Alexandria, VA 22314-3421 800-227-2732
Fax: 703-836-4413
e-mail: mmcleod@crfa.org
www.preventcancer.org
Prevention and early detection of cancer through research education and community outreach to all populations including children and the underserved.
Carolyn R Aldige, President and Founder
Marcia Myers Carlucci, Chairman

2274 **Virginia Commonwealth University: Massey Cancer Center**
401 College Street 804-828-0450
Richmond, VA 23298-5017 877-4MA-SSEY
Fax: 804-828-8453
e-mail: massey@vcu.edu
www.massey.vcu.edu
The mission of the University of Central Arkansas is to maintain the highest academic quality and to ensure that its programs remain current and responsive to the diverse needs of those it serves.
Gordon D Ginder MD, Director
Steven Grant MD, Associate Director

Washington

2275 **Fred Hutchinson Cancer Research Center**
1100 Fairview Avenue N 206-288-7222
Seattle, WA 98109-1024 800-804-8824
Fax: 206-288-1025
e-mail: hutchdoc@fhcrc.org
www.fhcrc.org
At Fred Hutchinson Cancer Research Center our interdisciplinary teams of world-renowned scientists and humanitarians work together to prevent diagnose and treat cancer HIV/AIDS and other diseases.
Lee Hartwell, Director/President
Mark Groudine, Executive Vice President and Deputy Dire

West Virginia

2276 **West Virginia University: Mary Babb Randolph Cancer Center**
Mary Babb Randolph Cancer Center Clinic
One Medical Center Drive 304-293-4500
Morgantown, WV 26506 877-427-2894
Fax: 304-598-4553
www.hsc.wvu.edu/mbrcc
Premier cancer facility with a national reputation of excellence in cancer treatment prevention and research.
Scot C Remick MD, Director

Wisconsin

2277 **Eastern Cooperative Oncology Group**
1818 Market Street 215-789-3645
Philadelphia, PA 19103 Fax: 267-256-5291
ecog.dfci.harvard.edu
Studies into cancer including biological response modifiers and cancer studies.

2278 **University of Wisconsin Paul P Carbone Comprehensive Cancer Center**
600 Highland Avenue 608-263-8600
Madison, WI 53792-6164 800-622-8922
Fax: 608-263-8613
e-mail: gxw@medicine.wisc.edu
www.cancer.wisc.edu
The University of Wisconsin Paul P. Carbone Comprehensive Cancer Center is the only comprehensive cancer center in Wisconsin as designated by the National Cancer Institute. An integral part of the UW School of Medicine and public Health this cancer center unites more than 250 physicians and scientists who work together in translating discoveries from research laboratories into new treatments that benefit cancer patients.
George Wildi MD, Director
Kelly Sitkin, Development Director

Support Groups & Hotlines

2279 **Alliance for Lung Cancer Advocacy Support and Education**
88 16th Street NW 202-463-2080
Washington, DC 20006 800-298-2436
e-mail: info@lungcanceralliance.org
www.lungcanceralliance.org
Dedicated solely to providing patient support and advocacy for people living with or at risk for the disease.
Laurie Fenton Ambrose, President/CEO

2280 **American Cancer Society: San Jose Prostate Cancer Support Group**
3369 Union Avenue
San Jose, CA 95124-2033 408-559-8553
www.cancer.org

2281 **American Foundation for Urologic Disease: Us Too Line**
1128 N Charles Street 301-727-2908
Baltimore, MD 21201-5506 800-828-7866
e-mail: admin@afud.org
www.afud.org
Provides information and referrals for family members, victims and other individuals concerned with prostate cancer.

2282 **American Institute for Cancer Research**
1759 R Street NW
Washington, DC 20009-2552 800-843-8114
Fax: 202-328-7226
www.aicr.org
Maryland Gentry, President

2283 **Cancer Information Service**
National Cancer Institute
Fhch 1100 Fairview Avenue North J24 206-667-4675
Seattle, WA 98109-1024 800-422-6237
Fax: 206-667-7792
TTY: 800-332-8615
www.cancer.gov
A nationwide phone service that answers questions from cancer patients and their families, health care professionals and the public. Information specialists can answer questions and provide booklets on all aspects of cancer. Spanish-speaking members are available during daytime hours.
Nancy Zbaren, Program Director

2284 **Cancer Support Community**
401 Laurel Street 415-929-7400
San Francisco, CA 94118-1909
Offers understanding, support and guidance to people with cancer and those who care about them.
Victoria Wells, Executive Director

2285 **Cancervive**
11636 Chayote Street 310-203-9232
Los Angeles, CA 90049 800-486-2873
Fax: 310-471-4618
e-mail: cancervive@aol.com
www.cancervive.org
This nonprofit organization helps cancer survivors deal with the challenges of life after cancer. They offer support groups and an

extensive library of educational materials for patients, survivors, family members and healthcare professionals.
Julie Brennglass MA/MFCC, Social Services Director
Clare Buie Chaney Ph.D/LPC, Support Group Facilitator

2286 **Center for Cancer Survival**
104 W Anapamu Street 805-962-6221
Santa Barbara, CA 93101-3126
Nonprofit, nonmedical outreach education program teaching specific emotional, mental and spiritual skills for survival on their journey of recovery from cancer.
Richard Sheldon, Founder

2287 **Collaborative Medicine Center**
10 Willow Street 415-383-3197
Mill Valley, CA 94941-2895
Not specifically a cancer treatment center but works with cancer patients by using a variety of supportive modalities. The emphasis at the center is on helping people learn to support and activate their own healing processes.
Martin L Rossman MD

2288 **Commonwealth Cancer Help Program**
451 Mesa Road 415-868-0970
Bolinas, CA 94924 Fax: 415-868-2230
e-mail: commonweal@commonweal.org
www.commonweal.org/programs/cancer-help/
An educational program designed to help participants reduce the stress of cancer, explore health habits, be with others experiencing the same difficulties and consider information on established and complementary therapeutic options.
Michael Lerner, President
Susan Braun, Executive Director

2289 **Corporate Angel Network**
One Loop Road 914-328-1313
White Plains, NY 10604-1215 866-328-1313
Fax: 914-328-3938
e-mail: info@corpangelnetwork.org
www.corpangelnetwork.org
A service which fills available space on corporate airplanes with cancer patients in need of transportation to recognized cancer treatment centers in the Continental U.S..
Peter H. Fleiss, Executive Director

2290 **Exceptional Cancer Patients/ECaP**
532 Jackson Park Drive 814-337-8192
Meadville, CT 16335 Fax: 814-337-0699
e-mail: info@ecap-online.org, info@mind-body.org
www.ecap-online.org/home.htm
The mission of EcaP/Exceptional Cancer Patients is to provide exceptional resources, comprehensive professional training programs and extraordinary interdisciplinary retreats that help people facing the challenges of cancer and other chronic illnesses discover their inner healing resources.
Bernie Siegal MD, Founder
Barry Bittman MD, Chief Executive Officer

2291 **Gilda's Club: Grand Rapids**
1806 Bridge Street NW 616-453-8300
Grand Rapids, MI 49504 Fax: 616-453-8355
e-mail: info@gildasclubgr.org
www.gildasclubgr.org/
Provides a place where people with cancer and their families can join with others to actively involve themselves in building social and emotional support as a supplement to regular medical care. Facility offers groups, lectures, workshops and social events in a conveniently located, non-residential home-like setting - free of charge and non-profit.
Leann Arkem, President/Chief Executive Officer

2292 **Gilda's Club: New York City**
502 Eigth Avenue 718-788-1600
Brooklyn, NY 11215 Fax: 718-788-0322
e-mail: info@gildasclubnyc.org
www.gildasclubnyc.org
Free cancer support community names for the late comedienne, Gilda Radner. It is a non-residential, home-like meeting leave place where people with every type of cancer and their families and friends join with others to build social and emotional support in living with cancer, whatever the outcome. The program is for men, women and children. Free of charge and non-profit, it offers support and networking groups, workshops, lectures, and social events plus Noogieland, program for children.
Robert Easton, Chairman of the Board
Migdalia Torres, Program Manager

2293 **Gilda's Club: Quad Cities**
4500 N Brady Street 319-326-7504
Davenport, IA 52806-4061 e-mail: gildasclub@qconline
www.qconline.com
Free, non-residential, social and emotional support community for men, women and children living with all types of cancer and for their families and friends.
Claudia Robinson, Director

2294 **Gilda's Club: South Florida**
119 Rose Drive 954-763-6776
Fort Lauderdale, FL 33316-1043 Fax: 954-763-6761
e-mail: barbara@gildasclubsouthflorida.org
www.gildasclubsouthflorida.org/
Free, non-residential, social and emotional support community for men, women and children living with all types of cancer and for their families and friends.
Barbara Wilson, President/Chief Executive Officer
Hilde Johnson, Director of Operations

2295 **I Can Cope**
American Cancer Society
1599 Clifton Road NE 404-320-3333
Atlanta, GA 30329-4250 800-227-2345
www.cancer.org
An educational program for people facing cancer, either personally, or as a friend or family caregiver. Helps dispel cancer myths by presenting straightforward facts and answers to your cancer-related questions

2296 **International Association of Cancer Victors and Friends**
7740 W Manchester Avenue 310-822-5032
Playa del Rey, CA 90293-8449 Fax: 310-822-4193
e-mail: IACUF@Inetworld.net
Offers reports and information on alternative therapies and recent cancer studies.
Ann Cinquina

2297 **JamesCare For Life Support Groups & Servic es**
Arthur James Cancer Hospital & Research Institute
300 West 10th Avenue 614-293-6428
Columbus, OH 43210 800-293-5066
Fax: 614-293-2565
e-mail: cancerinfo@jamesline.com
www.jamesline.com/
JamesCare for Life Cancer Support Groups and Services provides a wide range of resources and services to assist patients and families on their journey. This group offers support for patients and families to share experiences, express concerns, and learn more about the impact of cancer and available treatments.
Diana Blue MSW/LISW, Support Group Facilitator
Joyce Hendershott MSW/LISW, Support Group Facilitator

2298 **Look Good... Feel Better**
American Cancer Society
1599 Clifton Road NE 404-320-3333
Atlanta, GA 30329-4250 800-227-2345
A community-based, free, national service. Teaches female cancer patients beauty tips to look better and feel good about how they look during chemotherapy and radiation treatments

2299 **National Foundation for Cancer Research Hotline**
4600 E W Highway 301-654-1250
Bethesda, MD 20814 800-321-2873
Fax: 301-654-5824
www.nfcr.org/
Franklin Salisbury Jr, President

2300 **National Health Information Center**
PO Box 1133 310-565-4167
Washington, DC 20013 800-336-4797
Fax: 301-984-4256
e-mail: info@nhic.org
www.health.gov/nhic

Offers a nationwide information referral service, produces directories and resource guides.

2301 National Hospice Helpline
1700 Diagonal Road
Alexandria, VA 22314
703-837-1500
800-658-8898
Fax: 703-525-5762
e-mail: nhcpo_info@nhpco.org
www.nhpco.org
Offers more information on hospice in general and offers referrals to a hospice program in your area.
Scott Vickers, Director

2302 PDQ
National Cancer Institute
Building 31
Bethesda, MD 20892-0001
301-402-5874
www.cancer.gov
NCI's comprehensive cancer database. Contains peer-reviewed summaries on cancer treatment, screening, prevention, genetcis, and supportive care, and complementary and alternative medicine; a registry of more than 6,000 open and 17,000 closed cancer clinical trials from around the world; and a directory of professionals who provide genetics services
Mark Greene MD, Editor-in-Chief

2303 Reach to Recovery
American Cancer Society
1599 Clifton Road NE
Atlanta, GA 30329-4250
404-320-3333
800-227-2345
www.cancer.org
Provides support for people recentlry diagnosed with breast cancer; people facing a possible diagnosis of breast cancer; those interested in or who have undergone a lumpectomy or mastectomy; those considering breast reconstruction; those who have lymphedema; those who are undergoing or who have completed treatment such as chemotherapy and radiation therapy; people facing breast cancer recurrence or metastasis

2304 United Ostomy Associations of America Advocacy Hotline
United Ostomy Associations of America, Inc.
PO Box 66
Fairview, TN 37062-0066
800-826-0826
e-mail: info@uoaa.org
www.uoaa.org
A strong advocate for ostomy and alternative procedure patients. Answers questions ranging from employment issues to insurability. Avialable online through advocacy@uoaa.org
Ken Aukett, President

2305 Wainwright House Cancer Support Programs
260 Stuyvesant Avenue
Rye, NY 10580-3115
914-967-6080
Weeklong residential retreats offered four times a year to cancer patients. Retreats are devoted to cancer patient education, health promotion and stress management.
Richard Grossman, Program Director

2306 Women's Suffrage for Prostate Cancer Awareness
743 Caribou Court
Sunnyvale, CA 94087-4229
800-776-2262
e-mail: info@pcawomen.org
www.pcawomen.org
Women have banded together here to help people cope with the effects of prostate cancer on their lives and educate others about it. Members understand problems of patients and families and are here to support and educate.

Books

2307 3rd Opinion: International Directory to Complementary Therapy Centers
Avery Publishing Group
120 Old Broadway
New Hyde Park, NY 11040-5000
516-741-2155
Discusses over 300 alternative treatment cancer centers, educational centers, support groups and other research services.

2308 A Breast Cancer Journey: Your Personal Guidebook
American Cancer Society
1599 Clifton Road NE
Atlanta, GA 30329-4250
404-320-3333
800-227-2345
Helps women steer through the maze of information, empowering them to take control of their disease, treatment choices, health care team and life. Guidebook format encourages the reader to organize her information in a logical, easily accessible manner, record personal feelings and concerns and understand the details of practical matters such as paperwork and insurance, legal and sexual issues, side effects of treatment, and helping the entire family with support.
440 pages paperback
ISBN: 0-944235-20-4

2309 American Cancer Society Cancer Book
Doubleday & Company
666 5th Avenue
New York, NY 10103-0001
212-765-6500
www.randomhouse.com
Publishes 135 cancer organizations, centers, support services and various programs.

2310 American Cancer Society's Guide to Complementary/Alternative Cancer Methods
American Cancer Society
1599 Clifton Road NE
Atlanta, GA 30329-4250
404-320-3333
800-227-2345
Helps the public, the consumer and patients and their families understand what works, what's dangerous, and how best to evaluate the hundreds of claims that can be found on the internet and in the popular press. Each entry is researched and based on scientific evidence. Possible problems or complications are identified and clearly highlighted for easy reference. Covers a broad range, including herbs, vitamins, minerals, diet, manual healing and biological methods. Clear, understandable language.
464 pages hardcover
ISBN: 0-944235-20-4

2311 American Cancer Society's Guide to Pain Control
American Cancer Society
1599 Clifton Road NE
Atlanta, GA 30329-4250
404-320-3333
800-227-2345
Provides a wealth of information, including talking to your health care team about pain, understanding what pain is and where it comes from, current drug and non-drug treatments and dealing with the financial burden of pain treatment. Includes information on how to record, chart and rate pain, guidelines for pain management, a comprehensive list of medications and other methods of pain relief and an informative resource guide.
400 pages paperback
ISBN: 0-944235-20-4

2312 American Cancer Society's Healthy Eating Cookbook: A Celebration of Food...
American Cancer Society
1599 Clifton Road NE
Atlanta, GA 30329-4250
404-320-3333
800-227-2345
More than 200 pages of irresistable recipes that turn healthy eating into a celebration of good food. Features photos and recipes from a host of the American Cancer Society's celebrity friends and fans. Includes hundreds of recipes, celebrity photos and essays, a handy Smart Substitution reference section and numerous tips for healthy cooking, including smart shopping, using leftovers and eating out.
216 pages hardcover
ISBN: 0-944235-20-4

2313 Bowel Cancer
Oxford University Press
2001 Evans Road
Cary, NC 27513-2010
212-726-6000
800-451-7556
Fax: 919-677-1303
www.oup-usa.org
Offers information and public awareness on the disease of bowel cancer.
152 pages

2314 Breast Cancer
Brandén Publishing Company

17 Station Street
Brookline Village, MA 02147
617-734-2045
Fax: 617-734-2046
www.branden.com

Paperback
ISBN: 0-828319-49-9

2315 **Cancer Dictionary**
Facts on File
11 Penn Plaza
New York, NY 10001
212-967-8800
800-322-8755
Fax: 800-678-3633

352 pages Paperback

2316 **Cancer Facts and Figures**
American Cancer Society
1599 Clifton Road NE
Atlanta, GA 30329-4250
404-320-3333
800-227-2345
Publishes over 57 treatment centers.

2317 **Cancer Rates and Risks**
National Cancer Institute
Building 31
Bethesda, MD 20892-0001
800-422-6237
This book is a compact guide to statistics, risk factors, and risks for major cancer sites.
136 pages

2318 **Cancer Sourcebook**
Karen Bellenir, author
Omnigraphics
Penobscot Building
Detroit, MI 48226-4105
313-961-1340
800-234-1340
Fax: 800-875-1340
www.omnigraphics.com/
Offers basic information on cancer types, symptoms, diagnostic methods, and treatments. Includes statistics on cancer occurrences worldwide and the risks associated with known carcinogens and activities.
2003 1119 pages
ISBN: 0-780806-33-6

2319 **Cancer Therapy: Ind. Consumer's Guide to Non-Toxic Treatment & Prevention**
Ralph W. Moss, author
Equinox Press
Cancer Decisions
Lemont, PA 16851
814-238-3367
800-980-1234
Fax: 814-238-5865
www.cancerdecisions.com
A must for cancer patients and their families who want: Practical information on the most promising non-toxic treatments; Scientific evidence in readable language; Well-documented resource lists and medical references.
523 pages
ISBN: 1-881025-06-3

2320 **Cancer in the Family: Helping Children Cope with a Parent's Illness**
American Cancer Society
1599 Clifton Road NE
Atlanta, GA 30329-4250
404-320-3333
800-227-2345
A diagnosis of cancer changes a family forever. Ordinary responsibilities become more demanding, and parents sometimes need assistance in balancing all of their children's needs. This book outlines steps to take to help children understand what happens when a parent has been diagnosed with cancer. Offers suggestions for talking to children, helping them cope, answering difficult questions, managing role changes and disruptions in routines, recognizing signs that your child needs help.
272 pages paperback
ISBN: 0-944235-20-4

2321 **Caregiving: A Step-By-Step Resource for Caring for the Person w/Cancer at Home**
American Cancer Society
1599 Clifton Road NE
Atlanta, GA 30329-4250
404-320-3333
800-227-2345
This practical guide offers manageable solutions to the myriad conditions and situations the caregiver may face, from physical to emotional conditions and dealing with health care providers and insurance carriers, to taking care of his or her own needs as well as those of the patient. East to use, this handy reference offers thorough, concise check-lists, questions to ask, signs and symptoms to note, and where to turn for more help.
336 pages paperback
ISBN: 0-944235-20-4

2322 **Celebrate! Healthy Entertaining for Any Occasion**
American Cancer Society
1599 Clifton Road NE
Atlanta, GA 30329-4250
404-320-3333
800-227-2345
You can celebrate in style without taking a break from healthy eating or delicious food. This book combines 20 festive, fun theme menus with easy recipes that don't sacrifice taste. Each menu offers a combination of approximately 8 manageable recipes, including appetizers, main dishes, side dishes, desserts and even beverages. Activities and decorating ideas in each section help make entertaining a breeze.
272 pages paperback
ISBN: 0-944235-20-4

2323 **Choices: Realistic Alternatives in Cancer Treatment**
Harper Collins
Avenue of the Americas
New York, NY 10019
800-331-3761
Fax: 800-822-4090
Covers a wide gamut of information that includes treatment centers, associations, research groups, and other facilities that are equipped to assist cancer patients and their families.

2324 **Colorectal Cancer: A Compassionate Resource for Patients and Their Families**
American Cancer Society
1599 Clifton Road NE
Atlanta, GA 30329-4250
404-320-3333
800-227-2345
Addresses the full range of issues that colorectal cancer patients and their families may face- from what to do when confronted with a diagnosis to the latest medical data, treatment and procedures. Describes the process of the digestive system and the organs involved when the body is affected by colorectal cancer. Dietary factors for preventing colorectal cancer are explained and information about surgery, chemotherapy and radiation treatment follows. Includes easy recipes and a diet plan.
290 pages paperback
ISBN: 0-944235-20-4

2325 **Consumer's Guide to Cancer Drugs**
American Cancer Society
1599 Clifton Road NE
Atlanta, GA 30329-4250
404-320-3333
800-227-2345
Created for patients, cancer survivors and caregivers. Provides detailed information for the more than 200 medicines used to treat cancer or the symptoms of cancer. Drugs are listed alphabetically by generic name and described in depth. Detailed descriptions include common side effects, precautions and other important facts. All generic and trade names are listed in the index for easy cross-reference. Easy-to-understand language.
448 pages paperback
ISBN: 0-944235-20-4

2326 **Coping: A Young Woman's Guide to Breast Cancer Prevention**
Rosen Publishing Group
29 E 21st Street
New York, NY 10010
212-777-3017
800-237-9932
Fax: 888-436-4643
e-mail: customerservice@rosenpub.com
www.rosenpublishing.com
Breast cancer research has revealed the genetic predisposition of some cancers. This guide explains the nature of cancer, the risk of cancer and the ways to reduce that risk, especially for young women with a family history of breast cancer.

ISBN: 0-825929-67-1

2327 **Everyone's Guide to Cancer Therapy**
Andrews McMeel Publishing, LLC

c/o Simon & Schuster, Inc.
Riverside, NJ 08075 800-943-9839
Fax: 800-943-9831
e-mail: MPrzybylski@amuniversal.com
www.andrewsmcmeel.com

How cancer is diagnosed, treated, and managed day to day.
2002 960 pages Paperback
ISBN: 0-740718-56-8

2328 **Health Consequences of Smoking: Cancer & Chronic Lung Disease in the Workplace**
DIANE Publishing Company
330 Pusey Avenue, Unit #3 Rear 610-461-6200
Darby, PA 19023 800-782-3833
Fax: 610-461-6130
e-mail: dianepublishing@gmail.com
www.dianepublishing.net

Examines the relationship between cigarette smoking and occupational exposures. Establishes that in order to protect the workers fully, forces of labor, management, insurers and government must become as engaged in attempts to reduce the prevalence of cigarette smoking as they are in occupational exposure. Tables and figure. Extensive bibliography, index.
542 pages Paperback
ISBN: 0-788123-11-4
Herman Baron, Publisher

2329 **Healthy and Hearty Diabetic Cooking**
Diabetes Self-Management Books
PO Box 11477
Des Moines, IA 50381-0001 800-664-9269
James Hazlett, Editor
Melissa Glim, Associate Editor

2330 **Home Care Guide for Cancer**
John's Hopkins University Press
2715 N Charles Street 410-516-6900
Baltimore, MD 21218-4319 800-537-5487
Fax: 410-516-6998
www.press.jhu.edu

This easy to use workbook was designed for home caregivers, patients, support groups and education programs; it features easy to read type and index for quick reference and advice on twenty common cancer caregiving problems.
1996 260 pages Paperback
ISBN: 0-943126-30-4

2331 **I Choose to Fight: Tom Harper's Courageous Victory Over Cancer**
Prentice Hall
15 Columbus Circle
New York, NY 10023-7707 212-373-8000
www.prenhall.com

A semi, auto-biographical account of Tom Harper's ordeal with testicular cancer, an afflication in young men.

2332 **Informed Decisions: The Complete Book of Cancer Diagnosis, Treatment and Recovery**
American Cancer Society
1599 Clifton Road NE 404-320-3333
Atlanta, GA 30329-4250 800-227-2345

Offers the latest information on every aspect of cancer, from detection to recovery. Covers everything from cancer causes and risk, screening and diagnotic tests, and treatment strategies to coping tips and questions to ask your doctor. Includes tips on how to effectively deal with the system and get the most advanced care in the country. Helps cancer patients and families make the right kinds of decisions- decisions that suit your particular needs and desires, and help you feel in control.
690 pages hardcover
ISBN: 0-944235-20-4

2333 **Kid's 1st Cookbook: Delicious-Nutritious Treats to Make Yourself**
American Cancer Society
1599 Clifton Road NE 404-320-3333
Atlanta, GA 30329-4250 800-227-2345

Do creepy spiders, sloppy dogs and tornado swirls sound edible to you? They will to kids. Inside this beautifully illustrated hardcover edition are activities, colorful recipes and cooking tips that will turn meal preparation into exciting family fun. Kids of all ages can take charge, don a chef's hat and create delicious and nutricious snacks and dishes for every meal.
96 pages hardcover
ISBN: 0-944235-20-4

2334 **Love Knot**
Jones & Bartlett Publishers
40 Tall Pine Drive 978-443-5000
Sudbury, MA 01776 800-832-0034
Fax: 978-443-8000
e-mail: aberry@jbpub.com
www.jbpub.com

232 pages Paperback
ISBN: 0-763714-12-7
Joy Stark, Associate Marketing Manager

2335 **My Prostate and Me: Dealing with Prostate Cancer**
Addison Books
2719 Houston Avenue
Houston, TX 77009-7607 800-829-9653

2336 **National Cancer Institute Fact Book**
National Cancer Institute
Building 31
Bethesda, MD 20892-0001 800-422-6237

This book presents general information about the National Cancer Institute including budget data, grants and contracts and historical information.

2337 **No Less a Woman**
Firestone Touchstone Paperbacks/Simon & Schuster
200 Old Tappan Road
Old Tappan, NJ 07675-7005 800-999-5479

Offers intimate interviews that explore the major issues of coping and surviving breast cancer, from diagnosis and treatment to physical and psychological recovery. In their own words, ten women describe how they successfully adjusted to the changes in their bodies and their feelings about themselves.
288 pages
ISBN: 0-671868-99-3

2338 **Organizing and Maintaining Support Groups for Parents**
Candlelighters' Childhood Cancer Foundation
7910 Woodmont Avenue 301-657-8401
Bethesda, MD 20814-3015 800-366-2223

Benefits of self-help support groups, activities, referral systems and parent/professional relations.

2339 **Prostate Cancer: A Survivor's Guide**
Don Kaltenbach and Tim Richards, author
Dattoli Cancer Foundation
2803 Fruitville Road 941-365-5599
Sarasota, FL 24237 800-915-1001
Fax: 941-366-3786
e-mail: info@dattolifoundation.org
www.dattolifoundation.org

Written with the aid of leading prostate cancer specialists, this book clearly explains tests, the latest statistics and how to interpret them.
updated 2003 256 pages
ISBN: 0-964008-89-0

2340 **Prostate Cancer: What Every Man and His Family Needs to Know**
American Cancer Society
1599 Clifton Road NE 404-320-3333
Atlanta, GA 30329-4250 800-227-2345

Written by a team of internationally known and respected medical experts, this newly revised edition explains everything a man needs to know about prostate cancer, the most common form of cancer (excluding skin cancer) among American men.
322 pages paperback
ISBN: 0-944235-20-4

2341 **Prostate Health Workbook**
Newton Malerman, author
Hunter House Publishing

PO Box 2194
Alameda, CA 94501
510-865-5282
800-266-5592
Fax: 510-865-4295
e-mail: ordering@hunterhouse.com
www.hunterhouse.com

A practical guide for the prostate cancer patients.
2002 160 pages Paperback
Cristina Sverdrup, Customer Service Manager

2342 **Singing from the Soul**
Bone Marrow Foundation
981 1st Avenue
New York, NY 10022-5102
212-838-3029
800-365-1336
e-mail: thebmf@aol.com
www.bonemarrow.org

Jose Carreras' autobiography describes in eloquent detail his bone marrow transplant experience.

2343 **Teratologies: A Cultural Study of Cancer**
Routledge
270 Madison Avenue
New York, NY 10016
212-216-7800
Fax: 212-563-2269
www.routledge.com

A distinctively feminist look at how cancer is perceived, experienced and theorized in contemporary society. Beginning with powerful personal accounts of her own illness, as well as self-help manuals and patients' personal stories, Jackie Stacey explores changing beliefs about the causes and treatments of cancer in both biomedecine and its increasingly popular alternative counterparts.
304 pages

2344 **The Mountain You've Climbed: A Parent's Guide to Childhood Cancer Survivorship**
1015 Locust Street
Saint Louis, MO 63101
314-241-1600
Fax: 314-241-1996
e-mail: krudd@children-cancer.org
www.nationalchildrenscancersociety.org

This guide is designed to answer parent's questions regarding childhood cancer, address issues related to diagnosis and offer suggestions on how to integrate the cancer experience into all areas of the family's life. It addresses issues beginning from the time of diagnosis through the completion of treatment and beyond.
Mark Slocomb, Chairman
Mark Stolze, President/CEO

2345 **Understanding Breast Cancer Genetics**
Barbara T Zimmerman, PhD, author
University Press of Mississippi
3825 Ridgewood Road
Jackson, MS 39211-6492
601-432-6205
Fax: 601-432-6217
e-mail: kburgess@ihl.state.ms.us
www.upress.state.ms.us

Clinical explanations for the genetic causes of the disease women most greatly fear.
2004 128 pages Paperback
ISBN: 1-578065-79-8
Kathy Burgess, Advertising/Marketing Services Manager

2346 **Understanding Cancer Therapies**
Helen S L Chan, MD, author
University Press of Mississippi
3825 Ridgewood Road
Jackson, MS 39211-6492
601-432-6205
Fax: 601-432-6217
e-mail: kburgess@ihl.state.ms.us
www.upress.state.ms.us

A practical and hopeful guide to the many treatments available.
2006 144 pages Paperback
ISBN: 1-578066-89-1
Kathy Burgess, Advertising/Marketing Services Manager

2347 **Understanding Colon Cancer**
A Richard Adrouny, MD; FACP, author
University Press of Mississippi
3825 Ridgewood Road
Jackson, MS 39211-6492
601-432-6205
Fax: 601-432-6217
e-mail: kburgess@ihl.state.ms.us
www.upress.state.ms.us

For the general reader a concise manual of facts, warnings, prevention, treatments, and forecasts.
2002 168 pages Paperback
ISBN: 1-578062-03-9
Kathy Burgess, Advertising/Marketing Services Manager

2348 **When a Parent Has Cancer: A Guide to Caring for Your Children**
Harper Collins
10 E 53rd Street
New York, NY 10022
212-207-7000
www.harpercollins.com

ISBN: 0-060187-09-3

2349 **Women and Cancer: A Compassionate Reource for Patients and Their Families**
American Cancer Society
1599 Clifton Road NE
Atlanta, GA 30329-4250
404-320-3333
800-227-2345

Concise, thorough and up-to-date, this book provides women who have been diagnosed with cancer information about the four most common cancers of the reproductive system- breast, cervical, endometrial and ovarian cancer. Each chapter describes how each organ is structured and how it functions, and the risks and benefits of new drug therapies, radiation and chemotherapy, and surgical procedures. Includes patient stories and addresses the full range of issues faced by patients and their families.
290 pages paperback
ISBN: 0-944235-20-4

2350 **Young People with Cancer: A Handbook for Parents**
Barry Leonard, author
DIANE Publishing Company
330 Pusey Avenue, Unit #3 Rear
Darby, PA 19023
610-461-6200
800-782-3833
Fax: 610-461-6130
e-mail: dianepublishing@gmail.com
www.dianepublishing.net

Gives you information on all stages of your child's cancer. It tells you what to expect and suggests ways to prepare for different situations.
109 pages Paperback
ISBN: 0-756736-59-5
Herman Baron, Publisher

Children's Books

2351 **Cancer**
Franklin Watts Grolier
90 Old Sherman Turnpike
Danbury, CT 06816-0001
203-797-3500
800-621-1115
Fax: 203-797-3197
www.grolier.com

Discusses causes such as chemicals, viruses, radiation and oncogenes, as well as diagnosis, types of cancers, immune defenses and common treatments.
96 pages Grades 7-12
ISBN: 0-531108-03-1

2352 **Cancer: Overview Series**
Lucent Books
Thomson Gale
Farmington Hills, MI 48333-9187
800-877-4253
Fax: 800-414-5043
e-mail: gale.customerservice@thomson.com
www.gale.com/lucent

Questions are answered for young adults on the issues of cancer prevention and treatment.
1999 112 pages
ISBN: 1-560063-63-7

2353 **Help Yourself: Tips for Teenagers with Cancer**
National Cancer Institute
Building 31
Bethesda, MD 20892-0001
800-422-6237

This magazine-style booklet is designed to provide information and support adolescents with cancer.
37 pages

2354 Hospital Days: Treatment Ways
National Cancer Institute
Building 31
Bethesda, MD 20892-0001 800-422-6237
Coloring book helping to orient children with cancer to hospital and treatment procedures.
26 pages

2355 Kathy's Hats: A Story of Hope
Trudy Krisher, author
Albert Whitman & Company
6340 Oakton Street 847-581-0033
Morton Grove, IL 60053-2723 800-255-7675
Fax: 847-581-0039
e-mail: mail@awhitmanco.com
www.albertwhitman.com
When Kathy turns nine she learns she has cancer. When she loses her hair due to the chemotherapy, she feels ugly and awkward. This is a matter-of-fact book about a tough time and subject, and its calm and respectable treatment well serves a story that is indeed one of hope.
32 pages Hardcover
ISBN: 0-807541-16-6
Pat McPartland, Sales
Joe Campbell, Customer Service

2356 Kemo Shark
Kidscope
3400 Peachtree Road NE
Atlanta, GA 30326-1107 404-233-0001
www.kidscope.org
Color comic book designed to help children with the psychological and physiological changes in a family where a parent has cancer and chemotherapy.

2357 Living with Cancer
Franklin Watts Grolier
90 Old Sherman Turnpike 203-797-3500
Danbury, CT 06816-0001 800-621-1115
Fax: 203-797-3197
www.grolier.com
Shows how persons with cancer can overcome their illness and lead productive lives.
32 pages Grades 5-7
ISBN: 0-531108-59-7

2358 My Book for Kids with Cancer
Waterfront Books
98 Brookes Avenue
Burlington, VT 05401-3326 800-639-6063
www.waterfrontbooks.com/
Frustrated because he couldn't find any books about kids who survived cancer, Jason decided to write his own.
32 pages

2359 Our Mom Has Cancer
American Cancer Society
1599 Clifton Road NE 404-320-3333
Atlanta, GA 30329-4250 800-227-2345
When Abigail and Adrienne's mom told them she had cancer, they were afraid. But when the girls couldn't find any books that explained what might happen to their mother and what they might expect, they wrote one themselves. The girls, ages 9 and 11, tell readers that when their mother was tired during treatment, friends and family pitched in to help cook and to push her in her wheelchair. When chemotherapy made their mom's hair fall out, they threw a hat party for her.
32 pages hardcover
ISBN: 0-944235-20-4

2360 Sammie's New Mask: A Coloring Book for Friends of Children with Cancer
1015 Locust Street 314-241-1600
Saint Louis, MO 63101 Fax: 314-241-1996
e-mail: krudd@children-cancer.org
www.nationalchildrenscancersociety.org
Sammie's New Mask is about a young girl named Sammie and her friend, Jack, who has cancer. This story addresses Sammie's concerns and common misconceptions about cancer. This coloring book is designed for children in kindergarten through third grade.
K-3rd Grade
Mark Slocomb, Chairman
Mark Stolze, President/CEO

2361 Sammy's Mommy Has Cancer: For Children Who Have a Loved One with Cancer
Sherry Kohlenberg, author
Magination Press (American Psychological Assoc.)
750 First Street NE 202-336-5510
Washington, DC 20002-4242 800-374-2721
Fax: 202-336-5502
TDD: 202-336-6123
e-mail: magination@apa.org
www.apamaginationpress.apa.org
Sherry Kohlenberg wrote this book after she was diagnosed with breast cancer for her son. It is a warm, sensitive, straightforward story that will help young children understand and accept the changes in their lives when a parent is diagnosed with a life threatening illness. Parents will welcome this valuable aid in explaining the illness to their children. Both the story and the introduction offer useful suggestions for involving children in the jiys and sorrows of good and bad days.
1993 32 pages Softcover
ISBN: 0-945354-55-X

2362 Silver Kiss
Delacorte
1540 Broadway 212-354-6500
New York, NY 10036-4039
This moving tale describes the feelings of Zoe as her mother dies of cancer and her family attempts to shield her from seeing the slow decline in her mother.
Grades 8-12

2363 Silver Linings: Living with Cancer
Vantage Press
516 W 34th Street 212-736-1767
New York, NY 10001-1395 Fax: 212-736-2273
Highly personal journey of one woman's battle with breast cancer for over thirty-five years. From operations, radiation treatments, and hormone therapy and her faith and hope while induring them.

ISBN: 0-533113-52-0

2364 The Mountain You've Climbed: A Young Adult Guide to Childhood Cancer Survivorship
1015 Locust Street 314-241-1600
Saint Louis, MO 63101 Fax: 314-241-1996
e-mail: krudd@children-cancer.org
www.nationalchildrenscancersociety.org
This guide is designed to answer questions and address issues related to cancer survivorship for people ages 15 to 24. As survivorship rates continue to increase, the knowledge regarding late-effects also continues to increase. This survivorship guide will answer questions as well as address healthy living styles for your future.
Ages 15-24
Mark Slocomb, Chairman
Mark Stolze, President/CEO

2365 They Never Want to Tell You: Children Talk About Cancer
Harvard University Press
79 Garden Street 617-495-2480
Cambridge, MA 02138 800-448-2242
Fax: 800-962-4983
www.hup.harvard.edu
A comprehensive book that focuses on eight children who share their various experiences with cancer.
Grades 7-12
ISBN: 0-674883-70-5

2366 Waiting for Johnny Miracle
Harper & Row
10 E 53rd Street 212-207-7000
New York, NY 10022-5299

This powerful book focuses on Becky, a 17-year-old girl who must face the fear of cancer after being diagnosed with a malignant tumor. This book brings up the painful issues that come with the pain, treatment and death of cancer.
Grades 8-12

2367 Why God Gave Me Pain
Loyola University Press
3441 N Ashland Avenue 773-281-1818
Chicago, IL 60657-1355
Using a girl's diary entries, this book expounds on the side effects of cancer as well as the psychological ramifications of the debilitating disease.

Magazines

2368 American Journal of Clinical Oncology: Cancer Clinical Trials
Raven Press
1185 Avenue of the Americas 212-930-9500
New York, NY 10036-2601 800-777-2295
Offers outstanding coverage of ongoing research in cancer treatment. This journal is the primary source for timely updates covering all aspects of cancer management.
BiMonthly
ISBN: 0-277373-2 -
Luther W Brady, Editor

2369 Cancer Detection and Prevention Journal
Elsevier
Journals Customer Service Dept.
Orlando, FL 32887-4800 877-839-7126
Fax: 407-363-1354
e-mail: usjcs@elsevier.com
www.elsevier.com
A peer-refereed journal devoted to cancer prevention by predictive and preventitive oncology. It is uniquely focused on advances in genetics, molecular medicine and biotechnologies that have an impact on clinical oncology modalities.
2002-present

2370 Cancer Nursing: An International Journal for Cancer Care
Lippincott Williams & Wilkins
PO Box 1600
Hagerstown, MD 21741-1600 800-638-3030
Fax: 301-223-2400
e-mail: orders@lww.com
www.lww.com
Addresses the whole spectrum of problems arising in the care and support of cancer patients- prevention and early detection, geriatric and pediatric cancer nursing, medical and surgical oncology, ambulatory care, nutritional support, psychosocial aspects of cancer, patient responces to all treatment modalities, and specific nursing interventions.
BiMonthly
ISBN: 0-162220-X -

2371 Diseases of the Colon and Rectum
American Society of Colon and Rectal Surgeons
85 W Algonquin Road 847-290-9184
Arlington Heights, IL 60005 Fax: 847-290-9203
e-mail: ascrs@fascrs.org
www.fascrs.org
Diseases of the Colon and Rectum (DCR) is the official journal of the American Society of Colon and Rectal Surgeons and is mailed to all members on a mothly basis as a member benefit. Non-member subscribers have access to the online version of DCR.
journal

2372 Pancreas
Raven Press
1185 Avenue of the Americas 212-930-9500
New York, NY 10036-2601 800-777-2295
Provides a central forum for communication of original works involving both basic and clinical research on the exocrine and endocrine pancreas and their consequences in the disease state.
8x Year
ISBN: 0-885317-7 -
Vay Liang W Go, Editor

2373 Practice Parameters
American Society of Colon and Rectal Surgeons
85 W Algonquin Road 847-290-9184
Arlington Heights, IL 60005 Fax: 847-290-9203
e-mail: ascrs@fascrs.org
www.fascrs.org
Parameters that have been published in the scientific journal Diseases of the Colon and Rectum, along with other scientific journals. They can be found on the website under Professionals.

2374 Skin Cancer Foundation Journal
Skin Cancer Foundation
245 5th Avenue 212-725-5176
New York, NY 10016-8728 800-754-6490
Fax: 212-725-5751
e-mail: info@skincancer.org
www.skincancer.org
A collection of articles by physicians, scientists and lay writers on the subject.

Newsletters

2375 Candlelighters' Quarterly
Childhood Cancer Foundation
7910 Woodmont Avenue 301-657-8401
Bethesda, MD 20814 800-366-2223
Artlices on living with and treating pediatric/adolescent cancer, written by and for parents and professionals in the field. Includes reviews, resources, pen pal column, and more.

2376 Candlelighters' Youth Newsletter
Childhood Cancer Foundation
7910 Woodmont Avenue 301-657-8401
Bethesda, MD 20814-3015 800-366-2223
Offers information to teenagers and young adults on cancer issues, medical information, camps and programs.
Quarterly

2377 Melanoma Newsletter
Skin Cancer Foundation
245 5th Avenue 212-725-5176
New York, NY 10016-8728 800-754-6490
Fax: 212-725-5751
e-mail: info@skincancer.org
www.skincancer.org
For medical investigators and practitioners.

2378 Nutrition Action Healthletter
Center for Science in the Public Interest
1875 Connecticut Avenue NW 202-332-9110
Washington, DC 20009-5736 Fax: 202-265-4954
e-mail: cspi@cspinet.org
www.cspinet.org
The nation's leading consumer group concerned with food and nutrition issues. Focuses on diseases that result from consuming too many calories, too much fat, sodium and sugar such as cancer and heart disease.
16 pages 10 per year
Stephen Schmidt, Editor

2379 Oncology Times: The News Center for the Cancer Care Team
Lippincott Williams & Wilkins
PO Box 1600
Hagerstown, MD 21741-1600 800-638-3030
Fax: 301-223-2400
e-mail: orders@lww.com
www.lww.com
Reports on breaking clinical news in oncology, radiology, surgery, chemotherapy, and biological and gene therapy, as well as the professional, political, reimbursement, and practice management issues that affect those treating cancer patients.
2x Monthly

2380 Options: New Directions in the War on Cancer
People Against Cancer
614 E Street 515-972-4444
Otho, IA 50569-0010 Fax: 515-972-4415
e-mail: info@peopleagainstcancer.com
www.peopleagainstcancer.com

Published by People Against Cancer.
8 pages
Frank Wiewel, Executive Director

2381 **Phoenix: Newsletter**
Candlelighters' Childhood Cancer Foundation
7910 Woodmont Avenue 301-657-8401
Bethesda, MD 20814-3015 800-366-2223
For adult survivors of childhood cancer.

2382 **Sun and Skin News**
Skin Cancer Foundation
245 5th Avenue 212-725-5176
New York, NY 10016-8728 800-754-6490
Fax: 212-725-5751
e-mail: info@skincancer.org
www.skincancer.org
Deals with skin cancer and related subjects in nontechnical terms.

2383 **Support for People with Oral and Head and Neck Cancer**
PO Box 53 516-759-5333
Locust Valley, NY 11560-0053 800-377-0928
Fax: 516-671-8794
e-mail: info@spohnc.org
www.spohnc.org
This a patient run support program. Other services include patient networking oportunities, a national newsletter, a resource library and insurance information and assistance.
Nancy E Leupold, President/Founder

2384 **The Phoenix**
United Ostomy Associations of America, Inc.
The Phoenix Magazine 949-600-7296
Mission Viejo, CA 92690 800-826-0826
e-mail: publisher@uoaa.org
www.uoaa.org
The Phoenix magazine is the official publication of the United Ostomy Associations of America, Inc. and is published four times a year- December, March, June, and September.
Quarterly

2385 **Voice of Hope**
National Children's Cancer Society
1015 Locust Street 314-241-1600
Saint Louis, MO 63101 Fax: 314-241-1996
e-mail: krudd@children-cancer.org
www.nationalchildrenscancersociety.org
It educates donors on how their support is furthering the N.C.C.S. mission, and acknowledges supporters. Distributed to donors of the N.C.C.S.
3x/year
Mark Slocomb, Chairman
Mark Stolze, President/CEO

Pamphlets

2386 **Advanced Cancer: Living Each Day**
National Cancer Institute
Building 31
Bethesda, MD 20892-0001 800-422-6237
Booklet delving into all aspects of everyday living with cancer. Offers information on coping, how children react, facing the unknown, living wills, additional resources and making treatment decisions.
30 pages

2387 **After Breast Cancer: A Guide to Followup Care**
National Cancer Institute
Building 31
Bethesda, MD 20892-0001 800-422-6237
Explains the importance of checking for possible signs of recurring cancer by receiving regular mammograms, getting breast exams from a doctor, and continuing monthly breast self-exams.
15 pages

2388 **Basic Family Library**
Candlelighters' Childhood Cancer Foundation
7910 Woodmont Avenue 301-657-8401
Bethesda, MD 20814-3015 800-366-2223
A bibliography of materials on childhood cancers, medical support, death and bereavement and materials for children.

2389 **Brachytherapy and IMRT**
Michael Dattoli, Jennifer Cash, and Don Kaltenbach, author
Dattoli Cancer Foundation
2803 Fruitville Road 941-365-5599
Sarasota, FL 34237 800-915-1001
Fax: 941-366-3786
e-mail: info@dattolifoundation.org
www.dattolifoundation.org
A primer on seed implants and Intensity Modulated Radiation Therapy (IMRT). This booklet provides a comprehensive overview of prostate cancer treatment protocols that utilize brachytherapy and IMRT either with or without hormonal therapy.
50 pages Booklet

2390 **Breast Biopsy: What You Should Know**
National Cancer Institute
Building 31 301-496-4000
Bethesda, MD 20892-0001
Offers information on what happens before, during and after a breast biopsy.

2391 **Breast Cancer: Understanding Treatment Options**
National Cancer Institute
Building 31
Bethesda, MD 20892-0001 800-422-6237
Summarizes the biopsy procedure and examines the pros and cons of various types of breast surgery. It discusses lumpectomy and radiation therapy as primary treatment.
19 pages

2392 **Breast Exams: What You Should Know**
National Cancer Institute
Building 31
Bethesda, MD 20892-0001 800-422-6237
Provides answers to questions about breast cancer and breast screening methods.
10 pages

2393 **Camps for Children with Cancer and their Siblings**
Candlelighters' Childhood Cancer Foundation
7910 Woodmont Avenue 301-657-8401
Bethesda, MD 20814-3015 800-366-2223
A listing by state of day and overnight camp programs, children served and programs.

2394 **Cancer Tests You Should Know About: A Guide for People 65 and Over**
National Cancer Institute
Building 31
Bethesda, MD 20892-0001 800-422-6237
Describes the cancer tests important for people age 65 and older. Informs men and women of the exams they should be requesting when they schedule checkups with their doctors.
14 pages

2395 **Cancer of the Bladder: Research Report**
National Cancer Institute
Building 31
Bethesda, MD 20892-0001 800-422-6237
Offers information on the types of bladder cancer, mortality rates, diagnosis, symptoms, therapies, rehabilitation, clinical trials, and selected references.

2396 **Cancer of the Colon and Rectum: Research Report**
National Cancer Institute
Building 31
Bethesda, MD 20892-0001 800-422-6237
Informative pamphlet offering factual statistics on causes and prevention, detection, diagnosis, staging, treatment, followup, clinical trials and selected references.

2397 **Cancer of the Ovary: Research Report**
National Cancer Institute
Building 31
Bethesda, MD 20892-0001 800-422-6237

2398 **Cancer of the Pancreas: Research Report**
National Cancer Institute
Building 31
Bethesda, MD 20892-0001 800-422-6237
Offers information on the various types of pancreatic cancer, treatments, surgical procedures, chemotherapy, biological therapy, hormone therapy, clinical trials and selected references.

2399 **Cancer of the Uterus: Endometrial Cancer**
National Cancer Institute
Building 31
Bethesda, MD 20892-0001 800-422-6237
Offers information on the description and function of the uterus, incidence and mortality, possible causes and prevention, detection, diagnosis, staging, treatment, clinical trials and selected references.

2400 **Cancer of the Uterus: Research Report**
National Cancer Institute
Building 31
Bethesda, MD 20892-0001 800-422-6237

2401 **Candlelighters Guide to Bone Marrow Transplants in Children**
Candlelighters' Childhood Cancer Foundation
7910 Woodmont Avenue 301-657-8401
Bethesda, MD 20814-3015 800-366-2223
For parents who are contemplating a BMT or harvest for their child or whose child is undergoing the procedure.

2402 **Chemotherapy and You: A Guide to Self-Help During Treatment**
National Cancer Institute
Building 31
Bethesda, MD 20892-0001 800-422-6237
Explains chemotherapy and addresses problems and concerns of patients undergoing this treatment.

2403 **Chew or Snuff is Real Bad Stuff**
National Cancer Institute
Building 31 301-435-3848
Bethesda, MD 20892-2580 800-422-6237
www.nci.nih.gov
Designed for young adults, this brochure describes the health and social effects of using smokeless tobacco products.

2404 **Clearing the Air: A Guide to Quitting Smoking**
National Cancer Institute
Building 31
Bethesda, MD 20892-0001 800-422-6237
Offers hints on quitting smoking and cancer prevention.
24 pages

2405 **Cutaneous Melanoma of the Head and Neck**
American Academy of Otolaryngology
1 Prince Street 703-836-4444
Alexandria, VA 22314-3357 Fax: 703-683-5100
www.entnet.org

Self-instruction package.
Paperback
ISBN: 1-567720-22-6

2406 **Diet, Nutrition and Cancer Prevention: The Good News**
National Cancer Institute
Building 31
Bethesda, MD 20892-0001 800-422-6237
Provides an overview of dietary guidelines that may assist individuals in reducing their risks for some cancers.
16 pages

2407 **Diet, Nutrition and Cancer Prevention: A Guide to Food Choices**
National Cancer Institute
Building 31
Bethesda, MD 20892-0001 800-422-6237
Describes what is known about diet, nutrition and cancer prevention. Provides information about foods that contain components like fiber, fat and vitamins that may affect a person's risk of getting certain cancers.

2408 **Dilemmas of Providing Help in a Crisis: The Role of Friends & Parents**
Candlelighters' Childhood Cancer Foundation
7910 Woodmont Avenue 301-657-8401
Bethesda, MD 20814-3015 800-366-2223

2409 **Do the Right Thing: Get a Mammogram**
National Cancer Institute
Building 31
Bethesda, MD 20892-0001 800-422-6237
Targets black women age 40 and older. Describes the importance of regular mammograms in the early detection of breast cancer.

2410 **Eating Hints: Recipes and Tips for Better Nutrition During Cancer Treatment**
National Cancer Institute
Building 31
Bethesda, MD 20892-0001 800-422-6237
Provides recipes that help patients meet their needs for good nutrition during treatment.

2411 **Facing Forward: A Guide for Cancer Survivors**
National Cancer Institute
Building 31
Bethesda, MD 20892-0001 800-422-6237
Presents a concise overview of important survivor issues, including ongoing health needs, psychosocial concerns, insurance and employment.
43 pages

2412 **Facts About Lung Cancer**
American Lung Association
1740 Broadway 212-315-8700
New York, NY 10019-4315

2413 **Facts About Radon**
American Lung Association
1740 Broadway 212-315-8700
New York, NY 10019-4315

2414 **Help, Hope, Believe**
National Children's Cancer Society
1015 Locust Street 314-241-1600
Saint Louis, MO 63101 Fax: 314-241-1996
e-mail: krudd@children-cancer.org
www.nationalchildrenscancersociety.org
N.C.C.S. Informational Brochure
3x/year
Mark Slocomb, Chairman
Mark Stolze, President/CEO

2415 **Helping Children Cope While a Sibling Undergoes Bone Marrow Transplant**
Bone Marrow Foundation
981 1st Avenue 212-838-3029
New York, NY 10022-5102 e-mail: thebmf@aol.com
www.bonemarrow.org
Discusses the wide array of emotions felt by the entire family as a child receives a bone marrow transplant.

2416 **If You've Thought About Breast Cancer**
Rose Kushner Breast Cancer Advisory Center
PO Box 224
Kensington, MD 20895-0224 Fax: 301-897-3444

2417 **Immune System: How it Works**
National Cancer Institute
Building 31
Bethesda, MD 20892-0001 800-422-6237
Written for the high school level, this booklet explains the human immune system for the general public. It describes the sophistication of the body's immune responses, the impact of immune disorders and the relation of the immune system to cancer therapies.
28 pages

2418 **Informed Consent: Does the Current Process Reflect Current Treatments**
Candlelighters' Childhood Cancer Foundation
7910 Woodmont Avenue 301-657-8401
Bethesda, MD 20814-3015 800-366-2223

2419 **Insurance Articles**
Candlelighters' Childhood Cancer Foundation
7910 Woodmont Avenue 301-657-8401
Bethesda, MD 20814-3015 800-366-2223

Includes: Tips on securing health insurance for childhood cancer survivors and patients, Stay a step ahead of you insuruer, and others.

2420 Interpreting Your PSA and Related Prostate Cancer Blood Tests
Michael Dattoli, Jennifer Cash, and Don Kaltenbach, author
Dattoli Cancer Foundation
2803 Fruitville Road 941-365-5599
Sarasota, FL 34237 800-915-1001
Fax: 941-366-3786
e-mail: info@dattolifoundation.org
www.dattolifoundation.org
Provides a comprehensive overview of the PSA (prostate specific antigen) blood test and other related lab tests including the PSA velocity, free and bound PSA, and the PAP (prostatic Acid Phosphatase) blood test.
2006 50 pages Booklet

2421 Leading Self-Help Groups: Report on Workshop for Leaders of Groups
Candlelighters' Childhood Cancer Foundation
7910 Woodmont Avenue 301-657-8401
Bethesda, MD 20814-3015 800-366-2223

2422 Letter to a Friend Whose Child is Newly Diagnosed with Cancer
Candlelighters' Childhood Cancer Foundation
7910 Woodmont Avenue 301-657-8401
Bethesda, MD 20814-3015 800-366-2223

2423 Managing Your Child's Eating Problems During Cancer Treatment
National Cancer Institute
Building 31
Bethesda, MD 20892-0001 800-422-6237
Contains information about the importance of nutrition, side effects of cancer and its treatment.
32 pages

2424 Mastectomy: A Treatment for Breast Cancer
National Cancer Institute
Building 31
Bethesda, MD 20892-0001 800-422-6237
Presents information about the different types of breast surgery, explains what to expect at the hospital and during the recovery period.
25 pages

2425 Melanoma: Research Report
National Cancer Institute
Building 31
Bethesda, MD 20892-0001 800-422-6237
Offers information on types of skin cancer, detection, diagnosis, staging, treatment, clinical trials, selected references and additional information for patients with skin cancer.

2426 Nutrition for Patients Receiving Chemotherapy/Radiation Treatment
National Cancer Institute
Building 31
Bethesda, MD 20892-0001 800-422-6237
Describes the importance of maintaining nutritional intake while receiving chemotherapy and radiation.

2427 Once a Year for a Lifetime
National Cancer Institute
Building 31
Bethesda, MD 20892-0001 800-422-6237
Targets all women age 40 and older describing the importance of regular mammograms in the early detection of breast cancer.

2428 Oral Cancers: Research Report
National Cancer Institute
Building 31
Bethesda, MD 20892-0001 800-422-6237
Describes types of oral cancer, causes and risk factors, symptoms, prevention, detection, diagnosis, treatment, staging, methods of treatments, followup care, clinical trials and selected references for more information.

2429 Pap Test: It Can Save Your Life
National Cancer Institute
Building 31
Bethesda, MD 20892-0001 800-422-6237
Easy-to-read pamphlet tells women of the importance of getting a Pap test, how often to get it done and where to go to get it.

2430 Preparing your Child for a Bone Marrow Transplant
Bone Marrow Foundation
981 1st Avenue 212-838-3029
New York, NY 10022-5102 e-mail: thebmf@aol.com
www.bonemarrow.org
Discusses the wide array of emotions felt by the entire family as a child receives a bone marrow transplant.

2431 Questions and Answers About Breast Lumps
National Cancer Institute
Building 31
Bethesda, MD 20892-0001 800-422-6237
Describes some of the most common noncancerous breast lumps and what can be done about them.
22 pages

2432 Questions and Answers About Choosing a Mammography Facility
National Cancer Institute
Building 31
Bethesda, MD 20892-0001 800-422-6237
Lists questions to ask in selecting a quality mammography facility.

2433 Questions and Answers About DES Exposure During Pregnancy and Before Birth
National Cancer Institute
Building 31
Bethesda, MD 20892-0001 800-422-6237

2434 Questions and Answers About Metastatic Cancer
National Cancer Institute
Building 31
Bethesda, MD 20892-0001 800-422-6237
Presents information on detection, treatment methods and common areas of reoccurrence.

2435 Questions and Answers About Pain Control
National Cancer Institute
Building 31
Bethesda, MD 20892-0001 800-422-6237
Discusses pain control using both medical and nonmedical methods.

2436 Radiation Therapy and You: A Guide To Self-Help During Treatment
National Cancer Institute
Building 31
Bethesda, MD 20892-0001 800-422-6237
Explains radiation therapy and addresses concerns of patients receiving radiation treatment.

2437 Recurrence: What Do I Do Now?
Dattoli Cancer Foundation
2803 Fruitville Road 941-365-5599
Sarasota, FL 34237 800-915-1001
Fax: 941-366-3786
e-mail: info@dattolifoundation.org
www.dattolifoundation.org
This booklet offers comprehensive information on the issues surrounding ruccurence: detection, risk categories, treatment options including radiation, brachytherapy, and hormone therapy.
58 pages Booklet

2438 Research Report: Adult Kidney Cancer and Wilms' Tumor
National Cancer Institute
Building 31
Bethesda, MD 20892-0001 800-422-6237

2439 Skin Cancers, Basal Cell and Squamous Cell Carcinomas: Research Report
National Cancer Institute
Building 31
Bethesda, MD 20892-0001 800-422-6237

Offers information on types of skin cancer, incidence and mortality, risk factors, prevention, symptoms, detection, diagnosis, staging, treatment, followup care and clinical trials.

2440 **Students with Cancer: A Resource for the Educator**
National Cancer Institute
Building 31
Bethesda, MD 20892-0001 800-422-6237
Designed for teachers who have students with cancer in their classrooms or schools.
22 pages

2441 **Sunlight, Ultraviolet Radiation and the Skin**
National Cancer Institute
Building 31
Bethesda, MD 20892-0001 800-422-6237

2442 **Support Systems for Parents of Children with Cancer**
Candlelighters' Childhood Cancer Foundation
7910 Woodmont Avenue 301-657-8401
Bethesda, MD 20814-3015 800-366-2223

2443 **Taking Time: Support for People with Cancer & People Who Care for Them**
National Cancer Institute
Building 31
Bethesda, MD 20892-0001 800-422-6237
Discusses the emotional sides of cancer. how to deal with the disease and learn to talk with friends, family members and others about cancer.

2444 **Talking with Your Child About Cancer**
National Cancer Institute
Building 31
Bethesda, MD 20892-0001 800-422-6237
Designed for the parent whose child has been diagnosed with cancer.
16 pages

2445 **Testicular Cancer: Research Report**
National Cancer Institute
Building 31
Bethesda, MD 20892-0001 800-422-6237

2446 **Testicular Self-Examination**
National Cancer Institute
Building 31
Bethesda, MD 20892-0001 800-422-6237
Contains information about risks and symptoms of testicular cancer and provides instructions on how to perform testicular self-examination.

2447 **What You Need to Know About Bladder Cancer**
National Cancer Institute
Building 31 301-496-4000
Bethesda, MD 20892-0001
Offers information on the history, symptoms, diagnosis, treatment, followup care, support groups, medical terms and resources for more information.

2448 **What You Need to Know About Cancer**
National Cancer Institute
Building 31
Bethesda, MD 20892-0001 800-422-6237
Offers information on signs and symptoms, diagnosis, treatment, early detection and advances in medical technology.

2449 **What You Need to Know About Cancer of The Colon and Rectum**
National Cancer Institute
Building 31
Bethesda, MD 20892-0001 800-422-6237
Offers information on symptoms, diagnosis, treatments, and support for cancer patients.

2450 **What You Need to Know About Cervical Cancer**
National Cancer Institute
Building 31
Bethesda, MD 20892-0001 800-422-6237
Areas covered include early detection, symptoms, treatments, diagnosis, followup care, support, medical terms and resources.

2451 **What You Need to Know About Esophagal Cancer**
National Cancer Institute
Building 31
Bethesda, MD 20892-0001 800-422-6237
Offers information on symptoms, causes, preventions, diagnosis, support, medical terms and available resources.

2452 **What You Need to Know About Kidney Cancer**
National Cancer Institute
Building 31
Bethesda, MD 20892-0001 800-422-6237
Offers factual information on diagnosis, symptoms, prevention, treatment and referral sources.

2453 **What You Need to Know About Larynx Cancer**
National Cancer Institute
Building 31
Bethesda, MD 20892-0001 800-422-6237
Offers information on what cancer is, symptoms, diagnosis, treatment options, side effects of medication, rehabilitation, learning to speak again, living with cancer, causes and preventions, medical terms and resources.

2454 **What You Need to Know About Lung Cancer**
National Cancer Institute
Building 31
Bethesda, MD 20892-0001 800-422-6237
Offers information on types of lung cancer, symptoms, diagnosis, treatments, support, medical terms and resources.

2455 **What You Need to Know About Oral Cancers**
National Cancer Institute
Building 31
Bethesda, MD 20892-0001 800-422-6237
Offers information on symptoms, diagnosis, treatments, rehabilitation, followup care, support, medical terms and resources for cancer patients.

2456 **What You Need to Know About Ovarian Cancer**
National Cancer Institute
Building 31
Bethesda, MD 20892-0001 800-422-6237
Early detection, symptoms, diagnosis, treatments, medical terms and resources for further information.

2457 **What You Need to Know About Pancreatic Cancer**
National Cancer Institute
Building 31
Bethesda, MD 20892-0001 800-422-6237
Offers information on symptoms, diagnosis, treatment, support, medical terms and resources.

2458 **What You Need to Know About Prostate Cancer**
National Cancer Institute
Building 31
Bethesda, MD 20892-0001 800-422-6237
Offers information on symptoms, diagnosis, treatment options, side effects of medications, followup care, living with cancer and support resources for patients.

2459 **What You Need to Know About Skin Cancer**
National Cancer Institute
Building 31
Bethesda, MD 20892-0001 800-422-6237
Offers information on types of skin cancer, symptoms, causes, prevention, treatment planning, treating skin cancer, research and medical terms.

2460 **What You Need to Know About Testicular Cancer**
National Cancer Institute
Building 31
Bethesda, MD 20892-0001 800-422-6237
Offers information on the symptoms, diagnosing of testicular cancer, side effects of treatments, followup care, support for patients, cancer research, medical terms and resources.

2461 **What You Need to Know About Uterine Cancer**
National Cancer Institute
Building 31
Bethesda, MD 20892-0001 800-422-6237

Offers information on symptoms, diagnosing cancer of the uterus, treatments, followup care, support for patients, medical terms and resources.

2462 **What You Need to Know About...**
National Cancer Institute
Building 31
Bethesda, MD 20892-0001 800-422-6237
This is a series of booklets, broken down in this directory. Each provides information about a specific type of cancer. These booklets discuss emotional issues, treatment, diagnosis, symptoms and questions to ask the doctor about cancer.

2463 **What are Clinical Trials All About?**
National Cancer Institute
Building 31
Bethesda, MD 20892-0001 800-422-6237
Explains clinical trials (studies of new cancer treatments) to help patients decide if they want to take part in a trial.

2464 **When Cancer Recurs: Meeting the Challenge Again**
National Cancer Institute
Building 31
Bethesda, MD 20892-0001 800-422-6237
Offers information on why cancer can recur, where cancers can recur, diagnosing recurrent cancer, treatment methods and resources that offer more help.

2465 **When Someone in Your Family Has Cancer**
National Cancer Institute
Building 31
Bethesda, MD 20892-0001 800-422-6237
Written for young people whose parent or sibling has cancer.
28 pages

2466 **Who is This Person Who Helped Save My Life**
Bone Marrow Foundation
981 1st Avenue 212-838-3029
New York, NY 10022-5102 e-mail: thebmf@aol.com
www.bonemarrow.org
Discusses the wide range of emotions for a patient in the process of searching for and identifying a donor.

2467 **Why Do You Smoke?**
National Cancer Institute
Building 31
Bethesda, MD 20892-0001 800-422-6237
Contains a self-test to determine why people smoke and suggest alternatives that can help them stop and prevent cancer.

2468 **Wish Fulfillment Organizations**
Candlelighters' Childhood Cancer Foundation
7910 Woodmont Avenue 301-657-8401
Bethesda, MD 20814-3015 800-366-2223
A list of groups granting wishes of children with life-threatening, chronic or terminal illnesses, with criteria and contacts.

2469 **Young People with Cancer: A Handbook for Parents**
National Cancer Institute
Building 31
Bethesda, MD 20892-0001 800-422-6237
Discusses the most common types of childhood cancer, treatments, and side effects and issues that may arise when a child is diagnosed with cancer.
86 pages

Audio & Video

2470 **Beyond the Loss of the Breast**
Sherry Thomas-Zon, author
Fanlight Productions
4196 Washington Street 617-469-4999
Boston, MA 02131-1731 800-937-4113
Fax: 617-469-3379
e-mail: fanlight@fanlight.com
www.fanlight.com
This video addresses breast cancer throught the personal narratives and poetry of two women living with recurrent breast cancer and the film maker, whose mother died from metastatic disease.
1994 25 Minutes
ISBN: 1-572951-68-0

2471 **Living with Ovarian Cancer**
National Ovarian Cancer Coalition
500 NE Spanish River Blvd 561-393-0005
Boca Raton, FL 33431 888-682-7426
Fax: 561-393-7275
e-mail: nocc@ovarian.org
www.ovarian.org
Videotape for women who have been recently diagnosed with ovarian cancer. Created to orient and inform patients and their families; describes the experiences of individuals intimately connected with the disease.
Suzy Lockwood-Rayermann RN, Chair
Julene Fabrizio, President

2472 **Not Just a Cancer Patient**
Fanlight Productions
4196 Washington Street 617-469-4999
Boston, MA 02131-1731 800-937-4113
Fax: 617-469-3379
e-mail: fanlight@fanlight.com
www.fanlight.com
Focuses on several articulate teenagers who are undergoing cancer treatment to help caregivers understand the needs and feelings of this population.
1991 23 Minutes
ISBN: 1-572950-86-2

2473 **Skin Cancer: Preventable and Curable**
Skin Cancer Foundation
245 5th Avenue 212-725-5176
New York, NY 10016-8728 800-754-6490
Fax: 212-725-5751
e-mail: info@skincancer.org
www.skincancer.org

Web Sites

2474 **American Academy of Dermatology**
www.aad.org
An organization of doctors who specialize in diagnosing and treating skin problems.

2475 **American Cancer Society**
www.cancer.org
Provides free printed materials, offers a range of services to patients and their families.

2476 **American Lung Association**
www.lungusa.org
A voluntary organization interested in the prevention and control of lung disease.

2477 **American Prostate Society**
www.ameripros.org
Organization dedicated exclusively to using existing medical capabilities to reduce death due to prostate cancer and to reduce unnecessary or ineffective prostate surgery.

2478 **American Society of Colon and Rectal Surgeons**
www.fascrs.org
Represents more than 1000 board certified colon and rectal surgeons and other surgeons dedicated to advancing and promoting the science and practice of the treatment of patients with diseases and disorders affecting the colon, rectum and anus.

2479 **Association for the Cure of Cancer of the Prostate**
www.capcure.org

2480 **Bone Marrow Foundation**
www.bonemarrow.org

2481 **Healing Well**
www.healingwell.com

An online health resource guide to medical news, chat, information and articles, newsgroups and message boards, books, disease-related web sites, medical directories, and more for patients, friends, and family coping with disabling diseases, disorders, or chronic illnesses.

2482 **Health Finder**

www.healthfinder.gov

Searchable, carefully developed web site offering information on over 1000 topics. Developed by the US Department of Health and Human Services, the site can be used in both English and Spanish.

2483 **Healthlink USA**

www.healthlinkusa.com

Health information concerning treatment, cures, prevention, diagnosis, risk factors, research, support groups, email lists, personal stories and much more. Updated regularly.

2484 **Helios Health**

www.helioshealth.com

Online resource for your health information. Detailed information about specific health topics, access to expert advice from our Medical Advisory Board, and up-to-date health news.

2485 **International Association of Eating Disorders Professionals**

www.iaedp.com

Supplies printed information and sponsors meetings and other activities. Publishes a directory of speech instructors and maintains a list of sources for supplies for laryngectomee.

2486 **Leukemia Society of America**

www.leukemia.org

A national voluntary health agency dedicated to curing leukemia, lymphoma, Hodgkin's disease and myeloma and to improving the quality of life of patients and their families.

2487 **MedicineNet**

www.medicinenet.com

An online resource for consumers providing easy-to-read, authoritative medical and health information.

2488 **Medscape**

www.mywebmd.com

Medscape offers specialists, primary care physicians, and other health professionals the Web's most robust and integrated medical information and educational tools.

2489 **National Alliance of Breast Cancer Organizations**

www.nabco.org

A network of breast cancer organizations that provides information, assistance and referral to anyone with questions about breast cancer and acts as a voice for the interests and concerns of breast cancer survivors and women at risk.

2490 **National Ovarian Cancer Coalition**

www.ovarian.org

Our mission is to raise awareness about ovarian cancer and to promote education about the disease.

2491 **Support for People with Oral and Head and Neck Cancer**

www.spohnc.org

Nonprofit organization founded in 1991 to address the broad emotional, physical and humanistic needs of oral and head and neck cancer patients.

2492 **United Ostomy Association**

Produces and distributes materials about ostomy care and management; through trained UOA members, offers practical assistance and emotional support to ostomy patients; sponsors annual youth rally and state and regional conferences for local affiliates; has 500 chapters to serve people locally.

2493 **WebMD**

www.webmd.com

Information on Cancer, including articles and resources.

2494 **Webhelp**

www.webhelp.com

Provides links to information, including research, treatment, prevention, support, and more.

Description

2495 **Carpal Tunnel Syndrome**

Carpal Tunnel Syndrome, CTS, is a painful, often debilitating condition caused by compression of the median nerve as it passes through the wrist (carpal tunnel) to the hand. CTS most commonly occurs in women aged 30 to 50 years. The incidence is highest among keyboard users, secretaries, musicians, assembly-line workers, and others who engage in repetitive handwork.

An initial indication of CTS is a feeling that the hand is asleep. Typically, the patient wakes at night with numbness and tingling of the affected hand. The most serious functional problem occurs when it becomes difficult or impossible to move the thumb into a grasping position with the other fingers. In advanced cases, pain associated with CTS may radiate up the arm to the shoulder. While job-related movement is the most common cause of CTS, people with underlying conditions, such as diabetes, gout, rheumatoid arthritis, obesity and pregnancy, are more prone to experience symptoms. Although less common, the onset of CTS can stem from trauma, such as a blow to the hand or wrist.

Diagnosis involves the Phalen Test, in which the hands are placed together, back to back and the wrist is flexed. This maneuver generally produces tingling of the hand in a patient with CTS. Diagnosis is confirmed by testing how quickly an impulse is transmitted along the median nerve.

The condition can most often be successfully treated based on an understanding of workplace movement issues—ergonomics. Keyboard users, and those engaged in similar activities, should adjust their seats and backrests to assure that their arms are positioned comfortably during work sessions. For mild cases of CTS, a lightweight brace, especially worn at night, can decrease symptoms by holding the wrist stable. Marked improvement may arise from wearing a brace for a week or two. However, in many cases, it is recommended that the sufferer cease working until symptoms have improved. Exercises and deep-tissue massage can strengthen the wrist and hand.

Over-the-counter anti-inflammatory medications, such as ibuprofen and aspirin, can also reduce symptoms of mild Carpal Tunnel Syndrome. In more acute conditions, cortisone injections may be administered. When symptoms are severe and persistent, surgery may be required to reduce pressure on the nerves. The most common surgery is an open incision technique called open carpal tunnel release, which usually improves the condition dramatically. A newer and less invasive procedure is endoscopic carpal tunnel release, which uses a smaller incision and visualizes the operative field using a fiberoptic camera.

National Agencies & Associations

2496 **American Academy of Orthopaedic Surgeons**
6300 N River Road 847-823-7186
Rosemont, IL 60018-4262 800-346-2267
Fax: 847-823-8125
e-mail: custserv@aaos.org
www.aaos.org

The American Academy of Orthopaedic Surgeons provides education and practice management services for orthopaedic surgeons and allied health professionals. The Academy also serves as an advocate for improved patient care and to inform the public.
Karen L Hackett FACHE CAE, CEO
Richard J Stewart, Chief Financial Officer

2497 **American Chronic Pain Association**
PO Box 850
Rocklin, CA 95677 800-533-3231
Fax: 916-632-3208
e-mail: ACPA@pacbell.net
www.theacpa.org

ACPA mission is: (1) to facilitate peer support and education for individuals with chronic pain and their families so that these individuals may live more fully in spite of their pain; (2) to raise awareness among the health care community and policy makers.
Penny Cowan, Executive Director

2498 **American Society for Surgery of the Hand**
6300 N River Road 847-384-8300
Rosemont, IL 60018 Fax: 847-384-1435
e-mail: info@assh.org
www.assh.org

The mission of the ASSH is to advance the science and practice of hand and upper extremity surgery through education research and advocacy on behalf of patients and practitioners.
Mark C Anderson CAE, Executive Director
Dawn Briskey CAE, Director Strategic Operations

2499 **Arthritis Trust of America**
7376 Walker Road 615-799-1002
Fairview, TN 37602-8141 e-mail: admin@arthritistrust.org
www.arthritistrust.org

The Arthritis Trust of America provides information about auto-immune or collagen tissue diseases such as Rheumatoid Arthritis and related diseases. They provide publications and physician referrals and when funds are available they fund research.
Perry A Chapdelaine BA MA, Executive Director
Cheryl Jacobsen, President

2500 **National Institute of Arthritis and Musculoskeletal and Skin Disease (NIAMS)**
1 AMS Circle 301-495-4484
Bethesda, MD 20892 888-226-4267
Fax: 301-718-6366
TTY: 301-565-2966
e-mail: niamsinfo@mail.nih.gov
www.niams.nih.gov

The NIAMS Information Clearinghouse provides information about various forms of arthritis and rheumatic disease and bone, muscle, and skin diseases. It distributes patient and professional education materials and refers people to other sources of information.
Stephen I Katz MD, PhD, Director

Research Centers

2501 **Center for Neurology & Stroke Baptist Hospital Office**
Baptist Hospital Office
333 West Thomas Road 602-335-0300
Pheonix, AZ 85015 Fax: 602-249-3118
e-mail: info@cnsaz.com
www.cnsaz.com

Providing comprehensive testing and consulting for neurological disorders.

2502 **Michigan Hand Center**
1111 Leffingwell Avenue NE 616-957-4263
Grand Rapids, MI 49525 800-582-7244
Fax: 616-957-0444
e-mail: info@michiganhandcenter.com
www.michiganhand.com
Janid Pike, Director

2503 **National Institute of Arthritis & Musculoskeletal Skin Diseases**
National Institutes of Health
I AMS Circle 301-495-4484
Bethesda, MD 20892-3675 Fax: 301-718-6366
TTY: 301-565-2966
e-mail: niamsinfo@mail.nih.gov
www.niams.nih.gov

Support Groups & Hotlines

2504 **National Health Information Center**
PO Box 1133 310-565-4167
Washington, DC 20013 800-336-4797
Fax: 301-984-4256
e-mail: info@nhic.org
www.health.gov/nhic
Offers a nationwide information referral service, produces directories and resource guides.

Books

2505 **Occupational Therapy Practice Guidelines for Adults with Carpal Tunnel Syndrome**
American Occupational Therapy Association
4720 Montgomery Lane 301-652-2682
Bethesda, MD 20824-1220 Fax: 301-652-7711
TDD: 800-377-8555
www.aota.org
13 pages Paperback
ISBN: 1-569001-47-2

2506 **Pain Free Typing Techniques: Simple Solutions to Prevent Strain Injury**
Howard Richman, author
Sound Feelings Publishing
18375 Ventura Boulevard 818-757-0600
Tarzana, CA 91356 e-mail: information@soundfeelings.com
www.soundfeelings.com
This 12 page booklet provides drug-free treatments and suggestions for repetitive motion disorder and cumulative trauma disorders. Unconventional concepts for increasing human performance are revealed, which help prevent computer-related illnesses including hand pain, wrist pain, and other keyboard ergonomics. Most repetitive motion disorders and overuse injuries can be improved by correcting certain angles and positions.
1999 12 pages Booklet
ISBN: 1-882060-80-6

Pamphlets

2507 **Carpal Tunnel Syndrome**
Arthritis Foundation
PO Box 7669 404-872-7100
Atlanta, GA 30357-0669 800-283-7800
Fax: 404-872-0457
Offers an introduction to Carpal Tunnel, causes, symptoms, diagnosis and resources.

Web Sites

2508 **Avoiding Carpal Tunnel Syndrome**
www.indiana.edu/~ucsstaff/cts.html
A guide for computer keyboard users, by Mark Sheehan, reprinted from the University Computing Times.

2509 **CTD Resource Network**
www.ctdrn.org
This is an organization providing educational material and charitable assistance related to the prevention and treatment of cumulative trauma disorders, also known as repetitive strain injuries.

2510 **Carpal Tunnel Syndrome Home Page**
www.ctsplace.com
Information about carpal tunnel syndrome (CTS) and how to prevent it.

2511 **Computer-Related Repetitive Strain Injury**
www.unl.edu/ee/eeshop/rsi.html#PREVENT
Contains advice on proper posture and equipment from Paul Marxhausen, an engineering electronics technician.

2512 **Health Finder**
www.healthfinder.gov
Searchable, carefully developed web site offering information on over 1000 topics. Developed by the US Department of Health and Human Services, the site can be used in both English and Spanish.

2513 **MedicineNet**
www.medicinenet.com
An online resource for consumers providing easy-to-read, authoritative medical and health information.

2514 **Neurology Channel**
www.neurologychannel.com
Find clearly explained, medically accurate information regarding conditions, including an overview, symptoms, causes, diagnostic procedures and treatment options. On this site it is possible to ask questions and get information from a neurologist and connect to people who have similar health interests.

2515 **RSI Resources**
www.geocities.com/HotSprings/1702
Information on carpal tunnel and other repetitive strain injuries.

Description

2516 **Celiac Disease**

Celiac disease, also called celiac sprue, is a chronic disease in which the small bowel cannot absorb most nutrients. This inability, called malabsorption, is caused by inflammation of the bowel triggered by a sensitivity to gluten, a cereal protein found in wheat and rye, and less so in barley and oats.

The disease may appear when a child is first given wheat products, generally in the second year of life. Some cases, however, do not appear until a person is in their twenties, or later, with women showing symptoms 10 to 15 years earlier than men. Affected children will fail to grow normally. Adults may lose weight despite a voracious appetite. There is no typical presentation of celiac disease. However, painful abdominal distention and passage of large, loose stools are common; iron deficiency anemia and vitamin deficiencies may appear.

Family incidence is a valuable clue. Celiac disease is more common in people with Type I diabetes and certain forms of thyroid and skin disease. Blood tests are helpful in making the diagnosis, but the most definitive test is examination of a small sample of the inflamed bowel.

Withdrawal of dietary gluten is the treatment for celiac disease; eating even small amounts of gluten-containing foods can prevent remission and cause relapse. Vitamins and minerals may also have to be supplemented. See also *Gastrointestinal Disorders* and *Crohn's Disease.*

National Agencies & Associations

2517 **American Celiac Society**
PO Box 23455 504-737-3293
New Orleans, LA 70183 Fax: 973-669-8808
e-mail: info@americanceliacsociety.org
www.americanceliacsociety.org
Nonprofit tax exempt organization that supports efforts in education research and mutual support. Helps to set up support groups sponsors conferences seek funding for education and research identify ingredients in foods and educate the public.
News, V&A cass.
Annette Bentley, President
Jim Bentley Vice President

2518 **Canadian Celiac Association**
5170 Dixie Road 905-507-6208
Mississauga, ON, L4W-1E3 800-363-7296
Fax: 905-507-4673
www.celiac.ca
A national organization dedicated to providing services and support to persons with celiac disease and dermatitis herpetiformis through programs of awareness, advocacy, education and research.
Kenn Tuckey, President
Janet Dalziel, VP

2519 **Celiac Sprue Association: USA**
PO Box 31700 402-558-0600
Omaha, NE 68131 877-CSA-4CSA
Fax: 402-643-4108
e-mail: celiacs@csaceliacs.org
www.csaceliacs.org
Member based nonprofit support organization dedicated to helping individuals with celiac disease and dermatitis herpetiformis worldwide through education information and research. Includes over 150 support contacts nationwide and Cel-Kids Network.
Mary Schluckebier, Executive Director
Bill Eyl, President

2520 **Gluten Intolerance Group: GIG**
31214 124th Avenue SE 253-833-6655
Auburn, WA 98092-3667 Fax: 253-833-6675
e-mail: info@gluten.net
www.gluten.net
Provides instructional and general information materials as well as counseling and access to gluten-free products and ingredients to persons with celiac sprue and their families, operates telephone information and referral service and conducts educational seminars.
Cynthia Kupp RDCD, Executive Director

Support Groups & Hotlines

2521 **American Celiac Society Hotline**
Dietary Support Coalition
PO BOX 23455 504-737-3293
New Orleans, LA 70183-4e-mail: americanceliacsociety@yahoo.com
Provides practical assistance to members and individuals with celiac disease and information about the disease to the public.
Annette Bentley, President
James Bentley, Vice President

2522 **Celiac Disease Foundation**
13251 Ventura Boulevard 818-990-2354
Studio City, CA 91604-1838 Fax: 818-990-2379
e-mail: cdf@celiac.org
www.celiac.org/
Provides services and support to persons with celiac disease and dermatitis herpetiformis, through programs of awareness, education, advocacy and research; telephone information and referral services; medical advisory board annual educational conference and quarterly newsletters.
Elaine Monarch, Executive Director

2523 **National Health Information Center**
PO Box 1133 310-565-4167
Washington, DC 20013 800-336-4797
Fax: 301-984-4256
e-mail: info@nhic.org
www.health.gov/nhic
Offers a nationwide information referral service, produces directories and resource guides.

Books

2524 **CSA/USA Cookbook Series**
Celiac Sprue Association/USA
PO Box 31700 402-558-0600
Omaha, NE 68131 877-272-4272
Fax: 402-643-4108
e-mail: celiacs@csaceliacs.org
www.csaceliacs.org
Three cookbooks compiled from CSA members' contributions. Each contains a section of cooking hints, information on adapting recipes and a variety of special topics related to cooking gluten-free.
34 pages Annual
Mary Schluckebier, Executive Director

2525 **Cooperative Gluten-Free Commercial Products Listing**
Celiac Sprue Association/USA
PO Box 31700 402-558-0600
Omaha, NE 68131 877-272-4272
Fax: 402-643-4108
e-mail: celiacs@csaceliacs.org
www.csaceliacs.org
Listing of gluten-free products compiled from written documentation recieved by the Celiac Sprue Association from manufacturers and distributors. Also includes vendor information for companies

specializing in gluten-free products and phone numbers of companies.
2006 Annual
Mary Schluckebier, Executive Director

2526 Diets to Help Gluten and Wheat Allergy
HarperCollins Canada Limited/Order Department
1995 Markham Road
Scarborough, M1B 5M8, 800-387-0117
Fax: 800-668-5788
This book offers sound and practical advice on gluten allergy wheat sensitivity and Celiac disease.
96 pages
ISBN: 0-722529-10-4

2527 Gluten Intolerance
American Dietetic Association
1120 Connecticut Avenue NW 202-775-8277
Washington, DC 20036 800-877-1600
www.eatright.org
Resource and recipe book.

2528 The Gluten-Free Gourmet
Bette Hagman, author
Gluten Intolerance Group: GIG
31214 124th Avenue SE 253-833-6655
Auburn, WA 98092-3667 Fax: 253-833-6675
e-mail: info@gluten.net
www.gluten.net
225 recipes.
272 pages
ISBN: 0-805064-84-2
Cynthia Kupper RDCD, Executive Director

Newsletters

2529 GIG Quarterly Magazine
Gluten Intolerance Group: GIG
31214 124th Avenue SE 253-833-6655
Auburn, WA 98092-3667 Fax: 253-833-6675
e-mail: info@gluten.net
www.gluten.net
Member magazine. Offers updated medical and technological information for patients with celiac disease, their families and healthcare professionals.
Quarterly
Cynthia Kupper RDCD, Executive Director

2530 Lifeline
Celiac Sprue Association/USA
PO Box 31700 402-558-0600
Omaha, NE 68131 877-272-4272
Fax: 402-643-4108
e-mail: celiacs@csaceliacs.org
www.csaceliacs.org
Quarterly newsletter for members; contains up-to-date research information, personal stories from celiacs, cooking tips, recipes and contact information for support chapters and resource units.
Mary Schluckebier, Executive Director

2531 Whooo's Report
American Celiac Society
PO Box 23455 504-737-3293
New Orleans, LA 70183 e-mail: amerceliacsoc@netscape.net
Provides practical assistance to members and individuals with celiac disease and information about the disease to the public.

Pamphlets

2532 Celiac Disease
Gluten Intolerance Group: GIG
31214 124th Avenue SE 253-833-6655
Auburn, WA 98092-3667 Fax: 253-833-6675
e-mail: info@gluten.net
www.gluten.net
Offers facts and statistics on celiac disease.
Cynthia Kupper RDCD, Executive Director

2533 Celiac Disease: A Hidden Epidemic
Peter Greene, MD, author
Harper Collins Publishers
10 East 53rd Street
New York, NY 10022 212-207-7000
www.harpercollins.com
An "inside-out" examination and explanation of Celiac Disease.
2006 352 pages
ISBN: 0-060766-93-X
Cynthia Kupper RDCD, Executive Director

2534 Dermatitis Herpetiformis
Gluten Intolerance Group: GIG
31214 124th Avenue SE 253-833-6655
Auburn, WA 98092-3667 Fax: 253-833-6675
e-mail: info@gluten.net
www.gluten.net
Offers facts and statistics on dermatitis herpetformis.
Cynthia Kupper RDCD, Executive Director

2535 Grains and Flours
Celiac Sprue Association/USA
PO Box 31700 402-558-0600
Omaha, NE 68131 877-272-4272
Fax: 402-643-4108
e-mail: celiacs@csaceliacs.org
www.csaceliacs.org
A variety of different gluten-free flour mixtures, to experiment with and discover your favorite!
Mary Schluckebier, Executive Director

2536 Guide to Gluten-Free Diets
American Allergy Association
PO Box 7273 650-322-1663
Menlo Park, CA 94026-7273
Offers information on safe substitutes for baking and cooking. Differentiates celiac disease from wheat allergy. Sources of gluten in diet with warnings on when to check with the manufacturer.

2537 Patient Packet
Celiac Sprue Association/USA
PO Box 31700 402-558-0600
Omaha, NE 68131 877-272-4272
Fax: 402-643-4108
e-mail: celiacs@csaceliacs.org
www.csaceliacs.org
A basic information packet for the newly-diagnosed celiac. Provided free of charge to individuals, physicians, dietitians, and family members.
Mary Schluckebier, Executive Director

2538 Quick Start Diet Guide
Gluten Intolerance Group: GIG
31214 124th Avenue SE 253-833-6655
Auburn, WA 98092-3667 Fax: 253-833-6675
e-mail: info@gluten.net
www.gluten.net
Packet available to download on website.
Cynthia Kupper RDCD, Executive Director

Audio & Video

2539 CD-A NIH Consensus Conference
Celiac Sprue Association/USA
PO Box 31700 402-558-0600
Omaha, NE 68131 877-272-4272
Fax: 402-643-4108
e-mail: celiacs@csaceliacs.org
www.csaceliacs.org
Celiac Disease - A NIH Consensus Conference - Reaching Out to Improve the Health of Millions.
Mary Schluckebier, Executive Director

Web Sites

2540 Celiac Disease & Gluten-Free Diet Online Resource Center
www.celiac.com

Internet based support organization that provides important resources and information for people on gluten-free diets due to celiac disease, gluten intolerance or wheat allergy.

2541 Celiac Disease Foundation

www.celiac.org/

Provides services and support to persons with celiac disease and dermatitus herpetiformis, through programs of awareness, education, advocacy and research; telephone information and referral services; medical advisory board; and special educational seminars and quarterly meetings.

2542 Celiac Sprue Association: USA

www.csaceliacs.org

Member based, nonprofit support organization dedicated to helping individuals with celiac disease and dermatitis herpetiformis worldwide through education, information and research. Includes over 90 support chapters, 50 resource units, and Cel-Kids Network. Sponsors an annual conference, publishes educational materials, conducts a summer youth camp and provides phone and on-line counseling.

2543 Gluten Intolerance Group: GIG

www.gluten.net

Provides instructional and general information materials, as well as counseling and access to gluten-free products and ingredients to persons with celiac sprue and their families, operates telephone information and referral service, conducts educational seminars for health professionals, conducts and supports research, offers leadership and assistance to contacts and provides for a gluten-free kids camp.

2544 Healing Well

www.healingwell.com

An online health resource guide to medical news, chat, information and articles, newsgroups and message boards, books, disease-related web sites, medical directories, and more for patients, friends, and family coping with disabling diseases, disorders, or chronic illnesses.

2545 Health Finder

www.healthfinder.gov

Searchable, carefully developed web site offering information on over 1000 topics. Developed by the US Department of Health and Human Services, the site can be used in both English and Spanish.

2546 Healthlink USA

www.healthlinkusa.com

Health information concerning treatment, cures, prevention, diagnosis, risk factors, research, support groups, email lists, personal stories and much more. Updated regularly.

2547 Helios Health

www.helioshealth.com

Online resource for your health information. Detailed information about specific health topics, access to expert advice from our Medical Advisory Board, and up-to-date health news.

2548 MedicineNet

www.medicinenet.com

An online resource for consumers providing easy-to-read, authoritative medical and health information.

2549 Medscape

www.mywebmd.com

Medscape offers specialists, primary care physicians, and other health professionals the Web's most robust and integrated medical information and educational tools.

2550 WebMD

www.webmd.com

Provides links to over 20 articles involving Celiac disease.

Description

2551 # Cerebral Palsy

Cerebral palsy, CP, applies to disorders of voluntary movement resulting from damage to areas in the brain. CP can be caused by birth trauma, insufficient oxygen supplied to the infant at or before birth, premature birth or a severe systemic disease, such as meningitis, during early infancy. However, the exact cause is often difficult to establish.

Children with cerebral palsy may not be identified until they reach 1-2 years of age and may show only lagging motor development. Therefore, children known to be at risk should be followed closely. Increased spastic movements is the most common symptom, but children may also show weakness, poor sense of balance, involuntary movements and abnormal walking. In more severe cases, difficulty in speaking and mental retardation may also be present.

Since there is no known cure for cerebral palsy, the goal of treatment is to develop maximal independence. Therapy may include physical and occupational rehabilitation, the use of leg braces, speech training and special orthopedic surgery. Parents need assistance and guidance in understanding their child's status and potential.

National Agencies & Associations

2552 **American Academy for Cerebral Palsy and Developmental Medicine**
555 E Wells
Milwaukee, WI 53202
414-918-3014
Fax: 414-276-2146
e-mail: info@aacpdm.org
www.aacpdm.org

A multidisciplinary scientific society devoted to the study of cerebral palsy and other childhood onset disabilities, promoting professional education for the treatment and management of these conditions and to improving the quality of life for people with the condition.
1550 members

2553 **American Academy for Cerebral Palsy and De velopmental Medicine**
555 E Wells Street
Milwaukee, WI 53202
414-918-3014
e-mail: info@aacpdm.org
www.aacpdm.org

A multidisciplinary scientific society devoted to the study of cerebral palsy and other childhood onset disabilities, to promoting professional education for the treatment and management of these conditions, and to improving the quality of life for people with these disabilities.

2554 **Canadian Cerebral Palsy Sports Association**
305-1376 Bank Street
Ottawa, Ontario, K1H-7Y3
613-748-1430
866-247-9934
Fax: 613-748-1355
e-mail: info@ccpsa.ca
www.ccpsa.ca

Is an athelete focused national organization administering and governing sport opportunities targeted to athletes with CP and related disabilities.
Sandy Hermiston, President

2555 **Easter Seals**
233 S Wacker Drive
Chicago, IL 60606
312-726-6200
800-221-6827
Fax: 312-726-1494
TTY: 312-726-4258
e-mail: info@easter-seals.org
www.easter-seals.org

Provides services to children and adults with disabilities as well as support to their families.
Reenie Kavalar, VP Medical/Rehabilitation Services

2556 **Independent Living Research Utilization Project**
2323 S Shepherd
Houston, TX 77019
713-520-0232
Fax: 713-520-5785
TTY: 713-520-0232
e-mail: ilru@ilru.org
www.ilru.org

A national center for information training research and technical assistance in independent living. Goal is to expand the body of knowledge in independent living and to improve utilization of results of research programs and demonstration projects.
Lex Frieden, Director
Linda CoVan, Grant Coordinator

2557 **National Rehabilitation Information Center**
4200 Forbes Boulevard
Lanham, MD 20706
301-459-5900
800-346-2742
Fax: 301-459-5984
e-mail: narincinfo@heitechservices.com
www.naric.com/

One of the three components of the office of Special Education and Rehabilitative Services. Operates in concert with the Rehabilitation Services Administration and the Office of Special Education Programs.
Mark Odum, Director

2558 **United Cerebral Palsy Associations**
1660 L Street NW
Washington, DC 20036
202-776-0406
800-872-5827
Fax: 202-776-0414
TTY: 202-973-7197
e-mail: info@ucp.org
www.ucp.org

A network of approximately 119 state and local voluntary agencies which provide services conduct public and professional education programs and support research in cerebral palsy.
Bruce Merlin Fried, Chair
Keith Green, Vice Chair

State Agencies & Associations

Alabama

2559 **United Cerebral Palsy of Alabama**
301 EA Darden Drive
Anniston, AL 36202
256-237-8203
Fax: 256-235-2388
e-mail: executivedirector@ecaucp.org
www.ecaucp.org

United Cerebral Palsy provides information, advocacy, referral services for persons with disabilities and/or their families. UCP also operates an equipment loan program, conducts parent workshops, disseminates written literature on topics of interest.
Linda Johns, Executive Director
Shannon Priddy, Development Director

2560 **United Cerebral Palsy of East Central Alabama**
301 EA Darden Drive
Anniston, AL 36202
256-237-8203
Fax: 256-235-2388
e-mail: executivedirector@ecaucp.org
www.ucpa.org

United Cerebral Palsy provides information, advocacy, referral services for persons with disabilities and/or their families. UCP also operates an equipment loan program, conducts parent workshops, disseminates written literature on topics of interest to people with disabilities.

2561 United Cerebral Palsy of Greater Birmingha m
120 Oslo Circle 205-944-3900
Birmingham, AL 35211 800-654-4483
Fax: 205-944-3990
e-mail: gedwards@ucpbham.com
www.ucpbham.com
United Cerebral Palsy provides information, advocacy, referral services for persons with disabilities and/or their families. UCP also operates an equipment loan program, conducts parent workshops, disseminates written literature on topics of interest to people with disabilities.
Gary Edwards, Executive Director
Jennifer H Ellison, Chief Development Officer

2562 United Cerebral Palsy of Huntsville & Tennessee Valley
2075 Max Luther Drive 256-852-5600
Huntsville, AL 35810 Fax: 256-852-6722
e-mail: tracyc@ucphuntsville.org
www.ucp.org
United Cerebral Palsy provides information, advocacy, referral services for persons with disabilities and/or their families. UCP also operates an equipment loan program, conducts parent workshops, disseminates written literature on topics of interest.
Cheryl Smith, Executive Director
Tim Reeves, President

2563 United Cerebral Palsy of Mobile
3058 Dauphin Square Connector 251-479-4900
Mobile, AL 36607 Fax: 251-479-4998
e-mail: info@ucpmobile.org
www.ucp.org
United Cerebral Palsy provides information, advocacy, referral services for persons with disabilities and/or their families. UCP also operates an equipment loan program, conducts parent workshops, disseminates written literature on topics of interest.
Glenn Harger, President/CEO
Susan Watson, VP/COO

2564 United Cerebral Palsy of Northwest Alabama
4212 Jackson Highway 256-381-4310
Sheffield, AL 35660 Fax: 256-381-4378
e-mail: alison@ucpshoals.org
www.ucpshoals.org
United Cerebral Palsy provides information, advocacy, referral services for persons with disabilities and/or their families. UCP also operates an equipment loan program, conducts parent workshops, disseminates written literature on topics of interest.
Alison Isbell, Director
Linda Williamson, Development Director/WEE-CARE Director

2565 United Cerebral Palsy of West Alabama
1100 UCP Parkway 205-345-3031
Northport, AL 35476 Fax: 205-345-3035
e-mail: lisasucp@comcast.net
www.ucpa.org
United Cerebral Palsy provides information, advocacy, referral services for persons with disabilities and/or their families. UCP also operates an equipment loan program, conducts parent workshops, disseminates written literature on topics of interest.
Lisa D Skelton, Executive Director
Brenda Ewart, Development Director

Alaska

2566 United Cerebral Palsy of Alaska/PARENTS
4743 E Northern Lights Boulevard 907-337-7678
Anchorage, AK 99508 800-478-7678
Fax: 907-337-7671
TTY: 907-337-7629
e-mail: parents@parentsinc.org
www.ucpa.org
Provides information, advocacy, referral services for persons with disabilities and/or their families. UCP also operates an equipment loan program, conducts parent workshops, disseminates written literature on topics of interest to people with disabilities.

Arizona

2567 United Cerebral Palsy of Central Arizona
1802 Parkside Lane 602-943-5472
Phoenix, AZ 85027 Fax: 602-943-4936
e-mail: info@ucpofaz.org
www.ucpa.org
United Cerebral Palsy provides information, advocacy, referral services for persons with disabilities and/or their families. UCP also operates an equipment loan program, conducts parent workshops, disseminates written literature on topics of interest.
Dan Rossi, Executive Director
Perry Bramlett, Chief Human Resources Officer

2568 United Cerebral Palsy of Southern Arizona
635 N Craycroft Road 520-795-3108
Tucson, AZ 85711 Fax: 520-795-3196
e-mail: staff@ucpsa.org
www.ucpsa.org
United Cerebral Palsy provides information, advocacy, referral services for persons with disabilities and/or their families. UCP also operates an equipment loan program, conducts parent workshops, disseminates written literature on topics of interest.
Cindy Mars, Executive Director
Gary Bahman, Finance Director

Arkansas

2569 United Cerebral Palsy of Central Arkansas
9720 N Rodney Parham Road 501-224-6067
Little Rock, AR 72227 Fax: 501-227-5591
e-mail: general@ucpcark.org
www.ucpark.org
United Cerebral Palsy provides information, advocacy, referral services for persons with disabilities and/or their families. UCP also operates an equipment loan program, conducts parent workshops, disseminates written literature on topics of interest.

2570 United Cerebral Palsy of South Arkansas
9720 N Rodney Parham Road 501-224-6067
Little Rock, AR 72227 800-228-6174
Fax: 501-227-5591
e-mail: general@ucpcark.org
www.ucpark.org
United Cerebral Palsy provides information, advocacy, referral services for persons with disabilities and/or their families. UCP also operates an equipment loan program, conducts parent workshops, disseminates written literature on topics of interest.

California

2571 United Cerebral Palsy of Central California
4224 North Cedar Avenue 559-221-8272
Fresno, CA 93726-3700 Fax: 559-221-9347
e-mail: lauriea@ccucp.org
www.ucpa.org
United Cerebral Palsy provides information, advocacy, referral services for persons with disabilities and/or their families. UCP also operates an equipment loan program, conducts parent workshops, disseminates written literature on topics of interest to people with disabilities.

2572 United Cerebral Palsy of Greater Sacrament o
191 Lathrop Way 916-565-7700
Sacramento, CA 95815 Fax: 916-565-7773
e-mail: ucp@ucpsacto.org
www.ucpsacto.org
UCP provides programs and services for people with all types of developmental disabilities. These services include: day programs for adults, an in-home respite service, transportation, independent living services, information and referral services.
Doug Bergman, President/CEO
Tanya Hartle, COO

2573 United Cerebral Palsy of Los Angeles & Ventura Counties
6430 Independence Avenue 818-782-2211
Woodland Hills, CA 91367 Fax: 818-909-9106
e-mail: mail@ucpla.com
www.ucpla.org

United Cerebral Palsy provides information, advocacy, referral services for persons with disabilities and/or their families. UCP also operates an equipment loan program, conducts parent workshops, disseminates written literature on topics of interest to people with disabilities.
Ronald S Cohen, Chief Executive Officer
Clark Jensen, Chief Operating Officer

2574 United Cerebral Palsy of Orange County
980 Roosevelt
Irvine, CA 92602
949-333-6400
Fax: 949-333-6400
e-mail: info@ucp-oc.org
www.ucp-oc.org
United Cerebral Palsy provides information, advocacy, referral services for persons with disabilities and/or their families. UCP also operates an equipment loan program, conducts parent workshops, disseminates written literature on topics of interest.
Paul Pulver, Executive Directorÿ
Lauren Mille Beeler, Director of Therapy Services

2575 United Cerebral Palsy of San Diego County
8525 Gibbs Drive
San Diego, CA 92123
858-571-7803
Fax: 858-571-0919
e-mail: ucp@ucpsd.org
www.ucpa.org
United Cerebral Palsy provides information, advocacy, referral services for persons with disabilities and/or their families. UCP also operates an equipment loan program, conducts parent workshops, disseminates written literature on topics of interest.
David Carucci, Executive Director
Mary Krieger, Associate Executive Director

2576 United Cerebral Palsy of San Joaquin, Calaveras & Amador Counties
333 W Benjamin Holt Drive
Stockton, CA 95207
209-956-0290
Fax: 209-956-0294
e-mail: slarson@ucpsj.org
www.ucp.org
United Cerebral Palsy provides information, advocacy, referral services for persons with disabilities and/or their families. UCP also operates an equipment loan program, conducts parent workshops, disseminates written literature on topics of interest to people with disabilities.
Leslie Heier, Interim Executive Director
Theresa Galano-Burke, Executive Assistant

2577 United Cerebral Palsy of San Luis Obispo
3620 Sacramento Drive
San Luis Obispo, CA 93401
805-543-2039
877-UCP-CAR1
Fax: 805-543-2045
e-mail: shaftmt@aol.com
www.ucp-slo.org
United Cerebral Palsy provides information, advocacy, referral services for persons with disabilities and/or their families. UCP also operates an equipment loan program, conducts parent workshops, disseminates written literature on topics of interest to people with disabilities.
Mark Shaffer, UCP Executive Director
Karl Winkler, UCPÿAdministrative Assistant

2578 United Cerebral Palsy of Santa Barbara County
6430 Independence Avenue
Woodland Hills, CA 91367
818-782-2211
888-733-4227
Fax: 818-909-9106
e-mail: mail@ucpla.org
www.ucpla.org
United Cerebral Palsy provides information, advocacy, referral services for persons with disabilities and/or their families. UCP also operates an equipment loan program, conducts parent workshops, disseminates written literature on topics of interest.
Ellen Kessler, Chairperson
Nick Roxborough, President

2579 United Cerebral Palsy of Santa Clara & San Mateo Counties
512 E Maude Avenue
Sunnyvale, CA 94085-4431
650-917-6900
Fax: 650-948-8503
e-mail: info@ucpscsm.org
www.ucpscsm.org/
United Cerebral Palsy provides information, advocacy, referral services for persons with disabilities and/or their families. UCP also operates an equipment loan program, conducts parent workshops, disseminates written literature on topics of interest.
Stephen Bennett, President/CEO National Office (DC)
Armetta Parker, Marketing/Communications Director (DC)

2580 United Cerebral Palsy of Stanislaus County
1213 13th Street
Modesto, CA 95353
209-577-2122
Fax: 209-577-2392
e-mail: rlonczak@ucpstan.org
www.ucpstan.org
United Cerebral Palsy provides information, advocacy, referral services for persons with disabilities and/or their families. UCP also operates an equipment loan program, conducts parent workshops, disseminates written literature on topics of interest to people with disabilities.
Robert S Lonczak, Executive Director
Jeanette Jones, ProgramÿCoordinator

2581 United Cerebral Palsy of the Golden Gate
1970 Broadway
Oakland, CA 94612
510-832-7430
Fax: 510-839-1329
e-mail: info@ucpgg.org
www.ucp.org
United Cerebral Palsy provides information, advocacy, referral services for persons with disabilities and/or their families. UCP also operates an equipment loan program, conducts parent workshops, disseminates written literature on topics of interest.
Karen Glatze, Administrator
Dori Maxon, SNAP Program Director

2582 United Cerebral Palsy of the Inland Empire
35-325 Date Palm Drive
Cathedral City, CA 92234
760-321-8184
877-512-2224
Fax: 760-321-8284
e-mail: info@ucpie.org
www.ucpie.org
United Cerebral Palsy provides information, advocacy, referral services for persons with disabilities and/or their families. UCP conducts parent workshops, disseminates written literature on topics of interest to people with disabilities.
Roger M Alexander, Chair
Micki James, Vice Chair

2583 United Cerebral Palsy of the North Bay
3835 Cypress Drive
Petaluma, CA 94954
707-766-9990
800-872-5827
Fax: 202-776-0414
e-mail: info@ucpnb.org
www.ucp.org
United Cerebral Palsy's mission is to advance the independence, productivity and full citizenship of people with disabilities through an affiliate network.
Margaret Farman, Executive Director
Ron Hamilton, Chief of Operations

Colorado

2584 United Cerebral Palsy of Colorado
801 Yosemite Street
Denver, CO 80230-5708
303-691-9339
866-701-2277
Fax: 303-691-0846
www.cpco.org
United Cerebral Palsy provides information, advocacy, referral services for persons with disabilities and/or their families. UCP also operates an equipment loan program, conducts parent workshops, disseminates written literature on topics of interest.
Jim Reuter, Chairman of the Board
Judith I Ham, President/CEO

Connecticut

2585 United Cerebral Palsy of Eastern Connecticut
42 Norwich Road
Quaker Hill, CT 06375
860-447-3800
Fax: 860-443-8272
e-mail: email@ucpect.org
www.ucp.org
United Cerebral Palsy provides information, advocacy, referral services for persons with disabilities and/or their families. UCP also operates an equipment loan program, conducts parent work-

shops, disseminates written literature on topics of interest to people with disabilities.
Margaret Morrison, Executive Director
Patricia Mansfield, Executive Director

2586 **United Cerebral Palsy of Greater Hartford**
80 Whitney Street 860-236-6201
Hartford, CT 06105 Fax: 860-218-2454
e-mail: jmcmahon@sunrisegroup.org
www.ucp.org
United Cerebral Palsy provides information, advocacy, referral services for persons with disabilities and/or their families. UCP also operates an equipment loan program, conducts parent workshops, disseminates written literature on topics of interest to people with disabilities.

2587 **United Cerebral Palsy of Southern Connecticut**
94-96 South Turnpike Road 203-269-3511
Wallingford, CT 06492 Fax: 203-269-7411
e-mail: ucpasouthernct@yahoo.com
www.ucpa.org
United Cerebral Palsy provides information, advocacy, referral services for persons with disabilities and/or their families. UCP also operates an equipment loan program, conducts parent workshops, disseminates written literature on topics of interest to people with disabilities.

Delaware

2588 **United Cerebral Palsy of Delaware**
700 A River Road 302-764-2400
Wilmington, DE 19809-2746 Fax: 302-764-8713
e-mail: wmccool@ucpde.org
www.ucp.org/ucp_local.cfm/52
United Cerebral Palsy provides information, advocacy, referral services for persons with disabilities and/or their families. UCP also operates an equipment loan program, conducts parent workshops, disseminates written literature on topics of interest.
Michelle Welch, President
D Bruce McClenathan, Vice President

District of Columbia

2589 **United Cerebral Palsy of Washington DC & Northern Virginia**
1818 New York Avenue NE 202-526-0146
Washington, DC 20002 Fax: 202-526-0519
e-mail: webmaster@ucpdcnova.org
www.ucpa.org
United Cerebral Palsy provides information, advocacy, referral services for persons with disabilities and/or their families. UCP also operates an equipment loan program, conducts parent workshops, disseminates written literature on topics of interest to people with disabilities.

Florida

2590 **United Cerebral Palsy of Central Florida**
3305 S Orange Avenue 407-852-3300
Orlando, FL 32806 Fax: 407-852-3301
e-mail: mbetts@ucpcdc.org
www.ucpcfl.org
United Cerebral Palsy provides information, advocacy, referral services for persons with disabilities and/or their families. UCP also operates an equipment loan program, conducts parent workshops, disseminates written literature on topics of interest.
Ilene E Wilkins, President & Chief Executive Officer
Jill Wisth, Chief Financial Officer

2591 **United Cerebral Palsy of East Central Florida**
1100 Jimmy Ann Drive 386-274-6474
Daytona Beach, FL 32117 Fax: 386-274-6532
e-mail: info@ucpecf.org
www.ucp.org

Barry Pollack, President/CEO
Kelly Johanessen, VP of Operations

2592 **United Cerebral Palsy of Florida**
1830 Buford Court 850-922-5630
Tallahassee, FL 32308 Fax: 850-922-1258
e-mail: gloriawe@earthlink.net
www.ucp.org
United Cerebral Palsy provides information, advocacy, referral services for persons with disabilities and/or their families. UCP also operates an equipment loan program, conducts parent workshops, disseminates written literature on topics of interest.

2593 **United Cerebral Palsy of North Florida: Tender Loving Care**
1241 NE Avenue 850-769-7960
Panama City, FL 32401 Fax: 850-769-1060
e-mail: kimberly.mcmanus@comcast.net
www.ucp.org
United Cerebral Palsy provides information, advocacy, referral services for persons with disabilities and/or their families. UCP also operates an equipment loan program, conducts parent workshops, disseminates written literature on topics of interest to people with disabilities.

2594 **United Cerebral Palsy of Northeast Florida**
3311 Beach Boulevard 904-396-1462
Jacksonville, FL 32207 Fax: 904-396-1199
e-mail: cpnefagency@hotmail.com

2595 **United Cerebral Palsy of Northwest Florida**
2912 North East Street 850-432-1596
Pensacola, FL 32501-1324 Fax: 850-432-1930
e-mail: information@ucpnwfl.org
www.ucp.org
The number one service provider in Northwest Florida for individuals with cerebral palsy and other developmental disabilities, UCP provides information ,advocacy and referral services for persons with disabilities and/or their families. Additionally, UCP offers individuals assistance with daily living skills training, computer training, basic education, speech, physical and occupational therapy, residential, supported living and finding long-term employment.

2596 **United Cerebral Palsy of Sarasota-Manatee**
1090 S Tamiami Trail 941-957-3599
Sarasota, FL 34236 Fax: 947-957-3499
e-mail: ucpwendy@aol.com
www.ucpsarasota.org
United Cerebral Palsy provides information, advocacy, referral services for persons with disabilities and/or their families. UCP also operates an equipment loan program, conducts parent workshops, disseminates written literature on topics of interest.
Barnett A Greenberg, Chairperson
Mark Famiglio, President

2597 **United Cerebral Palsy of South Florida**
2700 W 81st Street 305-325-1080
Hialeah, FL 33016 Fax: 305-325-1313
e-mail: info@ucpsouthflorida.org
www.ucp.org
United Cerebral Palsy provides information, advocacy, referral services for persons with disabilities and/or their families. UCP also operates an equipment loan program, conducts parent workshops, disseminates written literature on topics of interest.
Joseph Aniello, President & CEO
Linda Gluck, Vice President & CFO

2598 **United Cerebral Palsy of Tallahassee**
1830 Buford Court 850-878-2141
Tallahassee, FL 32308 Fax: 850-922-1258
e-mail: gloriawe@earthlink.net
www.ucp.org
United Cerebral Palsy provides information, advocacy, referral services for persons with disabilities and/or their families. UCP also operates an equipment loan program, conducts parent workshops, disseminates written literature on topics of interest.

2599 **United Cerebral Palsy of Tampa Bay**
2215 E Henry Avenue 813-239-1179
Tampa, FL 33610 800-749-5155
Fax: 813-237-3091
e-mail: kryals@advanceability.org
www.achievetampabay.org

United Cerebral Palsy provides information, advocacy, referral services for persons with disabilities and/or their families. UCP also operates an equipment loan program, conducts parent workshops, disseminates written literature on topics of interest to people with disabilities.
David W Brooks, Executive Director
William Chisholm, Program Director

Georgia

2600 United Cerebral Palsy of Georgia
3300 NE Expressway
Atlanta, GA 30341
770-676-2000
Fax: 770-455-8040
e-mail: info@ucpga.org
www.ucp.org
United Cerebral Palsy provides information, advocacy, referral services for persons with disabilities and/or their families. UCP also operates an equipment loan program, conducts parent workshops, disseminates written literature on topics of interest to people with disabilities.
Diane Wilush, Executive Director
Kevin Walton, Associate Executive Director

Hawaii

2601 United Cerebral Palsy of Hawaii
414 Kuwili Street
Honolulu, HI 96817-5050
808-532-6744
800-606-5654
Fax: 808-532-6747
e-mail: ucpa@diverseabilities.org
www.ucpahi.org
United Cerebral Palsy provides information, advocacy, referral services for persons with disabilities and/or their families. UCP also operates an equipment loan program, conducts parent workshops, disseminates written literature on topics of interest.
Jerry Pupillo, President
Stephen Hink, 1st Vice President

Idaho

2602 United Cerebral Palsy of Idaho
5420 W Franklin Road
Boise, ID 83705
208-377-8070
888-289-3281
Fax: 208-322-7133
e-mail: info@ucpidaho.org
www.ucp.org
United Cerebral Palsy provides information, advocacy and referral services for persons with disabilities and/or their families.
Kim Kane, Executive Director
Kathy Griffin, Program Director

Illinois

2603 United Cerebral Palsy Land of Lincoln
101 N 16th Street
Springfield, IL 67203
217-525-6522
Fax: 217-525-9017
e-mail: info@ucpll.org
www.ucp.org
United Cerebral Palsy provides information, advocacy, referral services for persons with disabilities and/or their families. UCP also operates an equipment loan program, conducts parent workshops, disseminates written literature on topics of interest.
Brenda L Yarnell, President/CEO
Kathy Leuelling, Chief Operating Officer

2604 United Cerebral Palsy of East Central Illinois
1023 N Water
Decatur, IL 62523
217-428-5033
Fax: 217-428-5094
ww.ucpa.org
United Cerebral Palsy provides information, advocacy, referral services for persons with disabilities and/or their families. UCP also operates an equipment loan program, conducts parent workshops, disseminates written literature on topics of interest.

2605 United Cerebral Palsy of Greater Chicago
547 W Jackson
Chicago, IL 60661
312-765-0419
Fax: 312-765-0503
TTY: 312-368-0179
e-mail: pdulle@ucpnet.org
www.ucpnet.org
United Cerebral Palsy provides information, advocacy, referral services for persons with disabilities and/or their families. UCP also operates an equipment loan program, conducts parent workshops, disseminates written literature on topics of interest to people with disabilities.
Paul J Dulle, President/CEO
Peggy Childs, Executive Vice President

2606 United Cerebral Palsy of Illinois
310 E Adams
Springfield, IL 62701
877-550-8274
877-550-8274
Fax: 217-528-9739
TTY: 877-550-8274
e-mail: cpil@sbcglobal.net
www.ucpillinois.org
United Cerebral Palsy provides information, advocacy, referral services for persons with disabilities and/or their families. UCP also operates an equipment loan program, conducts parent workshops, disseminates written literature on topics of interest to people with disabilities.
Don Moss, Executive Director
Alice Foss, Associate Director

2607 United Cerebral Palsy of Southern Illinois
9 Cusumano Professional Plaza Drive
Mount Vernon, IL 62864
618-244-2505
Fax: 618-244-3568
e-mail: ucpsi@onemain.com
www.ucpa.org
United Cerebral Palsy provides information, advocacy, referral services for persons with disabilities and/or their families. UCP also operates an equipment loan program, conducts parent workshops, disseminates written literature on topics of interest to people with disabilities.

2608 United Cerebral Palsy of Will County
311 S Reed Street
Joliet, IL 60436
815-744-3500
Fax: 815-744-3504
e-mail: ucpwill@ucpwill.org
www.ucp.org
United Cerebral Palsy provides information, advocacy, referral services for persons with disabilities and/or their families. UCP also operates an equipment loan program, conducts parent workshops, disseminates written literature on topics of interest to people with disabilities.
Samuel Mancuso, President & Chief Executive Officer
Stephanie Bergner, Family Support/Respite Administrator

2609 United Cerebral Palsy of the Blackhawk Region
7399 Forest Hills Road
Rockford, IL 61111
815-636-7132
Fax: 815-282-8835
e-mail: ucpbr@aol.com
www.ucpa.org
United Cerebral Palsy provides information, advocacy, referral services for persons with disabilities and/or their families. UCP also operates an equipment loan program, conducts parent workshops, disseminates written literature on topics of interest to people with disabilities.

2610 United Cerebral Palsy: Eastern Seals
230 W Monroe Street
Chicago, IL 60606
312-726-6200
800-221-6827
Fax: 312-726-1494
stsweb.indstate.edu
United Cerebral Palsy provides information, advocacy, referral services for persons with disabilities and/or their families. UCP also operates an equipment loan program, conducts parent workshops, disseminates written literature on topics of interest.

Indiana

2611 **United Cerebral Palsy Association of Indiana**
1915 West 18th Street 317-632-3561
Indianapolis, IN 46202-1016 Fax: 317-632-3338
e-mail: donnar@ucpaindy.org
www.ucpa.org
United Cerebral Palsy provides information, advocacy, referral services for persons with Cerebal Palsy and/or their families. UCP also provides funding for equipment and operates an equipment loan program, disseminates written literature on topics of interest to people with disabilities.
Donna L Roberts, Executive Director

2612 **United Cerebral Palsy Associations**
6100 N Keystone Avenue 317-632-3561
Indianapolis, IN 46220 Fax: 317-632-3338
e-mail: donnar@ucpaindy.org
www.ucpaindy.org
United Cerebral Palsy provides information, advocacy, referral services for persons with Cerebral Palsy and/or their families. UCP also provides funding for equipment and operates an equipment loan program, disseminates written literature on topics of interest.
Donna L Roberts, Executive Director
Beth Allison, Case Manager

2613 **United Cerebral Palsy of the Wabash Valley**
621 Poplar Street 812-232-6305
Terre Haute, IN 47807 Fax: 812-234-3683
e-mail: ucp.wv@verizon.net
stsweb.indstate.edu
United Cerebral Palsy provides information, advocacy, referral services for persons with disabilities and/or their families. UCP also operates an equipment loan program, conducts parent workshops, disseminates written literature on topics of interest to people with disabilties.
Jacquie Denehie, Executive Director

Kansas

2614 **United Cerebral Palsy of Kansas**
5111 E 21st Street 316-688-1888
Wichita, KS 67208 Fax: 316-688-5687
e-mail: davej@cprf.org
www.ucp.org
United Cerebral Palsy provides information, advocacy, referral services for persons with disabilities and/or their families. UCP also operates an equipment loan program, conducts parent workshops, disseminates written literature on topics of interest.
Dave Jones, Executive Director
Amelia Ornelas, Office Manager

Louisiana

2615 **United Cerebral Palsy of Baton Rouge McMains Children's Developmental Center**
1805 College Drive 225-923-3420
Baton Rouge, LA 70808 Fax: 225-922-9316
e-mail: jketcham@mcmainscdc.org
www.mcmainscdc.org
United Cerebral Palsy provides information, advocacy, referral services for persons with disabilities and/or their families. UCP also operates an equipment loan program, conducts parent workshops, disseminates written literature on topics of interest.
Janet Ketcham, Director
Norman Landry, President

2616 **United Cerebral Palsy of Greater New Orleans**
1000 Leonidas St & Leake Avenue 504-865-0003
New Orleans, LA 70118 Fax: 504-865-0300
e-mail: info@ucpgno.com
www.ucpa.org
United Cerebral Palsy provides information, advocacy, referral services for persons with disabilities and/or their families. UCP also operates an equipment loan program, conducts parent workshops, disseminates written literature on topics of interest to people with disabilities.

Maine

2617 **United Cerebral Palsy of Northeastern Maine**
700 Mount Hope Avenue 207-941-2952
Bangor, ME 04401 877-603-0030
Fax: 207-941-2955
e-mail: office@ucpofmaine.org
www.ucp.org
United Cerebral Palsy provides information, advocacy, referral services for persons with disabilities and/or their families. UCP also operates an equipment loan program, conducts parent workshops, disseminates written literature on topics of interest to people with disabilities.
Bobbi-Jo Yeager, Executive Director
Tricia Kail, Director of Services

Maryland

2618 **United Cerebral Palsy of Central Maryland**
1700 Reistertown Road 410-484-4540
Baltimore, MD 21208-2935 Fax: 410-484-1807
TTY: 800-451-2452
e-mail: info@ucp-cm.org
www.ucp.org
United Cerebral Palsy provides information, advocacy, referral services for persons with disabilities and/or their families. UCP also operates an equipment loan program, conducts parent workshops, disseminates written literature on topics of interest.
Diane Coughlin, President and CEO
Judy Cox, Assistant to the President

2619 **United Cerebral Palsy of Prince Georges & Montgomery Counties**
4409 Forbes Boulevard 301-459-0566
Lanham, MD 20706 Fax: 301-459-7691
TTY: 301-459-7691
TDD: 301-262-4982
e-mail: ucppgmc@aol.com
www.ucppgmc.com
Provides information, advocacy, referral services for persons with disabilities and/or their families. UCP also operates an equipment loan program, conducts parent workshops, disseminates written literature on topics of interest to people with disabilities.
Charles McNelly, Executive Director
Diane Dekoladenu, Program Director

2620 **United Cerebral Palsy of Southern Maryland**
221 Chinquapin Round Road 410-280-2003
Annapolis, MD 21401 Fax: 410-269-5757
e-mail: ucpinfo@ucpsm.org
www.ucpsm.org
United Cerebral Palsy provides information, advocacy, referral services for persons with disabilities and/or their families. UCP also operates an equipment loan program, conducts parent workshops, disseminates written literature on topics of interest to people with disabilities.

Massachusetts

2621 **United Cerebral Palsy of Berkshire County**
208 W Street 413-442-1562
Pittsfield, MA 01201 Fax: 413-499-4077
e-mail: info@ucpberkshire.org
www.ucp.org
United Cerebral Palsy provides information, advocacy, referral services for persons with disabilities and/or their families. UCP also operates an equipment loan program, conducts parent workshops, disseminates written literature on topics of interest to people with disabilities.
Christine Singer, Executive Director
Joni Thomas, Director of Development

2622 **United Cerebral Palsy of MetroBoston**
71 Arsenal Street 617-926-5480
Watertown, MA 02472 Fax: 617-926-3059
e-mail: ucpboston@ucpboston.org
www.ucp.org
United Cerebral Palsy provides information, advocacy, referral services for persons with disabilities and/or their families. UCP

also operates an equipment loan program, conducts parent workshops, disseminates written literature on topics of interest.
Todd Kates, Executive Director
Roberta Jaro, Associate Executive Director

Michigan

2623 **United Cerebral Palsy of Metropolitan Detroit**
23077 Greenfield
Southfield, MI 48075
248-557-5070
Fax: 248-557-0224
e-mail: main@ucpdetroit.org
www.ucp.org
United Cerebral Palsy provides information, advocacy, referral services for persons with disabilities and/or their families. UCP also operates an equipment loan program, conducts parent workshops, disseminates written literature on topics of interest.
Leslynn Angel, President & CEO
Latoya Jones, Chief Financial Officer

2624 **United Cerebral Palsy of Michigan**
4970 Northwind Drive
E Lansing, MI 48823
517-203-1200
800-828-2714
Fax: 517-203-1203
e-mail: ucp@ucpmichigan.org
www.ucp.org
United Cerebral Palsy provides information, advocacy, referral services for persons with disabilities and/or their families. UCP also operates an equipment loan program, conducts parent workshops, disseminates written literature on topics of interest.
Linda Potter, Executive Director
Linda Carey, Office Manager

Minnesota

2625 **United Cerebral Palsy of Central Minnesota**
510 25th Avenue North
St. Cloud, MN 56303-3255
320-253-0765
Fax: 320-253-6753
e-mail: info@ucpcentralmn.org
www.ucpcentralmn.org
Provides information, advocacy, referral services for persons with disabilities and/or their families. UCP conducts parent workshops, disseminates free newsletter. Computers go round recycles quality used computers to persons with disabilities. UCP awards scholarship for post secondary education.

2626 **United Cerebral Palsy of Central Ohio**
510 25th Avenue N
St Cloud, MN 56303
320-253-0765
Fax: 320-253-6753
TTY: 320-253-0765
e-mail: info@ucpcentralmn.org
www.ucpcentralmn.org
Provides information, advocacy, referral services for persons with disabilities and/or their families. UCP conducts parent workshops, disseminates information in a free newsletter.
Judy K Moening, Executive Director
Alison Pauly, Program & Development Coordinator

2627 **United Cerebral Palsy of Minnesota**
1821 University Avenue W
St Paul, MN 55104-2892
651-646-7588
877-528-5678
Fax: 651-646-3045
e-mail: ucpmnStacey@hotmail.com
www.ucp.org
United Cerebral Palsy provides information, advocacy, referral services for persons with disabilities and/or their families. UCP also operates an equipment loan program, conducts parent workshops, disseminates written literature on topics of interest.
Stacey Vogele, Executive Director
Ramsey Lee, Events Coordinator

Missouri

2628 **United Cerebral Palsy of Greater Kansas City**
1044 Main Street
Kansas City, MO 64105
816-531-4454
Fax: 816-531-3383
e-mail: bscott@ucpkc.org
www.ucp.org
Provides information, advocacy, referral services for persons with disabilities and/or their families. UCP also operates residential programs and care management for seniors.
Bruce A Scott, President & CEO
Sam T Switzer, Senior Vice President & CFO

2629 **United Cerebral Palsy of Greater St. Louis**
8645 Old Bonhomme Road
St. Louis, MO 63132-3999
314-994-1600
Fax: 314-994-0179
e-mail: forkoshr@ucpstl.org
www.ucpa.org
United Cerebral Palsy provides information, advocacy, referral services for persons with disabilities and/or their families. UCP also operates an equipment loan program, conducts parent workshops, disseminates written literature on topics of interest to people with disabilities.

2630 **United Cerebral Palsy of Northwest Missouri**
3303 Frederick Avenue
St. Joseph, MO 64506
816-364-3836
Fax: 816-390-8546
e-mail: ucpnwmo@ccp.com
www.ucpa.org
United Cerebral Palsy provides information, advocacy, referral services for persons with disabilities and/or their families. UCP also operates an equipment loan program, conducts parent workshops, disseminates written literature on topics of interest to people with disabilities.

2631 **United Cerebral Palsy of Northwestern**
3303 Frederick Avenue
St Joseph, MO 64506
816-364-3836
Fax: 816-390-8546
e-mail: ucp@ucpnwmo.org
www.ucp.org
United Cerebral Palsy provides information, advocacy, referral services for persons with disabilities and/or their families. UCP also operates an equipment loan program, conducts parent workshops, disseminates written literature on topics of interest to people with disabilities.
Teresa Gagliano, Executive Director
Carmen Bartlett, Program Director

Nebraska

2632 **United Cerebral Palsy of Nebraska**
920 S 107th Avenue
Omaha, NE 68114
402-502-3572
800-729-2556
Fax: 402-502-6791
e-mail: jennyh@ucpnebraska.org
www.ucp.org
United Cerebral Palsy provides information, advocacy, referral services for persons with disabilities and/or their families. UCP also operates an equipment loan program, conducts parent workshops, disseminates written literature on topics of interest.
Carol Hahn, Executive Director
Anne Brodin, Financial & Services Director

Nevada

2633 **United Cerebral Palsy of Northern Nevada**
4068 S McCarran Boulevard
Reno, NV 89502-7532
775-331-3323
Fax: 775-331-7913
e-mail: upcnn@ucpnn.org
www.ucpa.org
United Cerebral Palsy provides information, advocacy, referral services for persons with disabilities and/or their families. UCP also provides employment and supported living services and disseminates written literature on topics of interest.

New Jersey

2634 **United Cerebral Palsy of Hudson County**
721 Broadway
Bayonne, NJ 07002
201-436-2200
Fax: 201-436-6642
e-mail: kkearney@ucpofhudsoncounty.org
www.ucp.org
United Cerebral Palsy provides information, advocacy, referral services for persons with disabilities and/or their families. UCP also operates an equipment loan program, conducts parent work-

shops, disseminates written literature on topics of interest to people with disabilities.
Nick Starita, Executive Director
Keith J Kearney, Associate Executive Director

2635 **United Cerebral Palsy of Morris-Somerset**
245 Main Street 908-879-2243
Chester, NJ 07930 Fax: 908-879-8363
e-mail: info@ucpnj.org
www.ucpa.org
United Cerebral Palsy provides information, advocacy, referral services for persons with disabilities and/or their families. UCP also operates an equipment loan program, conducts parent workshops, disseminates written literature on topics of interest.

2636 **United Cerebral Palsy of New Jersey**
1005 Whitehead Road Extension 609-392-4004
Ewing, NJ 08638 888-322-1918
Fax: 609-882-4054
TTY: 609-882-0620
e-mail: info@cpofnj.org
www.cpofnj.org
United Cerebral Palsy provides information, advocacy, referral services for persons with disabilities and/or their families. UCP also operates an equipment loan program, conducts parent workshops, disseminates written literature on topics of interest.

New York

2637 **Center for the Disabled**
314 S Manning Boulevard 518-437-5700
Albany, NY 12208 e-mail: bulgaro@cftd.org
www.cfdsny.org
United Cerebral Palsy provides information, advocacy, referral services for persons with disabilities and/or their families. UCP also operates an equipment loan program, conducts parent workshops, disseminates written literature on topics of interest to people with disabilities.
Alan Krafchin, CEO/President
Patrick J Rielly, Chief Operating Officer

2638 **Cerebral Palsy Associations of New York State**
90 State Street 518-436-0178
Albany, NY 12207 Fax: 518-436-8619
e-mail: AffiliateServices@cpofnys.org
www.cpofnys.org
Provides information, advocacy, referral services for persons with disabilities and/or their families. CP also operates an equipment loan program, conducts parent workshops and disseminates written literature on topics of interest to people with disabilities.
Michael Alvaro, Executive Vice President
Susan Constantino, President & CEO

2639 **Niagara Cerebral Palsy**
9812 Lockport Road 716-297-0798
Niagara Falls, NY 14304 Fax: 716-297-0998
e-mail: info@niagaracp.org
www.ucpaofniagara.com
Provides educational, residential, vocational and recreational programs.

2640 **Prospect Child And Family Center**
133 Aviation Road 518-798-0170
Queensbury, NY 12804 Fax: 518-798-0533
e-mail: pcfccent@prospectcenter.com
www.prospectcenter.com
United Cerebral Palsy provides information, advocacy, referral services for persons with disabilities and/or their families. UCP also operates an equipment loan program, conducts parent workshops, disseminates written literature on topics of interest to people with disabilties.

2641 **United Cerebral Palsy of Chemung County**
1118 Charles Street 607-734-7107
Elmira, NY 14901 Fax: 607-734-7334
www.chemungcp.com
United Cerebral Palsy provides information, advocacy, referral services for persons with disabilities and/or their families. UCP also operates an equipment loan program, conducts parent workshops, disseminates written literature on topics of interest to people with disabilities.
Mark Peters, Executive Director
Leisa Alger, Associate Executive Director

2642 **United Cerebral Palsy of Fulton & Montgomery Counties**
67 Division Street 518-842-3511
Amsterdam, NY 12010 Fax: 518-843-6042
www.ucpa.org
United Cerebral Palsy provides information, advocacy, referral services for persons with disabilities and/or their families. UCP also operates an equipment loan program, conducts parent workshops, disseminates written literature on topics of interest to people with disabilities.

2643 **United Cerebral Palsy of Greater Suffolk**
250 Marcus Boulevard 631-232-0011
Hauppauge, NY 11788 Fax: 631-232-4422
e-mail: info@ucp-suffolk.org
www.ucp-suffolk.org
United Cerebral Palsy provides information, advocacy, referral services for persons with disabilities and/or their families. UCP also operates an equipment loan program, conducts parent workshops, disseminates written literature on topics of interest.
Stephen H Friedman, President & CEO
James Monnier, Board of Directors

2644 **United Cerebral Palsy of Nassau County**
380 Washington Avenue 516-378-2000
Roosevelt, NY 11575 Fax: 516-868-4089
e-mail: info@ucpn.org
www.ucpn.org
United Cerebral Palsy provides information, advocacy, referral services for persons with disabilities and/or their families. UCP also operates an equipment loan program, conducts parent workshops, disseminates written literature on topics of interest to people with disabilities.
Robert Masterson, President
Thomas Connolly, Executive Vice President

2645 **United Cerebral Palsy of New York City**
80 Maiden Lane 212-683-6700
New York, NY 10038-4811 800-GIV-EUCP
Fax: 212-685-8394
e-mail: info@ucpnyc.org
www.ucpnyc.org
United Cerebral Palsy provides information, advocacy, referral services for persons with disabilities and/or their families. UCP also operates an equipment loan program, conducts parent workshops, disseminates written literature on topics of interest.

2646 **United Cerebral Palsy of Orange County**
980 Roosevelt 949-333-6400
Irvine, CA 92620 Fax: 949-333-6440
e-mail: info@ucp-oc.org
www.ucp-oc.org
United Cerebral Palsy provides information, advocacy, referral services for persons with disabilities and/or their families. UCP also operates an equipment loan program, conducts parent workshops, disseminates written literature on topics of interest.
Paul Pulver, Executive Directorÿ
Lauren Mille Beeler, Director of Therapy Services

2647 **United Cerebral Palsy of Putnam & Southern Dutchess Counties**
40 John Barrett Road 845-878-9078
Patterson, NY 12563 Fax: 845-878-3203
e-mail: hvcs@aol.com
www.ucpa.org
United Cerebral Palsy provides information, advocacy, referral services for persons with disabilities and/or their families. UCP also operates an equipment loan program, conducts parent workshops, disseminates written literature on topics of interest to people with disabilties.

2648 **United Cerebral Palsy of Queens: Queens Centers for Progress**
81-15 164th Street 718-380-3000
Jamaica, NY 11432 Fax: 718-380-0483
TTY: 718-969-0270
e-mail: info@queenscp.org
www.queenscp.org

Provides information advocacy and referral services for persons with disabilities and/or their families. Offers an equipment loan program parent workshops and written literature on topics of interest to people with disabilities. Comprehensive services i
Charles Houston, Executive Director

2649 **United Cerebral Palsy of Westchester County**
1186 King Street 914-937-3800
Rye Brook, NY 10573 Fax: 914-937-0967
www.cpwestchester.org
United Cerebral Palsy provides information advocacy referral services for persons with disabilities and/or their families. UCP also operates an equipment loan program conducts parent workshops disseminates written literature on topics of interest to p
Richard Osterer, President
Richard Eising, Executive Vice President

2650 **United Cerebral Palsy of Western New York**
7 Community Drive 716-894-0130
Buffalo, NY 14225 Fax: 716-894-8257
e-mail: ucpawny1@aol.com
www.ucpa.org
United Cerebral Palsy provides information advocacy referral services for persons with disabilities and/or their families. UCP also operates an equipment loan program conducts parent workshops disseminates written literature on topics of interest to p

2651 **United Cerebral Palsy of the North Country**
4 Commerce Lane 315-379-9667
Canton, NY 13617 Fax: 315-379-9388
e-mail: ucpa@imcnet.net
www.ucpa.org
United Cerebral Palsy provides information advocacy referral services for persons with disabilities and/or their families. UCP also operates an equipment loan program conducts parent workshops disseminates written literature on topics of interest to p

North Carolina

2652 **United Cerebral Palsy of North Carolina**
2315 Myron Drive 919-783-8898
Raleigh, NC 27607 800-662-7119
Fax: 919-782-5486
e-mail: QM@nc.eastersealsucp.com
nc.easterseals.com
United Cerebral Palsy provides information advocacy referral services for persons with disabilities and/or their families. UCP also operates an equipment loan program conducts parent workshops disseminates written literature on topics of interest to p

Ohio

2653 **United Cerebral Palsy of Central Ohio**
440 Industrial Mile Road 614-279-0109
Columbus, OH 43228-2411 Fax: 914-279-2527
e-mail: tfitch@ucpofcentralohio.org
www.ucpofcentralohio.org
United Cerebral Palsy provides information advocacy referral services for persons with disabilities and/or their families. UCP also operates an equipment loan program conducts parent workshops disseminates written literature on topics of interest to p
Charles Dyas, President/Executive Committee Chair
Diane Dierna, Vice-President

2654 **United Cerebral Palsy of Cincinnati**
3601 Victory Parkway 513-221-4606
Cincinnati, OH 45229 Fax: 513-872-5262
e-mail: sschiller@ucp-cincinnati.org
www.ucp-cincinnati.org
United Cerebral Palsy provides information advocacy referral services for persons with disabilities and/or their families. UCP also operates an equipment loan program conducts parent workshops disseminates written literature on topics of interest to p
Susan Schiller, Executive Director, Development Director

2655 **United Cerebral Palsy of Greater Cleveland**
10011 Euclid Avenue 216-791-8363
Cleveland, OH 44106 Fax: 216-721-3372
e-mail: sdean@ucpcleveland.org
www.ucpa.org
United Cerebral Palsy provides information, advocacy, referral services for persons with disabilities and/or their families. UCP also operates an equipment loan program, conducts parent workshops, disseminates written literature on topics of interest to people with disabilities.

2656 **United Cerebral Palsy of Greater Dane**
10011 Euclid Avenue 216-791-8363
Cleveland, OH 44106 Fax: 216-721-3372
e-mail: sdean@ucpcleveland.org
www.ucpcleveland.org
United Cerebral Palsy provides information advocacy referral services for persons with disabilities and/or their families. UCP also operates an equipment loan program conducts parent workshops disseminates written literature on topics of interest to p
Robert J Darden, President
Douglas A Neary, Vice President

Oklahoma

2657 **United Cerebral Palsy of Oklahoma**
10400 Greenbriar Place 405-759-3562
Oklahoma City, OK 73159 Fax: 405-917-7082
e-mail: info@ucpok.org
www.ucpok.org
United Cerebral Palsy provides information advocacy referral services for persons with disabilities and/or their families. UCP also operates an equipment loan program conducts parent workshops disseminates written literature on topics of interest to p

Oregon

2658 **United Cerebral Palsy of Oregon & SW Washington**
11731 NE Glenn Widing Drive 503-777-4166
Portland, OR 97220 800-473-4581
Fax: 503-771-8048
e-mail: ucpa@ucpaorwa.org
www.ucp.org
United Cerebral Palsy provides information advocacy referral services for persons with disabilities and/or their families. UCP also operates an equipment loan program conducts parent workshops disseminates written literature on topics of interest to p
Bud Thoune, Executive Director
Doug Taylor, Development and Marketing Director

Pennsylvania

2659 **United Cerebral Palsy Central PA**
44 S 38th Street 717-975-0611
Camp Hill, PA 17011 Fax: 717-975-0839
e-mail: kidscenter@ucpcentralpa.org
www.ucp.org
United Cerebral Palsy provides information advocacy referral services for persons with disabilities and/or their families. UCP also operates an equipment loan program conducts parent workshops disseminates written literature on topics of interest to p
Jeffrey W Cooper, President/CEO
Jennifer Brubakerÿÿ, Director of Administrative Services

2660 **United Cerebral Palsy of Beaver, Butler & Lawrence Counties**
101 Hindman Lane 724-482-4765
Butler, PA 16001 Fax: 724-283-5945
www.ucpa.org
United Cerebral Palsy provides information, advocacy, referral services for persons with disabilities and/or their families. UCP also operates an equipment loan program, conducts parent workshops, disseminates written literature on topics of interest to people with disabilities.

2661 **United Cerebral Palsy of Northwestern Pennsylvania**
3745 W 12th Street 814-836-9113
Erie, PA 16505 Fax: 814-833-3919
e-mail: leaton@mecaup.com
www.ucpa.org
United Cerebral Palsy provides information advocacy referral services for persons with disabilities and/or their families. UCP also operates a wheelchair ramp building program conducts parent workshops offers adaptive recreation activities disseminat
Laura Eaton, Executive Director

2662 **United Cerebral Palsy of Pennsylvania**
908 N Second Street
Harrisburg, PA 17102
717-441-6044
866-761-6129
Fax: 717-236-2046
e-mail: kimberlycossar@wannarassoc.com
www.ucp.org

United Cerebral Palsy provides information advocacy referral services for persons with disabilities and/or their families. UCP also operates an equipment loan program conducts parent workshops disseminates written literature on topics of interest to p
Joan Martin, Executive Director
Vini Portzline, Policy Information Exchange

2663 **United Cerebral Palsy of Philadelphia Vicinity**
102 E Mermaid Lane
Philadelphia, PA 19118
215-242-4200
Fax: 215-247-4229
TTY: 215-248-7620
e-mail: ucpkravitz@aol.com
www.ucpphila.org

United Cerebral Palsy provides information advocacy referral services for persons with disabilities and/or their families. UCP also operates an equipment loan program conducts parent workshops disseminates written literature on topics of interest to p
Gary J Weyhmuller, President
David J Barnhart, Vice President

2664 **United Cerebral Palsy of Pittsburgh**
4638 Centre Avenue
Pittsburgh, PA 15213
412-683-7100
Fax: 412-683-4160
e-mail: info@ucppittsburgh.org
www.ucp.org

United Cerebral Palsy provides information advocacy referral services for persons with disabilities and/or their families. UCP also operates an equipment loan program conducts parent workshops disseminates written literature on topics of interest to p
Al Condeluci, CEO
Joyce Redmerski, Chief Financial Officer

2665 **United Cerebral Palsy of South Central Pennsylvania**
788 Cherry Tree Court
Hanover, PA 17331
717-632-5552
800-333-3873
Fax: 717-632-2315
e-mail: phoughton@ucpsouthcentral.org
www.ucp.org

Provides early intervention, in home personal care and community integration services for children and adults with disabilities in York, Adams and Franklin counties.
Paulette Houghton, Executive Director
William Long, Director of Operations

2666 **United Cerebral Palsy of Southern Alleghenies Region**
119 Jari Drive
Johnstown, PA 15904
814-262-9600
877-371-1110
Fax: 814-262-9650
e-mail: info@ucpsar.org
www.alucp.org

United Cerebral Palsy provides information, advocacy, referral services for persons with disabilities and/or their families. UCP also operates an equipment loan program, conducts parent workshops, disseminates written literature on topics of interest.
Marie Polinsky, CEO
Mark Malzi, CFO

2667 **United Cerebral Palsy of Southwestern Pennsylvania**
190 N Main Street
Washington, PA 15301
724-229-0851
Fax: 724-229-9252
e-mail: info@ucpswpa.org
www.ucp.org

United Cerebral Palsy provides information, advocacy, referral services for persons with disabilities and/or their families. UCP also operates an equipment loan program, conducts parent workshops, disseminates written literature on topics of interest.

2668 **United Cerebral Palsy of Western Pennsylvania**
2904 Seminary Drive
Greensburg, PA 15601
724-832-8272
Fax: 724-837-8278
e-mail: ucp@ucpofwesternpa.org
www.ucpa.org

United Cerebral Palsy provides information, advocacy, referral services for persons with disabilities and/or their families. UCP also operates an equipment loan program, conducts parent workshops, disseminates written literature on topics of interest.

Rhode Island

2669 **United Cerebral Palsy of Rhode Island**
200 Main Street
Pawtucket, RI 02862
401-728-1800
Fax: 401-728-0182
e-mail: ucprisupport@ucpri.org
www.ucpa.org

United Cerebral Palsy provides information, advocacy, referral services for persons with disabilities and/or their families. UCP also operates an equipment loan program, conducts parent workshops, disseminates written literature on topics of interest to people with disabilities.

Tennessee

2670 **United Cerebral Palsy of Middle Tennessee**
1200 9th Avenue N
Nashville, TN 37208
615-242-4091
Fax: 615-242-3582
e-mail: request@ucpnashville.org
www.ucpa.org

United Cerebral Palsy provides information, advocacy, referral services for persons with disabilities and/or their families. UCP also operates an equipment loan program, conducts parent workshops, disseminates written literature on topics of interest to people with disabilities.

2671 **United Cerebral Palsy of the Mid-South**
4189 Leroy
Memphis, TN 38108
901-761-4277
Fax: 901-761-7876
e-mail: ucp@ucpmemphis.org
www.ucpa.org

United Cerebral Palsy provides information, advocacy, referral services for persons with disabilities and/or their families. UCP also operates an equipment loan program, conducts parent workshops, disseminates written literature on topics of interest to people with disabilties

Texas

2672 **United Cerebral Palsy of Greater Houston**
4500 Bissonet
Bellaire, TX 77401
713-838-9050
Fax: 713-838-9098
e-mail: ucp@ucphouston.org
www.ucpa.org

United Cerebral Palsy provides information, advocacy, referral services for persons with disabilities and/or their families. UCP also operates an equipment loan program, conducts parent workshops, disseminates written literature on topics of interest to people with disabilities.

2673 **United Cerebral Palsy of Metropolitan Dallas**
8802 Harry Hines Boulevard
Dallas, TX 75235
214-247-4505
800-999-1898
Fax: 214-351-2610
e-mail: billknudsen@ucpdallas
www.ucpdallas.org

United Cerebral Palsy provides information, advocacy, referral services for persons with disabilities and/or their families. UCP also operates an equipment loan program, conducts parent workshops, disseminates written literature on topics of interest to people with disabilities.
Bill Knudsen, President / Chief Executive Officer
Becky Adams, Chief Operations Officer

2674 **United Cerebral Palsy of Tarrant County**
1555 Merrimac Circle
Fort Worth, TX 76107
817-332-7171
Fax: 817-332-7601
e-mail: info@ucptc.org
www.ucpa.org

United Cerebral Palsy provides information, advocacy, referral services for persons with disabilities and/or their families. UCP also operates an equipment loan program, conducts parent workshops, disseminates written literature on topics of interest to people with disabilities.

2675 **United Cerebral Palsy of Texas**
1016 La Posada Drive 512-472-8696
Austin, TX 78752 800-798-1492
Fax: 512-472-8026
e-mail: info@ucptexas.org
www.ucpa.org
United Cerebral Palsy provides information, advocacy, referral services for persons with disabilities and/or their families. UCP also operates an equipment loan program, conducts parent workshops, disseminates written literature on topics of interest.

Utah

2676 **United Cerebral Palsy of Utah**
PO Box 65219 801-266-1805
S Salt Lake, UT 84165 Fax: 801-266-2404
e-mail: shellyp@ucputah.org
www.ucpa.org
United Cerebral Palsy provides information, advocacy, referral services for persons with disabilities and/or their families. UCP also operates an equipment loan program, conducts parent workshops, disseminates written literature on topics of interest.

Virginia

2677 **Cerebral Palsy of Virginia**
5825 Arrowhead Drive 757-497-7474
Virginia Beach, VA 23462 Fax: 757-497-0868
e-mail: kap@cerebralpalsyofvirginia.org
www.cerebralpalsyofvirginia.org
Cerebral Palsy provides information, advocacy, referral services for persons with disabilities and/or their families. Cerebral Palsy also operates an equipment loan program, summer computer camp, art works job training program and much more.
Kathy Prendergast, Executive Director
Michelle Majority, Associate Executive Director

2678 **United Cerebral Palsy of Washington DC**
1818 New York Avenue 202-526-0146
Washington, DC 20002 Fax: 202-526-0519
e-mail: dcarter@ucpdc.org
www.ucpdc.org
United Cerebral Palsy provides information, advocacy, referral services for persons with disabilities and/or their families. UCP also operates an equipment loan program, conducts parent workshops, disseminates written literature on topics of interest.
Mark A Simione ÿ, ÿBoard President
Roderick Johnson, ÿBoard Secretary

Washington

2679 **United Cerebral Palsy of Pierce County**
6315 S 19th Street 253-565-1463
Tacoma, WA 98466-6217 Fax: 253-565-1463
e-mail: info@ucp-sps.org
www.ucpa.org
United Cerebral Palsy provides information, advocacy, referral services for persons with disabilities and/or their families. UCP also operates an equipment loan program, conducts parent workshops, disseminates written literature on topics of interest to people with disabilities.

Wisconsin

2680 **United Cerebral Palsy of Greater Dane County**
2801 Coho Street 608-273-4434
Madison, WI 53713 Fax: 608-273-3426
e-mail: ucpgdc@ucpdane.org
www.ucpa.org
Provides information, advocacy, referral services for persons with disabilities and/or their families. UCP also conducts parent workshops and disseminates written literature on topics of interest to people with disabilities.
Susan Knox, Administrative Assistant

2681 **United Cerebral Palsy of North Central Wisconsin**
108 Scott Street 715-842-8700
Wausau, WI 54401 800-472-4408
www.ucpa.org
United Cerebral Palsy provides information, advocacy, referral services for persons with disabilities and/or their families. UCP also operates an equipment loan program, conducts parent workshops, disseminates written literature on topics of interest to people with disabilities.

2682 **United Cerebral Palsy of Southeastern Wisconsin**
7519 W Oklahoma Avenue 414-329-4500
Milwaukee, WI 53219 888-482-7739
Fax: 414-329-4510
TTY: 414-329-4511
e-mail: info@ucpsew.org
www.ucpa.org
United Cerebral Palsy provides information, advocacy, referral services for persons with disabilities and/or their families. UCP also operates an equipment loan program, conducts parent workshops, disseminates written literature on topics of interest to people with disabilities.

2683 **United Cerebral Palsy of West Central Wisconsin**
206 Water Street 715-832-1782
Eau Claire, WI 54703 Fax: 715-832-8203
e-mail: ucp1ruth@sbcglobal net
www.ucpa.org
United Cerebral Palsy provides information, advocacy, referral services for persons with disabilities and/or their families. UCP also operates an equipment loan program, conducts parent workshops, disseminates written literature on topics of interest to people with disabilities.

2684 **United Cerebral Palsy of Wisconsin**
206 Water Street 715-832-1782
Eau Claire, WI 54703 800-261-1895
Fax: 715-832-8203
e-mail: ucp1ruth@sbcglobal net
www.ucpa.org
United Cerebral Palsy provides information, advocacy, referral services for persons with disabilities and/or their families. UCP also operates an equipment loan program, conducts parent workshops, disseminates written literature on topics of interest.

Research Centers

2685 **Orthopaedic Biomechanics Laboratory Shriners Hospital for Crippled Children**
Shriners Hospital for Crippled Children
2181 Westlawn Building 319-335-7529
Iowa City, IA 52242-1100 Fax: 319-335-7530
Offers research and studies into cerebral palsy.
Stephen R Skinner, Clinical Director

Support Groups & Hotlines

2686 **Family Support Network**
215 Centennial Mall S 402-477-2992
Lincoln, NE 68508-1813 800-245-6081

2687 **National Health Information Center**
PO Box 1133 310-565-4167
Washington, DC 20013 800-336-4797
Fax: 301-984-4256
e-mail: info@nhic.org
www.health.gov/nhic
Offers a nationwide information referral service, produces directories and resource guides.

Books

2688 **An Introduction to Your Child Who Has Cerebral Palsy**
Medic Publishing Company
PO Box 89 425-881-2883
Redmond, WA 98073-0089
Information and answers to questions for parents of children with cerebral palsy.

2689 **Children with Cerebral Palsy**
Woodbine House

6510 Bells Mill Road
Bethesda, MD 20817-1636 301-897-3570
800-843-7323
Fax: 301-897-5838
e-mail: info@woodbinehouse.com
www.woodbinehouse.com

Explains what Cerebral Palsy is, and discusses its diagnosis and treatment. Also offers information and advice concerning daily care, early intervention, therapy, educational options and family life.
432 pages Paperback
ISBN: 0-933149-15-8

2690 **Discovery Book**
United Cerebral Palsy Association
1660 L Street NW 202-776-0406
Washington, DC 20036-5602 800-872-5827
Fax: 202-776-0414
ucpnatl@ucpa.org

2691 **Individuals with Cerebral Palsy**
Mainstream
1030 5th Street NW 202-898-1400
Washington, DC 20001-2504 e-mail: info@mainstreaminc.org
www.mainstreaminc.org

Mainstreaming individuals with cerebral palsy into the workplace.
12 pages

2692 **Occupational Therapy Practice Guidelines for Adults with Cerebral Palsy**
American Occupational Therapy Association
4720 Montgomery Lane 301-652-2682
Bethesda, MD 20824-1220 Fax: 301-652-7711
TDD: 800-377-8555
www.aota.org

15 pages
ISBN: 1-569001-59-6

Children's Books

2693 **Can't You Be Still?**
Gemma B Publishing
776 Corydon Avenue 204-452-7566
Winnipeg, MB, R3M 0Y1, Fax: 204-475-9903
e-mail: gempub@mts.net
www.gemmab.mb.ca

On Ann's first day at school, the other students are both fascinated and horrified by her cerebral palsy. She wins them over by helping them jump into the water and swim. Available in Braille.
24 pages Paperback
ISBN: 0-969647-70-0
Sarah Yates, President

2694 **Cerebral Palsy**
Franklin Watts Grolier
90 Old Sherman Tpke 203-797-3500
Danbury, CT 06816-0001 800-621-1115
Fax: 203-797-3197
www.grolier.com

A look at the causes, detection, prevention, effects and treatment of Cerebral Palsy.
112 pages Grades 7-12
ISBN: 0-531125-29-7

2695 **Here's What I Mean To Say**
Gemma B Publishing
776 Corydon Avenue 204-452-7566
Winnipeg, MB, R3M 0Y1, Fax: 204-475-9903
e-mail: gempub@mts.net
www.gemmab.mb.ca

In this books Ann's battle to read is assisted by an angel, who helps her read the directions in Jay's computer game. Is the angel read or is this the magic of reading? Available in Braille.
32 pages Paperback
ISBN: 0-969647-72-7
Sarah Yates, President

2696 **Mine for Keeps**
Little, Brown & Company
34 Beacon Street 617-227-0730
Boston, MA 02108-1415 800-343-9204

Sarah Jean Copeland was born with cerebral palsy. At four years of age she was placed in a school for handicapped children but made such good progress that she could return home. Coming home for Sarah meant a new school, and new adjustments to her parents, two sisters, and her brother. At first Sarah was scared and didn't think she could do all the things she needed to do, but she soon learned her fears were not well-founded.
186 pages Hardcover

2697 **My Brother Matthew**
Woodbine House
6510 Bells Mill Road
Bethesda, MD 20817-1636 800-843-7323

A book written from the point of view of the brother of Matthew, a boy with multiple disabilities, David describes the incidents characterizing how life in his family changes.
28 pages Grades K-5
Sarah Strickler

2698 **Nobody Knows!**
Gemma B Publishing
776 Corydon Avenue 204-452-7566
Winnipeg, MB, R3M 0Y1, Fax: 204-475-9903
e-mail: gempub@mts.net
www.gemmab.mb.ca

Is an adventure during which a frustrated Ann goes out to find someone who understand what she wants. She meets a turtle and an alligator, who like her don't use words to communicate. Available in Braille.
24 pages Paperback
ISBN: 0-969647-71-9
Sarah Yates, President

Newsletters

2699 **Family Support Bulletin**
United Cerebral Palsy Associations
1660 L Street NW 202-842-1266
Washington, DC 20036-1202 800-872-5827

Pamphlets

2700 **Cerebral Palsy: Facts & Figures**
United Cerebral Palsy Associations
1660 L Street NW
Washington, DC 20036 800-872-5827
Fax: 202-776-0414
www.ucp.org

Offers information on what cerebral palsy is, the effects, causes, types, and prevention.

Audio & Video

2701 **A Day At A Time**
Filmakers Library
124 E 40th Street 212-808-4980
New York, NY 10016-1798 Fax: 212-808-4983
e-mail: info@filmakers.com
www.filmakers.com

The story of twin girls with Cerebral Palsy, whose family is determined that they have every opportunity to participate in and lead normal lives. Winner of a number of awards. DVD or VHS $195, Classroom Rental $75
VHS or DVD
Sue Oscar, Co-President

Web Sites

2702 **American Academy for Cerebral Palsy and Developmental Medicine**
AACPDM.org

A multidisciplinary scientific society devoted to the study of cerebral palsy and other childhood onset disabilities, to promoting professional education for the treatment and management of these conditions, and to improving the quality of life for people with these disabilities.

2703 **Healing Well**

www.healingwell.com

An online health resource guide to medical news, chat, information and articles, newsgroups and message boards, books, disease-related web sites, medical directories, and more for patients, friends, and family coping with disabling diseases, disorders, or chronic illnesses.

2704 **Health Finder**

www.healthfinder.gov

Searchable, carefully developed web site offering information on over 1000 topics. Developed by the US Department of Health and Human Services, the site can be used in both English and Spanish.

2705 **Healthlink USA**

www.healthlinkusa.com

Health information concerning treatment, cures, prevention, diagnosis, risk factors, research, support groups, email lists, personal stories and much more. Updated regularly.

2706 **Helios Health**

www.helioshealth.com

Online resource for your health information. Detailed information about specific health topics, access to expert advice from our Medical Advisory Board, and up-to-date health news.

2707 **MedicineNet**

www.medicinenet.com

An online resource for consumers providing easy-to-read, authoritative medical and health information.

2708 **Medscape**

www.mywebmd.com

Medscape offers specialists, primary care physicians, and other health professionals the Web's most robust and integrated medical information and educational tools.

2709 **National Institute of Neurological Disorders and Stroke**

www.ninds.nih.gov

Conducts, fosters, coordinates, and guides research on the causes, prevention, diagnosis, and treatment of neurological disorders and stroke, and supports basic research in related scientific areas. Operates a program of contracts for the funding of research and research support efforts in selected areas of institute needed. Collects and disseminates research information related to neurological disorders.

2710 **National Rehabilitation Information Center**

www.naric.com/

One of the three components of the office of Special Education and Rehabilitative Services.

2711 **Neurology Channel**

www.neurologychannel.com

Find clearly explained, medically accurate information regarding conditions, including an overview, symptoms, causes, diagnostic procedures and treatment options. On this site it is possible to ask questions and get information from a neurologist and connect to people who have similar health interests.

2712 **United Cerebral Palsy Associations**

www.ucpa.org

A network of approximately 119 state and local voluntary agencies which provide services, conduct public and professional education programs and support research in cerebral palsy.

2713 **WebMD**

www.webmd.com

Provides links to over 20 articles involving cerebral palsy.

Description

2714 **Chronic Fatigue Syndrome**

Chronic Fatigue Syndrome, CFS, is an illness characterized by longstanding fatigue that impairs daily functioning. It may be accompanied by sore throat, swollen glands, muscle and joint pain, headaches, sleeplessness, and impaired memory or concentration. Profound or life-altering fatigue—the disease's hallmark—usually comes on suddenly and persists for at least six months, and often for years.

The cause of CFS is controversial. One theory is that a chronic viral infection is involved. Allergic reactions have also been proposed, and various immunologic abnormalities have been reported. Another theory involves proposed disturbances in the hormonal (endocrine) system. Psychological factors may be the cause, although CFS is distinct from typical depression or anxiety. Because the cause is unknown, there is no single test or group of tests that can diagnose CFS. Therefore, the goal in evaluating an individual with presumed CFS is to exclude other treatable illnesses.

Given the difficulty in proving a diagnosis or understanding the cause of CFS, it is not surprising that many treatments have been offered for it. Antidepressants appear to be the most successful treatment studied so far; as many as 80 percent of patients report benefit. Other therapies, including nutritional supplements, hormones, antiviral drugs and steroids have been mostly disappointing.

Patients with CFS need emotional support from physicians and family, due to the debilitating nature of the disease. Individual and group therapy may help some individuals. See also *Fibromyalgia*.

National Agencies & Associations

2715 **American Academy of Sleep Medicine**
One Westbrook Corporate Center 708-492-0930
Westchester, IL 60154 Fax: 708-492-0943
www.aasmnet.org

A unique multi-disciplinary organization for both individual members and center members. The individual member branch includes clinicians involved in the diagnosis and treatment of patients with disorders of sleep and alertness.
Jerome Barrett, Executive Director

2716 **International Association for Chronic Fatigue**
27 N Wacker Drive 847-258-7248
Chicago, IL 60606 Fax: 847-579-0975
e-mail: Admin@iacfs.net
www.IACFS.net

A nonprofit organization of research scientists, physicians, licensed medical healthcare professionals and other individuals and institutions interested in promoting the stimulation, coordination and exchange of ideas for CFS research and patient care.
Newsletter
Fred Friedbe PhD, President

2717 **National CFS Association**
PO Box 18426 816-737-1343
Kansas City, MO 64133 e-mail: information@ncfsa.org
www.ncfsfa.org

Provides information on different brochures journals books magazines and pamphlets on the Chronic Fatigue Syndrome.

2718 **National Chronic Fatigue Syndrome and Fibromyalgia Association**
PO Box 18426 816-313-2000
Kansas City, MO 64133-8426 e-mail: information@ncfsfa.org
www.ncfsfa.org

Compiles and provides peer reviewed, scientifically accurate educational materials to inform the public, health professionals, patients and their families about the nature and impact of chronic fatigue syndrome, fibromyalgia and related disorders. Offers a support group.

2719 **National Chronic Fatigue Syndrome and Fibr**
PO Box 18426 816-737-1343
Kansas City, MO 64133 Fax: 816-524-6782
e-mail: information@ncfsfa.org
www.ncfsfa.org

Compiles and provides peer reviewed scientifically accurate educational materials to inform the public health professionals, patients and their families about the nature and impact of chronic fatigue syndrome, fibromyalgia and related disorders.

2720 **National Institute of Allergy and Infectious Diseases**
Office of Communications
6610 Rockledge Drive 301-496-5717
Bethesda, MD 20892-6612 Fax: 301-402-0120
e-mail: af10r@nih.gov
www.niaid.nih.gov

Offers information and educational materials on Chronic Fatigue Syndrome and other disorders.
Anthony S Fauci, MD, Director

2721 **Option Institute**
2080 South Undermountain Road 413-229-2100
Sheffield, MA 01257 800-714-2779
Fax: 413-229-8931
e-mail: correspondence@option.org
www.option.org

Self-defeating beliefs, along with attitudes and judgments, can lead to a host of physical and psychological challenges, including Chronic Fatigue Syndrome. The Option Institute offers programs designed to help you gain new perspectives on the attitudes and judgments that may be affecting your life, especially those regarding and surrounding Chronic Fatigue Syndrome.
Barry Kaufman, Co-Founder
Samahria Ltye Kaufman, Co-Founder

Foundations

2722 **National CFIDS Foundation**
103 Aletha Road 781-449-3535
Needham, MA 02492 Fax: 781-449-8606
e-mail: info@ncf-net.org
www.ncf-net.org

The goals of the Foundation are to help fund medical research to find a cause, expedite treatments and eventually a cure for this devastating disease. The NCF also strives to provide information, education, and support to those people who have CFIDS (also known as chronic fatigue syndrome (CFS), myalgic encephalomyelitis (ME) and many other names)— as well as related illnesses such as Gulf War Illness (GWI) and Multiple Chemical Sensitivities (MCS). Provides guides, articles, and newsletters.
Gail Kansky, President
Prof. Alan Cocchetto, Medical Advisor

Support Groups & Hotlines

2723 **CDC AIDS/STD Hotline**
404-639-3534
800-342-2437
TTY: 800-243-7889
www.cdc.gov

Hotline

2724 **Centers for Disease Control**
1600 Clifton Road NE
Atlanta, GA 30329-4018
404-639-3534
800-311-3435
Fax: 404-639-7394
e-mail: in.the.news@cdc.gov
www.cdc.gov/
Offers information and educational materials on CFS.
Julie Gerberding, Director

2725 **Chronic Fatigue Syndrome & Fibromyalgia Support**
7250 Clearvista Dr
Indianapolis, IN 46256
317-252-9223
Offers emotional support, education and information about CFS and FMS through statewide monthly meetings and a quarterly newsletter. Provides 24-hour hotline and physician/attorney referrals. Financial assistance for members. Support group meets twice a month at Community Hospital North Professional Building and at other locations throughout Indiana.

2726 **National Chronic Fatigue Syndrome and Fibr omyalgia Association Group**
PO Box 18426
Kansas City, MO 64133
816-313-2000
Fax: 816-524-6782
e-mail: information@ncfsfa.org
www.ncfsfa.org
Support group meetings are held on the second Saturday of each month from 2-4 p.m. in the second floor board room of the Helen F Spencer Center for Education. The Center is part of St. Luke's Hospital and is located at 4400 Wornall Road, Kansas City, MO 64111.
Michelle Banks, Author

2727 **National Health Information Center**
PO Box 1133
Washington, DC 20013
310-565-4167
800-336-4797
Fax: 301-984-4256
e-mail: info@nhic.org
www.health.gov/nhic
Offers a nationwide information referral service, produces directories and resource guides.

Books

2728 **CFIDS in Children Packet**
CFIDS Association of America
PO Box 220398
Charlotte, NC 28222-0398
800-442-3437
This packet contains articles about CFIDS and children.
60 pages

2729 **CFS Cookbook**
CFIDS Association of America
PO Box 220398
Charlotte, NC 28222-0398
800-442-3437
Gourmet recipes designed to combat the monotony associated with CFIDS, allergy and immune-compromised diets.
218 pages

2730 **Chronic Fatigue Syndrome Cookbook: Delicious & Wellness-Enhancing Recipes**
DIANE Publishing Company
330 Pusey Avenue, Unit #3 Rear
Darby, PA 19023
610-461-6200
800-782-3833
Fax: 610-461-6130
e-mail: dianepublishing@gmail.com
www.dianepublishing.net
These recipes help combat the boredom of the CFS diet usually recommended and still satisfy all of your nutritional requirements as a CFS sufferer. In addition, the book includes a comprehensive look at the do's and don't's of a CFS diet, quick recipes for those days when you are too tired to cook and an insightful medical introduction.
218 pages Hardcover
ISBN: 0-756753-28-7
Herman Baron, Publisher

2731 **Chronic Fatigue Syndrome and the Yeast Connection**
CFIDS Association of America
PO Box 220398
Charlotte, NC 28222-0398
800-442-3437
Dr. Crook explains the possible role of multiple entities, including yeast overgrowth, allergies and chemical sensitivities, in CFS and how each contributes to immune dysregulation.
386 pages

2732 **Chronic Fatigue Syndrome: Information for Physicians**
Barry Leonard, author
DIANE Publishing Company
330 Pusey Avenue, Unit #3 Rear
Darby, PA 19023
610-461-6200
800-782-3833
Fax: 610-461-6130
e-mail: dianepublishing@gmail.com
www.dianepublishing.net
Includes a historical perspective on chronic fatigue syndrome; epidemiology; clinical picture; evaluation of patients; patient management; etiologic theories; public health service resources; fact sheet; resources for patients, overview of the CFS research program; NIAID and NIAID/Johns Hopkins hospital study, which seeks volunteers, management strategies for CFS; the relationship between nuerally mediatec hypotension and CFS and fibromyalgia and CFS; solving diagnostic and therapeutic dilemmas.
60 pages Paperback
ISBN: 0-788143-78-6
Herman Baron, Publisher

2733 **Chronic Fatigue Syndrome: The Limbic Hypothesis**
CFIDS Association of America
PO Box 220398
Charlotte, NC 28222-0398
800-442-3437
A detailed thesis proposing CFS as a limbic system encephalopathy in the context of a dysregulated neuroimmune system.
259 pages

2734 **Chronic Fatigue: Your Complete Exercise Guide**
Human Kinetics Press
PO Box 5076
Champaign, IL 61825-5076
217-351-5076
800-747-4457
Fax: 217-351-2674
www.humankinetics.com
1993 144 pages Paperback
ISBN: 0-873223-93-4
Steve Ruhlig, Marketing Director

2735 **Coping With CFS**
CFIDS Association of America
PO Box 220398
Charlotte, NC 28222-0398
704-365-2343
800-442-3437
Fax: 704-365-9755
e-mail: info@cfids.org
www.cfids.org
Offers practical, established coping strategies for living better with CFIDS. Based on Dr. Friedberg's experiences as a person with CFIDS and a counselor to PWCs.
176 pages
Jon Sterling, Chairman
Kim Kenny, President/CEO

2736 **Disability and Chronic Fatigue Syndrome**
The Haworth Press
10 Alice Street
Binghamton, NY 13904-1580
607-722-5857
800-429-6784
Fax: 800-895-0582
e-mail: getinfo@haworthpressinc.com
www.haworthpressinc.com
Discusses the difficult subject of how to diagnose disability in chronic fatigue syndrome patients, how to determine the severity of a patient's disability, and how new disability guidelines would make more chronic fatigue patients eligible to apply for disability benefits.
121 pages Paperback
ISBN: 0-789005-01-8
Bill Cohen, Publisher
Sandy Jones, VP Marketing

2737 **Doctor's Guide to Chronic Fatigue Syndrome**
CFIDS Association of America
PO Box 220398
Charlotte, NC 28222-0398
800-442-3437

Written by one of the world's leading experts on CFIDS.
275 pages

2738 Fifty Things You Should Know About the Chronic Fatigue Syndrome Epidemic
St. Martin's Press
175 5th Avenue 212-674-5151
New York, NY 10010-7848 800-221-7945
Fax: 212-420-9314
1993
ISBN: 0-312950-43-8

2739 Hope and Help for Chronic Fatigue Syndrome
CFIDS Association of America
PO Box 220398 704-365-2343
Charlotte, NC 28222-0398 800-442-3437
Fax: 704-365-9755
e-mail: info@cfids.org
www.cfids.org
Insight into the experience of having CFIDS, the physical and emotional impact, difficulty in obtaining a diagnosis, available methods of treatment and key strategies for regaining control over your life.
216 pages
Jon Sterling, Chairman
Kim Kenny, President/CEO

2740 International Classification of Sleep Disorders
American Academy of Sleep Medicine
One Westbrook Corporate Center 708-492-0930
Westchester, IL 60154 Fax: 708-492-0943
www.aasmnet.org
A comprehensive manual for physicians and other healthcare professionals containing information on 84 sleep disorders. The extensive text describes the diagnostic features of each disorder and includes specific diagnostic and severity criteria for each disorder.
396 pages Paperback

2741 Living with CFS: A Personal Story of the Struggle for Recovery
CFIDS Association of America
PO Box 220398
Charlotte, NC 28222-0398 800-442-3437
Describes the pain associated with the author's loss of livelihood, impaired physical and mental functioning and the strain on his marriage and friendships, while maintaining hope for recovery.
224 pages
ISBN: 1-560250-75-5

2742 Living with ME
CFIDS Association of America
PO Box 220398
Charlotte, NC 28222-0398 800-442-3437
Fax: 704-365-9755
The author describes M.E. (mylagic encephalomyelitis - the British term for chronic fatigue syndrome), and discusses practical methods for coping and comments on various treatments.

2743 Music Appreciation
CFIDS Association of America
PO Box 220398
Charlotte, NC 28222-0398 800-442-3437
A full-length collection of poems by Skloot who has been disabled by CFIDS since 1988.
105 pages

2744 Night-Side: CFS and the Illness Experience
CFIDS Association of America
PO Box 220398 704-365-2343
Charlotte, NC 28222-0398 800-442-3437
Fax: 704-365-9755
e-mail: info@cfids.org
www.cfids.org
An honest and ultimately hopeful exploration of what it means to have your life shattered by disease.
190 pages
Jon Sterling, Chairman
Kim Kenny, President/CEO

2745 Recovering From the Chronic Fatigue Syndrome: A Guide to Self-Empowerment
Berkley Books
200 Madison Avenue
New York, NY 10016-3903 212-951-8800
www.penguinputman.com
This book teaches persons with CFIDS to take control of their illness and to help themselves find the road to recovery.
1993 224 pages Paperback
ISBN: 0-399518-07-0

2746 Running on Empty
CFIDS Association of America
PO Box 220398 704-365-2343
Charlotte, NC 28222-0398 800-442-3437
Fax: 704-365-9755
e-mail: info@cfids.org
www.cfids.org
Landmark guide to CFIDS has just been revised and re-released. A must read for the newly disgnosed.
315 pages
Jon Sterling, Chairman
Kim Kenny, President/CEO

2747 Self-Caring Fatigue
Rodale Press
33 E Minor Street 610-967-5171
Emmaus, PA 18098-0099 800-441-7761
Fax: 610-967-8963
e-mail: info@rodale.com
www.rodale.com
A step-by-step plan to uncover and eliminate the causes of chronic fatigue.
1993 320 pages
ISBN: 0-875961-61-4

2748 Solving the Puzzle of CFS
2730 Wilshire Boulevard 310-453-4424
Santa Monica, CA 90403-4724 Fax: 310-966-9196

Magazines

2749 CFIDS Chronicle
CFIDS Association of America
PO Box 220398 704-362-2343
Charlotte, NC 28222-0398 800-442-3437
Fax: 704-365-9755
The largest and most comprehensive periodical specifically pertaining to chronic fatigue syndrome information in the world.

2750 Feel Good Catalog
2895 W Oxford Avenue 303-790-1045
Englewood, CO 80110-4370 800-997-6789
Variety of items to ease pain.

2751 Journal SLEEP
American Academy of Sleep Medicine
One Westbrook Corporate Center 708-492-0930
Westchester, IL 60154 Fax: 708-492-0943
www.journalsleep.org
Publishes articles ranging from clinical investigations of sleep/wake disorders and medical problems during sleep, to investigations of the basic physiological and biochemical events and anatomical structures involved in normal and abnormal sleep. Includes psychological and psycho-physiological research, as well as research in relevant areas of circadian and biological rhythms.
10x Year
ISBN: 0-161810-5 -

2752 Journal of the Chronic Fatigue Syndrome
Haworth Medical Press
10 Alice Street 607-722-5857
Binghamton, NY 13904-1503 800-429-6784
Fax: 607-722-0012
www.haworth.org
Peer reviewed medical journal containing CFIDS scientific abstract information. Appropriate for patients as well as medical professionals.
Quarterly
Nancy Klimas MD, Founding Co-Editor

Newsletters

2753 **Health Points**
TyH Publications
17007 E Colony Drive
Fountain Hills, AZ 85268 800-801-1406
e-mail: editor@e-tyh.com
National newsletter with articles on complementary therapy, latest nutrition news, disability issues and much more. Focus is on fibromyalgia, chronic fatigue, arthritis and chronic pain.
Quarterly

2754 **Heart of America News**
National Chronic Fatigue Syndrome & Fibromyalgia
PO Box 18426 660-313-2000
Kansas City, MO 64133-8426
Offers scientifically accurate information, medical updates, informational references, articles on coping and living with Chronic Fatigue Syndrome and more, based on peer-reviewed materials.
Quarterly

2755 **National Forum**
103 Aletha Road 781-449-3535
Needham, MA 02492 Fax: 781-449-8606
e-mail: info@ncf-net.org
www.ncf-net.org
The Forum's focus: CFIDS/ME, FMS, GWI, MCS and related illnesses.
Gail Kansky, President

2756 **Syndrome Sentinel**
Massachusetts CFIDS Association
808 Main Street
Waltham, MA 02451-8533 781-893-4415
www2.shore.net
This quarterly newsletter contains articles written by health-care professionals working with these conditions. Contributors include traditional and alternative experts, as well as personal stories from people with these chronic syndromes and their significant others.

2757 **The National Forum**
The National CFIDS Foundation
103 Aletha Road 781-449-3535
Needham, MA 02492 Fax: 781-449-8606
e-mail: info@ncf-net.org
www.ncf-net.org
Offers the latest information on CFIDS treatments being tried throughout the United States.

Pamphlets

2758 **Americans with Disabilities Act: CFS and Employment**
National Chronic Fatigue Syndrome & Fibromyalgia
PO Box 18426 660-313-2000
Kansas City, MO 64133-8426

2759 **CFIDS Membership Packet**
CFIDS Association of America
PO Box 220398
Charlotte, NC 28222-0398 800-442-3437
Fax: 704-365-9755
Offers pamphlets, brochures, information on local support groups for members.

2760 **CFIDS in Children**
CFIDS Association of America
PO Box 220398
Charlotte, NC 28222-0398 800-442-3437
Describes the special difficulties faced by children with CFIDS.

2761 **CFS in the Workplace**
National Chronic Fatigue Syndrome & Fibromyalgia
PO Box 18426 660-313-2000
Kansas City, MO 64133

2762 **Chronic Fatigue Syndrome & School Success**
National Chronic Fatigue Syndrome & Fibromyalgia
PO Box 18426 660-313-2000
Kansas City, MO 64133-8426

2763 **Chronic Fatigue Syndrome in Children**
National Chronic Fatigue Syndrome & Fibromyalgia
PO Box 18426 660-313-2000
Kansas City, MO 64133

2764 **Chronic Fatigue Syndrome in Men**
National Chronic Fatigue Syndrome & Fibromyalgia
PO Box 18426 660-313-2000
Kansas City, MO 64133-8426

2765 **Chronic Fatigue Syndrome: A Pamphlet for Physicians**
National Institute of Allergy & Infectious Disease
Building 31, Room 7A50
Bethesda, MD 20892-2520 301-496-5717
www.niaid.nih.gov
Offers information on epidemiology, clinical procedures, evaluations, patient management, neuropsychologic features and etiologic theories.

2766 **Chronic Fatigue Syndrome: The Thief of Vitality**
National Chronic Fatigue Syndrome & Fibromyalgia
PO Box 18426 660-313-2000
Kansas City, MO 64133-8426

2767 **Coping Skills**
National Chronic Fatigue Syndrome & Fibromyalgia
PO Box 18426 660-313-2000
Kansas City, MO 64133-8426

2768 **Disability Packet**
CFIDS Association of America
PO Box 220398
Charlotte, NC 28222-0398 800-442-3437
Includes nine Chronicle articles about disability benefits and how persons with CFIDS can secure Social Security Disability Insurance benefits.
42 pages

2769 **Facts About Chronic Fatigue Syndrome**
Centers for Disease Control & Prevention
Division of Viral Diseases 404-639-3311
Atlanta, GA 30333

2770 **Fibromyalgia**
National Chronic Fatigue Syndrome & Fibromyalgia
PO Box 18426 660-313-2000
Kansas City, MO 64133-8426

2771 **March is Chronic Fatigue Syndrome Awareness Month Tips**
National Chronic Fatigue Syndrome & Fibromyalgia
PO Box 18426 660-313-2000
Kansas City, MO 64133

2772 **Neuropsychological Rehabilitation Suggestions/Techniques**
National Chronic Fatigue Syndrome & Fibromyalgia
PO Box 18426 660-313-2000
Kansas City, MO 64133-8426

2773 **School's Guide for Students with CFS**
National Chronic Fatigue Syndrome & Fibromyalgia
PO Box 18426 660-313-2000
Kansas City, MO 64133-8426

2774 **Social Security Disability Benefits Information**
National Chronic Fatigue Syndrome & Fibromyalgia
PO Box 18426 660-313-2000
Kansas City, MO 64133-8426

2775 **Understanding CFIDS**
CFIDS Association of America
PO Box 220398
Charlotte, NC 28222-0398 800-442-3437
Provides an extensive overview of CFIDS and answers the most commonly asked questions about the disease.

2776 **Understanding the Emotions Surrounding CFS**
National Chronic Fatigue Syndrome & Fibromyalgia
PO Box 18426 660-313-2000
Kansas City, MO 64133-8426

Audio & Video

2777 **Behavioral and Circadian Sleep Problems of Infancy and Childhood**
American Academy of Sleep Medicine
One Westbrook Corporate Center 708-492-0930
Westchester, IL 60154 Fax: 708-492-0943
www.aasmnet.org
Addresses the problems of sleep disorders in children and outlines the types of disturbances, both of a medical and behavioral nature, that are commonly identified.
66 slides

2778 **CFS and Self-Esteem**
CFIDS Association of America
PO Box 220398
Charlotte, NC 28222-0398 800-442-3437
Addresses the sources of low self-esteem in persons with CFIDS and offers reassurance and practical techniques for increasing self-confidence.
Audiotape

2779 **CFS: Addressing the Realities of a Chronic Illness**
National Chronic Fatigue Syndrome & Fibromyalgia
PO Box 18426 660-313-2000
Kansas City, MO 64133-8426
This video offers reliable information featuring patients and a medical professional.

2780 **CFS: Unraveling the Mystery**
CFIDS Association of America
PO Box 220398
Charlotte, NC 28222-0398 800-442-3437
An excellent videotape for convincing skeptics that CFIDS is a real disease.
Videotape

2781 **Chronic Fatigue Syndrome: For Those Who Care**
CFIDS Association of America
PO Box 220398
Charlotte, NC 28222-0398 800-442-3437
An audiotape designed for friends and family of persons with CFIDS.
Audiotape

2782 **Chronic Fatigue Syndrome: Information, Relaxation/Healing Exercise**
CFIDS Association of America
PO Box 220398
Charlotte, NC 28222-0398 800-442-3437
Includes a comprehensive overview of CFS and relaxation/healing and imagery/stress reduction exercises for persons with CFIDS.
Audiotape

2783 **Fibromyalgia**
National Chronic Fatigue Syndrome & Fibromyalgia
PO Box 18426 660-313-2000
Kansas City, MO 64133
Videotape

2784 **HHS Satelite Video on Chronic Fatigue Syndrome and Fibromyalgia Association**
National Chronic Fatigue Syndrome and Fibromyalgia
PO Box 18426 660-313-2000
Kansas City, MO 64133-8426

2785 **Living Hell: The Real World of Chronic Fatigue Syndrome**
CFIDS Association of America
PO Box 220398
Charlotte, NC 28222-0398 800-442-3437
An emotional exposure of the tragedy of CFIDS.
Videotape

2786 **Neurocognitive Aspects of CFS**
CFIDS Association of America
PO Box 220398
Charlotte, NC 28222-0398 800-442-3437
A description of CFIDS-associated neurocognitive deficits and strategies for coping with them and the embarrassment and frustration they cause.
Audiotape

Web Sites

2787 **American Association for Chronic Fatigue Syndrome**
www.aacfs.org
A non profit organization of research scientists, physicians, licensed medical healthcare professionals, and other indviduals and institutions interested in promoting the stimulation, coordination, and exchange of ideas for CFS research and patient care.

2788 **CFIDS Association of America**
www.cfids.org
The nation's leading charitable organization devoted to conquering chronic fatigue syndrome by supporting research, education and public policy programs.

2789 **Centers for Disease Control and Prevention**
www.cdc.gov
Offers information and educational materials on CFS.

2790 **Healing Well**
www.healingwell.com
An online health resource guide to medical news, chat, information and articles, newsgroups and message boards, books, disease-related web sites, medical directories, and more for patients, friends, and family coping with disabling diseases, disorders, or chronic illnesses.

2791 **Health Finder**
www.healthfinder.gov
Searchable, carefully developed web site offering information on over 1000 topics. Developed by the US Department of Health and Human Services, the site can be used in both English and Spanish.

2792 **Healthlink USA**
www.healthlinkusa.com
Health information concerning treatment, cures, prevention, diagnosis, risk factors, research, support groups, email lists, personal stories and much more. Updated regularly.

2793 **Helios Health**
www.helioshealth.com
Online resource for your health information. Detailed information about specific health topics, access to expert advice from our Medical Advisory Board, and up-to-date health news.

2794 **Journal of Chronic Fatigue Syndrome**
www.cfs-news.org/jcfs.htm
Offers multidisciplinary original research, practical clinical management, case reports, and literature reviews to keep the entire health care delivery team well informed.

2795 **MedicineNet**
www.medicinenet.com
An online resource for consumers providing easy-to-read, authoritative medical and health information.

2796 **Medscape**
www.mywebmd.com
Medscape offers specialists, primary care physicians, and other health professionals the Web's most robust and integrated medical information and educational tools.

2797 **Option Institute**
www.option.org/cfs.shtml
Self-defeating beliefs, along with attitudes and judgments, can lead to a host of physical and psychological challenges, including Chronic Fatigue Syndrome. The Option Institute offers programs designed to help you gain new perspectives on the attitudes and judgments that may be affecting your life, especially those regarding and surrounding Chronic Fatigue Syndrome.

2798 **Sleepnet**
www.sleepnet.com
Links all the sleep information located on the internet. Provides a place for everyone to read and post questions, or responses.

2799 **WebMD**

www.webmd.com

Information on Chronic Fatigue Syndrome, including articles and resources.

Description

2800 **Chronic Pain**

Chronic pain is defined as pain persisting for more than one month after resolution of an acute injury or pain that persists or recurs for more than three months. The pain may begin for unknown reasons, or may begin with some injury or illness but persist long after the triggering event is gone. Human pain has physiological causes but also has psychological components differing for each person. Many Americans suffer from chronic pain. The annual cost, including treatment and lost work days, now hovers around $100 billion in the US.

Doctors and patients have tried almost every conceivable type of therapy for chronic pain. Drug treatments include narcotics (codeine and morphine), nonnarcotic painkillers such as acetaminophen, and nonsteroidal anti-inflammatory drugs such as ibuprofen. Use of antidepressants, either alone or in conjunction with pain medications, can be beneficial. Doctors may inject drugs to block the nerves that carry the pain signal, or may even cut the nerve. Physical measures include heat or cold application, application of electrical stimuli (TENS), stretching, and general conditioning exercises. Psychological treatment includes psychotherapy, meditation, hypnosis and biofeedback-relaxation. Because of the complexity of chronic pain and its treatment, some doctors have begun to specialize in management of pain, and have organized multidisciplinary pain clinics which offer expertise from anesthesiology, rheumatology, neurosurgery, psychology and physical therapy.

A realistic goal of therapy is to improve one's daily functioning; for instance, being able to return to work or pleasurable activities. Those able to achieve this status will often state that the pain is still there but that it does not bother them like it once did. Whatever the stage of one's condition, peer support is important, and is available from local in-person support groups or from Internet chat rooms and bulletin boards.

National Agencies & Associations

2801 **American Chronic Pain Association**
PO Box 850
Rocklin, CA 95677
800-533-3231
Fax: 916-632-3208
e-mail: ACPA@pacbell.net
www.theacpa.org
ACPA mission is: (1) to facilitate peer support and education for individuals with chronic pain and their families so that these individuals may live more fully in spite of their pain; and (2) to raise awareness among the health care community and policy makers.
Penny Cowan, Executive Director

2802 **American Pain Society**
4700 W Lake Avenue
Glenview, IL 60025
847-375-4715
Fax: 877-734-8758
e-mail: info@amipainsoc.org
www.ampainsoc.org
A multidisciplinary organization of basic and clinical scientists practicing clinicians policy analysts and others. Mission is to advance pain-related research education treatment and professional practice.
Richard Payn MD, Director
Patricia McG PhD, Scientific Director

2803 **International Association for the Study of Pain**
111 Queen Anne Avenue N
Seattle, WA 98109-4955
206-283-0311
Fax: 206-283-9403
e-mail: iaspdesk@iasp-pain.org
www.iasp-pain.org
The International Association for the Study of Pain is the leading professional forum for science practice and education in the field of pain.
Gerald F Gebhart PhD, President
Kathy Kreiter, Executive Director

2804 **International Pelvic Pain Society Women's Medical Plaza**
Women's Medical Plaza
1100 E Woodfield Road
Schaumburg, IL 60173
847-517-8712
800-624-9676
Fax: 847-517-7229
e-mail: info@pelvicpain.org
www.pelvicpain.org
Short range goal is to recruit organize and educate health care professionals actively involved with the treatment of patients who have chronic pelvic pain.
Fred Marion Howard, Chairman of the Board
Howard Taylo Sharp MD, President

2805 **Reflex Sympathetic Dystrophy Syndrome Association (RSDSA)**
PO Box 502
Milford, CT 06460
203-877-3790
877-662-7737
Fax: 203-882-8362
e-mail: info@rsds.org
www.rsds.org
Nonprofit professional and consumer organization founded to support research into the cause, treatment and cure of reflex sympathetic dystrophy syndrome. RSDSA also organizes support groups, promote awareness among health professionals and develop educational programs.
Paul R Charlesworth, President
James E Tyrrell Jr, Chairman of the Board

Support Groups & Hotlines

2806 **National Health Information Center**
PO Box 1133
Washington, DC 20013
310-565-4167
800-336-4797
Fax: 301-984-4256
e-mail: info@nhic.org
www.health.gov/nhic
Offers a nationwide information referral service, produces directories and resource guides.

Books

2807 **ACPA Facilitator Guide & Materials**
American Chronic Pain Association
PO Box 850
Rocklin, CA 95677
916-632-0922
800-533-3231
Fax: 916-632-3208
e-mail: acpa@pacbell.net
www.theacpa.org
This guide will help you and others in your community organize an ACPA chapter. The manual contains how-to information on organizing an ACPA chapter, sharing responsibility for the group with others, finding a meeting place, conducting the first meeting, and generating public interest in your area. You must be an ACPA member to purchase this manual.
Penny Cowan, Executive Director

2808 **ACPA Family Manual**
Penny Cowan, author
American Chronic Pain Association

PO Box 850
Rockin, CA 95677
916-632-0922
800-533-3231
Fax: 916-632-3208
e-mail: acpa@pacbell.net
www.theacpa.org

A manual designed with the needs of those who live with a person who has chronic pain.
149 pages
ISBN: 0-967387-82-5
Penny Cowan, Executive Director

2809 ACPA Journal Reflections of You
American Chronic Pain Association
PO Box 850
Rocklin, CA 95677
916-632-0922
800-533-3231
Fax: 916-632-3208
e-mail: acpa@pacbell.net
www.theacpa.org

A daily meditation and personal journal book which provides positive and motivating thoughts to stimulate your thinking and challenge you to personal growth. Your daily entries in the journal will help track your progress and show when you have reached your personal goal.
Penny Cowan, Executive Director

2810 ACSM's Exercise Management for Persons with Chronic Disease & Disabilities
Human Kinetics Press
PO Box 5076
Champaign, IL 61825-5076
217-351-5076
800-747-4457
Fax: 217-351-2674
www.humankinetics.com

1993 384 pages Hardcover
ISBN: 0-736038-72-8
Steve Ruhlig, Marketing Director

2811 Essential Guide to Chronic Illness: The Active Patient's Handbook
James W Long, author
DIANE Publishing Company
330 Pusey Avenue, Unit #3 Rear
Darby, PA 19023
610-461-6200
800-782-3833
Fax: 610-461-6130
e-mail: dianepublishing@gmail.com
www.dianepublishing.net

A comprehensive guide to dealing with nearly 50 chronic illness and conditions from acne to Zollinger-Ellison syndrome, including diabetes, menopause, migraines, rheumatoid arthritis and psoriasis.
625 pages Paperback
ISBN: 0-788169-03-3
Herman Baron, Publisher

2812 From Patient to Person: First Steps
American Chronic Pain Association
PO Box 850
Rocklin, CA 95677
916-632-0922
800-533-3231
Fax: 916-632-3208
e-mail: acpa@pacbell.net
www.theacpa.org

A workbook designed to help anyone who has a chronic pain problem to gain a better understanding of how one can begin to cope with all the problems that their pain creates.

ISBN: 0-967387-80-9
Penny Cowan, Executive Director

2813 Occupational Therapy Practice Guidelines for Adults with Low Back Pain
American Occupational Therapy Association
4720 Montgomery Lane
Bethesda, MD 20824-1220
301-652-2682
Fax: 301-652-7711
TDD: 800-377-8555
www.aota.org

15 pages
ISBN: 1-569001-49-9

2814 Occupational Therapy Practice Guidelines for Adults with Hip Fracture/Replacement
American Occupational Therapy Association
4720 Montgomery Lane
Bethesda, MD 20824-1220
301-652-2682
Fax: 301-652-7711
TDD: 800-377-8555
www.aota.org

10 pages
ISBN: 1-569001-48-0

2815 Staying Well: Advanced Pain Management for ACPA Members
American Chronic Pain Association
PO Box 850
Rocklin, CA 95677
916-632-0922
800-533-3231
Fax: 916-632-3208
e-mail: acpa@pacbell.net
www.theacpa.org

This workbook is designed for those who have a working knowledge of the basics of pain management. This workbook provides additional skills necessary to continue to move forward in the journey to wellness.

ISBN: 0-969387-81-7
Penny Cowan, Executive Director

2816 Understanding Chronic Pain
Angela Koestler, PhD; Ann Myers, MD, author
University Press of Mississippi
3825 Ridgewood Road
Jackson, MS 39211-6492
601-432-6205
Fax: 601-432-6217
e-mail: kburgess@ihl.state.ms.us
www.upress.state.ms.us

A handbook for people coping with chronic pain and suffering and for those who seek to understand and support them.
2002 184 pages Paperback
ISBN: 1-578064-40-6
Kathy Burgess, Advertising/Marketing Services Manager

2817 Your Pain is Real: Free Yourself from Chronic Pain, Breakthrough Med. Trtmnt.
DIANE Publishing Company
330 Pusey Avenue, Unit #3 Rear
Darby, PA 19023
610-461-6200
800-782-3833
Fax: 610-461-6130
e-mail: dianepublishing@gmail.com
www.dianepublishing.net

A complete, authoritative and hopeful book on the subject of chronic pain relief. Offers revolutionary ways to relieve all types and degrees of painful conditions. Also offers breakthrough medical treatments, clear guidelines for seeking expert care and the latest scientific findings on pain management.
252 pages Hardcover
ISBN: 0-756753-70-8
Herman Baron, Publisher

Newsletters

2818 American Chronic Pain Association
PO Box 850
Rocklin, CA 95677-0850
916-632-0922
800-533-3231
Fax: 916-632-3208
e-mail: ACPA@pacbell.net
www.theacpa.org

A nonprofit organization with over 400 chapters in the US, Canada, Australia, New Zealand and Russia. The purpose of this organization is to provide a support system for those suffering chronic pain through group activities.
Quart w/ mbrshp
Penny Cowan, Executive Founder & Director

2819 Health Points
TyH Publications
17007 E Colony Drive
Fountain Hills, AZ 85268
800-801-1406
e-mail: editor@e-tyh.com

National newsletter with articles on complementary therapy, latest nutrition news, disability issues and much more. Focus is on fibromyalgia, chronic fatigue, arthritis and chronic pain.
Quarterly

Pamphlets

2820 Suicide is Not an Option
National Chronic Fatigue Syndrome
PO Box 18426 — 660-313-2000
Kansas City, MO 64133-8426

Audio & Video

2821 ACPA Relaxation Tapes
American Chronic Pain Association
PO Box 850 — 916-632-0922
Rocklin, CA 95677 — 800-533-3231
Fax: 916-632-3208
e-mail: acpa@pacbell.net
www.theacpa.org
Audio tapes offering information on pain relief, breath relaxation and autogenic relaxation. These tapes are designed to help persons regain control of their bodies through exercises in relaxation techniques. $10.00-$25.00.
Audio Tapes
Penny Cowan, Executive Director

2822 ACPA Video: 10 Steps from Patient to Person
American Chronic Pain Association
PO Box 850 — 916-632-0922
Rocklin, CA 95677 — 800-533-3231
Fax: 916-632-3208
e-mail: acpa@pacbell.net
www.theacpa.org
The video, featuring Penny Cowan, founder of the ACPA, discussed the value of a multidisiplinary pain management program and what is necessary to maintain wellness long term.
Penny Cowan, Executive Director

2823 Affirmation Tape
American Chronic Pain Association
PO Box 850 — 916-632-0922
Rocklin, CA 95677 — 800-533-3231
Fax: 916-632-3208
e-mail: ACPA@pacbell.net
www.theacpa.org
Designed to help you focus on positive things about yourself and builds self-esteem.
Penny Cowan, Executive Director

2824 Relaxation Tape
American Chronic Pain Association
PO Box 850 — 916-632-0922
Rocklin, CA 95677 — 800-533-3231
Fax: 916-632-3208
e-mail: ACPA@pacbell.net
www.theacpa.org
Tape one includes pain relief and breath relaxation. Tape two includes general relaxation and autogenic relaxation.
Penny Cowan, Executive Director

Web Sites

2825 American Chronic Pain Association
www.theacpa.org
Facilitating peer support and education for individuals with chronic pain and their families so that these individuals may live more fully in spite of their pain.

2826 American Pain Society
ampainsoc.org
Multidisciplinary organization of basic and clinical scientists, practicing clinicians, policy analysts, and others.

2827 Discovery Health
health.discovery.com
A source of information on various health topics, including chronic pain and its symptoms and treatments.

2828 Healing Well
www.healingwell.com
An online health resource guide to medical news, chat, information and articles, newsgroups and message boards, books, disease-related web sites, medical directories, and more for patients, friends, and family coping with disabling diseases, disorders, or chronic illnesses.

2829 Health Finder
www.healthfinder.gov
Searchable, carefully developed web site offering information on over 1000 topics. Developed by the US Department of Health and Human Services, the site can be used in both English and Spanish.

2830 Healthlink USA
www.healthlinkusa.com
Health information concerning treatment, cures, prevention, diagnosis, risk factors, research, support groups, email lists, personal stories and much more. Updated regularly.

2831 Helios Health
www.helioshealth.com
Online resource for your health information. Detailed information about specific health topics, access to expert advice from our Medical Advisory Board, and up-to-date health news.

2832 International Pelvic Pain Society
www.pelvicpain.org/
Short range goal is to recruit, organizae, and educate health care professionals actively invlved with the treatment of patients who have chronic opelvic pain.

2833 MedicineNet
www.medicinenet.com
An online resource for consumers providing easy-to-read, authoritative medical and health information.

2834 Medscape
www.mywebmd.com
Medscape offers specialists, primary care physicians, and other health professionals the Web's most robust and integrated medical information and educational tools.

2835 WebMD
www.webmd.com
Information on chronic pain, including articles and resources.

Description

2836 **Congenital Heart Disease**

Congenital Heart Disease (CHD) represents the most common group of congenital (present from birth) anomalies. CHD can be thought of as a group of disorders that result from the abnormal formation of the heart in utero. The heart develops between the 2nd and 6th week of gestation, and may be affected by genetic mutation, maternal systemic medications or toxins (e.g. alcohol abuse). The incidence of CHD in the population is about 8 cases in 1,000 live births, or just under 1%. About half of these cardiac defects are considered to be minor and can be followed clinically while the other half fall into the categories of major CHD. This latter group often requires surgery early in life to either completely repair the heart defect or in some cases, to redirect blood through the cardiovascular system to palliate the structural abnormality.

CHD can be divided into three major categories: left to right shunting lesions, left heart obstructive lesions and those that lead to marked cyanosis (decreased oxygen delivery to the organs and tissues), the so called cyanotic heart diseases.

The left to right shunting lesions are the most common of the three groups and include the ventricular septal defect (VSD), the atrial septal defect (ASD), the atrioventricular septal defect (also referred to as the AV canal), and the patent ductus arteriosus. In all of these left to right shunting lesions, there is a progressive increase in the amount of blood sent from the left side of the heartacross the given defect (hole) into the right side that delivers blood to the lungs. There is as a result, too much blood entering the pulmonary circuit and this can lead to problems with breathing and feeding for infants in the first few months of life.

The more common left heart obstructive diseases include aortic stenosis, coarctation of the aorta and the hypoplastic left heart syndrome. Each of these can lead to a marked reduction in the amount of blood flow that is able to leave the left side of the heart and can be delivered to the organs and tissues. This leads to marked abnormalities in the way the organs and tissues function and can cause serious and emergent problems for infants in the first week or two of life.

Cyanotic heart disease are those cardiac malformations that lead to a bluish discoloration of the baby as there is insufficient oxygenated blood that is delivered to the body with or without inadequate blood delivered to the lungs to pick up oxygen. The more common disorders in this group are tetralogy of Fallot, Transposition of the great arteries, tricuspid atresia and truncus arteriosus.

With the remarkable advances in neonatal cardiac surgery and interventional cardiac catheterization, almost all of the cardiac malformations can be aggressively addressed with excellent results, even in the youngest and smallest of patients. Overall, survival from all cardiac surgeries in children with CHD is greater than 95%, and even for the most complex of CHD it is approaching 90%. These children often require long-term follow-up from a pediatric cardiologist, but the vast majority lead healthy active lives. See also *Birth Defects*.

National Agencies & Associations

2837 **Adult Congenital Heart Association**
6757 Greene Street
Philadelphia, PA 19119
215-849-1260
888-921-ACHA
Fax: 215-849-1261
e-mail: Info@achaheart.org
www.achaheart.org

The Adult Congenital Heart Association (ACHA) is a nonprofit organization which seeks to improve the quality of life and extend the lives of adults with congenital heart defects through education, outreach, advocacy and promotion of research.
Amy Verstappen, President
Paula Miller, Vice President

2838 **Congenital Heart Information Network**
101 N Washington Avenue
Margate City, NJ 08402
609-822-1572
Fax: 609-822-1574
e-mail: mb@tchin.org
www.tchin.org

C.H.I.N. is a national organization that provides reliable information support services, financial assistance and resources to families of children with congenital heart defects and acquired heart disease and adults with congenital heart defects.
Mona Barmash, President

2839 **Kids with Heart National Association for Children's Heart Disorders**
1578 Careful Drive
Green Bay, WI 54307
920-498-0058
800-538-5390
www.kidswithheart.org

Kids with Heart is a nonprofit organization founded in 1985 dedicated to providing support for families affected by congenital heart defects through surgical care packages.
Michelle Rin BA, President
Dean Rintamaki, Vice President

2840 **Schneeweiss Adult Congenital Heart Disease Center**
New York Presbyterian Hospital
161 Fort Washington Avenue
New York, NY 10032
212-305-6936
Fax: 212-305-0490
congenitalheart.hs.columbia.edu

We provide such diagnostic services such as echocardiography cardiac MRI and cardiac catheterization. Highly specialized care is provided by a team of physicians specifically interested in the problems of adults with congenital heart disease.
Marlon S Rosenbaum MD, Director

Web Sites

2841 **Heartpoint**
www.heartpoint.com

Heartpoint provides information about specific heart defects.

2842 **MedicineNet**
www.medicinenet.com

An online resource for consumers providing easy-to-read, authoritative medical and health information.

2843 **Medline Plus**
www.nlm.nih.gov/medlineplus

This website includes information about congenital heart disease and includes links regarding support and treatment.

2844 **Yale: Congenital Heart Disease**
info.med.yale.edu/intmed/cardio/chd

This web site provides in-depth information regarding various types of heart conditions.

Description

2845 **Cooley's Anemia (Thalassemia)**

Cooley's anemia, or beta-Thalassemia major, is an inherited disorder characterized by abnormal production of hemoglobin in the red blood cells. There are two forms of beta-Thalassemia: beta-Thalassemia minor, in which the person has no symptoms, and beta-Thalassemia major, or Cooley's anemia, which is a severe, debilitating disease. Although a baby who has Cooley's anemia appears normal at birth, growth rates are impaired, and puberty may be significantly delayed or absent. Without therapy, there is a general decline. The skin becomes pale or jaundiced, facial bones become more prominent and pronounced, and the spleen becomes enlarged.

While there is no cure for Cooley's anemia, there are treatments such as blood transfusions, which can reduce some symptoms of the disease. However, children with Cooley's anemia should receive as few transfusions as possible because of the danger of iron overload from the "heme" portion of hemoglobin. Chelation, or binding, of the excess iron associated with multiple, repetitive transfusions is important, and is accomplished with deferoxamine. Removal of the spleen may reduce transfusion requirements.

Because there is no cure for beta-Thalassemia major, genetic screening of at-risk populations is very important, notably for persons of Mediterranean, African and Southeast Asian ancestry. Prenatal diagnosis can also be performed.

National Agencies & Associations

2846 **American Hellenic Educational Progressive Association**
1909 Q Street NW 202-232-6300
Washington, DC 20009 Fax: 202-232-2140
e-mail: ahepa@ahepa.org
www.ahepa.org
The mission of the AHEPA Family is to promote Hellenism Education Philanthropy Civic Responsibility and Family and Individual Excellence.
Basil N Mossaidis, Executive Director

2847 **Fanconi Anemia Research Foundation**
1801 Willamette Street 541-687-4658
Eugene, OR 97401 888-FAN-CONI
Fax: 541-687-0548
e-mail: info@fanconi.org
www.fanconi.org
Funds research and provides education and support services worldwide to families affected with Fanconi anemia a rare genetic aplastic anemia that leads to bone marrow failure acute myelogenous leukemia and squamous cell carcinomas.

State Agencies & Associations

California

2848 **Cooley's Anemia Foundation (CAF): Californ ia**
2629 Foothill Boulevard
La Crescenta, CA 91214 800-601-2821
Fax: 212-279-5999
e-mail: info@cooleysanemia.org
www.cooleysanemia.org
The Cooley's Anemia Foundation (CAF) is dedicated to serving people afflicted with various forms of thalassemia, most notably the major form of this genetic blood disease, Cooley's anemia/thalassemia major. CAF's mission is advancing the treatment and curing the disease.
Christine Giannamore, Coordinator
Gina Cioffi Esq, National Office Executive Director

Illinois

2849 **Cooley's Anemia Foundation (CAF): Illinois Oakbrook Towers**
Oakbrook Towers
40 N Tower Road 847-602-2616
Altbrook, IL 62503 800-522-7222
Fax: 212-279-5999
e-mail: info@cooleysanemia.org
www.cooleysanemia.org
The Cooley's Anemia Foundation (CAF) is dedicated to serving people afflicted with various forms of thalassemia most notably the major form of this genetic blood disease Cooley's anemia/thalassemia major. CAF's mission is advancing the treatment and curing the disease.
Bruce Rod, President Illinois Office
Gina Cioffi, National Office Executive Director

Maryland

2850 **Cooley's Anemia Foundation (CAF): Capital Area**
15321 Peach Orchard Avenue 301-989-8947
Silver Spring, MD 20905 800-522-7222
Fax: 212-279-5999
e-mail: info@cooleysanemia.org
www.cooleysanemia.org
The Cooley's Anemia Foundation (CAF) is dedicated to serving people afflicted with various forms of thalassemia most notably the major form of this genetic blood disease Cooley's anemia/thalassemia major. CAF's mission is advancing the treatment and curing the disease.
Carl C Vitaliti, President Capital Area Office
Gina Cioffi Esq, National Office Executive Director

Massachusetts

2851 **Cooley's Anemia Foundation (CAF): Massachu setts Chapter**
44 Joseph Road 617-332-5952
Newton, MA 02460-1122 800-522-7222
Fax: 212-279-5999
e-mail: info@cooleysanemia.org
www.cooleysanemia.org
The Cooley's Anemia Foundation (CAF) is dedicated to serving people afflicted with various forms of thalassemia most notably the major form of this genetic blood disease Cooley's anemia/thalassemia major. CAF's mission is advancing the treatment and curing the disease.
Rudi Viscomi, President Massachusetts Office
Gina Cioffi, National Office Executive Director

New Jersey

2852 **Cooley's Anemia Foundation (CAF): New Jers sey Chapter**
29 Alyson Place 732-688-2279
Bloomfield, NJ 07003 800-522-7222
Fax: 212-279-5999
e-mail: info@cooleysanemia.org
www.cooleysanemia.org
The Cooley's Anemia Foundation (CAF) is dedicated to serving people afflicted with various forms of thalassemia most notably the major form of this genetic blood disease Cooley's anemia/thalassemia major. CAF's mission is advancing the treatment and curing the disaease.
Christine Somma, President New Jersey Office
Gina Cioffi, National Office Executive Director

New York

2853 **Cooley's Anemia Foundation (CAF): Buffalo**
135 Wellington Road 716-834-8903
Buffalo, NY 14216 800-522-7222
Fax: 212-279-5999
e-mail: info@cooleysanemia.org
www.cooleysanemia.org

The Cooley's Anemia Foundation (CAF) is dedicated to serving people afflicted with various forms of thalassemia most notably the major form of this genetic blood disease Cooley's anemia/thalassemia major. CAF's mission is advancing the treatment and curing the disease.
Dennis Locurto, President Buffalo Office
Gina Cioffi Esq, National Office Executive Director

2854 **Cooley's Anemia Foundation (CAF): Long Isl and**
111 Cherry Valley Avenue 516-358-9100
Garden City, NY 11530 800-522-7222
Fax: 516-358-9101
e-mail: info@cooleysanemia.org
www.cooleysanemia.org
The Cooley's Anemia Foundation (CAF) is dedicated to serving people afflicted with various forms of thalassemia most notably the major form of this genetic blood disease Cooley's anemia/thalassemia major. CAF's mission is advancing the treatment and curing the disease.
Thomas Rotolo, President Long Island Office
Janice Cenzoprano, Vice President Long Island Office

2855 **Cooley's Anemia Foundation (CAF): Queens**
157-26 9th Avenue 718-746-7677
Beachurst, NY 11357 800-522-7222
Fax: 718-746-7678
e-mail: info@cooleysanemia.org
www.cooleysanemia.org
The Cooley's Anemia Foundation (CAF) is dedicated to serving people afflicted with various forms of thalassemia most notably the major form of this genetic blood disease Cooley's anemia/thalassemia major. CAF's mission is advancing the treatment and curing the disease.
Paul Tucci, President Queen Office
Abbey Chakalis, Events Manager

2856 **Cooley's Anemia Foundation (CAF): Rocheste r**
585-482-5587
800-522-7222
Fax: 212-279-5999
e-mail: info@cooleysanemia.org
www.cooleysanemia.org
The Cooley's Anemia Foundation (CAF) is dedicated to serving people afflicted with various forms of thalassemia most notably the major form of this genetic blood disease Cooley's anemia/thalassemia major. CAF's mission is advancing the treatment and curing the disease.
Shirley Cammilleri, President Rochester Office
Gina Cioffi Esq, National Office Executive Director

2857 **Cooley's Anemia Foundation (CAF): Staten I sland**
16B Dreyer Avenue 718-761-5380
Staten Island, NY 10314 800-522-7222
Fax: 718-761-5381
e-mail: info@cooleysanemia.org
www.cooleysanemia.org
The Cooley's Anemia Foundation (CAF) is dedicated to serving people afflicted with various forms of thalassemia most notably the major form of this genetic blood disease Cooley's anemia/thalassemia major. CAF's mission is advancing the treatment and curing the disaese.
Gina Cioffi Esq, National Office Executive Director
Craig Butler, National Office Communications Director

2858 **Cooley's Anemia Foundation (CAF): Suffolk Chapter Office**
740 Smithtown Bypass 631-863-0532
Smithtown, NY 11787 800-522-7222
Fax: 631-863-0535
e-mail: info@cooleysanemia.org
www.cooleysanemia.org
The Cooley's Anemia Foundation (CAF) is dedicated to serving people afflicted with various forms of thalassemia most notably the major form of this genetic blood disease Cooley's anemia/thalassemia major. CAF's mission is advancing the treatment and curing the disease.
Gina Cioffi Esq, National Office Executive Director
Craig Butler, National Office Communications Director

2859 **Cooley's Anemia Foundation (CAF): Westches tchester/Rockland Chapter**
3 Samuel Purdy Lane 914-232-1808
Katonah, NY 10536 800-522-7222
Fax: 212-279-5999
e-mail: info@cooleysanemia.org
www.cooleysanemia.org
The Cooley's Anemia Foundation (CAF) is dedicated to serving people afflicted with various forms of thalassemia most notably the major form of this genetic blood disease Cooley's anemia/thalassemia major. CAF's mission is advancing the treatment and curing the disease.
Peter Chieco, President Westchester/Rockland Office
Janet Manning, Executive Director

Texas

2860 **Cooley's Anemia Foundation (CAF): Texas**
4504 Astor Road 214-324-6147
Mesquite, TX 75150-2320 800-522-7222
Fax: 214-324-0612
e-mail: info@cooleysanemia.org
www.cooleysanemia.org
The Cooley's Anemia Foundation (CAF) is dedicated to serving people afflicted with various forms of thalassemia most notably the major form of this genetic blood disease Cooley's anemia/thalassemia major.
Mateen Shah, President
Gina Cioffi Esq, National Office Executive Director

Foundations

2861 **Cooleys Anemia Foundation**
330 Seventh Avenue
New York, NY 10001 800-522-7222
Fax: 212-279-5999
e-mail: info@cooleysanemia.org
www.cooleysanemia.org
Our mission is advancing the treatment and cure for this fatal blood disease, enhancing the quality of life of patients and educating the medical profession, trait carriers and the public about Cooley's anemia/thalassemia major.
Gina Cioffi, Esq, National Executive Director
Craig Butler, Communications Director

Support Groups & Hotlines

2862 **National Health Information Center**
PO Box 1133 310-565-4167
Washington, DC 20013 800-336-4797
Fax: 301-984-4256
e-mail: info@nhic.org
www.health.gov/nhic
Offers a nationwide information referral service, produces directories and resource guides.

Books

2863 **Genes, Blood & Courage**
129-09 26th Avenue 212-598-0911
Flushing, NY 11354 800-522-7222
www.cooleysanemia.org

2864 **What is Cooley's Anemia**
129-09 26th Avenue 718-321-2873
Flushing, NY 11354 800-522-7222
Fax: 718-321-3340
e-mail: info@cooleysanemia.org
www.cooleysanemia.org
Patient and family handbook.
Jayne Restivo, National Executive Director

2865 **What is Thalassemia?**
Cooley's Anemia Foundation

129-09 26th Avenue 718-321-2873
Flushing, NY 11354 800-522-7222
Fax: 718-321-3340
e-mail: info@cooleysanemia.org
www.cooleysanemia.org

A guide to help thalassemics and their parents understand thalassemia, the reasons for treatment and the hope for the future.
Jayne Restivo, National Executive Director

Children's Books

2866 Coloring Book on Thalassemia
129-09 26th Avenue 718-321-2873
Flushing, NY 11354 800-522-7222
Fax: 718-321-3340
e-mail: info@cooleysanemia.org
www.cooleysanemia.org

Available in English, Italian, Greek and Chinese.
Jayne Restivo, National Executive Director

Magazines

2867 AHEPAN Magazine
American Hellenic Educational Progressive Assn
1909 Q Street NW 202-232-6300
Washington, DC 20009 Fax: 202-232-2140
e-mail: ahepa@ahepa.org
www.ahepa.org

This magazine includes all of the AHEPA organizations.
Quarterly
Basil N Mossaidis, Executive Director

Newsletters

2868 Lifeline
Cooley's Anemia Foundation
129-09 26th Avenue 718-321-2873
Flushing, NY 11354 800-522-7222
Fax: 718-321-3340
e-mail: info@cooleysanemia.org
www.cooleysanemia.org

A newsletter published by Cooley's Anemia Foundation.
Jayne Restivo, National Executive Director

Pamphlets

2869 Desferal Q&A
129-09 26th Avenue 718-321-2873
Flushing, NY 11354 800-522-7222
Fax: 718-321-3340
e-mail: info@cooleysanemia.org
www.cooleysanemia.org

Guideline for home infusion.
Jayne Restivo, National Executive Director

2870 What is Thalassemia Trait?
Cooley's Anemia Foundation
129-09 26th Avenue 718-321-2873
Flushing, NY 11354 800-522-7222
Fax: 718-321-3340
e-mail: info@cooleysanemia.org
www.cooleysanemia.org

This booklet offers information on the thalassemia trait.
1995
Jayne Restivo, National Executive Director

Audio & Video

2871 TAG Annual Patient/Family Conference Video
Cooley's Anemia Foundation
Thalassemia Action Group
New York, NY 10001 800-522-7222
Fax: 212-279-5999
e-mail: TAG@cooleysanemia.org
www.cooleysanemia.org/

Video from the Thalassemia Action Group/TAG Annual Patient/Family Conference held in March of each year.
Gina Cioffi Esq, National Executive Director
Craig Butler, Communications Director

2872 To Live
Cooley's Anemia Foundation
330 Seventh Avenue
New York, NY 10001 800-522-7222
Fax: 212-279-5999
e-mail: info@cooleysanemia.org
www.cooleysanemia.org/

An informative and educational video from Cooley's Anemia Foundation.
Gina Cioffi Esq, National Executive Director
Craig Butler, Communications Director

2873 You're Not Alone
Cooley's Anemia Foundation
330 Seventh Avenue
New York, NY 10004 800-522-7222
Fax: 212-279-5999
e-mail: info@cooleysanemia.org
www.cooleysanemia.org

An informative and educational video from Cooley's Anemia Foundation.
Gina Cioffi Esq, National Executive Director
Craig Butler, Communications Director

Web Sites

2874 Healing Well
www.healingwell.com

An online health resource guide to medical news, chat, information and articles, newsgroups and message boards, books, disease-related web sites, medical directories, and more for patients, friends, and family coping with disabling diseases, disorders, or chronic illnesses.

2875 Health Finder
www.healthfinder.gov

Searchable, carefully developed web site offering information on over 1000 topics. Developed by the US Department of Health and Human Services, the site can be used in both English and Spanish.

2876 Healthlink USA
www.healthlinkusa.com

Health information concerning treatment, cures, prevention, diagnosis, risk factors, research, support groups, email lists, personal stories and much more. Updated regularly.

2877 Helios Health
www.helioshealth.com

Online resource for your health information. Detailed information about specific health topics, access to expert advice from our Medical Advisory Board, and up-to-date health news.

2878 MedicineNet
www.medicinenet.com

An online resource for consumers providing easy-to-read, authoritative medical and health information.

2879 Medscape
www.mywebmd.com

Medscape offers specialists, primary care physicians, and other health professionals the Web's most robust and integrated medical information and educational tools.

2880 WebMD
www.webmd.com

Information on Cooley's Anemia (Thalassemia), including articles and resources.

Description

2881 **Crohn's Disease**

Crohn's disease is a chronic inflammation in the lining of the digestive tract, generally in the small bowel or part of the colon. The cause is unknown, although the disease is more common in some families and racial groups. Although not a proven cause, periods of emotional stress have been linked with flare-ups of the disease. Onset is typically before age 30, with the peak incidence between 14 and 24 years.

Common symptoms include diarrhea, weight loss, fever, abdominal pain and loss of appetite. If the disease is extensive it may cause deficiencies of essential vitamins and other nutrients. Sometimes inflammation occurs outside the gut, attacking the eyes, joints or skin. Local complications include bowel perforation with formation of abscesses or fistulas which drain out to the skin. Established chronic Crohn's disease is characterized by lifelong exacerbations. These patients carry an increased risk of cancer of the small bowel and colon/rectum.

Therapy depends on the location of the disease and on its severity. Although no specific therapy is known, drug treatment can range from simple anti-diarrheal medications to anti-inflammatory drugs and immunosuppressives. Surgery may be necessary to treat complications. In all cases, careful attention should be paid to the patient's nutritional status and psychological well-being. See also *Gastrointestinal Disorders* and *Celiac Disease.*

National Agencies & Associations

2882 **CCFA Camps Across America Crohn's & Colitis Foundation of America**
Crohn's & Colitis Foundation of America
386 Park Avenue S
New York, NY 10016
212-685-3440
800-932-2423
Fax: 212-779-4098
e-mail: info@ccfa.org
www.ccfa.org

A chance for children with Crhon's disease or ulcerative colitis to have a camping experience. Because CCFA camps are offered by chapters across the country every camp has its own flavor and style. Activities, as well as the length of stay may vary from child to child.

2883 **Crohn's & Colitis Foundation of America**
386 Park Avenue S
New York, NY 10016
212-685-3440
800-932-2423
Fax: 212-779-4098
e-mail: info@ccfa.org
www.ccfa.org

CCFA's mission is to cure and prevent Crohn's disease and ulcerative colitis through research and to improve the quality of life of children and adults affected by this disease through education and support. The foundation offers patient and professional support.
Barbara Rosenstein, Director Communication

2884 **Ileitis and Colitis Educational Foundation**
Central DuPage Hospital
25 N Winfield Road
Winfield, IL 60190
630-933-1600
Fax: 630-933-1300
TTY: 630-933-4833
e-mail: cdh_information@cdh.org
www.cdh.org

Offers support groups fund-raising activities educational materials and public awareness campaigns pertaining to these disorders.
C William Pollard, Chair
Richard A Mark, Vice Chair

2885 **International Foundation for Functional Gastrointestinal Disorders (IFFGD)**
PO Box 170864
Milwaukee, WI 53217-8076
414-964-1799
888-964-2001
Fax: 414-964-7176
e-mail: iffgd@iffgd.org
www.iffgd.org

Nonprofit education, support and research organization devoted to increasing awareness and understanding of functional gastrointestinal disorders, including irritable bowel syndrome (IBS), constipation, diarrhea, pain, and incontinence. Mission is to inform, assist and support people affected by these disorders.

2886 **National Institute of Diabetes, Digestive & Kidney Diseases**
National Institutes of Health
31 Center Drive, MSC 2560
Bethesda, MD 20892-2560
301-496-4000
e-mail: NIHInfo@OD.NIH.GOV
www.diabetes.niddk.nih.gov

Conducts and supports research on many of the most serious diseases affecting public health. The Institute supports much of the clinical research on the diseases of internal medicine and related subspecialty fields as well as many basic science disiplines.
Dr. Griffin Rodgers, Acting Director

2887 **Pediatric Crohn's and Colitis Association**
PO Box 188
Newton, MA 02468
617-489-5854
e-mail: questions@pcca.hypermart.net
www.pcca.hypermart.net

Focuses on all aspects of pediatric and adolescent Crohn's disease and ulcerative colitis, including medical, nutritional, psychological and social factors. Activities include information sharing, educational forums, newsletters and hospital outreach programs.

2888 **Reach Out for Youth with Ileitis and Colitis**
84 Northgate Circle
Melville, NY 11747
631-293-3102
e-mail: reachoutforyouth@reachoutforyouth.org
www.reachoutforyouth.org

Provides educational seminars and individual and group support to patients and their families. Fundraising efforts support the center's programs, clinical and laboratory research, and purchase of state-of-the-art equipment.

2889 **United Ostomy Association**
PO Box 66
Fairview, TN 37062-0066
800-826-0826
e-mail: info@uoa.org
www.uoa.org

Volunteer based health organization dedicated to providing education, information, support and advocacy for those who have or will have an intestinal or urinary diversion. We provide patient visiting services, 800 number referral and information service, over 425 local chapters, the Ostomy quarterly magazine and the UOA web site, www.uoa.org.
Nancy Italia, Executive Director

2890 **World Ostomy and Continence Nurses Society**
15000 Commerce Parkway
Mt Laurel, NJ 08054
888-224-9626
Fax: 856-439-0525
e-mail: info@wocn.org

Membership comprises nurses that specialize in enterostomal therapy.
Margaret T Goldberg MSN RN, President
Janice C Colwell MSN R, President-Elect

State Agencies & Associations

Alabama

2891 **CCFA Alabama Chapter**
244 Goodwin Crest Drive
Birmingham, AL 35209
205-941-9900
800-249-1993
Fax: 205-941-1411
e-mail: ptalty@ccfa.org OR info@ccfa.org
www.ccfa.org/chapters/alabama

Crohn's and Colitis Foundation of America is a non-profit, volunteer-driven organization dedicated to finding the cure for Crohn's disease and ulcerative colitis.
Pat Talty, Executive Director

Arizona

2892 **CCFA Southwest Chapter: Arizona**
8098 Via de Negocio
Scottsdale, AZ 85258
480-246-3676
877-259-2104
Fax: 480-246-3679
e-mail: southwest@ccfa.org
www.ccfa.org/chapters/southwest

Crohn's and Colitis Foundation of America is a non-profit volunteer-driven organization dedicated to finding the cure for Crohn's disease and ulcerative colitis.
Kathie Gadberry, Executive Director
Bernadette Sewer, Development Coordinator

California

2893 **CCFA California: Greater Bay Area Chapter**
386 Park Avenue S
New York, NY 10016-2722
650-578-6590
800-932-2423
Fax: 650-578-6599
e-mail: ccfagba@pacbell.net
www.ccfa.org

To cure and prevent Crohn's disease and ulcerative colitis through research, and to improve the quality of life of children and adults affected by these digestive diseases through education and support.
Carol Gerstein, Executive Director
Bernadette Sewer, Development Coordinator

2894 **CCFA California: Greater Los Angeles Chapt er**
1640 S Sepulveda Boulevard
Los Angeles, CA 90025
310-478-4500
866-831-9157
Fax: 310-478-4546
e-mail: losangeles@ccfa.org
www.ccfa.org/chapters/losangeles

Crohn's and Colitis Foundation of America is a non-profit volunteer-driven organization dedicated to finding the cure for Crohn's disease and ulcerative colitis.
Iyad Zabaneh, Development Coordinator
Kerri Yoder, Education Manager

Colorado

2895 **CCFA Rocky Mountain Chapter: Colorado**
1777 S Bellaire Street
Denver, CO 80222
303-639-9163
866-768-2232
Fax: 303-693-9166
e-mail: rockymountain@ccfa.org
www.ccfa.org/chapters/rockymountain

Crohn's and Colitis Foundation of America is a non-profit volunteer-driven organization dedicated to finding the cure for Crohn's disease and ulcerative colitis.
Nancy Freimuth, Walk Manager
Mackenzie Lyle, Interim Executive Director

Connecticut

2896 **CCFA Central Connecticut Chapter**
P O Box 275
Branford, CT 06405
203-208-3130
e-mail: mgrande@ccfa.org
www.ccfa.org/chapters/centralct

Crohn's and Colitis Foundation of America is a non-profit volunteer-driven organization dedicated to finding the cure for Crohn's disease and ulcerative colitis.
Sally Connolly, Board President

2897 **CCFA Northern Connecticut Affiliate Chapte r**
PO Box 370614
W Hartford, CT 06137-0614
212-679-1570
800-932-2423
Fax: 212-679-3567
e-mail: info@ccfa.org
www.ccfa.org/chapters/northernct

Crohn's and Colitis Foundation of America is a non-profit volunteer-driven organization dedicated to finding the cure for Crohn's disease and ulcerative colitis.
Marilyn Hagg Blohm, Executive Director National Headquarters
Jeff Neale, Public Relations National Headquarters

Florida

2898 **CCFA Florida Chapter**
21301 Powerline Road
Boca Raton, FL 33433-2391
561-218-2929
877-664-2929
Fax: 516-218-2240
e-mail: kkeohane@ccfa.org
www.ccfa.org/chapters/florida

Crohn's and Colitis Foundation of America is a non-profit volunteer-driven organization dedicated to finding the cure for Crohn's disease and ulcerative colitis.
Deborah Barnard, Development Manager
Lacy Woods, Administrator

Georgia

2899 **CCFA Georgia Chapter**
2250 N Druid Hills Road
Atlanta, GA 30329
404-982-0616
800-472-6795
Fax: 404-982-0656
e-mail: georgia@ccfa.org
www.ccfa.org/chapters/georgia

Crohn's and Colitis Foundation of America is a non-profit volunteer-driven organization dedicated to finding the cure for Crohn's disease and ulcerative colitis.
Marcia Greenburg, Executive Director
Karen Rittenbaum, Development Director

Illinois

2900 **CCFA Illinois: Carol Fisher Chapter**
2250 E Devon Avenue
Des Plaines, IL 60018
847-827-0404
800-886-6664
Fax: 847-827-6563
e-mail: Illinois@ccfa.org
www.ccfa.org/chapters/illinois

Crohn's and Colitis Foundation of America is a non-profit volunteer-driven organization dedicated to finding the cure for Crohn's disease and ulcerative colitis.
Marianne Floriano, Executive Director
Kristina Sickles, Development Coordinator

Indiana

2901 **CCFA Indiana Chapter**
931 E 86th Street
Indianapolis, IN 46240
317-259-8071
800-332-6029
Fax: 317-259-8091
e-mail: indiana@ccfa.org
www.ccfa.org/chapters/indiana

Crohn's and Colitis Foundation of America is a non-profit volunteer-driven organization dedicated to finding the cure for Crohn's disease and ulcerative colitis.
Scott Baumruck, Development Director
Dawn Drinkut, Development Assistant

Iowa

2902 **CCFA Iowa Chapter**
PO Box 1184
Johnston, IA 50131-0016
515-664-8961
Fax: 319-277-6293
e-mail: iowa@ccfa.org
www.ccfa.org/chapters/iowa

Crohn's and Colitis Foundation of America is a non-profit volunteer-driven organization dedicated to finding the cure for Crohn's disease and ulcerative colitis.
Tony Kline, Chapter President
Abbie Hansen, Vice President Communications

Kansas

2903 **CCFA Mid-America Chapter: Kansas**
1034 S Brentwood
St Louis, MO 63117
314-863-4747
800-783-8006
Fax: 314-863-4749
e-mail: sskodak@ccfa.org
www.ccfa.org/chapters/midamerica

Crohn's and Colitis Foundation of America is a non-profit volunteer-driven organization dedicated to finding the cure for Crohn's disease and ulcerative colitis.
Steve Skodak, Executive Director
Andi Harrington, Development Manager

Kentucky

2904 **CCFA Kentucky Chapter c/o CCFA Indiana Chapter**
c/o CCFA Indiana Chapter
95 White Bridge Road
Nashville, TN 37205
615-356-0444
866-814-CCFA
Fax: 615-356-0445
e-mail: tennessee@ccfa.org
www.ccfa.org/chapters/kentucky

Crohn's and Colitis Foundation of America is a non-profit volunteer-driven organization dedicated to finding the cure for Crohn's disease and ulcerative colitis.
Steve Picton, President
Erskine Courtenay, Vice President

Louisiana

2905 **CCFA Louisiana Chapter**
7611 Maple Street
New Orleans, LA 70118
504-861-3433
866-382-2232
Fax: 504-861-3466
e-mail: lams@ccfa.org
www.ccfa.org/chapters/louisiana

Crohn's and Colitis Foundation of America is a non-profit volunteer-driven organization dedicated to finding the cure for Crohn's disease and ulcerative colitis.
David Lee Thomas, Development Director
Gail C Smith, Development Assistant

Maryland

2906 **CCFA Maryland Chapter**
10400 Little Patuxent Parkway
Columbia, MD 21044
443-276-0861
800-618-5583
Fax: 443-276-0865
e-mail: maryland@ccfa.org
www.ccfa.org/chapters/md-southdc

Crohn's and Colitis Foundation of America is a non-profit volunteer-driven organization dedicated to finding the cure for Crohn's disease and ulcerative colitis.
Robert J Milanchus, Regional Executive Director
Mary Glagola, President

Massachusetts

2907 **CCFA New England Chapter: Massachusetts**
280 Hillside Avenue
Needham, MA 02494
781-449-0324
800-314-3459
Fax: 781-449-0325
e-mail: ne@ccfa.org
www.ccfa.org/chapters/ne

Crohn's and Colitis Foundation of America is a non-profit volunteer-driven organization dedicated to finding the cure for Crohn's disease and ulcerative colitis.
Jess Adani, Development Manager
Kristin Patmos, Education Manager

Michigan

2908 **CCFA Michigan Chapter: Farmington Hills**
31313 N Western Highway
Farmington Hills, MI 78334
248-737-0900
Fax: 248-737-0904
e-mail: michigan@ccfa.org
www.ccfa.org/chapters/michigan

Crohn's and Colitis Foundation of America is a non-profit volunteer-driven organization dedicated to finding the cure for Crohn's disease and ulcerative colitis.
Bernard L Riker, Executive Director
Gilda Hauser, Development Manager

Minnesota

2909 **CCFA Minnesota Chapter**
1885 University Avenue W
Saint Paul, MN 55104
651-917-2424
888-422-3266
Fax: 651-917-2425
e-mail: Minnesota@ccfa.org
www.ccfa.org/chapters/minnesota

Crohn's and Colitis Foundation of America is a non-profit volunteer-driven organization dedicated to finding the cure for Crohn's disease and ulcerative colitis.
Maggie Brown, Take Steps Manager
Ruby Lanoux, Development Manager

Mississippi

2910 **CCFA Mississippi Chapter c/o Louisiana Chapter**
c/o Louisiana Chapter
7611 Maple Street
New Orleans, LA 70118
504-861-3433
866-382-2232
Fax: 504-861-3466
e-mail: lams@ccfa.org
www.ccfa.org/chapters/louisiana

Crohn's and Colitis Foundation of America is a non-profit volunteer-driven organization dedicated to finding the cure for Crohn's disease and ulcerative colitis.
David Lee Thomas, Development Director Louisiana Office
Gail C Smith, Development Assistant Louisiana Office

Missouri

2911 **CCFA Mid-America Chapter: Missouri**
1034 S Brentwood
Saint Louis, MO 63117
314-863-4747
800-783-8006
Fax: 314-863-4749
e-mail: info@ccfa.org
www.ccfa.org/chapters/midamerica

Crohn's and Colitis Foundation of America is a non-profit volunteer-driven organization dedicated to finding the cure for Crohn's disease and ulcerative colitis.
Steve Skodak, Executive Director
Andi Harrington, Development Manager

New Jersey

2912 **CCFA New Jersey Chapter**
45 Wilson Avenue
Manalapan, NJ 07726
732-786-9960
Fax: 732-786-9964
e-mail: newjersey@ccfa.org
www.ccfa.org/chapters/newjersey

Crohn's and Colitis Foundation of America is a non-profit volunteer-driven organization dedicated to finding the cure for Crohn's disease and ulcerative colitis.
Rosemarie Golombos, Executive Director
Barbara Fedorchak, Chapter Development Manager

New York

2913 CCFA Greater New York Chapter: National He adquarters
386 Park Avenue S 800-932-2423
New York, NY 10016-8804 800-932-2423
Fax: 212-679-3567
e-mail: info@ccfa.org
www.ccfa.org
Crohn's and Colitis Foundation of America is a non-profit volunteer-driven organization dedicated to finding the cure for Crohn's disease and ulcerative colitis.
Marilyn Hagg Blohm, Executive Director
Jeff Neale, Public Relations/Media Director

2914 CCFA Long Island Chapter
585 Stewart Avenue 516-222-5530
Garden City, NY 11530 Fax: 516-222-5535
e-mail: longisland@ccfa.org
www.ccfa.org/chapters/longisland
Crohn's and Colitis Foundation of America is a non-profit volunteer-driven organization dedicated to finding the cure for Crohn's disease and ulcerative colitis.
Marilyn Hagg Blohm, Executive Director National Office
Jeff Neale, Public Relations/Media National Office

2915 CCFA Rochester/Southern Tier Chapter
2117 Buffalo Road 585-617-4771
Rochester, NY 14624 800-932-2423
e-mail: rochester@ccfa.org
www.ccfa.org/chapters/rochester
Crohn's and Colitis Foundation of America is a non-profit volunteer-driven organization dedicated to finding the cure for Crohn's disease and ulcerative colitis.
Marilyn Hagg Blohm, Executive Director National Headquarters
Jeff Neale, Public Relations

2916 CCFA Upstate/Northeastern New York Chapter
4 Normanskill Boulevard 518-439-0252
Delmar, NY 12054 e-mail: upstateny@ccfa.org
www.ccfa.org/chapters/upstateny
Crohn's and Colitis Foundation of America is a non-profit volunteer-driven organization dedicated to finding the cure for Crohn's disease and ulcerative colitis.
Linda Winston, Chapter President
Peter Purcel MD, Medical Advisory Chair

2917 CCFA Western New York Chapter
2714 Sheridan Drive 716-833-2870
Tonawanda, NY 14150-0224 800-932-2423
e-mail: jpetri@ccfa.org
www.ccfa.org/chapters/westernny
Crohn's and Colitis Foundation of America is a non-profit volunteer-driven organization dedicated to finding the cure for Crohn's disease and ulcerative colitis.
Marilyn Hagg Blohm, Executive Director National Headquarters
Jeff Neale, Public Relations

North Carolina

2918 CCFA Carolinas Chapter
2901 N Davidson Street 704-332-1611
Charlotte, NC 28205 877-332-1611
Fax: 704-332-1612
e-mail: carolinas@ccfa.org
www.ccfa.org/chapters/carolinas
Crohn's and Colitis Foundation of America is a non-profit volunteer-driven organization dedicated to finding the cure for Crohn's disease and ulcerative colitis.
Angela Parks, Development Director
Julie Perkins, Special Events/Development Manager

Ohio

2919 CCFA Central Ohio Chapter
5008 Pine Creek Drive 614-865-1933
Westerville, OH 43081 800-625-5977
Fax: 614-865-1934
e-mail: centralohio@ccfa.org
www.ccfa.org/chapters/centralohio
Crohn's and Colitis Foundation of America is a non-profit volunteer-driven organization dedicated to finding the cure for Crohn's disease and ulcerative colitis.
Janelle Gasaway, Take Steps Manager
Kelly Bush, Development Coordinator

2920 CCFA Northeast Ohio Chapter
23775 Commerce Park Road 216-831-2692
Beachwood, OH 44122 866-345-2232
Fax: 216-831-2792
e-mail: neohio@ccfa.org
www.ccfa.org/chapters/neohio
Crohn's and Colitis Foundation of America is a non-profit volunteer-driven organization dedicated to finding the cure for Crohn's disease and ulcerative colitis.
Kristin Knipp, Development Coordinator
Patty Kaplan, Development Manager NE Ohio Chapter

2921 CCFA Southwest Ohio Chapter
8 Triangle Park Drive 513-772-3550
Cincinnati, OH 45246 877-283-7513
Fax: 513-772-7599
e-mail: SWOhio@ccfa.org
www.ccfa.org/chapters/swohio
Crohn's and Colitis Foundation of America is a non-profit volunteer-driven organization dedicated to finding the cure for Crohn's disease and ulcerative colitis.
Rachel Spradlin, Take Steps Manager
Jenny Southers, Development Manager SE Ohio Chapter

Oklahoma

2922 CCFA Oklahoma Chapter
4504 E 67th Street 918-523-8540
Tulsa, OK 74136 800-658-1533
Fax: 918-523-8560
e-mail: jsummers@ccfa.org
www.ccfa.org/chapters/oklahoma
Crohn's and Colitis Foundation of America is a non-profit volunteer-driven organization dedicated to finding the cure for Crohn's disease and ulcerative colitis.
Judy Summers, Regional Executive Director
Christopher Woods, President

Pennsylvania

2923 CCFA Philadelphia/Delaware Valley Chapter
367 E Street Road 215-396-9100
Trevose, PA 19053 888-340-4744
Fax: 215-396-1170
e-mail: Philadelphia@ccfa.org
www.ccfa.org/chapters/philadelphia
Crohn's and Colitis Foundation of America is a non-profit volunteer-driven organization dedicated to finding the cure for Crohn's disease and ulcerative colitis.
Barbara Berman, Executive Director
Suzanne Rhodeside, Development Director

2924 CCFA Western Pennsylvania/West Virginia Ch apter
300 Penn Center Boulevard 412-823-8272
Pittsburgh, PA 15235 877-823-8272
Fax: 412-823-8276
e-mail: wpawv@ccfa.org
www.ccfa.org/chapters/wpawv
Crohn's and Colitis Foundation of America is a non-profit volunteer-driven organization dedicated to finding the cure for Crohn's disease and ulcerative colitis.
10-12 pages
Jamie Rhoades, Development Manager
Susan Kukic, Executive Director

South Carolina

2925 CCFA South Carolina Chapter
2901 N Davidson Street 704-332-1611
Charlotte, NC 28205 877-632-1611
Fax: 704-332-1612
e-mail: carolinas@ccfa.org
www.ccfa.org/chapters/carolinas

Crohn's and Colitis Foundation of America is a non-profit volunteer-driven organization dedicated to finding the cure for Crohn's disease and ulcerative colitis.
Angela Parks, Development Manager
Tewanna Sanders, Education & Support Manager

Tennessee

2926 CCFA Tennessee Chapter
95 White Bridge Road
Nashville, TN 37205
615-356-0444
866-814-2232
Fax: 615-356-0445
e-mail: tennessee@ccfa.org
www.ccfa.org/chapters/tennessee
Crohn's and Colitis Foundation of America is a non-profit volunteer-driven organization dedicated to finding the cure for Crohn's disease and ulcerative colitis.
Michelle J Chianese, Education & Support Manager
Nicole Boisvert, Walk Manager

Texas

2927 CCFA Houston Gulf Coast/South Texas Chapte r
5120 Woodway
Houston, TX 77056
713-572-2232
800-785-2232
Fax: 713-572-2433
e-mail: infohouston@ccfa.org
www.ccfa.org/chapters/houston
Crohn's and Colitis Foundation of America is a non-profit volunteer-driven organization dedicated to finding the cure for Crohn's disease and ulcerative colitis.
Brandy Bendele, Walk Manager
Erin Fagan, Development Manager

2928 CCFA North Texas Chapter
12801 N Central Expressway
Dallas, TX 75243
972-386-0607
Fax: 972-386-0509
e-mail: ntexas@ccfa.org
www.ccfa.org/chapters/ntexas
Crohn's and Colitis Foundation of America is a non-profit volunteer-driven organization dedicated to finding the cure for Crohn's disease and ulcerative colitis.
Rachel Wallace, Development Manager
Sharon Seagraves, Executive Director

Virginia

2929 CCFA Greater Washington DC/Virginia Chapte r
4085 Chain Bridge Road
Fairfax, VA 22314
703-865-6130
877-807-5271
Fax: 703-865-8873
e-mail: washingtondc@ccfa.org
www.ccfa.org/chapters/washingtondc
Crohn's and Colitis Foundation of America is a non-profit volunteer-driven organization dedicated to finding the cure for Crohn's disease and ulcerative colitis.
Eileen Pugh, Executive Director
Stephanie Campbell, Development Coordinator

Washington

2930 CCFA Washington State Chapter
9 Lake Bellevue Drive
Bellevue, WA 98005
425-451-8455
877-703-6900
Fax: 425-451-1708
e-mail: northwest@ccfa.org
www.ccfa.org/chapters/northwest
Crohn's and Colitis Foundation of America is a non-profit volunteer-driven organization dedicated to finding the cure for Crohn's disease and ulcerative colitis.
Linda Huse, Executive Director
Jennifer Simmons, Development Manager

Wisconsin

2931 CCFA Wisconsin Chapter
1126 S 70th Street
W Allis, WI 53214
414-475-5520
877-586-5588
Fax: 414-475-5502
e-mail: wisconsin@ccfa.org
www.ccfa.org/chapters/wisconsin
Crohn's and Colitis Foundation of America is a non-profit volunteer-driven organization dedicated to finding the cure for Crohn's disease and ulcerative colitis.
Jan Lenz, Executive Director
Nadine Davis, Development Coordinator

Libraries & Resource Centers

2932 National Digestive Diseases Information Clearinghouse
2 Information Way
Bethesda, MD 20892-3570
800-891-5389
Fax: 703-738-4929
e-mail: nddic@info.niddk.nih.gov
http://digestive.niddk.nih.gov/
Established to increase knowledge and understanding about digestive diseases among people with these conditions and their families, health care professionals, and the general public. To carry out this mission, NDDIC works closely with a coordinating panel of representatives from Federal agencies, voluntary organizations on the national level, and professional groups to identify and respond to informational needs about digestive diseases.
Kathy Kranzfelder, Director

Research Centers

2933 Hahnemann University, Krancer Center for Inflammatory Bowel Disease Research
Broad & Vine Streets
Philadelphia, PA 19102
215-854-8100
Fax: 215-448-3417
Research into the causes and treatments of ulcerative colitis and Crohn's disease.
Dr. Harris Clearfield, Director

Support Groups & Hotlines

2934 Crohn's & Colitis Foundation of America Hotline
Crohn's & Colitis Foundation of America
386 Park Avenue S
New York, NY 10016-8804
212-685-3440
800-932-2423
Fax: 212-779-4098
e-mail: info@ccfa.org
www.ccfa.org
Our mission is to cure and prevent Crohn's disease and ulcerative colitis through research and to improve the quality of life of children and adults affected by these digestive disease through education and support. Known collectively as inflammatory bowel disease (IBD), these painful chronic illnesses affect up to one million Americans, including approximately 100,000 children under the age of 18.

2935 National Health Information Center
PO Box 1133
Washington, DC 20013
310-565-4167
800-336-4797
Fax: 301-984-4256
e-mail: info@nhic.org
www.health.gov/nhic
Offers a nationwide information referral service, produces directories and resource guides.

Books

2936 Crohn's Disease and Ulcerative Colitis Fact Book
Crohn's & Colitis Foundation of America

386 Park Avenue S 212-685-3440
New York, NY 10016-8804 800-932-2423
Fax: 212-779-4098
e-mail: info@ccfa.org
www.ccfa.org

Written in layman's language, this first complete guide is helpful in understanding and coping with inflammatory bowel diseases.

2937 Managing Your Child's Crohn's Disease or Ulcerative Colitis

Crohn's & Colitis Foundation of America
386 Park Avenue S 212-685-3440
New York, NY 10016-8804 800-932-2423
Fax: 212-779-4098
e-mail: info@ccfa.org
www.ccfa.org

Full-length book on Crohn's disease and ulcerative colitis, specifically targeted for parents of children and teenagers; includes topics on cause and diagnosis, treatment, surgery, hospitalization, diet and nutrition, school and social issues and resources for the patient.
$16.95 Members

2938 Ostomy Book: Living Comfortably with Colostomies, Ileostomies and Urostomies

Barbara Dorr Mullen and Kerry Anne McGinn, author

Bull Publishing Company
PO Box 1377thur Boulevard
Boulder, CO 80306 800-676-2855
Fax: 303-545-6354
www.bullpub.com

This book provides complete information on everything from details of surgery to the management of the appliances. Just as importantly, it is a beautifully told story of the entire expereince from diagnosis through rehabilitation to looking forward to a full and happy life.

ISBN: 0-923521-12-7

2939 People...Not Patients: Source Book for Living with Bowel Disease

Chron's & Colitis Foundation of America
386 Park Avenue S 212-685-3440
New York, NY 10016-8804 800-932-2423
Fax: 212-779-4098
e-mail: info@ccfa.org
www.ccfa.org

Contains the essential information you need to help you cope with Chron's disease and ulcerative colitis after you leave the doctor's office.

2940 Special Kind of Cookbook

Canadian Foundation for Ileitis and Colitis
Box 961, Sta T, Calgary 403-263-2425
Alberta, Canada, T2H 2H4,

Presents guidelines for good nutrition to help maintain one's body during a period of inflammatory bowel disease and to maintain health during periods of remission.

2941 Treating IBD

Crohn's & Colitis Foundation of America
386 Park Avenue S 212-685-3440
New York, NY 10016-8804 800-932-2423
Fax: 212-779-4098
e-mail: info@ccfa.org
www.ccfa.org

Patient's guide to the medical and surgical management of Inflammatory Bowel Disease, this book gives information on treating crohn's disease and ulcerative colitis, including drug therapies, advances in nutritional care, and recently developed surgical alternatives.

2942 Understanding Crohn Disease and Ulcerative Colitis

Jon Zonderman, Ronald S Vender, MD, author

University Press of Mississippi
3825 Ridgewood Road 601-432-6205
Jackson, MS 39211-6492 Fax: 601-432-6217
e-mail: kburgess@ihl.state.ms.us
www.upress.state.ms.us

For patients and caregivers an overview of the nature and treatments of inflammatory bowel disease.
2000 128 pages Paperback
ISBN: 1-578062-03-9
Kathy Burgess, Advertising/Marketing Services Manager

Magazines

2943 Colon and Rectal Surgery

International Academy of Proctology
PO Box 1716 765-342-3686
Martinsville, IN 46151 Fax: 765-342-4173

Information for professionals involved with colon and rectal surgery.
George Donnally MD

2944 Digestive Health Matters

Intl. Foundation for Gastrointestinal Disorders
PO Box 170864 414-964-1799
Milwaukee, WI 53217-0864 888-964-2001
Fax: 414-964-7176
e-mail: iffgd@iffgd.org
www.iffgd.org

Quarterly journal focuses on upper and lower gastrointestinal disorders in adults and children. Educational pamphlets and factsheets are available. Patient and professional membership.

2945 Foundation Focus

Crohn's & Colitis Foundation of America
386 Park Avenue S 212-685-3440
New York, NY 10016-8804 800-932-2423
Fax: 212-779-4098
e-mail: info@ccfa.org
www.ccfa.org

Magazine for CCFA supporters.

Newsletters

2946 Crohn's Disease, Ulcerative Colitis, and School

Pediatric Crohn's & Colitis Association
PO Box 188 617-489-5854
Newton, MA 02468 e-mail: questions@pcca.hypermart.net
pcca.hypermart.net

Information on Crohn's Disease and Ulcerative Colitis, including medical, nutritional, psychological and social factors.

2947 IBD File

Crohn's & Colitis Foundation of America
386 Park Avenue S 212-685-3440
New York, NY 10016-8804 800-932-2423
Fax: 212-779-4098
e-mail: info@ccfa.org
www.ccfa.org

Offers updated information and the latest medical news about Crohn's Disease and Colitis.

2948 Inflammatory Bowel Disease

Gastro-Intestinal Research Foundation
70 E Lake Street 312-332-1350
Chicago, IL 60601 Fax: 312-332-4757
e-mail: girf@girf.org
www.girf.org

Newsletter and patient pamphlet.

2949 Inner Circle

Reach Out for Youth with Ileitis and Colitis
84 Northgate Circle 516-293-3102
Melville, NY 11747 Fax: 516-293-3103

Provides information to patients with ileitis and colitis and their families.

2950 Inside Story

Reach Out for Youth with Ileitis and Colitis
84 Northgate Circle 516-293-3102
Melville, NY 11747 Fax: 516-293-3103

Provides information to patients with ileitis and colitis and their families.

Pamphlets

2951 ABC's of Pediatric Inflammatory Bowel Disease
Pediatric Crohn's & Colitis Association
PO Box 188
Newton, MA 02468
617-489-5854
e-mail: questions@pcca.hypermart.net
pcca.hypermart.net
Information on Pediatric Inflammatory Disease, including medical, nutritional, psychological and social factors.

2952 CCFA: A Case for Support
Crohn's & Colitis Foundation of America
386 Park Avenue S
New York, NY 10016-8804
212-685-3440
800-932-2423
Fax: 212-779-4098
e-mail: info@ccfa.org
www.ccfa.org
Reviews the work of the Crohn's and Colitis Foundation of America, sponsors a nationally recognized research program, which seeks to improve treatment and ultimately find the cure for inflammatory bowel disease.

2953 Coping with Crohn's and Colitis is Tough
Crohn's & Colitis Foundation of America
386 Park Avenue S
New York, NY 10016-8804
212-685-3440
800-932-2423
Fax: 212-779-4098
e-mail: info@ccfa.org
www.ccfa.org
Offers information on the Crohn's and Colitis Association. Also offers factual information and statistics on the diseases.

2954 Crohn's Disease
NDDIC
2 Information Way
Bethesda, MD 20892-0001
301-654-3810
800-891-5389
Fax: 301-907-8906
e-mail: nddic@info.niddlc.nin.gov
www.niddk.nih.gov
October 1992

2955 Guide for Children and Teenagers to Crohn's Disease/Ulcerative Colitis
Crohn's & Colitis Foundation of America
386 Park Avenue S
New York, NY 10016-8804
212-685-3440
800-932-2423
Fax: 212-779-4098
e-mail: info@ccfa.org
www.ccfa.org
Offers important information on these illnesses to children and teens.

2956 Ileostomy Guide
United Ostomy Associations of America, Inc.
PO Box 66
Fairview, TN 37062-0066
800-826-0826
e-mail: info@uoaa.org
www.uoaa.org
Written for persons who have recently had an ileostomy, this guidebook covers a spectrum of topics including basic facts about ileostomies, information for patients, helpful ideas and practical tips.
28 pages

2957 Questions & Answers About Diet and Nutrition
Crohn's & Colitis Foundation of America
386 Park Avenue S
New York, NY 10016-8804
212-685-3440
800-932-2423
Fax: 212-779-4098
e-mail: info@ccfa.org
www.ccfa.org
Raises important facts about how diet and nutrition affect persons with Crohn's Disease.

2958 Questions and Answers About Complications
Crohn's & Colitis Foundation of America
386 Park Avenue S
New York, NY 10016-8804
212-685-3440
800-932-2423
Fax: 212-779-4098
e-mail: info@ccfa.org
www.ccfa.org
Medical facts and complications from surgery.

2959 Questions and Answers About Crohn's Disease & Ulcerative Colitis
Crohn's & Colitis Foundation of America
386 Park Avenue S
New York, NY 10016-8804
212-685-3440
800-932-2423
Fax: 212-779-4098
e-mail: info@ccfa.org
www.ccfa.org
Offers information on the illness and answers the most frequently asked questions about Crohn's Disease. Also includes a glossary of IBD terms.

2960 Questions and Answers About Emotional Factors in Ileitis and Colitis
Crohn's & Colitis Foundation of America
386 Park Avenue S
New York, NY 10016-8804
212-685-3440
800-932-2423
Fax: 212-779-4098
e-mail: info@ccfa.org
www.ccfa.org
Answers some of the most commonly asked questions about ileitis and colitis and the role of emotional factors in their cause and course.

2961 Questions and Answers About Pregnancy in Ileitis and Colitis
Crohn's & Colitis Foundation of America
386 Park Avenue S
New York, NY 10016-8804
212-685-3440
800-932-2423
Fax: 212-779-4098
e-mail: info@ccfa.org
www.ccfa.org
Answers questions about inflammatory bowel disease concerning conception, pregnancy, delivery and nursing.

2962 Questions and Answers About Surgery
Crohn's & Colitis Foundation of America
386 Park Avenue S
New York, NY 10016-8804
212-685-3440
800-343-3637
Fax: 212-779-4098
e-mail: info@ccfa.org
www.ccfa.org
Answers questions and offers basic facts about surgery for persons suffering from Crohn's Disease and Ulcerative Colitis.

2963 Teacher's Guide to Crohn's Disease and Ulcerative Colitis
Crohn's & Colitis Foundation of America
386 Park Avenue S
New York, NY 10016-8804
212-685-3440
800-932-2423
Fax: 212-779-4098
e-mail: info@ccfa.org
www.ccfa.org
The purpose of this brochure is to increase the support and encouragement given to young people with Crohn's disease and ulcerative colitis by teachers who understand their illness.

2964 Crohn's Disease, Ulcerative Colitis and Your Child
Crohn's & Colitis Foundation of America
386 Park Avenue S
New York, NY 10016-8804
212-685-3440
800-932-2423
Fax: 212-779-4098
e-mail: info@ccfa.org
www.ccfa.org
Answers questions about IBD in children, providing information on early signs, growth and developments, treatments and special problems in school.

Web Sites

2965 Crohn's & Colitis Foundation of America
www.ccfa.org

CCFA provides educational and patient support services to both the lay and medical communities and plans to provide grants dedicated to pediatric research.

2966 Healing Well

www.healingwell.com

An online health resource guide to medical news, chat, information and articles, newsgroups and message boards, books, disease-related web sites, medical directories, and more for patients, friends, and family coping with disabling diseases, disorders, or chronic illnesses.

2967 Health Finder

www.healthfinder.gov

Searchable, carefully developed web site offering information on over 1000 topics. Developed by the US Department of Health and Human Services, the site can be used in both English and Spanish.

2968 Healthlink USA

www.healthlinkusa.com

Health information concerning treatment, cures, prevention, diagnosis, risk factors, research, support groups, email lists, personal stories and much more. Updated regularly.

2969 MedicineNet

www.medicinenet.com

An online resource for consumers providing easy-to-read, authoritative medical and health information.

2970 Medscape

www.mywebmd.com

Medscape offers specialists, primary care physicians, and other health professionals the Web's most robust and integrated medical information and educational tools.

2971 National Digestive Diseases Information Clearinghouse

www.niddk.nih.gov

Offers various educational information, resources and reprints focusing on Colitis, Ulcerative Colitis and Crohn's disease.

2972 Pediatric Crohn's and Colitis Association

pcca.hypermart.net/

Focuses on all aspects of pediatric and adolescent Crohn's disease and ulcerative colitis, including medical, nutritional, psychological and social factors. Activities include information sharing, educational forums, newsletters and hospital outreach programs, as well as support of research.

2973 United Ostomy Association

www.uoa.org

Extensive information about ostomy surgery, support, products and advocacy for Medicaid/Insurance reimbursement. Interactive discussion board to post and answer questions, weekly updates on ostomy-related news items.

2974 WebMD

www.webmd.com

Information on Crohn's disease, including articles and resources.

Description

2975 **Cystic Fibrosis**

Cystic fibrosis, CF, is an inherited disease of the exocrine (mucus-producing) glands, primarily affecting the gastrointestinal and respiratory tracts. The mucus that is secreted by persons with the disease is especially thick, thus blocking, rather than lubricating, passageways in the lungs and digestive tract. CF is the most common life-shortening genetic disease in the white population, occurring in 1 in 3,000 live births in the United States, but it occurs in people of all ethnic and racial backgrounds.

In the newborn with CF, thick fecal material may cause partial obstruction of the intestine, which then may contort and rupture. Later in life, blockage of secretions from the pancreas results in frequent, foul-smelling, fatty stools, distention of the abdomen and slowed growth. Damage to the lung occurs as thick mucus secretions plug airways. Fifty percent of all patients develop breathing problems marked by a chronic cough, wheezing and repeated lung infections.

The course of CF is usually determined by the degree to which the lungs are affected, and varies greatly from patient to patient. The prognosis is poor, but advances in therapy have helped many survive well into adulthood. Treatment usually includes aggressive use of antibiotics and other drugs to prevent lung complications, physical therapy, adequate nutrition and psychosocial support.

The first CF gene therapy research began in 1993, and scientists have identified mutations in a CF regulator genethat cause cells to produce abnormally thick mucus. Gene therapy to replace the defective gene with a functional copy is currently under study. Genetic screening is now available.

National Agencies & Associations

2976 **Cystic Fibrosis Worldwide**
50 Elm Street
Southbridge, MA 01550
508-764-2730
Fax: 508-765-8883
e-mail: information@cfww.org
www.cfww.org

IACFA is a non profit organization headquartered in Zurich Switzerland. The purpose and direction of the organization is to assist in improving the quality of life by identifying common problems and attempting to define possible solutions.
Christine Noke, Executive Director
Mitch Messer, President

Foundations

2977 **Cystic Fibrosis Foundation**
6931 Arlington Road
Bethesda, MD 20814
301-951-4422
800-344-4823
Fax: 301-951-6378
e-mail: info@cff.org
www.cff.org

The mission of the Cystic Fibrosis Foundation is to assure the development of the means to cure and control cystic fibrosis and to improve the quality of life for those with the disease.
Robert J Beall, PhD, President/CEO

Libraries & Resource Centers

2978 **Children's Hospital of Orange County**
455 S Main Street
Orange, CA 92868-3874
714-997-3000
e-mail: mail@choc.org
www.choc.org

Our mission is to nuture, advance and protect the health and well-being of children.
Kimberly C Cripe, President/CEO

Research Centers

Alabama

2979 **Cystic Fibrosis Foundation**
6931 Arlington Road
Bethesda, MD 20814
301-951-4422
800-344-4823
Fax: 301-951-6378
e-mail: info@cff.org
www.cff.org

The mission of the Cystic Fibrosis Foundation a nonprofit donor-supported organization is to assure the development of the means to cure and control cystic fibrosis and to improve the quality of life for those with the disease.
Robert J Beall, President and CEO

Arizona

2980 **Cystic Fibrosis Center: Phoenix Childrens Hospital**
A, author
1919 E Thomas Road
Phoenix, AZ 85016
602-546-1000
888-908-5437
Fax: 602-460-23
www.phoenixchildrens.com

Robert Meyer, President and Chief Executive Officer
Bruce Morgenstern, Medical Staff President

Arkansas

2981 **Arkansas Cystic Fibrosis Center Arkansas Children's Hospital**
Arkansas Children's Hospital
800 Marshall Street
Little Rock, AR 72202
501-364-1006
Fax: 501-364-3930
e-mail: pedspulmonary@uams.edu
www.uams.edu/pediatrics/cf

Provide high-quality specialized care to patients from comprehensive diagnosis to ongoing treatment.
John L Carroll MD, Division Chief
Dennis E Schellhase, Director

California

2982 **Children's Hospital of Los Angeles**
4650 Sunset Boulevard
Los Angeles, CA 90027
323-660-2450
e-mail: webmaster@chla.usc.edu
www.childrenshospitalla.org

Provides the highest quality healthcare for children who are the sickest and most seriously injured in our region and beyond.
Richard D Cordova, President/CEO
Rodney B Hanners, Senior Vice President & Chief Operating

2983 **Childrens Hospital at Oakland**
747 52nd Street
Oakland, CA 94609
510-428-3000
www.childrenshospitaloakland.org

The mission of Children's Hospital Oakland is to ensure the delivery of the highest quality pediatric care for all children through regional primary and subspecialty networks; a strong education and teaching program a diverse workforce state of the art research programs and facilities; and nationally recognized child advocacy efforts.
Frank Tiedemann, President and Chief Executive Officer
Douglas T Myers, Chief Operating Officer and Chief Financ

2984 **Cystic Fibrosis Center: Cedars-Sinai Medical Center**
Cedars-Sinai Medical Center

8700 Beverly Boulevard
Los Angeles, CA 90048
310-423-4431
800-233-2771
Fax: 310-423-4131
www.cedarsinai.edu

2985 Cystic Fibrosis Center: Cedars-Sinai Medic Cedars-Sinai Medical Center
8700 Beverly Boulevard
Los Angeles, CA 90048
310-423-3277
800-233-2771
Fax: 310-423-4131
www.cedars-sinai.edu

2986 Cystic Fibrosis Center: University of California at San Francisco
400 Parnassus Avenue
San Francisco, CA 94143-0106
415-353-7337
Fax: 415-476-9278
e-mail: maryellen.kleinhenz@ucsf.edu
pulmonary.ucsf.edu

Provides comprehensive evaluation as well as inpatient and outpatient care for patients with cystic fibrosis.
Mary Ellen Kleinhenz MD, Adult CF Director
Dennis Niels MD, Pediatric CF Director

2987 Cystic Fibrosis Research
2672 Bayshore Parkway
Mountain View, CA 94043
650-404-9975
Fax: 650-404-9981
e-mail: cjenkins@cfri.org
www.cfri.org

Cystic Fibrosis Research exists to fund research to provide educational and personal support and spread awareness of Cystic Fibrosis a life threatening genetic disease.
Carroll Jenkins, Executive Director
David Soohoo, Director of Programs

2988 Memorial Miller Children's Hospital Cystic Fibrosis Center
2801 Atlantic Avenue
Long Beach, CA 90806
562-933-8521
Fax: 562-933-8501
e-mail: enussbaum@memorialcare.org
www.memorialcare.org/miller

provides a multidisciplinary approach to asthma cystic fibrosis sleep disorders and the entire spectrum of chronic and acute lung and airway disorders in children.
Eliezer Nuss MD, Medical Director

2989 Stanford CF Center Packard Children's Hospital At Stanford
Packard Children's Hospital At Stanford
770 Welch Road
Palo Alto, CA 94304-1601
650-497-8841
e-mail: jkirby@leland.stanford.edu
cfcenter.stanford.edu

Colorado

2990 Denver Childrens Hospital
1056 E 19th Avenue
Denver, CO 80218-1007
303-837-2522
800-624-6553
Fax: 303-832-9245
TTY: 720-777-6050
www.thechildrenshospital.org

Frank Accurs MD, Director

Connecticut

2991 University of Connecticut Health Center
263 Farmington Avenue
Farmington, CT 06030-0001
860-679-2000
TTY: 860-679-2242
TDD: 860-679-2242
e-mail: president@uconn.edu
www.uchc.edu

Michael J Hogan, President
Cato T Laurencin MD, Vice President for Health Affairs

2992 Yale University Cystic Fibrosis Research Center
Yale Pediatrics
PO Box 208064
New Haven, CT 06520-8064
203-785-2480
e-mail: sheila.rivera@yale.edu
www.yalepediatrics.org

One of only two in the state of Connecticut the CF Center in the Children's Hospital at the Yale-New Haven Hospital offers a multidisciplinary team approach to provide the most comprehensive "state of the art" care of CF patients.
Marie Egan MD, Director

District of Columbia

2993 Metropolitan DC Cystic Fibrosis Center Children s Hospital National Medical Cen
Children s Hospital National Medical Center
111 Michigan Avenue NW
Washington, DC 20010-2970
202-884-5000
e-mail: cgeorge@cnmc.org
www.dcchildrens.com

An active clinical and basic science research program that exists within the center.

Florida

2994 Cystic Fibrosis Center: All Children's Hospital
Department of Pulmonology
801 6th Street S
Saint Petersburg, FL 33701
727-767-4146
800-456-4543
Fax: 727-767-4218
www.allkids.org

Anthony D Kriseman MD, Pulmonology

2995 Miami Childrens Hospital Division of Pulmonology
3100 SW 62nd Avenue
Miami, FL 33155-3309
305-662-8380
800-432-6837
Fax: 305-663-8417
e-mail: info@mch.com
www.mch.com

Division evaluates and treats many respiratory disorders including asthma chronic lung disease cystic fibrosis pneumonia and tuberculosis. The Division is strongly committed to a multidisciplinary medical approach to these complex disorders.
Moises Simps MD, Director
Antonio M Rodriguez MD, Associate Director

2996 Nemours Childrens Clinic
PO Box 5720
Jacksonville, FL 32247
904-390-3600
Fax: 904-390-3699
www.nemours.org

Nemours Children's Clinic is one integrated multispecialty group practice with locations in four states seeing patients from across the US and the world.

Georgia

2997 Department of Pediatrics Medical College of Georgia
1120 15th Street
Augusta, GA 30912
706-721-3466
Fax: 706-721-7311
www.mcg.edu/pediatrics

Dr William Kanto Jr, Chairperson Pediatrics

2998 Emory University: Cystic Fibrosis Center
1547 Clifton Road NE
Atlanta, GA 30322-1028
404-727-5728
Fax: 404-727-4828
e-mail: lwolfen@emory.edu
www.emory.edu

Lindy Wolfen MD, Director

Illinois

2999 Comer Children's Hospital at the University of Chicago
5721 S Maryland Avenue
Chicago, IL 60637
773-702-1000
888-824-0200
www.uchospitals.edu

3000 Comer Children's Hospital at the Universit
5721 S Maryland Avenue
Chicago, IL 60637
773-702-1000
888-824-0200
www.uchicagokidshospital.org

To provide superior healthcare in a compassionate manner ever mindful of each patient's dignity and individuality.

3001 Cystic Fibrosis Center: Childrens Memorial Hospital
2300 Childrens Plaza
Chicago, IL 60614
773-880-4382
800-543-7362
e-mail: cf@childrensmemorial.org
www.childrensmemorial.org

The Cystic Fibrosis Center at Children's Memorial Hospital has been a CFF-accredited CF care center since 1963. It is committed to providing exemplary care to each patient and family focused on

individualized preventative care active management of lung health and nutrition and patient family education.
Susanna McCo MD, Director

3002 Cystic Fibrosis Center: Park Ridge Lutheran General Children's Hospital
Lutheran General Children's Hospital
1775 Dempster Street
Park Ridge, IL 60068
847-723-5437
www.advocatehealth.com/lgch

3003 Loyola University Medical Center: Department of Pediatrics
2160 S 1st Avenue
Maywood, IL 60153
708-327-9120
www.luhs.org/depts/peds/institution

3004 Loyola University Medical Center: Departme
2160 S 1st Avenue
Maywood, IL 60153
708-327-9120
www.stritch.luc.edu
Provides a comprehensive array of general tertiary and subspecialty care for children.

3005 Saint Francis Medical Center Peoria Pulmonary Association
214 NE Glen Oak Avenue
Peoria, IL 61603
309-672-5682
www.osfsaintfrancis.org

3006 Saint Francis Medical Center Peoria Pulmon
530 NE Glen Oak Avenue
Peoria, IL 61637
309-672-5682
www.osfsaintfrancis.org

Indiana

3007 The Riley Cystic Fibrosis Center
702 Barnhill Drive
Indianapolis, IN 46202
317-274-4071
800-248-1199
www.rileychildrenshospital.com
The Riley Cystic Fibrosis Center is the only Cystic Fibrosis Foundation accredited Cystic Fibrosis Center in the state. The Center provides state-of-the-art CF care at Riley and across the state.

Iowa

3008 Blank Childrens Hospital Pediatric Pulmonology Clinic
Children's Health Center 1
1212 Pleasant Street
Des Moines, IA 50309
515-241-6548
www.blankchildrens.org
Steve Stephenson, Executive Vice President

3009 Pediatric Allergy & Pulmonary Division University of Iowa Healthcare
University of Iowa Healthcare
200 Hawkins Drive
Iowa City, IA 52242
319-356-1828
e-mail: allerpulm@uiowa.edu
www.uihealthcare.com/depts/med/pediatric
The Division of Allergy and Pulmonology offers evaluation and management of allergic disorders in children with too many infections and acute and chronic breathing disorders of childhood and adolescence.
Miles Weinbe MD, Director

Kansas

3010 Kansas University Medical Center: Cystic Fibrosis Center
3901 Rainbow Boulevard
Kansas City, KS 66160
913-588-6377
800-332-4199
Fax: 913-588-6280
e-mail: gperry@kumc.edu
www2.kumc.edu
Gayln Perry MD, Director

3011 St. Joseph Medical Center Cystic Fibrosis Care and Teaching Center
707 North Emporia
Wichita, KS 67214
316-858-3470
Fax: 316-583-90
e-mail: contact@viachristi.org
www.viachristi.org
Kay Glasner, Director
Maria Loving, Public Relations Specialist

Kentucky

3012 Kentucky University: Cystic Fibrosis Center
740 S Limestone
Lexington, KY 40536-0298
859-323-6211
800-333-8874
Fax: 859-257-7706
www.ukhealthcare.uky.edu
The cystic fibrosis team works with more than 175 patients and is dedicated to working with the most advanced therapies to improve the life of every patient.
Jamshed F Kanga MD, Director

3013 Kosair Childrens Cystic Fibrosis Center
231 E Chestnut Street
Louisville, KY 40202-2021
502-629-8060
e-mail: contactcenter@nortonhealthcare.org
www.nortonhealthcare.com
The Cystic Fibrosis Center is one of 120 centers in the United States accredited by the National Cystic Fibrosis Foundation. Specialists provide diagnosis and multidisciplinary care for cystic fibrosis patients of all ages. Professional education and training is also provided.
Nemie Eid, Medical Director

Louisiana

3014 Ernest N Morial Asthma, Allergy & Respiratory Disease Center
Louisiana State University School of Medicine
1901 Perdido Street
New Orleans, LA 70112-3932
504-568-4634
888-695-8647
Fax: 504-568-4295
e-mail: dthoma2@lsumc.edu
www.lsuhsc.edu
Warren R Summer MD, Director

Maine

3015 Central Maine Cystic Fibrosis Center
300 Main Street
Lewiston, ME 04240-7027
207-795-0111
Fax: 207-795-2303
www.cmhc.org
Ralph V Harder, Director
Peter Chkale, Chief Executive Officer

3016 Maine Medical Center: Cystic Fibrosis Clinical Center
887 Congress Street
Portland, ME 04102-6674
207-828-8226
Fax: 207-775-6024
www.mmc.org
Anne Marie Cairns, Director

3017 Maine Medical Center: Cystic Fibrosis Clin
887 Congress Street
Portland, ME 04102
207-828-8226
877-339-3107
Fax: 207-775-6024
TTY: 207-662-4900
www.mmc.org

Maryland

3018 Cystic Fibrosis Center: National Institute of Health NIDDK
Building 31 Room 9A06
Bethesda, MD 20892-2560
www2.niddk.nih.gov
Dr Griffin Rodgers, Acting Director

Massachusetts

3019 Baystate Medical Center Wesson Memorial Unit
Wesson Memorial Unit
759 Chestnut Street
Springfield, MA 01199
413-794-0000
e-mail: Marian.Panto@bhs.org
www.baystatehealth.com

BMC serves as a regional resource for specialty medical care and research while providing comprehensive primary medical services to the community.
Mark R Tolosky, President & Chief Executive Officer
Paula S Dennison, Senior Vice President Human Resources

3020 **Childrens Hospital Medical Center Cystic Fibrosis Center**
300 Longwood Avenue 617-355-1900
Boston, MA 02115 Fax: 617-730-0373
TTY: 617-730-0152
www.childrenshospital.org
The Cystic Fibrosis Center at Children's Hospital Boston is one of the oldest and largest cystic fibrosis centers in the United States and was founded by Dr. Harry Schwachman one of the earliest physician investigators to help characterize the disorder.
Terry Spence MD, Director

3021 **Cystic Firbrosis Center: Tufts New England Medical Center**
Pediatric Pulmonology and Allergy Department
800 Washington Street
Boston, MA 02111 617-636-5000
www.nemc.org
We strive to heal to comfort to teach to learn and to seek the knowledge to promote health and prevent disease.
Ellen Zane, President and Chief Executive Officer
Margaret Vosburgh, Chief Operating Officer

3022 **Massachusetts General Hospital**
55 Fruit Street 617-726-2000
Boston, MA 02114-2622 Fax: 617-726-6989
TTY: 617-724-8800
TDD: 617-724-8800
www.massgeneral.org
Peter L Slavin MD, President
David Torchi MD, Chairman and Chief Executive Officer

3023 **University of Massachusetts Memorial Medical Center**
55 Lake Avenue N
Worcester, MA 01655 508-334-1000
www.umassmemorial.org
UMass Memorial Medical Center is the region's trusted academic medical center committed to improving the health of the people of Central New England through excellence in clinical care service teaching and research.
John O'Brien, President/CEO
George Brenckle, Senior Vice President and Chief Informat

Michigan

3024 **East Lansing Cystic Fibrosis Center Michigan State University**
Michigan State University
1200 E Michigan Avenue 517-364-5440
Lansing, MI 48910-2819 Fax: 517-364-5413
phd.msu.edu
Eliane F Eakin MD, Director

3025 **Kalamazoo Center for Medical Studies Michigan State University**
Michigan State University
1000 Oakland Drive 269-337-6400
Kalamazoo, MI 49008-1202 800-275-5267
Fax: 269-337-4234
e-mail: programs@kcms.msu.edu
www.kcms.msu.edu

3026 **University of Michigan: Cystic Fibrosis Center**
A Alfred Taubman Health Care Center
1500 E Medical Center Drive 734-936-4000
Ann Arbor, MI 48109-0318 Fax: 734-936-7635
TTY: 800-649-3777
TDD: 800-649-3777
www.med.umich.edu
Samya Z Nasr MD, Director

Minnesota

3027 **University of Minnesota: Cystic Fibrosis Center**
University of Minnesota Hospital
420 Delaware Street SE 612-624-0962
Minneapolis, MN 55455 800-688-5252
Fax: 612-624-0696
e-mail: cfcenter@umn.edu
www.med.umn.edu/peds/cfcenter/home.html
The mission was to develop approaches to understanding and treating the complications of CF.
Warren E Regelmann MD, Co-Director
Jordan M Dunitz MD, Co-Director

Mississippi

3028 **University of Mississippi Medical Center**
2500 N State Street 601-984-5046
Jackson, MS 39216-4500 Fax: 601-984-1973
www.umc.edu
Suzanne Mill MD, Director

Missouri

3029 **Children's Mercy Hospital Children's Mercy Hospitals & Clinics**
Children's Mercy Hospitals & Clinics
2401 Gilham Road 816-234-3000
Kansas City, MO 64108 Fax: 816-842-6107
TTY: 816-234-3816
e-mail: webmaster@cmh.edu
www.childrensmercy.org
Children's Mercy Hospital provides the highest level of medical care technology services equipment and facilities in promoting the health and well-being of children in the region from birth through adolescence.
Randall L O'Donnell PhD, President/CEO
V Fred Burry MD, Executive Medical Director/Executive Vic

3030 **University of Missouri Columbia Cystic Fibrosis Center**
University of Missouri/Dept of Child Health
One Hospital Drive N712 573-882-6882
Columbia, MO 65212-1 Fax: 573-821-54
e-mail: clarksonb@health.missouri.edu
www.ch.missouri.edu/cysticfibrosis.htm
Peter Konig, Director

3031 **Washington University: Cystic Fibrosis Center**
St. Louis Children's Hospital
One Children's Place 314-454-2694
Saint Louis, MO 63110 888-678-4357
Fax: 314-454-2515
peds.wustl.edu
Dedicated to the treatment of patients with cystic fibrosis (CF) for more than 4 decades. The Cystic Fibrosis Clinical Center and affiliated programs has developed into a premier clinical and research program.
Thomas Ferko MD, Director

Nebraska

3032 **University of Nebraska Medical Center Cystic Fibrosis Center**
985190 Nebraska Medical Center 402-559-6275
Omaha, NE 68198-5190 Fax: 402-559-7062
e-mail: necfcntr@unmc.edu
www.unmc.edu
John L Colombo MD, Chief
Hari Bandla MD, Associate Professor

Nevada

3033 **Children's Lung Specialists**
3838 Meadow Lane 702-598-4411
Las Vegas, NV 89107 Fax: 702-598-1988
e-mail: cls@childrens-lung-specialists.com
www.childrens-lung-specialists.com
The certified Cystic Fibrosis Center of Southern Nevada.
Ruben Diaz MD, Director/President/Owner
Craig Nakamu MD, Assistant Director

New Hampshire

3034 **New Hampshire Cystic Fibrosis Care Teaching and Research Center**
DarthmouthHitchcock Medical Center
One Medical Center Drive
Lebanon, NH 03756-1
603-653-9884
Fax: 603-500-07
TTY: 603-650-8034
www.dhmc.org

William Boyl Jr MD, Director
Dennis Stoke MD, Director

New Jersey

3035 **Monmouth Medical Center: Cystic Fibrosis & Pediatric Pulmonary Center**
Monmouth Medical Center
300 Second Avenue
Long Branch, NJ 07740-6300
732-222-5200
Fax: 908-222-4472
e-mail: info@sbhcs.com
www.sbhcs.com

3036 **Monmouth Medical Center: Cystic Fibrosis & Monmouth Medical Center**
300 Second Avenue
Long Branch, NJ 07740
732-222-5200
Fax: 908-222-4472
e-mail: info@sbhcs.com
www.sbhcs.com

3037 **New Jersey Medical School**
185 S Orange Avenue
Newark, NJ 07101-2757
973-972-4595
Fax: 973-972-5965
e-mail: webnjms@umdnj.edu
njms.umdnj.edu

The mission of New Jersey Medical School is to educate students physicians and scientists to meet society's current and future healthcare needs through patient-centered education; pioneering research; innovative clinical rehabilitative and preventive care; and collaborative community outreach.
Maria Soto-G MD, Vice Dean
Robert L Johnson MD, Interim Dean

New York

3038 **Albany Medical College Pediatric Pulmonary & Cystic Fibrosis Center**
Department of Pediatrics
43 New Scotland Avenue
Albany, NY 12208
518-262-3125
877-262-8008
Fax: 518-262-6884
www.amc.edu

Scott Scroed MD, Division Chief

3039 **Armond V Mascia Cystic Fibrosis Center NY Medical College**
Division of Pediatrics Pulmonology
New York Medical College
Valhalla, NY 10595
914-493-7585
Fax: 914-594-4336
e-mail: pedpulm@nymc.edu
www.nycmc.edu

Provides comprehensive inpatient and outpatient consultation and management for children suffering from a broad variety of respiratory problems. They are the only accredited Cystic Fibrosis center in the Hudson Valley. The center is dedicated to teaching research and patient care.
Allen Dozer MD, Chief

3040 **CF & Pediatric Pulmonary Care Center The Pediatric Pulmonary Care Center at M**
The Pediatric Pulmonary Care Center at Mount Sinai
One Gustave L Levy Place
New York, NY 10029
212-241-7788
800-637-4624
Fax: 212-876-3255
www.mssm.edu/peds/pulmonary_center

Center staff perform outpatient and inpatient consultations with an integrated multidisciplinary team of professionals who are dedicated specifically to the practice of Pediatric Pulmonary Medicine.

3041 **Childrens Lung and Cystic Fibrosis Center**
Women and Children' s Hospital of Buffalo
140 Hodge Avenue
Buffalo, NY 14222-2099
716-878-7561
Fax: 716-888-3945
e-mail: AMTaylor@kaleidahealth.org

Services for infants children and teenagers with cystic fibrosis and other chronic respiratory conditions.
Annise Taylor, Manager

3042 **Cystic Fibrosis Center St. Vincent's Hospital & Medical Center**
St. Vincent's Hospital & Medical Center of NY
36 7th Avenue
New York, NY 10011-6600
212-604-8895
Fax: 212-604-3899
www.svcmc.org

Maria Berdel MD, Co-Director
Patricia Wal MD, Co-Director

3043 **Pulomonolgy Morgan Stanley Children's Hospital**
Morgan Stanley Children's Hospital
3959 Broadway
New York, NY 10032-3702
212-305-5122
877-NYP-WELL
www.childrensnyp.org

Meyer Kattan MD, Director

3044 **State University of NY Hospital: Upstate Medical Center**
750 E Adams Street
Syracuse, NY 13210-1834
315-464-5540
877-464-5540
TDD: 315-464-5769
www.upstate.edu/uh

3045 **State University of NY Hospital: Upstate M**
750 E Adams Street
Syracuse, NY 13210
315-464-5540
877-464-5540
TTY: 315-464-5769
www.upstate.edu/uh

North Carolina

3046 **Duke University Medical Center: Division of Pulmonary and Critical Care Medicine**
106 Research Drive
Durham, NC 27705
919-681-0355
888-275-3853
Fax: 919-684-5266
www.pulmonary.duke.edu

Provides primary and consultative care for patients with various lung diseases on an inpatient and outpatient basis.
Paul Noble, Chief

3047 **UNC Cystic Fibrosis Center Department of Pediatrics**
Department of Pediatrics
7011 Thurston-Bowles Building
Chapel Hill, NC 27599-7248
919-966-1077
Fax: 919-966-7524
www.med.unc.edu/cystfib/CFcent.htm

A large multidisciplinary group focused on the pathogenesis and other lung diseases.
Richard C Boucher MD, Director
Margaret Lei MD, Director

North Dakota

3048 **St. Alexius Medical Heart and Lung Clinic**
10th & Rosser
Bismarck, ND 58501
701-530-7500
877-530-5550
Fax: 701-530-8984
TTY: 701-530-5555
TDD: 701-530-5555
www.st.alexius.org

Specializes in services such as cardiac consultation cardiac surgery cardiac catheterization electrophysiology angioplasty intracoronary stents rotoblade asthma emphysema cystic fibrosis chronic lung disease. lung cancer allergy and anesthesia.
Richard Shider, Director

Ohio

3049 **Case Western Reserve University: Cystic Fibrosis Center**
2101 Adelbert Road
Cleveland, OH 44106-2624
216-844-2391
Fax: 216-844-5916
e-mail: Mds11@case.edu
www.case.edu

3050 **Case Western Reserve University: Cystic Fi**
2101 Adelbert Road 216-844-2391
Cleveland, OH 44106 Fax: 216-844-5916
e-mail: Mds11@case.edu
www.case.edu

3051 **Columbus Children's Hospital: Cystic Fibrosis Center**
700 Childrens Drive 614-722-4766
Columbus, OH 43205-0296 Fax: 614-722-4755
www.nationwidechildrens.org
Karen S McCoy MD, Chief
Elizabeth D Allen MD, Physician

3052 **Lewis H Walker MD: Cystic Fibrosis Center Children's Hospital Medical Center of Ak**
Children's Hospital Medical Center of Akron
Considine Professional Building 330-543-3249
Akron, OH 44308-1062 800-262-0333
TTY: 330-543-8080
www.akronchildrens.org/respiratory
One of six CF centers in the state of Ohio providing comprehensive care for patients who suffer from this disease. The center which is part of the Robert T. Stone Respiratory Center actively participates in clinical trials to research new drug therapies to manage cystic fibrosis.
Nathan Krayn MD, Director Cystic Fibrosis Center

3053 **Pediatric Pulmonary Center The Children's Medical Center of Dayton**
The Children's Medical Center of Dayton
1 Children's Plaza 937-641-3000
Dayton, OH 45404-1815 Fax: 937-641-4500
www.childrensdayton.org
Robert Fink MD, Medical Director

3054 **University of Cincinnati College of Medicine Division of Pediatrics**
Children s Hospital Medical Center
3333 Burnet Avenue 513-636-4588
Cincinnati, OH 45229-3039 800-344-2462
Fax: 513-636-0345
TTY: 513-636-4900
e-mail: thomas.boat@cchmc.org
www.cincinnatichildrens.org
The University of Cincinnati Department of Pediatrics consists entirely of staff members from Cincinnati Children's Hospital Medical Center one of the nation's leading pediatric research and teaching institutions.
Thomas F Boat MD, Professor of Pediatrics
Arnold W Strauss MD, Department Head

Oklahoma

3055 **University of Oklahoma: Cystic Fibrosis Center**
Department of Pediatrics
940 NE 13th Street 405-271-6390
Oklahoma City, OK 73104 Fax: 405-271-2873
e-mail: brenda-freese@ouhsc.edu
pediatrics.ouhsc.edu
James A Royall MD, Professor/Chief Pediatric Pulmonology
Terrence L Stull MD, Chairman

Oregon

3056 **Oregon Health & Science University**
3181 SW Sam Jackson Park Road 503-494-8311
Portland, OR 97239 e-mail: contactus@ohsuhealth.com
www.ohsuhealth.com
Oregon Health & Science University is a leading health and research university that strives for excellence in patient care education research and community service.
Joseph Rober Jr MD MBA, President
Steven D Stadum JD, Executive Vice President

Pennsylvania

3057 **Cystic Fibrosis Center: Polyclinic Medical Center**
Polyclinic Medical Center
2501 N 3rd Street 717-782-4790
Harrisburg, PA 17110-2098 800-334-1007
Fax: 717-782-4679
www.pinnaclehealth.org
Muttiah Gane MD, Director

3058 **Pediatric Pulmonary and Cystic Fibrosis Center**
St. Christopher's Hospital for Children
E Erie Avenue & N Front Street
Philadelphia, PA 19134 215-427-5183
www.stchristophershospital.com
A team of pediatric pulmonary medicine experts treats children with a wide range of acute and chronic lung diseases such as cystic fibrosis bronchopulmonary dysplasia apnea respiratory infections bronchiolitis congenital malformations including chest wall deformities and pneumonia.
Laurie Varlo MD, Director

3059 **University of Pennsylvania: Penn Lung Center**
Hospital of The University of Pennsylvania
3 Ravdin Suite F
Philadelphia, PA 19104 800-789-7366
www.pennhealth.com
Penn Lung Center of the University of Pennsylvania Health System is a multidisciplinary resource for consultation second opinion diagnosis and ongoing treatment of patients with lung disease.
Leslie A Litzky MD, Associate Professor of Pathology and Lab
Maryl Kreide MD MSCE, Assistant Professor of Medicine

3060 **University of Pittsburgh Cystic Fibrosis Center: Children's Hospital**
Department of Cell Biology And Physiology
S362 BST 412-648-9362
Pittsburgh, PA 15261 Fax: 412-648-8330
e-mail: cdpweb@pitt.edu
www.cbp.pitt.edu/centers/cfrc.html
The primary goal of the Center is to focus the attention of new and established investigators on multidisciplinary approaches designed to improve the understanding and treatment of cystic fibrosis (CF).
Raymond A Frizzell PhD, Director
Carol A Bertrand PhD, Research Assistant Professor

Rhode Island

3061 **Rhode Island Hospital: Cystic Fibrosis Center**
Department of Pediatrics
593 Eddy Street 401-793-8560
Providence, RI 02903 Fax: 401-444-2168
e-mail: mschechter@lifespan.org
www.lifespan.org
Michael S Schechter MD, Director
Mary Anne Passero MD, Co-Director

South Carolina

3062 **Medical University of South Carolina: Cystic Fibrosis Center**
Department of Pediatrics
135 Rutledge Avenue Suite 279 803-792-1414
Charleston, SC 29425 800-424-6872
Fax: 843-876-1435
www.musc.edu/cfcenter

3063 **Medical University of South Carolina: Cyst Department of Pediatrics**
135 Rutledge Avenue Suite 279 803-792-1414
Charleston, SC 29425 800-424-6872
Fax: 843-876-1435
www.musc.edu/cfcenter
The objectives of the Cystic Fibrosis Center at MUSC are to offer unsurpassed care to patients with cystic fibrosis to teach medical students house staff medical care providers and general public about cystic fibrosis and to learn about cystic fibrosis through clinical and laboratory research.

Tennessee

3064 **Memphis Cystic Fibrosis Center LeBonheur Children's Medical Center**
LeBonheur Children's Medical Center

50 N Dunlap Street
Memphis, TN 38103
901-287-5437
e-mail: info@lebonheur.org
www.lebonheur.org

3065 Vanderbilt Children's Hospital
2200 Childrens Way
Nashville, TN 37232
615-936-1000
866-936-7811
www.vanderbiltchildrens.com
Children's Hospital provides top-level care while including the family as an essential element of a child's treatment plan.
Kevin B Churchwell MD, Chief Executive Officer
Patricia Giv RN EdM, Chief Nursing Officer

Texas

3066 Cook Children's Medical Center: Cystic Fibrosis Clinic
801 7th Avenue
Fort Worth, TX 76104
682-885-6299
www.cookchildrens.org
James C Cunningham MD, Director
Paula Webb RN MSN CNAA B, Vice President of Nursing Services

3067 Cystic Fibrosis Care and Teaching Center Children's Medical Center
Children's Medical Center
1935 Motor Street
Dallas, TX 75235-7701
214-456-2361
Fax: 214-456-2563
www.childrens.com
The Dallas Cystic Fibrosis Care and Teaching Center manages the outpatient and inpatient care of approximately 400 infants children adolescents and adults.
Claude Prest MD, Director
Brenda Urbanczyk, Practice Administrator

3068 Cystic Fibrosis-Lung Disease Center: Santa Rosa Children's Hospital
CHRISTUS Center for Children and Families
333 N Santa Rosa
San Antonio, TX 78207-3900
210-704-4100
Fax: 210-704-2651
www.santarosahealth.org
Serving more than 150 000 children each year CSRCH is a 200-plus bed facility and is the only academic Children's hospital in San Antonio partnering with The University of Texas Health Science Center at San Antonio while collaborating with private pediatricians to provide comprehensive pediatric services at one location since 1959.
Donna Beth Willey-Courand MD, Director
Melanie Drum BSN RN, Nurse Coordinator

3069 Texas Childrens Cystic Fibrosis Care Center
Texas Children's Clinical Care Center
6701 Fannin Street
Houston, TX 77030
832-822-3300
Fax: 832-825-3072
e-mail: pulmonarymedicine@texaschildrenshospital
www.texaschildrenshospital.org
Provides comprehensive clinical services to help patients families and referring physicians deal with the many problems cystic fibrosis causes.
Dan K Seilheimer MD, Director
Peter W Hiatt MD, Chief of Service

3070 Tri-Services Military Cystic Fibrosis Center
Brooke Army Medical Center/Pediatrics Department
3851 Roger Brooke Drive
Fort Sam Houston, TX 78234-6320
210-916-3400
Fax: 210-916-3076
e-mail: ted.cieslak@cen.amedd.army.mil
www.bamc.amedd.army.mil
COL Ted Cieslak, Chief of Pediatrics

Utah

3071 University of Utah Intermountain Cystic Fibrosis Center
University Hospital & Clinics
26 N 1900 E
Salt Lake City, UT 84132-1
801-585-2804
800-824-2073
Fax: 801-585-5350
e-mail: judy.carle@hsc.utah.edu
www.med.utah.edu
Barbara A Chatfield MD, Director Pediatric Program
Theodore G Liou MD, Director Adult Program

Vermont

3072 Medical Center Hospital of Vermont Cystic Fibrosis Center
Cystic Fibrosis Center
111 Colchester Avenue
Burlington, VT 05401-7152
802-847-8600
Fax: 802-847-5805
www.fahc.org
Tom Lahiri MD, Director

Virginia

3073 Eastern Virginia Medical School Children's Hospital of The King's Daught
Children's Hospital of The King's Daughters
601 Children's Lane
Norfolk, VA 23507
757-668-7000
e-mail: healthinfo@chkd.org
www.chkd.org
Provider of quality children's health services
Leslie Acakpo-Satchi, Neurosurgery
Maria Aguiar, Pathology

3074 University of Virginia School of Medicine Cystic Fibrosis Center
Department of Pediatrics
PO Box 800386
Charlottesville, VA 22908
434-924-2250
800-251-3627
Fax: 434-243-6618
www.healthsystem.virginia.edu
Comprehensive care for children and adults with cystic fibrosis.
Deborah K Froh MD, Director Children S Of Program
Mark Robbins MD, Director Adult Of Program

Washington

3075 University of Washington: Cystic Fibrosis Center
University of Washington Medical Center/Adult Prog
1959 NE Pacific Street
Seattle, WA 98195
206-598-6116
Fax: 206-598-4610
www.washington.edu
UW Medicine works to improve the health of the public by advancing medical knowledge
Ronald Gibson, Center Director
Ronald Gibson, Professor and Center Director

West Virginia

3076 West Virginia University Cystic Fibrosis Center
Pediatrics Department
PO Box 9100
Morgantown, WV 26506-9214
304-293-6607
Fax: 304-293-6627
e-mail: gpiedimonte@hsc.wvu.edu
www.hsc.wvu.edu
The Hospital providing the full range of services including allergy/immunology cardiology child development critical care cystic fibrosis endocrinology adolescent medicine gastroenterology genetics and metabolic disease hematology/oncology neonatology nephrology neurology and apnea evaluation. Services provided by faculty with joint appointments include ophthalmology urology orthopedics psychiatry surgery and cardiothoracic surgery.
Kathryn S Moffett MD, Director
Giovanni Piedimonte, Chair

Wisconsin

3077 Medical College of Wisconsin: Cystic Fibrosis Clinic
Children's Hospital of Wisconsin
PO Box 1997
Milwaukee, WI 53201-1997
414-607-5280
877-607-5280
www.chw.org
Children's Hospital and Health System is an independent health care system dedicated solely to the health and well-being of children.
M Susan Jay, Adolescent Medicine
Peter J Bartz, Cardiology Pediatric

3078 University of Wisconsin-Madison: Cystic Fibrosis/Pulmonary Center
Clinical Science Center
600 Highland Avenue
Madison, WI 53792
608-263-6400
800-323-8942
www.uwhealth.org

UW Health represents the academic medical care providers of the University of Wisconsin-Madison and its affiliated organizations.
Michael J Rock, Faculty
Prasad S Dalvie, Radiology

Support Groups & Hotlines

3079 **National Health Information Center**
PO Box 1133
Washington, DC 20013
310-565-4167
800-336-4797
Fax: 301-984-4256
e-mail: info@nhic.org
www.health.gov/nhic
Offers a nationwide information referral service, produces directories and resource guides.

Books

3080 **Cystic Fibrosis: A Guide for Patient and Family**
Raven Press
1185 Avenue of the Americas
New York, NY 10036-2601
212-930-9500
800-777-2295
253 pages Softcover
ISBN: 0-397516-53-3

3081 **Understanding Cystic Fibrosis**
Karen Hopkin, PhD, author
University Press of Mississippi
3825 Ridgewood Road
Jackson, MS 39211-6492
601-432-6205
Fax: 601-432-6217
e-mail: kburgess@ihl.state.ms.us
www.upress.state.ms.us
A useful guide for families and patients.
1998 128 pages Paperback
ISBN: 0-878059-67-9
Kathy Burgess, Advertising/Marketing Services Manager

Children's Books

3082 **Give Me One Wish**
Norton Publishers
500 5th Avenue
New York, NY 10110-0002
212-354-5500
800-233-4830
www.scholastic.com/
This book reads like a novel because it re-enacts the author's daughter's bout with cystic fibrosis.
Grades 10-12

3083 **Robyn's Book: A True Diary**
Scholastic
730 Broadway
New York, NY 10003-9511
212-505-3000
800-325-6149
This book chronicles the life of the author and her battle with cystic fibrosis.
Grades 7-12

3084 **Toothpick**
Holiday
40 E 49th Street
New York, NY 10017-1105
212-688-0085
This book uses relationships between two different teenagers to parallel the life of a person with cystic fibrosis.
Grades 6-9

Newsletters

3085 **Better Breathing Bulletin**
American Lung Association of Connecticut
45 Ash Street
East Hartford, CT 06108-3294
860-289-5401
800-586-4872
Fax: 860-289-5405
www.alact.org
This newsletter is aimed at persons with chronic lung problems.
John E Zinn, President/CEO

3086 **Commitment**
Cystic Fibrosis Foundation
6931 Arlington Road
Bethesda, MD 20814-5231
301-951-4422
800-344-4823
Fax: 301-951-6378
e-mail: info@cff.org
www.cff.org
Offers general information on cystic fibrosis, fund-raising features, public policy and news from across the nation on cystic fibrosis.

Pamphlets

3087 **Consumer Fact Sheet**
Cystic Fibrosis Foundation
6931 Arlington Road
Bethesda, MD 20814-5231
301-951-4422
800-344-4823
Fax: 301-951-6378
e-mail: info@cff.org
www.cff.org
Offers a brief introduction to cystic fibrosis, symptoms, causes, treatments and offers illustrations pertaining to drainage positions.

3088 **Cystic Fibrosis: A Guide for Parents**
American Lung Association
1740 Broadway
New York, NY 10019-4315
212-315-8700
Comprehensive booklet covering topics such as treatment, social aspects, inheritance, genetics and outlook for the future.
24 pages

3089 **For Adults with Cystic Fibrosis: Facts on Reproduction**
National Maternal and Child Health Clearinghouse
2070 Chain Bridge Road
Vienna, VA 22182-2588
703-442-9051
888-275-4772
Fax: 703-821-2098
e-mail: ask@hrsa.gov
www.ask.hrsa.gov
The purpose of this booklet is to review the reproductive issues that are unique to individuals with cystic fibrosis.

3090 **Foundation Facts**
Cystic Fibrosis Foundation
6931 Arlington Road
Bethesda, MD 20814-5231
301-951-4422
800-344-4823
Fax: 301-951-6378
e-mail: info@cff.org
www.cff.org
Offers information on the fund-raising and grants offered and supported by the foundation.

3091 **Here's Everything You'll Need to Save Money with the CFF Health Services**
CFF Home Health & Pharmacy Services
6931 Arlington Road
Bethesda, MD 20814-5223
800-342-6967
Fax: 800-233-3504
Offers information on the Cystic Fibrosis Foundation's home health services.

3092 **Home Line**
Cystic Fibrosis Foundation
6931 Arlington Road
Bethesda, MD 20814-5231
301-951-4422
800-344-4823
Fax: 301-951-6378
e-mail: info@cff.org
www.cff.org
Offers information on services and programs offered by the foundation.

Audio & Video

3093 **Alex: The Life of a Child**
Cystic Fibrosis Foundation

6931 Arlington Road
Bethesda, MD 20814
301-951-4422
800-344-4823
Fax: 301-951-6378
e-mail: info@cff.org
www.cff.org

The story of Alexandra Deford, a young girl who lost her battle with CF at the age of 8, has touched the hearts of millions and has helped to put a "face" to this disease. Alex's courage and strength is a true inspiration, and in the decades since her death, much progress has been made in the fight against CF. VHS only.

1986 1 Hr 35 Minutes

Robert J Beall, PhD, President/CEO

3094 **Embers of the Fire**

Mary Kondrat, author

Fanlight Productions
4196 Washington Street
Boston, MA 02131-1731
617-469-4999
800-937-4113
Fax: 617-469-3379
e-mail: fanlight@fanlight.com
www.fanlight.com

Offers a straight forward explanation of the disease with a primary focus on the stories of several courageous young people with cystic fibrosis during a week at summer camp. Addresses their fears of rejection, isolation and death while demonstrating the ways they have learned to lead fulfilling lives.

1992 28 Minutes

ISBN: 1-572950-98-6

3095 **Expanding the Horizon of Hope: 50 Years of Progress**

Cystic Fibrosis Foundation
6931 Arlington Road
Bethesda, MD 20814
301-951-4422
800-344-4823
Fax: 301-951-6378
e-mail: info@cff.org
www.cff.org

This film highlights the progress that has been made in CF research and care over the past 50 years, as well as the challenges that still lie ahead. It pays tribute to all who are involved in the CF effort—from researchers and clinicians, to patients and their families, to volunteers, donors and staff. DVD only.

2005 60 Minutes

Robert J Beall, PhD, President/CEO

3096 **Faces of Cystic Fibrosis**

Cystic Fibrosis Foundation
6931 Arlington Road
Bethesda, MD 20814
301-951-4422
800-344-4823
Fax: 301-951-6378
e-mail: info@cff.org
www.cff.org

Through the words of people with CF and their family members, hear the story of how the fight against CF has evolved into a story of hope and optimism that was never possible before...and how none of this would be possible without the dedication and efforts of volunteers. Available in VHS/DVD.

2001 11 Minutes

Robert J Beall, PhD, President/CEO

3097 **Information About the Sweat Test**

Cystic Fibrosis Foundation
6931 Arlington Road
Bethesda, MD 20814
301-951-4422
800-344-4823
Fax: 301-951-6378
e-mail: info@cff.org
www.cff.org

See and hear some basic information about the sweat test, the standard diagnostic test for CF. It is intended to help families better understand the sweat testing procedure and what to expect when the test is conducted. VHS only.

3.47 Minutes

Robert J Beall, PhD, President/CEO

Web Sites

3098 **Healing Well**

www.healingwell.com

An online health resource guide to medical news, chat, information and articles, newsgroups and message boards, books, disease-related web sites, medical directories, and more for patients, friends, and family coping with disabling diseases, disorders, or chronic illnesses.

3099 **Health Finder**

www.healthfinder.gov

Searchable, carefully developed web site offering information on over 1000 topics. Developed by the US Department of Health and Human Services, the site can be used in both English and Spanish.

3100 **Healthlink USA**

www.healthlinkusa.com

Health information concerning treatment, cures, prevention, diagnosis, risk factors, research, support groups, email lists, personal stories and much more. Updated regularly.

3101 **Helios Health**

www.helioshealth.com

Online resource for your health information. Detailed information about specific health topics, access to expert advice from our Medical Advisory Board, and up-to-date health news.

3102 **MedicineNet**

www.medicinenet.com

An online resource for consumers providing easy-to-read, authoritative medical and health information.

3103 **Medscape**

www.mywebmd.com

Medscape offers specialists, primary care physicians, and other health professionals the Web's most robust and integrated medical information and educational tools.

3104 **WebMD**

www.webmd.com

Provides links to over 45 articles involving cystic fibrosis.

Description

3105 **Diabetes Mellitus**

Diabetes mellitus is a condition in which the body lacks enough insulin to control its own blood glucose (sugar) level. Ordinarily, the pancreas releases enough of this hormone to let the body's cells absorb and metabolize glucose. In Type I diabetes (formerly called juvenile-onset diabetes and affecting 10 percent of diabetic patients), the pancreas simply stops producing insulin. In Type II, commonly affecting overweight individuals older than 40, the pancreas might release normal, reduced, or even elevated levels of insulin, but the body's cells are resistant to the insulin's action. In either case, blood glucose levels rise (hyperglycemia) until the kidney starts to dump sugar into the urine. The patient may experience excessive thirst and urination, hunger, weakness and weight loss. In extreme cases, when there is either insufficient insulin or the body undergoes stress, or strenuous exercise, some components of the blood become seriously altered and the patient may lapse into a coma. Long-term complications include an increased risk of coronary heart disease and other vascular diseases, such as stroke, vision loss and kidney failure.

Type I appears to be caused by a genetic predisposition that may express itself after an acute insult, often a viral infection. Genetic factors are important in Type II diabetes which runs strongly in families. It is much more common in obese people, as well as among African-Americans, Hispanics and Native Americans.

Prevention ofacute and long-term complications requires careful management including maintaining the proper diet and exercise, blood glucose monitoring and medications. Thorough education of the patient and relevant family members is absolutely critical.

Some individuals with Type II diabetes can control their disease through diet, exercise and weight loss alone. Some will have to take oral medication that helps the pancreas make more insulin or makes the body more sensitive to insulin. Some Type II diabetics, and all Type I diabetics, need to take insulin. Research has shown that tight control of diabetes through frequent blood testing and proper adjustment of the dosage of insulin is most beneficial. Insulin is generally given in multiple injections throughout the day, with preparations varying by length of effectiveness. Closest control of glucose levels is achieved by giving insulin through a continuously-connected insulin pump. Pancreas transplantation is considered only for patients who also need some other organ, generally a kidney.

National Agencies & Associations

3106 **American Association of Diabetes Educators**
200 W Madison Street
Chicago, IL 60606
800-338-3633
e-mail: aade@aadenet.org
www.aadenet.org

An independent multidisciplinary organization of health professionals involved in teaching persons with diabetes. The mission is to enhance the competence of health professionals who teach persons with diabetes and advance the specialty practice of diabetes.
Marcia Draheim, President

3107 **American Diabetes Association**
1701 N Beauregard Street
Alexandria, VA 22311
804-225-8038
888-342-2383
Fax: 804-225-8211
e-mail: askada@diabetes.org
www.diabetes.org

The nation's leading voluntary organization concerned with diabetes and its complications. The mission of the organization is to prevent and cure diabetes and to improve the lives of persons with diabetes. Offers a network of offices nationwide.
Julie Heverly, Area Director
Ellsabeth King, Associate Manager

3108 **Diabetes Exercise and Sports Association**
10216 Taylorsville Road
Louisville, KY 40299
800-898-4322
Fax: 502-261-8346
e-mail: desa@diabetes-exercise.org
www.diabetes-exercise.org

Exists to enhance the quality of life for people with diabetes through exercise and physical fitness.
Paula Harper, Founder

3109 **Juvenile Diabetes Foundation: International**
120 Wall Street
New York, NY 10005-4001
800-533-2873
Fax: 212-785-9595
e-mail: info@jdrf.org
www.jdf.org

Focuses energies on fund-raising, referrals, educational materials and information pertaining to juvenile diabetes.
Stephen H Leeper DDS, President

3110 **National Certification Board for Diabetes Educators**
330 E Algonquin Road
Arlington Heights, IL 60005
847-228-9795
Fax: 847-228-8469
e-mail: info@ncbde.org
www.ncbde.org

The Board for Diabetes Educators is dedicated to promoting excellence in the field of diabetes education through the development maintenance and protection of the certified Diabetes Educator credential and the certification process.
Karen Bolderman, Chair
Lance Hoxie, Chief Executive Officer

3111 **National Diabetes Action Network for the Blind**
National Federation of the Blind
1800 Johnson Street
Baltimore, MD 21230
410-659-9314
Fax: 410-685-5653
e-mail: nfb@nfb.org
www.nfb.org

Leading support and information organization of persons losing vision due to diabetes. Provides personal contact and resource information with other blind diabetics about non-visual techniques of independently managing diabetes and monitoring glucose levels.
Marc Maurer, President
Fredric Schroeder, First Vice President

3112 **National Institute of Diabetes, Digestive & Kidney Diseases**
National Institutes of Health
31 Center Drive, MSC 2560
Bethesda, MD 20892-2560
301-496-4000
e-mail: NIHInfo@OD.NIH.GOV
www.diabetes.niddk.nih.gov

Conducts and supports research on many of the most serious diseases affecting public health. The Institute supports much of the clinical research on the diseases of internal medicine and related subspecialty fields as well as many basic science disiplines.
Dr. Griffin Rodgers, Acting Director

State Agencies & Associations

Alabama

3113 **American Diabetes Association: Alabama**
3918 Montclair Road
Birmingham, AL 35213
205-870-5172
888-DIA-BETE
Fax: 205-879-2903
e-mail: acasey@diabetes.org
www.diabetes.org

Aimee Casey, Executive Director
Stephanie Willis, Director

3114 **Juvenile Diabetes Research Foundation: Bir mingham**
14 Office Park Circle
Birmingham, AL 35223
205-871-0333
Fax: 205-871-0355
e-mail: alabama@jdf.org
www.jdrf.org/alabama

Karin Scott, Executive Director
Sarah Hendren, Special Events Manager

Alaska

3115 **American Diabetes Association: Alaska**
801 W Fireweed Lane
Anchorage, AK 99503
907-272-1424
888-DIA-BETE
Fax: 907-272-1428
e-mail: mcassano@diabetes.org
www.diabetes.org

Michelle Cassano, Executive Director
Phoebe O'Connell, Manager

Arizona

3116 **American Diabetes Association: Arizona**
8125 N 23rd Avenue
Phoenix, AZ 85021
602-861-4731
Fax: 602-995-1344
www.diabetes.org

3117 **American Diabetes Association: Arizona, Bo rder Area**
333 W Ft Lowell Rd
Tucson, AZ 85705
520-795-3711
888-DIA-BETE
Fax: 520-795-1179
e-mail: fgomez@diabetes.org
www.diabetes.org

Fred Gomez, Executive Director
Heidi Goldsmith, Manager

3118 **American Diabetes Association: Atlanta Met**
8125 N 23rd Avenue
Phoenix, AZ 85021
602-861-4731
Fax: 602-995-1344
e-mail: kbisko@diabetes.org
www.diabetes.org

Karen Bisko, Executive Director
Suzanne Miller, Director

3119 **Juvenile Diabetes Research Foundation: Pho enix Chapter**
4343 E Camelback Road
Phoenix, AZ 85018
602-224-1800
Fax: 602-224-1801
e-mail: desertsouthwest@jdrf.org
www.jdrf.org/arizona

Marci Zimmerman, Executive Director
Valerie Jones, Associate Executive Director

3120 **Juvenile Diabetes Research Foundation: Sou thern Arizona/Tucson Chapter**
4560 E Broadway Boulevard
Tucson, AZ 85711
520-327-9900
Fax: 520-327-9906
e-mail: southernarizona@jdrf.org
www.jdrf.org/tucsonwalk

Christina Stucki, Tucson Branch Manager

Arkansas

3121 **American Diabetes Association: Arkansas**
320 Executive Court
Little Rock, AR 72205
501-221-7444
888-DIA-BETE
Fax: 501-221-3138
e-mail: rselig@diabetes.org
www.diabetes.org

Rick Selig, Director
Charlotte Williams, Associate Manager

3122 **Juvenile Diabetes Research Foundation: Nor thwest Arkansas Branch**
440 N College Avenue
Fayetteville, AR 72701
479-443-9190
Fax: 479-443-2692
e-mail: nwarkansas@jdrf.org
www.jdrf.org/nwark

Deb Euculano, Special Events Manager

California

3123 **American Diabetes Association: California**
2720 Gateway Oaks Drive
Sacramento, CA 95833
916-924-3232
888-DIA-BETE
Fax: 916-924-0529
e-mail: AskADA@diabetes.org
www.diabetes.org/

The American Diabetes Association is a nonprofit health organization providing diabetes research, information and advocacy. Founded in 1940, the American Diabetes Association conducts programs in all 50 states and the District of Columbia.
Michael D Farley CFRE, Chief Community Relations Officer
Richard Kahn PhD, Chief Scientific/Medical Officer

3124 **Diabetes Society of Santa Clara Valley**
4040 Moorpark Avenue
San Jose, CA 95117
408-241-1922
888-DIA-BETE
Fax: 408-241-1972
e-mail: Info@thediabetessociety.org
www.diabetes.org

The Diabetes Society is dedicated to providing education and information to those who have diabetes educating the general public about the seriousness of this disease, and supporting research aimed at preventing complications and finding a cure.
Douglas Metz DPM/MPH, Executive Director
Thomas Smith, Program/Camp Director

3125 **Juvenile Diabetes Research Foundation: Bak ersfield Chapter**
712 19th Street
Bakersfield, CA 93301
661-636-1305
Fax: 661-636-1307
e-mail: Bakersfield@jdrf.org
www.jdrf-bakersfield.org

The Juvenile Diabetes Research Foundation International (JDRF) is a charitable funder and advocate of type 1 (juvenile) diabetes research worldwide. The mission of JDRF is to find a cure for diabetes and its complications through the support of research.
Allison Perkins Thomas, Bakersfield Branch Manager
Arnold Donald, President/CEO Corporate Office (NY)

3126 **Juvenile Diabetes Research Foundation: Gre ater Bay Area Chapter**
49 Stevenson Street
San Francisco, CA 94105
415-977-0360
Fax: 415-977-0355
e-mail: greaterbay@jdf.org
www.jdrf.org/greaterbay

The Juvenile Diabetes Research Foundation International (JDRF) is a charitable funder and advocate of type 1 (juvenile) diabetes research worldwide. The mission of JDRF is to find a cure for diabetes and its complications through the support of research.
Vicki Weiland, Executive Director
Mavie Mendelson, Special Events Director

3127 **Juvenile Diabetes Research Foundation: Inl and Empire Chapter**
1001 East Cooley Drive
Colton, CA 92324
909-424-0100
Fax: 909-424-0044
e-mail: inlandempire@jdrf.org
www.jdrf.org/index.cfm?page_id=100614

The Juvenile Diabetes Research Foundation International (JDRF) is a charitable funder and advocate of type 1 (juvenile) diabetes re-

search worldwide. The mission of JDRF is to find a cure for diabetes and its complications through the support of research.
Jamie Brunelle, Board of Directors
Evelyn Edinin, Board of Directors

3128 Juvenile Diabetes Research Foundation: Los Angeles Chapter
800 West Sixth Street 213-233-9901
Los Angeles, CA 90017 Fax: 213-622-6276
e-mail: losangeles@jdrf.org
www.jdrf.org/losangeles
The Juvenile Diabetes Research Foundation International (JDRF) is a charitable funder and advocate of type 1 (juvenile) diabetes research worldwide. The mission of JDRF is to find a cure for diabetes and its complications through the support of research.
Mark Rieck, Executive Director
Dennis Ellman Esq, Board of Directors President

3129 Juvenile Diabetes Research Foundation: Nor thern California Inland Chapter
1329 Howe Avenue 916-920-0790
Sacramento, CA 95825 Fax: 916-920-0367
e-mail: northernca@jdrf.org
www.jdrf.org/norcal
The Juvenile Diabetes Research Foundation International (JDRF) is a charitable funder and advocate of type 1 (juvenile) diabetes research worldwide. The mission of JDRF is to find a cure for diabetes and its complications through the support of research.
Victoria Webster, Executive Director
Molly Atkinson, Special Events Coordinator

3130 Juvenile Diabetes Research Foundation: Ora nge County Chapter
17872 Mitchell North 949-553-0363
Irvine, CA 92614 Fax: 949-553-8813
e-mail: orangecounty@jdrf.org
www.jdf.org/chapters/CA/Orange-County
The Juvenile Diabetes Research Foundation International (JDRF) is a charitable funder and advocate of type 1 (juvenile) diabetes research worldwide. The mission of JDRF is to find a cure for diabetes and its complications through the support of research.
Louise Cummings, Executive Director
Jennifer Walker, Special Events Manager

3131 Juvenile Diabetes Research Foundation: San Diego Chapter
5677 Oberlin Drive 858-597-0240
San Diego, CA 92121 Fax: 858-597-2072
e-mail: sandiego@jdrf.org
www.jdrf-sandiego-news.org
The Juvenile Diabetes Research Foundation International (JDRF) is a charitable funder and advocate of type 1 (juvenile) diabetes research worldwide. The mission of JDRF is to find a cure for diabetes and its complications through the support of research.
Linda Riley, Executive Director
Katherine Griswold, Special Events Manager

Colorado

3132 American Diabetes Association: Denver
2480 W 26th Avenue 720-855-1102
Denver, CO 80211 Fax: 720-855-1302
e-mail: AskADA@diabetes.org
www.diabetes.org/
The American Diabetes Association is a nonprofit health organization providing diabetes research, information and advocacy. Founded in 1940 the American Diabetes Association conducts programs in all 50 states and the District of Columbia.
Michael D Farley CFRE, Chief Community Relations Officer
Richard Kahn PhD, Chief Scientific/Medical Officer

3133 Juvenile Diabetes Research Foundation: Col orado Springs Chapter
3710 Sinton Road 719-633-8110
Colorado Springs, CO 80907 Fax: 719-633-8155
e-mail: lpage@jdrf.org
www.jdrfcoloradosprings.org
The Juvenile Diabetes Research Foundation International (JDRF) is a charitable funder and advocate of type 1 (juvenile) diabetes research worldwide. The mission of JDRF is to find a cure for diabetes and its complications through the support of research.
Lynn Page, Branch Manager
Andi Chernushin, President

3134 Juvenile Diabetes Research Foundation: Roc ky Mountain Chapter
5613 DTC Parkway 303-779-0525
Greenwood Village, CO 80111 Fax: 303-720-1630
e-mail: RockyMountain@jdrf.org
www.jdrf.org/rockymountain
The Juvenile Diabetes Research Foundation International (JDRF) is a charitable funder and advocate of type 1 (juvenile) diabetes research worldwide. The mission of JDRF is to find a cure for diabetes and its complications through the support of research.
James Buckles, Executive Director
Nancy L Walters, Special Events Director

Connecticut

3135 American Diabetes Association: Connecticut
306 Industrial Park Road 203-639-0385
Middletown, CT 06457 888-DIA-BETE
Fax: 860-632-5098
e-mail: AskADA@diabetes.org
www.diabetes.org
The American Diabetes Association is a nonprofit health organization providing diabetes research, information and advocacy. Founded in 1940 the American Diabetes Association conducts programs in all 50 states and the District of Columbia.
Michael D Farley CRFE (Corpora, Chief Community Relations Officer
Richard Kahn PhD, Chief Scientific/Medical Officer

3136 Juvenile Diabetes Research Foundation: Greater New Haven Chapter
2969 Whitney Avenue 203-248-1880
Hamden, CT 06518 Fax: 203-248-1820
e-mail: newhaven@jdf.org
www.jdrf.org/greaternewhaven
The Juvenile Diabetes Research Foundation International (JDRF) is a charitable funder and advocate of type 1 (juvenile) diabetes research worldwide. The mission of JDRF is to find a cure for diabetes and its complications through the support of research.
Mary K Kessler, Executive Director
Will Martinez, Board of Directors President

3137 Juvenile Diabetes Research Foundation: Fai rfield County Chapter
200 Connecticut Avenue 203-854-0658
Norwalk, CT 06854 Fax: 203-854-0798
e-mail: fairfield@jdrf.org
www.jdrf.org/fairfieldcounty
The Juvenile Diabetes Research Foundation International (JDRF) is a charitable funder and advocate of type 1 (juvenile) diabetes research worldwide. The mission of JDRF is to find a cure for diabetes and its complications through the support of research.
Barbara Rose, Executive Director
Michelle Tighe, Special Events Coordinator

3138 Juvenile Diabetes Research Foundation: Nor th Central CT and Western MA
18 North Main Street 860-561-1153
West Hartford, CT 06107 Fax: 860-561-3440
e-mail: northcentralct@jdrf.org
www.jdrf.org/index.cfm?page_id=100619
The Juvenile Diabetes Research Foundation International (JDRF) is a charitable funder and advocate of type 1 (juvenile) diabetes research worldwide. The mission of JDRF is to find a cure for diabetes and its complications through the support of research.
Mary Ann Slomski, Executive Director
Ellen Kellie, Special Events Coordinator

Delaware

3139 **American Diabetes Association: Delaware**
100 W 10th Street
Wilmington, DE 19801
302-656-0030
888-342-2383
Fax: 302-656-7331
e-mail: AskADA@diabetes.org
www.diabetes.org
The American Diabetes Association is a nonprofit health organization providing diabetes research, information and advocacy. Founded in 1940 the American Diabetes Association conducts programs in all 50 states and the District of Columbia.
Michael D Farley CFRE (Corpora, Chief Community Relations Officer
Richard Kahn PhD, Chief Scientific/Medical Officer

3140 **Juvenile Diabetes Research Foundation: Del aware**
100 West 10th Street
Wilmington, DE 19801
302-888-1117
Fax: 302-888-1878
e-mail: delaware@jdrf.org
www.jdrf.org/delaware
The Juvenile Diabetes Research Foundation International (JDRF) is a charitable funder and advocate of type 1 (juvenile) diabetes research worldwide. The mission of JDRF is to find a cure for diabetes and its complications through the support of research.
Ellen Rubesin, Executive Director
Stephanie Bucksner, Special Events Coordinator

District of Columbia

3141 **American Diabetes Association: District of Columbia**
1025 Connecticut Avenue NW
Washington, DC 20036
202-331-8303
888-342-2383
Fax: 202-331-1402
e-mail: AskADA@diabetes.org
www.diabetes.org
The American Diabetes Association is a nonprofit health organization providing diabetes research, information and advocacy. Founded in 1940 the American Diabetes Association conducts programs in all 50 states and the District of Columbia.
Michael D Farley CFRE (Corpora, Chief Community Relations Officer
Richard Kahn PhD, Chief Scientific/Medical Officer

3142 **Juvenile Diabetes Research Foundation: Cap itol Chapter**
1400 K Street NW
Washington, DC 20005
202-371-0044
Fax: 202-371-0046
e-mail: capitol@jdrf.org
www.jdrfcapitol.org
The Juvenile Diabetes Research Foundation International (JDRF) is a charitable funder and advocate of type 1 (juvenile) diabetes research worldwide. The mission of JDRF is to find a cure for diabetes and its complications through the support of research.
Pam Gatz, Executive Director
Carrie Hamilton, Special Events Director

Florida

3143 **American Diabetes Association: Northeast F lorida/Southeast Georgia**
8384 Baymeadows Road
Jacksonville, FL 32256
904-730-7200
888-342-2383
Fax: 940-730-7933
e-mail: AskADA@diabetes.org
www.diabetes.org
The American Diabetes Association is a nonprofit health organization providing diabetes research, information and advocacy. Founded in 1940 the American Diabetes Association conducts programs in all 50 states and the District of Columbia.
Sheri Criswell, Executive Director
Richard Kahn PhD, Chief Scientific/Medical Officer

3144 **American Diabetes Association: Seattle**
1101 N Lake Destiny Road
Maitland, FL 32751
407-660-1926
Fax: 407-660-1080
e-mail: AskADA@diabetes.org
www.diabetes.org
The American Diabetes Association is a nonprofit health organization providing diabetes research, information and advocacy. Founded in 1940 the American Diabetes Association conducts programs in all 50 states and the District of Columbia.
Pauline Lowe, Executive Director
Richard Kahn PhD, Chief Scientific/Medical Officer

3145 **American Diabetes Association: South Coast Regional/Central Florida**
1101 North Lake Destiny Road
Maitland, FL 32751
407-660-1926
888-342-2383
Fax: 407-660-1080
e-mail: AskADA@diabetes.org
www.diabetes.org
The American Diabetes Association is a nonprofit health organization providing diabetes research, information and advocacy. Founded in 1940, the American Diabetes Association conducts programs in all 50 states and the District of Columbia, reaching hundreds of communities.
Michael D Farley CFRE (Corporate), Chief Community Relations Officer
Richard Kahn Ph.D (Corporate), Chief Scientific/Medical Officer

3146 **Juvenile Diabetes Research Foundation: Cen tral Florida Chapter**
279 Douglas Avenue
Altamonte Springs, FL 32714
407-774-2166
Fax: 407-774-2168
e-mail: centralflorida@jdrf.org
www.jdrf.org/centralflorida
The Juvenile Diabetes Research Foundation International (JDRF) is a charitable funder and advocate of type 1 (juvenile) diabetes research worldwide. The mission of JDRF is to find a cure for diabetes and its complications through the support of research.
Kendra Presley, Special Events Manager
Gwen Bell, Office Manager

3147 **Juvenile Diabetes Research Foundation: Flo rida Sun Coast Chapter**
3333 Clark Road
Sarasota, FL 34231
941-929-0621
Fax: 941-929-0602
e-mail: floridasuncoast@jdrf.org
www.jdrf.org/index.cfm
The Juvenile Diabetes Research Foundation International (JDRF) is a charitable funder and advocate of type 1 (juvenile) diabetes research worldwide. The mission of JDRF is to find a cure for diabetes and its complications through the support of research.
Sara Rankin, Executive Director
Jeannie Kawcak, Special Events Coordinator

3148 **Juvenile Diabetes Research Foundation: Gre ater Palm Beach County Chapter**
1450 Centrepark Boulevard
West Palm Beach, FL 33401
561-686-7701
Fax: 561-686-7702
e-mail: greaterpalmbeach@jdrf.org
www.jdrf.org/greaterpalmbeach
The Juvenile Diabetes Research Foundation International (JDRF) is a charitable funder and advocate of type 1 (juvenile) diabetes research worldwide. The mission of JDRF is to find a cure for diabetes and its complications through the support of research.
Lora Hazelwood, Executive Director
Esther Swann, Special Events Coordinator

3149 **Juvenile Diabetes Research Foundation: Nor th Florida Chapter**
8400 Baymeadows Way
Jacksonville, FL 32256
904-739-2101
Fax: 904-739-2693
e-mail: northflorida@jdrf.org
www.jdrf.org/northflorida
The Juvenile Diabetes Research Foundation International (JDRF) is a charitable funder and advocate of type 1 (juvenile) diabetes research worldwide. The mission of JDRF is to find a cure for diabetes and its complications through the support of research.
Brooks Biagini, Executive Director
Wendy Smit, Special Events Assistant

3150 **Juvenile Diabetes Research Foundation: Sou th Florida Chapter**
3411 NW 9th Avenue
Fort Lauderdale, FL 33309
954-565-4775
Fax: 954-565-4767
e-mail: southflorida@jdrf.org
www.jdrf.org/chapters/FL/South-Florida
The Juvenile Diabetes Research Foundation International (JDRF) is a charitable funder and advocate of type 1 (juvenile) diabetes re-

search worldwide. The mission of JDRF is to find a cure for diabetes and its complications through the support of research.
Ingrid Velarde, Special Events Coordinator
Katelyn Tolzien, Special Events Coordinator

3151 Juvenile Diabetes Research Foundation: Tam pa Bay Chapter
5959 Central Avenue 727-344-2873
Saint Petersburg, FL 33710 Fax: 727-384-9009
e-mail: tampabay@jdrf.org
www.jdf.org
The Juvenile Diabetes Research Foundation International (JDRF) is a charitable funder and advocate of type 1 (juvenile) diabetes research worldwide. The mission of JDRF is to find a cure for diabetes and its complications through the support of research.
Arnold Donald, President/CEO Corporate Office
Robin Harding, EVP Development & COO

Georgia

3152 American Diabetes Association: Atlanta Met ro
17 Executive Park 404-320-7100
Atlanta, GA 30329 888-342-2383
Fax: 404-320-0025
e-mail: AskADA@diabetes.org
www.diabetes.org
The American Diabetes Association is a nonprofit health organization providing diabetes research, information and advocacy. Founded in 1940 the American Diabetes Association conducts programs in all 50 states and the District of Columbia, reaching hundreds of communities
Michael Gault, Senior Executive Director
Richard Kahn PhD, Chief Scientific/Medical Officer

3153 American Diabetes Association: Savannah
5105 Paulsen Street 912-353-8110
Savannah, GA 31405 888-343-2383
Fax: 912-353-9114
e-mail: AskADA@diabetes.org
www.diabetes.org
The American Diabetes Association is a nonprofit health organization providing diabetes research, information and advocacy. Founded in 1940 the American Diabetes Association conducts programs in all 50 states and the District of Columbia.
Maria Center, Director
Richard Kahn PhD, Chief Scientific/Medical Officer

3154 Juvenile Diabetes Research Foundation: Geo rgia Chapter
400 Perimeter Center Terrace 404-420-5990
Atlanta, GA 30346 Fax: 404-420-5995
e-mail: georgia@jdrf.org
www.jdrfgeorgia.org/
The Juvenile Diabetes Research Foundation International (JDRF) is a charitable funder and advocate of type 1 (juvenile) diabetes research worldwide. The mission of JDRF is to find a cure for diabetes and its complications through the support of research.
Rob Shaw, Executive Director
Scott Whiteside, EVP/General Manager

Hawaii

3155 American Diabetes Association: Hawaii
1500 S Beretania Street 808-947-5979
Honolulu, HI 96826 888-342-2383
Fax: 808-947-5978
e-mail: AskADA@diabetes.org
www.diabetes.org
The American Diabetes Association is a nonprofit health organization providing diabetes research, information and advocacy. Founded in 1940 the American Diabetes Association conducts programs in all 50 states and the District of Columbia.
Majken Mechling, Executive Director
Richard Kahn PhD, Chief Scientific/Medical Officer

3156 Juvenile Diabetes Research Foundation: Haw aii Chapter
1019 Waimanu Street 808-988-1000
Honolulu, HI 96814 Fax: 808-597-8758
e-mail: hawaii@jdrf.org
www.jdf.org
The Juvenile Diabetes Research Foundation International (JDRF) is a charitable funder and advocate of type 1 (juvenile) diabetes research worldwide. The mission of JDRF is to find a cure for diabetes and its complications through the support of research.
Arnold Donald, President/CEO Corporate
Robin Harding, EVP/Develpment & COO Corporate

Illinois

3157 American Diabetes Association: Greater Ill inois
2580 Federal Drive 217-875-9011
Decatur, IL 62526 888-342-2383
Fax: 217-875-6849
e-mail: AskADA@diabetes.org
www.diabetes.org
The American Diabetes Association is a nonprofit health organization providing diabetes research, information and advocacy. Founded in 1940 the American Diabetes Association conducts programs in all 50 states and the District of Columbia, reaching hundreds of communities.
Donna Scott, Executive Director
Richard Kahn PhD, Chief Scientific/Medical Officer

3158 American Diabetes Association: Northern Il linois
30 North Michigan Avenue 312-346-1805
Chicago, IL 60602 888-343-2383
Fax: 312-346-5342
e-mail: AskADA@diabetes.org
www.diabetes.org
The American Diabetes Association is a nonprofit health organization providing diabetes research, information and advocacy. Founded in 1940, the American Diabetes Association conducts programs in all 50 states and the District of Columbia, reaching hundreds of communities.
Michael D Farley CFRE (Corporate), Chief Community Relations Officer
Richard Kahn Ph.D (Corporate), Chief Scientific/Medical Officer

3159 Juvenile Diabetes Research Foundation: Gre ater Chicago Chapter
500 North Dearborn Street 312-670-0313
Chicago, IL 60610 Fax: 312-670-0250
e-mail: illinois@jdrf.org
www.jdrfillinois.org
The Juvenile Diabetes Research Foundation International (JDRF) is a charitable funder and advocate of type 1 (juvenile) diabetes research worldwide. The mission of JDRF is to find a cure for diabetes and its complications through the support of research.
Amy Franze, Executive Director
Janine Tobola, Director Office Operations

Indiana

3160 American Diabetes Association: Northern In diana/Northern Ohio
6415 Castleway W Drive 317-352-9226
Indianapolis, IN 46250 888-342-2383
Fax: 317-594-0748
e-mail: AskADA@diabetes.org
www.diabetes.org
The American Diabetes Association is a nonprofit health organization providing diabetes research, information and advocacy. Founded in 1940 the American Diabetes Association conducts programs in all 50 states and the District of Columbia.
Jennifer Pferrer, Executive Director
Richard Kahn PhD, Chief Scientific/Medical Officer

3161 Diabetes Youth Foundation of Indiana
7311 Tousley Drive 317-750-9310
Indianapolis, IN 46256-9212 Fax: 317-243-4418
e-mail: dyfjulie@yahoo.com
www.dyfofindiana.org
This nonprofit group whose mission is to improve the lives of children with diabetes and their families.
Julie Shutt, Executive Director
Rick Crosslin, Camp Director

3162 Juvenile Diabetes Research Foundation: Ind iana State Chapter
8465 Keystone Crossing 317-202-0352
Indianapolis, IN 46240 Fax: 317-202-0357
e-mail: indianastate@jdrf.org
www.jdrf.org/indiana

The Juvenile Diabetes Research Foundation International (JDRF) is a charitable funder and advocate of type 1 (juvenile) diabetes research worldwide. The mission of JDRF is to find a cure for diabetes and its complications through the support of research.
Henry Rodriguez MD, Chapter President

3163 Juvenile Diabetes Research Foundation: Nor thern Indiana Chapter
2004 Ironwood Circle
South Bend, IN 46635
574-273-1810
Fax: 574-273-1870
e-mail: northernindiana@jdrf.org
www.jdrf.org
The Juvenile Diabetes Research Foundation International (JDRF) is a charitable funder and advocate of type 1 (juvenile) diabetes research worldwide. The mission of JDRF is to find a cure for diabetes and its complications through the support of research.
Arnold Donald, President/CEO Corporate
Robin Harding, EVP/Development & COO Corporate

Iowa

3164 American Diabetes Association: Cedar Rapid s District
St Luke's Resource Center
Cedar Rapids, IA 52406
319-247-5124
888-342-2383
Fax: 319-247-5125
e-mail: AskADA@diabetes.org
www.diabetes.org
The American Diabetes Association is a nonprofit health organization providing diabetes research, information and advocacy. Founded in 1940 the American Diabetes Association conducts programs in all 50 states and the District of Columbia.
Jennifer Petsche, Manager
Richard Kahn PhD, Chief Scientific/Medical Officer

3165 Juvenile Diabetes Research Foundation: Eas tern Iowa Chapter
701 10th Street SE
Cedar Rapids, IA 52403
319-393-3850
Fax: 319-393-3852
e-mail: easterniowa@jdrf.org
www.jdrf.org/easterniowa
The Juvenile Diabetes Research Foundation International (JDRF) is a charitable funder and advocate of type 1 (juvenile) diabetes research worldwide. The mission of JDRF is to find a cure for diabetes and its complications through the support of research.
Ann Elise Walsh, Special Events Manager
Mary Henry, Special Events Coordinator

3166 Juvenile Diabetes Research Foundation: Gre ater Iowa Chapter
5444 NW 96th Street
Johnston, IA 50131
515-986-1512
Fax: 515-986-1513
e-mail: greateriowa@jdif.org
www.jdrf.org/greateriowa
The Juvenile Diabetes Research Foundation International (JDRF) is a charitable funder and advocate of type 1 (juvenile) diabetes research worldwide. The mission of JDRF is to find a cure for diabetes and its complications through the support of research.
Jean Howieson, Special Events Director
Judy Greaves, Office Administrator

Kansas

3167 American Diabetes Association: Kansas
837 S Hillside
Wichita, KS 67211
316-684-6091
888-342-2383
Fax: 316-684-5675
e-mail: AskADA@diabetes.org
www.diabetes.org
The American Diabetes Association is a nonprofit health organization providing diabetes research, information and advocacy. Founded in 1940 the American Diabetes Association conducts programs in all 50 states and the District of Columbia.
Sarah Beth Webb, Director
Richard Kahn PhD, Chief Scientific/Medical Officer

Kentucky

3168 American Diabetes Association: Kentucky
161 St Matthews Avenue
Louisville, KY 40207
502-452-6072
888-342-2383
Fax: 502-893-2698
e-mail: AskADA@diabetes.org
www.diabetes.org
The American Diabetes Association is a nonprofit health organization providing diabetes research, information and advocacy. Founded in 1940 the American Diabetes Association conducts programs in all 50 states and the District of Columbia.
Samantha Carroll, Associate Director
Richard Kahn PhD, Chief Scientific/Medical Officer

3169 Juvenile Diabetes Research Foundation: Kentuckiana Chapter
133 Evergreen Road
Louisville, KY 40243
502-485-9397
866-485-9397
Fax: 502-485-9591
e-mail: kentuckiana@jdrf.org
www.jdf.org/chapters/ky/kentuckiana
The Juvenile Diabetes Research Foundation International (JDRF) is a charitable funder and advocate of type 1 (juvenile) diabetes research worldwide. The mission of JDRF is to find a cure for diabetes and its complications through the support of research.
Twynette S Davidson, Executive Director
Joe Salvagne, Chapter President

Louisiana

3170 American Diabetes Association: Louisana
2644 S Sherwood Forest Boulevard
Baton Rouge, LA 70816
225-216-3980
888-342-2383
Fax: 225-295-7005
e-mail: AskADA@diabetes.org
www.diabetes.org
Paige Grogan, Associate Manager
Lori Koonce, Associate Manager

3171 Juvenile Diabetes Research Foundation: Bat on Rouge Chapter
9457 Brookline Avenue
Baton Rouge, LA 70809
225-932-9511
Fax: 225-932-9514
e-mail: batonrouge@jdrf.org
www.jdrf.org/batonrouge
Kristy Andries, President/Development Chair
Danielle Graham, Special Events Assistant

3172 Juvenile Diabetes Research Foundation: Lou isiana Chapter
2201 Veterans Memorial Bouelvard
Metairie, LA 70002
504-828-2873
Fax: 504-828-4922
e-mail: louisiana@jdrf.org
www.jdrf.org/louisiana
Sam Robinson, President Board of Directors
Becky Spinnato, Vice President Fundraising

3173 Juvenile Diabetes Research Foundation: Shr eveport Chapter
2001 East 70th Street
Shreveport, LA 71105
318-798-1195
Fax: 318-798-1194
e-mail: jburns@jdrf.org
www.jdrf.org/shreveport
Jeff Knutson, President Board of Directors
Craig Floyd, Vice President Fundraising

Maine

3174 American Diabetes Association: Maine
80 Elm Street
Portland, ME 04101
207-774-7717
888-342-2383
Fax: 207-774-7714
e-mail: AskADA@diabetes.org
www.diabetes.org
Emily Silevinac, Associate Manager
Ryan Williams, Associate Manager

3175 **Juvenile Diabetes Research Foundation: New England/Maine Chapter**
33 Silver Street 207-761-0133
Portland, ME 04101 Fax: 207-761-1687
e-mail: maine@jdrf.org OR eburgo@jdrf.org
www.jdrf.org/maine
Heidi Daniels, New England Chapter Executive Director
Emily Hampton Burgo, Branch Manager

Maryland

3176 **American Diabetes Association: Maryland**
800 Wyman Park Drive 410-265-0075
Baltimore, MD 21211 888-342-2383
Fax: 410-235-4048
e-mail: AskADA@diabetes.org
www.diabetes.org
Kathy Rogers, Executive Director
Dotty Raynor, Director

3177 **Juvenile Diabetes Research Foundation: Mar yland Chapter**
200 East Joppa Road 410-823-0073
Towson, MD 21286 Fax: 410-823-0416
e-mail: maryland@jdrf.com
www.jdrf.org/maryland/
Rebecca Maude, Executive Director
Dotty Raynor, Outreach Manager

Massachusetts

3178 **American Diabetes Association: Boston**
330 Congress Street 617-482-4580
Boston, MA 02210 888-342-2383
Fax: 617-482-1824
e-mail: AskADA@diabetes.org
www.diabetes.org
Christopher Boynton, Executive Director
Lori Glowacki, Director of Special Events

3179 **Juvenile Diabetes Research Foundation: New England/Bay State Chapter**
20 Walnut Street 781-431-0700
Wellesley, MA 02481 Fax: 781-431-8836
e-mail: baystate@jdrf.org
www.jdrf.org/baystate
Heidi Daniels, New England Chapter Executive Director
Virginia Irving, Associate Executive Director

Michigan

3180 **American Diabetes Association: Michigan**
3940 Broadmoor Avenue SE 616-458-9341
Grand Rapids, MI 49512 888-342-2383
Fax: 616-575-9930
e-mail: AskADA@diabetes.org
www.diabetes.org
Darla Hill, Coordinator
Sharice Purman, Director

3181 **Juvenile Diabetes Research Foundation: Metropolitan Detroit/SE Michigan**
24359 Northwestern Highway 248-355-1133
Southfield, MI 48075-2020 Fax: 248-355-1188
e-mail: metrodetroit@jdrf.org
www.jdrfdetroit.org
Rita L Combest, Development Director
Susan Kossik, Development Manager

3182 **Juvenile Diabetes Research Foundation: Wes t Michigan Chapter**
5075 Cascade Road SE 616-957-1838
Grand Rapids, MI 49546 Fax: 616-957-1169
e-mail: westmichigan@jrdf.org
www.jdrf.org/westmichigan
Annette Guilfoyle, Executive Director
Maxine Gray, Special Events Coordinator

Minnesota

3183 **American Diabetes Association: Minnesota**
Parkdale Center 763-593-5333
Saint Louis Park, MN 55416 888-342-2383
Fax: 952-582-9000
e-mail: AskADA@diabetes.org
www.diabetes.org
Jenni Hargraves, Executive Director
Becky Barnett, Associate Manager

3184 **Juvenile Diabetes Research Foundation: Min nesota Chapter**
2626 East 82nd Street 952-851-0770
Bloomington, MN 55425 800-663-1860
Fax: 952-851-0766
e-mail: minnesota@jdrf.org
www.jdrf.org/minnesota
Jackie Casey, Executive Director
Angie McCarthy, Special Events Manager

Mississippi

3185 **American Diabetes Association: Mississippi**
16 Northtown Drive 601-932-1118
Jackson, MS 39211 888-342-2383
Fax: 601-932-1988
e-mail: AskADA@diabetes.org
www.diabetes.org
The nation's leading voluntary health organization providing diabetes research, information and advocacy. Our mission is to prevent and cure diabetes and to improve the lives of all people affected by diabetes.
Mary D Fortune, Executive Vice President
Stephanie J Coghlan MBA, Senior Regional Director

Missouri

3186 **American Diabetes Association: Missouri**
1944-A Sunshine 417-890-8400
Springfield, MO 65804 888-342-2383
Fax: 417-890-8484
e-mail: AskADA@diabetes.org
www.diabetes.org
Renee Paulsell, Executive Director
Jennifer Cotner-Jone, Associate Director

3187 **Juvenile Diabetes Research Foundation: St. Louis Chapter**
225 S Meramec Avenue 314-726-6778
Clayton, MO 63105 Fax: 314-726-6778
e-mail: metrostlouis@jdrf.org
www.jdrfstl.org
M Marie Davis, Executive Director
William Schmitt, Corporate Development

Montana

3188 **American Diabetes Association: Montana**
3203 3rd Avenue N 406-256-0616
Billings, MT 59101 888-342-2383
Fax: 406-896-0289
e-mail: AskADA@diabetes.org
www.diabetes.org
Trina Adams, Associate Manager

Nebraska

3189 **American Diabetes Association: Nebraska**
14216 Dayton Circle 402-571-1101
Omaha, NE 68137 888-342-2383
Fax: 402-572-8141
e-mail: AskADA@diabetes.org
www.diabetes.org
Shawn Murphy, Executive Director
Kortney Krill, Associate Manager

3190 Juvenile Diabetes Research Foundation: Lin coln Chapter
1540 S 70th Street
Lincoln, NE 68506
402-484-8300
Fax: 402-484-8302
e-mail: lincoln@jdrf.org
www.jdrf.org/lincoln

Deb Gokie, Executive Director
Maggie Pavelka, Special Events Assistant

3191 Juvenile Diabetes Research Foundation: Oma ha Council Bluffs Chapter
9202 W Dodge Road
Omaha, NE 68114
402-397-2873
Fax: 402-572-3343
e-mail: omaha@jdrf.org
www.jdrf.org/omaha

Shawn Reynolds, Executive Director
Melissa Shapiro, Special Events Coordinator

Nevada

3192 American Diabetes Association: Nevada
2785 E Desert Inn Road
Las Vegas, NV 89121
702-369-9995
888-342-2383
Fax: 702-369-3717
e-mail: AskADA@diabetes.org
www.diabetes.org

Mary Stokes, Manager
Carly Rohrer, Associate Manager

3193 Juvenile Diabetes Research Foundation: Nevada Chapter
5542 S Fort Apache Road
Las Vegas, NV 89148
702-732-4795
Fax: 702-732-1635
e-mail: nevada@jdf.org
www.jdrf.org/nevada

Stuart Mason, Nevada Chapter Co-Founder
Flora Mason, Nevada Chapter Co-Founder

3194 Juvenile Diabetes Research Foundation: Nor thern Nevada Branch
5335 Kietzke Lane
Reno, NV 89511
775-786-1881
Fax: 775-827-0131
e-mail: northernnevada@jdrf.org
www.jdrf.org/northernnevada

Molly Dillon, Branch Manager
Arnie Pitts MD, Board of Directors President

New Hampshire

3195 American Diabetes Association: New Hampshire
249 Canal Street
Manchester, NH 03101
603-627-9579
888-342-2383
Fax: 603-669-1477
www.diabetes.org

3196 Juvenile Diabetes Research Foundation: New England/New Hampshire Chapter
2 Wellman Avenue
Nashua, NH 03064
603-595-2595
Fax: 603-595-2073
e-mail: newhampshire@jdrf.org
www.jdrf.org/newhampshire

Brooke Edwards, Special Events Coordinator
Heidi Daniels, New England Chapter Executive Director

New Jersey

3197 American Diabetes Association: New Jersey
CentrePoint II Suite 103
Bridgewater, NJ 08807
732-469-7979
888-342-2383
Fax: 732-469-4887
e-mail: AskADA@diabetes.org
www.diabetes.org

James Roberts, Executive Director
Pamela Hooper, Director

3198 Juvenile Diabetes Research Foundation: South Jersey Chapter
1415 Route 70 E
Cherry Hill, NJ 08034
856-429-1101
Fax: 856-429-1105
e-mail: southjersey@jdrf.org
www.jdrf.org/southjersey

Stephen Blocher, Executive Director
Robin Berger, Special Events Coordinator

3199 Juvenile Diabetes Research Foundation: Cen tral Jersey Chapter
740 Broad Street
Shrewsbury, NJ 07702
732-219-6654
Fax: 732-219-8722
e-mail: centraljersey@jdrf.org
www.jdrf.org/chapters/NJ/Central-Jersey

Lori McLane, Executive Director
Beckie Burlew, Special Events Coordinator

3200 Juvenile Diabetes Research Foundation: Mid -Jersey Chapter
28 Kennedy Boulevard
East Brunswick, NJ 08816
732-296-7171
Fax: 732-296-1433
e-mail: midjersey@jdrf.org
www.jdrf.org/NJ/Mid-Jersey

Elizabeth Giardina Preston, Chapter Executive Director
Sandra Hilsenrath, Special Events Coordinator

3201 Juvenile Diabetes Research Foundation: Roc kland County/Northern New Jersey
560 Sylvan Avenue
Englewood Cliffs, NJ 07632
201-568-4838
Fax: 201-568-5360
e-mail: rockland@jdrf.org
www.jdrf.org/northernnj

Douglas Rouse, Executive Director
Allison Hartstone, Special Events Coordinator

New Mexico

3202 American Diabetes Association: New Mexico
2625 Pennsylvania NE
Albuquerque, NM 87110
505-266-5716
888-342-2383
Fax: 505-268-4533
e-mail: AskADA@diabetes.org
www.diabetes.org

Betsey Robinson, Associate Director
Lisa Johnson, Manager

3203 Juvenile Diabetes Research Foundation: Albuquerque
2501 San Pedro NE
Albuquerque, NM 87110
505-255-4005
Fax: 505-260-1430
e-mail: newmexico@jdrf.org
www.jdrf.org/newmexico

Joann Perrine, Branch Manager
Elizabeth Romero, Fundraising Assistant

New York

3204 American Diabetes Association: New York
Pine W Plaza Building 2
Albany, NY 12205
518-218-1755
888-342-2383
Fax: 518-218-0114
e-mail: AskADA@diabetes.org
www.diabetes.org

Amy R Young, District Director
Karen Dooley, Associate Manager

3205 Juvenile Diabetes Research Foundation Executive Office/Corporate Headquarters
Executive Office/Corporate Headquarters
120 Wall Street
New York, NY 10005-4001
212-725-4925
800-533-2873
Fax: 212-785-9595
e-mail: info@jdrf.org
www.jdrf.org/

Allan J Lewis, President/Chief Executive Officer
Amy C Franze, EVP Development

3206 Juvenile Diabetes Research Foundation: Long Island/South Shore Chapter
532 Broadhollow Road
Melville, NY 11747
631-414-1126
Fax: 631-414-1133
e-mail: longisland@jdrf.org
www.jdrf.org/longisland

Barbara Rogus, Executive Director
Christina Colandro, Special Events Manager

3207 **Juvenile Diabetes Research Foundation: Buf falo/Western New York Chapter**
331 Alberta Drive 716-833-2873
Buffalo, NY 14226 Fax: 716-833-0199
e-mail: westernny@jdrf.org
www.jdrf.org/westernny

Karen Swierski, Executive Director
Jennifer Hickok, Special Events Manager

3208 **Juvenile Diabetes Research Foundation: Hud son Valley Chapter**
Hollowbrook Office Park 845-297-8600
Wappinger Falls, NY 12590 Fax: 845-297-7887
e-mail: hudsonvalley@jdrf.org
www.letscurediabetes.com

Charlie Lawrence, Branch Manager
Linda Delia, Events Assistant

3209 **Juvenile Diabetes Research Foundation: New York Chapter**
432 Park Avenue S 212-689-2860
New York, NY 10016 Fax: 212-689-4038
e-mail: newyorkchapter@jdrf.org
www.jdrf.org/nyc

Mania Boyder, New York City Chapter Executive Director

3210 **Juvenile Diabetes Research Foundation: Nor theastern New York**
6 Greenwood Drive 518-477-2873
East Greenbush, NY 12061 Fax: 518-477-7004
e-mail: northeastny@jdrf.org
www.jdrf.org/NortheasternNY

Bev Kennedy, Executive Director
Darlene Robbiano, Special Events Manager

3211 **Juvenile Diabetes Research Foundation: Roc hester Branch/Western New York Chapter**
1200-A Scottsville Road 585-546-1390
Rochester, NY 14624 Fax: 585-546-1404
e-mail: rochester@jdrf.org
www.jdrf.org/rochester

Mary Anne Fox, Executive Director
Anne Blythe, Special Events Coordinator

3212 **Juvenile Diabetes Research Foundation: Wes tchester County Chapter**
30 Glenn Street 914-686-7700
White Plains, NY 10603 Fax: 914-686-7701
e-mail: westchester@jdrf.org
www.jdrf.org/westchester

Katherine Cintron, Executive Director
Dejan Popovich, Special Events Coordinator

North Carolina

3213 **American Diabetes Association: Eastern North Carolina**
1701 N Beauregard Street 919-743-5400
Alexandria, VA 22311 888-342-2383
Fax: 919-783-7838
e-mail: AskADA@diabetes.org
www.diabetes.org

The American Diabetes Association is the nation's leading non-profit health organization providing diabetes research, information and advocacy.
Larry Hausner, CEO
Richard Kahn PhD, Chief Scientific & Medical Officer

3214 **American Diabetes Association: North Carolina**
222 South Church Street 704-373-9111
Charlotte, NC 28202 888-342-2383
Fax: 704-373-9113
www.diabetes.org

Dianne Roth, Executive Director

3215 **Juvenile Diabetes Research Foundation: Triangle/Eastern North Carolina Chapter**
2210 Millbrook Road 919-431-8330
Raleigh, NC 27604 Fax: 919-431-8373
e-mail: triangle@jdrf.org
www.jdrftriangle.org

Jim Burson, Chapter President
Courtney Davies, Executive Director

3216 **Juvenile Diabetes Research Foundation: Cha rlotte Chapter**
9140 ArrowPoint Boulevard 704-561-0828
Charlotte, NC 28273 Fax: 704-561-9920
e-mail: charlotte@jdrf.org
www.jdrf.org/charlotte

Brenning Johnston, Volunteer Coordinator

3217 **Juvenile Diabetes Research Foundation: Pie dmont Triad Chapter**
1401-B Old Mill Circle 336-768-1027
Winston-Salem, NC 27103 Fax: 336-768-1029
e-mail: piedmont@jdrf.org
www.jdrf.org/triad

Brad Calloway, President Board of Directors
Tom Brinkley, VP Fundraising & Development

North Dakota

3218 **American Diabetes Association: Nashville**
1323 23rd Street S 701-234-0123
Fargo, ND 58103 Fax: 701-235-3080
e-mail: AskADA@diabetes.org
www.diabetes.org

Stephanie Chimeziri, Associate Director

3219 **American Diabetes Association: North Dakota**
1323 23rd Street South 701-234-0123
Fargo, ND 58103 888-342-2383
Fax: 701-235-3080
www.diabetes.org

Ohio

3220 **American Diabetes Association: Ohio**
4500 Rockside Road 216-328-9989
Independence, OH 44131 888-342-2383
Fax: 216-328-0007
e-mail: AskADA@diabetes.org
www.diabetes.org

Jill Pupa, Executive Director
Patti Clair, Associate Director

3221 **Juvenile Diabetes Research Foundation/JDRF**
1293-H Lyons Road 937-439-2873
Dayton, OH 45458 Fax: 937-439-4086
e-mail: dayton@jdrf.org
www.jdrf.org/dayton

Karen Myers, Executive Director
Vicky Williams, Office Manager

3222 **Juvenile Diabetes Research Foundation: Mid-Ohio Chapter**
950 Michigan Avenue 614-464-2873
Columbus, OH 43215 Fax: 614-464-2877
e-mail: midohio@jdrf.org
www.jdrf.org/midohio

Staci Perkins, Executive Director
Roberta Smedes, Office Manager

3223 **Juvenile Diabetes Research Foundation: Akr on/Canton Chapter**
5000 Rockside Road
Canton, OH 44131 888-718-3061
Fax: 216-328-8340
e-mail: jcallahan@jdrf.org
www.jdrf.org/chapters/OH/Northeast-Ohio

Laura E Maciag, Executive Director
Danielle Thompson, Special Events Manager

3224 **Juvenile Diabetes Research Foundation: Gre ater Cincinnati Chapter**
8041 Hosbrook Road 513-793-3223
Cincinnati, OH 45236-3830 Fax: 513-936-5333
e-mail: cincinnati@jdrf.org
www.jdrf.org/cincinnati

Bill Rice, Executive Director
Bethe Ferguson, Special Events Coordinator

3225 **Juvenile Diabetes Research Foundation: Tol edo/Northwest Ohio Chapter**
3450 W Central Avenue 419-873-1377
Toledo, OH 43606 800-533-2873
Fax: 419-720-6339
e-mail: northwestohio@jdrf.org
www.jdrf.org/northwestohio
Megan Meyer, Executive Director
Marna Cousino, Special Events Coordinator

Oklahoma

3226 **American Diabetes Association: Oklahoma**
3000 United Founders Boulevard 405-840-3881
Oklahoma City, OK 73112 888-342-2383
Fax: 405-840-3899
e-mail: AskADA@diabetes.org
www.diabetes.org
Diane Sarantakos, Executive Director
Andrea Barnett, Associate Manager

3227 **Juvenile Diabetes Research Foundation: Cen tral Oklahoma Chapter**
2601 NW Expressway 405-810-0070
Oklahoma City, OK 73112 888-533-9255
Fax: 405-810-0078
e-mail: oklahoma@jdrf.org
www.jdrf.org/centralok
Renee MacDonald, Executive Director
Shannon Scott, Special Events Coordinator

3228 **Juvenile Diabetes Research Foundation: Tul sa Green County Chapter**
4606 E 67th Street 918-481-5807
Tulsa, OK 74136 Fax: 918-481-5823
e-mail: tulsa@jdrf.org
www.jdrf.org/tulsa-green
Brandi Sullivan, Executive Director
Angela Peterson, Special Events Coordinator

Oregon

3229 **American Diabetes Association: Oregon**
2350 Oakmont Way 541-343-0735
Eugene, OR 97401 888-342-2383
Fax: 541-342-1491
e-mail: AskADA@diabetes.org
www.diabetes.org
Cynthia Benton, Associate Director

3230 **Juvenile Diabetes Research Foundation: Ore gon/SW Washington Chapter**
7460 SW Hunziker Street 503-643-1995
Portland, OR 97223 866-598-9074
Fax: 503-598-9087
e-mail: oregon-washington@jdrf.org
www.jdrf.org/oregon
Ashleigh Farleigh, Special Events Manager
Debbie Secor, Special Events Assistant

Pennsylvania

3231 **American Diabetes Association: Pennsylvania**
3544 Progress Avenue 717-657-4310
Harrisburg, PA 17110 888-342-2383
Fax: 717-657-4320
www.diabetes.org

3232 **American Diabetes Association: Western Pennsylvania**
300 Penn Center Boulevard 412-824-1181
Pittsburgh, PA 15235 888-342-2383
Fax: 412-824-2191
e-mail: AskADA@diabetes.org
www.diabetes.org
Terri Seidman, Area Manager
Steven Shivak, Executive Director

3233 **Juvenile Diabetes Research Foundation: Central Pennsylvania Chapter**
119 Aster Drive 717-901-6489
Harrisburg, PA 17112 Fax: 717-901-6573
e-mail: centralpa@jdrf.org
www.jdrf.org/centralpa
Susan Harral, Executive Director
Kate Severs, Special Events Assistant

3234 **Juvenile Diabetes Research Foundation: Ber ks County Chapter**
619 Wellington Avenue 610-775-4169
West Lawn, PA 19609
Tammy A. Edwards, Contact

3235 **Juvenile Diabetes Research Foundation: Nor thwestern Pennsylvania Chapter**
1030 State Street 814-452-0635
Erie, PA 16501 Fax: 814-452-0645
e-mail: northwestpa@jdrf.org
www.jdrf.org/northwestpa
Douglas K White, Executive Director
Amy Bement, Special Events Assistant

3236 **Juvenile Diabetes Research Foundation: Phi ladelphia Chapter**
225 City Line Avenue 610-664-9255
Bala Cynwyd, PA 19004 Fax: 610-664-9585
e-mail: philadelphia@jdrf.org
www.jdrf.org/philadelphia
Ellen Rubesin, Executive Director
Kathy Farren, Special Events Director

3237 **Juvenile Diabetes Research Foundation: Wes tern Pennsylvania**
960 Penn Avenue 412-471-1414
Pittsburgh, PA 15222 888-528-8788
Fax: 412-471-1417
e-mail: westernpa@jdrf.org
www.jdrf.org/westernpa
David R Donahue, Executive Director
Kimberly A McElroy, Office Manager

Rhode Island

3238 **American Diabetes Association: Rhode Island**
222 Richmond Street 401-351-0498
Providence, RI 02903 888-342-2383
Fax: 401-351-1674
www.jdf.org

3239 **American Diabetes Association: Richmond**
222 Richmond Street 401-351-0498
Providence, RI 02903 Fax: 401-351-1674
e-mail: AskADA@diabetes.org
www.diabetes.org
Liana Ahrens, Associate Manager
Matthew Netto, Associate Manager

South Carolina

3240 **American Diabetes Association: South Carolina**
2711 Middleburg Drive 803-799-4246
Columbia, SC 29204 888-342-2383
Fax: 803-799-5792
www.diabetes.org

3241 **American Diabetes Association: South Coast**
2711 Middleburg Drive 803-799-4246
Columbia, SC 29204 Fax: 803-799-5792
e-mail: AskADA@diabetes.org
www.diabetes.org

3242 **Juvenile Diabetes Research Foundation: Palmetto Chapter**
3608 Landmark Drive 803-782-1477
Columbia, SC 29204 Fax: 803-782-8975
e-mail: palmetto@jdrf.org
http://palmettojdrf.org
Jack Douglas, President Executive Committee
David Campbell, Vice President Executive Committee

3243 Juvenile Diabetes Research Foundation: Low Country Chapter
520 Folly Road 843-345-0369
Charleston, SC 29412 Fax: 843-406-7957
e-mail: dmenefee@jdrf.org
www.jdrf.org/lowcountry
Pam Nestor McAdams, Events/Walk Director South Coastal Chptr

South Dakota

3244 Juvenile Diabetes Research Foundation: Sio ux Falls Chapter
PO Box 88540 605-338-2295
Sioux Falls, SD 57109-8540

Tennessee

3245 American Diabetes Association: Nashville
4205 Hillsboro Road 615-298-3066
Nashville, TN 37215 888-342-2383
Fax: 615-292-5357
e-mail: AskADA@diabetes.org
www.diabetes.org
Glenda Berry, Executive Director
Harlyn Hardin, Director of Programs

3246 American Diabetes Association: Tennessee
5583 Murray Road 901-682-8232
Memphis, TN 38119 888-342-2383
Fax: 901-682-8170
e-mail: AskADA@diabetes.org
www.diabetes.org
John Carroll, Director
Daniele Cain, Coordinator

3247 Juvenile Diabetes Research Foundation: East Tennessee Chapter
6701 Baum Drive 865-544-0768
Knoxville, TN 37919 Fax: 865-544-4312
e-mail: EastTennessee@jdrf.org
www.jdf.org/chapters/tn/ecsh-tennessee

3248 Juvenile Diabetes Research Foundation: Mid dle Tennessee Chapter
2200 Hillsboro Road 615-383-6781
Nashville, TN 37212 Fax: 615-383-4284
e-mail: MidTennessee@jrdf.org
www.jdf.org/chapters/tn/middle-tennessee

Texas

3249 American Diabetes Association: Texas
4150 International Plaza 817-332-7110
Fort Worth, TX 76109 888-342-2383
Fax: 817-732-6244
www.diabetes.org

3250 Juvenile Diabetes Research Foundation: South Central Texas Chapter
8700 Crownhill Boulevrad 210-822-5336
San Antonio, TX 78209 Fax: 210-822-1443
e-mail: scentraltexas@jdrf.org
www.jdf.org

3251 Juvenile Diabetes Research Foundation: Dal las Chapter
9400 North Central Expressway 214-373-9808
Dallas, TX 75231-5063 Fax: 214-373-6337
e-mail: dallas@jrdf.org
www.jdf.org/chapters/tx/

3252 Juvenile Diabetes Research Foundation: Gre ater Fort Worth/ Arlington Chapter
550 Bailey Avenue 817-332-2601
Fort Worth, TX 76107-2127 Fax: 817-332-5641
e-mail: grfortworth@jdrf.org
www.jdf.org

3253 Juvenile Diabetes Research Foundation: Hou ston/Gulf Coast Chapter
2425 Fountain View 713-334-4400
Houston, TX 77057 Fax: 713-334-4040
e-mail: houston@jdrf.org
www.jdf.org

3254 Juvenile Diabetes Research Foundation: Wes t Texas Chapter
Clay Desta Towers, 10 Desta Drive 432-570-5643
Midland, TX 79705 Fax: 432-682-0765
e-mail: westtexas@jdrf.org
www.jdf.org

Utah

3255 American Diabetes Association: Utah
1245 E Brickyard Road 801-363-3024
Salt Lake City, UT 84106 888-342-2383
Fax: 801-363-3031
www.diabetes.org

Vermont

3256 American Diabetes Association: Vermont
1 Kennedy Drive 802-654-7716
S Burlington, VT 05403 888-342-2383
Fax: 802-658-9145
www.diabetes.org

Virginia

3257 American Diabetes Association: Richmond
4335 Cox Road 804-225-8038
Glen Allen, VA 23060 888-342-2383
Fax: 804-270-4742
www.diabetes.org

3258 American Diabetes Association: Virginia
870 Greenbrier Circle 757-424-6662
Chesapeake, VA 23320 888-342-2383
Fax: 757-420-0490
www.diabetes.org

3259 Juvenile Diabetes Research Foundation: Gre ater Blue Ridge Chapter
3959 Electric Road 540-772-1975
Roanoke, VA 24018 888-849-0510
Fax: 540-772-6672
e-mail: greaterblueridge@idrf.org
www.jdf.org

Washington

3260 American Diabetes Association: Seattle
Metropolitan Park E 206-282-4616
Seattle, WA 98101 888-342-2383
Fax: 206-903-8107
www.diabetes.org
Linda Henderson, Executive Director
Andrew Willmer, Director

3261 American Diabetes Association: Washington
1200 Sixth Avenue 509-624-7478
Spokane, WA 99204 888-342-2383
Fax: 509-624-7212
www.diabetes.org

3262 Juvenile Diabetes Research Foundation: Seattle Guild
1001 4th Avenue 206-343-0873
Seattle, WA 98154-1101 Fax: 206-343-7015

3263 Juvenile Diabetes Research Foundation: Sea ttle Chapter
1333 N Northlake Way 206-545-1510
Seattle, WA 98103-8900 Fax: 206-545-1511
www.jdf.org

3264 Juvenile Diabetes Research Foundation: Spo kane County Area Chapter
9 South Washington 509-459-6307
Spokane, WA 99201 Fax: 509-459-6392
e-mail: inlandnw@jdrf.org
Kay C Dightman, Contact

West Virginia

3265 American Diabetes Association: West Virginia
PO Box 238
Hurricane, WV 25526
304-768-2596
888-342-2383
Fax: 304-562-1887
e-mail: rahearn@diabetes.org
diabetes.org
Roberta Ahearn, Executive Director

3266 American Diabetes Association: Wisconsin
PO Box 238
Hurricane, WV 25526
304-768-2596
Fax: 304-562-1887
e-mail: rahearn@diabetes.org
www.diabetes.org
Roberta Ahearn, Executive Director

3267 Juvenile Diabetes Research Foundation: Hun tington Chapter
PO Box 2903
Huntington, WV 25728
304-525-4533

Wisconsin

3268 American Diabetes Association: Wisconsin
S Towne Office Park Building 4
Monona, WI 53713
608-222-7785
888-342-2383
Fax: 608-222-7795
e-mail: bfolco@diabetes.org
www.diabetes.org
Barb Folco, Manager
Jay Kemp, Coordinator

3269 Juvenile Diabetes Research Foundation: Southeastern Chapter
2825 North Mayfair Road
Wauwatosa, WI 53222
414-453-4673
Fax: 414-453-4919
e-mail: southeastwi@jdrf.org

3270 Juvenile Diabetes Research Foundation: Gre ater Madison Chapter
PO Box 46039
Madison, WI 53744-6039
608-836-4408

3271 Juvenile Diabetes Research Foundation: Nor theast Wisconsin Chapter
1800 Appleton Road
Menasha, WI 54952-0101
920-997-0038
Fax: 920-997-0039
e-mail: northeastwi@jdrf.org
www.jdrf.org
Julie Kersten, Executive Director
Dana Paschen, Special Events Coordinator

Libraries & Resource Centers

3272 Diabetes Control Program
California Department of Health Services
PO Box 997413
Sacramento, CA 95899-7413
916-552-9888
Fax: 916-552-9988
http://www.caldiabetes.org/
Our mission is to prevent diabetes and its complications in California's diverse communities.
Susan Lopez-Payan, Interim Chief

3273 Division of Diabetes Translation
National Center for Chronic Disease Prevention
4770 Buford Highway NE
Atlantia, GA 30341-3717
770-488-5000
Fax: 770-488-5966
e-mail: cdcinfo@cdc.gov
www.cdc.gov/diabetes
The Division of Diabetes Translation's (DDT) goal is to reduce the burden of diabetes in the United States. The division works to achieve this goal by combining support for public health-oriented diabetes prevention and control programs (DPCPs) and translating diabetes research findings into widespread clinical and public health practice.

3274 Health Science Library
Marshall University
1600 Medical Center Drive
Huntington, WV 25701
304-691-1700
www.musom.marshall.edu/library
The Health Sciences Library's primary mission is serving the informational needs of the students, faculty, and staff at Marshall University and the Cabell-Huntington Hospital. The Library also plays an important role in providing information services to hospitals and healthcare professionals in the Huntington and the Tri-State area.
Edward Dzierzak, Director

3275 Joslin Center at University of Maryland Medicine
22 S Greene Street
Baltimore, MD 21201
800-492-5538
TDD: 800735225800
e-mail: joslin@umms001.ab.umd.edu
www.umm.edu/joslindiabetes
The Joslin Center at University of Maryland Medicine meets the highest standards of care for people with diabetes. Its programs reflect a philosophy which have been the hallmark of Joslin's care — a comprehensive team approach to diabetes treatment with programs designed to help children and adults with diabetes take charge of their own health and well-being.
Thomas W Donner, MD, Director

3276 Naomi Berrie Diabetes Center at Columbia University Medical Center
Russ Berrie Medical Science Pavillion
1150 St. Nicholas Avenue
New York, NY 10032
212-851-5494
Fax: 212-851-5459
e-mail: diabetes@columbia.edu
nbdiabetes.org
The special focus of the Naomi Berrie Diabetes Center is on families — a concept that differentiates it from almost every other diabetes treatment facility in America. People with diabetes are strongly encouraged to involve their entire families in the treatment process.
Robin Goland, MD, Co-Director
Rudolph Liebel, MD, Co-Director

3277 National Diabetes Information Clearinghouse
One Information Way
Bethesda, MD 20892-3560
800-860-8747
Fax: 703-738-4929
e-mail: ndic@info.niddk.nih.gov
diabetes.niddk.nih.gov
To serve as a diabetes informational, educational, and referral resource for health professionals and the public. NDIC is a service of the NIDDK.

3278 Schulze Diabetes Institute
University of Minnesota
420 Delaware Street SE
Minneapolis, MN 55455
612-626-3016
e-mail: diitinfo@umn.edu
www.med.umn.edu
Formerly the Diabetes Institute for Immunology and Transplantation
David Sutherland MD, PhD, Director
Bernard Hering MD, Director

3279 Tallahassee Memorial Diabetes Center
Tallahassee Memorial Health Care
1981-2 Capital Circle NE
Tallahassee, FL 32308
850-431-5404
800-662-4278
Fax: 850-431-6325
www.tmh.org/diabetes
TMH provides comprehensive, patient-centered services to both children and adults. The Diabetes Center uses a team approach that involves the patient, physicians, nurse educators, registered dietitians with access to a diabetes counselor and registered pharmacists and social worker.
Richard M Bergenstal, MD, Medical Director

Research Centers

3280 Barbara Davis Center for Childhood Diabetes
1775 Aurora Street
Aurora, CO 80045-6511
303-724-2323
Fax: 303-724-6839
e-mail: george.eisenbarth@uchsc.edu
www.uchsc.edu/misc/diabetes

Research and educational organization.
Marian Rewers, Clinical Director
George S Eisenbarth, Executive Director

3281 **Baylor College of Medicine: Children's General Clinical Research Center**
One Baylor Plaza 713-798-4780
Houston, TX 77030 Fax: 713-790-1345
e-mail: pedi-webmaster@bcm.edu
www.bcm.edu/pediatrics
Offers research into juvenile aspects of immunology and infectious diseases including diabetes research activities.
Lisa Bomgaars, Medical Director
Dennis M Bier, Program Director

3282 **Benaroya Research Institute Virginia Mason Medical Center**
Virginia Mason Medical Center
1201 9th Avenue 206-583-6525
Seattle, WA 98101-2795 Fax: 206-223-7543
e-mail: info@benaroyaresearch.org
www.benaroyaresearch.org
Immunology and diabetes research.
Robert B Lemon, Chair
Gerald Nepom, Director

3283 **Diabetes Education and Research Center The Franklin House**
The Franklin House
PO Box 897 215-829-3426
Philadelphia, PA 19105 Fax: 215-829-5807
e-mail: webmaster@dibeteseducationandresearchcen
www.diabeteseducationandresearchcenter.o
Is a non-profit organization serving the needs of people living in Philadelphia PA and surrounding communities. The goal of the Foundation is to improve the health of people with diabetes.

3284 **Diabetes Research and Training Center: University of Alabama at Birmingham**
Department of Medicine
1530 3rd Avenue S 205-996-7433
Birmingham, AL 35294-0001 Fax: 205-934-4389
www.main.uab.edu/Sites/drtc/
The DRTC works to develop and evaluate new models of diabetes care and to facilitate translational diabetes research.
Jeffrey Kudlow, Director
Hussein Abdullatif, Associate Professor

3285 **Division on Endocrinology Northwestern University Feinberg School**
Northwestern University Feinberg School of Medicin
303 E Chicago Avenue 312-503-0340
Chicago, IL 60611 Fax: 312-503-7757
e-mail: help@medicine.northwestern.edu
www.medicine.northwestern.edu
Nonprofit organization focusing research activities on endocrinology metabolism nutrition and specializing in diabetes.
Andrea Dunaif, Professor Division of Endocrinology
J Larry Jameson, Professor Division of Endocrinology

3286 **Endocrinology Research Laboratory Cabrini Medical Center**
Cabrini Medical Center
227 E 19th Street 212-222-7464
New York, NY 10003-7457 e-mail: info@cabrininty.org
www.cabrininy.org
Focuses on the effects of insulin and insulin-like growth factors on human body functions.
Dr Leonid Poretsky, Director

3287 **Indiana University: Area Health Education Center**
1110 W Michigan Street 317-278-8893
Indianapolis, IN 46202 Fax: 317-274-4444
e-mail: ahec@iupui.edu
www.ahec.iupui.edu
A collaborative statewide system for community-based primary health care professions education that fosters the continuing improvement of health care services for all citizens in Indiana.
Richard D Kiovsky, Director
Jonathan C Barclay, Associate Director

3288 **Indiana University: Center for Diabetes Research**
545 Barnhill Drive 317-274-8438
Indianapolis, IN 46202-5111 Fax: 317-274-1437
e-mail: rconsidi@iupui.edu
www.medicine.iu.edu/body.cfm?id=4472&oTo
Our goal is to promote the training of scientists whose research will develop new understandings of the basis of the disease and its complications and to cultivate basic science research that can speed the discovery of more effective therapies.
Robert Considine, Associate Professor of Medicine
Michael J Econs, Division Chief

3289 **Indiana University: Pharmacology Research Laboratory**
Division of Clinical Pharmacology
1001 W 10th Street 317-630-8795
Indianapolis, IN 46202 Fax: 317-630-8185
e-mail: tamllewi@iupui.edu
www.medicine.iupui.edu/clinpharm
We will train highly skilled compassionate and altruistic professionals both generalists and specialists to be future leaders in medical practice academia and industry.
David A Flockhart, Division Director
John T Callaghan, Associate Professor of Medicine

3290 **International Diabetes Center at Nicollet**
3800 Park Nicollet Boulevard 952-993-3393
Saint Louis Park, MN 55416-2533 888-825-6315
Fax: 952-993-1302
e-mail: idcdiabetes@parknicollet.com
www.parknicollet.com/diabetes
Research center which improves the quality of life of individuals with diabetes and those at risk of developing diabetes by undertaking clinical care education research and outreach activities that stimulate and support health.
Richard Berg MD, Executive Director

3291 **Joslin Diabetes Center**
One Joslin Place 617-732-2400
Boston, MA 02215-5306 800-567-5461
Fax: 617-322-40
e-mail: diabetes@joslin.harvard.edu
www.joslin.org
An internationally recognized leader in diabetes and endocrine disease treatment research and patient and professional education affiliated with Harvard Medical School. In addition to its headquarters in Boston's Longwood Medical area Joslin has affiliated treatment centers across the nation. Established in 1898.
C Ronald Kahn, Board of Trustee
Ranch C Kimball, President and CEO Joslin Diabetes Cente

3292 **Metabolic Research Institute**
1515 N Flagler Drive 561-802-3060
West Palm Beach, FL 33401 Fax: 561-802-3260
e-mail: moreinformation@metabolic-institute.com
www.metabolic-institute.com
The Metabolic Research Institute specializes in clinical studies involving endocrinology disorders complications of endocrinology disorders metabolic problems and selected renal disease.
William A Kaye, Co-Director
Barry Horowitz, Co-Director

3293 **Sansum Diabetes Research Institute**
2219 Bath Street 805-682-7638
Santa Barbara, CA 93105-4321 Fax: 805-682-3332
e-mail: info@sansum.org
www.sansum.org
A research institute devoted to the prevention treatment and cure of diabetes.
Lois Jovanovich, CEO & Chief Scientific Officer of Sansum
Wendy Bevier, Associate Investigator

3294 **University of Chicago: Comprehensive Diabetes Center**
5841 S Maryland Avenue 773-702-2371
Chicago, IL 60637 800-989-6740
e-mail: diabetes@uchospitals.edu
www.kovlerdiabetescenter.org
The University of Chicago Kovler Diabetes Center offers a unique fully comprehensive approach to diagnosing and treating diabetes.

Focuses on children adolescents and adults with diabetes as well as individuals at the highest risk for serious complications.
Louis H Philipson, Medical Director
Elizabeth Littlejohn, Kovler Diabetes Center Pediatric Program

3295 **University of Colorado: General Clinical Research Center, Pediatric**
13123 E 16th Avenue — 720-777-2957
Aurora, CO 80045 — Fax: 72- 77- 727
e-mail: CTRCAdmin@tchden.org
www.uchsc.edu/pedsgcrc
Focuses on developmental studies and diabetes research.
Ronald J Sokol, Program Director
Philip S Zeitler, Associate Program Director

3296 **University of Iowa: Diabetes Research Center**
Department of Internal Medicine
200 Hawkins Drive
Iowa City, IA 52242 — 319-353-7842
www.int-med.uiowa.edu/research/DRC.htm
The Diabetes Research Center combines the talents of experienced clinical investigators molecular biologists and vascular physiologists in an integrated multidisciplinary approach toward the study and treatment of abnormalities of vascular reactivity which characterize diabetes mellitus.
Ken Kates, Associate Vice President and Chief Execu
John Swenning, Associate Director

3297 **University of Kansas Cray Diabtetes Center**
3901 Rainbow Boulevard — 913-588-5000
Kansas City, KS 66160-7376 — Fax: 913-588-4023
TTY: 913-588-7963
e-mail: geaks@kumc.edu
www.kumc.edu
The KU Medical Center is a complex institution whose basic functions include research education patient care and community service involving multiple constituencies at state and national levels.
Timothy Kestermont, Division of Clinical Research Administra
Ben Duncan, Internal Medicine

3298 **University of Massachusetts: Diabetes and Endocrinology Research Center**
55 Lake Avenue N — 508-856-8989
Worcester, MA 01655 — e-mail: evelyn.vignola@umassmed.edu
www.umassmed.edu
UMMS has exploded onto the national scene as a major center for research, and in the past four decades, UMMS researchers have made pivotal advances in HIV, cancer, diabetes, infectious disease and in understanding the molecular basis of disease.
Aldo Rossini MD, Professor
Michael P Czech PhD, Professor and Chair

3299 **University of Miami: Diabetes Research Institute**
1450 NW 10th Avenue — 305-243-5300
Miami, FL 33136 — Fax: 954-964-7036
e-mail: info@drif.org
www.diabetesresearch.org
The Diabetes Research Institute (DRI) is an innovator in many fields of diabetes research but one of its primary strengths lies in islet cell transplantation, a cellular therapy that restores insulin production to normalize blood sugar control.
Hirohito Ich MD, Researcher
Camillo Ricordi, DRI Scientific Director

3300 **University of New Mexico General Clinical Research Center**
University of New Mexico Hospital
The University of New Mexico — 505-277-0111
Albuquerque, NM 87131-2240 — Fax: 505-272-0266
e-mail: mburge@salud.unm.edu
hsc.unm.edu/som/gcrc
Diabetes research.
Mark Burge MD, GCRC Program Director
Mark Schuyle MD, Associate Program Director

3301 **University of Pennsylvania Diabetes and Endocrinology Research Center**
700 Clinical Research Building (CRB — 215-898-4365
Philadelphia, PA 19104 — Fax: 215-898-5408
e-mail: neavesst@mail.upenn.edu
www.med.upenn.edu/idom/derc
The Penn Diabetes and Endocrinology Research Center (DERC) participates in the nationwide inter-disciplinary program established over two decades ago by the NIDDK to foster research and training in the areas of diabetes and related endocrine and metabolic disorders.
Elizabeth Ne Straw, DERC Administrative Coordinator
Heather Yavil, DERC Coordinator

3302 **University of Pittsburgh: Department of Molecular Genetics and Biochemistry**
200 Lothrop Street — 412-648-9570
Pittsburgh, PA 15261 — Fax: 412-624-8997
e-mail: info@mmg.pitt.edu
www.mgb.pitt.edu
MMG students and fellows routinely publish their research in outstanding journals, present their science at international conferences and go on to achieve positions at prestigious laboratories and institutions.
J Richard Chaillet, Associate Professor
Bruce A McClane, Professor

3303 **University of Tennessee: General Clinical Research Center**
1265 Union Avenue — 901-516-2212
Memphis, TN 38104 — Fax: 901-516-7013
e-mail: bsalpert@utmem.edu
www.utmem.edu/crc
Congress directed the National Institutes of Health to establish clinical research centers throughout the United States to launch an all-out attack on human diseases.
Bruce S Alpert MD, Program Director
Teresa Carr, Research Nurses

3304 **University of Texas General Clinical Research Center**
7400 Merton Minter Boulevard — 409-772-1950
San Antonio, TX 78229 — Fax: 409-772-8097
e-mail: public.affairs@utmb.edu
www.utmb.edu/gcrc
Focuses on diabetes and infectious disease research.
Michael Lich MD, Program Director
Garland D Anderson, Principal Investigator

3305 **University of Washington Diabetes: Endocrinology Research Center**
DVA Puget Sound Health Care System
1660 S Columbian Way — 206-616-4860
Seattle, WA 98108 — Fax: 206-764-2693
e-mail: derc@u.washington.edu
www.depts.washington.edu/diabetes
The primary purpose of the DERC is to facilitate and enhance the diabetes-related research of approximately 100 Affiliate Investigators at the University of Washington
Jerry P Palmer MD, Director
David E Cummings MD, Deputy Director and Associate Director f

3306 **Vanderbilt University Diabetes Center**
707 Light Hall — 615-322-7004
Nashville, TN 37232-0615 — Fax: 615-936-1667
e-mail: dc.brown@vanderbilt.edu
www.mc.vanderbilt.edu/diabetes/vdc
The Vanderbilt Diabetes Center provides complete care for children and adults with diabetes under one roof
Joe C Davis, Chair in Biomedical Sciences
Alvin C Powers, Director Vanderbilt Diabetes Center

3307 **Veterans Affairs Medical Center: Research Service**
500 Foothill Drive — 801-582-1565
Salt Lake City, UT 84148 — Fax: 801-584-1289
www.va.gov
Diabetes and cancer research.
James Floyd, Director
Byron Bair, Director

3308 **Warren Grant Magnuson Clinical Center**
National Institute of Health
9000 Rockville Pike
Bethesda, MD 20892 — 800-411-1222
Fax: 301-480-9793
TTY: 866-411-1010
e-mail: prpl@mail.cc.nih.gov
www.clinicalcenter.nih.gov

Established in 1953 as the research hospital of the National Institutes of Health. Designed so that patient care facilities are close to research laboratories so new findings of basic and clinical scientists can be quickly applied to the treatment of patients. Upon referral by physicians, patients are admitted to NIH clinical studies.
John Gallin, Director
David Henderson, Deputy Director for Clinical Care

3309 **Washington University: Diabetes Research and Training Center**
School of Medicine
660 S Euclid Avenue 314-362-0558
Saint Louis, MO 63110 Fax: 314-747-2692
e-mail: apermutt@wustl.edu
drtc.im.wustl.edu
DRTC investigators were involved in conducting 60 investigator-initiated diabetes-related clinical research protocols on the WU GCRC
M Alan Permutt MD, Professor of Medicine
Kristin E Mondy MD, Medicine/Infectious Diseases

Support Groups & Hotlines

3310 **American Diabetes Association National Center**
1701 N Beauregard Street
Alexandria, VA 22311 800-342-2383
Fax: 703-549-6995
www.diabetes.org
Lawrence T Smith, Chairman of the Board
Robert A Rizza, President

3311 **Diabetes Society of Santa Clara Valley**
1165 Lincoln Avenue 408-287-3785
San Jose, CA 95125 Fax: 408-287-2701
e-mail: ruth@diabetesscv.org
www.diabetesscv.org
The Diabetes Society was organized in 1963 as the result of efforts by a group of mothers of children with diabetes. Today, the Diabetes Society offers its services to the estimated 140,000 people with diabetes in the Santa Clara Valley.
Bernie Blegen, Board President
Douglas Metz Ph.D, Executive Director

3312 **Juvenile Diabetes International Hotline**
120 Wall Street
New York, NY 10005 800-533-2873
Fax: 212-785-9595
e-mail: info@jdrs.org
www.jdf.org
Gary Fiet, Manager Public Information

3313 **National Health Information Center**
PO Box 1133 310-565-4167
Washington, DC 20013 800-336-4797
Fax: 301-984-4256
e-mail: info@nhic.org
www.health.gov/nhic
Offers a nationwide information referral service, produces directories and resource guides.

Books

3314 **101 Tips for Improving Your Blood Sugar**
American Diabetes Association
1660 Duke Street
Alexandria, VA 22314-3447 800-232-3472
Fax: 703-549-6995
www.diabetes.org
Tips for 101 common situations and questions to reduce the risk of complications from blood sugar at the wrong level.
122 pages

3315 **Balance Your Act: A Book for Adults with Diabetes**
Pritchett & Hull
3440 Oakcliff Road
Atlanta, GA 30340-3079 800-774-1124
1993 96 pages Paperback
ISBN: 0-939838-14-1

3316 **Buyer's Guide**
American Diabetes Association
1660 Duke Street
Alexandria, VA 22314-3447 800-232-3472
Fax: 703-549-6995
www.diabetes.org
A catalog listing all manufacturers of insulin, syringes, pumps, test strips, monitors and more.

3317 **Caring for the Diabetic Soul**
American Diabetes Association
1660 Duke Street
Alexandria, VA 22314-3447 800-232-3472
Fax: 703-549-6995
www.diabetes.org
Restoring emotional balance for yourself and your family.
213 pages

3318 **Clinical Practice Recommendations**
American Diabetes Association
1660 Duke Street
Alexandria, VA 22314-3447 800-232-3472
Fax: 703-549-6995
www.diabetes.org
Features all current position and consensus statements of the American Diabetes Association.

3319 **Complete Weight Loss Workbook**
American Diabetes Association
1660 Duke Street
Alexandria, VA 22314-3447 800-232-3472
Fax: 703-549-6995
www.diabetes.org
A unique, brisk, practical workbook that offers a series of fresh, memorable tests, checklists, worksheets, mini-cases, calculation exercises, mental reminders, and other practical aids to losing weight and staying fit for good.
252 pages

3320 **Computer Planned Menus for Health Professionals**
American Diabetes Association
1660 Duke Street
Alexandria, VA 22314-3447 800-232-3472
Fax: 703-549-6995
www.diabetes.org
Input a patient's dietary prescription, food preferences, and budget, and the program produces individualized menus. Professional version includes license to distribute these customized menus.

3321 **Control Diabetes the Easy Way**
Random House Trade Books
400 Hahn Road
Westminster, MD 21157-4663 800-733-3000
Fax: 800-659-2436
ISBN: 0-679778-03-9

3322 **Convenience Food Facts**
American Diabetes Association
1660 Duke Street
Alexandria, VA 22314-3447 800-232-3472
Fax: 703-549-6995
www.diabetes.org
Helps to serve appetizing convenience foods low in sodium, cholesterol, and fat.
459 pages Softcover

3323 **Cooking a la Heart**
American Diabetes Association
1660 Duke Street
Alexandria, VA 22314-3447 800-232-3472
Fax: 703-549-6995
www.diabetes.org
Recipes that include a complete nutrient profile with diabetic exchanges.

3324 **Diabetes & Pregnancy: What to Expect**
American Diabetes Association

1660 Duke Street
Alexandria, VA 22314-3447
800-232-3472
Fax: 703-549-6995
www.diabetes.org

Information concerning an unborn baby's development, tests to expect, labor and delivery, birth control, and more.

3325 **Diabetes A to Z**
American Diabetes Association
1660 Duke Street
Alexandria, VA 22314-3447
800-232-3472
Fax: 703-549-6995
www.diabetes.org

Dictionary-style guidebook discussing basic terms and issues concerning diabetes. Third edition.
202 pages

3326 **Diabetes Care Made Easy**
Chronimed Publishing
PO Box 59032
Minneapolis, MN 55459-0032
612-513-6475
800-848-2793
Fax: 612-443-2806

Written and designed for both adults and for children with limited reading skills, this easy-to-read book explains how to exercise and eat for better health, prevent foot problems, test blood sugar, cope with emotions, take insulin, and more. Also available in Spanish.
180 pages Paperback
ISBN: 1-885115-31-8

3327 **Diabetes Education Goals**
American Diabetes Association
1660 Duke Street
Alexandria, VA 22314-3447
800-232-3472
Fax: 703-549-6995
www.diabetes.org

Features advice on how to assess, plan, and evaluate patient education and counseling programs. Covers both short-term and in-depth goals. Focuses on the education process and assessing the unique needs of each patient.
64 pages Softcover

3328 **Diabetes Low-Fat & No-Fat Meals in Minutes**
John Wiley and Sons, Inc.
Customer Service-Consumer Accounts
Indianapolis, IN 46256
877-762-2974
Fax: 800-597-3299
e-mail: consumers@wiley.com
www.wiley.com

Includes more than 250 recipes, 60 days of diabetic menus, and 16 pages of full-color photographs. Each recipe features a complete nutrition analysis, including diabetic exchanges.
1998 352 pages
ISBN: 1-565610-84-9

3329 **Diabetes Medical Nutrition Therapy**
American Diabetes Association
1660 Duke Street
Alexandria, VA 22314-3447
800-232-3472
Fax: 703-549-6995
www.diabetes.org

A professional guide to management and nutrition education resources. Provides in-depth coverage of nutrition assessment, goal setting, intervention, and outcome evaluation. Information is provided on specific resources and case studies are cited for practical examples.
Softcover

3330 **Diabetes Mellitus: A Practical Handbook**
Bull Publishing Company
PO Box 1377
Boulder, CO 80306
800-676-2855
Fax: 303-545-6354
www.bullpub.com

This helpful and user friendly practical guide adresses the everyday concerns of all diabetics.
2002 Paperback
ISBN: 0-923521-72-0

3331 **Diabetes Self-Management**
RA Rapaport Publishing
150 W 22nd Street
New York, NY 10011-2421
212-989-0200
800-234-0923
Fax: 212-989-4786
e-mail: editor@diabetes-self-mgmt-com

Publishes practical, how to information, focusing on the day-to-day and long term aspects of diabetes in a positive and upbeat style. Gives subscribers up-to-date news, facts and advice to help them maintain their wellness and make informed decisions regarding their health.
Ingird Strauch, Executive
Richard A. Rapaport, Publisher

3332 **Diabetes Sourcebook**
Dawn D Matthews, author
Omnigraphics
615 Griswold
Detroit, MI 48226-4105
313-961-1340
800-234-1340
Fax: 800-875-1340
www.omnigraphics.com

This Sourcebook contains information for people seeking to understand the risk factors, complications, and management of the different types of diabetes. It includes information about testing, diagnosis, medications, and other topics related to living with diabetes.
2003 622 pages
ISBN: 0-780806-29-8

3333 **Diabetes Teaching Guide for People Who Use Insulin**
Joslin Diabetes Center
1 Joslin Place
Boston, MA 02215-5306
617-732-2400
Fax: 617-732-2562
e-mail: diabetes@joslin.harvard.edu
www.joslin.org

Discusses the causes of diabetes, the role of diet and exercise, meal planning and complications. Also provide information on drawing blood, mixing and injecting insulin.

3334 **Diabetes Youth Curriculum: A Toolbox for Educators**
Chronimed Publishing
PO Box 59032
Minneapolis, MN 55459-0032
612-513-6475
800-848-2793
Fax: 612-443-2806

Program consisting of two volumes: the Curriculum and the Resource and Activities Guide (listed separately). Divided into sections dealing with general development concepts and specific guidelines for ages 6 to 8, 9 to 11, and 12 to 16.
136 pages Paperback
ISBN: 0-937721-49-2

3335 **Diabetes: A Guide to Living Well**
American Diabetes Association
7 Washington Square
Albany, NY 12205
518-218-1755
888-342-2383
Fax: 518-218-0114
e-mail: ADAorders@pbd.com
www.diabetes.org

Offers a guide to helping the person with diabetes design a program of individualized self-care and gain the willingness to follow it. Also tells how to deal with diet, exercise, stress, emotions, negative beliefs, and self-image.
242 pages Paperback
ISBN: 1-580402-09-7

3336 **Diabetes: Your Complete Exercise Guide**
Human Kinetics Publishers
PO Box 5076
Champaign, IL 61825-5076
217-351-1549
800-747-4457
Fax: 217-351-5076

Part of the Cooper Clinic and Research Institute Fitness Series providing exercise rehabilitation for persons with diabetes.
144 pages Paperback
ISBN: 0-873224-27-2

3337 **Diabetes: Your Questions Answered**
Paul Drury and Wendy Gatling, author
Elsevier

Book Customer Service Department
St. Louis, MO 63146 800-545-2522
Fax: 800-535-9935
e-mail: usbkinfo@elsevier.com
www.elsevier.com

This new volume in the popular "Your Questions Answered" series uses a question-and-answer format to provide easy access to hands-on guidance on the management of diabetes. Its succinct, practical coverage explores the latest evidence-based practice guilines and their interpretation. Case vignettes illustrate the clinical relevance of the material.
2004 380 pages Softcover
ISBN: 0-443073-89-9

3338 **Diabetic Gourmet**
Diabetes Self-Management Books
PO Box 10676
Des Moines, IA 50336-0676 800-664-9269

3339 **Diabetic's Guide to Health and Fitness**
Human Kinetics Publishers
PO Box 5076 217-351-1549
Champaign, IL 61825-5076 800-747-4457
Fax: 217-351-5076

272 pages Paperback
ISBN: 0-880113-47-2

3340 **Direct and Indirect Costs of Diabetes in the US**
American Diabetes Association
1660 Duke Street
Alexandria, VA 22314-3447 800-232-3472
Fax: 703-549-6995
www.diabetes.org

Examines the specific costs of diabetes, as well as all the costs of health care for people with diabetes and compares those costs with the total cost of health care for the US population without diabetes.
32 pages Softcover

3341 **Dr. Bernstein's Diabetes Solution**
Richard K Bernstein, MD, author
Little, Brown and Company
Publicity Department
New York, NY 10020 800-759-0190
e-mail: publicity@littlebrown.com
www.hachettebookgroupusa.com

A complete guide to achieving normal blood sugars with strong emphasis on diet and up-to-date information on products, insulins, and oral agents.
512 pages Hardcover
ISBN: 0-316099-06-6

3342 **Easy & Elegant Entrees**
American Diabetes Association
1660 Duke Street
Alexandria, VA 22314-3447 800-232-3472
Fax: 703-549-6995
www.diabetes.org

Recipes that are low in fat and calories.

3343 **Exchanges for All Occasions**
American Diabetes Association
1660 Duke Street
Alexandria, VA 22314-3447 800-232-3472
Fax: 703-549-6995
www.diabetes.org

Meal planning suggestions for traveling, entertaining, camping, dining out, and more.

3344 **Family Cookbook: Volumes I-IV**
American Diabetes Association
1660 Duke Street
Alexandria, VA 22314-3447 800-232-3472
Fax: 703-549-6995
www.diabetes.org

Unforgettable recipes for the whole family. Great for diabetics.

3345 **Fitness Book: For People with Diabetes**
American Diabetes Association
1660 Duke Street
Alexandria, VA 22314-3447 800-232-3472
Fax: 703-549-6995
www.diabetes.org

Advice on learning to exercise to lose weight, exercise safely, increase your competitive edge, get your mind and body ready to exercise, and more.
149 pages

3346 **Great Starts & Fine Finishes**
American Diabetes Association
1660 Duke Street
Alexandria, VA 22314-3447 800-232-3472
Fax: 703-549-6995
www.diabetes.org

Healthy select cookbook offering great meals in minutes.

3347 **Healthy Eater's Guide to Family & Chain Restaurants**
American Diabetes Association
1660 Duke Street
Alexandria, VA 22314-3447 800-232-3472
Fax: 703-549-6995
www.diabetes.org

Advice on safe choices from fast-food menus, complete with nutrition values and exchanges.

3348 **Healthy Homestyle Cookbook**
American Diabetes Association
1660 Duke Street
Alexandria, VA 22314-3447 800-232-3472
Fax: 703-549-6995
www.diabetes.org

Lay-flat binding for hands-free reference.
181 pages

3349 **How to Cook for People with Diabetes**
American Diabetes Association
1660 Duke Street
Alexandria, VA 22314-3447 800-232-3472
Fax: 703-549-6995
www.diabetes.org

One hundred and fifty recipes featuring unusual techniques.
205 pages

3350 **If Your Child Has Diabetes: An Answer Book for Parents**
Putnam Publishing Group
200 Madison Avenue 212-951-8400
New York, NY 10016-3903

Provides information and recommendations for parents of children with diabetes on subjects such as school, recreation, medical and life insurance and employment as well as general information about diabetes.

3351 **Intensified Insulin Management for You**
Chronimed Publishing
PO Box 59032 612-513-6475
Minneapolis, MN 55459-0032 800-848-2793
Fax: 612-443-2806

Manual helping those with diabetes to understand and use an intensified insulin regimen under the guidance of their health care provider. A personalized program for advanced diabetes self-care that focuses on emotional and intellectual goals as well as on how diet and exercise fit into an intensified regimen.
85 pages Paperback
ISBN: 0-937721-84-0

3352 **Intensive Diabetes Management**
American Diabetes Association
1660 Duke Street
Alexandria, VA 22314-3447 800-232-3472
Fax: 703-549-6995
www.diabetes.org

Delivers practical advice on how to help your patients achieve better glucose control through intensified management.
128 pages Softcover

3353 **Learning to Live Well with Diabetes**
Chronimed Publishing
PO Box 59032 612-513-6475
Minneapolis, MN 55459-0032 800-848-2793
Fax: 612-443-2806

Updated and revised edition reflects the latest medical advances, technologies, and research. In straight-forward language, it explains how to take charge of your diabetes and live an active, healthy life.
525 pages Paperback
ISBN: 0-937721-79-4

3354 **Life with Diabetes: A Series of Teaching Outlines**
American Diabetes Association
1660 Duke Street
Alexandria, VA 22314-3447 800-232-3472
Fax: 703-549-6995
www.diabetes.org
Presents a comprehensive curriculum for diabetes education. Each outline includes a statement of purpose, prerequisites for attending the session, materials needed for teaching the session, recommended teaching method, a content outline, instructor notes, an evaluation and documentation plan, and suggested readings related to each topic.

3355 **Managing Type II Diabetes**
Chronimed Publishing
PO Box 59032 612-513-6475
Minneapolis, MN 55459-0032 800-848-2793
Fax: 612-443-2806
Revised and updated guide for people with Type II diabetes. Offers the latest medical advances and practical advice. Includes tips on dealing with emotions, finding motivation to manage diabetes, preventing and treating complications, monitoring blood glucose, and more.
192 pages Paperback
ISBN: 1-885115-26-1

3356 **Managing Your Gestational Diabetes**
Chronimed Publishing
PO Box 59032 612-513-6475
Minneapolis, MN 55459-0032 800-848-2793
Fax: 612-443-2806
Gives answers to questions on weight gain, injecting insulin, and preventing complications.
128 pages Paperback
ISBN: 1-565610-52-0

3357 **Manual of Pediatric Nutrition**
Kristy Hendricks RD, MS, ScD (Editor), author
B.C Decker, Inc.
50 King Street E, Floor 2 PO Box620 905-522-7017
Ontario, Canada L8N 3K7, 800-568-7281
Fax: 905-522-7839
e-mail: info@bcdecker.com
www.bcdecker.com
A comprehensive guide that provides an overview of nutritional care for both healthy and ill pediatric patients.
2005 500 pages
ISBN: 1-550093-08-8

3358 **Maximizing the Role of Nutrition in Diabetes Management**
American Diabetes Association
1660 Duke Street
Alexandria, VA 22314-3447 800-232-3472
Fax: 703-549-6995
www.diabetes.org
Integrates medical, nutritional, and behavioral sciences and recognizes the importance of each in total diabetes care.
64 pages Softcover

3359 **Medical Management of Pregnancy Complicated by Diabetes**
American Diabetes Association
1660 Duke Street
Alexandria, VA 22314-3447 800-232-3472
Fax: 703-549-6995
www.diabetes.org
Information on every aspect of pregnancy and diabetes, providing precise protocols for treatment. Techniques for managing blood glucose levels from the time of conception through every stage of pregnancy.
136 pages Softcover

3360 **Medical Management of Type I Diabetes**
American Diabetes Association
1660 Duke Street
Alexandria, VA 22314-3447 800-232-3472
Fax: 703-549-6995
www.diabetes.org
Instruction on all issues impacting patients with Type 1 diabetes, including: blood glucose regulation, nutrition, exercise, blood pressure, blood lipid levels, and other key elements.
176 pages Softcover

3361 **Medical Management of Type II Diabetes**
American Diabetes Association
1660 Duke Street
Alexandria, VA 22314-3447 800-232-3472
Fax: 703-549-6995
www.diabetes.org
Complete overview of Type II diabetes, including diagnosis and classification, pathogenesis, and prevention/treatment of complications.
112 pages Softcover

3362 **Month of Meals Set of 5**
American Diabetes Association
1660 Duke Street
Alexandria, VA 22314-3447 800-232-3472
Fax: 703-549-6995
www.diabetes.org
Each planner offers twenty-eight day's worth of tasty selections including a holiday planner, ethnic meals, fast foods, meat and potatoes, and vegetarian dishes. Available individually.
5 planners

3363 **Outsmarting Diabetes**
Richard S Beaser, author
John Wiley and Sons, Inc.
Customer Service-Consumer Accounts
Indianapolis, IN 46256 877-762-2974
Fax: 800-597-3299
e-mail: consumers@wiley.com
www.wiley.com
Shows how intensive control can dramatically reduce the effects of insulin-dependent diabetes and the risk of long-term complications.
256 pages Paperback
ISBN: 0-471346-94-4

3364 **Pumping Insulin**
John Walsh PA, CDE and Ruth Roberts, MA, author
Torrey Pines Publishing
The Diabetes Mall 619-497-0900
San Diego, CA 92103 800-988-4772
Fax: 619-497-0900
www.diabetesnet.com
Features information for achieving excellent blood sugar control, correcting pump problems quickly, and lowering risks for complications.
322 pages Paperback

3365 **Quick and Easy Meals and Menus**
Diabetes Self-Management Books
PO Box 11066
Des Moines, IA 50380-0001 800-664-9269

3366 **Quick and Healthy Recipes & Ideas**
American Diabetes Association
1660 Duke Street
Alexandria, VA 22314-3447 800-232-3472
Fax: 703-549-6995
www.diabetes.org
More than 190 recipes with complete nutrition information for each.

3367 **Quick and Hearty Main Dishes**
American Diabetes Association
1660 Duke Street
Alexandria, VA 22314-3447 800-232-3472
Fax: 703-549-6995
www.diabetes.org
Offers recipes for main courses.

3368 Raising a Child with Diabetes: A Guide for Parents
American Diabetes Association
1660 Duke Street
Alexandria, VA 22314-3447
800-232-3472
Fax: 703-549-6995
www.diabetes.org

You'll learn how to help your child adjust to insulin to allow for favorite foods, have a busy schedule and still feel healthy and strong, negotiate the twists and turns of being different, and much more.

3369 Real Life Parenting of Kids with Diabetes
Virginia Nasmyth Loy, author
McGraw-Hill Companies
Returns Department
Dubuque, IA 52002
877-833-5524
Fax: 609-308-4484
e-mail: pbg.ecommerce_custserv@mcgraw-hill.com
www.mcgraw-hill.com

Virginia Loy had engineered successful management of her two sons' diabetes for 12 years at the time of publication. She is offering her organized, experienced, and practical advice to parents, for helping children to cope with and manage their diabetes from elementary school through college.
2001 188 pages Paperback
ISBN: 1-580400-83-3

3370 Resource and Activities Guide
Chronimed Publishing
PO Box 59032
Minneapolis, MN 55459-0032
612-513-6475
800-848-2793
Fax: 612-443-2806

For use with the Diabetes Youth Curriculum. Contains 300 educational activities that correspond with the text in the Curriculum and can easily be removed for photocopying.
260 pages Loose Leaf
ISBN: 0-937721-50-6

3371 Right from the Start
American Diabetes Association
1660 Duke Street
Alexandria, VA 22314-3447
800-232-3472
Fax: 703-549-6995
www.diabetes.org

Addresses issues such as: learning to take charge, coping, changing one's eating habits, getting fit, self-testing, family issues, preventive care, finances, as well as resources to turn to for further information and support. Available for both Type 1 and Type 2.
Pkg. of 25

3372 Savory Soups and Salads
American Diabetes Association
1660 Duke Street
Alexandria, VA 22314-3447
800-232-3472
Fax: 703-549-6995
www.diabetes.org

Offers exciting recipes for quick and healthy side dishes.

3373 Simple and Tasty Side Dishes
American Diabetes Association
1660 Duke Street
Alexandria, VA 22314-3447
800-232-3472
Fax: 703-549-6995
www.diabetes.org

Healthy recipes for the diabetic.

3374 Special Celebrations and Parties Cookbook
American Diabetes Association
1660 Duke Street
Alexandria, VA 22314-3447
800-232-3472
Fax: 703-549-6995
www.diabetes.org

Offers a list of more than 150 holiday recipes.

3375 Take-Charge Guide to Type I Diabetes
American Diabetes Association
1660 Duke Street
Alexandria, VA 22314-3447
800-232-3472
Fax: 703-549-6995
www.diabetes.org

Offers answers to the most important questions regarding Type 1 diabetes.

3376 Therapy for Diabetes Mellitus and Related Disorders
American Diabetes Association
1660 Duke Street
Alexandria, VA 22314-3447
800-232-3472
Fax: 703-549-6995
www.diabetes.org

Guides through the treatment of specific problems of persons with diabetes. Represents the views and experience of leading clinicians in a concise, practical approach to treatment.
384 pages

3377 Type 2 Diabetes: Your Healthy Living Guide
American Diabetes Association
1660 Duke Street
Alexandria, VA 22314-3447
800-232-3472
Fax: 703-549-6995
www.diabetes.org

A thorough guide to staying healthy with Type 2. Includes everything from choosing a health care team and eating and exercising properly to self-monitoring, insulin, dealing with complications, and keep mentally fit.
180 pages

3378 Using Insulin
Torrey Pines Press
The Diabetes Mall
San Diego, CA 92103
619-497-0900
800-988-4772
Fax: 619-497-0900
www.diabetesnet.com

How to take charge of your blood sugars in diabetes. Information on feeling better, improving your health, and achieving peace of mind.
316 pages Paperback

3379 Voice of the Diabetic
811 Chern Street
Columbia, MO 65201
573-875-8911
e-mail: epc@roudley.com
www.nfb.org

Personal stories and practical guidelines by blind diabetics and medical professionals, medical news, resource column and a recipe corner.

3380 Weight Management for Type II Diabetes
John Wiley and Sons, Inc.
Customer Service-Consumer Accounts
Indianapolis, IN 46256
877-762-2974
Fax: 800-597-3299
e-mail: consumers@wiley.com
www.wiley.com

An interactive, personalized guide that helps you manage your weight and your diabetes by making gradual lifestyle changes. Details how to set reasonable goals, keep pace with an exercise program, design your own meal plan, manage stress, and more.
1997 224 pages Paperback
ISBN: 0-471347-50-7

3381 When Diabetes Complicates Your Life
Chronimed Publishing
PO Box 59032
Minneapolis, MN 55459-0032
612-513-6475
800-848-2793
Fax: 612-443-2806

Directly addresses the subject of diabetic complications. This revised edition includes chapters on nerves and circulation, kidneys, and eyes. Enhancements to the new edition include a chapter on vitamins, herbs, and supplements, and reference to the latest research.
Feb 1998 208 pages Paperback
ISBN: 1-565611-27-6

Children's Books

3382 Diabetes
Franklin Watts Grolier

90 Old Sherman Turnpike
Danbury, CT 06816-0001
203-797-3500
800-621-1115
Fax: 203-797-3197
www.grolier.com

Looks at the differences between juvenile and adult-onset diabetes, discusses the history of the disease, causes, complications and treatments.
128 pages Grades 7-12
ISBN: 0-531108-82-1

3383 **Dinosaur Tamer**
American Diabetes Association
1660 Duke Street
Alexandria, VA 22314-3447
800-232-3472
Fax: 703-549-6995
www.diabetes.org

Twenty-five fictional stories that will entertain, enlighten, and ease your child's frustrations about having diabetes. Each tale evaporates the fear of insulin shots, blood tests, going to diabetes camp, and more.
Ages 8-12

3384 **Even Little Kids Get Diabetes**
Connie Pirner, author
Albert Whitman & Company
6340 Oakton Street
Morton Grove, IL 60053-2723
847-581-0033
800-255-7675
Fax: 847-581-0039
e-mail: mail@awhitmanco.com
www.albertwhitman.com

A preschooler tells how it was discovered when she was only two, that she has this common disease and describes her daily treatment and the precautions her family must observe.
24 pages Hardcover
ISBN: 0-807521-58-8
Pat McPartland, Sales
Joe Campbell, Customer Service

3385 **Everyone Likes to Eat**
John Wiley and Sons, Inc.
Customer Service-Consumer Accounts
Indianapolis, IN 46256
877-762-2974
Fax: 800-597-3299
e-mail: consumers@wiley.com
www.wiley.com

Revised and up-to-date second edition. How children can eat most of the foods they enjoy and still take care of their diabetes. Intended for elementary-school-age children, this guide is filled with activities, puzzles, and problem-solving exercises.
128 pages Paperback
ISBN: 0-471346-82-1

3386 **Grilled Cheese**
American Diabetes Association
1660 Duke Street
Alexandria, VA 22314-3447
800-232-3472
Fax: 703-549-6995
www.diabetes.org

Story designed to ease children's fears and frustrations of having diabetes.

3387 **Kiss the Candy Days Good-bye**
Delacorte Press
1540 Broadway
New York, NY 10036-4039
212-354-6500

This book focuses on Jimmy who is surprised to learn he has diabetes after seeming so healthy and fit. The story contains information on symptoms and the dangers of untreated diabetes.
Grades 6-8

3388 **Living with Diabetes**
Franklin Watts Grolier
90 Old Sherman Turnpike
Danbury, CT 06816-0001
203-797-3500
800-621-1115
Fax: 203-797-3197
www.grolier.com

Shows how persons with diabetes can control their illness and lead productive lives.
32 pages Grades 5-7
ISBN: 0-531108-44-9

3389 **Shira: A Legacy of Courage**
Doubleday
666 5th Avenue
New York, NY 10103-0001
212-354-6500

A biographical account of Shira Putter's fight with a rare form of diabetes. Using the victim's diary, this book is both powerful and poignant, as well as an educational resource for all people struggling with diabetes.
Grades 4-9

3390 **Sun, the Rain and the Insulin**
American Diabetes Association
1660 Duke Street
Alexandria, VA 22314-3447
800-232-3472
Fax: 703-549-6995
www.diabetes.org

Author chronicles a week at a summer diabetes camp, using her expertise and experience to capture the journey and the fight to cope that all people go through when diabetes hits the family.

Magazines

3391 **Countdown**
Juvenile Diabetes Foundation International
432 Park Avenue S
New York, NY 10016-8013
212-889-7575
Fax: 212-725-7259

Offers the latest news and information in diabetes research and treatment to everyone from an international arena of diabetes investigators to parents of small children with diabetes, from physicians to school teachers, from pharmacists to corporate executives.
Sandy Dylak, Editor

3392 **Diabetes**
American Diabetes Association
1660 Duke Street
Alexandria, VA 22314-3447
800-232-3472
Fax: 703-549-6995
www.diabetes.org

A peer-reviewed journal focusing on laboratory research.
Monthly

3393 **Diabetes Care**
American Diabetes Association
1660 Duke Street
Alexandria, VA 22314-3447
800-232-3472
Fax: 703-549-6995
www.diabetes.org

A peer-reviewed journal emphasizing reviews, commentaries and original research on topics of interest to clinicians.
Monthly

3394 **Diabetes Forecast**
American Diabetes Association
1660 Duke Street
Alexandria, VA 22314-3447
800-232-3472
Fax: 703-549-6995
www.diabetes.org

The monthly lifestyle magazine for people with diabetes, featuring complete, in-depth coverage of all aspects of living with diabetes.
Monthly

3395 **Diabetes Spectrum: From Research to Practice**
American Diabetes Association
1701 N Beauregard Street
Alexandria, VA 22311
800-232-3472
Fax: 703-549-6995
www.diabetes.org

A journal translating research into practice and focusing on diabetes education and counseling.
Quarterly

3396 **Joslin Magazine**
Joslin Diabetes Center
1 Joslin Place
Boston, MA 02215-5306
617-732-2400
Fax: 617-732-2562
e-mail: diabetes@joslin.harvard.edu
www.joslin.org

3397 **Voice of the Diabetic**
Ed Bryant, author
National Federation of the Blind
1800 Johnson Street 410-659-9314
Baltimore, MD 21230-4998 Fax: 410-685-5653
e-mail: subscribe@diabetes.nfb.org
www.nfb.org
The leading publication in the diabetes field. Each issue addresses the problems and concerns of diabetes, with a special emphasis for those who have lost vision due to diabetes. Available in print and on cassette.
28 pages Quarterly
Eileen Ley, Director of Publishing
Elizabeth Lunt, Editor

Newsletters

3398 **Clinical Diabetes**
American Diabetes Association
1660 Duke Street
Alexandria, VA 22314-3447 800-232-3472
Fax: 703-549-6995
www.diabetes.org
A bimonthly newsletter providing practical treatment information for primary care physicians.
BiMonthly

3399 **Diabetes Advisor**
American Diabetes Association
1701 N Beauregard Street 703-549-1500
Alexandria, VA 22311 800-232-3472
Fax: 703-836-7439
e-mail: askada@diabetes.org
www.diabetes.org
Offers informative articles and research in the area of diabetes for professionals and patients. Offers facts and research on diagnosis, symptoms, technology and the newest devices for persons with diabetes, as well as referral and hotline numbers.
Bi-Monthly
John G Graham IV, CEO

3400 **Diabetes Dateline**
National Diabetes Information Clearinghouse
1 Information Way 301-654-3327
Bethesda, MD 20205 800-860-8747
Fax: 301-907-8906
e-mail: ndic@info.niddck.nih.gov
www.niddk.nih.gov
BiAnnually

3401 **Diabetes Educator**
American Association of Diabetes Educators
444 N Michigan Avenue 312-644-2233
Chicago, IL 60611-3959 Fax: 312-644-4411
Offers information to health professionals working with persons with diabetes.
James J Balija, Executive Director

3402 **Kid's Corner**
American Diabetes Association
1660 Duke Street
Alexandria, VA 22314-3447 800-232-3472
Fax: 703-549-6995
www.diabetes.org
A mini-magazine for kids that offers word searches, puzzles and jokes - plus an encouraging story in each issue about kids with diabetes.
8 pages Quarterly

Pamphlets

3403 **Dental Tips for Diabetics**
National Diabetes Information Clearinghouse
1 Information Way 301-654-3327
Bethesda, MD 20892-0001 800-860-8747
Fax: 301-907-8906
e-mail: ndic@info.niddk.nih.gov
www.niddk.nih.gov
Discusses the relationship between diabetes and periodontal disease. Describes the symptoms of periodontal problems and preventive measures.

3404 **Diabetes Dateline**
National Diabetes Information Clearinghouse
1 Information Way 301-654-3327
Bethesda, MD 20892-0001 Fax: 301-907-8906
e-mail: ndic@aeric.com
This bulletin features news about current issues in diabetes research and control, special events, patient and professional meeting, and new publications available from NDIC and other organizations.
Quarterly

3405 **Diabetes and Brief Illness**
Chronimed Publishing
PO Box 59032 612-513-6475
Minneapolis, MN 55459-0032 800-848-2793
Fax: 612-443-2806
This booklet gives self-care instructions and eating suggestions to prevent development of ketoacidosis during brief illness that disrupts normal eating.
12 pages 10-pack

3406 **Diabetes and Exercise**
Chronimed Publishing
PO Box 59032 612-513-6475
Minneapolis, MN 55459-0032 800-848-2793
Fax: 612-443-2806
Exercise and weight loss tips and precautions for those with both insulin and non-insulin-dependent diabetes.
36 pages Pack of 10

3407 **Diabetes in Pregnancy**
March of Dimes
233 Park Avenue South 212-353-8353
New York, NY 10003 Fax: 212-254-3518
e-mail: NY639@marchofdimes.com
www.marchofdimes.com
Fact Sheets: one or two page review written for the general public. Also available electronically on the website: www.marchofdimes.com.

3408 **Diabetic Foot Care**
American Diabetes Association
1660 Duke Street
Alexandria, VA 22314-3447 800-232-3472
Fax: 703-549-6995
www.diabetes.org
Booklet discussing early detection and prompt treatment of diabetic foot problems.
12 pages

3409 **Gestational Diabetes: What To Expect**
American Diabetes Association
7 Washington Square 518-218-1755
Albany, NY 12205 888-342-2383
Fax: 518-218-0114
e-mail: ADAorders@pbd.com
www.diabetes.org
A complete comprehensive guide for women with gestational diabetes. Explains the stages in your baby's development, the types of prenatal testing you may recieve, and what to expect during labor, delivery, and beyond.
100 pages
ISBN: 1-580402-33-X

3410 **Healthy Eating**
Chronimed Publishing
PO Box 59032 612-513-6475
Minneapolis, MN 55459-0032 800-848-2793
Fax: 612-443-2806

Offers simple guidelines for choosing healthful foods, lowering fat intake, and timing meals and snacks. Available in Spanish.
Pack of 10

3411 Healthy Food Choices
American Diabetes Association
1660 Duke Street
Alexandria, VA 22314-3447
800-232-3472
Fax: 703-549-6995
www.diabetes.org
Pamphlet containing the basics of good nutrition.

3412 Hypoglycemia The Other Sugar Disease
Anita Flegg, author
Book Coach Press
3-390 MacKay Street
Ontario, Canada K1M 2C4,
613-746-3334
e-mail: info@bookcoachpress.com
www.bookcoachpress.com
This book is filled with dozens of real-life practical tips and will give you the tools to feel better and take control of your life.

3413 Insulin-Dependent Diabetes
National Diabetes Information Clearinghouse
1 Information Way
Bethesda, MD 20892-0001
301-654-3327
Fax: 301-654-3327
e-mail: ndic@aerie.com
Explains diabetes and how it develops and describes the differences between the two major forms of diabetes, insulin-dependent and noninsulin-dependent.

3414 Low Blood Sugar
Chronimed Publishing
PO Box 59032
Minneapolis, MN 55459-0032
612-513-6475
800-848-2793
Fax: 612-443-2806
Pack of 10

3415 Noninsulin-Dependent Diabetes
National Diabetes Information Clearinghouse
1 Information Way
Bethesda, MD 20892-0001
301-654-3327
Fax: 301-907-8906
e-mail: ndic@aerie.com
Describes the symptoms and diagnosis of noninsulin-dependent diabetes; diabetes management, including diet, oral drugs, and insulin; glucose monitoring; and complications.
1992 35 pages

3416 Recognizing and Treating Low Blood Sugar (Hypoglycemia)
Chronimed Publishing
PO Box 59032
Minneapolis, MN 55459-0032
612-513-6475
800-848-2793
Fax: 612-443-2806
The causes, symptoms, and treatment of low blood sugar are clearly presented in this booklet, including guidelines for using glucagon.
12 pages Pack of 10

3417 Taking Care of Gestational Diabetes
International Diabetes Center at Park Nicollet
3800 Park Nicollet Boulevard
Minneapolis, MN 55416-2699
952-993-3874
888-637-2675
Fax: 952-993-0501
e-mail: idccustsvc@parknicollet.com
www.idcpublishing.com
Available in Spanish. Empowering women to make healthy choices for a healthy pregnancy, a healthy baby, and a healthy lifestyle. This book covers food planning, testing, targets, medications and more.
242 pages

3418 Understanding Gestational Diabetes
National Diabetes Information Clearinghouse
1 Information Way
Bethesda, MD 20892-0001
301-654-3327
Fax: 301-907-8906
e-mail: ndic@aerie.com
A guide for women who develop diabetes during pregnancy. It discusses symptoms and diagnosis of gestational diabetes, risk factors, tests during pregnancy and daily management including the use of insulin and blood gluclose monitoring.
44 pages

Audio & Video

3419 ADA Clinical Education Series on CD-Rom
American Diabetes Association
1660 Duke Street
Alexandria, VA 22314-3447
800-232-3472
Fax: 703-549-6995
www.diabetes.org
Features complete texts of Medical Management of Type 1 Diabetes, Medical Management of Type 2 Diabetes, Therapy for Diabetes Mellitus and Related Disorders, 2nd Ed., and Medical Management of Pregnancy Complicated by Diabetes, 2nd Ed.
CD-Rom

3420 Black Experience
American Diabetes Association
300 Research Parkway
Meriden, CT 06450-7137
203-639-0385
800-342-2383
Fax: 203-639-0292
www.diabetes.org/
Designed to increase awareness of diabetes in the black community.
L Butcher, District Director

3421 Diabetes & Exercise Video
American Diabetes Association
1660 Duke Street
Alexandria, VA 22314-3447
800-232-3472
Fax: 703-549-6995
www.diabetes.org
A video offering information on how to maintain good health and exercise in controlling diabetes.

3422 Label Reading and Shopping
American Diabetes Association/Conn. Affiliate
300 Research Parkway
Meriden, CT 06450-7137
203-639-0385
800-842-6323
Fax: 203-639-0292
www.diabetes.org/
Provides practical information on how to shop and what to look for on labels.
Videotape

3423 Living Well with Diabetes
American Diabetes Association/Conn. Affiliate
300 Research Parkway
Meriden, CT 06450-7137
203-639-0385
800-842-6323
Fax: 203-639-0292
www.diabetes.org/
Presents two patient role models who are successfully following a treatment plan for noninsulin dependent diabetes.
Videotape

3424 On Top of My Game: Living with Diabetes
American Diabetes Association/Conn. Affiliate
300 Research Parkway
Meriden, CT 06450-7137
203-639-0385
800-842-6323
Fax: 203-639-0292
www.diabetes.org/
Six patients and their families share their day-to-day frustrations and successes in managing diabetes.
Videotape

3425 Physicians Guide to Type I Diabetes
American Diabetes Association/Conn. Affiliate
300 Research Parkway
Meriden, CT 06450-7137
203-639-0385
800-842-6323
Fax: 203-639-0292
www.diabetes.org/
Principles of good care in the diagnosis and management of Type I.
Videotape

3426 Survival Skills for Diabetic Children
Ajn Company
555 W 57th Street
New York, NY 10019-2961
212-582-8820
800-226-6256
Fax: 212-586-5462
How to provide insulin-dependent children with education, supervision, and support.
1988 28 minutes

3427 **Understanding Diabetes: A User's Guide to Novolin**
American Diabetes Association/Conn. Affiliate
300 Research Parkway 203-639-0385
Meriden, CT 06450 800-842-6323
Fax: 203-639-0292
www.diabetes.org/
Basic information about diabetes and the role insulin plays in blood glucose control.
Videotape

Web Sites

3428 **American Association of Diabetes Educators**
www.aabenet.org
The mission is to enhance the competence of health professionals who teach persons with diabetes, advance the specialty practice of diabetes education, and to improve the quality of diabetes education and care for all those affected by diabetes.

3429 **American Diabetes Association**
www.diabetes.org
Offers a network of 52 affiliates with over 55,000 volunteers, including a professional membership of more than 10,000 physicians, social workers, nutritionists, educators and nurses.

3430 **Diabetes Dictionary**
www.niddk.nih.gov
Provides research funding and support for basic and clinical research in the areas of type 1 and type 2 diabetes and other metabolic disprders.

3431 **Diabetes Exercise and Sports Association**
www.diabetes-exercise.org
Exists to enhance the quality of life for people with diabetes through exercise and physical fitness.

3432 **Healing Well**
www.healingwell.com
An online health resource guide to medical news, chat, information and articles, newsgroups and message boards, books, disease-related web sites, medical directories, and more for patients, friends, and family coping with disabling diseases, disorders, or chronic illnesses.

3433 **Health Finder**
www.healthfinder.gov
Searchable, carefully developed web site offering information on over 1000 topics. Developed by the US Department of Health and Human Services, the site can be used in both English and Spanish.

3434 **Healthlink USA**
www.healthlinkusa.com
Health information concerning treatment, cures, prevention, diagnosis, risk factors, research, support groups, email lists, personal stories and much more. Updated regularly.

3435 **Helios Health**
www.helioshealth.com
Online resource for your health information. Detailed information about specific health topics, access to expert advice from our Medical Advisory Board, and up-to-date health news.

3436 **MedicineNet**
www.medicinenet.com
An online resource for consumers providing easy-to-read, authoritative medical and health information.

3437 **Medscape**
www.mywebmd.com
Medscape offers specialists, primary care physicians, and other health professionals the Web's most robust and integrated medical information and educational tools.

3438 **National Diabetes Information Clearinghouse**
www.niddk.nih.gov/health/diabetes/ndic
Offers various materials, resources, books, pamphlets and more for persons and families in the area of diabetes.

3439 **WebMD**
www.webmd.com
Information on diabetes, including articles and resources.

Description

3440 **Down Syndrome**

Down syndrome is a collection of inherited abnormalities caused by an extra chromosome. Instead of having the normal number of chromosomes (46), children with Down syndrome have an extra chromosome 21. (Because there are three copies of chromosome 21 instead of the normal two, Down syndrome is often called trisomy 21). This chromosomal abnormality results in altered growth and development. Approximately 4,000 children are born with Down syndrome every year in the United States. The overall incidence is about 1 in every 700 live births, but there is a marked variability depending on maternal age. In the early childbearing years, the incidence is about 1/2000 live births; for mothers over 40, it rises to at least 1/100 if not more frequent with advancing age.

Down syndrome is associated with a wide variety of clinical signs, although most individuals do not possess all of them. Common findings include decreased muscle tone, slanting eyes with folds of skin in the inside corners, white spots appearing in the irises of the eyes, and single creases across the palms of one or both hands. Physically, children with Down syndrome have broad feet with short toes, short ears and necks, small heads and small oral cavities. Mental development in the child with Down syndrome is impaired; the mean IQ is approximately 50. Hearing and speech abilities may also be hampered. However, many children with Down syndrome can reach surprisingly high levels of achievement. Congenital heart disease is found in nearly half of patients, and there is an increased susceptibility to acute leukemia. Today, most patients survive well into adulthood, although problems such as Alzheimer's Disease and psychiatric illness may increase with age.

It is essential that parents enroll their with Down syndrome in an infant development program. These programs advise parents on how to help a child with Down syndrome in language, cognitive, social and motor skills.

National Agencies & Associations

3441 **ARC The ARC of the United States**
The ARC of the United States
1010 Wayne Avenue
Silver Spring, MD 20910
301-565-3842
800-433-5255
Fax: 301-565-3843
e-mail: info@thearc.org
www.thearc.org

Works to include all children and adults with cognitive intellectual and developmental disabilities in every community.
Lynne Cleveland, President
Michael Mack, Vice President

3442 **Aleh Foundation Aleh Institustions USA**
Aleh Institustions USA
5317 13th Avenue
Brooklyn, NY 11219
718-851-4596
877-453-9170
Fax: 718-851-4597
e-mail: shlomo@alehfoundation.com
www.alehfoundation.org

Founded in 1983, the Aleh Rehabilitation Center has served as a residential facility to close to 200 children with multiple, physical and mental disabilities. These children and their families benefit from a wide range of services in a caring, supportive atmosphere.

3443 **Canadian Down Syndrome Society**
811-14 Street NW
Calgary Alberta, T2N 2-2A4
403-270-8500
800-883-5608
Fax: 403-270-8291
e-mail: info@cdss.ca
www.cdss.ca

Resource linking parents and professionals through advocacy education and providing information.
Krista J Flint, Executive Director

3444 **National Association for Down Syndrome**
PO Box 206
Wilmette, IL 60091
630-325-9112
e-mail: info@nads.org
www.nads.org

A non-for-profit organization founded in Chicago in 1961 by parents of children with Down syndrome who felt a need to create a better environment and bring about understanding and acceptance of people with Down syndrome.
Diane Gomboz, President
M Sheila Hebein, Executive Director

3445 **National Dissemination Center for Children with Disabilities**
PO Box 1492
Washington, DC 20013
202-884-8200
800-695-0285
Fax: 202-884-8441
e-mail: nichcy@aed.org
www.nichcy.org

Publishes free, fact filled newsletters. Arranges workshops. Advises parents on the laws entitling children with disabilities to special education and other services.
Dr Suzanne Ripley, Contact

3446 **National Down Syndrome Congress**
1370 Center Drive
Atlanta, GA 30338
770-604-9500
800-232-6372
Fax: 770-604-9898
e-mail: info@ndsccenter.org
www.NDSCcenter.org

The mission of the NDSC is to provide information, advocacy, and support concerning all aspects of life for individuals with Down Syndrome.
David Tolleson, Executive Director
Sue Joe, Resources Specialist

3447 **National Down Syndrome Society**
666 Broadway
New York, NY 10012
212-460-9330
800-221-4602
Fax: 212-979-2873
e-mail: info@ndss.org
www.ndss.org

NDSS supports researchers seeking the causes of and answers to many of the medical genetic behavioral and learning problems associated with Down syndrome. Also sponsors symposia and conferences for parents and professionals provides advocacy.
Jon Colman, President
Betsy Goodwin, Founder

3448 **National Early Childhood Technical Assistance System**
University of North Carolina, Chapel Hill
Campus Box 8040 UNC-CH
Chapel Hill, NC 27599-0001
919-962-2001
Fax: 919-966-7463
e-mail: nectac@unc.edu
www.nectac.org

Assists states and other entities in developing comprehensive services for children with special needs through the age of eight and their families.
Lynne Kahn, Director & Principal Investigator
Joan Danaher, Associate Director Information Resources

State Agencies & Associations

California

3449 Down Syndrome Association of Los Angeles
315 Arden Avenue 818-242-7871
Glendale, CA 91203 Fax: 818-242-7819
e-mail: info@dsala.org
www.dsala.org

Offers information on Down syndrome, counseling, resources, facts, laws and other forms of information.
Gail Williamson, Executive Director
Sandra Baker, Office Administrator/Spanish Coordinator

Colorado

3450 Mile High Down Syndrome Association
2121 S Oneida Street 303-797-1699
Denver, CO 80224 Fax: 303-756-6144
e-mail: info@mhdsa.org
www.mhdsa.org

Mac Macsovits, Executive Director
Melissa Davis, Volunteer Coordinator

Connecticut

3451 Connecticut Down Syndrome Congress
263 Farmington Avenue 205-351-1157
Farmington, CT 06030-0485 888-486-8537
e-mail: manager@ctdownsyndrome.org
www.ctdownsyndrome.org

Sheryl Knapp, Secretary
Walter Glomb, President

Florida

3452 Gold Coast Down Syndrome Organization
2255 Glades Road 561-912-1231
Boca Raton, FL 33431 Fax: 561-912-1232
e-mail: gcdso@bellsouth.net
www.goldcoastdownsyndrome.org

Gold Coast Down syndrome Organization is a private nonprofit corporation dedicated to making the future brighter for people with Down syndrome in Palm Beach County, Florida.

3453 Goodwill Industries-Suncoast
Goodwill Industries-Suncoast
10596 Gandy Boulevard 727-523-1512
St. Petersburg, FL 33733 Fax: 727-577-2749
e-mail: gw.marketing@goodwill-suncoast.rog
www.goodwill-suncoast.org

A nonprofit community based organization whose purpose is to improve the quality of life for people who are disabled, disadvantaged and/or aged. This mission is accomplished through a staff of over 1,200 employees providing independent living skills, affordable housing, career assessment and planning, job skills, training, placement, and job retention assistance with useful employment. Annually, Goodwill Industries-Suncoast serves over 30,000 people in Citrus, Hernando, Levy, Marion and more.
Martin W Gladysz, Chair
R Lee Waits, President/CEO

Georgia

3454 Down Syndrome Association of Atlanta
4355 J Cobb Parkway 404-320-3233
Atlanta, GA 30339 Fax: 770-946-9687
e-mail: contactus@down-syndrome-atlanta.org
www.atlantadsaa.org

Hawaii

3455 Hawaii Down Syndrome Congress
419 Keoniana Street 808-949-1999
Honolulu, HI 96815 e-mail: Conkay@AOL.com
www.downscity.com

Constance K Smith, President

Indiana

3456 Indiana Down Syndrome Foundation
3050 N Meridian Street 317-925-7617
Indianapolis, IN 46208 888-989-9255
Fax: 317-925-7619
e-mail: info@indianadsf.org
www.indianadsf.org

Lisa Tokarz-Guiterre, Executive Director
Steve Simpson, President

Massachusetts

3457 Massachusetts Down Syndrome Congress
PO Box 866
Melrose, MA 02176 800-664-MDSC
e-mail: mdsc@mdsc.org
www.mdsc.org

Maureen Gallagher, Executive Director
Sarah Cullen, Outreach Coordinator

Minnesota

3458 Down Syndrome Association of Minnesota
656 Transfer Road 651-603-0720
St Paul, MN 55114 800-511-3696
e-mail: dsam@dsam.org
www.dsamn.org

A non-profit organization dedicated to ensuring that all individuals with Down syndrome and their families receive the support necessary to participate in, contribute to and achieve the fulfillment of life in their community.
Teresa Yira, President
Kathleen Forney, Executive Director

New York

3459 Association for Children with Down Syndrome
4 Fern Place 516-933-4700
Plainview, NY 11803 Fax: 516-933-9524
e-mail: msmith@acds.org
www.acds.org

Nonprofit educational program that combines national information and research dissemination with direct services at the local level. Services include early intervention, pre-school, recreation programs and residential homes.
Michael M Smith, Executive Director
Cecilia Barry, Principal

Ohio

3460 Down Syndrome Association of Greater Cinci nnati
644 Linn Street 513-761-5400
Cincinnati, OH 45203-1734 Fax: 513-761-5401
e-mail: dsagc@dsagc.com
www.dsagc.com

The mission of the Down Syndrome Association of Greater Cincinnati is to provide information resources and support to individuals with Down syndrome, their families, and their communities.
Janet Gora, Executive Director
Nora Lindsay Quinn, Event Coordinator

Tennessee

3461 Down Syndrome Association of Middle Tennessee
111 N Wilson Boulevard 615-386-9002
Nashville, TN 37205-2411 Fax: 615-386-9754
e-mail: dsamt@bellsouth.net
www.dsamt.org

A nonprofit organization of families whose mission is to enhance the quality of life for all individuals with Down Syndrome by providing information and support to families professionals and the community.

Texas

3462 **Down Syndrome Guild of Dallas**
701 N Central Expressway 214-267-1374
Richardson, TX 75080-1174 Fax: 972-234-2510
www.downsyndromedallas.org
Kelly Drablos, President
Tamara White, Secretary

3463 **Texas Association on Mental Retardation**
TAMR Headquarters 512-349-7470
Austin, TX 78755 Fax: 512-349-2117
e-mail: pat.holder@tamr-web.com
www.tamr-web.com
An organization made up of professionals, parents, consumers and advocates. Our goal is to create an accessible system of services and resources which support personal choice and promotes lives of dignity and self-determination.
Pat Holder

Virginia

3464 **Down Syndrome Association of Hampton Roads**
The Endependence Center 757-466-3696
Norfolk, VA 23502 e-mail: DSAHR@verizon.net
www.dsahr.org
The Down Syndrome Association of Hampton Roads is a not-for-profit organization serving the needs of individuals with Down Syndrome and their families. The association is supported by a board of directors, an advisory board and dedicated volunteers.
Andrea Anderson, President
Florence Thacker, Secretary

Wisconsin

3465 **Down Syndrome Association of Wisconsin**
9401 W Beloit Road 414-327-3729
Milwaukee, WI 53227 866-327-3729
Fax: 414-327-1329
e-mail: info@dsaw.org
www.dsaw.org
An organization created by families for families of individuals and for individuals with Down Syndrome. Our primary mission is to provide each person with Down Syndrome the support needed to achieve personal goals and develop self-esteem.
Heidi Dauer, President
Angie Fech, Interim Executive Director

Libraries & Resource Centers

3466 **Adult Down Syndrome Center of Lutheran General Hospital**
1999 Dempster Street
Park Ridge, IL 60068 847-318-2303
www.advocatehealthc.com
The Adult Down Syndrome Center is a comprehensive medical resource providing multidisciplinary medical and psychosocial care for adults with Down syndrome, with an emphasis on health promotion.
Brian Chicoine MD, Medical Director

3467 **Ann Whitehill Down Syndrome Program**
Riley Hospital for Children
702 Barnhill Drive
Indianapolis, IN 46202 800-248-1199
rileychildrenshospital.com
Brings together specialists from many areas to address the medical and psychosocial needs of children with Down Syndrome. We also refer the family to local resources for therapy and developmental programs.

3468 **Blick Clinic for Developmental Disabilities**
640 W Market Street 330-762-5425
Akron, OH 44303-1465 Fax: 330-762-4019
e-mail: blickclinic@blickclinic.com
www.blickclinic.com
Blick Clinic is a private, non-profit outpatient clinic which began by a group of parents of children with developmental disabilities and a few volunteer professionals. Together, they developed the Clinic into a single, comprehensive source of diagnostic, evaluation, treatment, and support group services to persons with developmental disabilities.

3469 **Dartmouth-Hitchcock Medical Center - Genetics and Development**
One Medical Center Drive 603-653-6044
Lebanon, NH 03756-0001 Fax: 603-653-3585
www.dhmc.org
Dartmouth-Hitchcock Clinic is committed to a regional, integrated, comprehensive healthcare system, which can evolve under physician leadership, lay administrative support and public trustee guidance. DHC and its partnering DHMC organizations are recognized as leaders in using scientific methods to improve health care delivery.
Carol B Andrew EdD, MS
Mary Beth Dinulos, MD

3470 **Developmental Evaluation Clinic**
Westchester Institute for Human Development
Cedarwood Hall 914-493-8150
Valhalla, NY 10595-1681 e-mail: wihd@wihd.org
www.wihd.org
WIHD envisions a future where all people, including children and adults living with disabilities, fully participate in society, live healthy and productive lives, and have access to culturally appropriate services and supports, emerging technologies, competent professionals, caring families, caregivers, and communities.

3471 **Developmental Medicine Center (DMC)**
Children's Hospital Boston
300 Longwood Avenue
Boston, MA 02115 617-355-7025
www.childrenshospital.org
Provides developmental evaluation and treatment services for children aged birth to adolescence with a wide range of developmental, behavioral and learning difficulties
Leonard A Rappaport MD, MS, Program Director

3472 **Down Syndrome Center of Western Pennsylvania**
3420 5th Avenue 412-692-7963
Pittsburgh, PA 15213-2524 Fax: 412-692-5723
www.chp.edu
The Down Syndrome Center of Western Pennsylvania has a lending library of books, videos, audio cassettes and periodicals; provides current information about Down syndrome to families and professionals; maintains a file of articles on issues relating to Down Syndrome and publishes a quarterly newsletter in conjunction with the Down Syndrome Group of Western Pennsylvania.
Dr William Cohen, MD, Director

3473 **Down Syndrome Clinic of Houston**
6701 Fannin Street, 16th Floor 832-822-3478
Dallas, TX 75235-7701 Fax: 832-825-3399
e-mail: downsyndrome@texaschildrenshospital.org
www.texaschildreshospital.org
The mission of the Down Syndrome Clinic of Houston is to help individuals with Down syndrome reach his or her fullest potential. We accomplish our goal by offering a clinic where children receive complete evaluations by a multidisciplinary team. Families will obtain needed strategies for management of common concerns.
Nirupama Madduri, MD, Chief of Service
Jennifer Chung, Clinic Coordinator

3474 **Dr. Gertrude A Barber National Institute**
136 E Avenue 814-453-7661
Erie, PA 16507-1899 Fax: 814-455-1132
e-mail: BNIeric@barberinstitute.org
www.barberinstitute.org
We believe that all persons have the capacity for growth and fulfillment, and to that end they must be afforded every opportunity to attain the greatest use of thier potential within themselves and their community.
John Barber, JD, President/CEO
Maureen Barber-Carey, EdD, Executive Vice President

3475 **Jane and Richard Thomas Center for Down Syndrome**
Cincinnati Center for Developmental Disorders
3333 Burnet Avenue 513-636-0520
Cincinnati, OH 45229-3039 Fax: 513-636-0527
www.cincinnatichildrens.org

The Jane and Richard Thomas Center for Down Syndrome conducts research and offers interdisciplinary evaluations and intervention for infants, children, adolescents and young adults with Down syndrome. By providing a range of comprehensive services within one center, families can now spend less time pursuing services through multiple agencies and professionals.
David J Schonfeld MD, Division Head

3476 **Kennedy Krieger Institute**
707 N Broadway 443-923-9200
Baltimore, MD 21205-1888 800-873-3377
Fax: 410-550-9292
e-mail: info@kennedykrieger.org
www.kennedykrieger.org
Kennedy Krieger Institute is an internationally recognized facility located in Baltimore, Maryland dedicated to improving the lives of children and adolescents with pediatric developmental disabilities through patient care, special education, research, and professional training. Our clinical programs offer an interdisciplinary approach in treatment tailored to the individual needs of each child.
Gary W Goldstein, President

3477 **Marcus Institute for Development and Learning**
1920 Briarcliff Road 404-727-9450
Atlanta, GA 30329 Fax: 404-727-9598
e-mail: Marcus_Info@MarcusInstitute.org
www.marcus.org
Our mission is to provide information, services and programs to people with developmental disabilities and their families, as well as those who live and work with them. We offer integrated state-of-the-art clinical, behavioral, educational and family support services through a single organization to reduce the stress and aggravation for families who may have a child with mild to severe disabilities.
Charles M Shaffer, Jr, President/CEO
Dr Claire Coles, Director Fetal Alcohol Center

3478 **MeritCare Children's Hospital Down Syndrome Outpatient Service**
Coordinated Treatment Center
736 Broadway 701-234-6600
Fargo, ND 58122-4420 800-828-2901
Fax: 701-234-6965
www.meritcare.com
MeritCare Children's Hospital offers a multidisciplinary outpatient service to help accommodate the special medical developmental, behavioral, family and community needs of patients with Down Syndrome.

3479 **Santa Rosa Medical Center**
PO Box 7330 210-228-2386
San Antonio, TX 78207-0330
Dr. Robert Clayton

3480 **UCSF Children's Hospital Health Library**
505 Parnassus Avenue
San Francisco, CA 94143 415-476-1000
www.ucsfhealth.org
This Health Library is an online resource to supplement information your doctors, nurses and pharmacists may provide. Our library includes a medical dictionary and an online calendar of our health events. We have news about our research advances and treatments, patient education materials and listings of other helpful Web sites.

3481 **University of Maryland: Department of Pediatrics**
22 South Greene Street 410-328-8667
Baltimore, MD 21201 Fax: 410-328-3981
http://www.umm.edu/pediatrics/
Recognized throughout Maryland and the mid-Atlantic region as a valuable resource for critically and chronically ill children, the University of Maryland Hospital for Children combines state-of-the-art medicine with family-centered care.

3482 **University of Washington: Experimental Education Unit**
Box 357925 206-543-4011
Seattle, WA 98195-7925 Fax: 206-543-8480
www.eeuweb.org
The Experimental Education Unit (EEU) is a state-certified special education school that serves children from birth to age 7 with diverse abilities. Faculty at the EEU conduct research projects, and provide training opportunties to undergraduate and graduate students, educators, and other professionals.
Rick Neel, Director

Illinois

3483 **LaRabida Children's Hospital: Developmental Disabilities & Delays**
East 65th Street at Lake Michigan 773-363-6700
Chicago, IL 60649 e-mail: info@larabida.org
www.larabida.org
La Rabida Children's Hospital is dedicated to excellence in caring for children with chronic illness, disabilities, or who have been abused, allowing them to achieve their fullest potential through expertise and innovation within the health care and academic communities.
Paula Kienberger Jaudes, MD, President/CEO

Iowa

3484 **Center for Disabilities and Development**
University of Iowa Hospitals and Clinics
100 Hawkins Drive 319-353-6900
Iowa City, IA 52242-1011 877-686-0031
Fax: 319-356-8284
TTY: 877-686-0032
e-mail: CDD-Webmaster@uiowa.edu
www.healthcare.uiowa.edu/cdd
Provides comprehensive health care and services to people with disabilities of all ages and their families through a combination of outpatient, impatient, and community based programs. UHS provides information, evaluation, treatment recommendations, and training related to aging and disabilities. UHS provides both preservice and inservice training programs for service providers and others who provide services to individuals with disabilities.

Maryland

3485 **Mt. Washington Pediatric Clinic**
1708 W Rogers Avenue 410-578-8600
Baltimore, MD 21209-4596 Fax: 410-466-1715
www.mwph.org
The primary purpose of the Mt. Washington Pediatric Hospital and its affiliates is to sponsor and promote the provision of the highest quality pediatric health care services in a nurturing environment.
Sheldon J Stein, President/CEO
Robert H Imhoff, III, VP Development

Pennsylvania

3486 **Children's Hospital of Philadelphia**
34th St & Civic Center Boulevard
Philadelphia, PA 19104-4399 215-590-1000
www.chop.edu
The oldest hospital dedicated exclusively to pediatrics, strives to be the world leader in the advancement of healthcare for children by integrating excellent patient care, innovative research and quality professional education into all of its programs.

Rhode Island

3487 **Children's Neurodevelopment Center**
Hasbro Children's Hospital
593 Eddy Street
Providence, RI 02903 401-444-5685
www.hasbrochildrenshosptial.org
The Children's Neurodevelopment Center (CNDC) at Hasbro Children's Hospital provides evaluation and treatment of children with neurological, genetic, developmental, metabolic and behavioral disorders.
David Mandelbaum MD, PhD, Director

Research Centers

3488 **Institute for Basic Research in Developmental Disabilities**
1050 Forest Hill Road 718-494-0600
Staten Island, NY 10314-6330 Fax: 718-494-0833
www.omr.state.ny.us

Conducts research into neurodegenerative diseases Alzheimer's disease developmental disabilities fragile X syndrome Down's Syndrome autism epilepsy and basic science issues underlying all developmental disabilities.
W Ted Brown, Director
Raju K Pullarkat PhD, Chair Developmental Biochemistry

3489 **Kennedy Krieger Institute - Down Syndrome**
707 N Broadway
Baltimore, MD 21205
443-923-9200
888-554-2080
Fax: 443-923-9138
TTY: 443-923-2645
e-mail: webmaster@kennedykrieger.org
www.kennedykrieger.org
Dedicated to improving the lives of children and adolescents with pediatric developmental disabilities through patient care special education research and professional training.
George Capon MD, Director
Char Koller, Research

3490 **National Institute of Child Health and Human Development**
PO Box 3006
Rockville, MD 20847
800-370-2943
Fax: 301-984-1473
TTY: 888-320-6942
e-mail: NICHDInformationResourceCenter@mail.nih.
www.nih.gov/nichd

Support Groups & Hotlines

3491 **Down Syndrome Association of Greater Cinci nnati**
644 Linn Street
Cincinnati, OH 45203-1734
513-761-5400
Fax: 513-761-5401
e-mail: dsagc@dsagc.com
http://www.dsagc.com
The DSAGC offers regular meetings to provide education and support for parents and families of children with Down syndrome. We have several support groups to meet the needs of our families. These are informal get togethers that allow individuals and families an opportunity to share experiences while creating new friendships.
Janet Gora, Executive Director
Debbie Baker, Event/Public Relations Coordinator

3492 **National Down Syndrome Congress**
1370 Center Drive
Atlanta, GA 30338
770-604-9500
800-232-6372
Fax: 770-604-9898
e-mail: info@ndsccenter.org
www.NDSCcenter.org
The mission of the NDSC is to provide information, advocacy, and support concerning all aspects of life for individuals with Down Syndrome.
David Tolleson, Executive Director

3493 **National Down Syndrome Society Hotline**
666 Broadway
New York, NY 10012-2317
212-460-9330
800-221-4602
Fax: 212-979-2873
www.ndss.org
NDSS supports researchers seeking the causes of and answers to many of the medical, genetic, behavioral and learning problems associated with Down syndrome; sponsors symposia and conferences for parents and professionals; performs advocacy; provides information and refferal through a toll-free number; and develops and disseminates educational materials.
Andrea Lack, Director

3494 **Parents of Children with Down Syndrome**
Arc of Montgomery County
11600 Nebel Street
Rockville, MD 20852-2538
301-984-5777
Fax: 301-816-2429
TTY: 301-881-1548
e-mail: asachs@arcmontmd.org
www.arcmontmd.org/
Activities include formal and informal meetings, parent-to-parent support, contacting new parents of down syndrome children to offer support and information on community resources, providing information on doctors, hospitals and professionals.
Petere Holden, Executive Director
John Slavcoff, President of the Board

Books

3495 **ACDS Infant, Toddler & Pre-school Curriculum for Children**
Association for Children with Down Syndrome
4 Fern Place
Plainview, NY 11803
516-933-4700
Fax: 516-933-9524
e-mail: msmith@acds.org
www.acds.org
This curriculum is user friendly for parents, educators, related service professionals and other caregivers. It provides checklists and teaching strategies to facilitate aquisition of skills in cognition, self-help, socialization, speech and language, gross and fine motor skills plus much more.
Michael M. Smith, Executive Director

3496 **Babies with Down Syndrome**
Woodbine House
6510 Bells Mill Road
Bethesda, MD 20817-1636
800-843-7323
Praised as the finest book ever written for new parents, this book covers everything they need to know about rearing these beautiful and special children in a loving environment.
237 pages Paperback
ISBN: 0-933149-02-6

3497 **Bethy and the Mouse: God's Gifts in Special Packages**
Faith and Life Press
718 Main Street
Newton, KS 67114-0344
316-283-5100
A father's account of his special children, Bethy with Down Syndrome and The Mouse who has been born with microcephaley. A tender story of a father's love.
164 pages Paperback
ISBN: 0-873031-11-3

3498 **Breast Feeding the Baby with Down Syndrome**
LaLeche League International
957 Plum Grove Road
Schaumburg, IL 60173-4048
847-519-7730
Fax: 847-963-0460
e-mail: llli@llli.org
www.llli.org
16 pages Pamphlet

3499 **Cara: Growing with a Retarded Child**
Temple University Press
USB Room 305, Broad & Oxford
Philadelphia, PA 19122
215-204-8787
www.temple.edu/tempress
The author offers information and experiences on raising her daughter, Cara, who has Down syndrome.

3500 **Communication Skills in Children with Down Syndrome**
Woodbine House
6510 Bells Mill Road
Bethesda, MD 20817
800-843-7323
Offers parents a chance to learn what to expect as communication skills progress from infancy through early teenage years. Discussions are included on speech and language therapy, hearing problems, school performance and intelligibility issues.
150 pages Paperback
ISBN: 0-933149-53-0

3501 **Current Approaches to Down's Syndrome**
Greenwood Publishing Group, Inc/Praeger Publishers
PO Box 6926
Portsmouth, NH 03802-6926
800-225-5800
Fax: 877-231-6980
e-mail: service@greenwood.com
www.greenwood.com

An exploration of current initiatives relating to Down syndrome in the medical, educational and social fields.
447 pages
ISBN: 0-275902-12-9
David Lane, Editor
Brian Stratford, Editor

3502 Differences in Common: Straight Talk on Mental Retardation/Down Syndrome
Woodbine House
6510 Bells Mill Road
Bethesda, MD 20817 800-843-7323
A collection of essays by the mother of an adult son who has Down syndrome. Focuses on mainstreaming, terminology, parent groups and advocacy.
M Trainer, Editor

3503 Down Syndrome: A Review of Current Knowledge
Jean-Adolphe Rondal, Juan Perera, and Lynn Nadek, author
John Wiley and Sons, Inc.
Customer Service-Consumer Accouts
Indianapolis, IN 46256 877-762-2974
Fax: 800-597-3299
e-mail: consumers@wiley.com
www.wiley.com
1999 350 pages Hardcover
IT Lott, Editor
E McCoy, Editor

3504 Down Syndrome: An Update and Review for Primary Care Physicians
Dartmouth-Hitchcock Medical Center
1 Medical Center Drive 603-650-5000
Lebanon, NH 03756-0001
An excellent medical review of Down syndrome intended for physicians.
WC Cooley, Editor

3505 Down Syndrome: The Facts
Oxford University Press
2001 Evans Road 212-726-6000
Cary, NC 27513-2010 800-451-7556
Fax: 919-677-1303
www.oup-usa.org
A book for parents who have a child with Down syndrome written by a pediatrician who works with Down syndrome children.
M Selikowitz, Editor

3506 From 17 Months to 17 Years...A Look at Down Syndrome
Bonnie Lavender
RR-1, Box 102C 315-287-2973
Richville, NY 13681
Includes profiles of six families who have children with Down syndrome. Offers photographs and accompanying text that detail each family's experiences with Down syndrome.
B Lavender, Editor
GJ Lega, Editor

3507 Medical and Surgical Care for Children with Down Syndrome
Woodbine House
6510 Bells Mill Road
Bethesda, MD 20817-1636 800-843-7323
Provides detailed and easy-to-understand information for parents on a wide range of medical conditions and treatments including: heart disease, recurrent infections, thyroid problems, eye problems, skin conditions, ear, nose and throat problems, orthopedic conditions, leukemia, facial and dental concerns and neurological problems.
320 pages Paperback
ISBN: 0-933149-54-9

3508 Parent's Guide to Down Syndrome: Toward a Brighter Future
Siegfried M Pueschel, MD, PhD, JD, MPH, author
Brookes Publishing Company
Customer Service Department
Baltimore, MD 21285-0624 800-638-3775
Fax: 410-337-8539
e-mail: custserv@brookespublishing.com
www.brookespublishing.com
A comprehensive reference book especially for new parents but useful and informative to seasoned parents as well. Range of topics include a history of Down syndrome, physical characterisitcs, developmental expectations, early intervention, feeding the young child and the school years.
2001 338 pages Paperback
ISBN: 1-557664-52-8

3509 Parents of Children with Down Syndrome
11600 Nebel Street 301-984-5792
Rockville, MD 20852-2538 Fax: 301-816-2429
Activities include formal and informal meetings, parent-to-parent support, contacting new parents of down syndrome children to offer support and information on community resources, providing information on doctors, hospitals and professionals.

3510 Paul
Miriam Perrone
440 Park Avenue 912-638-8551
Saint Simons Island, GA 31522-4357
How a determined mother carved a semi-independent life for her now-grown Down's syndrome child.

3511 Show Me No Mercy
Cokesbury
PO Box 801
Nashville, TN 37202-0801
A father of a young adult man with Down syndrome relates the experiences of his attempt to be reunited with his son after a family tragedy separates them.
R Perske, Editor

3512 Since Owen
Johns Hopkins University Press
2715 N Charles Street 410-516-6900
Baltimore, MD 21211-2105 Fax: 410-516-6968
www.press.jhu.edu
A well written book displaying understanding from a veteran parent communicating with other parents of children with disabilities.
466 pages
Charles R Callanan, Editor

3513 Teaching the Infant with Down Syndrome: A Guide for Parents & Professionals
Pro-Ed, Inc.
8700 Shoal Creek Boulevard 512-451-3246
Austin, TX 78757-6897 800-897-3202
Fax: 800-397-7633
e-mail: info@proedinc.com
www.proedinc.com
A manual providing teaching ideas and activities that can be used to assist an infant's development.
MJ Hanson, Editor

3514 To Give an Edge: A Guide for New Parents of Children with Down's Syndrome
Viking Press
7000 Washington Avenue S 612-941-8780
Eden Prairie, MN 55344-3580
A guide for new parents designed to provide information about the disorder and how other parents of children with Down syndrome have coped.
JE Rynders, Editor
JM Horrobin, Editor

3515 Understanding Down's Syndrome An Introduction for Parents
Brookline Books
PO Box 1209 617-734-6772
Brookline, MA 02445 800-666-2665
Fax: 617-734-3952
www.brooklinebooks.com
The author provides answers and explanations to the countless questions directed to him during his twenty years' involvement with Down syndrome individuals and their families.
Softcover
ISBN: 1-571290-09-5

Children's Books

3516 **Our Brother Has Down's Syndrome: An Introduction for Children**
Firefly Books
250 Sparks Avenue 416-499-8412
Willowdale, M2H 2S4, e-mail: service@fireflybooks.com
www.fireflybooks.com
Two young sisters tell about their little brother with Down syndrome in this color picture book.
21 pages
S Cairo, Editor

3517 **Secret Place of the Stairs**
Harper & Row
10 E 53rd Street 212-207-7000
New York, NY 10022-5299
A story that weaves many themes, including the institutionalizing of the protagonist's sister, her parents' divorce and her own expectations.
Grades 7-10

3518 **We Can Do It!**
Macmillan
866 3rd Avenue
New York, NY 10022-6221 212-702-7865
www.macmillan.com
A colorful book of photographs that show the daily activities of young children with different developmental delays, including Down syndrome.
L Dwight, Editor

Magazines

3519 **Down Syndrome, Papers and Abstracts for Professionals**
200 Rabbit Road 301-963-1857
Gaithersburg, MD 20878
Quarterly review of research literature pertaining to Down syndrome.
Monthly

3520 **Exceptional Parent Magazine**
209 Harvard Street 617-730-5800
Brookline, MA 02446-5071 Fax: 617-730-8742
A publication dealing with many issues affecting exceptional children and their families.
Monthly

Newsletters

3521 **Down Syndrome News**
National Down Syndrome Congress
7000 Peachtree Dunwoody Rd NE 770-604-9500
Atlanta, GA 30328-1655 800-232-6372
e-mail: NDSC.center@aol.com
www.ndsccenter.org
Contains book reviews, articles and items of interest to those touched by Down syndrome.
10x Annually
Frank J Murphy, Executive Director

3522 **Down Syndrome Today**
Down Syndrome Today Publications
PO Box 212 516-654-3242
Holtsville, NY 11742-0212
Offers information, articles, resources and materials for the parent and professional working and nurturing patients and persons with Downs syndrome.
Debra Hoeft, Publisher

3523 **National Down Syndrome Society Update**
666 Broadway 212-460-9330
New York, NY 10012-2317 800-221-4602
Fax: 212-979-2873
www.ndss.org
Offers information on the activities of the society, new breakthroughs in medical technology, articles offering state of the art information to families and individuals with Down syndrome, and answers to questions about the illness.
12 pages Quarterly
Fran Goldstein, Editor

3524 **On the Up with Down Syndrome**
Carole Shafer, author
Down Syndrome Association of Wisconsin
9401 West Beloit Road 414-327-3729
Milwaukee, WI 53227 866-327-3729
Fax: 414-327-1329
e-mail: thomtalent@aol.com
www.dsaw.org
Offers the exchange of ideas and experiences. Free to our members. Membership is $20.00/year.
Quarterly
Ron Irwin, Board President
Robbin Lyons, Newsletter Contact

Pamphlets

3525 **Alzheimer's Disease and Down Syndrome**
National Down Syndrome Society
666 Broadway 212-460-9330
New York, NY 10012-2317 800-221-4602
www.ndss.org
1995

3526 **Down Syndrome**
March of Dimes
233 Park Avenue South 212-353-8353
New York, NY 10003 Fax: 212-254-3518
e-mail: NY639@marchofdimes.com
www.marchofdimes.com

3527 **Heart and Down Syndrome**
National Down Syndrome Society
666 Broadway 212-460-9330
New York, NY 10012-2317 800-221-4602
www.ndss.org
1995

3528 **Life Planning and Down Syndrome**
National Down Syndrome Society
666 Broadway 212-460-9330
New York, NY 10012-2317 800-221-4602
www.ndss.org

3529 **Neurology of Down Syndrome**
National Down Syndrome Society
666 Broadway 212-460-9330
New York, NY 10012-2317 800-221-4602
www.ndss.org
1995

3530 **New Parents**
Association for Children with Down Syndrome
4 Fern Place 516-933-4700
Plainview, NY 11803 Fax: 516-933-9524
e-mail: msmith@acds.org
www.acds.org
Bibliography compiled for parents who have just given birth to a child with Down syndrome. Free upon reciept of a stamped, self-addressed envelope.
Michael Smith, Executive Director

3531 **Sexuality in Down Syndrome**
National Down Syndrome Society
666 Broadway 212-460-9330
New York, NY 10012-2317 800-221-4602
www.ndss.org
1995

3532 **Speech and Language in Children and Adolescents with Down Syndrome**
National Down Syndrome Society

666 Broadway
New York, NY 10012-2317
212-460-9330
800-221-4602
www.ndss.org

1995

Audio & Video

3533 **Adaptation to the Initial Crisis**
Lawren Productions
930 Pitner Avenue 847-328-6700
Evanston, IL 60202-1556 800-421-2363
A family learns to adapt to the birth of a child with a handicap.

3534 **Bernardsville Beginnings**
National Down Syndrome Society
666 Broadway 212-460-9330
New York, NY 10012-2317 800-221-4602
Fax: 212-979-2873
www.ndss.org
Follows Alison through her first full year in a first grade inclusion program. Step-by-step account of teaching staff preparation, classroom experiences, a portrayal of one girl's successful adjustment, and a whole class matured by the experience.
23 minutes

3535 **Bittersweet Waltz**
National Down Syndrome Society
666 Broadway 212-460-9330
New York, NY 10012-2317 800-221-4602
Fax: 212-979-2873
e-mail: info@ndss.org
www.ndss.org
Experience of Alec and his first year included in a regular fifth grade class. From a point of view of a parent, a child, and the school administration.
18 minutes

3536 **Colin and Ricky**
Lawren Productions
930 Pitner Avenue 847-328-6700
Evanston, IL 60202-1556 800-421-2363
A young boy comes to deal with his disappointment surrounding the birth of his baby brother with Down syndrome.

3537 **Congratulations: An Introduction to Down Syndrome for Parents/Family/Friends**
New Challenges
96 Ogden Avenue 914-287-0723
White Plains, NY 10605
Film for parents which addresses some of the most commonly asked questions about raising a child with Down syndrome.

3538 **Daddy's Girl**
Carle Media
110 W Main Street 217-384-4838
Urbana, IL 61801-2715
A film starring a twelve-year-old actress with Down syndrome, dealing with her divorced father's inability to accept the fact that his daughter has Down syndrome.
Carolyn Baxley

3539 **Down Syndrome: See the Potential**
Down Syndrome Association of Charlotte
PO Box 3136
Charlotte, NC 28210 800-232-6372
Video highlighting the capability of children with Down syndrome.

3540 **Gifts of Love**
National Down Syndrome Society
666 Broadway 212-460-9330
New York, NY 10012-2317 800-221-4602
Fax: 212-979-2873
www.ndss.org
Four families of children with Down syndrome talk about their feelings and experiences with their children, particularly during the first six years. All the children live at home and attend programs in their communities.
25 minutes

3541 **Infant Motor Development: A Look at the Phases**
Communication Skill Builders/Therapy Skill Builder
3830 E Bellevue 520-323-7500
Tucson, AZ 85733
A video depicting development in and activities for infants birth through 12 months.

3542 **New Expectations**
Lawren Productions
930 Pitner Avenue
Evanston, IL 60202-1556 800-421-2363
Focuses on the emotional and technical aspects of Down syndrome. Highlights four persons at various life stages from infancy to adulthood in the areas of education and employment.

3543 **New Set of Fears, a New Set of Hopes**
Meyer Children's Rehabilitation Institute
Resource Center, 444 S 44th Street 402-559-7467
Omaha, NE 68131 800-232-6372
Explores the way a family adjusts as they go through the life cycle with their child who has Down syndrome.

3544 **Opportunities to Grow**
National Down Syndrome Society
666 Broadway 212-460-9330
New York, NY 10012-2317 800-221-4602
Fax: 212-979-2873
e-mail: info@ndss.org
www.ndss.org
Sequel to Gifts of Love video shows how people with Down syndrome, ages 6 to 26, participate equally in all phases of community life. Vignettes of 15 young men and women illustrate how inclusion, education, computer facilitation, socialization programs, and employment training help them to fulfill their potential.
25 minutes

3545 **Stepping Stones**
AIT
PO Box A
Bloomington, IN 47402-0120 800-457-4509
Series of video programs on teaching basic skills to at-risk, special needs and normally developed children.

3546 **Thanks Mom and Dad: Profiles of Patrick**
University of Washington
CDMRC Mail Stop WJ-10 206-543-4011
Seattle, WA 98195-0001 800-232-6372
Documentary on the life of Patrick, a young man with Down syndrome from birth through his graduation from high school.

3547 **You Don't Outgrow Down Syndrome**
National Association for Down Syndrome
PO Box 4542 630-325-9112
Oak Brook, IL 60522-4542 800-232-6372
www.nads.org
Winner of the second annual International Rehabilitation Film Festival.

Web Sites

3548 **Aleh Foundation**
www.aleh.org
Aleh Rehabilitation Center has served as a residential facility to close to 200 children with multiple, physical and mental disabilities.

3549 **Down Syndrome**
www.downsyn.com
A resource for new paretns of children with Down syndrome. Provides a personnel perspective from parents who also have children with Down syndrome.

3550 **Healing Well**
www.healingwell.com
An online health resource guide to medical news, chat, information and articles, newsgroups and message boards, books, disease-related web sites, medical directories, and more for patients, friends, and family coping with disabling diseases, disorders, or chronic illnesses.

3551 **Health Finder**

www.healthfinder.gov

Searchable, carefully developed web site offering information on over 1000 topics. Developed by the US Department of Health and Human Services, the site can be used in both English and Spanish.

3552 **Healthlink USA**

www.healthlinkusa.com

Health information concerning treatment, cures, prevention, diagnosis, risk factors, research, support groups, email lists, personal stories and much more. Updated regularly.

3553 **Helios Health**

www.helioshealth.com

Online resource for your health information. Detailed information about specific health topics, access to expert advice from our Medical Advisory Board, and up-to-date health news.

3554 **MedicineNet**

www.medicinenet.com

An online resource for consumers providing easy-to-read, authoritative medical and health information.

3555 **Medscape**

www.mywebmd.com

Medscape offers specialists, primary care physicians, and other health professionals the Web's most robust and integrated medical information and educational tools.

3556 **National Down Syndrome Society**

www.ndss.org

NDSS works to obtain a better understanding of Down syndrome, the potential of people with Down syndrome, to support research about the condition, and to provide information and referral services for families and professionals.

3557 **WebMD**

www.webmd.com

Information on Down Syndrome, including articles and resources.

Description

3558 **Eating Disorders (Anorexia Nervosa, Bulimia)**

Anorexia nervosa and bulimia nervosa are eating disorders characterized by a disturbed sense of body image and an irrational fear of obesity. They are manifested by abnormal patterns relating to food and by self-induced, marked weight loss.

Anorexia is a psychiatric disorder in which dieting and a desire for thinness leads to excessive weight loss. About 95 percent of persons with this disorder are female, although males can be affected. The onset usually occurs during adolescence and some sufferers are in their 60s. Anorexia nervosa is characterized by self-starvation, food preoccupation and rituals, compulsive exercising, and often a resulting absence of menstrual cycles. The cause is unknown, although social factors appear to play an important role, including advertisements that equate thinness with desirability. Denial is a prominent feature, and sufferers usually resist treatment.

Bulimia is characterized by recurring episodes of binge eating followed by efforts to avoid weight gain, such as purging through self-induced vomiting or abuse of laxatives and/or diuretics (water pills). Unlike patients with anorexia, those with bulimia usually have normal weight. Binges are often triggered by psychological stress and carried out in secret. Warning signs of bulimia include eating uncontrollably, frequent use of the bathroom, erosion of dental enamel of the front teeth (from vomiting), and painless swollen salivary glands. Bulimia may coexist with anorexia.

Anorexia nervosa is associated with a 10 percent death rate, generally from a sudden disturbance of heart rhythm. Fortunately, most sufferers will eventually return to a normal or near-normal body weight, although many continue to struggle with body image and unhealthy eating patterns. Treatment for both illnesses is similar, beginning with the need to restore body weight. Initial treatment may require hospitalization for physical stabilization. Long-term psychological treatment and behavior modification is often necessary and focuses on behavioral and emotional growth for both the individual with the eating disorder and their family. See also *Obesity*.

National Agencies & Associations

3559 **Academy for Eating Disorders**
111 Deer Lake Road 847-498-4274
Deerfield, IL 60015-1577 Fax: 847-480-9282
e-mail: info@aedweb.org
www.aedweb.org
AED is an association of multidisciplinary professionals promoting effective treatment, developing prevention initiatives, advocating for the field, stimulating research and sponsoring an annual conference.
Judith Banker, President
Greg Schultz, Interim Executive Director

3560 **American Dietetic Association**
120 S Riverside Plaza 312-899-0040
Chicago, IL 60606-6995 800-877-1600
e-mail: media@eatright.org
www.eatright.org
ADA offers nutrition information consumer tips nutrition fact sheets consumer frequently asked questions and referrals to registered dieticians.
Patricia M Babjak, Chief Executive Officer
Martin M Yadrick, President

3561 **Anna Westin Foundation**
PO Box 268 952-361-3051
Chaska, MN 55318 e-mail: kitty@annawestinfoundation.org
www.annawestinfoundation.org
The Anna Westin Foundation is dedicated to the prevention and treatment of eating disorders. They are committed to preventing the tragic loss of life to anorexia nervosa and bulimia and to raising public awareness of those dangerous illnesses.
Kitty Westin, President

3562 **Anorexia Nervosa & Bulimia Association**
767 Bayridge Drive
Kingston Ontario, K7P-1C0 www.phe.queensu.ca
Facilitate advocate and coordinate support for any individual directly or indirectly affected by eating disorders and to raise public awareness through improved communication and the provision of education within our community.

3563 **Dads and Daughters**
34 E Superior Street 218-772-3942
Duluth, MN 55802 888-824-DADS
Fax: 218-728-0314
e-mail: info@dadsanddaughters.org
www.thedadman.com
Provides tools to strengthen father-daughter relationships and transform pervasive cultural messages that value daughters more for how they look than who they are.
Gregg Rutter, Development Director

3564 **Eating Disorders Action Group**
6156 Quinpool Road 902-443-9944
Halifax Nova Scotia, B3L 1-3Z9 e-mail: reception@edag.ca
www.edag.ca
A community based charitable organization dedicated to promoting healthy body image and self esteem and to supporting individuals who experience disordered eating.

3565 **Eating Disorders Anonymous**
PO Box 55876
Phoenix, AZ 85078-5876 e-mail: info@eatingdisordersanonymous.org
www.4eda.org
EDA provides information about local support group meetings.

3566 **Eating Disorders Coalition for Research, Policy and Action**
720 7th Street NW 202-543-9570
Washington, DC 20001-4303 Fax: 202-543-9570
e-mail: manager@eatingdisorderscoalition.org
www.eatingdisorderscoalition.org
Advocates at the federal level on behalf of people with eating disorders their families and professionals working with these populations. Promotes federal support for improved access to care.
David Jaffe, Executive Director
Jeanine Cogan, Policy Director

3567 **Healthy Weight Network**
402 S 14th Street 701-567-2646
Hettinger, ND 58639 Fax: 701-567-2602
e-mail: hwj@healthyweight.net
www.healthyweight.net
Promotes information and resources pertaining to the Health at Any Size paradigm.
Frances M Berg MS, Founder/Editor

3568 **International Association of Eating Disorders Professionals**
PO Box 1295 309-346-3341
Pekin, IL 61555-1295 800-800-8126
Fax: 309-346-2874
e-mail: iaedpmembers@earthlink.net
www.iaedp.com

IAEDP Offers professional counseling and assistance to the medical community, courts, law enforcement officials and social welfare agencies.
Andrea Penni MD, President
Emmett R Bishop MD CEDS, Immediate Past President

3569 **Jessie's Hope Society**
11739 23rd Street
Maple Ridge, BC, V2X-5X8
604-466-4877
877-288-0877
Fax: 604-466-4897
e-mail: info@jessieshope.org
www.jessieshope.org
Promote positive body image by fostering in youth within communities and across cultures throughout British Columbia.
Brian W Chittock, Executive Director

3570 **National Association of Anorexia Nervosa and Associated Disorders**
PO Box 7
Highland Park, IL 60035
847-831-3438
Fax: 847-433-4632
e-mail: anadhelp@anad.org
www.anad.org
Works to prevent eating disorders and provides numerous programs — all free — to help victims and families including hotlines, support groups, referrals, information packets and newsletters. Educational/prevention programs include presentations and early detection.
Vivian Hanse Meehan, Founder/President
Dawn Ries, Administrator

3571 **National Eating Disorder Information Centr e**
ES 7-421, 200 Elizabeth Street
Toronto, Ontario, M5G-2C4
416-340-4156
866-633-4220
Fax: 416-340-4736
e-mail: nedic@uhn.on.ca
www.nedic.ca
Promotes healthy lifestyles, including both healty eating and appropriate, enjoyable exercise.
Merryl Bear MEd, Director
Jessica Rust, Administrative Coordinator

3572 **National Eating Disorders Association**
603 Stewart Street
Seattle, WA 98101
206-382-3587
800-931-2237
Fax: 206-829-8501
e-mail: info@NationalEatingDisorders.org
www.nationaleatingdisorders.org
Our mission is to eliminate eating disorders and body dissatisfaction through prevention efforts education referral and support services advocacy training and research.
Lynn S Grefe MA, Chief Executive Officer
Molly Bauthues, Communications Manager

3573 **National Eating Disorders Screening Program**
One Washington Street
Wellesley Hills, MA 02481
781-239-0071
Fax: 781-431-7447
e-mail: smhinfo@mentalhealthscreening.org
www.mentalhealthscreening.org
Offers eating disorders screening.
Douglas G Jacobs MD, President & CEO

3574 **National Women's Health Information Center**
8270 Willow Oaks Corporate Drive
Fairfax, VA 22031
800-994-9662
Fax: 703-560-6598
TTY: 888-220-5446
TDD: 888-220-5446
e-mail: Wanda.jones@hhs.gov
www.4woman.gov
Government agency with free health information for women.
Wanda K Jones PhD, Deputy Assistant Secretary for Health
Frances E Ashe-Goins RN, Deputy Director

3575 **Weight-control Information Network National Institutes of Health**
National Institutes of Health
1 WIN Way
Bethesda, MD 20892-3665
202-828-1025
877-946-4627
Fax: 202-828-1028
e-mail: win@info.niddk.nih.gov
www.win.niddk.nih.gov/index.htm
Information on obesity weight-control and nutrition.
BiAnnual

State Agencies & Associations

Connecticut

3576 **Renfrew Center of Connecticut**
436 Danbury Road
Wilton, CT 06897
800-REN-FREW
Fax: 203-563-9936
e-mail: foundation@renfrew.org
www.renfrewcenter.com

Florida

3577 **Renfrew Center of Miami**
151 Majorca Avenue
Coral Gables, FL 33134
800-REN-FREW
Fax: 305-445-2729
e-mail: info@renfrewcenter.com
www.renfrewcenter.com

3578 **Renfrew Center of South Florida**
7700 Renfrew Lane
Coconut Creek, FL 33073
800-REN-FREW
Fax: 954-698-9007
e-mail: info@renfrewcenter.com
www.renfrewcenter.com

Maryland

3579 **St. Joseph's Medical Center**
7601 Osler Drive
Towson, MD 21204
410-337-1000
www.sjmcmd.org
John Tolmie, President/CEO

Massachusetts

3580 **Massachusetts Eating Disorder Association**
92 Pearl Street
Newton, MA 02458
617-558-1881
866-343-MEDA
Fax: 617-558-1771
e-mail: info@medainc.com
www.medainc.org
A nonprofit organization dedicated to the treatment and prevention of eating disorders. MEDA provides helpline resource and referral, assessments, client consultations, individual therapy, support groups and an intensive evening treatment program.
100+ Members
Rebecca Manley, Founder
Beth Mayer, CEO

New Jersey

3581 **American Anorexia Bulimia Association: New Jersey Chapter**
10 Station Place
Metuchen, NJ 09940
732-549-6886
800-522-2230
Fax: 609-688-1544
e-mail: njaaba@NJAABA.org
www.njaaba.org

3582 **Renfrew Center of Northern New Jersey**
174 Union Street
Ridgewood, NJ 07450
800-REN-FREW
Fax: 201-652-6253
e-mail: info@renfrewcenter.org
www.renfrewcenter.com

New York

3583 **National Eating Disorders Association Long Island**
603 Stewart Street 206-382-3587
Seattle, WA 98101 800-931-2237
Fax: 206-829-8501
e-mail: info@NationalEatingDisorders.org
www.nationaleatingdisorders.org
Nonprofit organization devoted to prevention, education and support on the issue of eating disorders. As the number of eating disorder sufferers has grown significantly in our local community, the council was developed to deal with the needs of those suffering with eating disorders.
Lynn S Grefe MA, CEO
Tracy L Kahlo MNPL, Vice President

3584 **Renfrew Center of New York**
11 E 36th Street
New York, NY 10016 800-REN-FREW
Fax: 212-686-1865
e-mail: info@renfrewcenter.org
www.renfrewcenter.com

3585 **Westchester Task Force on Eating Disorders/American Anorexia Bulimia**
3 Mount Joy Avenue 914-472-3701
Scarsdale, NY 10583-2632

Pennsylvania

3586 **American Anorexia Bulimia Association of Philadelphia**
PO Box 1287 215-221-1864
Langhorne, PA 19047 Fax: 215-702-8944
www.aabaphila.org

3587 **American Anorexia Bulimia Association:**
PO Box 1287 215-221-1864
Langhorne, PA 19047 Fax: 215-702-8944
www.aabaphila.org

3588 **Pennsylvania Educational Network for Eating Disorders**
4801 McKnight Road
Pittsburgh, PA 15101 412-215-7967
www.pened.org
PENED is a nonprofit organization providing education, support, and referral information to the general and professional public.

3589 **Renfrew Center of Bryn Mawr**
735 Old Lancaster Road
Bryn Mawr, PA 19010 800-736-3739
Fax: 610-527-9361
e-mail: info@renfrewcenter.org
www.renfrewcenter.com

3590 **Renfrew Center of Philadelphia**
475 Spring Lane
Philadelphia, PA 19128 800-REN-FREW
Fax: 215-482-7390
e-mail: info@renfrew.org
www.renfrewcenter.com

Research Centers

3591 **Academy for Eating Disorders**
111 Deer Lake Road 847-498-4274
Deerfield, IL 60015-1577 Fax: 847-480-9282
e-mail: info@aedweb.org
www.aedweb.org
Disseminate knowledge regarding eating disorders to members of the Academy other professionals and the general public
Judith Banker, President
Susie Orbach, Board of Advisor

3592 **Center for the Study of Anorexia and Bulimia**
1841 Broadway at 60th Street 212-333-3444
New York, NY 10023 Fax: 212-333-5444
www.icpnyc.org/CenterForStudy.nxg
The Institute is composed of a group of 150 professionally trained licensed psychotherapists who offer a full range of psychotherapeutic services including individual and group psychotherapy and psychoanalysis in addition to more specialized treatment services
Jim M Pollack CSW, Executive Director/Director of Treatment
Ron Taffel PhD, Chair

3593 **Division of Digestive & Liver Diseases of Cloumbia University**
630 W 168th Street 212-305-8156
New York, NY 10032 e-mail: hjw14@columbia.edu
www.cumc.columbia.edu/dept/gi
The Division's faculty members are devoted to research and the clinical care of patients with gastrointestinal liver and nutritional disorders. The Division is also responsible for the Gastroenterology Training Program at the medical center and for teaching medical students interns residents fellows and attending physicians aspects of gastrointestinal and liver diseases
Howard J Worman MD, Division Director
Nora V Bergasa MD, Associate Professor of Clinical Medicine

3594 **Harris Center for Education and Advocacy in Eating Disorders**
2 Longfellow Place 617-726-8470
Boston, MA 02114 Fax: 617-726-1595
e-mail: dherzog@partners.org
www.harriscentermgh.org
Conducts research provides a newsletter and information.
David B Herzog MD, Director
David B Herzog MD, Director

Support Groups & Hotlines

3595 **AABA Support Group**
Tucker Pavilion 804-320-3911
Richmond, VA 23225
Chippenham Medical Center, Tucker Pavillion, 7101 Jahnke Road. Every 1st and 3rd Tuesday of the month, 7:30 p.m.
Elliot Spanier, Contact

3596 **About Kids GI Disorders**
158 Pleasant Street 978-685-4477
North Andover, MA 01845-2797 800-394-2747
Fax: 508-685-4488
e-mail: aphs@tiac.net
www.aboutkidsgi.org/
ABOUT KIDS is the pediatric branch of the International Foundation for Functional Gastrointestinal Disorders (IFFGD), a registered nonprofit education and research organization founded in 1991. Their mission is to inform, assist, and support those affected by gastrointestinal (GI) disorders, addressing issues of digestive health in children through support of education and research. IFFGD promotes awareness among the public, health care providers, researchers, and regulators.
Douglas Drossman MD, Director
Nancy Norton, President of the Board

3597 **Association of Gastrointestinal Motility D isorders**
AGMD International Corporate Headquarters
12 Roberts Drive 781-861-3874
Bedfored, MA 01730 Fax: 781-275-1304
e-mail: gimotility@msn.com
www.agmd-gimotility.org/
Support and education for persons affected by digestive motility disorders. Serves as educational resource and information base for medical professionals. Physician referrals, video tapes, educational materials, networking support, symposiums and several publications.
Mary Angela DeGrazia-DiTucci, President/Patient/Founder

3598 **Coconut Creek Eating Disorders Support Group**
Renfrew Center
7700 NW 48th Avenue 954-698-9222
Coconut Creek, FL 33073-3508 877-367-3383
Fax: 954-698-9007
www.renfrew.org
Samuel Menagad, Director

3599 **Eating Disorder Resource Center**
330 W 58th Street 212-989-3987
New York, NY 10019 e-mail: drjbris@gmail.com
www.edrcnyc.org

Develops and offers specialized treatment programs for the eating-disordered population. Provide a psychotherapy referral service which offers the most up-to-date, professional treatment available for problematic eating behaviors, food obsessions, and body image concerns.
Judith Brisman PhD, Director

3600 Eating Disorders Association of New Jersey
10 Station Place
Metuchen, NJ 08840
800-522-2230
Fax: 732-906-9307
e-mail: info@edanj.org
www.edanj.org
A non-profit state organization whose mission is to provide supportive services and resources to indivudals affected by eating disorders, including family members and friends.

3601 First Presbyterian Church in the City of N ew York Support Groups
First Presbyterian Church in the City of New York
12 West 12th Street
New York, NY 10011
212-675-6150
Fax: 212-625-4321
e-mail: info@fpcnyc.org
www.fpcnyc.org/
The First Presbyterian Church in the City of New York provides numerous programs and supports groups for both adults and children including an educational program for autistic children.
Jon M Walton, Senior Pastor
Eugene Rogers, Business Manager

3602 Holliswood Hospital Psychiatric Care, Serv ices and Self-Help/Support Groups
87-37 Palermo Street
Holliswood, NY 11423
718-776-8181
800-486-3005
Fax: 718-776-8572
e-mail: HolliswoodInfo@libertymgt.com
www.holliswoodhospital.com/
The Holliswood Hospital, a 110-bed private psychiatric hospital located in a quiet residential Queens community, is a leader in providing quality, acute inpatient mental health care for adult, adolescent, geriatric and dually diagnosed patients. Holliswood Hospital treats patients with a broad range of psychiatric disorders. Additionally, specialized services are available for patients with psychiatric diagnoses compounded by chemical dependency, or a history of physical or sexual abuse.
Susan Clayton, Support Group Coordinator
Angela Hurtado, Support Group Coordinator

3603 National Health Information Center
PO Box 1133
Washington, DC 20013
310-565-4167
800-336-4797
Fax: 301-984-4256
e-mail: info@nhic.org
www.health.gov/nhic
Offers a nationwide information referral service, produces directories and resource guides.

3604 Pedicatric/Adolescent Gastroesophageal Reflux Association
PO Box 466
Garrett Park, MD 20896-0466
301-601-9541
e-mail: gergroup@aol.com
www.reflux.org
Provides information and support to parents, patients and doctors about Gastroesophageal Reflux.
Beth Anderson, Director

3605 Richmond Support Group
Warwick Medical & Professional Ctr
Richmond, VA
804-320-7881

Books

3606 Anorexia Nervosa & Recovery: A Hunger for Meaning
The Haworth Press
10 Alice Street
Binghamton, NY 13904
607-722-5857
800-429-6784
e-mail: getinfo@haworth.com
www.haworth.com
1993 146 pages Paperback
ISBN: 0-918393-95-7

3607 Bearly Any Fat Cookbook
Obesity Foundation
5600 S Quebec Street
Englewood, CO 80111-2202
303-850-0328
e-mail: editor@obesity.org
www.obesity.org
Perfect cookbook to assist anyone in a weight reduction program.

3608 Body Betrayed
American Psychiatric Press
1400 K Street NW
Washington, DC 20005-2403
202-682-6268
Fax: 202-789-2648
A book concentrating on women, eating disorders and treatments.
440 pages Hardcover
ISBN: 0-880485-22-1

3609 Bulimia: A Guide to Recovery
Gurze Books
PO Box 2238
Carlsbad, CA 92018-9883
800-756-7533
Fax: 760-434-5476
e-mail: gzcatl@aol.com
www.bulimia.com
This intimate guidebook offers a complete understanding of bulimia and a plan for recovery. It includes a two-week program to stop bingeing, things-to-do instead of bingeing, a two-week guide for support groups, specific advice for loved ones and Eating Without Fear, Hall's story of self-cure which has inspired thousands of other bulimics.
280 pages Paperback
ISBN: 0-936077-31-X

3610 Conversations with Anorexics
Jason Aronson
PO Box 15100
York, PA 17405-7100
800-782-0015
Fax: 201-840-7242
www.aronson.com
A Compassionate and Hopeful Journey through the Therapeutic Process.
238 pages
ISBN: 1-568212-61-5

3611 Coping with Eating Disorders
Rosen Publishing Group
29 E 21st Street
New York, NY 10010
212-777-3017
800-237-9932
Fax: 888-436-4643
e-mail: customerservice@rosenpub.com
www.rosenpublishing.com
This book offers practical suggestions on coping with eating disorders.

ISBN: 0-823929-74-4
Barbara Moe, Author

3612 Cult of Thinness
Oxford University Press
2001 Evans Road
Cary, NC 27513-2010
212-726-6000
800-451-7556
Fax: 919-677-1303
www.oup-usa.org
1996 256 pages
ISBN: 0-195082-41-9

3613 Deadly Diet: Recovering from Anorexia & Bulimia
New Harbinger Publications
5674 Shattuck Avenue
Oakland, CA 94609-1662
800-748-6273
Fax: 510-652-5472
www.newharbinger.com
1993 265 pages Paperback
ISBN: 1-879237-42-3

3614 Eating Diorders Resource Catalogue
Gurze Books
PO Box 2238
Carlsbad, CA 92018-9883
800-756-7533
Fax: 760-434-5476
www.bulimia.com

This catalogue of resources contains over 140 books, videos and audiotapes, lists of national organizations and treatment facilities and basic facts about eating disorders. It is widely distributed by individuals who are suffering, their loved ones, the health care professionals who treat them and educators who are working towards prevention.
24 pages Annual

3615 Eating Disorder Sourcebook
Gurze Books
PO Box 2238
Carlsbad, CA 92018-2238
800-756-7533
Fax: 760-434-5476
e-mail: gzcatl@aol.com
www.bulimia.com
An ideal book for someone with a loved one who has an eating disorder but who knows little about this subject, this new release presents a clear overview of basic issues.
222 pages Paperback

3616 Eating Disorders Resource Catalogue
Gurze Books
PO Box 2238
Carlsbad, CA 92018-9883
800-756-7533
Fax: 760-434-5476
www.bulimia.com
This catalogue of resources contains over 140 books, videos and audiotapes, lists of national organizations and treatment facilities and basic facts about eating disorders. It is widely distributed by individuals who are suffering, their loved ones, the health care professionals who treat them and educators who are working towards prevention.
28 pages Annual

3617 Eating Disorders-Overview Series
Lucent Books
Thomson Gale
Farmington Hills, MI 48333-9187
800-877-4253
Fax: 800-414-5043
e-mail: gale.customerservice@thomson.com
www.gale.com/lucent
This book examines how eating disorders can be identified, who is affected by them, and how they can be treated.
2001
ISBN: 1-560066-59-8

3618 Eating Disorders: When Food Turns Against You
Franklin Watts Grolier
90 Old Sherman Tpke
Danbury, CT 06816-0001
203-797-3500
Fax: 203-797-3197
www.grolier.com
1993 96 pages
ISBN: 0-531111-75-0

3619 Emotional Eating: A Practical Guide to Taking Control
Free Press
866 3rd Avenue
New York, NY 10022
800-223-7445
Fax: 800-943-9831
www.simonsays.com
1003 200 pages
ISBN: 0-029002-15-0

3620 Encyclopedia of Obesity and Eating Disorders
Facts on File
11 Penn Plaza
New York, NY 10001
212-967-8800
800-322-8755
Fax: 800-678-3633
From abdominoplasty to Zung Rating Scale, this volume defines and explains these disorders, along with medical and other problems associated with them.
272 pages Hardcover

3621 Endorphins: Eating Disorders & Other Addictive Behavior
WW Norton & Company
500 5th Avenue
New York, NY 10110-0054
212-354-5500
800-233-4830
Fax: 800-458-6515
www.wwnorton.com
1993 320 pages
ISBN: 0-393701-56-5

3622 Etiology and Treatment of Bulimia Nervosa
Jason Aronson
PO Box 15100
York, PA 17405-7100
800-782-0015
Fax: 201-767-1576
www.aronson.com
352 pages Softcover
ISBN: 1-568213-39-5

3623 Evaluation and Management of Eating Disorders
Human Kinetics Publishers
PO Box 5076
Champaign, IL 61825-5076
217-351-1549
800-747-4457
Fax: 217-351-5076
368 pages Cloth
ISBN: 0-873229-11-8

3624 Fear of Being Fat
Jason Aronson
PO Box 15100
York, PA 17405-7100
800-782-0015
Fax: 201-840-7242
www.aronson.com
366 pages
ISBN: 0-876688-99-7

3625 Getting Better Bit(e) by Bit(e)
Gurze Books
PO Box 2238
Carlsbad, CA 92018-2238
800-756-7533
Fax: 760-434-5476
e-mail: gzcatl@aol.com
www.bulimia.com
This practical book on recovery from bulimia and binge eating is packed with lists, exercises, case studies, discussions, insights and specific things to do. This book also addresses the day-to-day problems faced by eating disorder sufferers and concentrates on key behavior changes necessary for progress.
143 pages Paperback

3626 Going Backwards
Scholastic
730 Broadway
New York, NY 10003-9511
212-505-3000
800-325-6149
A story that weaves the themes of acceptance, death, mortality and family loyalty to present a controversial plot.
Grades 7-10

3627 Golden Cage: The Enigma of Anorexia Nervosa
Gurze Books
PO Box 2283
Carlsbad, CA 92018-2283
800-756-7533
Fax: 760-434-5476
e-mail: gzcatl@aol.com
www.bulimia.com

3628 Group Psychotherapy for Eating Disorders
American Psychiatric Press
1400 K Street NW
Washington, DC 20005-2403
202-682-6268
Fax: 202-789-2648
The first book to fully explore the use of group therapy in the treatment of eating disorders.
353 pages Hardcover
ISBN: 0-880484-19-5

3629 Helping Athletes with Eating Disorders
Human Kinetics Publishers
PO Box 5076
Champaign, IL 61825-5076
217-351-1549
800-747-4457
Fax: 217-351-5076

Gives readers the information they need to identify and address major eating disorders such as: anorexia, bulimia nervosa, and eating disorders not otherwise specified.
208 pages Cloth
ISBN: 0-873223-83-7

3630 Hope and Recovery: A Mother-Daughter Story About Anorexia Nervosa & Bulimia
Franklin Watts Grolier
90 Old Sherman Tpke
Danbury, CT 06816-0001 800-621-1115
Fax: 800-374-4329
Mother and daughter tell a story of a young woman's recovery from the horror of an eating disorder. This compelling account shows how anorexia and bulimia can affect an entire family.
192 pages
ISBN: 0-531111-40-7

3631 Hungry Self: Women, Eating and Identity
Gurze Books
PO Box 2283
Carlsbad, CA 92018-2283 800-756-7533
Fax: 760-434-5476
e-mail: gzcatl@aol.com
www.bulimia.com

3632 Insights in the Dynamic Psychotherapy of Anorexia and Bulimia
Jason Aronson
400 Keystone Industrial Park
Dunmore, PA 18512-1523 800-782-0015
Fax: 201-840-7242
www.aronson.com
320 pages Hardcover
ISBN: 0-876685-68-8

3633 It's Not Your Fault
Gurze Books
PO Box 2238
Carlsbad, CA 92018-2238 800-756-5476
Fax: 760-434-5476
e-mail: gzcatl@aol.com
www.bulimia.com
In this comprehensive, medically sound guide to overcoming eating disorders, Dr. Marx defines the warnings signs of eating disorders, explores causes, at risk populations, the role of drug therapy and advises patients and families where and how they can find help.

3634 Making Peace with Food
Gurze Books
PO Box 2238
Carlsbad, CA 92018-2238 800-756-7533
Fax: 760-434-5476
e-mail: gzcatl@aol.com
www.bulimia.com
This unique, full sized workbook is designed to help anyone who experienced compulsive eating, yo-yo dieting, food and body anxiety, or associated eating disorders. Filled with ideas, workbook pages, exercises and resources, Kano's book is an excellent aid to clarifying and overcoming your personal diet/weight struggle.
224 pages Paperback

3635 Meals Without Squeals Sense
Bull Publishing
PO Box 1377
Boulder, CO 80306 800-676-2855
Fax: 303-545-6354
www.bullpub.com
Straight forward information on childrens growth accompanies age specific, child tested recipes. Explained is how common feeding problems can be solved and show ways to offer children positive experiences with food.
2006 288 pages
ISBN: 1-933503-00-4

3636 My Name is Caroline
Doubleday
666 Fifth Avenue 212-354-6500
New York, NY 10103
A poignant tale of one woman's battle with bulimia throughout her life as a successful student, athlete, scholar and musician.
Grades 10-12

3637 Obesity: Theory and Therapy
Raven Press
1185 Avenue of the Americas 212-930-9500
New York, NY 10036-2601 800-777-2295
A classic reference for clinicians dealing with obesity, this volume provides the most up-to-date research, preclinical and clinical information.
500 pages
ISBN: 0-881678-84-8

3638 Practice Guidelines for Eating Disorders
American Psychiatric Press
1400 K Street NW 202-682-6268
Washington, DC 20005-2403 Fax: 202-789-2648
Designed for health care professionals, this guideline includes information on all aspects of anorexia nervosa and bulimia nervosa, including self-induced vomiting, use of laxatives and vigorous exercise to prevent weight gain.
38 pages Paperback
ISBN: 0-890423-00-8

3639 Psychodynamic Technique in the Treatment of the Eating Disorders
Jason Aronson
PO Box 15100
York, PA 17405-7100 800-782-0015
Fax: 201-840-7242
www.aronson.com
440 pages Hardcover
ISBN: 0-876686-22-6

3640 Self-Starvation
Jason Aronson
PO Box 15100
York, PA 17405-7100 800-782-0015
Fax: 201-840-7242
www.aronson.com
312 pages Softcover
ISBN: 1-568218-22-2

3641 Starving to Death in a Sea of Objects
Jason Aronson
PO Box 15100
York, PA 17405-7100 800-782-0015
Fax: 201-840-7242
www.aronson.com
How emancipation becomes security for anorexics.
464 pages Softcover
ISBN: 0-876684-35-5

3642 Surviving an Eating Disorder: Perspectives & Strategies
Gurze Books
PO Box 2238
Carlsbad, CA 92018-2238 800-756-7533
Fax: 760-434-5476
e-mail: gzcatl@aol.com
www.bulimia.com
Parents, spouses and friends of individuals with food problems will find practical guidelines in this book for helping themselves and their loved ones.
222 pages Paperback

3643 Treating Bulimia: A Psychoeducational Approach
American Anorexia/Bulimia Association
165 W 46th Street 212-575-6200
New York, NY 10036-2501 e-mail: amanbu@aol.com
www.members.aol.com/amanbu

3644 When Food is Love
Gurze Books
PO Box 2238
Carlsbad, CA 92018-2238 800-756-7533
Fax: 760-434-5467
e-mail: gzcatl@aol.com
www.gurze.com
Drawing on her own personal experience, Roth explores similarities between eating and loving such as fantasizing, wanting the for-

bidden, creating drama, control issues, and the experience of relationship.
205 pages Paperback

3645 **Withering Child**
University of Georgia Press
330 Research Drive 404-542-2830
Athens, GA 30602 800-266-5842
Fax: 709-369-6131
e-mail: books@ugapress.uga.edu
www.uga.edu/ugapress

1993 288 pages
ISBN: 0-820315-60-5

Children's Books

3646 **Billy's Story**
Metro Intergroup of Overeaters Anonymous
117 W 26th Street 212-206-8621
New York, NY 10001

3647 **I Was a Fifteen-Year-Old Blimp**
Harper & Row
10 E 53rd Street 212-207-7000
New York, NY 10022-5299
This story focuses on Gabby, a teenage girl who overhears others discuss her weight and takes radical steps to become popular.
Grades 6-9

Magazines

3648 **BASH Magazine**
Bulimia Anorexia Self-Help/Behavior Adaptation
PO Box 39903
Saint Louis, MO 63139-8903 800-762-3334
A journal of eating and mood disorders.
Monthly

Newsletters

3649 **AABA Newsletter**
American Anorexic and Bulemic Association
165 W 46th Street 212-575-6200
New York, NY 10036-2501
This newsletter is published three times a year and is mailed to the members of the AABA. The AABA is a tax-exempt, nonprofit organization with a membership of professionals, sufferers of eating disorders, and their family and friends.

3650 **Eating Disorders Review**
Gurze Books
PO Box 2238
Carlsbad, CA 92018-9883 800-756-7533
Fax: 760-434-5476
e-mail: gzcatl@aol.com
www.bulimia.com
Presents current clinical information for the professional treating eating disorders. Features summeries of relevant research from journals and unpublished studies, abstracts, nutritional notes, questions and answers, book reviews and reproducible client handouts.
8 pages BiMonthly
Joel Yager MD, Editor-in-Chief
Liegh Cohn, Publisher

3651 **National Association of Anorexia Nervosa and Associated Disorders Newsletter**
PO Box 7 847-831-3438
Highland Park, IL 60035 Fax: 847-433-4632
e-mail: anad20@aol.com
www.anad.org

2 pages Quarterly
Vivian Hansen Meehan, President
Dawn Ries, Administrator

3652 **WIN Notes**
Weight-control Information Network
1 WIN Way 202-828-1025
Bethesda, MD 20892-3665 877-946-4627
Fax: 202-828-1028
e-mail: win@mathewsgroup.com
www.niddk.nih.gov/health/nutrit/win.htm
Addresses the health information needs of individuals with weight-control problems. Available on the WIN web site.
BiAnnual

3653 **Working Together**
Anorexia Nervosa and Associated Disorders
PO Box 7 847-831-3438
Highland Park, IL 60035-0007 Fax: 847-433-4632
Designed for individuals, families, group leaders and professionals concerned with eating disorders. Provides updates on treatments, resources, conferences, programs, articles by therapists, recovered victims, group members and leaders.
Quarterly
Dawn Ries, Administrator

Pamphlets

3654 **Applying New Attitudes & Directions**
Anorexia Nervosa and Associated Disorders
PO Box 7 847-831-3438
Highland Park, IL 60035-0007 Fax: 847-433-4632
e-mail: anad20@aol.com
Self-help booklet offering an eight-step program to recovery with suggestions, information and recovery stories.
Dawn Ries, Administrator

Audio & Video

3655 **Bulimia: A Guide to Recovery**
Gurze Books
PO Box 2238
Carlsbad, CA 92018-2238 800-756-7533
Fax: 760-434-5476
e-mail: gzcatl@aol.com
www.bulimia.com
This newly rediscovered tape is an inspirational talk by Lindsey Hall on the relationship between bulimia, self-esteem and love. This was one of Lindsey's last public appearances, where she addressed a 1991 eating disorers conference in Colorado Springs.
Audio tape

Web Sites

3656 **Anorexia Nervosa & Related Eating Disorders**
www.anred.com
Comprehensive site on eating disorders and related issues.

3657 **GERD Information Resource Center**
www.gerd.com
A resource center with educational resources on Gastroesophageal Reflux Disease ("GERD").

3658 **Gastroenterology Therapy Online**
www.gastrotherapy.com
An informational website with resources for many kinds of diseases.

3659 **Healing Well**
www.healingwell.com
An online health resource guide to medical news, chat, information and articles, newsgroups and message boards, books, disease-related web sites, medical directories, and more for patients, friends, and family coping with disabling diseases, disorders, or chronic illnesses.

3660 **Health Finder**
www.healthfinder.gov
Searchable, carefully developed web site offering information on over 1000 topics. Developed by the US Department of Health and Human Services, the site can be used in both English and Spanish.

3661 **Healthlink USA**

www.healthlinkusa.com

Health information concerning treatment, cures, prevention, diagnosis, risk factors, research, support groups, email lists, personal stories and much more. Updated regularly.

3662 **Helios Health**

www.helioshealth.com

Online resource for your health information. Detailed information about specific health topics, access to expert advice from our Medical Advisory Board, and up-to-date health news.

3663 **MedicineNet**

www.medicinenet.com

An online resource for consumers providing easy-to-read, authoritative medical and health information.

3664 **Medscape**

www.mywebmd.com

Medscape offers specialists, primary care physicians, and other health professionals the Web's most robust and integrated medical information and educational tools.

3665 **National Association for Anorexia Nervosa and Associated Disorders**

www.anad.org

ANAD provides educational/prevention programs include presentations and early detection packets for schools and community groups, sponsoring local and national training conferences for health professionals, and working with electronic and print media. Undertakes and encourages research, fights insurance discrimination.

3666 **National Eating Disorders Association**

www.NationalEatingDisorders.org

National nonprofit organization dedicated to increasing the awareness and prevention of eating disorders.

3667 **WebMD**

www.webmd.com

Information on Eating Disorders, including articles and resources.

3668 **Weight-control Information Network**

www.niddk.nih.gov/health/nutrit/win.htm

WIN addresses the health information needs of individuals through the production and dissemination of educational materials. In addition, WIN is developing communication strategies for a pilot program to encourage at-risk individuals to achieve and maintain a healthy weight by making changes in their lifestyle.

Description

3669 **Endometriosis**

Endometriosis is a hormonal condition in which the tissue that normally lines the inside of the uterus (endometrium) is also found outside the uterus, generally on the outer surface of pelvic organs. These cells respond to the woman's hormonal cycles, and swell and bleed at the time of menses. This causes pain, generally worse with each period, pelvic masses and alterations of the menstrual cycle. The pain may be aggravated by intercourse or defecation. Although the reported incidence varies, endometriosis is commonly found in 10 to 15 percent of women between the ages of 25 and 44 years. It is estimated that 25 to 50 percent of infertile women have this disorder.

Treatment depends on the severity of the symptoms and the age and reproductive wishes of the patient. The pain associated with mild cases may be treated with non-steroidal anti-inflammatory drugs. More severe cases may respond to suppression of ovarian function. Laparoscopic surgery may destroy some of the collection of tissue, and is often used in hopes of improving fertility. Hysterectomy (removal of the uterus) is used for intractable cases, especially in women who do not desire future pregnancy.

National Agencies & Associations

3670 **American Association of Gynecologic Laproscopists**
6757 Katella Avenue 714-503-6200
Cypress, CA 90630-4505 800-554-2245
Fax: 714-503-6201
e-mail: lmichels@aagl.org
www.aagl.com
Our global commitment to women's healthcare is embodied in our continuing medical education of physicians and professionals to further promote the well documented high standards of minimally invasive gynecologic surgery.
Linda Michels, Executive Director
Franklin D Loffer MD, EVP/Medical Director

3671 **American Society for Reproductive Medicine**
1209 Montgomery Highway 205-978-5000
Birmingham, AL 35216-2809 Fax: 205-978-5005
e-mail: asrm@asrm.com
www.asrm.com
A private, nonprofit medical organization devoted to advancing the knowledge, understanding and expertise in all phases of reproductive medicine and biology. Offers patient education brochures, recommended readings and support. Publishes professional journal and consumer publications.
Robert W Rebar, MD, Executive Director
Andrew LaBarbera, PhD, Scientific Director

3672 **Endometriosis Association**
630 Ibis Drive 561-274-7442
Delray Beach, FL 33444 800-992-3636
Fax: 561-274-0931
e-mail: exec-comm@endocenter.org
www.endocenter.org
Nonprofit international organization dedicated to helping women and girls suffering from endometriosis. Services include chapter and support groups, crisis/counseling assistance, education of the public and medical community materials including books and videos.
Ann Koerner, Operations Manager

3673 **Endometriosis Association International**
8585 N 76th Place 414-355-2200
Milwaukee, WI 53223 800-992-3636
Fax: 414-355-6065
www.endometriosisassn.org
Offers a 24 hour crisis call hotline, support groups, education in the form of literature including fact sheets, brochures, newsletters, articles educational videos, books and research.
Mary Lou Ballweg, President/Executive Director
Carolyn Keith, Co-Founder

3674 **Hysterectomy Educational Resources & Services (HERS) Foundation**
422 Bryn Mawr Avenue 610-667-7757
Bala Cynwyd, PA 19004 888-750-4377
Fax: 610-677-8096
e-mail: hersfdn@earthlink.net
www.hersfoundation.com
A nonprofit foundation which provides information about the alternatives to hysterectomy, the risks of the alternatives, and the consequences of the surgery. HERS provides telephone counseling by appointment for a fee of $5.00 per quarter hour. The fee can be waived if necessary. HERS also provides copies of a medical journals, a quarterly newsletter, and a free lending library of books, videos and audio tapes.

3675 **International Pelvic Pain Society Women's Medical Plaza**
Women's Medical Plaza
1100 E Woodfield Road 847-517-8712
Schaumburg, IL 60173 800-624-9676
Fax: 847-517-7229
e-mail: info@pelvicpain.org
www.pelvicpain.org
Short range goal is to recruit organize and educate health care professionals actively involved with the treatment of patients who have chronic pelvic pain.
Fred Marion Howard, Chairman of the Board
Howard Taylo Sharp MD, President

3676 **National Women's Health Network**
1413 K Street 202-682-2640
Washington, DC 20005 Fax: 202-682-2648
e-mail: nwhn@nwhn.org
www.womenshealthnetwork.org
Nonprofit organization that does not accept financial support from pharmaceutical or tobacco companies or medical device manufacturers. Advocates for national policies that protect and promote all women's health and provides evidence-based independent information.
Bindiya Patel, Chairperson
Malika Redmond, Action Vice Chair

Foundations

3677 **Fertility Research Foundation**
877 Park Avenue 212-744-5500
New York, NY 10021 Fax: 212-744-6536
e-mail: info@frfbaby.com
www.frfbaby.com
Offers information on treatment and the latest research on male and female infertility.
Masood Khatamee MD, Executive Director

Libraries & Resource Centers

3678 **National Womens Health Resource Center**
157 Broad Street
Red Bank, NJ 07701 877-986-9472
Fax: 732-249-4671
e-mail: info@healthywomen.org
www.healthywomen.org
The not-for-profit National Women's Health Resource Center (NWHRC) is the leading independent health information source for women. NWHRC develops and distributes up-to-date and ob-

jective women's health information based on the latest advances in medical research and practice.
Elizabeth Battaglino Cahill, Executive Vice President
Amber McCracken, Director Communications

Research Centers

3679 Dartmouth Medical School: Microbiology Department
Department of Microbiology & Immunology
1 Rope Ferry Road
Hanover, NH 03755
603-650-1200
877-DMS-1797
Fax: 603-650-1202
e-mail: microbiology@dartmouth.edu
www.dms.dartmouth.edu/microbiology
Dartmouth Medical School is a beacon of discovery and learning stimulating inquiry and harnessing ingenuity for new solutions and better health
Marcia Ingalls, Administrative Assistant
Gregory J MacDonald MD, Assistant Professor of Medicine

3680 Endometriosis Association Research Program : Vanderbuilt University
1211 22nd Avenue S
Nashville, TN 37232
615-322-4927
Fax: 615-343-8881
www.mc.vanderbilt.edu
Heather Arnold, Senior Secretary

3681 Endometriosis Reseach Center and Women's Hospital
The Endometriosis Research Center
630 Ibis Drive
Delray Beach, FL 33444
561-274-7442
800-239-7280
Fax: 561-274-0931
www.endocenter.org
A nonprofit organization dedicated to establishing a center to conduct research and provide women education and treatment.

3682 Endometriosis Reseach Center and Women's H The Endometriosis Research Center
630 Ibis Drive
Delray Beach, FL 33444
561-274-7442
800-239-7280
Fax: 561-274-0931
e-mail: exec-comm@endocenter.org
www.endocenter.org
A nonprofit organization dedicated to establishing a center to conduct research and provide women education and treatment.

3683 Endometriosis Research Center 0
630 Ibis Drive
Delray Beach, FL 33444
561-274-7442
800-239-7280
Fax: 561-274-0931
e-mail: endofl@aol.com
www.endocenter.org
Endometriosis is a reproductive and immunological illness affectingmillions of women and girls around the world Mistakenly stigmatized as merely painful periods, Endometriosis is a far more than i killer cramp the far- reaching feects of this Endometriosis can negatively impact all of society.

3684 Endometriosis Research Center 0
630 Ibis Drive
Delray Beach, FL 33444
561-274-7442
800-239-7280
Fax: 561-274-0931
e-mail: exec-comm@endocenter.org
www.endocenter.org
Endometriosis is a reproductive and immunological illness affectingmillions of women and girls around the world Mistakenly stigmatized as merely painful periods Endometriosis is a far more than i killer cramp the far- reaching feects of this Endometriosis can negatively impact all of society.

3685 University of Tennessee: Division of Reproductive Endocrinology
956 Court Avenue
Memphis, TN 38163
901-528-5859
www.utmem.edu/obgyn/reproductive.htm
Studies into endometriosis.
Dr. Jon Buster, Chief

Support Groups & Hotlines

3686 National Health Information Center
PO Box 1133
Washington, DC 20013
310-565-4167
800-336-4797
Fax: 301-984-4256
e-mail: info@nhic.org
www.health.gov/nhic
Offers a nationwide information referral service, produces directories and resource guides.

3687 RESOLVE Helpline
1760 Old Meadow Road
McLean, VA 22102
703-556-7172
Fax: 703-506-3266
www.resolve.org
A community for women and men with infertility and provides information, support and opportunities to take action.

Books

3688 Alternatives for Women with Endometriosis Guide by Women for Women
Third Side Press
225 W Farragut
Chicago, IL 60625-1863
773-271-3029
Fax: 773-271-0459
e-mail: thirdside@aol.com
174 pages
ISBN: 1-879427-12-5

3689 Coping with Endometriosis
Avery Putnam Penguin
375 Hudson Street
New York, NY 10014
212-366-2000
800-847-5515
Fax: 800-775-4829
e-mail: online@penguinputnam.com
www.penguinputnam.com
Educates readers about the disease, focusing on the particular psychological and emotional concerns that those suffering from endometriosis may have.
322 pages
ISBN: 1-583330-74-7

3690 Endometriosis Sourcebook
Endometriosis Association
8585 N 76th Place
Milwaukee, WI 53223
414-355-2200
800-992-3636
Fax: 414-355-6065
e-mail: endo@endometriosisassn.org
www.EndometriosisAssn.org
Comprehensive, authorative and up-to-date resource that includes information about treatment options, strategies for coping with the disease and its effects on you and those around you.
473 pages Paperback
ISBN: 0-809232-63-4
Mary Lou Ballweg, Founder/Executive Director

3691 Endometriosis and Infertility and Traditio nal Chinese Medicine
Blue Poppy Press
5441 Western Avenue
Boulder, CO 80301
303-447-8372
800-487-9296
Fax: 303-245-8362
e-mail: honora@bluepoppy.com
www.bluepoppy.com/press
An easy to understand guide to Chinese medicine as it relates to endometriosis and infertility.
105 pages Paperback
ISBN: 0-936185-14-7
Honora Wolfe, Marketing Director

3692 Endometriosis: A Key to Healing through Nutrition
Endometriosis Association
8585 N 76th Place
Milwaukee, WI 53223
414-355-2200
800-992-3636
Fax: 414-355-6065
e-mail: endo@endometriosisassn.org
www.endometriosisassn.org

An excellent resource tool to help patients begin making changes in their diets.
Mary Lou Ballweg, Founder/Executive Director

3693 **Endometriosis: A Natural Approach**
Ulysses Press
PO Box 3440 510-601-8301
Berkeley, CA 94703 800-377-2542
Fax: 510-601-8307
e-mail: ulysses@ulyssespress.com
www.ulyssespress.com
This is a solid resource, written in a clear, basic tone, for anyone who needs information about the widespread disease known as endometriosis. Chapters cover all aspects of endometriosis, from what it is and what causes it, to diagnosis, natural therapies, and conventional treatments.
120 pages
ISBN: 1-569750-88-2

3694 **Endometriosis: Advanced Management and Surgical Techniques**
Springer Verlag
175 5th Avenue 212-460-1500
New York, NY 10010 800-777-4643
Fax: 212-473-6272
e-mail: service@springer-ny.com
www.springer-ny.com
This book provides a practical, clinical, and thorough examination of both the medical and surgical treatment of this disease.

3695 **Endometriosis: Complete Reference for Taking Charge of Your Health**
Contemporary Books/McGraw-Hill Companies
130 E Randolf Street 312-233-7596
Chicago, IL 60601 Fax: 312-233-7570
An authoritative guide on endometriosis, including its prevention and relationship with other diseases. Special sections are dedicated to endo and menopause, endo and teenagers, endo and nutrition, endo and cancer as well as endo and environmental toxins.

Newsletters

3696 **Endometriosis Association Newsletter**
Endometriosis Association
8585 N 76th Place 414-355-2200
Milwaukee, WI 53223 800-992-3636
Fax: 414-355-6065
e-mail: endo@endometriosisassn.org
www.EndometriosisAssn.org
Contains research updates and latest health news that affects women and girls with endometriosis. Regular features such as crisis call helpers, news and announcements, and request for contact provide networking and support assistance.
10 pages Bi-Monthly
Mary Lou Ballweg, Executive Director

Pamphlets

3697 **Infertility: Causes and Treatment**
American College/Obstetricians and Gynecologists
409 12th Street SW 304-725-8410
Washington, DC 20024 800-762-2264
Fax: 304-728-2171
www.acog.com
To obtain a free copy of this publication, please send a self-addressed stamped #10 envelope and request by title.

Audio & Video

3698 **Monroe Institute Surgical Support Tapes**
Endometriosis Association
8585 N 76th Place 414-355-2200
Milwaukee, WI 53223-2633 800-992-3636
Fax: 414-355-6065
e-mail: endo@endometriosisassn.org
www.EndometriosisAssn.org
Anxiety is normal for women before surgery, so women with endometriosis will be happy to hear this wonderful series of audiotapes specifically developed for relaxation.
Audiotape
Mary Lou Ballweg, Founder/Executive Director

Web Sites

3699 **American Society for Reproductive Medicine**
www.asrm.com
Devoted to advancing the knowledge, understanding and expertise in all phases of reproductive medicine and biology. Offers patient education brochures, recommended readings and support.

3700 **Endometriosis Association**
www.EndometriosisAssn.org
Nonprofit organization dedicated to helping women and girls suffering from endometriosis. Services include chapter and support groups, crisis/counseling assistance, education of the public and the medical community. Materials, including books, video/audiotapes, CDs, newsletters and articles mostly based on data from the Association's research registries and its extensive research program, including a flagship scientific team at Vanderbuilt University School of Medicine.

3701 **Endometriosis Research Center**
www.endocenter.org
Maintain and offer a vast database of unbased and fact-based materials on every aspect of Endometriosis to practitioners, researchers, patients and all those interested in the disease.

3702 **Endometriosis Support Group**
www.geocities.com/HotSprings/5422
Online support group and question forum for endometriosis.

3703 **Healing Well**
www.healingwell.com
An online health resource guide to medical news, chat, information and articles, newsgroups and message boards, books, disease-related web sites, medical directories, and more for patients, friends, and family coping with disabling diseases, disorders, or chronic illnesses.

3704 **Health Finder**
www.healthfinder.gov
Searchable, carefully developed web site offering information on over 1000 topics. Developed by the US Department of Health and Human Services, the site can be used in both English and Spanish.

3705 **Healthlink USA**
www.healthlinkusa.com
Health information concerning treatment, cures, prevention, diagnosis, risk factors, research, support groups, email lists, personal stories and much more. Updated regularly.

3706 **Helios Health**
www.helioshealth.com
Online resource for your health information. Detailed information about specific health topics, access to expert advice from our Medical Advisory Board, and up-to-date health news.

3707 **International Pelvic Pain Society**
www.pelvicpain.org/
Short range goal is to recruit, organize, and educate health care professionals actively involved with the treatment of patients who have chronic pelvic pain.

3708 **MedicineNet**
www.medicinenet.com
An online resource for consumers providing easy-to-read, authoritative medical and health information.

3709 **Medscape**
www.mywebmd.com
Medscape offers specialists, primary care physicians, and other health professionals the Web's most robust and integrated medical information and educational tools.

3710 **Universe of Women's Health**
www.obgyn.net

A comprehensive website dedicated to women's health.

3711 WebMD

www.webmd.com

Information on Endometriosis, including articles and resources.

Description

3712 **Fabry Disease**

Fabry disease is an inherited fat storage disorder caused by deficiency of an enzyme involved in the biodegradation of lipids (fats). As abnormal storage of the fatty compound increases with time, blood vessels become narrowed, leading to decreased blood flow. The problem occurs in all blood vessels in the body, but affects in particular the skin, kidneys, heart, brain and nerves.

In children, Fabry begins with pain and burning sensations in hands and feet that is worse with exercise and hot weather. Other symptoms include a dark red rash around the waist, decreased ability to prespire and cloudiness of the cornea, which usually does not affect vision.

As those with Fabry's grow older, they may have impaired circulation, leading to early heart attacks and strokes. As kidneys become more involved, many patients require kidney transplants or dialysis. Gastrointestinal symptoms include frequent bowel movements shortly after eating. Patients with Fabry disease usually survive into adulthood but have a reduced life expentancy.

Currently, there is no cure for Fabry disease and treatment typically deals with controlling its symptoms. Pain in hands and feet respons to several medications. Gastrointestinal hyperactivity may be controlled by taking a nutritional supplement. Enzyme replacement therapy was given a dramatic boost in 2003 when the FDA approved a new synthetic enzyme. It is given intravenously and reduces lipid (fat) accumulation in many types of cells.

National Agencies & Associations

3713 **Association for Neuro-Metabolic Disorders**
5223 Brookfield Lane — 419-885-1809
Sylvania, OH 43560 — 800-334-7980
e-mail: VOLK4OLKS@aol.com
www.kumc.edu

Serves as an advocate organization for families of patients with neuro-methabolic disorders such as phenylketonuria, maple syrup urine disease, galactosemia and biotinidase. Provides educational information for parents and children and provides networking.

3714 **Genetic and Rare Diseases Information Center**
PO Box 8126 — 301-519-3194
Gaithesburg, MD 20898-8126 — 888-205-2311
Fax: 240-632-9164
TTY: 888-205-3223
e-mail: GARDinfo@nih.gov
www.rarediseases.info.nih.gov/GARD

Provides free and immediate access to accurate, reliable information about genetic and rare diseases. Also provides assistance to patients and families, health professionals and other interested parties.

3715 **International Center for Fabry Disease Mt. Sinai School of Medicine**
Mt. Sinai School of Medicine
5th Avenue at 100th Street
New York, NY 10029 — 866-322-7963
e-mail: fabry.disease@mssm.edu
www.mssm.edu/genetics/fabry/index.shtml

Clinical research center attended by a staff of physicians and nurses specially trained to understand and meet the needs of individuals with Fabry disease. Services offered to both men and women of all ages include diagnosis, evaluation and treatment consultation.
Robert J Desnick PhD MD, Professor and Chair

3716 **National Institute of Neurological Disorders and Stroke (NINDS)**
PO Box 5801 — 301-496-5751
Bethesda, MD 20824 — 800-352-9424
Fax: 301-496-0296
TTY: 301-468-5981
e-mail: braininfo@ninds.nih.gov
www.ninds.nih.gov

Conducts, foster, coordinates, and guides research on the causes, prevention, diagnosis, and treatment of neurological disorders and stroke, and supports basic research in related scientific areas. Provides grants-in-aid to public and private institutions and individuals in fields related to its areas of interest, including research project, program project, and research center grants.
Story C Landis, Director
Audrey S Penn, Deputy Director

3717 **National Organization for Rare Disorders (NORD)**
55 Kenosia Avenue — 203-744-0100
Danbury, CT 06813-1968 — 800-999-6673
Fax: 203-798-2291
TDD: 203-797-9590
e-mail: orphan@rarediseases.org
www.rarediseases.org

The National Organization for Rare Disorders(NORD), a 501(c)3 organization, is a unique federation of voluntary health organizations dedicated to helping people with rare orphan diseases and assisting the organizations that serve them. NORD is committed to the identification, treatment, and cure of rare disorders through programs of education, advocacy, research, and service.
Carolyn Asbury, PhD, Chair
Frank Sasinowski, Vice Chair

3718 **National Tay-Sachs and Allied Disease Association**
2001 Beacon Street — 800-906-8723
Brighton, MA 02135 — 800-906-8723
Fax: 617-277-0134
e-mail: info@ntsad.org
www.ntsad.org

A mutual support group coordinated by staff and volunteers who are parents of affected children of affected adults. One of several programs supported and sponsored by the association.
Bradley L Campbell, President
Stewart Altman, Vice President

Research Centers

3719 **Lysosomal Disease Center at the University of Pittsburgh**
E1650 Biomedical Science Tower
Pittsburgh, PA 15261 — 800-334-7980
pitt.edu/~geneorb/ctr-lyso.html

Offers diagnosis management treatment and genetic counseling for people with or at risk for lysosomal storage disease and their families.
John A Barrenger MD PhD, Director
Erin O'Rourk MS CGC, Manager

3720 **National Gaucher Disease Foundation**
2227 Idlewood Road — 770-934-2910
Tucker, GA 30084 — 800-504-3189
Fax: 770-934-2911
e-mail: rhonda@gaucherdisease.org
www.gaucherdisease.org

Provides information and assistance for those affected by Gaucher disease.
Rhonda P Buyers, CEO/Executive Director
Barbara Lichtenstein, Programs Director National Gaucher Care

Support Groups & Hotlines

3721 Fabry Support & Information Group
108 NE 2nd Street Suite C
Concordia, MO 64020-510
660-463-1355
Fax: 660-463-1356
e-mail: info@fabry.org
www.fabry.org

Nonprofit organization. Its mission is to educate, support and raise awareness of Fabry disease and its symtoms.
Jack Jackson, Executive Director
J Johnson, Founder

Web Sites

3722 A World of Genetic Societies
www.faseb.org/genetics
Listing of genetic professional societies, many with searchable databases.

3723 Alliance of Genetic Support Groups
www.geneticalliance.org
Coalition of individuals, professionals and genetic support organizations.

3724 Fabry Support & Information Group
www.fabry.org
Discussion page, information about disease, newsletters, patient biographies, links.

3725 Gene Clinics
www.geneclinics.org
Searchable, expert-authored, peer reviewed disease database.

3726 International Center for Fabry Disease
www.mssm.edu/crc/Fabry/fabry.html
Associated with Mt. Sinai, with information about Fabry including a program to family tree.

3727 International Storage Disease Collaborative
www.pediatrics.med.umn/edu/isdcsg/
This study group focuses on stem cell and bone marrow transplantation. Has discussion page/general information.

3728 MedicineNet
www.medicinenet.com
An online resource for consumers providing easy-to-read, authoritative medical and health information.

3729 Morbus Fabry
home.t-online.de
Fabry information and links to other sites.

3730 NIH's National Institute of Neurological Disorders & Strokes
www.ninds.nih.gov
Description of disease, therapies.

3731 National Organization for Rare Disorders (NORD)
www.rarediseases.org
The NORD is a unique federation of voluntary health organizations dedicated to helping people with rare "orphan" diseases and assisting the organization that serve them.

3732 National Society of Genetic Counselors
nsgc.org
Society website with searchable membership database.

3733 OMIM: Fabry Disease
www.ncbi.nlm.nih.gov
Description of disease and links to research papers written.

3734 Pediatric Database: Fabry Disease
www.icondata.com
Description of disease.

3735 Support-Group.Com: Fabry Disease
www.support-group.com
Fabry Disease discussion forum.

Description

3736 **Fibromyalgia Syndrome**

Fibromyalgia syndrome, FMS, also called fibrositis or fibromyositis, is a condition of widespread muscular pain and fatigue. It strikes mostly women between the ages of 20 and 50, and may affect as many as one in 20 adult females. The pain ranges from mild discomfort to complete disability and may vary from day to day. Physical over-exertion, changes in weather, drafty environments, stress, depression, and hormonal changes can all contribute to flare-ups in FMS symptoms.

In addition to widespread pain, FMS also causes a decreased sense of energy, disturbances of sleep, and varying degrees of anxiety and depression. Other medical conditions sometimes associated with fibromyalgia include tension headaches, migraine, irritable bowel syndrome, premenstrual tension syndrome, chronic fatigue syndrome, cold intolerance, and restless leg syndrome.

A physician's diagnosis of FMS is usually based on the following criteria: widespread musculoskeletal pain; tenderness at 11 or more of 18 specific tender points, which are exquisitely more tender than adjacent sites; and scans of the brain. Fibromyalgia may remit spontaneously with decreased stress but can recur at frequent intervals or become chronic.

There is currently no commonly accepted cure for this condition. Aspirin and other drugs used to treat musculoskeletal pain partially improve symptoms. Antidepressant drugs, taken in low doses, have been shown to provide restorative sleep. Patients may also benefit from regular aerobic exercises, local applications of heat, gentle massage and reduced stress in their lives. See also *Chronic Fatigue Syndrome*.

National Agencies & Associations

3737 **American Fibromyalgia Syndrome Association**
6380 East Tanque Verde — 520-733-1570
Tucson, AZ 85715 — Fax: 520-290-5550
e-mail: kthorson@afsafund.org
www.afsafund.org
Nonprofit organization whose primary mission is to seed research in FMS and CFS. We acknowledge that patient and physician education, public awareness and advocacy are all important ingredients in aiding the lives of people with FMS and CFS.
Kristen Thorson, President
Steve Thorson, VP

3738 **FM-CFS Canada**
99 Fifth Avenue
Ottawa, Ontario, K1S-5P5 — www.fm-cfs.ca
Dedicated to advancing Fibromyalgia (FM) and Chronic Fatigue Syndrome (CFS) education, research and treatment.
David Mann, President/Director
Ed Napke MD PhD, VP/Director

3739 **National Chronic Fatigue Syndrome and Fibromyalgia Association**
PO Box 18426 — 816-313-2000
Kansas City, MO 64133 — Fax: 816-524-6782
e-mail: information@ncfsfa.org
www.ncfsfa.org
Offering a support group, medical and patient information plus research.

3740 **National Chronic Fatigue Syndrome and Fibr**
PO Box 18426 — 816-737-1343
Kansas City, MO 64133 — Fax: 816-524-6782
e-mail: information@ncfsfa.org
www.ncfsfa.org
Offering a support group medical and patient information plus research.

3741 **National Fibromyalgia Association**
2121 S Towne Centre Place — 714-921-0150
Anaheim, CA 92806 — Fax: 714-921-6920
e-mail: kfox@fmaware.org
www.fmaware.org
Develops and extends programs dedicated to improving the quality of life for people with Fibromyalgia by increasing the awareness of the public media government and medical communities. Supports an ongoing media presence and assist local support groups.
Lynne Matallana, Founder/President
Rae Marie Gleason, Executive Director

3742 **National Fibromyalgia Partnership (NFP)**
PO Box 160
Linden, VA 22642 — 866-725-4404
Fax: 866-666-2727
e-mail: mail@fmpartnership.org
www.fmpartnership.org
The NFP is a 501(c)(3) non-profit, membership organization which publishes medically accurate information on fibromyalgia to patients, health care professionals and the public. Information and resources not listed in this volume are available in print and/or on the NFP website. It also provides support and start-up informaiton to support groups. Additional website: www.frontiersnews.org
Tamara K Liller, President & Director of Publications
Jacqueline M Yencha, Vice-President, Asst Dir of Publications

3743 **National Hemophilia Foundation/Hemophilia and AIDS/HIV Network (HANDI)**
116 W 23nd Street — 212-328-3700
New York, NY 10001 — Fax: 212-219-8180
www.hemophilia.org
Dedicated to the treatment and the cure of hemophilia AIDS and other blood related disorders. This foundation wished to improve the quality of life of all those affected through promotion and support of research education and other services.

3744 **National ME/FM Action Network**
3836 Carling Avenue — 613-829-6667
Nepean, Ontario, K2K-2Y6 — Fax: 613-829-6667
www.mefmaction.net
A non-profit organization dediced to advancing the recognition and understanding of Myalgic Encephalomyelitis/Chronic Fatigue Syndrome (ME/CFS) and Fibromyalgia Syndrome (FMS) through education, advocacy, support, and research.
Lydia Neilson, Contact

3745 **Option Institute**
2080 S Undermountain Road — 413-229-2100
Sheffield, MA 01257 — 800-714-2779
Fax: 413-229-8931
e-mail: participantsupport@option.org
www.option.org
Self-defeating beliefs along with attitudes and judgments can lead to a host of physical and psychological challenges, including Fibromyalgia. The Option Institute offers programs designed to help you gain new perspectives on the attitudes and judgments that can hamper progress.
Barry Kaufman, Co-Founder
Samahria Lyt Kaufman, Co-Founder

Libraries & Resource Centers

3746 **Fibromyalgia Resources Group**
103 Sherwood Hill Road — 845-278-5944
Brewster, NY 10509 — Fax: 845-278-2641
e-mail: kindness@fibrobetsy.com

Personalized patient service searches and distributes information on patient recommended, fibromyalgia literate doctors world wide. Information packet is included with each doctor list emailed. Doctor recommendations are welcome.
Betsy Jacobson, President

Support Groups & Hotlines

3747 **National Chronic Fatigue Syndrome and Fibr omyalgia Association Support Group**
PO Box 18426
Kansas City, MO 64133
816-737-1343
Fax: 816-524-6782
e-mail: information@ncfsfa.org
www.ncfsfa.org/
Support group meetings are held on the second Saturday of each month from 2-4 p.m. in the second floor board room of the Helen F Spencer Center for Education. The Center is part of St. Luke's Hospital and is located at 4400 Wornall Road, Kansas City, MO 64111.
Michelle Banks, Author

3748 **National Health Information Center**
PO Box 1133
Washington, DC 20013
310-565-4167
800-336-4797
Fax: 301-984-4256
e-mail: info@nhic.org
www.health.gov/nhic
Offers a nationwide information referral service, produces directories and resource guides.

3749 **Rocky Mountain CFIDS/FMS Association**
7020 E Girard Avenue
Denver, CO 80224
303-423-7367
e-mail: link@rmcfa.org
www.rmcfa.org
Promotes and conducts activities which furhter education, support awareness, advocacy and research for Chronic Fatigue Immune Dysfunction syndrome and Fibromyalgia
Tim Smith, President

Arizona

3750 **Fibromyalgia Network**
PO Box 31750
Tucson, AZ 85751-1750
520-290-5508
800-853-2929
Fax: 520-290-5550
e-mail: inquiry@fmnetnews.com
www.fmnetnews.com
Aim to educate and assist patients with ad-free, patient-focused information that they can put to use today. An organization that attends medical conferences, interviews the experts, and sifts through the details in the medical journals for members, so they can recieve up-to-date objective reporting and information that can't be found anywhere else.

Books

3751 **All About Fibromyalgia**
Oxford University Press
198 Madison Avenue
New York, NY 10016-4314
212-726-6033
800-451-7556
Fax: 212-726-6447
www.oup-usa.org

ISBN: 0-195147-53-7

3752 **Delicate Balance: Living Successfully with Chronic Illness**
Perseus Books Group
5500 Central Avenue
Boulder, CO 80301
800-386-5656
Fax: 303-449-3356
e-mail: info@perseuspublishing.com
www.perseuspublishing.com
Up to date and practical advice and inspiration for the millions of Americans who struggle daily against chronic illness. From locating a suitable healthcare provider and making sense of the powerful emotions that accompany chronic illness, to seeking accomodations from the Americans with Disabilities Act, this book is helpful and hopeful.
312 pages
ISBN: 0-738203-23-8

3753 **Fibromyalgia**
NAMSIC/National Institutes of Health
1 AMS Circle
Bethesda, MD 20892-0001
301-495-4484
877-226-4267
Fax: 301-718-6366
TTY: 301-565-2966
e-mail: niamsinfo@mail.nih.gov
www.nih.gov/niams

3754 **Fibromyalgia & Other Central Pain Syndromes**
Daniel Wallace, Daniel Clauw, author
Lippincott Williams & Wilkins
16522 Hunters Green Parkway
Hagerstown, MD 21740-2116
800-638-3030
Fax: 301-223-2400
www.lww.com
Devoted to fibromyalgia and other centrally mediated chronic pain syndromes. Leading experts examine the latest research findings on these syndromes and present evidence-based reviews of current controversies.
2005
ISBN: 0-781752-61-2

3755 **Fibromyalgia Guidelines: The Concensus Diagnosis & Treatment Protocols**
FM-CFS Canada
99 Fifth Avenue
Ottawa ON CANADA K1S 5P5,
www.fm-cfs.ca/fm
This entire special issue of the Journal of Musculoskeletal Pain [JMP] is devoted to presentation of what will likely to be called the Canadian Consensus Document on Fibromyalgia Syndrome (FMS). The document encompasses a very broad scope, involving a clinical case definition, diagnosis, and management of FMS.
130 pages Volume 11, #4

3756 **Fibromyalgia Relief Book: 213 Ideas for Improving Your Quality of Life**
Walker & Company
435 Hudson Street
New York, NY 10014
212-727-8300
Fax: 212-727-0984
e-mail: orders@walkerbooks.com
www.walkerbooks.com

208 pages Paperback
ISBN: 0-802775-53-5
Josh Wood, Sales Director

3757 **Fibromyalgia Supporter**
Anadem Publishing Company
3620 N High Street
Columbus, OH 43214
800-633-0055
Fax: 614-262-6630
e-mail: anadem@anadem.com
www.anadem.com

3758 **Fibromyalgia Survivor**
Anadem Publishing Company
3620 N High Street
Columbus, OH 43214
800-633-0055
Fax: 614-262-6630
e-mail: anadem@anadem.com
www.anadem.com

ISBN: 0-964689-12-X

3759 **Fibromyalgia Syndrome and Chronic Fatigue Syndrome in Young People**
Fibromyalgia Network
PO Box 31750
Tucson, AZ 85751-1750
800-853-2929
Fax: 520-290-5550
www.fmnetnews.com

Guide for parents.

3760 **Fibromyalgia and Chronic Myofascial Pain Syndrome: a Survivor Manual**
New Harbinger Publishers
5674 Shattuck Avenue
Oakland, CA 94609
800-748-6273
Fax: 510-652-5472
www.newharbinger.com

Written from the perspective of myofacial pain syndrome.
432 pages

3761 **Fibromyalgia, Managing the Pain**
Anadem Publishing Company
3620 N High Street
Columbus, OH 43214-3611
800-633-0055
Fax: 614-262-6630
e-mail: anadem@anadem.com
www.anadem.com

Comprehensive guide to the syndrome, including chapters on diagnosis, medication, physical medicine treatments, occupational adjustments, advice on flare ups and some medical and legal aspects of FMS.

3762 **Inside Fibromyalgia**
Anadem Publishing Company
3620 N High Street
Columbus, OH 43214
614-262-2539
800-633-0055
Fax: 614-262-6630
e-mail: anadem@anadem.com
www.anadem.com

Written by a physician who has fibromyalgia. From the newest medications to alternative therapies and everything in between, Dr. Pellegrino helps you develop a plan for healing today and tomorrow.
Paperback
ISBN: 1-890018-36-8

3763 **Laugh at Your Muscles**
Anadem Publishing Company
3620 N High Street
Columbus, OH 43214-3611
800-633-0055
Fax: 614-262-6630
e-mail: anadem@anadem.com
www.anadem.com

3764 **Occupational Therapy Practice Guidelines for Adults with Rheumatoid Arthritis**
American Occupational Therapy Association
4720 Montgomery Lane
Bethesda, MD 20824-1220
301-652-2682
Fax: 301-652-7711
TDD: 800-377-8555
www.aota.org

20 pages
ISBN: 1-569001-12-X

3765 **Taking Charge of Fibromyalgia**
FMS Educational Systems
500 Bushway Road
Wayzata, MN 55391
419-841-3435
Fax: 419-841-3435
e-mail: info@fmsedsys.com
www.fmsedsys.com

Written by three professionals who have fibromyalgia and who often update the book.

3766 **Taking Control of TMJ: Your Total Wellness Program**
Robert O Uppgaard, DDS, author
New Harbinger Publications
5674 Shattuck Avenue
Oakland, CA 94609
800-748-6273
Fax: 510-652-5472
www.newharbinger.com

Six-step wellness program helps readers understand what TMJ is and provides exercises to improve jaw functioning, relieve pain and deal with trigger points, eliminate harmful habits, deal with contributing stress, and evaluate and improve your diet and exercise habits. Additional chapters cover the connection between TMJ, whiplash, and fibromyalgia.
2004 200 pages Paperback
ISBN: 1-572241-26-8

3767 **Understanding Post-Traumatic Fibromyalgia**
Anadem Publishing Company
3620 N High Street
Columbus, OH 43214-3611
800-633-0055
Fax: 614-262-6630
e-mail: anadem@anadem.com
www.anadem.com

Anyone with post-traumatic fibromyalgia will benefit from reading this book focusing exclusively on this condition.

Magazines

3768 **FM Monograph**
National Fibromyalgia Partnership
PO Box 160
Linden, VA 22642
866-725-4404
Fax: 866-666-2727
e-mail: mail@fmpartnership.org
www.fmpartnership.org

Publishes a print quarterly (available online and in booklet form in English, Spanish, and French) which provides information on fibromyalgia symptoms, diagnosis, treatment, and research. Comprehensive resource packets and reprints are also available on a variety of subjects. Technical support is provided to fibromyalgia support organizations worldwide.
Quarterly
Tamara Liller, President

3769 **Fibromyalgia AWARE**
National Fibromyalgia Association
2238 N Glassell Street
Orange, CA 92865
714-921-0150
Fax: 714-921-6920
e-mail: nfa@FMaware.org
www.FMaware.org

Official publication of the National Fibromyalgia Association. Available to members and contributors.

3770 **Fibromyalgia Frontiers**
National Fibromyalgia Partnership (NFP)
PO Box 160
Linden, VA 22642
866-725-4404
Fax: 866-666-2727
e-mail: mail@fmpartnership.org
www.fmpartnership.org

Publishes a print quarterly (available online and in booklet form in English, Spanish, and French) which provides information on fibromyalgia symptoms, diagnosis, treatment, and research. Comprehensive resource packets and reprints are also available on a variety of subjects. Technical support is provided to fibromyalgia support organizations worldwide. Included with membership into NFP.
Quarterly
Tamara Liller, President

3771 **Journal of Musculoskeletal Pain**
Haworth Medical Press
10 Alice Street
Binghamton, NY 13904-1503
607-722-5857
800-429-6784
Fax: 607-722-0012
e-mail: getinfo@haworthpress.com
www.haworthpress.com

Peer reviewed medical journal containing FMS scientific abstract information. Appropriate for medical professionals as well as amateur.
Quarterly

Newsletters

3772 **Fibromyalgia Clinic Kentfield Rehabilitation Newsletter**
Fibromyalgia Clinic
25 Sir Francis Drake Boulevard
415-485-3530
Kentfield, CA 94904

3773 **Florida Fibromyalgia News**
FMS Association of Florida
PO Box 14848
352-371-2750
Gainesville, FL 32604-4848
Quarterly newsletter.

3774 **Health Points**
TyH Publications
17007 E Colony Drive
Fountain Hills, AZ 85268 800-801-1406
e-mail: editor@e-tyh.com
National newsletter with articles on complementary therapy, latest nutrition news, disability issues and much more. Focus is on fibromyalgia, chronic fatigue, arthritis and chronic pain.
Quarterly

3775 **Healthwatch**
CFIDS and Fibromyalgia Health Resource
2040 Alameda Padre Serra
Santa Barbara, CA 93103 800-366-6056
Fax: 805-965-0042
e-mail: cutomerservice@prohealthinc.com
www.immunesupport.com
Healthwatch serves fibromyalgia and chronic fatigue syndrome sufferers by focusing on reporting the latest news in research and treatment, making hard-to-find nutritional supplements available at low prices, and raising needed funds for medical research.

3776 **Journal of Musculoskeletal Medicine**
Cliggott Publishing Company
55 Holly Hill Lane 203-661-0600
Greenwich, CT 06830-6074
This journal provides a unique and efficient monthly update on the management of musculoskeletal disorders. Offers articles regarding orthopedics, rheumatology, sports medicine, etc.

3777 **Tender Points**
The Arthritis Society
393 University Avenue 416-979-7228
Ontario, Canada M5G 1E6, 800-321-1433
Fax: 416-979-8366
e-mail: info@on.erthritis.ca
Newsletter of The Arthritis Society.
Quarterly

3778 **To Your Health and Healthpoints**
To Your Health
17007 E Colony Drive
Fountain Hills, AZ 85268 800-801-1406
Fax: 480-837-1875
www.e-tyh.com
Resource catalogue and newspaper for FMS, CFIDS, arthritis, and chronic pain. Features vitamins and health products developed specifically for FMS and CFIDS making hard-to-find, recommended nutritional supplements available to fibromyalgia and chronic fatigue syndrome sufferers at a manufacturer-direct low price.

Audio & Video

3779 **Audio Cassette Program on Fibromyalgia**
Arthritis Foundation/Research Cassettes
111 E Wacker Drive 312-616-3470
Chicago, IL 60601-3713
Covers treatment and research taped during a patient education forum.

3780 **Fibromyalgia Interval Training**
Arthritis Foundation Distribution Center
PO Box 6996
Alpharetta, GA 30023-6996 800-207-8633
Fax: 770-442-9742
www.arthritis.com
Designed for people with fibromyalgia, the video features warm water exercises in shallow and deep water, including warmup, stretching, upper and lower body exercises, aerobics, strengthing, cool-down and relaxation. Designed to help you manage the pain, stiffness and fatigue of fibromyalgia.

3781 **Fibromyalgia Stretch Video & Strength and Toning Video**
Oregon Fibromyalgia Foundation
1221 SW Yamhill
Portland, OR 97205 503-228-3217
www.myalgia.com
These videos offer comprehensive stretching and strength and toning regimens developed by exercise physiologist Sharon Clark PhD, FNP, specifically for people with FMS. Fibromyalgia patients are shown demonstrating these unique stretching and strength and toning programs. Prices are per video and do not include shipping and handling.

3782 **Fibromyalgia: Face to Face**
Ontario Fibromyalgia Association
250 Cloor Street E 416-979-7228
Toronto, Ontario, M4W
A 14 minute insight into living with FMS from people, including children, who are coping with this syndrome.

3783 **Improving Muscle Tone and Strength**
Oregon Fibromyalgia Foundation
1221 SW Yamhill 503-228-3217
Portland, OR 97205
A video developed by exercise physiologist Sharon Clark, PhD, RN, specifically for people with fibromyalgia.

Web Sites

3784 **American Fibromyalgia Research Association**
www.afsafund.org
Charitable organization whose primary mission is to seed research in FMS and CFS. We acknowledge that patient and physician education, public awareness and advocacy are all important ingredients in aiding the lives of people with FMS and CFS.

3785 **FM/CFS Canada**
www.fm-cfs.ca
Dedicated to advancing Fibromyalgia (FM) and Chronic Fatigue Syndrome (CFS) education, research and treatment.

3786 **Healing Well**
www.healingwell.com
An online health resource guide to medical news, chat, information and articles, newsgroups and message boards, books, disease-related web sites, medical directories, and more for patients, friends, and family coping with disabling diseases, disorders, or chronic illnesses.

3787 **Health Finder**
www.healthfinder.gov
Searchable, carefully developed web site offering information on over 1000 topics. Developed by the US Department of Health and Human Services, the site can be used in both English and Spanish.

3788 **Healthlink USA**
www.healthlinkusa.com
Health information concerning treatment, cures, prevention, diagnosis, risk factors, research, support groups, email lists, personal stories and much more. Updated regularly.

3789 **Helios Health**
www.helioshealth.com
Online resource for your health information. Detailed information about specific health topics, access to expert advice from our Medical Advisory Board, and up-to-date health news.

3790 **MedicineNet**
www.medicinenet.com
An online resource for consumers providing easy-to-read, authoritative medical and health information.

3791 **Medscape**
www.mywebmd.com
Medscape offers specialists, primary care physicians, and other health professionals the Web's most robust and integrated medical information and educational tools.

3792 **My Fibromyalgia & Chronic Fatigue Syndrome**
www.fms-help.com
A woman's personal story about her battle with fibromyalgia.

3793 **National Fibromyalgia Association**
www.fmaware.org
Information for fibromyalgia patients and the general public.

3794 **National Fibromyalgia Partnership (NFP)**
PO Box 160
Linden, VA 22642
866-725-4404
Fax: 866-666-2727
e-mail: mail@fmpartnership.org
www.fmpartnership.org

The NFP is a 501(c)(3) non-profit, membership organization which publishes medically accurate information on fibromyalgia to patients, health care professionals and the public. Information and resources not listed in this volume are available in print and/or on the NFP website. It also provides support and start-up informaiton to support groups. Additional website: www.frontiersnews.org

Tamara K Liller, President & Director of Publications
Jacqueline M Yencha, Vice-President, Asst Dir of Publications

3795 **Neurology Channel**
www.neurologychannel.com

Find clearly explained, medically accurate information regarding conditions, including an overview, symptoms, causes, diagnostic procedures and treatment options. On this site it is possible to ask questions and get information from a neurologist and connect to people who have similar health interests.

3796 **Option Institute**
Option Institute
www.option.org/fibromyalgia.html

Self-defeating beliefs, along with attitudes and judgments, can lead to a host of physical and psychological challenges, including Fibromyalgia. The Option Institute offers programs designed to help you gain new perspectives on the attitudes and judgments that may be affecting your life, especially those regarding and surrounding Fibromyalgia.

3797 **WebMD**
www.webmd.com

Information on Fibromyalgia Syndrome, including articles and resources.

Description

3798 **Gastrointestinal Disorders**

The digestive tract is responsible for taking food into the body, processing it into simple chemicals that can be absorbed to nourish the body, and expelling the remainder.

Motility disorders of the gastrointestinal (GI) tract are conditions in which there is a failure of normal top-to-bottom movement of gastric contents. In reflux, the food content moves from the stomach back into the esophagus, irritating that organ and causing heartburn,the most common symptom. This is known as GERD, or gastro-esophageal reflux disease, and sometimes causes choking or coughing. Complications include inflammation and even ulceration of the esophagus. It is a problem in infants, but also occurs in adults especially with advancing age. Occasionally, an ulcer may develop in a segment of the GI tract, typically in the stomach or duodenum. An infectious agent, H. pylori, plays a central role in peptic ulcer disease. In achalasia, the normal movement of food down the GI tract by peristalsis is disrupted, and contents of the esophagus are unable to move into the stomach. As a result, the person chokes on food or liquid. Chest pain and coughing at night may also occur.

Other motility disorders reflect the bowel's inability to move its contents forward properly. Children may be born with Hirschprung's disease in which peristalsis is absent or abnormal in the large bowel, resulting in partial or complete obstruction. The most common motility disorder in adults is called irritable bowel syndrome; also known as functional bowel or spastic colitis, it causes variable degrees of abdominal pain and bloating, diarrhea and/or constipation.

Outpouchings in the walls of the lower GI tract, called diverticula, sometimes trap nutrient waste, and may become infected, bleed, and rupture. Finally, the digestive tract may fail in its primary task of absorbing nutrients, known as malabsorption syndromes. Rarely it will absorb too much of something. In hemochromatosis, for instance, the bowel takes in too much iron from the diet, and the excess is stored in and damages the liver, pancreas, heart, and gonads. More commonly, the body absorbs too little nutrient rather than too much. For instance, celiac disease, or sprue, is a disorder caused by intolerance to gluten, a cereal protein in wheat rye, barley, and oats. Lactose intolerance is an inability to digest a carbohydrate in dairy products. Treatment for malabsorption syndromes includes dietary modifications and, in more serious cases, supplementation with intravenous feedings known as parenteral nutrition.

National Agencies & Associations

3799 **American College of Gastroenterology**
PO Box 342260
Bethesda, MD 20827-2260
301-263-9000
www.acg.gi.org

ACG serves clinical and scientific information needs of member physicians and surgeons who specialize in digestive and related disorders. Emphasis is on scholarly practice, teaching and research.
Eamonn M M Quigley MD FACG, President
Delbert L Chumley MD FAC, VP

3800 **American Dietetic Association**
120 S Riverside Plaza
Chicago, IL 60606-6995
312-899-0040
800-877-1600
e-mail: media@eatright.org
www.eatright.org

ADA serves the public through the promotion of optimal nutrition health and well-being.
Patricia M Babjak, Chief Executive Officer
Martin M Yadrick, President

3801 **American Gastroenterological Association National Office**
National Office
4930 Del Ray Avenue
Bethesda, MD 20814
301-654-2055
Fax: 301-654-5920
e-mail: member@gastro.org
www.gastro.org

AGA fosters the development and application of the science of gastroenterology by providing leadership and aid including patient care, research, teaching, continuing education, scientific communication and matters of national health policy.
Robert B Greenberg JD, Executive Vice President
Michael H Stolar PhD, Senior VP

3802 **American Hemochromatosis Society**
4044 W Lake Mary Boulevard
Lake Mary, FL 32746-2012
407-829-4488
888-655-4766
Fax: 407-333-1284
e-mail: mail@americanhs.org
www.americanhs.org

Educates the public, the medical community and the media by distributing the most current information available on hereditary hemochromatosis (HH) including DNA screening for HH and pediatric HH; also facilitates patient empowerment through an online network.
Sandra Thomas, President/Founder

3803 **American Motility Society**
45685 Harmony Lane
Belleville, MI 48111
734-699-1130
Fax: 734-699-1136
e-mail: admin@motilitysociety.org
www.motilitysociety.org

Promotes research and sponsors professional education seminars about gastrointestinal motility topics including disorders of esophageal, gastric, small intestinal, and colonic function; and sponsors biennial meetings (even years), syposia and courses.
Michael Cami MD, President

3804 **American Pancreatic Association**
45 High Valley Drive
Chesterfield, MO 63017
314-210-2904
Fax: 314-754-9515
e-mail: american-pancreatic-association@lettucep
www.american-pancreatic-association.org

Provides forum for presentation of scientific research related to the pancreas.
Ashok K Saluja PhD, President

3805 **American Pseudo-Obstruction and Hirschsprung's Disease Society**
158 Pleasant Street
N Andover, MA 01845
978-685-4477
Fax: 978-685-4488
e-mail: aphs@tiac.net
www.nichcy.org

Promotes public awareness of gastrointestinal motility disorders in particular intestinal pseudo-obstruction and Hirschsprung's disease; provides education and support to individuals and families of children who have been diagnosed with these disorders.

3806 **American Society for Gastrointestinal Endoscopy**
1520 Kensington Road
Oak Brook, IL 60523
630-573-0600
800-353-2743
Fax: 630-573-0691
e-mail: info@asge.org
www.asge.org

ASGE provides information training and practice guidelines about gastrointestinal endoscopic techniques.
John L Petrini MD FASGE, President
Jacques Van Dam MD PhD FAS, President-Elect

3807 American Society for Parenteral and Enteral Nutrition (ASPEN)
8630 Fenton Street 301-587-6315
Silver Spring, MD 20910-3805 Fax: 301-587-2365
e-mail: aspen@nutr.org
www.nutritioncare.org
Offers information and continuing medical education to professionals involved in the care of parenterally and enterally fed patients. Membership includes complimentary subscriptions to two peer reviewed journals.
Debra Ben Avram CAE, Chief Executive Officer
Paula Bowen, Research Program Administrator

3808 American Society of Adults with Pseudo-Obstruction
International Corporate Headquarters
19 Carrol Road 781-935-9776
Woburn, MA 01801-6161 Fax: 781-933-4151
ASAP educates the general public and medical community about chronic intestinal pseudo-obstruction (CIP) and other related digestive motility disorders; serves as an integral source of information for patients of all ages with CIP and related disorders.

3809 Center for Digestive Disorders: Central DuPage Hospital
25 N Winfield Road 630-933-1600
Winfield, IL 60190 877-933-4234
Fax: 630-933-1300
TTY: 630-933-4833
e-mail: cdh_information@cdh.org
www.cdh.org
Multifaceted program to meet the needs of people who suffer from gastrointestinal problems; offers literature, videotapes and educational meetings and, if medical care is needed, appropriate referrals are made.
Luke McGuinness, President/CEO
Jim Spear, Executive Vice President/CFO

3810 Cyclic Vomiting Syndrome Association
2819 W Highland Boulevard 414-342-7880
Milwaukee, WI 53208 Fax: 414-342-8980
e-mail: cvsa@cvsaonline.org
www.cvsaonline.org
CVSA provides opportunities for patients, families and professionals to offer and receive support and share knowledge about cyclic vomiting syndrome; actively promotes and facilitates medical research about nausea and vomiting.

3811 Digestive Disease National Coalition
507 Capitol Court NE 202-544-7497
Washington, DC 20002 Fax: 202-546-7105
e-mail: ddnc@hmcw.org
www.ddnc.org
Informs the public and the health care community about digestive disorders; seeks Federal funding for research education and training; and represents members' interests regarding Federal and State legislation that affects digestive diseases research.
Linda Aukett, Chairperson
Peter Banks, President

3812 International Academy of Proctology
2209 John R Wooden Drive 765-342-3686
Martinsville, IN 46151 Fax: 765-342-4173
Encourages study of diseases of the colon and accessory organs of digestion and conducts seminars.
George Donna MD

3813 International Foundation for Functional Gastrointestinal Disorders
PO Box 170864 414-964-1799
Milwaukee, WI 53217-8076 888-964-2001
Fax: 414-964-7176
e-mail: iffgd@iffgd.org
www.iffgd.org
IFFGD is a nonprofit education support and research organization devoted to increasing awareness and understanding of functional gastrointestinal disorders, including irritable bowel syndrome (IBS), constipation, diarrhea, pain, and incontinence.
Nancy J Norton, President

3814 Iron Overload Diseases Association
PO Box 15857 561-586-8246
W Palm Beach, FL 33416-5123 866-768-8629
Fax: 561-842-9881
e-mail: iod@ironoverload.org
www.ironoverload.org
Conducts professional education symposiums and exhibits at medical meetings; serves and counsels hemochromatosis patients and families; offers doctor referrals; promotes patient advocacy concerning insurance, Medicare, blood banks, and the FDA.
Roberta Crawford, Founder/President

3815 National Digestive Diseases Information Clearinghouse
Two Information Way
Bethesda, MD 20892-3570 800-891-5389
Fax: 703-738-4929
TTY: 866-569-1162
e-mail: nddic@info.niddk.nih.gov
www.digestive.niddk.nih.gov
Offers various educational information, public resources and reprints, public awareness materials and more on digestive disorders.
Griffin P Rodgers MD MACP, Director

3816 North American Society for Pediatric Gastroenterology and Nutrition
PO Box 6 215-233-0808
Flourtown, PA 19031 Fax: 215-233-3918
e-mail: naspghan@naspghan.org
www.naspgn.org/
Promotes research and provides a forum for professionals in the areas of pediatric GI liver disease, gastroenterology, and nutrition. Associated with fellow organizations in Europe and Australia (ESPGAN, AUSPGAN).
Margaret K Stallings, Executive Director
Philip M Sherman, MD, FRCPC, President

3817 Pediatric Adolescent Gastroesophageal Reflux Association
PO Box 486 301-601-9541
Buckeystown, MD 21717 888-887-7729
e-mail: gergroup@aol.com
www.reflux.org
PAGER's mission is to: (1) gather and disseminate information on pediatric gastroesophageal reflux (GER) and related disorders; (2) provide educational and emotional support to patients with GER, their families, and professionals; (3) promote awareness of GER within both the medical community and the general public; and (4) promote research into the causes, treatments and eventual cure for pediatric GER.
Beth Anderson, Director

3818 Pediatric Adolescent Gastroesophageal Asso ciation
PO Box 486 301-601-9541
Buckeystown, MD 21717 e-mail: gergroup@aol.com
www.reflux.org
PAGER's mission is to: (1) gather and disseminate information on pediatric gastroesophageal reflux (GER) and related disorders; (2) provide educational and emotional support to patients with GER, their families and professionals; (3) promote awareness.
Beth Anderson, Director
Jennifer Rackley, Associate Director

3819 Pediatric/Adolescent Gastroesophageal Reflux Association
PO Box 466 301-601-9541
Garrett Park, MD 20896-1153 888-887-7729
e-mail: gergroup@aol.com
www.reflux.org
PAGER gathers and disseminates information on pediatric gastroesophageal reflux and related disorders; provides support and education to patients their families and the public; promotes the general welfare of patients, their families and the public.
Beth Anderson, Director
Jennifer Rackley, Associate Director

3820 **Society for Surgery of the Alimentary Tract**
900 Cummings Center
Beverly, MA 01915
978-927-8330
Fax: 978-524-8890
www.ssat.com
SSAT provides a forum for exchange of information among physicians specializing in alimentary tract surgery.
David W McFadden MD, President
David M Mahvi MD, President-Elect

3821 **Society of American Gastrointestinal Endoscopic Surgeons**
11300 W Olympic Boulevard
Los Angeles, CA 90064
310-437-0544
Fax: 310-437-0585
www.sages.org
SAGES encourages study and practice of gastrointestinal endoscopy laparoscopy and minimal access surgery.
Mark A Talamini MD, President
C Daniel Smith MD, President-Elect

3822 **Society of Gastroenterology Nurses and Associates**
401 N Michigan Avenue
Chicago, IL 60611-4267
312-321-5165
800-245-7462
Fax: 312-673-6694
e-mail: sgna@smithbucklin.com
www.sgna.org
SGNA provides members with continuing education opportunities practice and training guidelines and information about trends and development in the field of gastroenterology.
Lisa Heard BSN RN CGRN, President
Theresa Vos MS BSN RN CGRN, President-Elect

3823 **United Ostomy Association**
PO Box 66
Fairview, TN 37062
949-660-8624
800-826-0826
Fax: 949-660-9262
e-mail: info@uoaa.org
www.uoaa.org
Volunteer based health organization dedicated to providing education, information, support and advocacy for those who have or will have an intestinal or urinary diversion. We provide patient visiting services, 800 number referral and information services.
Ken Aukett, President
Kristin Knipp, President-Elect

Foundations

3824 **American Porphyria Foundation**
PO Box 22712
Houston, TX 77227
713-266-9617
Fax: 713-840-9552
e-mail: porphyrus@aol.com
www.porphyriafoundation.com
The APF is dedicated to improving the health and well-being of individuals and families affected by porphyria. Our mission is to enhance public awareness about porphyria, develop educational programs and distributing educational material for patients and physicians and support research to improve treatment and ultimately lead to a cure.
Desiree H Lyon, Executive Director

3825 **Gastro-Intestinal Research Foundation**
70 East Lake Street
Chicago, IL 60601-5907
312-332-1350
Fax: 312-332-4757
e-mail: girf@girf.org
www.girf.org
Provides funds for equipment, laboratories and the support of investigators and young physicians in the University of Chicago Gastroenterology Section, a group of full-time dedicated doctors who seek solutions to all kinds of gastrointestinal illnesses, affecting the esophagus, the stomach, the small intestine, the large intestine, the liver, the gallbladder, and the pancreas.
Jennifer Wright, Executive Director

3826 **Oley Foundation**
Albany Medical Center
Albany, NY 12208-3478
518-262-5079
800-776-6539
Fax: 518-262-5528
www.oley.org
Promotes and advocates education and research in home parenteral and enteral nutrition; provides support and networking to patients through information clearinghouse and regional volunteer networks; sponsors meetings and conferences, including annual patient/clinician conference; maintains speakers bureau.
Joan Bishop, Executive Director

Research Centers

3827 **Baylor College of Medicine: General Clinical Research Center for Adults**
TXWT 10th Floor
Houston, TX 77030
713-798-7022
e-mail: dbier@bcm.edu
www.bcm.edu/pediatrics
Endocrinology, genetics and gastroenterology research.
Dennis M Bier MD, Program Director

3828 **Digestive Disorders Associates Ridgely Oaks Professional Center**
Ridgely Oaks Professional Center
621 Ridgely Avenue
Annapolis, MD 21401
41- 22- 363
800-273-0505
Fax: 410-224-6971
TTY: 800-735-2258
www.dda.net
Specialize in the diagnosis and treatment of diseases of the entire digestive system including esophagus stomach small and large intestine colon liver pancreas and gall bladder.
Michael S Epstein, Founder
Charles E King, Doctor

3829 **Gastrointestinal Research Foundation**
70 E Lake Street
Chicago, IL 60601-5915
312-332-1350
Fax: 312-332-4757
e-mail: info@girf.org
www.girf.org
Founded to help combat gastrointestinal diseases. Raises funds to support research at the Center for study of the Digestive Diseases at the University of Chicago Medical Center and to support advanced training for scientists. Sponsors educational activities for the public.
Martin N Sandler, Co-Founder
Steven R Davidson, Co-Chairman

3830 **University of California: Davis Gastroenterology & Nutrition Center**
Pediatric GI Medical Center
4301 X Street
Sacramento, CA 95817-2214
916-453-3750
Research into gastrointestinal mobility and electro-physiology nutrition support and references for the public and patient evaluations.
Robert A Cannon MD, Director

3831 **University of California: Los Angeles Center for Ulcer Research**
LA Medical Center
Building 115 Room 117
Los Angeles, CA 90073
310-312-9284
Fax: 310-268-4963
e-mail: cureadmn@mednet.ucla.edu
www.cure.med.ucla.edu
Offers basic and clinical research related to peptic ulcer disease including causes checks and balances and stress-ulcer relationships.
Enrique Rozengurt, Director
Emeran Mayer, Co-Director

3832 **University of Michigan Michigan Gastrointestinal Peptide Research Ctr.**
U-M Health System
1150 W Medical Center
Ann Arbor, MI 48109
734-936-4000
Fax: 734-763-2535
e-mail: GutPeptide@umich.edu
www.med.umich.edu/mgpc
Research into gastroenterology including chemistry of gut hormones is studied.
Chung Owyang MD, Director
Juanita Merc MD PhD, Associate Director

3833 **University of Pennsylvania: Harrison Department of Surgical Research**
3400 Spruce Street 215-662-3000
Philadelphia, PA 19104 800-789-PENN
Fax: 215-615-0471
e-mail: julie.koehler@uphs.upenn.edu
www.uphs.upenn.edu/surgery/res/harrisonr
Offers research and studies on surgical transplantations gastrointestinal physiology.
Julie Hagan Koehler MBA, Business Director
Georgina Suarez, Administrative Assistant

Support Groups & Hotlines

3834 **National Health Information Center**
PO Box 1133 310-565-4167
Washington, DC 20013 800-336-4797
Fax: 301-984-4256
e-mail: info@nhic.org
www.health.gov/nhic
Offers a nationwide information referral service, produces directories and resource guides.

3835 **Pull-thru Network**
2312 Savoy Street 205-978-2930
Hoover, AL 35226-1528 e-mail: ptnmail@charter.net
www.pullthrough.org
Dedicated to the needs of those born wutith anorectal malformation or colon disease and any of the associated diagnoses.

Magazines

3836 **ASAP Forum**
ASAP International Corporate Headquarters
19 Carroll Road 781-935-9776
Woburn, MA 01801 Fax: 781-933-4151
e-mail: asapgi@sprynet.com
Educates the general public and medical community about chronic intestinal pseudo-obstruction (CIP) and other related digestive motility disorders; serves as an integral source of information for patients of all ages with CIP and related disorders, their families, and members of the medical community.

3837 **American Journal of Gastroenterology**
American College of Gastroenterology
4900B 31st St S 703-820-7400
Arlington, VA 22206-1656 Fax: 703-931-4520
www.acg.gi.org
Serves clinical and scientific information needs of member physicians and surgeons, who specialize in digestive and related disorders. Emphasis is on scholarly practice, teaching, and research.
Thomas F Fise, Executive Director

3838 **American Journal of Gastrointestinal Surgery**
Society for Surgery of the Alimentary Tract
13 Elm Street 978-526-8330
Manchester, MA 01944 Fax: 978-526-4018
e-mail: ssat@prri.com
www.ssat.com
Provides information for physicians specializing in gastrointestinal surgery.

3839 **Clinical Perspectives in Gastroenterology**
American Gastroenterological Association
7910 Woodmont Avenue 301-654-2055
Bethesda, MD 20814 Fax: 301-654-5920
e-mail: aga001@801.com
www.gastro.org
Focuses on research, medical and professional developments in the science of gastroenterology.
Robert Greenberg, Executive VP

3840 **Digestive Health Matters**
Intl. Foundation for Gastrointestinal Disorders
PO Box 170864 414-964-1799
Milwaukee, WI 53217-0864 888-964-2001
Fax: 414-964-7176
e-mail: iffgd@iffgd.org
www.iffgd.org
Quarterly journal focuses on upper and lower gastrointestinal disorders in adults and children. Educational pamphlets and factsheets are available. Patient and professional membership.

3841 **Gastroenterology**
American Gastroenterological Association
7910 Woodmont Avenue 301-654-2055
Bethesda, MD 20814-3002 Fax: 301-654-5920
e-mail: aga001@801.com
www.gastro.org
Focuses on research, medical and professional developments in the science of gastroenterology.
Robert Greenberg, Executive VP

3842 **Gastroenterology Nursing**
Society of Gastroenterology Nurses and Associates
401 N Michigan Avenue 312-321-5165
Chicago, IL 60611 800-245-7462
Fax: 312-321-5194
e-mail: sgna@sba.com
www.sgna.org
Provides members with information about trends and development in the field of gastroenterology nursing.

3843 **Gastrointestinal Endoscopy**
American Society for Gastrointestinal Endoscopy
1520 Kensington Road 630-573-0600
Oak Brook, IL 60523 Fax: 630-573-0691
www.asge.org
Provides information, training, and practice guidelines about gastrointestinal endoscopic techniques.

3844 **Journal of Parenteral and Enteral Nutrition**
ASPEN
8630 Fenton Street 301-587-6315
Silver Spring, MD 20910-3805 Fax: 301-587-2365
e-mail: aspen@nutr.org
www.nutritioncare.org
Offers information to professionals involved in the care of parenterally and enterally fed patients.
100 pages BiMonthly
Adrian Nickel, Director Communications/Marketing

3845 **Journal of Pediatric Gastroenterology and Nutrition**
N American Society for Pediatric Gastroenterology
6900 Grove Road 609-848-1000
Thorofare, NJ 08086 Fax: 609-848-5274
www.jpgn.org/
Provides information for professionals in the areas of pediatric GI liver disease, gastroenterology, and nutrition.

3846 **Journal of the American Dietetic Association**
American Dietetic Association
216 W Jackson Boulevard 312-899-0040
Chicago, IL 60606-6995 800-877-1600
Fax: 312-899-1979
www.eatright.org
Professional journal of the ADA.

3847 **Nutrition in Clinical Practice**
ASPEN
8630 Fenton Street 301-587-6315
Silver Spring, MD 20910-3805 Fax: 301-587-2365
e-mail: aspen@nutr.org
www.nutritioncare.org
Offers information to professionals involved in the care of parenterally and enterally fed patients.
100 pages BiMonthly
Adrian Nickel, Director Communications/Marketing

3848 **Pancreas**
American Pancreatic Association
10833 LeConte Avenue 310-825-4976
Los Angeles, CA 90095-6904 Fax: 310-206-2472
e-mail: hreber@surgery.medch.ucla.edu

Provides information on scientific research related to the pancreas.
Howard A Reber MD

Newsletters

3849 **ADA Courier**
American Dietetic Association
216 W Jackson Boulevard
Chicago, IL 60606-6995
312-899-0040
800-877-1600
Fax: 312-899-1979
www.eatright.org
Information for the public on the promotion of optimal nutrition, health, and well-being.

3850 **APF Newsletter**
PO Box 22712
Houston, TX 77227
713-266-9617
Fax: 713-840-9552
e-mail: porphyrus@aol.com
www.porphyriafoundation.com
Provides updates on treatment and research, as well as informative articles on patients and specialists who treat porphyria. It's mailed to all Sponsors of the APF.
Desiree H Lyon, Executive Director

3851 **ASAP Capsule**
ASAP International Corporate Headquarters
19 Carroll Road
Woburn, MA 01801
781-935-9776
Fax: 781-933-4151
e-mail: asapgi@sprynet.com
Professional membership newsletter for ASAP, an organization which educates the general public and medical community about chronic intestinal pseudo-obstruction (CIP) and other related digestive motility disorders; serves as an integral source of information for patients of all ages with CIP and related disorders, their families, and members of the medical community.

3852 **ASAP Digest**
ASAP International Corporate Headquarters
19 Carroll Road
Woburn, MA 01801
781-935-9776
Fax: 781-933-4151
e-mail: asapgi@sprynet.com
General membership newsletter for ASAP. Educates the general public and medical community about chronic intestinal pseudo-obstruction (CIP) and other related digestive motility disorders; serves as an integral source of information for patients of all ages with CIP and related disorders, their families, and members of the medical community.

3853 **Clinical Updates**
American Society for Gastrointestinal Endoscopy
1520 Kensington Road
Oak Brook, IL 60523
630-573-0600
Fax: 630-573-0691
www.asge.org
Provides information, training, and practice guidelines about gastrointestinal endoscopic techniques.
Quarterly

3854 **Code V**
Cyclic Vomiting Syndrome Association (CVSA)
13180 Caroline Court
Elm Grove, WI 53122-1732
614-837-2586
Fax: 614-837-6543
e-mail: drwaites@infinet.com
www.beaker.iupui.edu/cvsa
Newsletter for members of the CVSA.

3855 **Hemochromatosis Awareness**
Hemochromatosis Foundation
PO Box 8569
Albany, NY 12208
518-489-0972
Fax: 518-489-0227
www.hemochromatosis.org
Provides information to the public, families, professionals and government agencies about hereditary hemochromatosis (HH); conducts and raises funds for research; encourages early screening for HH; holds symposiums and meetings; and offers genetic counseling along with support for patients, families, and professionals.
Margit Krikker MD, Medical Director

3856 **Ironic Blood**
Iron Overload Diseases Association
433 Westward Drive
North Palm Beach, FL 33408-5123
561-840-8512
Fax: 561-842-9881
e-mail: iod@ironoverload.org
www.ironoverload.org
Information for hemochromatosis patients and families.

3857 **Lifeline Letter**
Oley Foundation
Albany Medical Center
Albany, NY 12208-3478
518-262-5079
800-776-6539
Fax: 518-262-5528
e-mail: bishopj@mail.amc.edu
www.oley.org
Information on home parenteral and enteral nutrition for patients and the public.
16 pages Bi-Monthly
Joan Bishop, Executive Director

3858 **Ostomy Quarterly**
United Ostomy Association
PO Box 66
Fairview, TN 37062
800-826-0826
e-mail: info@uoa.org
www.uoa.org
First person stories, ostomy management advice from an ET and MD, organization news and ostomy product information.
72 pages Quarterly

3859 **Pull-thru Network News**
Pull-thru Network
4 Woody Lane
Westport, CT 06880
203-221-7530
e-mail: Pullthrunw@aol.com
members.aol.com/pullthrunw/Pullthru.html
Provides information to patients and families of children who have had or will have pull-through surgery to correct an imperforate anus or associated malformation, Hirschsprung's disease, or other fecal incontinence problems.

3860 **SGNA News**
Society of Gastroenterology Nurses and Associates
401 N Michigan Avenue
Chicago, IL 60611
312-321-5165
800-245-7462
Fax: 312-321-5194
e-mail: sgna@sba.com
www.sgna.org
Provides members with information about trends and development in the field of gastroenterology.

3861 **WIN Notes**
Weight-control Information Network
1 WIN Way
Bethesda, MD 20892-3665
202-828-1025
877-946-4627
Fax: 202-828-1028
e-mail: win@mathewsgroup.com
www.niddk.nih.gov/health/nutrit/win.htm
Addresses the health information needs of individuals with weight-control problems. Available on the WIN web site.
BiAnnual

Pamphlets

3862 **Acute Intermittent Porphyria**
American Prophyria Foundation
PO Box 22712
Houston, TX 77227
713-266-9617
www.enterprise.net
An informational brochure published by the American Porphyria Foundation.

3863 **Common Questions About Porphyria**
American Prophyria Foundation
PO Box 22712
Houston, TX 77227
713-266-9617
www.enterprise.net
An informational brochure published by the American Porphyria Foundation.

3864 **Diet and Nutrition in Porphyria**
American Prophyria Foundation

PO Box 22712
Houston, TX 77227 713-266-9617
www.enterprise.net
An informational brochure published by the American Porphyria Foundation.

3865 Drugs and Porphyria
American Prophyria Foundation
PO Box 22712
Houston, TX 77227 713-266-9617
www.enterprise.net
An informational brochure published by the American Porphyria Foundation.

3866 Erythropoietic Protoporphyria
American Prophyria Foundation
PO Box 22712
Houston, TX 77227 713-266-9617
www.enterprise.net
An informational brochure published by the American Porphyria Foundation.

3867 Hematin
American Prophyria Foundation
PO Box 22712
Houston, TX 77227 713-266-9617
www.enterprise.net
An informational brochure published by the American Porphyria Foundation.

3868 Iron Overload Alert
Iron Overload Diseases Association
433 Westward Drive 561-840-8512
North Palm Beach, FL 33408-5123 Fax: 561-842-9881
e-mail: iod@ironoverload.org
www.ironoverload.org
Information for hemochromatosis patients and families.

3869 Issues in Women's Gastrointestinal Health
Gastro-Intestinal Research Foundation
70 E Lake Street 312-332-1350
Chicago, IL 60601 Fax: 312-332-4757
e-mail: girf@girf.org
www.girf.org
Patient education pamphlet.

3870 Porphyria Cutanea Tarda
American Prophyria Foundation
PO Box 22712
Houston, TX 77227 713-266-9617
www.enterprise.net
An informational brochure published by the American Porphyria Foundation.

Audio & Video

3871 A Day in the Life of a Child
Albany Medical Center 518-262-5079
Albany, NY 12208-3478 800-776-6539
Fax: 518-262-5528
www.oley.org
In this video you are welcomed into the household of the Miller family. The Millers have three children, one of whom is tube fed. Jessica has been dependent on tube-feedings since birth, and her family is prepared to show you just what that means. They share tips for keeping a sterile environment in a house with three children, and tips for helping Jessica fit in with her peers.
Joan Bishop, Executive Director

3872 Cleveland Clinic Teaching Conference
Hemochromatosis Foundation
PO Box 8569 518-489-0972
Albany, NY 12208 Fax: 518-489-0227
www.hemochromatosis.org
Provides information to the public, families, and professionals about hereditary hemochromatosis.

3873 Family Teaching Conference
Hemochromatosis Foundation
PO Box 8569 518-489-0972
Albany, NY 12208 Fax: 518-489-0227
www.hemochromatosis.org
Provides information to the public, families, and professionals about hereditary hemochromatosis.
2 3/4 hours

3874 Life with Mic-Key
Albany Medical Center 518-262-5079
Albany, NY 12208-3478 800-776-6539
Fax: 518-262-5528
www.oley.org
Serves as an informative and introductory guide for adapting to life with a Mic-key low profile feeding tube. "Low profile" means that the Mic-key tube lies very close to the patient's body and does not stick out. It's slim design allows more air to circulate around the stoma site and makes it easy to care for. The Mic-key tube uses a balloon to hold it in place and comes with several important accessories, including two types of extensions sets and an anti-reflux valve.
10 Minutes
Joan Bishop, Executive Director

3875 Mealtime Notions - The 'Get Permission' Approach to Mealtimes and Oral Motor
Marsha Dunn Klein, MED, OTR/L, author
Albany Medical Center 518-262-5079
Albany, NY 12208-3478 800-776-6539
Fax: 518-262-5528
www.oley.org
This video explores the development of trusting feeding relationships, understanding the child's pace, and strategies for increasing permissive behavior. Tools discussed in this video include an introduction to the "sensory continuum," a description of the "around the bowl technique," and tips for removing the stress from your child's mealtime.
10 Minutes
Joan Bishop, Executive Director

Web Sites

3876 American College of Gastroenterology (ACG)
www.acg.gi.org
Serves clinical and scientific information needs of member physicians and surgeons, who specialize in digestive and related disorders. Emphasis is on scholarly practice, teaching, and research.

3877 American Gastroenterological Association (AGA)
www.gastro.org
Fosters the development and application of the science of gastroenterology by providing leadership and aid, including patient care, research, teaching, continuing education, scientific communication, and matters of national health policy pertaining to gastroenterology.

3878 American Hemochromatosis Society
www.americanhs.org
Educates the public, the medical community, and the media by distributing the most current information available on hereditary hemochromatosis (HH), including DNA screening for HH and pediatric HH; also facilitates patient empowerment through an online network.

3879 American Porphyria Foundation
PO Box 22712 713-266-9617
Houston, TX 77227 Fax: 713-840-9552
e-mail: porphyrus@aol.com
www.porphyriafoundation.com
Advances awareness, research, and treatment of the porphyrias; provides self-help services for members; and provides referrals to porphyria treatment specialists.
Karl E Anderson, MD, Chairman

3880 American Pseudo-Obstruction and Hirschsprung's Disease Society
Promotes public awareness of gastrointestinal motility disorders, in particular intestinal pseudo-obstruction and Hirschsprung's Disease; provides education and support to individuals and families of children who have been diagnosed with these disorders

through parent-to-parent contact, publications, and educational symposia; and encourages and supports medical research in the area of gastrointestinal motility disorders.

3881 **American Society for Gastrointestinal Endoscopy**
www.asge.org
ASGE provides information, training, and practice guidelines about gastrointestinal endoscopic techniques.

3882 **American Society of Abdominal Surgeons**
www.gis.net/~absurg/
ASAS sponsors extensive continuing education program for physicians in the field of abdominal surgery and maintains library.

3883 **Background on Functional Gastrointestinal Disorders**
www.med.unc.edu
Statistical background information on gastrointestinal disorders.

3884 **Children's Motility Disorder Foundation**
www.motility.org
CMDF works to increase awareness of pediatric motility disorders in the general public and among the physicians most likely to encounter children suffering from these conditions, such as pediatricians and family practice doctors. Supports medical research regarding the causes, treatment, and potentially life-threatening disorders.

3885 **Cyclic Vomiting Syndrome Association**
www.cvsaonline.org/
CVSA provides opportunities for patients, families, and professionals to offer and receive support and share knowledge about cyclic vomiting syndrome; actively promotes and facilitates medical research about nausea and vomiting; increases worldwide public and professional awareness; and serves as a resource center for information.

3886 **Gastrointestinal Research Foundation**
www.girf.org
Founded to help combat gastrointestinal diseases. Raises funds to support research at the Center for the study of the Digestive Diseases at the University of Chicago Medical Center and to support advanced training for scientists. Sponsors educational activities for the public.

3887 **Healing Well**
www.healingwell.com
An online health resource guide to medical news, chat, information and articles, newsgroups and message boards, books, disease-related web sites, medical directories, and more for patients, friends, and family coping with disabling diseases, disorders, or chronic illnesses.

3888 **Health Finder**
www.healthfinder.gov
Searchable, carefully developed web site offering information on over 1000 topics. Developed by the US Department of Health and Human Services, the site can be used in both English and Spanish.

3889 **Healthlink USA**
www.healthlinkusa.com
Health information concerning treatment, cures, prevention, diagnosis, risk factors, research, support groups, email lists, personal stories and much more. Updated regularly.

3890 **Helios Health**
www.helioshealth.com
Online resource for your health information. Detailed information about specific health topics, access to expert advice from our Medical Advisory Board, and up-to-date health news.

3891 **Hemochromatosis Foundation**
www.hemochromatosis.org
Provides information to the public, families, and professionals about hereditary hemochromatosis (HH); conducts and raises funds for research; encourages early screening for HH; holds symposiums and meetings; and offers genetic counseling along with support for patients, families, and professionals.

3892 **International Foundation for Functional Gastrointestinal Disorders**
www.iffgd.org
IFFGD is a nonprofit education, support and research organization devoted to increasing awareness and understanding of functional gastrointestinal disorders, including irritable bowel syndrome (IBS), constipation, diarrhea, pain, and incontinence. Mission is to inform, assist and support people affected by these disorders.

3893 **MedicineNet**
www.medicinenet.com
An online resource for consumers providing easy-to-read, authoritative medical and health information.

3894 **Medscape**
www.mywebmd.com
Medscape offers specialists, primary care physicians, and other health professionals the Web's most robust and integrated medical information and educational tools.

3895 **National Digestive Diseases Information Clearinghouse**
www.niddk.nih.gov
Offers various educational information, public resources and reprints, public awareness materials and more on digestive disorders.

3896 **North American Society for Pediatric Gastroenterology and Nutrition**
www.naspgn.org
Promotes research and provides a forum for professionals in the areas of pediatric GI liver disease, gastroenterology, and nutrition. Associated with fellow organizations in Europe and Australia (ESPGAN, AUSPGAN).

3897 **Nutrition in Clinical Practice**
www.clinnutr.org
Offers information to professionals involved in the care of parenterally and enterally fed patients.

3898 **Oley Foundation**
www.wizvax.net/oleyfdn
Promotes and advocates education and research in home parenteral and enteral nutrition; provides support and networking to patients through information clearinghouse and regional volunteer networks; sponsors meetings and conferences, including annual patient/clinician conference; maintains speakers bureau.

3899 **Pediatric Adolescent Gastroesophageal Assn**
www.reflux.org
Discussions led by local experts, family medical histories and check swabs, supervised nap room and separate activity room for kids, trained babysitters available.

3900 **Pediatric/Adolescent Gastroesophageal Reflux Association**
www.reflux.org
PAGER gathers and disseminates information on pediatric gastroesophageal reflux and related disorders; provides support and education to patients, their families, and the public; promotes the general welfare of patients, their families, and the public; promotes the general welfare of patients with gastroesophageal reflux and their families; and promotes public awareness of the condition.

3901 **Pull-thru Network**
members.aol.com/pullthrunw/Pullthru.html
Provides emotional support and information to patients and families of children who have had or will have pull-through surgery to correct an imperforate anus or associated malformation, Hirschsprung's disease, or other fecal incontinence problems; sponsors online discussion groups. A chapter of the United Ostomy Association.

3902 **Society for Surgery of the Alimentary Tract**
www.ssat.com
SSAT provides a forum for exchange of information among physicians specializing in alimentary tract surgery.

3903 **Society of American Gastrointestinal Endoscopic Surgeons**
www.sages.org
SAGES encourages study and practice of gastrointestinal endoscopy, laparoscopy, and minimal acces surgery.

3904 **WebMD**
www.webmd.com
Information on Gastrointestinal Disorders, including articles and resources.

Description

3905 **Gaucher's Disease**

Gaucher's disease is an inherited disorder of metabolism of fats. These metabolic products can not be broken down properly because of a deficiency of an enzyme called glucocerebroside. Symptoms can include fatigue, anemia, bleeding problems (such as nosebleeds and easy bruising), enlargement of the spleen and/or liver, bone pain, easily fractured bones and brown pigmentation of the skin. The degree of symptoms and complications vary by age of onset and the degree of involvement of the disorder's clinical forms. Diagnosis is based on finding Gaucher's typical cells in the bone marrow.

The treatment for Gaucher's disease is enzyme replacement, called Cerezyme, administered intravenously. Removal of the spleen and blood transfusions may be necessary. Current research is aimed at genetic therapy.

National Agencies & Associations

3906 **National Foundation for Jewish Genetic Diseases**
Fifth Avenue at 100th Street 212-659-6774
New York, NY 10029 Fax: 212-241-6947
www.mssm.edu/jewish_genetics
This foundation was created to raise funds for and to inform the public about genetic diseases which afflict descendants of eastern and central European Jews. It sponsors medical symposia from time to time.
R J Desnick PhD MD, Center Director

3907 **National Gaucher Foundation**
2227 Idlewood Road
Tucker, GA 30024 800-504-3189
Fax: 770-934-2911
e-mail: ngf@gaucherdisease.org
www.gaucherdisease.org
National foundation providing information and assistance for those affected by Gaucher disease as well as education and outreach to increase public awareness.
Robin A Ely MD, President/Medical Director
Rhonda P Buyers, CEO/Executive Director

3908 **National Organization for Rare Disorders (NORD)**
55 Kenosia Avenue 203-744-0100
Danbury, CT 06813-1968 800-999-6673
Fax: 203-798-2291
TDD: 203-797-9590
e-mail: orphan@rarediseases.org
www.rarediseases.org
The NORD is a unique federation of voluntary health organizations dedicated to helping people with rare orphan diseases and assisting the organizations that serve them.
Carolyn Asbury, PhD, Chair
Frank Sasinowski, Vice Chair

Research Centers

3909 **Children's Gaucher Research Fund**
PO Box 2123 916-797-3700
Granite Bay, CA 95746-2123 Fax: 916-797-3707
e-mail: research@childrensgaucher.org
www.childrensgaucher.org
A nonprofit organization that raises funds to coordinate support research to find a cure for Type 2 and Type 3 Gaucher Disease.
Roscoe Brady, Scientific Advisory Board
Gregory Grabowski, Scientific Advisory Board

3910 **Comprehensive Gaucher Treatment Center at Tower Hermatology Oncology**
9090 Wilshire Boulevard 310-888-8680
Beverly Hills, CA 90211 888-248-4456
Fax: 310-285-7298
e-mail: info@gaucherwest.com
www.gaucherwest.com
The Comprehensive Gaucher Treatment Center at Tower Hermatology Oncology under the direction of Dr. Barry Rosenbloom provides clinical evaluations for the diagnosis and treatment of patient's with Gaucher disease. We provide a multi-disciplinary program that includes Hermatology Genetics Orthopedics and Radiology. To ensure continuity of care we provide assistance to other physicians regarding testing diagnosis evaluation and management of the Gaucher patient.
Barry Rosenbloom, Director
Cheryl Elzinga, Gaucher Coordinator

3911 **LAC/USC Imaging Science Center**
1744 Zonal Avenue 323-221-2424
Los Angeles, CA 90033 Fax: 323-224-5118
e-mail: nestrada@usc.edu
www.usc.edu/schools/medicine
Provides a Gaucher Disease radiology consultant: Michael R Terk MD.and Muskuloskeletal Imaging.
Thomas Learc MD, Director
Jennifer Anorve, Administrative Contact

Support Groups & Hotlines

3912 **Brave Kids**
151 Sawgrass Corners Drive 904-280-1895
Ponte Vedra Beach, FL 32082 800-568-1008
Fax: 904-280-1897
e-mail: info@bravekids.org
www.bravekids.org
An organization that offers support for parents and children suffering from serious health problems.
Kristen Fitzgerald, Founder

3913 **National Health Information Center**
PO Box 1133 310-565-4167
Washington, DC 20013 800-336-4797
Fax: 301-984-4256
e-mail: info@nhic.org
www.health.gov/nhic
Offers a nationwide information referral service, produces directories and resource guides.

Newsletters

3914 **Gaucher Disease Newsletter**
National Gaucher Foundation
11140 Rockville Pike 301-816-1515
Rockville, MD 20852-3151 800-925-8885
Offers information on the latest research, treatments and technology for persons affected by Gaucher Disease. Also includes legislative and medical information.
Quarterly

Pamphlets

3915 **Gaucher Disease Fact Sheet**
National Gaucher Foundation
11140 Rockville Pike 301-816-1515
Rockville, MD 20852-3151 800-925-8885
Offers information on what Gaucher Disease is, the symptoms, risks, treatments and the workings of the National Gaucher Foundation.

3916 **Living with Gaucher Disease**
National Gaucher Foundation
11140 Rockville Pike 301-816-1515
Rockville, MD 20852-3151 800-925-8885

A guide for parents, families and relatives that teach them how to deal with and cope with a diagnosis of Gaucher Disease.
24 pages

Audio & Video

3917 **Pain & Hope**
National Gaucher Foundation
11140 Rockville Pike 301-816-1515
Rockville, MD 20852-3151 800-925-8885
A patient and family perspective on Gaucher Disease.

Web Sites

3918 **Gaucher Disease Homepage**
www.gaucherdisease.org
Information on Gaucher disease, including symptoms, treatment, prevalence, resources, support, and news.

3919 **Healing Well**
www.healingwell.com
An online health resource guide to medical news, chat, information and articles, newsgroups and message boards, books, disease-related web sites, medical directories, and more for patients, friends, and family coping with disabling diseases, disorders, or chronic illnesses.

3920 **Health Finder**
www.healthfinder.gov
Searchable, carefully developed web site offering information on over 1000 topics. Developed by the US Department of Health and Human Services, the site can be used in both English and Spanish.

3921 **Healthlink USA**
www.healthlinkusa.com
Health information concerning treatment, cures, prevention, diagnosis, risk factors, research, support groups, email lists, personal stories and much more. Updated regularly.

3922 **Helios Health**
www.helioshealth.com
Online resource for your health information. Detailed information about specific health topics, access to expert advice from our Medical Advisory Board, and up-to-date health news.

3923 **MedicineNet**
www.medicinenet.com
An online resource for consumers providing easy-to-read, authoritative medical and health information.

3924 **Medscape**
www.mywebmd.com
Medscape offers specialists, primary care physicians, and other health professionals the Web's most robust and integrated medical information and educational tools.

3925 **WebMD**
www.webmd.com
Information on Gaucher's disease, including articles and resources.

Description

3926 **Growth Disorders**

There are many conditions that make a child grow more slowly than average. Any sort of severe chronic illness, especially one involving the digestive system, may cause this. Certain genetic conditions such as Turner syndrome, a sex chromosome abnormality or achondroplasia (skeletal maldevelopment) will predictably limit growth and eventual adult height. Endocrine, or hormonal, causes of short stature include underactivity of the thyroid gland (hypothyroidism) or pituitary gland, where growth hormone (GH) is normally formed. Finally, there are many cases where the child's height is significantly below that of peers, yet none of these conditions is present. This may reflect two parents who are themselves quite short, or may be completely unexplained.

If slow growth is related to low levels of GH, therapy with synthetic GH is extremely effective. Regular injections will be necessary for a prolonged period until an acceptable height is reached.

Regardless of the underlying cause, a child whose disorder is recognized at birth or who is not growing as quickly as the rest of his or her peers should receive a complete evaluation by a pediatric endocrinologist or other growth specialist.

National Agencies & Associations

3927 **Alliance of Genetic Support Groups**
4301 Connecticut Avenue NW 202-966-5557
Washington, DC 20008-2369 Fax: 202-966-8553
e-mail: info@geneticalliance.org
www.geneticalliance.org

A coalition of voluntary genetic support groups consumers and professionals addressing the needs of individuals and families affected by genetic disorders from a national perspective.
Sharon F Terry MA, President/CEO
Lisa Wise MA BFA BA, COO

3928 **Dwarf Athletic Association of America**
708 Gravenstein Highway N 972-317-8299
Sebastopol, CA 95472 888-598-3222
Fax: 972-966-0184
e-mail: daaa@flash.net
www.daaa.org

Develops, promotes and provides quality amateur level athletic opportunities for dwarf athletes in the US. Our mission is to encourage people with dwarfism to participate in sports regardless of their level of skill.
Amy B Andrews, Board President
Mike Cekanor, Board VP

3929 **Little People of America**
250 El Camino Real 714-368-3689
Tustin, CA 92780 888-LPA-2001
Fax: 714-368-3367
e-mail: info@lpaonline.org
www.lpaonline.org

Focuses research, support and information on persons who are short in stature.
Lois Gerage-Lamb, President
Bill Bradford, Senior VP

3930 **Little People's Research Fund (LPRF)**
616 Old Edmondson Avenue 410-747-1100
Catonsville, MD 21228 800-232-LPRF
Fax: 410-747-1374
e-mail: lprf@lprf.org
www.lprf.org

LPRF supports research into the disabling conditions of skeletal dysplasia (dwarfism), promotes patient care and education of the medical community as well as the general public. It assists families by sponsoring clinics in various states.
Steven E Kopits MD, Medical Advisor

3931 **National Institute of Child Health and Human Development**
31 Center Drive
Bethesda, MD 20892-2425 800-370-2943
Fax: 301-984-1473
TTY: 888-320-6942
www.nichd.nih.gov

Duane Alexander MD, Director

Foundations

3932 **Human Growth Foundation**
997 Glen Cove Avenue 516-671-4041
Glen Head, NY 11545 800-451-6434
Fax: 516-671-4055
e-mail: hgf1@hgfound.org
www.hgfound.org

Our mission is to help children, and adults with disorders of growth and growth hormone through research, education, support, and advocacy. The Foundation is dedicated to helping medical science to better understand the process of growth. It is composed of concerned parents and friends of children, and adults, with growth problems; and, interested health professionals.
Patricia D Costa, Executive Director

3933 **MAGIC Foundation for Children's Growth**
6645 West North Avenue 708-383-0808
Oak Park, IL 60302 800-362-4423
Fax: 708-383-0899
e-mail: dianne@magicfoundation.org
www.magicfoundation.org

Provides support services for the families of children afflicted with a wide variety of chronic and/or critical disorders, syndromes and that affect a child's growth.
Dianne Tamburrino, Executive Director
Susan Smith, RN, Director Medical Education

3934 **March of Dimes Birth Defects Foundation**
1275 Mamaroneck Avenue
White Plains, NY 10605 914-997-4488
www.marchofdimes.com

Our mission is to improve the health of babies by preventing birth defects, premature birth, and infant mortality.

Research Centers

3935 **Case Western Reserve University: Bolton Brush Growth Study Center**
2123 Abington Road 216-368-4649
Cleveland, OH 44106-4905 Fax: 216-368-3204
e-mail: mgh4@po.cwru.edu
dental.cwru.edu/bolton-brush

Investigations and research into the growth and development of the human body. Extensive collection of longitudinal human growth data.
Mark G Hans, Director
Aaron Weinbe DMD PhD, Associate Professor and Chairman

3936 **International Skeletal Dysplasia Registry Medical Genetics Institute**
Medical Genetics Institute
8700 Beverly Boulevard 310-423-3277
Los Angeles, CA 90048 800-233-2771
Fax: 310-423-0462
www.csmc.edu

Provides patient services for skeletal dysplasia patients particularly research in dwarfism.
David L Rimoin MD PhD, Director
Xiao-Ning Chen, Research Scientist

3937 **New Jersey Institute of Technology Center for Biomedical Engineering**
University Heights 973-596-8449
Newark, NJ 07102-1982 Fax: 973-596-6056
e-mail: william.c.hunter@njit.edu
www.njit.edu
Offers research into facial and bone disorders.
William C Hunter, PhD BioMed Certification
Treena Arinzeh, Interim Chairman

3938 **WM Krogman Center for Research in Child Growth and Development**
4019 Irving Street 215-898-1470
Philadelphia, PA 19104-6003 e-mail: katz@kidshealth.org
www.upenn.edu/krogman/krogman.html
Focuses research and studies on growth disorders and birth defects.
Dr Solomon Katz, Director

Support Groups & Hotlines

3939 **National Health Information Center**
PO Box 1133 310-565-4167
Washington, DC 20013 800-336-4797
Fax: 301-984-4256
e-mail: info@nhic.org
www.health.gov/nhic
Offers a nationwide information referral service, produces directories and resource guides.

Books

3940 **Growing Children: A Parent's Guide**
Human Growth Foundation
997 Glen Cove Avenue 516-671-4041
Glen Head, NY 11545 800-451-6434
Fax: 516-671-4055
e-mail: hgf1@hgfound.org
www.hgfound.org
Offers parents information on the normal pattern of their child's growth, growth charts, recognition of growth problems, evaluation of growth problems and resources for more information.
Patricia D Costa, Executive Director

3941 **Short and OK**
Human Growth Foundation
997 Glen Cove Avenue 516-671-4041
Glen Head, NY 11545 800-451-6434
Fax: 516-671-4055
e-mail: hgf1@hgfound.org
www.hgfound.org
Guide for parents of short children offering information on behavior issues, medical issues and psychological warning signs.
54 pages
Patricia D Costa, Executive Director

Pamphlets

3942 **Achondroplasia**
Human Growth Foundation
997 Glen Cove Avenue 516-671-4041
Glen Head, NY 11545 800-451-6434
Fax: 516-671-4055
e-mail: hgf1@hgfound.org
www.hgfound.org
Signs, causes and prevention of achondroplasia.
Patricia D Costa, Executive Director

3943 **Growth Hormone Testing**
Human Growth Foundation
997 Glen Cove Avenue 516-671-4041
Glen Head, NY 11545 800-451-6434
Fax: 516-671-4055
e-mail: hgf1@hgfound.org
www.hgfound.org
What to expect during the testing period.
Patricia D Costa, Executive Director

3944 **Intrauterine Growth Retardation**
Human Growth Foundation
997 Glen Cove Avenue 516-671-4041
Glen Head, NY 11545 800-451-6434
Fax: 516-671-4055
e-mail: hgf1@hgfound.org
www.hgfound.org
Explains some of the reasons for an infant's failure to grow normally in intrauterine life.
Patricia D Costa, Executive Director

3945 **Most Frequently Asked Questions with Growth Hormone Deficiency**
Human Growth Foundation
997 Glen Cove Avenue 516-671-4041
Glen Head, NY 11545 800-451-6434
Fax: 516-671-4055
e-mail: hgf1@hgfound.org
www.hgfound.org
Provides a brief overview for parents about Growth Hormone Deficiency.
Patricia D Costa, Executive Director

3946 **Septo-Optic Dysplasia**
Human Growth Foundation
997 Glen Cove Avenue 516-671-4041
Glen Head, NY 11545 800-451-6434
Fax: 516-671-4055
e-mail: hgf1@hgfound.org
www.hgfound.org
Also known as DeMorsier Syndrome. Describes the disease and the different treatments that can lead to the significant improvement in the quality of life.
Patricia D Costa, Executive Director

Web Sites

3947 **Alliance of Genetic Support Groups**
A coalition of voluntary genetic support groups, consumers and professionals addressing the needs of individuals and families affected by genetic disorders from a national perspective.

3948 **Atomz**
www.pediatricservices.com
A search engine providing over 60 links to sites involving various growth disorders.

3949 **Healing Well**
www.healingwell.com
An online health resource guide to medical news, chat, information and articles, newsgroups and message boards, books, disease-related web sites, medical directories, and more for patients, friends, and family coping with disabling diseases, disorders, or chronic illnesses.

3950 **Health Finder**
www.healthfinder.gov
Searchable, carefully developed web site offering information on over 1000 topics. Developed by the US Department of Health and Human Services, the site can be used in both English and Spanish.

3951 **Healthlink USA**
www.healthlinkusa.com
Health information concerning treatment, cures, prevention, diagnosis, risk factors, research, support groups, email lists, personal stories and much more. Updated regularly.

3952 **Helios Health**
www.helioshealth.com
Online resource for your health information. Detailed information about specific health topics, access to expert advice from our Medical Advisory Board, and up-to-date health news.

3953 Human Growth Foundation

www.HGFound.org

Organization committed to expanding and accelerating research into growth hormone deficiency. Provides education and support to those affected by growth disorders and their families and fosters the exchange of information with the medical community.

3954 MedicineNet

www.medicinenet.com

An online resource for consumers providing easy-to-read, authoritative medical and health information.

3955 Medscape

www.mywebmd.com

Medscape offers specialists, primary care physicians, and other health professionals the Web's most robust and integrated medical information and educational tools.

3956 OHSU Homepage Search

www.ohsu.edu

A search which provides several links for information on growth disorders.

3957 WebMD

www.webmd.com

Information on growth disorders, including articles and resources.

Description

3958 **Head Injuries**

Head Injuries, or Traumatic Brain Injuries, cover a range of severity. Currently, there are 5.3 million Americans living with a disability because of a head or brain injury. Concussion, the most common injury, is the momentary loss of consciousness. It usually resolves without any major complications. Damage can result from penetration of the skull or from acceleration/deceleration of the brain that occurs in severe automobile accidents. Injuries can include brain bruising and bleeding into the brain, resulting in swelling that can be life threatening because the skull, as a rigid structure, cannot expand.

Postconcussion syndrome commonly follows a mild injury and can include temporary headaches, dizziness, mild mental slowing and sleepiness. A moderate head or brain injury results in loss of consciousness usually lasting from minutes to a few hours, followed by a few days or weeks of confusion. Loss of conciousness for greater than two minutes implies a worse outcome. Cognitive and psychological impairments lasting many months or even permanently are usual consequences of moderate injury. A severe injury almost always results in prolonged unconsciousness or coma lasting days to weeks or longer. People who sustain a severe head or brain injury often have brain contusions, hematomas (a collection of blood) and/or damage to the nerve fibers or axons. Many people who sustain a severe brain injury make significant improvements in the first year or two. After that improvement tends to slow down, but may continue for years. Some physical and/or cognitive impairments are permanent. See also *Brain Tumors*.

National Agencies & Associations

3959 **American Brain Tumor Association**
2720 River Road
Des Plaines, IL 60018-4117
847-827-9910
800-886-2282
Fax: 847-827-9918
e-mail: info@abta.org
www.abta.org
Services includes over 40 publications which address brain tumors their treatment and coping with the disease. Materials address brain tumors in all age groups. Provide free social service consultations and a mentorship program for new brain tumor support groups.
Elizabeth M Wilson, Executive Director
Geri Jo Duda RN, Patient Services

3960 **Brain Injury Association**
1608 Spring Hill Road
Vienna, VA 22182
703-761-0750
800-444-6443
Fax: 703-761-0755
e-mail: info@biausa.org
www.biausa.org
The BIA's mission is to create a better future through brain injury prevention research education and advocacy. Offers information on state and national offices treatment and rehabilitation conferences prevention financial development and more.
Susan H Connors, President/CEO
Mary S Reitter CAE, EVP/COO

3961 **Dynamic Rehab**
2637 Lazy Bend
Pearland, TX 77581
281-485-4144
Fax: 281-485-4196
e-mail: dynmaicrehab@sbcglobal.net
www.dynamicrehab.net
Primary focus is the production and distribution of motivational videotapes and workshops.
Greta Ludwig PT, Owner/Physical Therapist
Teresa Turner, Owner/Physical Therapist

3962 **FASST, Friends & Survivors Standing Together**
21100 W. Capitol Drive
Pewaukeeille, WI 53072
Fax: 262-790-9670
Nonprofit organization supporting brain injured people and their caregivers. Information, support groups and more.

3963 **Family Caregiver Alliance/National Center on Caregiving**
180 Montgomery Street
San Francisco, CA 94104
415-434-3388
800-445-8106
Fax: 415-434-3508
e-mail: info@caregiver.org
www.caregiver.org
Caregiver information and assistance via phone or e-mail; fact sheets and publications describing and documenting caregiver needs and services.
Kathleen Kelly, Executive Director
Jennifer Arthur, President

3964 **International Brain Injury Association**
PO Box 1804
Alexandria, VA 22313-8889
703-960-6500
Fax: 703-960-6603
e-mail: chaynes@hdipub.com
www.internationalbrain.org
Provides scientific and medical leadership worldwide in the field of brain injury.
Chas Haynes, Executive Director of Operations
Margaret Roberts, Executive Director/Administration

3965 **Rainbow House**
4149 W 26th Street
Chicago, IL 60623
773-521-1815
www.rainbow-house.org
Rainbow House is a Chicago-based nonprofit organization whose mission is to end domestic violence. Rainbow House has offered domestic violence prevention programs support and outreach services and resources to survivors across the City of Chicago.

3966 **TPN: The Perspective Network**
PO Box 121012
W Melbourne, FL 32912-1012
770-844-6898
Fax: 770-844-6898
e-mail: TPN@tbi.org
www.tbi.org
The Perspective Network provides forums and resources for persons with families, caregivers, friends and the professionals who serve them. Their goals are to promote a sense of community and to increase public awareness of brain injury.

State Agencies & Associations

Alabama

3967 **Alabama Head Injury Foundation**
3100 Lorna Road
Hoover, AL 5216-
205-823-3818
800-433-8002
Fax: 205-823-4544
e-mail: ahif1@bellsouth.net
www.ahif.org
Services provided to Alabamians with traumatic brain injury or spinal cord injury include information, housing, respite care, recreation programs, resource coordination.
Al Ellison, President
Charles D Priest, Executive Director

Alaska

3968 Brain Injury Association of America's National Family Helpline
1608 Spring Hill Road 703-761-0750
Vienna, VA 22182 800-444-6443
Fax: 703-761-0755
e-mail: FamilyHelpline@biausa.org
www.biausa.org
Marianna Abashian, Director of Professional Services
Gregory Ayotte, Director of Consumer Servicesÿÿ

Arizona

3969 Brain Injury Association of Arizona
777 E Missouri Avenue 602-508-8024
Phoenix, AZ 85014 888-500-9165
Fax: 602-508-8285
e-mail: info@biaaz.org
www.biaaz.org
Services provided by BIAAZ: camp for adults age 18+ with brain injuries; one-to-one phone and/or mail peer support program for individuals affected by brain injury and their families.
Mattie Cummins, Executive Director
Mary Bradley, Board President

Arkansas

3970 Brain Injury Association of Arkansas
PO Box 26236 501-374-3585
Little Rock, AR 72221-6236 800-444-6443
Fax: 501-918-6595
e-mail: info@brainassociation.org
www.brainassociation.org
Yousef A Fahoum, President
Dana Gonzales, Vice President

Colorado

3971 Brain Injury Association of Colorado
4200 W Conejos Place 303-355-9969
Denver, CO 80204 800-955-2443
Fax: 303-355-9968
e-mail: informationreferral@biacolorado.org
www.biacolorado.org
William Levis, President
Gavin Attwood, Executive Director

Connecticut

3972 Brain Injury Association of Connecticut
333 E River Drive 860-721-8111
E Hartford, CT 06108 800-278-8242
Fax: 860-721-9008
e-mail: general@biact.org
www.biact.org
500 Members
Paul A Slager, President
Julie Peters, Executive Director

Delaware

3973 Brain Injury Association of Delaware
840 Walker Road 302-346-2083
Dover, DE 19904 800-411-0505
Fax: 888-258-3694
e-mail: biadresourcecenter@cavtel.net
www.biausa.org/Delaware
Devon Dorman, President
Howard H Hitch, Vice President

Florida

3974 Brain Injury Association of Florida
1621 Metropolitan Boulevard 850-410-0103
Tallahassee, FL 32308 800-992-3442
Fax: 850-410-0105
e-mail: biaftalla@biaf.org
www.biaf.org
Frank Toral, President
Valerie Bree MSSA ACSW, Executive Director

3975 Choices for Work Program Goodwill Industries-Suncoast
Goodwill Industries-Suncoast
10596 Gandy Boulevard 727-523-1512
St Petersburg, FL 33702 888-279-1988
Fax: 727-563-9300
e-mail: gw.marketing@goodwill-suncoast.com
www.goodwill-suncoast.org
A nonprofit community based organization whose purpose is to improve the quality of life for people who are disabled, disadvantaged and/or aged. This mission is accomplished through a staff of over 1,200 employees providing independent living skills, affordable housing, career assessment and job skills training and opportunities.
R Lee Waits, President/Chief Executive Officer
Martin W Gladysz, Chair

3976 Goodwill Industries-Suncoast
Goodwill Industries-Suncoast
10596 Gandy Boulevard 727-523-1512
St. Petersburg, FL 33702 888-729-1988
Fax: 727-563-9300
e-mail: gw.marketing@goodwill-suncoast.org
www.goodwill-suncoast.org
A nonprofit community based organization whose purpose is to improve the quality of life for people who are disabled, disadvantaged and/or aged. This mission is accomplished through a staff of over 1,200 employees providing independent living skills, affordable housing, career assessment and planning, job skills, training, placement, and job retention assistance with useful employment. Annually, Goodwill Industries-Suncoast serves over 30,000 people in Citrus, Hernando, Levy, Marion and more.
R Lee Waits, President/CEO
Martin W Gladysz, Chair

3977 Pensacola Brain Injury TBI/ABI Support Group
TBI/ABI Support Group
2001 N E Street 850-457-2870
Pensacola, FL 32507 e-mail: hens8250@bellsouth.net
pensacolabrainnetwork.com/sys-tmpl/door
Survivors and caregivers oriented association. Publishes monthly magazine.
Peggy Henshall, Support Group Coordinator

Hawaii

3978 Brain Injury Association of Hawaii
420 Kuwili Street 808-791-6942
Honolulu, HI 96817-1474 Fax: 808-454-1975
e-mail: biahi@hawaiiantel.net
www.biausa.org/Hawaii
Ian Mattoch, President
Mary Wilson, Executive Director

Idaho

3979 Brain Injury Association of Idaho
PO Box 414 208-342-0999
Boise, ID 83701-0414 888-374-3447
Fax: 208-333-0026
e-mail: info@biaid.org
www.biaid.org
Michelle Featherston, President

Illinois

3980 **Brain Injury Association of Illinois**
PO Box 64420
Chicago, IL 60664-0420
312-726-5699
800-699-6443
Fax: 312-630-4011
e-mail: info@biail.org
www.biail.org

Philicia L Deckard, Executive Director
Irene Pedersen, Founder

Indiana

3981 **Brain Injury Association of Indiana**
9531 Valparaiso Court
Indianapolis, IN 46268
317-356-7722
866-854-4246
Fax: 317-808-7770
e-mail: info@biai.org
www.biausa.org/Indiana

Rebecca D Eberle, Chairperson of the Board
Laura C Trexler, TBI Grant Program Director

Iowa

3982 **Brain Injury Association of Iowa**
7025 Hickman Road
Urbandale, IA 50322
319-466-7455
800-444-6443
Fax: 800-381-0812
e-mail: info@biaia.org
www.biaia.org

Julie Dixon, President
Geoffrey Lauer, Executive Director

Kansas

3983 **Brain Injury Association of Kansas and Greater Kansas City**
6405 Metcalf Avenue
Overland Park, KS 66202
913-754-8883
800-444-6443
Fax: 816-842-1531
e-mail: info@biaks.org
www.biaks.org

Rob Flores, President
Betsy Johnson, Executive Director

Kentucky

3984 **Brain Injury Association of Kentucky**
7410 New Lagrange Roadd
Louisville, KY 40222
502-493-0609
800-592-1117
Fax: 502-426-2993
www.biak.us

Chell Austin, President
Melinda Mast, Executive Director

Maine

3985 **Brain Injury Association of Maine**
13 Washington Street
Waterville, ME 04901
207-861-9900
800-275-1233
Fax: 207-861-4617
e-mail: info@biame.org
www.biame.org

Mary Lombardo, President
Leslie DuVall, Director of Operations

Maryland

3986 **Brain Injury Association of Maryland**
2200 Kernan Drive
Baltimore, MD 21207
410-448-2924
800-221-6443
Fax: 410-448-3541
e-mail: info@biamd.org
www.biamd.org

Patricia Janus, President
Diane Tripplet, Executive Director

Massachusetts

3987 **Brain Injury Association of Massachusetts**
30 Lyman Street
Westborough, MA 01581
508-475-0032
800-242-0030
Fax: 508-475-0400
e-mail: biama@biama.org
www.biama.org

Shahriar Khaksari, President
Arlene Korab, Executive Director

Michigan

3988 **Brain Injury Association of Michigan**
7305 Grand River
Brighton, MI 48114-2334
810-229-5880
800-772-4323
Fax: 810-229-8947
e-mail: info@biami.org
www.biami.org

Our mission is to enhance the lives of those affected by brain injury through education, advocacy, research and local support groups and to reduce the incidence of brain injury through prevention.
Kevin Arnold, Chairperson
Michael F Dabbs, President

Minnesota

3989 **Brain Injury Association of Minnesota**
34 13th Avenue NE
Minneapolis, MN 55413
612-378-2742
800-669-6442
Fax: 612-378-2789
e-mail: info@braininjurymn.org
www.braininjurymn.org

20-24 pages
Paul Godlewski, ChairÿElect
David King, Executive Director

Mississippi

3990 **Brain Injury Association of Mississippi**
2727 Old Canton
Jackson, MS 39296-5912
601-981-1021
800-444-6443
Fax: 601-981-1039
e-mail: info@msbia.org
www.msbia.org

Howard T Katz, Chairman
Lee Jenkins, Executive Director

Missouri

3991 **Brain Injury Association of Missouri**
10270 Page Avenue
Saint Louis, MO 63132-1322
314-426-4024
800-377-6442
Fax: 314-426-3290
e-mail: info@biamo.org
www.biamo.org

Information and referral services and support groups through the state of Missouri.
Tom Martin, President of the Board
Scott Gee, Executive Director

Montana

3992 **Brain Injury Association of Montana**
1280 S 3rd W
Missoula, MT 59801
406-541-6442
800-241-6442
Fax: 406-541-4360
e-mail: biam@biamt.org
www.biamt.org

Luke Foust, President
Brenda Toner, Executive Director

New Hampshire

3993 Brain Injury Association of New Hampshire
109 N State Street
Concord, NH 03301
603-225-8400
800-773-8400
Fax: 603-228-6749
e-mail: mail@bianh.org
www.bianh.org

Brant Elkind, President
Steven Wade, Executive Director

New Jersey

3994 Brain Injury Association of New Jersey
825 Georges Road
N Brunswick, NJ 08902
732-745-0200
800-669-4323
Fax: 732-745-0211
e-mail: info@bianj.org
www.bianj.org

Glenn McCreesh, Committee Member
Barbara Geiger-Parke, Executive Director/President/CEO

New Mexico

3995 Brain Injury Association of New Mexico
121 Cardenas NE
Albuquerque, NM 87108
505-292-7414
888-292-7415
Fax: 505-271-8983
e-mail: braininjurnm@msn.com
www.braininjurynm.org

Dr. Mark Pedrotty, Board President
Clara Holguin, Executive Director

3996 Brain Injury Association of New Mexico Hel
121 Cardenas NE
Albuquerque, NM 87108
505-292-7414
Fax: 505-271-8983
e-mail: info@braininjurynm.org
www.braininjurynm.org

Kathleen Padilla, Board President
Rachel O'Connor, Executive Director

New York

3997 Brain Injury Association of New York State
10 Colvin Avenue
Albany, NY 12206-1242
518-459-7911
800-228-8201
Fax: 518-482-5285
e-mail: info@bianys.org
www.bianys.org

Marie Cavallo, President
Judith Avner, Executive Director

3998 RRTC on Community Integration of Persons with TBI
2323 S Shepherd
Houston, TX 77019
713-630-0526
800-732-8124
Fax: 713-630-0529
e-mail: terri.hudler-hull@memorialhermann.org
www.tbicommunity.org

Karen A Hart PhD, Director Of Training
Sunil Kothari, Medical Director

North Carolina

3999 Brain Injury Association of North Carolina
PO Box 748
Raleigh, NC 27601
919-833-9634
800-377-1464
Fax: 919-833-5415
e-mail: Sandra.farmer@bianc.net
www.bianc.net/

Marylin Lash, President
Sandra Farmer, Executive Director

4000 Brain Injury Association of North Dakota H
2113 Cameron Street
Raleigh, NC 27605
919-833-9634
Fax: 919-833-5415
e-mail: bianc@bianc.net
www.bianc.net/

Cindy Boyd, Board Chairman
Sandra Farmer, President

Ohio

4001 Brain Injury Association of Ohio
855 Grand View Avenue
Columbus, OH 43215-1123
614-481-7100
866-644-6242
Fax: 614-481-7103
e-mail: help@biaoh.org
www.biaoh.org

Jon Fishpaw, President
Suzanne Minnich, Executive Director

Oklahoma

4002 Brain Injury Association of Oklahoma
PO Box 88
Hillsdale, OK 73743-0088
580-233-4363
800-444-6443
Fax: 580-233-4546
e-mail: brainhelp@braininjuryoklahoma.orgÿ
www.braininjuryoklahoma.org

Tracy Grammer, President

Oregon

4003 Brain Injury Association of Oregon
2145 NW Overton Street
Portland, OR 97210
503-413-7707
800-544-5243
Fax: 503-413-6849
e-mail: biaor@biaoregon.org
www.biaoregon.org

Frank Bocci, President
Sherry Stock, Executive Director

Pennsylvania

4004 Brain Injury Association of Pennsylvania
950 Walnut Bottom Road
Carlisle, PA 17015
717-657-3601
866-635-7097
Fax: 717-776-4420
e-mail: info@biapa.org
www.biapa.org

Drew Nagele, Chairman of Board Development Committee
Stewart L Cohen, Chairman

Rhode Island

4005 Brain Injury Association of Rhode Island
935 Park Avenue
Cranston, RI 02910-2743
401-461-6599
Fax: 401-461-6561
e-mail: braininjuryctr@biaofri.org
www.biaofri.org

Paula O'Connor, President
Sharon Brinkworth, Executive Director

4006 Brain Injury Association of Rhode Island H
935 Park Avenue
Cranston, RI 02910
401-461-6599
Fax: 401-461-6561
e-mail: braininjuryctr@biaofri.org
www.biaofri.org

Paula O'Connor, President
Sharon Brinkworth, Executive Director

South Carolina

4007 Brain Injury Association of South Carolina
800 Dutch Square Boulevard
Columbia, SC 29210
803-731-9823
877-TBI-FACT
Fax: 803-731-4804
e-mail: scbraininjury@bellsouth.net
www.biausa.org/sc

Thomas Seastrunk, President
Joyce Davis, Director

Tennessee

4008 **Brain Injury Association of Tennessee**
15 Athens Way
Nashville, TN 37228
615-248-5878
877-757-2428
Fax: 615-248-5879
e-mail: biaoftn@yahoo.com
www.biaoftn.org

Guynn Edwards, President

4009 **Brain Injury Association of Tennessee Help**
151 Athens Way
Nashville, TN 37228
615-248-2541
Fax: 615-248-5879
e-mail: biaoftn@yahoo.com
www.biaoftn.org

Guynn Edwards, President
Pam Bryan, Executive Director

Texas

4010 **Brain Injury Association of Texas**
316 W 12th Street
Austin, TX 78701
512-326-1212
800-392-0040
Fax: 512-478-3370
e-mail: info@biatx.org
www.biatx.org

Jane Boutte, President

Utah

4011 **Brain Injury Association of Utah**
1800 S W Temple
Salt Lake City, UT 84115
801-484-2240
800-281-8442
Fax: 801-484-5932
e-mail: biau@sisna.com
www.biau.org

Teresa Such-Niebar, President
Ron S Roskos, Executive Director

Vermont

4012 **Brain Injury Association of Vermont**
92 S Main Street
Waterbury, VT 05676
802-244-6850
877-856-1772
Fax: 802-244-6850
e-mail: support1@biavt.org
www.biavt.org

Marsha Bancroft, President
Trevor Squirrell, Executive Director

Virginia

4013 **Brain Injury Association of Virginia**
1506 Willow Lawn Drive
Richmond, VA 23230
804-355-5748
800-334-8443
Fax: 804-355-6381
e-mail: info@biav.net
www.biav.net

Teresa Poole, President
Anne McDonnell, Executive Director

Washington

4014 **Brain Injury Association of Washington**
800 Jefferson Street
Seattle, WA 98104
206-388-0900
800-523-5438
Fax: 206-388-0901
e-mail: info@biawa.org
www.biawa.org

Richard Adler, President
Gene van den Bosch, Executive Director

4015 **Brain Injury Association of Washington Hel**
3516 S 47th Street
Tacoma, WA 98409
253-238-6085
Fax: 253-238-1042
e-mail: info@biawa.org
www.biawa.org

Richard Adler, President
Mary Spielma Chapman, Interim Executive Director

West Virginia

4016 **Brain Injury Association of West Virginia**
PO Box 574
Institute, WV 25112-0574
304-766-4892
800-356-6443
Fax: 304-766-4940
e-mail: mdavis@brainman.com
www.biausa.org/WVirginia

Michael W Davis, Board of Director
Linda Arthur, Board of Director

Wisconsin

4017 **Brain Injury Association of Wisconsin**
21100 W Capitol Drive
Pewaukee, WI 53072
262-790-9660
800-882-9282
Fax: 262-790-9670
e-mail: admin@execpc.com
www.biaw.org

Advocacy, education, prevention, information, resources, and support groups in regards to traumatic brain injury.
Kalli Reinheimer, President Wisconsin State Office
Mark Warhus, Executive Director

Wyoming

4018 **Brain Injury Association of Wyoming**
111 W 2nd Street
Casper, WY 82601
307-473-1767
800-643-6457
Fax: 307-237-5222
e-mail: biaw@tribcsp.com
www.biausa.org/Wyoming

Larry Plemmons, President
Dorothy Cronin, Director

Foundations

4019 **Brain Trauma Foundation**
708 Third Avenue
New York, NY 10017-4201
212-772-0608
Fax: 212-772-2035
e-mail: info@braintrauma.org
www.braintrauma.org

Our goal at the Brain Trauma Foundation is to improve the outcome of TBI patients through Guideline development, clinical research, professional education, and quality improvement programs.
Quarterly
Jamshid Ghajar, MD, President
Pamela Drexel, Executive Director

Research Centers

4020 **Brady Institute Jamaica Hospital Medical Center**
Jamaica Hospital Medical Center
8900 Van Wyck Expressway
Jamaica, NY 11418-2897
718-206-6000
Fax: 718-206-6559
www.jamaicahospital.org

The James and Sarah Brady Institute for Traumatic Brain Injury.
David P Rosen, President & CEO
Neil Foster Phillips, Chairman

4021 **Dana Alliance for Brain Initiatives**
745 Fifth Avenue
New York, NY 10151
212-223-4040
Fax: 212-317-8721
e-mail: danainfo@dana.org
www.dana.org

A non-profit organization of more than 250 neuroscientists which was formed to help provide information about the personal and public benefits of brain research.
William Safire, Chairman
Edward F Rover, President

4022 Institute for Rehabilitation and Research
1333 Moursund Avenue 713-704-4000
Houston, TX 77030-3405 800-447-3422
Fax: 713-874-1798
e-mail: tirr.referrals@memorialhermann.org
www.tirr.org
John Kajander, President

4023 New York University Medical Center Head Trauma Program
Rect 212-998-9819
New York, NY 10010-4020 Fax: 212-340-7158
Research pertaining to young adults suffering from head injuries.
Dr Yehuda Ben-Yishay, Coordinator

4024 Ohio State University Laboratory of Psychobiology
1885 Neil Avenue 614-292-8185
Columbus, OH 43210-1222 Fax: 614-292-4537
www.psy.ohio-state.edu/labs
Studies done on recovery of function after brain damage.
Laura Peterson, Lab Coordinator
James Walton, Research Associate

4025 Rehabilitation Institute of Michigan
261 Mack Avenue 313-745-1203
Detroit, MI 48201 Fax: 313-745-2376
www.rimrehab.org
Physical medicine and rehabilitation medicine.
William H Restum PhD, President
Horacio Varg Jr, Interim Executive Director

4026 Thomas Jefferson University Ischemia-Shock Research Center
1020 Locust Street 215-503-1272
Philadelphia, PA 19107-6731 Fax: 215-955-2073
Promotes research into head injuries and clinical studies.

4027 Thomas Jefferson University Ischemia-Shock
1020 Locust Street 215-503-1272
Philadelphia, PA 19107 Fax: 215-923-7932
www.jefferson.edu/main
Promotes research into head injuries and clinical studies.

4028 Tulane University: US-Japan Biomedical Research Laboratories
3705 Main Street 504-394-7199
Belle Chasse, LA 70037 Fax: 504-394-7169
e-mail: arimura@tulane.edu
www.som.tulane.edu/labs/usjamed
Focuses research efforts on neuroendocrinology and neurosciences.
L Lee Hamm MD, Professor and Greenberg Chair in Medicin
Patrice Dela MD, Vice Chair

4029 UCLA Neuropsychiatric Institute
760 Westwood Plaza 310-825-0511
Los Angeles, CA 90024 Fax: 310-825-9179
www.semel.ucla.edu
Devote to teach research and patient care in psychiatry neuroscience and related fields.
Peter C Whybrow MD, Professor and Executive Chair
James E Spar, Professor Director Psychiatry Residenc

4030 University of California: Irvine Brain Imaging Center
101 The City Drive S 949-824-5011
Irvine, CA 92697-3960 Fax: 949-824-7873
e-mail: BIC@msx.hsis.uci.edu
www.bic.uci.edu
Offers PET scan analysis of brain functions focusing on brain damage brain tumors and head injuries.
Steven G Potkin MD, Director

4031 University of California: San Francisco Laboratory for Neurotrauma
1001 Potrero Avenue 415-206-8313
San Francisco, CA 94110-3518
Research done into traumatic brain and head injuries.
Lawrence H Pitts MD

4032 University of Tennessee: Memphis State University of Neuropsychology Lab
Memphis State University
Psychology Department 901-678-4213
Memphis, TN 38152-0001 Fax: 901-678-2579
e-mail: g.mittleman@mail.psyc.memphis.edu
www.psyc.memphis.edu/capr/capr.shtml
Evaluation and development of assessment and treatment procedures for neurologically impaired persons.
Guy Mittleman, Professor Director of CAPR

4033 Virginia Commonwealth University: Rehab Research and Training Center
1314 W Main Street 804-828-1851
Richmond, VA 23284-2011 Fax: 804-828-2193
TTY: 804-828-2494
www.worksupport.com
Focuses research on traumatic brain and head injuries.
Paul Wehman, Director
Jeanne Dalton, Public Relations Assistant Specialist

Michigan

4034 Wayne State University: Gurdjian-Lissner Biomechanics Laboratory
Department of Neurological Surgery
4160 John R Street 313-831-0777
Detroit, MI 48201 Fax: 313-966-0368
e-mail: jont@med.wayne.edu
www.med.wayne.edu/neurosurgery
Head and neck injury research.
Murali Guthi MD FA CS, Professor (Clinician-Educator) and Chair
Kenneth Case MD, Associate Professor

Support Groups & Hotlines

4035 National Health Information Center
PO Box 1133 310-565-4167
Washington, DC 20013 800-336-4797
Fax: 301-984-4256
e-mail: info@nhic.org
www.health.gov/nhic
Offers a nationwide information referral service, produces directories and resource guides.

Alabama

4036 Alabama Head Injury Foundation Helpline
3100 Lorna Road 205-823-3818
Hoover, AL 35216-5451 800-433-8002
Fax: 205-823-4544
e-mail: ahif1@bellsouth.net
www.ahif.org/
The Alabama Head Injury Foundation (AHIF) was founded by professionals and families in 1983 to increase public awareness of Traumatic Brain Injury (TBI) and to stimulate the development of supportive services. AHIF provides accessible resources, services and programs that meet the unique needs of individuals with traumatic brain injury (TBI) as well as spinal cord injury (SCI) in certain programs.
Charles D Priest, Executive Director
Sandra Koplon, Director Community Outreach

Arizona

4037 Brain Injury Association of Arizona
777 E Missouri 602-508-8024
Phoenix, AZ 85014 888-500-9165
Fax: 602-508-8285
e-mail: info@biaaz.org
www.biaaz.org
Information and resources for brain injury survivors and their families. Support group listings available.
Mattie Cummins, Executive Director
Mary Bradley, Board President

Arkansas

4038 **Brain Injury Association of Arkansas Helpl ine**
PO Box 26236
North Little Rock, AR 72221-6236
501-374-3585
800-235-2443
Fax: 501-918-6595
e-mail: info@brainassociation.org
www.brainassociation.org
Founded in 1980, the Brain Injury Association of America (BIAA) is a national organization serving and representing individuals, families and professionals who are touched by a life-altering, often devastating, traumatic brain injury (TBI). BIAA provides information, education and support through its network of chartered state affiliates, local chapters and support groups across the country to assist the 5.3 million Americans currently living with traumatic brain injury and their families.
Dianne Gutierrez, President Arkansas State Office
Dana Gonzales Ph.D, Vice President

California

4039 **Brain Injury Association of California Hel pline**
2658 Mt Vernon Avenue
Bakersfield, CA 93306
661-872-4903
Fax: 661-873-2508
e-mail: calbiainfo@yahoo.com
www.calbia.org/
Founded in 1980, the Brain Injury Association of America (BIAA) is a national organization serving and representing individuals, families and professionals who are touched by a life-altering, often devastating, traumatic brain injury (TBI). BIAA provides information, education and support through its network of chartered state affiliates, local chapters and support groups across the country to assist the 5.3 million Americans currently living with traumatic brain injury and their families.
Paula Daoutis, Executive Director
Richard Adams MD, Board of Directors

4040 **Jodi House**
1235 C Veronica Springs Road
Santa Barbara, CA 93105
805-563-2882
Fax: 805-563-3982
e-mail: info@jodihouse.org
www.jodihouse.org
Jodi House is a community-based, post-rehabilitation day program that provides opportunities for social interaction, life skill training, recreation, and support for adults living with acquired brain injury (i.e. from head trauma, tumor, and stroke) and their families.
Jim Kearns, President
Luciana Cramer, Executive Director

Colorado

4041 **Brain Injury Association of Colorado Helpline**
6825 E Tennessee Avenue
Denver, CO 80224
303-355-9969
800-955-2443
Fax: 303-355-9968
e-mail: biacolo@aol.com
www.BIAColorado.org
Judy Dettmer, President
Helen O Kellogg, Exececutive Director

Connecticut

4042 **Brain Injury Association of Connecticut Helpline**
1800 Silas Deane Highway
Rocky Hill, CT 6067-1304
860-721-8111
800-278-8242
Fax: 860-721-9008
e-mail: general@biact.org
www.biact.org
Supports persons with brain injuries and their families by promoting services to facilitate full inclusion within their local community and to increase awareness and understanding of brain injury and its prevention through community education.
500 Members
David Bush, Chairman
Julia Peterson, Executive Director

4043 **TBI Support Group**
Gaylord Hospital
PO Box 400
Wallingford, CT 06492
203-284-2800
Christine Wilson

Delaware

4044 **Brain Injury Association of Delaware Helpl ine**
32 West Loockerman Street
Dover, DE 19904
302-346-2083
800-411-0505
Fax: 302-678-3183
e-mail: biadresourcecenter@cavdel.net
www.biausa.org/Delaware/bia.htm
Founded in 1980, the Brain Injury Association of America (BIAA) is a national organization serving and representing individuals, families and professionals who are touched by a life-altering, often devastating, traumatic brain injury (TBI). BIAA provides information, education and support through its network of chartered state affiliates, local chapters and support groups across the country to assist the 5.3 million Americans currently living with traumatic brain injury and their families.
John Goodier, President Delaware State Office
Howard H Hitch, Vice President

Florida

4045 **Brain Injury Association of Florida Helpline**
201 East Sample Road
Pompano Beach, FL 33064
954-786-2400
800-992-3442
Fax: 954-786-2437
e-mail: info@biaf.org
www.biaf.org
Doug Dennis, President
Elynor Kazuk, Executive Director

Hawaii

4046 **Brain Injury Association of Hawaii**
420 Kuwili Street
Honolulu, HI 96817
808-791-6942
e-mail: biahi@hawaiiantel.net
www.biausa.org/Hawaii
Dedicated to serving those affected by brain injury throughgh advocacy, prevention, and support
Mary Wilson, Executive Director

Illinois

4047 **American Brain Tumor Association Patient Line**
2720 S River Road
Des Plaines, IL 60018-4117
847-827-9910
800-886-2282
Fax: 847-827-9918
e-mail: info@abta.org
www.abta.org
Offers emergency support, information and referrals for patients and their families.
Naomi Berkowitz, Director

4048 **Brain Injury Association of Illinois Helpline**
Chicago, IL 60664-420
312-726-5699
800-699-6443
Fax: 312-630-4011
e-mail: info@biail.org
www.biail.org
Works with all people with brain inquiries and their families with professionals who serve them. Provides camp oppurtunities, support groups, educational seminars, information and referrals and a quarterly newsletter.
Irene Pedersen, Founder
Philicia Deckard, Executive Director

Indiana

4049 **Brain Injury Association of Indiana Helpli ne**
9531 Valparaiso Court
Indianapolis, IN 46268
317-356-7722
800-407-4246
Fax: 317-808-7770
e-mail: info@biai.org
www.biausa.org/Indiana
Founded in 1980, the Brain Injury Association of America (BIAA) is a national organization serving and representing individuals,

families and professionals who are touched by a life-altering, often devastating, traumatic brain injury (TBI). BIAA provides information, education and support through its network of chartered state affiliates, local chapters and support groups across the country to assist the 5.3 million Americans currently living with traumatic brain injury and their families.
Stacey Payne, Executive Director Indiana State Office
Laura C Trexler, TBI Grant Program Director

Iowa

4050 **Brain Injury Association of Iowa Helpline**
Brain Injury Association of America
2101 Kimball Avenue LL7 319-272-2312
Waterloo, IA 50702 800-475-4442
Fax: 319-272-2109
e-mail: diaia@cedarnet.org
www.biaia.org

Julie Dixon, President
Ed Boll, Program Manager

Kentucky

4051 **Brain Injury Association of Kentucky Helpl ine**
7410 New LaGrange Road 502-493-0609
Louisville, KY 40222 800-592-1117
Fax: 502-426-2993
e-mail: Melinda.Mast@biak.us
www.biak.us
Founded in 1980, the Brain Injury Association of America (BIAA) is a national organization serving and representing individuals, families and professionals who are touched by a life-altering, often devastating, traumatic brain injury (TBI). BIAA provides information, education and support through its network of chartered state affiliates, local chapters and support groups across the country to assist the 5.3 million Americans currently living with traumatic brain injury and their families.
Debbie Nelson, President Kentucky State Office
Melinda Mast, Executive Director

Louisiana

4052 **Brain Injury Association of Louisiana Help line**
c/o National Headquarters Office
8201 Greensboro Drive 703-761-0750
McLean, VA 22102 800-444-6443
Fax: 703-761-0755
e-mail: familyhelpline@biausa.org
www.biausa.org/
Founded in 1980, the Brain Injury Association of America (BIAA) is a national organization serving and representing individuals, families and professionals who are touched by a life-altering, often devastating, traumatic brain injury (TBI). BIAA provides information, education and support through its network of chartered state affiliates, local chapters and support groups across the country to assist the 5.3 million Americans currently living with traumatic brain injury and their families.
Susan H Connors, President/Chief Executive Officer (VA)
Mary S Reitter CAE, EVP/Chief Operations Officer (VA)

Maine

4053 **Brain Injury Association of Maine Helpline**
325 Main Street 207-681-9900
Waterville, ME 04901 800-275-1233
Fax: 207-861-4617
e-mail: info@biame.org
www.biame.org
Founded in 1980, the Brain Injury Association of America (BIAA) is a national organization serving and representing individuals, families and professionals who are touched by a life-altering, often devastating, traumatic brain injury (TBI). BIAA provides information, education and support through its network of chartered state affiliates, local chapters and support groups across the country to assist the 5.3 million Americans currently living with traumatic brain injury and their families.
Bev Bryant, President Maine State Office
John Bott, Executive Director

Maryland

4054 **Brain Injury Association of Maryland Helpl ine**
Kernan Hospital
2200 Kernan Drive 410-448-2924
Baltimore, MD 21207 800-221-6443
Fax: 410-448-3541
e-mail: info@biamd.org
www.biamd.org
Founded in 1980, the Brain Injury Association of America (BIAA) is a national organization serving and representing individuals, families and professionals who are touched by a life-altering, often devastating, traumatic brain injury (TBI). BIAA provides information, education and support through its network of chartered state affiliates, local chapters and support groups across the country to assist the 5.3 million Americans currently living with traumatic brain injury and their families.
Patricia Janus, President Maryland State Office
Dianne Tripp, Executive Director

Massachusetts

4055 **Brain Injury Association of Massachusetts Helpline**
30 Lyman Street 508-475-0032
Westborough, MA 01581 800-242-0030
Fax: 508-475-0400
e-mail: biama@biama.org
www.biama.org
Founded in 1980, the Brain Injury Association of America (BIAA) is a national organization serving and representing individuals, families and professionals who are touched by a life-altering, often devastating, traumatic brain injury (TBI). BIAA provides information, education and support through its network of chartered state affiliates, local chapters and support groups across the country to assist the 5.3 million Americans currently living with traumatic brain injury and their families.
Gregory L Zagloba, President Massachusetts State Office
Arlene Korab, Executive Director

4056 **VALT Support Group (Vital Active Life After Trauma)**
53 Linden Street 617-277-6327
Brookline, MA 02149

Michigan

4057 **Brain Injury Association of Michigan Helpline**
8619 W Grand River 810-229-5880
Brighton, MI 48116-2334 800-772-4323
Fax: 810-229-8947
e-mail: info@biami.org
www.biami.org

Jim Peterson, Chair
Michael F Dabbs, President

Minnesota

4058 **Brain Injury Association of Minnesota Helpline**
34 13th Avenue North East 612-378-2742
Minneapolis, MN 55413 800-669-6442
Fax: 612-378-2789
e-mail: biam@protocom.com
www.braininjurymn.org

Tom Gode, Executive Director

Mississippi

4059 **Brain Injury Association of Mississippi Helpline**
PO Box 55912 601-981-1021
Jackson, MS 39296-5912 800-641-6642
Fax: 601-981-1039
e-mail: biaofms@aol.com
www.members.aol.com/biaofms

Howard Katz PhD, Chair

Missouri

4060 **Brain Injury Association of Kansas and Greater Kansas City Helpline**
1100 Pennsylvania Avenue 816-842-8607
Kansas City, MO 64105 800-783-1356
Fax: 816-842-1531
www.braininjuryresource.org
Mark Thompson, President
Leigh Liggett, Executive Director

4061 **Brain Injury Association of Missouri Helpline**
10270 Page Avenue 314-426-4024
St Louis, MO 63132-1322 800-377-6442
Fax: 314-426-3290
e-mail: braininJry@aol.com
www.biausa.org/bia
Information and referral services and support groups throughout the state of Missouri.
Terrie Price, Board President
Scott Gee, Executive Director

Montana

4062 **Brain Injury Association of Montana Helpline**
52 Corbin Hall 406-243-5973
Missoula, MT 59812 800-241-6442
Fax: 406-243-2349
e-mail: biam@selway.umt.edu
Dr. MV Morton, President
Rose Davis, Office Manager

Nevada

4063 **Brain Injury Association of Nevada Helplin e**
c/o National Office Headquarters
8201 Greensboro Drive 703-761-0750
McLean, VA 22102 Fax: 702-591-0755
e-mail: FamilyHelpline@biausa.org
www.biausa.org/contactinfo.htm
Founded in 1980, the Brain Injury Association of America (BIAA) is a national organization serving and representing individuals, families and professionals who are touched by a life-altering, often devastating, traumatic brain injury (TBI). BIAA provides information, education and support through its network of chartered state affiliates, local chapters and support groups across the country to assist the 5.3 million Americans currently living with traumatic brain injury and their families.
Susan H Connors, President/Chief Executive Officer
Mary S Reitter CAE, EVP/Chief Operations Officer

New Hampshire

4064 **Brain Injury Association of New Hampshire**
Brain Injury Association of America
109 N State Street 603-225-8400
Concord, NH 3301-4447 800-773-8400
Fax: 603-228-6749
e-mail: mail@bianh.org
www.bianh.org
Newton Kersaw, President
Steven Wade, Executive Director

New Jersey

4065 **Brain Injury Association of New Jersey Helpline**
Brain Injury Association of America
1090 King George Post Road 732-738-1002
Edison, NJ 8837 800-669-4323
Fax: 732-738-1132
e-mail: info@bianj.org
www.bianj.org
Albert Pressler, President
Barbara Geigerparker, Executive Director

New Mexico

4066 **Brain Injury Association of New Mexico Hel pline**
121 Cardenas NE 505-292-7414
Albuquerque, NM 87108 888-292-7415
Fax: 505-271-8983
e-mail: braininjurynm@msn.com
www.braininjurynm.org
Founded in 1980, the Brain Injury Association of America (BIAA) is a national organization serving and representing individuals, families and professionals who are touched by a life-altering, often devastating, traumatic brain injury (TBI). BIAA provides information, education and support through its network of chartered state affiliates, local chapters and support groups across the country to assist the 5.3 million Americans currently living with traumatic brain injury and their families.
Mark Pedrotty Ph.D, Board President New Mexico State Office
Clara Holguin, Executive Director

New York

4067 **Brain Injury Association of New York State Helpline**
10 Colvin Avenue 518-459-7911
Albany, NY 12206-1242 800-228-8201
Fax: 518-482-5285
e-mail: info@bianys.org
www.bianys.org
Michael Kaplen, President
Judy Avner, Executive Director

4068 **Cafe Plus**
216 W Manlius Street
East Syracuse, NY 13057 315-446-3124
www.dreamscape.com/cafeplus
For people who have survived a head-injury or some type of head trauma.
David Listowski, Manager

4069 **Hy Feinstein Clubhouse**
Long Island Head Injury Association
65 Austin Boulevard 631-543-2245
Commack, NY 11725 Fax: 631-543-2261
www.lihia.org
The LIHIA provides a place for people with head injury to participate in meaningful work, to have the opportunity to meet and build friendships and ultimately seek employment within the community.

North Carolina

4070 **Brain Injury Association of North Carolina Helpline**
PO Box 748 919-833-9634
Raleigh, NC 27602 800-377-1464
Fax: 919-833-5415
e-mail: biaofnc@aol.com
www.bianc.net/
Bob Gauldin, President
Cecil Greene Jr, Executive Director

North Dakota

4071 **Brain Injury Association of North Dakota H elpline**
209 2nd Street SE 701-845-1124
Valley City, ND 58072 Fax: 701-845-1175
e-mail: FamilyHelpline@biausa.org
www.biausa.org/contactinfo.htm
Founded in 1980, the Brain Injury Association of America (BIAA) is a national organization serving and representing individuals, families and professionals who are touched by a life-altering, often devastating, traumatic brain injury (TBI). BIAA provides information, education and support through its network of chartered state affiliates, local chapters and support groups across the country to assist the 5.3 million Americans currently living with traumatic brain injury and their families.
Mary Simonson, President
Ken Moliter, Vice President

Ohio

4072 **Brain Injury Association of Ohio**
1335 Dublin Road
Columbus, OH 43215-1000
614-481-7100
866-644-6242
Fax: 614-481-7103
e-mail: help@biaoh.org
www.biaoh.org
Suzanne Minnich, Executive Director

Oklahoma

4073 **Brain Injury Association of Oklahoma Helpl ine**
PO Box 88
Hillsdale, OK 73743-0088
580-233-4363
800-765-6809
Fax: 580-233-4546
e-mail: information@braininjuryoklahoma.org
www.braininjuryoklahoma.org
Founded in 1980, the Brain Injury Association of America (BIAA) is a national organization serving and representing individuals, families and professionals who are touched by a life-altering, often devastating, traumatic brain injury (TBI). BIAA provides information, education and support through its network of chartered state affiliates, local chapters and support groups across the country to assist the 5.3 million Americans currently living with traumatic brain injury and their families.
Tracy Grammer, President Oklahoma State Office
Mary S Reitter CAE, COO/National Headquarters (703-761-0750)

Oregon

4074 **Brain Injury Association of Oregon Helpline**
Brain Injury Association of America
2145 NW Overton Street
Portland, OR 97210
503-413-7707
800-544-5243
Fax: 503-413-6849
e-mail: biaor@biaoregon.org
www.biaoregon.org
Non-profit providing information and referral, support groups, prevention, education, training, and advocacy for those with brain injury, families, and professionals.
Sherry Stock, Executive Director

Rhode Island

4075 **Brain Injury Association of Rhode Island H elpline**
935 Park Avenue
Cranston, RI 02910-2743
401-461-6599
Fax: 401-461-6561
e-mail: braininjuryctr@biaofri.org
biaofri.org
Founded in 1980, the Brain Injury Association of America (BIAA) is a national organization serving and representing individuals, families and professionals who are touched by a life-altering, often devastating, traumatic brain injury (TBI). BIAA provides information, education and support through its network of chartered state affiliates, local chapters and support groups across the country to assist the 5.3 million Americans currently living with traumatic brain injury and their families.
Paula O'Connor, President Rhode Island State Office
Sharon Brinkworth, Executive Director

Tennessee

4076 **Brain Injury Association of Tennessee Help line**
151 Athens Way
Nashville, TN 37228
615-248-5878
877-757-2428
Fax: 615-248-5879
e-mail: biaoftn@yahoo.com
www.biaoftn.org
Founded in 1980, the Brain Injury Association of America (BIAA) is a national organization serving and representing individuals, families and professionals who are touched by a life-altering, often devastating, traumatic brain injury (TBI). BIAA provides information, education and support through its network of chartered state affiliates, local chapters and support groups across the country to assist the 5.3 million Americans currently living with traumatic brain injury and their families.
Guynn Edwards, President Tennessee State Office
Stephanie Pruitt, Executive Director

Utah

4077 **Brain Injury Association of Utah Helpline**
Brain Injury Association of America
1800 SW Temple Suite 203
Salt Lake City, UT 84115
801-484-2240
800-281-8442
Fax: 801-484-5932
e-mail: biau@sisna.com
www.starpage.com/braininjury/
Barbara Hayward, President
Ron Roskos, Executive Director

Vermont

4078 **Brain Injury Association of Vermont Helpli ne**
PO Box 226
Shelburne, VT 05482
802-985-8440
877-856-1772
Fax: 802-985-8440
e-mail: biavtinfo@adelphia.net
www.biavt.org
Founded in 1980, the Brain Injury Association of America (BIAA) is a national organization serving and representing individuals, families and professionals who are touched by a life-altering, often devastating, traumatic brain injury (TBI). BIAA provides information, education and support through its network of chartered state affiliates, local chapters and support groups across the country to assist the 5.3 million Americans currently living with traumatic brain injury and their families.
Bob Luce, President Vermont State Office
Trevor Squirrell, Executive Director

Virginia

4079 **Brain Injury Association of Virginia Helpline**
3212 Cutshaw Avenue
Richmond, VA 23230-5018
804-355-5748
800-334-8443
Fax: 804-355-6381
e-mail: info@biav.net
www.biav.net
Nonprofit organization providing information and resources related to brain injury to individuals with brain injuries, their families and professionals who deal with brain injury.
Harry Weinstock, Executive Director

4080 **Brain Injury Association of Virginia Helpl ine**
3212 Cutshaw Avenue
Richmond, VA 23230
804-355-5748
800-334-8443
Fax: 804-355-6381
e-mail: info@biav.net
www.biav.net
Founded in 1980, the Brain Injury Association of America (BIAA) is a national organization serving and representing individuals, families and professionals who are touched by a life-altering, often devastating, traumatic brain injury (TBI). BIAA provides information, education and support through its network of chartered state affiliates, local chapters and support groups across the country to assist the 5.3 million Americans currently living with traumatic brain injury and their families.
Irv Cantor, President Virginia State Office
Anne McDonnell, Executive Director

Washington

4081 **Brain Injury Association of Washington Hel pline**
800 Jefferson Street
Seattle, WA 98104
206-388-0900
800-523-5438
Fax: 206-388-0901
e-mail: info@biawa.org
www.biawa.org
Founded in 1980, the Brain Injury Association of America (BIAA) is a national organization serving and representing individuals, families and professionals who are touched by a life-altering, often devastating, traumatic brain injury (TBI). BIAA provides information, education and support through its network of chartered state affiliates, local chapters and support groups across the country to assist the 5.3 million Americans currently living with traumatic brain injury and their families.
Richard Adler, President Washington State Office
Gene Van Den Bosch, Executive Director

4082 Head Injury Hotline
Brain Injury Resource Center
PO Box 84151 206-621-8558
Seattle, WA 98124-5451 Fax: 206-329-4355
e-mail: brain@headinjury.com
www.headinjury.com
Disseminates head injury information and provides referrals to facilitate adjustment to life following head injury. Organizes seminars for professionals, head injury survivors, and their families.
Constance Miller MA, Founder/President
B Parker Lindner MPA, Communications Specialist

West Virginia

4083 Brain Injury Association of West Virginia Helpline
Brain Injury Association of America
PO Box 574 304-766-4892
Institute, WV 25112-574 800-356-6443
Fax: 304-766-4940
e-mail: biawv@aol.com
Michael W Davis, President

Wisconsin

4084 Brain Injury Association of Wisconsin Help line
21100 W Capitol Drive 262-790-9660
Pewaukee, WI 53072 800-882-9282
Fax: 262-790-9670
e-mail: admin@execpc.com
www.biaw.org
Founded in 1980, the Brain Injury Association of America (BIAA) is a national organization serving and representing individuals, families and professionals who are touched by a life-altering, often devastating, traumatic brain injury (TBI). BIAA provides information, education and support through its network of chartered state affiliates, local chapters and support groups across the country to assist the 5.3 million Americans currently living with traumatic brain injury and their families.
Kalli Reinheimer, President Wisconsin State Office
Mark Warhus, Executive Director

Wyoming

4085 Brain Injury Association of Wyoming
111 West 2nd Street 307-473-1767
Casper, WY 82601 800-643-6457
Fax: 307-237-5222
www.biausa.org.wy
Dorothy Cronin, Director

Books

4086 An Educational Challenge: Meeting the Needs of Students with Brain Injury
Brain Injury Association
105 N Alfred Street 703-236-6000
Alexandria, VA 22314 800-444-6443
Fax: 703-236-6001

4087 Brain Injury Glossary
HDI Publishers
10600 NW Freeway, Suite 202
Houston, TX 77219 800-321-7037
Fax: 713-956-2288
Contains glossary and descriptions of health care providers.

4088 Brainlash
Demos Medical Publishing
386 Park Avenue S 212-683-0072
New York, NY 10016 Fax: 212-683-0118
e-mail: orderdept@demospub.com
www.demosmedpub.com
Maximize your recovery from mild brain injury.
376 pages
ISBN: 1-888799-37-4
Dr. Diana M Schneider

4089 Coming Home: A Discharge Manual for Families of Persons with a Brain Injury
HDI Publishers
10600 NW Freeway, Suite 202
Houston, TX 77219 800-321-7037
Fax: 713-956-2288

4090 Communication Disorders Following Traumatic Brain Injury
Pro-Ed, Inc.
8700 Shoal Creek Boulevard 512-451-3246
Austin, TX 78757-6897 800-897-3202
Fax: 800-397-7633
e-mail: info@proedinc.com
www.proedinc.com
For graduates and professionals, this text takes a holistic approach toward treating the client with traumatic brain injury.
439 pages Paperback
ISBN: 0-890792-95-X
Lindy Jordaan, Marketing Coordinator

4091 Dano Cerebral: Guia Para Familias y Cuidadores
Brain Injury Association/HDI Publishers/Catalogue
PO Box 131401
Houston, TX 77219 800-321-7037
Fax: 713-526-7787
This book, written in Spanish, is a thorough, well-researched guide for people with brain injury, their families and caregivers. Up-to-date information covers such topics as Intensive Care- admittance and discharge; Mechanics of brain injury; Coma; Consequences of brain injury; Mental and Emotional symptoms among many others.
158 pages 1994

4092 From the Ashes
Phoenix Project
PO Box 84151 206-329-1371
Seattle, WA 98124-5451
A self-help book that addresses the trauma that comes with a head injury and introduces methods of building a fulfilling and productive life.
108 pages

4093 Handbook of Head Truma: Acute Care to Recovery
Plenum Publishing Corporation
233 Spring Street 212-620-8000
New York, NY 10013-1522 800-221-9369
Fax: 212-463-0742
e-mail: books@plenum.com
466 pages
ISBN: 0-306439-47-6

4094 Head Injury and the Family: A Life and Living Perspective
St. Lucie Press
100 E Linton Boulevard 407-274-9906
Delary Beach, FL 33483 Fax: 407-274-9927
One of the best books written in this area. Easy to read, written with family, caregivers and patients in mind. Includes exercises and vignettes.

4095 Integrating Community Resources
HDI Publishers
10600 NW Freeway, Suite 202
Houston, TX 77219 800-321-7037
Fax: 713-956-2288

4096 Living with Brain Injury: A Guide for Families
Brain Injury Association/HDI Publishers/Catalogue
PO Box 131401
Houston, TX 77219 800-321-7037
Fax: 713-526-7787
This book will help readers- families, persons with brain injury and professionals alike- through this uncharted territory. topics include: How brain injury is caused and how it can be treated: Physical, cognitive and behavioral symptoms; Questions family members commonly ask.
145 pages 1998

4097 National Directory of Brain Injury Rehabilitatiom
Brain Injury Association

105 N Alfred Street 703-236-6000
Alexandria, VA 22314 800-444-6443
Fax: 703-236-6001
Desk reference for professionals listing brain injury rehabilitation programs and individual service providers nationwide.

4098 **National Directory of Head Injury Rehabilitation Services**
Brain Injury Association
105 N Alfred Street 703-236-6000
Alexandria, VA 22314 800-444-6443
Fax: 703-236-6001

4099 **Planning for the Future**
Brain Injury Association
105 N Alfred Street 703-236-6000
Alexandria, VA 22314 800-444-6443
Fax: 703-236-6001
This book provides a meaningful life for a child with a disability after your death.

4100 **Recovery from Brain Damage in the Elderly**
Aspen Publishers
PO Box 990
Frederick, MD 21705-0990 800-638-8437
Recovery and rehabilitation techniques in the area of brain damage in the elderly.

4101 **Sexuality and the Person with Traumatic Brain Injury**
Brain Injury Association
105 N Alfred Street 703-236-6000
Alexandria, VA 22314 800-444-6443
Fax: 703-236-6001

4102 **Stress Management Following Head Injury: Strategies for Families and Caregivers**
Brain Injury Association
105 N Alfred Street 703-236-6000
Alexandria, VA 22314 800-444-6443
Fax: 703-236-6001

4103 **TBI Tool Kit**
HDI Publishers
10600 NW Freeway, Suite 202
Houston, TX 77219 800-321-7037
Fax: 713-956-2288

4104 **Traumatic Brain Injury Rehabilitation: Brain Injury Consortium Monograph Series**
St. Lucie Press
100 E Linton Boulevard 407-274-9906
Delray Beach, FL 33483 Fax: 407-274-9927
Assistive technology, under the Americans with Disabilities Act, is that designed for and used by individuals with the intent of eliminating, ameliorating, or compensating for functional limitations. Coverage includes impaired functions that limit vocational outcome, behavior concerns in the workplace, maximizing a client's residual knowledge skills, use of computers and adapting work environments.

4105 **Traumatic Head Injury: Cause, Consequence and Challenge**
Brain Injury Association/HDI Publishers/Catalogue
PO Box 131401
Houston, TX 77219 800-321-7037
Fax: 713-526-7787
A resource book on traumatic brain injury which translates technical medical information on brain injury into simple, easy-to-understand language for persons with brain injury and their families. Covered topics: a general overview of brain injury; similarities and differences among people with brain injury; types and consequences of brain injury; recovery and rehabilitation; accepting and coping with change.
60 pages 1993

4106 **Why Did it Happen on a School Day: My Family's Experience with Brain Injury**
Brain Injury Association
105 N Alfred Street 703-236-6000
Alexandria, VA 22314 800-444-6443
Fax: 703-236-6001

4107 **Working After Brain Injury**
HDI Publishers
10600 NW Freeway, Suite 202
Houston, TX 77219 800-321-7037
Fax: 713-956-2288

Magazines

4108 **Journal of Head Trauma Rehabilitation**
Aspen Publishers
1600 Research Boulevard 301-251-8500
Rockville, MD 20850-3129 800-638-8437
www.aspenpub.com
Scholarly journal designed to provide information on clinical management and rehabilitation of the head-injured for the practicing professional.

4109 **Mouth Magazine**
PO Box 558 785-272-2578
Topeka, KS 66601-0558 Fax: 785-272-7348
www.mouthmag.org
Bi-monthly magazine with subscription.

Newsletters

4110 **Brain Injury Source**
Brain Injury Association
105 N Alfred Street 703-236-6000
Alexandria, VA 22314 Fax: 703-236-6001
e-mail: BIAV@visi.net
www.biausa.org
Written for and by professionals in the field. Blends professionally written articles on information and research in brain injury with a user friendly format that incorporates graphics and charts to effectively deliver the messages. Full color.
50+ pages Quarterly

4111 **TBI Challenge!**
Brain Injury Association of America
105 N Alfred Street 703-236-6000
Alexandria, VA 22314-3010 Fax: 703-236-6001
www.biausa.org
Exclusively for and about persons with brain injury. Provides information to individuals with brain injury and their families. Professionals will benefit from the perspectives provided in Kid's Corner, Relatively Speaking, Ask the Lawyer, Information and Resources and Ask the Doctor.
bimonthly

Arizona

4112 **Brainstorm**
Brain Injury Association of Arizona
777 E Missouri 602-323-9165
Phoenix, AZ 85014 888-500-9165
Fax: 602-508-8285
e-mail: info@biaaz.org
www.biaaz.org
A newsletter serving persons with brain injury, their families and professionals.
8 pages Quarterly
Mary Bradley, Board President
Mattie Cummins, Executive Director

Pamphlets

4113 **A Survey of Accredited and Other Rehabilitation Facilities**
Brain Injury Association
105 N Alfred Street 703-236-6000
Alexandria, VA 22314 800-444-6443
Fax: 703-236-6001
Education, training and cognitive rehabilitation in barin injury programs.

4114 **About Head Injuries**
Channing L Bete Company

200 State Road
South Deerfield, MA 01373 800-628-7733
Covers basic information including identifying the members of the treatment team and how to take care of yourself as a caregiver.

4115 Adolescents with Closed Head Injuries: A Report of Initial Cognitive Deficits
Brain Injury Association
105 N Alfred Street 703-236-6000
Alexandria, VA 22314 800-444-6443
Fax: 703-236-6001

4116 Basic Questions About Head Injury & Disability
Brain Injury Association
105 N Alfred Street 703-236-6000
Alexandria, VA 22314 800-444-6443
Fax: 703-236-6001

4117 Behavioral and Psychosocial Sequelae of Pediatric Head Injury
Brain Injury Association
105 N Alfred Street 703-236-6000
Alexandria, VA 22314 800-444-6443
Fax: 703-236-6001

4118 Brain Damage is a Family Affair
Brain Injury Association
105 N Alfred Street 703-236-6000
Alexandria, VA 22314 800-444-6443
Fax: 703-236-6001

4119 Brain Injuries: A Guide for Families & Caretakers
Brain Injury Association
105 N Alfred Street 703-236-6000
Alexandria, VA 22314 800-444-6443
Fax: 703-236-6001

4120 Brain Injury: A Home Based Cognitive Rehabilitation Program
HDI Publishers
10600 NW Freeway, Suite 202
Houston, TX 77219 800-321-7037
Fax: 713-956-2288

4121 Catastrophic Injury Cases: The Relationship of Traumatic Brain Injury
Brain Injury Association
105 N Alfred Street 703-236-6000
Alexandria, VA 22314 800-444-6443
Fax: 703-236-6001

4122 Children with Disabilities: Understanding Sibling Issues
Brain Injury Association
105 N Alfred Street 703-236-6000
Alexandria, VA 22314 800-444-6443
Fax: 703-236-6001

4123 Counseling Head Injured Patients: Guidelines for Community Health Workers
Brain Injury Association
105 N Alfred Street 703-236-6000
Alexandria, VA 22314 800-444-6443
Fax: 703-236-6001

4124 Education Concerns for the Traumatically Head Injured Student
Brain Injury Association
105 N Alfred Street 703-236-6000
Alexandria, VA 22314 800-444-6443
Fax: 703-236-6001

4125 From One Family Member to Another
Brain Injury Association
105 N Alfred Street 703-236-6000
Alexandria, VA 22314 800-444-6443
Fax: 703-236-6001
A mother tells the story of her son's injury and recovery. Gives suggestions for structuring the home environment.

4126 Guide to Selecting and Monitoring Head Injury Rehabilitation Services
Brain Injury Association
105 N Alfred Street 703-236-6000
Alexandria, VA 22314 800-444-6443
Fax: 703-236-6001

4127 Head Injury Survivor on Campus: Issues & Resources
Brain Injury Association
105 N Alfred Street 703-236-6000
Alexandria, VA 22314 800-444-6443
Fax: 703-236-6001

4128 Head Injury: A Booklet for Families
Brain Injury Association
105 N Alfred Street 703-236-6000
Alexandria, VA 22314 800-444-6443
Fax: 703-236-6001

4129 Head Injury: A Guide for Families
HDI Publishers
10600 NW Freeway, Suite 202
Houston, TX 77219 800-321-7037
Fax: 713-956-2288
Structured by problem with examples and practical coping strategies.

4130 Hearing Loss Following Head Injury
Brain Injury Association
105 N Alfred Street 703-236-6000
Alexandria, VA 22314 800-444-6443
Fax: 703-236-6001

4131 Hiring Persons with a Brain Injury: What to Expect
HDI Publishers
10600 NW Freeway, Suite 202
Houston, TX 77219 800-321-7037
Fax: 713-956-2288

4132 Individual Psychotherapy with the Brain Injured Adult
Brain Injury Association
105 N Alfred Street 703-236-6000
Alexandria, VA 22314 800-444-6443
Fax: 703-236-6001
Review of literature on substance abuse and head injury. Includes statistics, and treatment options, strategies and extensive bibliography.

4133 Information General Sobre: Lesion Cerebral
Brain Injury Association
105 N Alfred Street 703-236-6000
Alexandria, VA 22314 800-444-6443
Fax: 703-236-6001

4134 Introductory Information for Families
Brain Injury Association
105 N Alfred Street 703-236-6000
Alexandria, VA 22314 800-444-6443
Fax: 703-236-6001
A collection of readings on basic information about TBI and a guide for selecting rehabilitation facilities.

4135 Know Your Brain
Nat'l Institute of Neurological Disorders & Stroke
PO Box 5801
Bethesda, MD 20824 800-352-9424
Fax: 301-402-2186
www.ninds.nih.gov
Basic information about the brain, neuroscience research, and disorders of the brain.

4136 Legal and Financial Issues for Families
Brain Injury Association
105 N Alfred Street 703-236-6000
Alexandria, VA 22314 800-444-6443
Fax: 703-236-6001
Packet designed for families that explores some of the legal and financial issues faced after TBI.

4137 Life After Brain Injury: Who am I
HDI Publishers
10600 NW Freeway, Suite 202
Houston, TX 77219 800-321-7037
Fax: 713-956-2288
A well-structured book. Dicusses specific problems areas. Includes good examples and gives lists of practical coping strategies.

4138 Mild Brain Injury: Damage and Outcome
Brain Injury Association

105 N Alfred Street 703-236-6000
Alexandria, VA 22314 800-444-6443
Fax: 703-236-6001

4139 Neuropsychology of Attention and Memory
Brain Injury Association
105 N Alfred Street 703-236-6000
Alexandria, VA 22314 800-444-6443
Fax: 703-236-6001

4140 Persisting Problems After Mild Head Injury: A Review of the Syndrome
Brain Injury Association
105 N Alfred Street 703-236-6000
Alexandria, VA 22314 800-444-6443
Fax: 703-236-6001

4141 Post-Traumatic Headaches: Subtypes & Behavioral Treatments
Brain Injury Association
105 N Alfred Street 703-236-6000
Alexandria, VA 22314 800-444-6443
Fax: 703-236-6001

4142 Recovery and Cognitive Retraining After Craniocerebral Trauma
Brain Injury Association
105 N Alfred Street 703-236-6000
Alexandria, VA 22314 800-444-6443
Fax: 703-236-6001

4143 Relationships Between Personality Disorders
Brain Injury Association
105 N Alfred Street 703-236-6000
Alexandria, VA 22314 800-444-6443
Fax: 703-236-6001
Social Disturbances and physical disability following TBI.

4144 Resources List of Organizations
Brain Injury Association
105 N Alfred Street 703-236-6000
Alexandria, VA 22314 800-444-6443
Fax: 703-236-6001

4145 Severe Brain Injury
Brain Injury Association
105 N Alfred Street 703-236-6000
Alexandria, VA 22314 800-444-6443
Fax: 703-236-6001
This pamphlet is in hand out format and would be appropriate for use in clinic or hospital setting.

4146 Spouses of Persons Who Are Brain Injured: Overlooked Victims
Brain Injury Association
105 N Alfred Street 703-236-6000
Alexandria, VA 22314 800-444-6443
Fax: 703-236-6001

4147 Stress Management Following Head Injury: Strategies for Families & Caregivers
Brain Injury Association
105 N Alfred Street 703-236-6000
Alexandria, VA 22314 800-444-6443
Fax: 703-236-6001

4148 Subarachnoid Hemorrhage & Aneurysm
University Hospital & Clinics
One Hosptial Drive 314-882-4141
Columbia, MO 65212
This pamphlet includes easy to read, general information plus a glossary and schematic diagrams. This pamphlet would be most appropriate for use with recently head injured patients.

4149 Substance Abuse Task Force White Paper
Brain Injury Association
105 N Alfred Street 703-236-6000
Alexandria, VA 22314 800-444-6443
Fax: 703-236-6001
Review of literature on substance abuse and head injury. Includes statistics, and treatment options, strategies and extensive bibliography.

4150 Susan's Dad: A Child's Story of Head Injury
Brain Injury Association
105 N Alfred Street 703-236-6000
Alexandria, VA 22314 800-444-6443
Fax: 703-236-6001

4151 Teaching Persons with A Brain Injury: What to Expect
HDI Publishers
10600 NW Freeway, Suite 202
Houston, TX 77219 800-321-7037
Fax: 713-956-2288

4152 Unseen Injury: Minor Head Injury
Brain Injury Association
105 N Alfred Street 703-236-6000
Alexandria, VA 22314 800-444-6443
Fax: 703-236-6001

4153 What is Anoxic Brain Injury
Brain Injury Association
105 N Alfred Street 703-236-6000
Alexandria, VA 22314 800-444-6443
Fax: 703-236-6001

4154 When Your Child Goes to School After an Injury
Brain Injury Association
105 N Alfred Street 703-236-6000
Alexandria, VA 22314 800-444-6443
Fax: 703-236-6001

4155 When Your Child is Seriously Injured: The Emotional Impact on Families
Brain Injury Association
105 N Alfred Street 703-236-6000
Alexandria, VA 22314 800-444-6443
Fax: 703-236-6001

4156 Working After A Head Injury
HDI Publishers
10600 NW Freeway, Suite 202
Houston, TX 77219 800-321-7037
Fax: 713-956-2288

Audio & Video

4157 A Fate Better than Death
Brain Injury Association
105 N Alfred Street 703-236-6000
Alexandria, VA 22314 800-444-6443
Fax: 703-236-6001
Video features 4 young adults with traumatic brain injury. Focuses on support groups.

4158 Neuropsychological Assessment: What it Does & Does Not Do
Brain Injury Association
105 N Alfred Street 703-236-6000
Alexandria, VA 22314 800-444-6443
Fax: 703-236-6001
This pamphlet is in hand out format and would be appropriate for use in clinic or hospital setting.

4159 Peter Wegner Is Alive and Well and Living in Providence
Filmakers Library
124 E 40th Street 212-808-4980
New York, NY 10016-1798 Fax: 212-808-4983
e-mail: info@filmakers.com
www.filmakers.com
Peter Wegner was a professor at Brown University when he received an award in London and was hit by a bus there. The film follows the challenges and decisions faced by his family, in dealing with the serious brain injuries sustained. Comatose, brain surgery, how can a person decide the right path for their loved one? Winner of American Psychology Award. DVD or VHS $195, Classroom Rental $55
VHS or DVD
Sue Oscar, Co-President

4160 Unseen Injury: Minor Head Injury
Brain Injury Association
105 N Alfred Street 703-236-6000
Alexandria, VA 22314 800-444-6443
Fax: 703-236-6001

Designed specifically for viewing by family members.

4161 Surviving Coma: The Journey Back
Brain Injury Association
105 N Alfred Street
Alexandria, VA 22314
703-236-6000
800-444-6443
Fax: 703-236-6001

21 minutes

Web Sites

4162 Agency for Healthcare: Research Facility
www.ahcpr.gov
Mission is to improve quality, safety, efficiency, and effectiveness of healthcare for all Americans.

4163 American Brain Tumor Association
www.abta.org
Provides a mentorship program for new brain tumor support group leaders; a nationwide database of established support groups; the Connections pen-pal program; networking with organizations that provide services to patients and families; a resource listing of physicians offering investgative treatments.

4164 Brain Injury Association
www.biausa.org
Seeking to improve the quality of life for people with brain injuries and their families through information and resource referral, legislative advocacy, prevention awareness, and professional education. BIA's mission is to create a better future through brain injury prevention, research, education and advocacy.

4165 Brain Research Institute: Medicine School University of California, Los Angeles
medicine.ucsd.edu
BRI is an organized research unit.

4166 Headinjury.Com
www.headinjury.com
Maintained by the Head Injury Hotline, a non-profit clearinghouse founded and operated by head injury activist. The primary goal are to empower through education, resources and support. The basic premise is that the medical system is deeply flawed and that the brain injury rehab industry is no exception. The site integrates resources from diverse organizations including support groups, rehabilitation and research sites.

4167 Healing Well
www.healingwell.com
An online health resource guide to medical news, chat, information and articles, newsgroups and message boards, books, disease-related web sites, medical directories, and more for patients, friends, and family coping with disabling diseases, disorders, or chronic illnesses.

4168 Health Finder
www.healthfinder.gov
Searchable, carefully developed web site offering information on over 1000 topics. Developed by the US Department of Health and Human Services, the site can be used in both English and Spanish.

4169 Healthlink USA
www.healthlinkusa.com
Health information concerning treatment, cures, prevention, diagnosis, risk factors, research, support groups, email lists, personal stories and much more. Updated regularly.

4170 Helios Health
www.helioshealth.com
Online resource for your health information. Detailed information about specific health topics, access to expert advice from our Medical Advisory Board, and up-to-date health news.

4171 MedicineNet
www.medicinenet.com
An online resource for consumers providing easy-to-read, authoritative medical and health information.

4172 Medscape
www.mywebmd.com
Medscape offers specialists, primary care physicians, and other health professionals the Web's most robust and integrated medical information and educational tools.

4173 Neurology Channel
www.neurologychannel.com
Find clearly explained, medically accurate information regarding conditions, including an overview, symptoms, causes, diagnostic procedures and treatment options. On this site it is possible to ask questions and get information from a neurologist and connect to people who have similar health interests.

4174 Road Less Traveled
www.lesstravel.org
Dedicated to survivors and families of victims of Traumatic Brain Injury.

4175 TBI Help
www.tbihelp.com
Information concerning head injury.

4176 Traumatic Brain Injury
community-2.webtv.net
This site is dedicated to survivors and all who wish to learn more about traumatic brain injury.

Description

4177 **Hearing Impairment**

Approximately 21 million Americans have some degree of hearing impairment or Deafness. This commom problem affects people of all ages, and the loss can range from mild to severe.

Hearing loss is divided into four categories: conductive, sensorineural, mixed and central. Conductive hearing loss is caused by a defect in the external ear canal or middle ear, and can be helped by hearing aids, medical treatment or surgery. Sensorineural hearing loss results from damage to the inner ear and to the primary nerve that transmits sound waves to the brain. Mixed hearing loss is a combination of conductive and sensorineural defects. Central hearing loss results from impairment of brain function.

Hearing loss may be present at birth or begin later in life. Causes include infections (such as meningitis), injury, prolonged noise exposure, hereditary diseases and side effects of certain drugs. Amplification of sound with hearing aids helps almost all persons with mild-to-severe conductive or sensorineural hearing loss. Profoundly deaf persons who cannot be helped by hearing aids may benefit from a cochlear implant, a specialized device inserted into the inner ear. Children with hearing impairments may have slow or innaccurate speech development, or problems with concentration. Early diagnosis usually helps children improve their auditory ability, through the use of hearing aids, educational programs and speech therapy. Hearing loss in adults, if moderate or severe, is usually obvious to the patient family members. In young children, however, the problem is easily overlooked and the opportunity for early intervention can be lost.

National Agencies & Associations

4178 **ABLEDATA**
8630 Fenton Street
Silver Spring, MD 20910
301-608-8998
800-227-0216
Fax: 301-608-8958
TTY: 301-608-8912
e-mail: abledata@macrointernational.com
www.abledata.com

An information and referral service that uses computer listings and a large file system to answer requests related to assistive devices. Houses a large file system library and contacts with other sources which enables them to answer just about any question.
Katherine Belknap, Project Director
Steve Lowe, Associate Project Manager/Webmaster

4179 **ADARA**
PO Box 480
Myersville, MD 21773
501-224-6678
Fax: 501-868-8812
TTY: 501-868-8850
e-mail: adaraorg@comcast.net
www.adara.org

Professional networking for excellence in service delivery with individuals who are deaf or hard of hearing. A partnership of national organizations, local affiliates, professional sections and individual members working together to support social services.
David Tout, President
Doug H Dittfurth, Vice President

4180 **Academy of Dispensing Audiologists**
1020 Monarch Street
Lexington, KY 40513
866-493-5544
Fax: 859-977-7441
e-mail: cstone@audiologist.org
www.audiologist.org

Encourages audiology training programs to include pertinent aspects of hearing aid dispensing in their curriculum.
Charles Ston AuD, President
Tabitha Pare Buck AuD, President-Elect

4181 **Academy of Rehabilitative Audiology**
PO Box 952
DeSoto, TX 75123
e-mail: ara@audrehab.org
www.audrehab.org

Provides professional education research and interest in programs for hearing handicapped persons.
Jill E Preminger, President

4182 **Alexander Graham Bell Association for the Deaf and Hard of Hearing**
3417 Volta Place NW
Washington, DC 20007
202-337-5220
Fax: 202-337-8314
TTY: 202-337-5221
e-mail: info@agbell.org
www.agbell.org

The world's oldest and largest membership organization promoting the use of spoken language by children and adults who are hearing impaired. Members include parents of children with hearing loss, adults who are deaf or hard of hearing and educators.
Alexander T Graham, Executive Director/CEO
John R Wyant, President

4183 **American Academy of Audiology**
11730 Plaza America Drive
Reston, VA 20190
703-790-8466
800-222-2336
Fax: 703-790-8631
e-mail: nfo@audiology.org
www.audiology.org

A professional organization of individuals dedicated to providing high quality hearing care to the public. Provides professional development education and research and provides increased public awareness of hearing disorders and audiologic services.
Cheryl Kreid Carey CAE, Executive Director
Edward A M Sullivan, Deputy Executive Director

4184 **American Academy of Otolaryngology: Head**
1650 Diagonal Road
Alexandria, VA 22314-3357
703-836-4444
TTY: 703-519-1585
e-mail: executiveservices@entnet.org
www.entnet.org

The missions of the AAO-HNS and its foundation are to advance the art and science of otalaryngology-head and neck surgery through state-of-the-art education, research and learning; and to unite, serve and represent the interests of its members and their families.
Megan Schagrin, Director of Corporate Relations

4185 **American Association of the Deaf-Blind**
8630 Fenton Street
Silver Spring, MD 20910-4500
301-495-4403
Fax: 301-495-4404
TTY: 301-495-4402
e-mail: AADB-Info@aadb.org
www.aadb.org

Promotes better opportunities and services for deaf-blind people. The mission of this organization is to assure that a comprehensive, coordinated system of services is accessible to all deaf-blind people, enabling them to achieve their maximum potential.
600 Members
Arthur Roehrig, President
Jamie McNama Pope, Executive Director

4186 **American Auditory Society**
352 Sundial Ridge Circle
Dammeron Valley, UT 84783
435-574-0062
Fax: 435-574-0063
e-mail: amaudsoc@aol.com
www.amauditorysoc.org

Publishes Ear & Hearing and The Bulletin of the American Auditory Society.
Michael Gorg PhD, President

4187 **American Hearing Research Foundation**
8 S Michigan Avenue 312-726-9670
Chicago, IL 60603-4539 Fax: 312-726-9695
e-mail: sparmet@american-hearing.org
www.american-hearing.org
Supports medical research and education into the causes prevention and cures of deafness, hearing losses and balance disorders. Also keeps physicians and the public informed of the latest developments in hearing research and education.
William L Lederer, Executive Director
Sharon Parmet, Associate Director

4188 **American Society for Deaf Children**
3820 Hartzdale Drive 717-703-0073
Camp Hill, PA 17011 800-942-2732
Fax: 717-909-5599
TTY: 717-334-8808
e-mail: asdc@deafchildren.org
www.deafchildren.org
A nonprofit parent-helping-parent organization promoting a positive attitude toward signing and deaf culture. Also provides support encouragement and current information about deafness to families with deaf and hard of hearing children.
Beth S Benedict PhD, President
Joseph Finnegan, VP

4189 **American Speech-Language-Hearing Association**
2200 Research Boulevard 301-296-5700
Rockville, MD 20850 800-498-2071
Fax: 301-296-5650
TTY: 301-296-8580
e-mail: actioncenter@asha.org
www.asha.org
A professional and scientific organization for speech-language pathologists and audiologists concerned with communication disorders. Provides informational materials and a toll-free HELPLINE number for consumers to inquire about speech, language or hearing disorders.
Arlene A Pietranton PhD CAE, Executive Director
Sue T Hale, President

4190 **American Tinnitus Association**
522 SW Fifth Avenue 503-248-9985
Portland, OR 97204-0005 800-634-8978
Fax: 503-248-0024
e-mail: tinnitus@ata.org
www.ata.org
Provides information about tinnitus and referrals to local contacts/support groups nationwide. Also provides a bibliography service, funds scientific research related to tinnitus and offers workshops to professionals. Works to promote public education.
Gary Reul EdD, Chief Executive Officer
Terri Baltus, Chief Development Officer

4191 **Association of Late-Deafened Adults**
8038 MacIntosh Lane 815-332-1515
Rockford, IL 61107 866-402-2532
Fax: 877-907-1738
TTY: 815-332-1515
e-mail: info@alda.org
www.alda.org
Serves as a resource and information center for late-deafened adults and works to increase public awareness of the special needs of late-deafened adults.
Kathy Schleuter, President
Linda Dratell, President-Elect

4192 **Auditory-Verbal International**
1390 Chain Bridge Road 703-739-1049
McLean, VA 22101 Fax: 703-739-0395
TTY: 703-739-0874
e-mail: audiverb@aol.com
www.auditory-verbal.org
Dedicated to helping children who have hearing losses learn to listen and speak. Promotes the Auditory-Verbal Therapy approach which is based on the belief that the overwhelming majority of these children can hear and talk by using their residual hearing ability.
Chellie Lisenby, Executive Director
Steven R Rech, President

4193 **Better Hearing Institute**
1444 I Street NW 202-449-1100
Washington, DC 20005 800-327-9355
Fax: 202-216-9646
TTY: 703-642-0580
e-mail: mail@betterhearing.org
www.betterhearing.org
A nonprofit educational organization that implements national public information programs on hearing loss and available medical, surgical, hearing aid and rehabilitation assistance for millions with uncorrected hearing problems.
Sergei Kochk PhD, Executive Director
Renee La Mura, Administrative Director

4194 **CAPCOM**
6707 Old Dominion Drive 202-363-0535
McLean, VA 22101 800-241-2232
TTY: 703-749-1876
Conducts research on the special needs of the hearing impaired including senior citizens. Presents workshops on law and the deaf and on promoting productive working relationships for the hearing impaired employees of agencies and corporations.

4195 **Canine Assistance for the Disabled CADI**
CADI
3958 Union Road 314-892-2554
Saint Louis, MO 63125 e-mail: supportdogs@MSN.com
The mission of Support Dogs Inc. is to give people with disabilities greater independence and improve lives through the help of a support or touch dog and promote canines as partners through abilities education.

4196 **Center on Employment: Rochester Institute of Technology**
National Technical Institute for the Deaf
52 Lomb Memorial Drive 505-475-6219
Rochester, NY 14623-5604 Fax: 585-475-7570
TTY: 505-475-6219
e-mail: ntidcoe@rit.edu
www.rit.edu/ntid/coops/jobs
Operated by the National Technical Institute for the Deaf at Rochester Institute of Technology, the NTIC Center on employment was established to promote successful employment of RIT's deaf students and graduates.
John Macko, Director
Lorie Fidurko, Office Assistant

4197 **Cochlear Implant Association**
5335 Wisconsin Avenue NW 202-895-2781
Washington, DC 20015-2052 Fax: 202-895-2782
e-mail: CIAIinfo@cici.org
www.cici.org
Provides information and support to implant users and their families, professionals and the general public.
John McCelland, President
Lorie Singer, VP

4198 **Convention of American Instructors of the Deaf**
PO Box 377 817-354-8414
Bedford, TX 76095-0377 TTY: 817-354-8414
e-mail: caid@swbell.net
www.caid.org
An organization that promotes professional development communication and information among educators of deaf individuals and other interested people.
Helen Lovato, Office Manager

4199 **Council on Education of the Deaf College of Education**
College of Education
800 Florida Avenue NE 330-672-0735
Washington, DC 20002-0001 Fax: 330-672-2498
TTY: 330-672-2396
e-mail: ced@gallaudet.edu
www.deafed.net/PageText.asp?hdnPageId=58
Offers information and referral services to the hearing impaired.
Dr Karen Dilka, Executive Director
Dr Carmel Collum Yarger, President

4200 **Deaf Artists of America**
302 Goodman Street N
Rochester, NY 14607-1148
Fax: 315-244-3690
TTY: 315-224-3460
Organized to bring support and recognition to deaf and hard of hearing artists. The goals are to publish information about deaf artists, provide cultural and educational opportunities, exhibit and market deaf artists' work and collect and disseminate information.
Tom Willard, Executive Director

4201 **Deaf REACH**
3521 12th Street NE
Washington, DC 20017
202-832-6681
Fax: 202-832-8454
TTY: 202-832-6681
www.deaf-reach.org
Offers group homes for mentally ill adults, day programs for the developmentally disabled deaf, referrals case management and housing placement. Serves adults with disabilities, specifically deaf and/or low-income.
Rudy Gawlik, President
Peter Goodman, VP

4202 **Deafness Research Foundation**
641 Lexington Avenue
New York, NY 10022
212-328-9480
866-454-3924
Fax: 212-328-9484
TTY: 888-435-6104
e-mail: info@drf.org
www.drf.org
The nation's largest voluntary health organization entirely committed to public awareness and support for basic and clinical research into deafness and hearing disabilities. Sponsors a broad program of innovative research and education.
Andrea Kardo Boidman, COO
Liz Saldana, Chief Development Officer

4203 **Deafness and Communicative Disorders Branch**
Department of Education
330 C Street SW
Washington, DC 20202-2736
202-205-8730
Fax: 202-205-8737
TTY: 202-205-8352
e-mail: annette.reichman@ed.gov
www.ed.gov/offices/OSERS/RSA.html
Promotes improved and expanded rehabilitation services for deaf and hard of hearing people and individuals with speech or language impairments.
Annette Reichman, Branch Chief

4204 **Dogs for the Deaf**
10175 Wheeler Road
Central Point, OR 97502
541-826-9220
Fax: 541-826-6696
TTY: 541-826-9220
TDD: 541-826-9220
e-mail: info@dogsforthedeaf.org
www.dogsforthedeaf.org
Trains ear dogs to alert deaf persons to certain sounds. Dogs are chosen from pet adoption shelters and assigned on the basis of a prioritized waiting list. Four to five months of training teaches them to alert their masters to a number of sounds.
Robin Dickson, President/CEO

4205 **EAR Foundation**
1817 Patterson Street
Nashville, TN 37203
615-627-2724
800-545-4327
Fax: 615-627-2728
TTY: 615-627-2724
TDD: 615-627-2724
e-mail: info@earfoundation.org
www.earfoundation.org
A national non-profit organization committed to the goal of better hearing and balance through public and professional education programs including The Meniere's Network and the Young Ears program. The Meniere's Network is a national network of patient outreach.
Amy Nielsen, Associate Director

4206 **Hands Organization: Advocacy Network for the Deaf and Hearing Impaired**
Advocacy Network For The Deaf And Hearing Impaired
PO Box 17755
Chicago, IL 60617-0755
773-978-8552
TTY: 773-978-8552
Advocacy for the deaf and hearing impaired; information and referrals educational events sign language summer youth camps and newsletters.

4207 **Hear Now: Starkey Hearin Foundation**
The Starkey Hearing Foundation
6700 Washington Avenue S
Eden Prairie, MN 55344
Fax: 952-828-6946
e-mail: shf_contact@starkey.com
www.sotheworldmayhear.org
Committed to making technology accessible to deaf and hard of hearing individuals throughout the United States. Also raises funds to provide hearing aids, cochlear implants and related services to children and adults who have hearing losses.
Brian Theiss, President
Debbie Wright, Executive Director

4208 **Hearing Education and Awareness for Rocker s**
1405 Lyon Street
San Francisco, CA 94115
415-409-3277
Fax: 415-552-4296
TTY: 415-476-7600
e-mail: hear@hearnet.com
www.hearnet.com
Educates the public about the real dangers of hearing loss resulting from repeated exposure to excessive noise levels.
Kathy Peck, Executive Director

4209 **Helen Keller National Center for Deaf/Blind Youth and Adults**
141 Middle Neck Road
Sands Point, NY 11050-1299
516-944-8900
Fax: 516-944-7302
TTY: 516-944-8637
e-mail: hkncinfo@hknc.org
www.hknc.org
The national center and its 10 regional offices providing diagnostic evaluations comprehensive vocational and personal adjustment training and job preparation and placement for people who are deaf/blind from every state and territory.

4210 **House Ear Institute**
2100 W 3rd Street
Los Angeles, CA 90057
213-483-4431
800-388-8612
Fax: 213-483-8789
TTY: 213-484-2642
TDD: 213-484-2642
e-mail: info@hei.org
www.hei.org
A national non-profit otologic research and educational institute that provides information on hearing and balance disorders.
John W House MD, President
James D Boswell, CEO

4211 **International Hearing Dog**
5901 E 89th Avenue
Henderson, CO 80640
303-287-3277
Fax: 303-287-3425
TTY: 303-287-3277
e-mail: ihdi@aol.com
www.ihdi.org
Trains dogs to hear for deaf persons - telephones, doorbells, babies etc.
Martha Foss, President

4212 **International Hearing Society**
16880 Middlebelt Road
Livonia, MI 48154
734-522-7200
800-521-5247
Fax: 734-522-0200
e-mail: amarkey@ihsinfo.org
www.ihsinfo.org
A nonprofit professional association which represents Hearing Instrument Specialists in the United States, Canada and several other countries. The society is recognized for promoting and maintaining the highest possible standards for its members.
Cindy Helms, Executive Director
Lee Martin, Marketing Communications & Membership

4213 John Tracy Clinic
806 W Adams Boulevard
Los Angeles, CA 90007-2505
213-748-5481
800-522-4582
Fax: 213-749-1651
TTY: 213-747-2924
www.johntracyclinic.org

An educational facility for preschool age children who have hearing losses and their families. In addition to on-site services worldwide correspondence courses in English and Spanish are offered to parents whose children are of preschool age and are hard of hearing.

Kevin Matthews, VP Finance and Administration
Mary Ann Bell, VP Development and Communications

4214 National Association of the Deaf
8630 Fenton Street
Silver Spring, MD 20910-4500
301-587-1788
Fax: 301-587-1791
TTY: 301-587-1789
e-mail: NADinfo@nad.org
www.nad.org

The nation's largest constituency organization safeguarding the accessibility and civil rights of 28 million deaf and hard of hearing Americans in education, employment, health care and telecommunications. A private, nonprofit organization.

Nancy J Bloch, CEO/Ex-Officio Board Member
Rosaline H Crawford, Director-Law and Advocacy Center

4215 National Association of the Deaf Law and Advocacy Center
8630 Fenton Street
Silver Spring, MD 20910-4500
301-587-1788
Fax: 301-587-1791
TTY: 301-587-1789
e-mail: NADinfo@nad.org
www.nad.org

Represents deaf and hard of hearing individuals in cases of discrimination on the basis of deafness under federal laws such as the ADA, IDEA and the Rehabilitation Act. Provides legal information about how these laws affect deaf people in jobs, education and more.

Nancy J Bloch, CEO/Ex-Officio Board Member
Rosaline H Crawford, Director-Law and Advocacy Center

4216 National Captioning Institute
1900 Gallows Road
Vienna, VA 22182
703-917-7600
Fax: 703-917-9853
TTY: 703-917-7600
e-mail: jagudelo@ncicap.org
www.ncicap.org

Advocates captioned television for people who want to see, as well as hear, the dialogue of a television program. It not only enables deaf and hard-of-hearing people to understand all of a program's content but it is also beneficial for new Americans learning English.

Juan Mario Agudelo, National Director Sales/Marketing
Elissa Sarna, Director of West Coast Sales/Marketing

4217 National Center for Voice and Speech: Univ ersity of Iowa
The University Of Iowa
200 Hawkins Drive
Iowa City, IA 52242
319-335-6600
Fax: 319-335-6603
e-mail: julie-ostrem@uiowa.edu
www.ncvs.org

This is a consortium of institutions focusing on voice and speech disorders. The members of this consortium are the University of Iowa, the Denver Center for Performing Arts, the University of Wisconsin-Madison and the University of Utah.

Richard Hurt PhD, Board Member
Ingo Titze PhD, Executive Director

4218 National Dissemination Center for Children
PO Box 1492
Washington, DC 20013
202-884-8200
800-695-0285
Fax: 202-884-8441
TTY: 202-884-8200
e-mail: nichcy@aed.org
www.nichcy.org

Publishes free fact filled newsletters. Arranges workshops. Advises parents on the laws entitling children with disabilities to special education and other services.

Dr Suzanne Ripley, Executive Director
Stephen D Luke, Director of Research

4219 National Family Association for Deaf-Blind
141 Middle Neck Road
Sands Point, NY 11050
800-225-0411
Fax: 516-883-9060
e-mail: NFADB@aol.com
www.nfadb.org

NFADB advocates for all persons who are deaf-blind of any chronological age and cognitive ability, supports national policy to benefit people who are deaf-blind, encourages the founding and strengthening of family organizations in each state and shares information.

Linda Syler, President

4220 National Fraternal Society of the Deaf
1118 S 6th Street
Springfield, IL 62703
217-289-7429
Fax: 217-789-7489
TTY: 217-789-7438
e-mail: thefrat@nfsd.com
www.nfsd.com

This organization is comprised of over 80 divisions across the country that work in the area of life insurance and advocacy for deaf people.

Al Van Nevel, Grand President

4221 National Information Clearinghouse on Children Who are Deaf-Blind
Teaching Research
345 N Monmouth Avenue
Monmouth, OR 97361
800-438-9376
Fax: 503-838-8150
TTY: 800-854-7013
e-mail: info@nationaldb.org
www.nationaldb.org

Collects organizes and disseminates information related to children and youth who are deaf-blind and connects consumers of deaf-blind information to sources of information about deaf-blindness assistive technology and deaf-blind people.

John Reiman PhD, Associate Research Professor
Kathy McNulty

4222 National Institute on Deafness and other Communication Disorders
National Institutes Of Heath
31 Center Drive
Bethesda, MD 20892-2320
301-496-7243
Fax: 301-402-0018
TTY: 301-402-0252
e-mail: nidcdinfo@nidcd.nih.gov
www.nidcd.nih.gov

A national resources center for information about hearing, balance, smell, taste, voice, speech and language.

James Battey Jr MD PhD, Director
Marin Allen PhD, Chief Office of Health Communication

4223 National Organization for Hearing Research
225 Haverford Avenue
Narberth, PA 19072
610-664-3135
Fax: 610-668-1428
TTY: 610-664-3135
e-mail: smsnohr@worldnet.att.net
www.nohrfoundation.org

This organization is a nonprofit private foundation seeking to fund exceptional researchers with $5 000 seed money grants.

4224 Rainbow Alliance of the Deaf
309 Millside Drive
Columbus, OH 43230
e-mail: president@rad.org
www.rad.org

A national organization serving the deaf gay and lesbian community. Represents approximately 24 chapters throughout the United States Canada and Europe.

Larry Pike, President
Steven Schumacher, Secretary

4225 Registry of Interpreters for the Deaf
333 Commerce Street
Alexandria, VA 22314
703-838-0030
Fax: 703-838-0454
TTY: 703-838-0459
e-mail: 72620.3143@compuserve.com
www.RID.org

A membership organization with almost 4 000 members including professional interpreters and translators persons with deafness or hearing impairments and professionals in related fields.
Clay Nettles, Executive Director
Cheryl Moose, President/Board of Directors

4226 **Self-Help for Hard of Hearing People**
7910 Woodmont Avenue 301-657-2248
Bethesda, MD 20814-3079 Fax: 301-913-9413
TTY: 301-657-2248
e-mail: info@hearingloss.org
www.hearingloss.org
Promotes awareness and information about hearing loss communication assistive devices and alternative communication skills through publications exhibits and presentations.
Brenda Battat, Executive Director
Christopher Sutton, Director of Development & Education

4227 **Society of Hearing Impaired Physicians**
1999 Mowry Avenue 510-797-2939
Fremont, CA 94538-1622 Fax: 510-797-0168
e-mail: fphship@aol.com
This Society aids and assists physicians medical students and prospective medical students whose hearing impairment may necessitate different tools and/or approaches to medical practice and training.
Frank Hochma MD, President

4228 **Telecommunications for the Deaf**
8630 Fenton Street 301-589-3786
Silver Spring, MD 20910 Fax: 301-589-3797
TTY: 301-589-3006
e-mail: info@tdi-online.org
www.tdi-online.org
A nonprofit consumer advocacy organization promoting full visual and other access to information and telecommunications for people who are deaf, hard of hearing, deaf-blind and speech impaired.
Claude Stout, Executive Director
Scott Recht, Business Manager

4229 **Tripod**
1727 W Burbank Boulevard 818-972-2080
Burbank, CA 91506 Fax: 818-972-2090
TTY: 818-972-2080
e-mail: info@tripod.org
www.tripod.org
TRIPOD is a nonprofit organization dedicated to providing support and services for deaf and hard of hearing children and their families. TRIPOD offers model local educational programs, Montessori, bilingual parent, infant, toddler and preschool programs.

4230 **USA Deaf Sports Federation**
102 N Krohn Place 605-367-5760
Sioux Falls, SD 57103-1800 Fax: 605-782-8441
TTY: 605-367-5761
e-mail: HomeOffice@usdeafsports.org
www.usdeafsports.org
A governing body for all deaf sports and recreation in the United States.
Lawrence R Fleischer, President
Robert C Steele, VP of Financial Affairs

State Agencies & Associations

Alabama

4231 **Alabama Association of the Deaf**
1002 Tomahawk Drive
Talladega, AL 35160 Fax: 256-362-1495
TTY: 256-362-1415
e-mail: kochie.matt@aidb.state.al.us
www.aldeaf.org
Judith Gilliam, Publicity Director
Jerry Smith, ALRID President

Arizona

4232 **Arizona Association of the Deaf**
5025 N Central Avenue
Phoenix, AZ 85012 e-mail: tposedly@aol.com
www.azadinc.org
This organization shall be organized and operated exclusively to promote the welfare of deaf and hard of hearing residents of the state of Arizona in education, economic, security, social equality, and just rights and privileges as citizens.
James Oster, President
Tom Buell, Vice President

Arkansas

4233 **Arkansas Association of the Deaf**
26 Corporate Hill Drive
Little Rock, AR 72205 e-mail: president@arkad.org
www.arkad.org
The mission of the Arkansas Association of the Deaf is to promote the educational, economic, and social welfare of Arkansans who are deaf or hard of hearing.
Holly Ketchum, President
Tommy Walker, Trustee

District of Columbia

4234 **Shiloh Senior Center for the Hearing Impaired**
913 P Street NW 202-232-1425
Washington, DC 20001 TTY: 202-667-9779
Senior programs, sponsored by the DC Office on Aging in co-ordination with grantee: Shiloh Baptist Church serving the entire Metro Washington area's deaf and hard-of-hearing senior citizens.

Florida

4235 **Florida Association of the Deaf**
PO BOX 971134
Boca Raton, FL 33497 e-mail: alange@fadcentral.org
www.fadcentral.org
The mission of the Florida Association of the Deaf is to promote, protect, and preserve the rights and quality of life of Deaf and hard of hearing individuals in the state of Florida.
Andy J Lange, President
Melissa A Watson, Vice President

4236 **Goodwill Industries-Suncoast**
Goodwill Industries-Suncoast
10596 Gandy Boulevard 727-523-1512
St. Petersburg, FL 33702 888-279-1988
Fax: 727-563-9300
e-mail: gw.marketing@goodwill-suncoast.com
www.goodwill-suncoast.org
A nonprofit community based organization whose purpose is to improve the quality of life for people who are disabled, disadvantaged and/or aged. This mission is accomplished through a staff of over 1,200 employees providing independent living skills, affordable housing, career assessment and planning, job skills, training, placement, and job retention assistance with useful employment. Annually, Goodwill Industries-Suncoast serves over 30,000 people in Citrus, Hernando, Levy, Marion and more.
R Lee Waits, President/Chief Executive Officer
Martin W Gladysz, Chair

Georgia

4237 **Georgia Association of the Deaf**
PO Box 1616
Stockbridge, GA 30281-1616 e-mail: turqcat9992000@yahoo.com
www.gadeaf.org
Dixie Blackwell, President
Sandra Dukes, Vice President

Illinois

4238 **Illinois Association of the Deaf**
PO Box 1275
Oak Park, IL 60304
773-237-1877
Fax: 847-740-2319
TTY: 847-740-2319
e-mail: info@iadeaf.org
www.iadeaf.org

The Illinois Association of the Deaf is a non-profit, political, educational, social economic, welfare of the deaf, and cultural organization made up of deaf, hard of hearing, and hearing members.
Sara Bianco, President
Marietta Coufal, Vice-President

Kansas

4239 **Kansas Association of the Deaf**
PO Box 10085
Olathe, KS 66051
785-273-0612
Fax: 785-273-9063
e-mail: legalnetwk@aol.com
www.deafkansas.org

The mission of the Kansas Association of the Deaf a state-wide, non-profit organization is to assure that an extensive, organized system of services is accessible to all deaf or hard of hearing people in Kansas.
Ann Cooper, President
Shane Dundas, Vice-President

Kentucky

4240 **Kentucky Association of the Deaf**
1707 Richmond Drive
Louisville, KY 40205-1407
Fax: 606-272-7747
TTY: 606-223-3999
e-mail: j.k.martin@insightbb.com
www.kydeaf.org

The mission of the Kentucky Association of the Deaf is to advocate for the deaf and hard of hearing in Kentucky by promoting equality, accessibility, and quality of life through employment, services, education and welfare.
Rick Pittman, Board of Director
J Kevin Martin, President

Louisiana

4241 **Louisiana Association of the Deaf**
3112 Valley Creek Drive
Baton Rouge, LA 70808
225-923-1266
800-947-5277
Fax: 225-923-1235
e-mail: kathylad@lad1908.org
www.lad1908.org

Randall Pipp Sr, President
Thelma Covello, Secretary

Massachusetts

4242 **Massachusetts State Association of the Deaf**
PO Box 276
Reading, MA 01867
781-388-9114
Fax: 781-388-9015
TTY: 781-388-9115
e-mail: MSADeaf@aol.com
www.msad.org

The Massachusetts State Association of the Deaf is a statewide nonprofit organization serving the estimated 350 000 deaf and hard of hearing Massachusetts citizens and their families.
Justine Barros, President
Michelle Donatello, Vice President

Michigan

4243 **Michigan Deaf Association**
PO Box 71501
Madison Heights, MI 48071-0501
Fax: 586-775-0906
e-mail: dimckitty@aol.com
www.mideaf.org

MDA is a non-profit, tax exempt organization with a mission to help improve the lives of Deaf and Hard of Heating citizens of Michigan. MDA is affiliated with he National Association of the Deaf whose mission is to promote, protect, and preserve the rights of the deaf and hearing impaired communities.
Diana McKittrick, President
Scott A Pott, 1st Vice-President

New York

4244 **League for the Hard of Hearing**
50 Broadway
New York, NY 10004
917-305-7700
Fax: 917-305-7888
TTY: 917-305-7999
e-mail: inf@lhh.org
www.lhh.org

A private not-for-profit rehabilitation agency for infants, children and adults who are hard of hearing and deaf. The League's mission is to improve the quality of life for people with all degrees of hearing loss.
Laurie Hanin PhD, Executive Director
Anita Stein-Meyers, Assistant Director Audiology

North Carolina

4245 **North Carolina Association of the Deaf**
1200 Revolution Mill Drive
Greensboro, NC 27405
919-773-2974
Fax: 919-834-0127
e-mail: lknelson2@msn.com
www.ncadeaf.org

Linda Nelson, President
Frank Griffin, Vice President

North Dakota

4246 **North Dakota Association of the Deaf**
101 2nd Street S
Fargo, ND 58103
e-mail: jeremy.sebelius@gmail.com
www.nddeaf.org

The North Dakota Association of the Deaf is actively involved in issues affecting Deaf citizens in North Dakota.
Michele Rolewitz, President
Jeremy Sebelius, Secretary

Oklahoma

4247 **Oklahoma Association of the Deaf**
2737 Sunnybrook Lane
Enid, OK 73703
www.ok-oad.org

The purpose of Oklahoma Association of the Deaf is to promote the interests of the deaf and to advance the social, educational, cultural and economic well-being of the deaf.
Chris Reagle, President
Glenna Cooper, Vice-President

Oregon

4248 **Oregon Association of the Deaf**
999 Locust Street NE
Salem, OR 97301
e-mail: contact@deaforegon.com
www.deaforegon.com

The Oregon Association of the Deaf is a non-profit organization working toward a better life for the deaf. Their mission is to create an opportunity for the Deaf of Oregon to join together in planning, devising, conducting and participating in activities.
Daniel Sloan, Committee
Wendy Stanley, Committee

Rhode Island

4249 **Rhode Island Association of the Deaf**
PO Box 40853
Providence, RI 02940
e-mail: CwFuller@aol.com
members.aol.com/EarnestO/RIAD.html

Nancy Fuller, President
Sharon Lane, VP

Texas

4250 **Texas Association of the Deaf**
PO Box 1982
Manchaca, TX 78652-3570
e-mail: steve@deaftexas.org
www.deaftexas.org

Texas Association of the Deaf is an organization for persons who are deaf or hard of hearing. It is a membership organization to provide information and education including surveys and studies to bring the viewpoint on various issues affecting the lives of the deaf and hearing impaired.
Steve C Baldwin, President
Chris Kearney, VP

Virginia

4251 **Virginia Association of the Deaf**
5251 College Drive
Dublin, VA 24084
757-587-9555
Fax: 757-461-5376
TTY: 757-461-7527
e-mail: rbavister@comcast.net
www.vad.org

Rachel Bavister, President
LaDonna Larsen, VP

Wisconsin

4252 **Wisconsin Association of the Deaf**
519 Heatherstone Ridge
Sun Prairie, WI 53590-4230
608-825-9791
TTY: 414-607-3297
e-mail: wad@wi-deaf.org
www.wi-deaf.org

The mission of the Wisconsin Association of the Deaf is to ensure that a comprehensive and coordinated system of resources is accessible to Wisconsin people who are deaf or hard of hearing, enabling them to achieve their maximum potential.
Jerrod Keim, President
Jeffrey Cucinotta, Vice President

Wyoming

4253 **Deaf Association of Wyoming**
PO Box 20107
Cheyenne, WY 82003
307-635-1125
e-mail: president@dawyoming.org
www.dawyoming.org

The Deaf Association of Wyoming is a state non-profit organizations; which is associated with the Association of the Deaf. Membership is open to all deaf persons, parents of deaf children, interpreters, professionals who work with deaf and all interested parties.
Heather Parsons, President
Bill Bitner, VP

Libraries & Resource Centers

4254 **Alexander Graham Bell Association for the Deaf and Hard of Hearing**
3417 Volta Place NW
Washington, DC 20007-2737
202-337-5220
Fax: 202-337-8314
TTY: 202-337-5221
e-mail: info@agbell.org
www.agbell.org

Contains one of the world's largest historical collections of publications, documents and information on deafness. In addition to the main collection, which includes books, periodicals and indexed clipping files dating from the turn of the century, the library also houses a significant archival collection dealing with the history of deafness since the 16th century.
Todd Houston, PhD, Executive Director/CEO
Jessica Ripper, Senior Dir Marketing/Communications

4255 **Captioned Films/Videos**
National Association of the Deaf
8630 Fenton Street
Silver Spring, MD 20910-4500
301-587-1788
Fax: 301-587-1791
TTY: 301-587-1789
www.nad.org

The mission of the National Association of the Deaf is to promote,protect,and preserve the rights and quality of life of eaf and hard of hearing individuals in the United States of America.
Bill Stark, Project Director
Donna Morris, Publications Manager

4256 **Captioned Media Program**
National Association of the Deaf
8630 Fenton Street
Spartanburgng, SC 29307-4500
301-587-1788
Fax: 301-587-1791
TTY: 301-587-1789
www.nad.org

Free loans of educational and entertainment captioned films and videos for deaf and hard of hearing people.
Bill Stark, Project Director
Donna Morris, Publications Manager

4257 **Friends of Libraries for Deaf Action USA**
2930 Craiglawn Road
Silver Spring, MD 20904-1816
202-727-2255
Fax: 301-572-5168
TTY: 301-572-5168
e-mail: folda86@aol.com
http://www.folda.net/

Library services for people with disabilities.
Alice L Hagemeyer, President

4258 **Wallace Memorial Library**
Rochester Institute of Technology
90 Lomb Memorial Drive
Rochester, NY 14623
585-475-2562
www.rit.edu

Information on physical disabilities and deafness.
Chandra McKenzie, Assistant Provost/Director

District of Columbia

4259 **Library Services to the Deaf Community**
District of Columbia Public Library
901 G Street NW
Washington, DC 20001
202-727-2145
TTY: 202-727-2255
e-mail: library_deaf_dc@yahoo.com
www.dclibrary.org

Assures that the deaf community is aware of existing library and information services by the District of Columbia Public Library; promotes public awareness about the deaf community, deaf history and culture, American Sign Language, and assistive technology for people with hearing loss.
John W Hill Jr, President
Bonnie R Cohen, VP

Research Centers

4260 **Boys Town National Research Hospital**
555 N 30th Street
Omaha, NE 68131
402-498-6511
800-320-1171
Fax: 402-498-6331
TTY: 800 320-1171
www.boystownhospital.org

An internationally recognized center for state-of-the-art research diagnosis treatment of patients with ear diseases hearing and balance disorders cleft lip and palate and speech/language problems. Also includes programs such as Parent/Child Workshops Center for Childhood Deafness Register for Heredity Hearing Loss Center for Hearing research Center for Abused Handicapped and summer programs for gifted deaf teens and college students.
Michael Gorg PhD, Program Coordinator
Walt Jestead PhD, Director of Research

4261 **Center for Hearing Loss in Children Boystown National Research Hospital**
Boystown National Research Hospital
555 N 30th Street
Omaha, NE 68131-2136
402-498-6511
800-282-6657
Fax: 402-498-6331
TTY: 800 320-1171
e-mail: chilic@boystown.org
www.boystown.org

The Center for Hearing Loss in Children unites professionals from a variety of disciplines to focus on research research training infor-

mation dissemination and continuing education in the area of childhood deafness.
Patrick Brookhouser, Director
Walt Jestead PhD, Director of Research

4262 Central Institute for the Deaf
825 S Taylor Avenue
Saint Louis, MO 63110-1502
314-977-0132
877-444-4574
Fax: 314-977-0023
TTY: 314-977-0037
e-mail: rfeder@cid.edu
www.cid.edu
Central Institute for the Deaf is a private nonprofit auditory-oral school for children who have hearing impairments. We teach children with hearing loss birth-12 to listen talk and succeed in the mainstream.
Robin Feder MS CFRE, Executive Director
Christine Cl MAEd CED, Joanne Parrish Knight Family Center Coor

4263 City University of New York Center for Research in Speech and Hearing
365 Fifth Avenue
New York, NY 10016-8003
212-817-8807
Fax: 212-817-1537
e-mail: strangepin@aol.com
www.gc.cuny.edu
Programmable research of digital and auditory hearing aids and sensory aids for the speech and hearing impaired person.
Winifred Strange, Director
James J Jenkins, Professor Emeritus

4264 Civitan International Research Center
1530 3rd Avenue S
Birmingham, AL 35294-0001
205-934-8900
800-822-2472
Fax: 205-975-6330
www.circ.uab.edu
Studies of deaf children.
Dr Harald Sontheimer, Director
Dr Alan Percy, Medical Director

4265 Cleveland Hearing and Speech Center
11206 Euclid Avenue
Cleveland, OH 44106
216-231-8787
Fax: 216-231-7141
TTY: 216-231-5266
e-mail: webmaster@chsc.org
www.chsc.org
Offers research and studies into speech language and hearing disorders.
Bernard P Henri PhD, Executive Director
Hilary F Beatrez, Director Finance

4266 David T Siegel Institute for Communicative Disorders
Humana Hospital-Michael Reese
3033 S Cottage Grove Avenue
Chicago, IL 60616-3346
773-791-2900
Fax: 773-791-4014
Conducts behavioral research on language development and sign language for the deaf.
Edward Applebaum, Chief Service

4267 Eaton-Peabody Laboratory of Auditory Physiology
Massachusetts Eye & Ear Institute
243 Charles Street
Boston, MA 02114-3002
617-573-3745
Fax: 617-720-4408
research.meei.harvard.edu/EPL
Auditory system and auditory information processing including ear-brain interactions in normal and pathologic hearing.
M Charles Liberman, Director
Thane Benson, Consultant

4268 Gallaudet University Cued Speech Team
800 Florida Avenue NE
Washington, DC 20002-3660
202-651-5000
Fax: 202-651-5508
TTY: 202-651-5005
e-mail: publicrelations@gallaudet.edu
www.gallaudet.edu
Transmission of spoken languages are researched.
I King Jordan, President
Dr Richard Lytle, Special Assistant to the President

4269 Gallaudet University: Center for Auditory and Speech Sciences
800 Florida Avenue NE
Washington, DC 20002-3660
202-651-5000
Fax: 202-651-5295
TTY: 202-651-5005
www.gallaudet.edu
Develops new hearing tests that use speech sounds to measure hearing loss.
Sally G Revoille, Director

4270 Hear Center
301 E Del Mar Boulevard
Pasadena, CA 91101
626-796-2016
Fax: 626-796-2320
e-mail: auditory@hearcenter.org
www.hearcenter.org
Auditory and verbal program designed to help hearing impaired children infants and adults lead normal and productive lives. Seeks to develop auditory techniques to aid people who have communication problems due to deafness.
Josephine Wilson, Executive Director

4271 Houston Ear Research Foundation
7737 SW Freeway
Houston, TX 77074-1867
713-771-9966
800-843-0808
Fax: 713-771-0546
TTY: 800-843-0807
e-mail: info@houstoncochlear.org
www.houstoncochlear.org
Aims to improve health care and education for deaf and hearing-impaired children.

4272 Loyola University of Children: Parmly Hearing Institute
6525 N Sheridan Road
Chicago, IL 60626-5385
773-274-3000
Fax: 773-508-2719
e-mail: rfay@luc.edu
www.luc.edu
Engage in the comparative study of sensory systems including hearing vision speech perception vestibular function and the special senses of the lateral-line organ and electroreception in fish.
Richard Fay PhD, Director
Dr William Yost, Professor of Psychology

4273 Memphis State University Center for the Communicatively Impaired
Memphis State University
807 Jefferson Avenue
Memphis, TN 38105-5042
901-678-5800
Fax: 901-251-82
www.memphis.edu/ausp
Offers research into hearing loss and deafness as well as speech impairments.
Maurice I Mendel, Dean
Walt Manning, Associate Director

4274 Northern Illinois University Research and Training Center
1425 W Lincoln Highway
DeKalb, IL 60115-2825
815-753-9999
Fax: 815-753-6520
www.niu.edu
Conducts research resource development and training/technical assistance projects geared toward enhancing the employment independent living and quality of life outcomes for traditionally underserved people who are deaf.
Sue E Ouellette PhD, Project Director

4275 Ohio State University Otological Research Laboratories
456 W 10th Avenue
Columbus, OH 43210-1240
614-293-8103
800-293-5123
Fax: 614-293-5506
www.medicalcenter.osu.edu
Clinical and basic research in otology.
Dr Thomas DeMaria, Acting Director

4276 Ohio University Therapy Associates: Hearing, Speech and Language Clinic
W218 Grover Center
Athens, OH 45701
740-593-1407
Fax: 740-593-0287
e-mail: hallowel@ohio.edu
www.ohio.edu/hearingspeech
Focuses on hearing and speech impairments.
Brooke Hallowell, Director
Davida Parsons, Clinical Director

4277 **Oregon Health Sciences University Oregon Hearing Research Center Tinnitus Clinic**
3181 S W Sam Jackson Park Road 503-494-7954
Portland, OR 97239 Fax: 503-945-5656
TTY: 503-494-0910
e-mail: ohrc@ohsu.edu
www.ohsu.edu/ohrc/tinnitusclinic
The first medical clinic in the world established exclusively for the treatment of chronic tinnitus. During the last 25 years we have successfully treated more than 7 000 patients with severe tinnitus. The Clinic also treats patients with hyperacusis (hypersensitivity to sounds).
William H Martin PhD, Director
John V Brigande, Faculty Member

4278 **Regional Resource Center on Deafness Western Oregon State College**
Western Oregon State College
345 N Monmouth Avenue 503-838-8000
Monmouth, OR 97361 877-877-1593
TTY: 503-838-8000
e-mail: wolfgram@wou.edu
www.wou.edu
Improve the employment and independent living status of deaf and hard-of-hearing people by increasing the number of rehabilitation professionals and their community partners nationwide who have the necessary knowledge and communication skills to serve this population.
John Freeburg, Professor
Cheryl Davis, Director

4279 **Rehabilitation Engineering Center for Technological Aids for the Deaf**
Lexington Center
800 Florida Avenue NE 202-651-5335
Washington, DC 20002 Fax: 202-651-5324
e-mail: RERC.HE@gmail.com
www.hearingresearch.org
A federally funded center that conducts research into hearing aid technology and alternate technologies.
Matthew H Bakke Ph D, Director
Arlene C Neuman Ph D, Director

4280 **Research and Training Center for Persons Who are Deaf or Hard of Hearing**
University of Arkansas
26 Corporate Hill Drive 501-686-9691
Little Rock, AR 72205-3822 Fax: 501-869-98
TTY: 501-686-9691
e-mail: dwatson@uark.edu
www.uark.edu/depts/rehabres
Rehabilitation of deaf and hearing impaired individuals.
Douglas Watson, Director
Glenn B Anderson, Professor Director of Training

4281 **Rochester Institute of Technology: Natn'l Technical Institute for the Deaf**
Lyndon Baines Johnson Building
52 Lomb Memorial Drive 716-475-6400
Rochester, NY 14623 Fax: 585-475-5978
TTY: 585-475-6700
e-mail: ntidmc@rit.edu
www.ntid.rit.edu
Provides technical and professional education and training for deaf students.
James J DeCaro, Director
T Alan Hurwitz, President

4282 **Scottish Rite Center for Childhood Language Disorders**
2800 - 16th Street NW 202-232-8155
Washington, DC 20009-3602 Fax: 209-483-8169
dcsr.org
Association offering speech-language evaluations and treatment hearing screening and consultation and referrals to children ages birth to 18 years with hearing or speech disorders.
Ronald A Seale, Sovereign Grand Commander/Supreme Counci
Leonard Proden, Sovereign Grand Inspector General

4283 **Speech Simulation Research Foundation**
PO Box 824 757-442-2755
Nassawadox, VA 23413-0824
Focuses on hearing and speech disorders.
Monte Penney, Director

4284 **State University College at Fredonia Youngerman Clinic**
E336B Thompson Hall 716-673-4813
Fredonia, NY 14063 Fax: 716-673-3332
e-mail: Business.School@fredonia.edu
www.fredonia.edu
Studies communication disorders including hearing and speech.
Dennis L Hefner, President
Denise Szalkowski, Assistant to the President

4285 **State University College at Plattsburgh Auditory Research Laboratory**
101 Broad Street
Plattsburgh, NY 12901-2170 518-564-2000
www.plattsburgh.edu
Roger Hamernik, Professor of Biological Sciences
Delbert Hart, Lecturer of Computer Science

4286 **Syracuse University Institute for Sensory Research**
Syracuse University
621 Skytop Road 315-443-4164
Syracuse, NY 13244-1 Fax: 315-443-1184
e-mail: rlsmith@syr.edu
www.isr.syr.edu
Sensory processing and hearing disorders.
Robert Smith, Director

4287 **Temple University Speech and Hearing Science Laboratories**
13th & Cecil B Moore Avenues
Philadelphia, PA 19122 215-204-7543
www.temple.edu
Speech and hearing studies.
Dr Aquilles Iglesias, Director
Brian Goldstein, Department Chair

4288 **Temple University: Section of Auditory Research**
3509 N Broad Street 215-707-3663
Philadelphia, PA 19140 Fax: 215-707-6417
www.temple.edu
Wasyl Szerem MD, Residency Program Director
Brian Goldstein, Brian Goldstein

4289 **Trace Center University of Wisconsin: Madison**
University of Wisconsin: Madison
1550 Engineering Drive 608-262-6966
Madison, WI 53706-2274 Fax: 608-262-8848
TTY: 608-263-5408
e-mail: info@trace.wisc.edu
trace.wisc.edu
Research and development center working with communication control and computer access technologies for people with disabilities.
Peter Borden, Communication Director
Gregg Vanderheiden, Center Director

4290 **University of Alabama Speech and Hearing Center**
2000 University Commons 251-380-2600
Mobile, AL 36688 Fax: 251-380-2699
e-mail: spaadmt@jaguar1.usouthal.edu
www.southalabama.edu/speechandhearing
Providing undergraduate master's and doctoral programs that challenge the student to achieve the highest standards of academic learning scientific inquiry and clinical excellence.
Robert E Moore, Chair
Elizabeth M Adams, Assistant Professor of Audiology

4291 **University of Chicago: Temporal Bone Laboratory for Ear Research**
5841 S Maryland Avenue 773-702-1000
Chicago, IL 60637-1463 Fax: 773-702-6809
www.uchospitals.edu
Focuses on hearing impairments and deafness research.
Dr Raul Hinojasa, Director

4292 **University of Maine: Conley Speech and Hearing Center**
5724 Dunn Hall 207-581-2006
Orono, ME 04469-5724 Fax: 207-581-2060
e-mail: mboyd@maine.edu
www.umaine.edu/comscidis
Speech disorders of adults and children including hearing impairments and deafness.
Judy Stickles, Clinic Director
Amy Engler Booth, Audiologist

4293 **University of Michigan Communicative Disorders Clinic**
412 Maynard Street 734-764-7260
Ann Arbor, MI 48109-2054 Fax: 734-764-7084
e-mail: kkellogg@chartermi.net
www.umich.edu/comdis
Focuses on communicative disorders including hearing impairments and speech disorders.
Holly Craig, Professor of Education
Joerg Lahann, Assistant Professor of Biomedical Engine

4294 **University of Michigan: Kresge Hearing Research Institute**
1150 W Medical Center Drive 734-764-8110
Ann Arbor, MI 48109-0500 Fax: 734-764-0014
TTY: 734-764-8110
e-mail: josef@umich.edu
www.khri.med.umich.edu
Focuses on hearing and auditory disorders.
Josef M Miller, Director
Sue Kelch, Research Administrator

4295 **University of Nebraska: Lincoln Barkley Memorial Center**
Barkley Center 301 402-472-2145
Lincoln, NE 68583 Fax: 402-472-7697
e-mail: jbernthal1@unl.edu
www.unl.edu
Focuses on hearing impairments and deaf research.
John Bernthal, Director
Evie Reiners, Assistant to the Director

4296 **University of North Carolina at Chapel Hill Division of Speech & Hearing**
CB 7190 919-966-1007
Chapel Hill, NC 27599-1 Fax: 919-966-0100
e-mail: jroush@med.unc.edu
www.med.unc.edu/ahs/sphs
The Division of Speech and Hearing Sciences prepares clinical practitioners in speech-language pathology and audiology to be scholars teachers and researchers in both the theoretical and applied aspects of human communication sciences and disorders.
Jackson Roush, Director
Joni Alberg, Executive Director

4297 **University of Oklahoma Speech & Hearing Center**
University of Oklahoma
1200 N Stonewall Avenue 405-271-4214
Oklahoma City, OK 73126-1 Fax: 405-713-60
www.ouhsc.edu
Glenda Ochan MD, Director

4298 **University of Texas at Dallas Callier Center for Communication Disorders**
1966 Inwood Road 214-905-3000
Dallas, TX 75235-7205 Fax: 214-905-3022
e-mail: roeser@callier.utdallas.edu
www.callier.utdallas.edu
Focuses on communication and behavioral disorders including hearing impairments and deafness research.
Tom Campbell, Executive Director
Phillip L Wilson, Head of Audiology

4299 **University of Washington Department of Speech & Hearing Sciences**
1417 NE 42nd Street 206-685-7400
Seattle, WA 98105-6246 Fax: 206-543-1093
e-mail: sphscadv@u.washington.edu
depts.washington.edu
Communication sciences and disorders.
Joan Hanson, Clinic Manager
Mary Wood, Assistant to the Chair

4300 **University of Washington Speech and Hearing Clinic**
4131 15th Avenue NE 206-543-5440
Seattle, WA 98105-0001 Fax: 206-616-1185
e-mail: shclinic@u.washington.edu
depts.washington.edu/sphsc/clinic.htm
Normal speech language and hearing processes development and disorders research.
Nancy B Alarcon, Clinic Director
Joan Hanson, Clinic Manager

4301 **University of Wisconsin: Auditory Physiology Center**
273 Medical Sciences Building
Madison, WI 53706 608-262-0818
www.wisc.edu
Activities include studies in hearing loss and deafness.
Dr John Brugge, Director

4302 **Yeshiva University: Institute of Communication Disorders**
Montefiore Medical Center
3400 Bainbridge Avenue 718-920-2991
Bronx, NY 10467-2401 Fax: 718-515-8235
e-mail: mfried@montefiore.org
www.yu.edu
Studies on communicative disorders including speech and hearing.
Ann Allowe, Administrator
Marvin P Fried MD, Chair

Support Groups & Hotlines

4303 **Aurora of Central New York**
518 James Street 315-422-7263
Syracuse, NY 13203-2282 Fax: 315-229-46
TDD: 315-422-4792
e-mail: auroracny@auroraofcny.org
Professional counseling services helps to assist individuals and their families deal with the trauma of hearing or vision loss.
Debra Chaken, Executive Director

4304 **Beginnings for Parents of Children Who are Deaf or Hard of Hearing**
3714 Benson Drive 919-850-2746
Raleigh, NC 27609 800-541-4327
Fax: 919-850-2804
TTY: 919-850-2746
e-mail: raleigh@beginningssvcs.com
www.ncbegin.org/
Beginnings provides support to parents of deaf and hard-of-hearing children in an unbiased, family-centered atmosphere. In addition, Beginnings also offers impartial information on communication options, placement and educational programs, and workshops for professional personnel who work with deaf and hard-of-hearing children. Advocacy and support for young people from birth to age 21 is available.
Joni Y Alberg Ph.D, Executive Director
Christene A Tashjian, Research/Development Asst Exec Director

4305 **Children of Deaf Adults**
PO Box 30715
Santa Barbara, CA 93130-0715 805-682-0997
www.coda-international.org
Promotes family awareness and individual growth in hearing children of deaf parents.
Carmel Batson, President
Millie Brother, Founder

4306 **Children's Rights Program**
Alexander Graham Bell Association
3417 Volta Place NW 202-337-5220
Washington, DC 20007 866-337-5220
Fax: 202-337-8314
e-mail: info@agbell.org
www.agbell.org
Actively advocates for the legal rights of children with hearing impairments and for legislation to upgrade the delivery of services to children and adults who are hearing impaired.
Gerri A Hanna, Director Advocacy/Policy

4307 Dial-a-Hearing Screening Test
PO Box 1880
Media, PA 19063
610-544-7700
800-222-3277
Fax: 610-543-2802
e-mail: dahst@aol.com
Hearing help information center. Provides local phone number for Dial-a-Hearing Screening Test and hearing information.
George Biddle, Executive Director

4308 Hearing Aid Helpline
International Hearing Society (IHS)
16880 Middlebelt Road
Livonia, MI 48154
734-522-7200
800-521-5247
Fax: 734-522-0200
e-mail: chelms@ihsinfo.org
http://ihsinfo.org/IhsV2/Home/Index.cfm
Hearing Aid Helpline, a service of International Hearing Society (IHS), provides a referral service for locating qualified hearing healthcare professionals. IHS is a professional association representing Hearing Instrument Specialists worldwide engaged in the practice of testing human hearing, selecting, fitting and dispensing of hearing instruments. Founded in 1951, the Society conducts programs in competency accreditation, education, training promoting specialty-level certification.
Cindy Helms, Executive Director
Phyllis Wilson, Associate Director

4309 John Tracy Clinic on Deafness
806 W Adams Boulevard
Los Angeles, CA 90007-2599
800-522-4582
Fax: 213-749-1651
www.jpc.org
Hotline.
Barbara Hecht, President
Eska Wilson, Vice President

4310 National Health Information Center
PO Box 1133
Washington, DC 20013
310-565-4167
800-336-4797
Fax: 301-984-4256
e-mail: info@nhic.org
www.health.gov/nhic
Offers a nationwide information referral service, produces directories and resource guides.

4311 Project Eyes and Ears
1844 T Street SE
Washington, DC 20020-4635
202-889-7045
Fax: 202-889-6312
Disseminates information about resources to families and service providers, provides transition services for pre-kindergarten children who are deaf-blind and integrates children into normalized settings.
Janice Wellborn

Books

4312 A Child with Hearing Loss in Your Classroom? Don't Panic!
Alexander Graham Bell Association
3417 Volta Place NW
Washington, DC 20007-2737
202-337-5220
Fax: 202-337-8270
TTY: 202-337-5220
Designed for mainstream teachers, this booklet discusses educational needs for students with hearing impairments. It especially focuses on students' language skills and their abilities to follow directions, learn new concepts, and comprehend reading. Candid advice about getting support from professionals, implementing and mantaining an IEP, improving classroom acoustic environments and using the PATERR approach.
1993 25 pages

4313 A New Civil Right: Telecommunications Equality for Deaf and Hard of Hearing
Karen Peltz Strauss, author
Hearing Loss Association of America
7910 Woodmont Avenue
Bethesda, MD 20814-3079
301-657-2248
Fax: 301-913-9413
TTY: 301-657-2249
e-mail: info@hearingloss.org
www.hearingloss.org
This book provides a compelling picture of the challenges and the realization that FCC regulation is required for people with hearing loss to receive the functional equivalence of what everyone else takes for granted.
2006 Hardcover
Jerry Portis, Executive Director
Brenda Battat, Assistant Executive Director

4314 A Quiet World: Living with Hearing Loss
David G Myers, author
Hearing Loss Association of America
7910 Woodmont Avenue
Bethesda, MD 20814-3079
301-657-2248
Fax: 301-913-9413
TTY: 301-657-2249
e-mail: info@hearingloss.org
www.hearigloss.org
A social psychologist, teacher, and author. The Author's gradual hearing loss caused serious trouble in his career and in his relationships with loved ones as he approached 50. He tells the story of his journey from denial to acceptance to an exploration of the technologies that offer help.
2000 Hardcover
Jerry Portis, Executive Director
Brenda Battat, Assistant Executive Director

4315 ASL PAH! Deaf Students' Essays About their Language
Sign Media
4020 Blackburn Lane
Burtonsville, MD 20866-1167
301-421-0268
800-475-4756
Fax: 301-421-0270
TTY: 301-421-4460
e-mail: signmedia@aol.com
www.signmedia.com
Tape/text combination featuring student essays on the role of ASL in their lives. The tape offers additional insights from the student authors. The text is not a transcript of the tape.
1979 Paperback/Video
ISBN: 0-932130-14-3
Barabara Olmert, Director Marketing

4316 ASL in Schools: Policies and Curriculum
Gallaudet University
11030 S Langley Avenue
Chicago, IL 60628-3819
800-621-2736
Fax: 800-621-8476
TTY: 888-630-9347
www.gallaudet.edu
Conference participants questioned experts on bilingual education for deaf students and discussed policy issues faced by educators across the United States.
139 pages

4317 Academic Acceptance of ASL
Gallaudet University
11030 S Langley Avenue
Chicago, IL 60628-3819
800-621-2736
Fax: 800-621-8476
TTY: 888-630-9347
www.gallaudet.edu
This monograph presents a dozen articles that demonstrate clearly and convincingly that the study of ASL affords the same educational values and the same intellectual rewards as the study of any other foreign language.
196 pages

4318 Access for All: Integrating Deaf, Hard of Hearing and Hearing Preschoolers
Gallaudet University
11030 S Langley Avenue
Chicago, IL 60628-3819
800-621-2736
Fax: 800-621-8476
TTY: 888-630-9347
www.gallaudet.edu

Describes a model program for integrating the Deaf and hard of hearing children in early education.
150 pages Book & Video

4319 **American Deaf Culture**
Gallaudet University
11030 S Langley Avenue
Chicago, IL 60628-3819
800-621-2736
Fax: 800-621-8476
TTY: 888-630-9347
www.gallaudet.edu
This book presents a collection of classic articles which have been selected to provide a variety of perspectives on language and culture of deaf people in America.
132 pages

4320 **American Deaf Culture: An Anthology**
Sign Media
4020 Blackburn Lane
Burtonsville, MD 20866-1167
301-421-0268
800-475-4756
Fax: 301-421-0270
TTY: 301-421-4460
e-mail: signmedia@aol.com
www.signmedia.com
Features deaf and hearing authors offering their experience and perspectives on cultural values, ASL, social interaction in the Deaf community, education, folklore and more.
Paperback
ISBN: 0-932130-09-7
Barbara Olmert, Director Marketing
Sherman Wilcox, Editor

4321 **American Sign Language: A Beginning Course**
National Association of the Deaf
8630 Fenton Street
Silver Spring, MD 20910-4500
301-587-1788
Fax: 301-587-1791
TTY: 301-587-1789
www.nad.org
An interactive approach to teaching and learning American Sign Language, with 700 sign illustrations, each accompanied by an object drawing.
199 pages Paperback
ISBN: 0-913072-64-8
Donna Morris, Publications Manager

4322 **An Invisible Condition: The Human Side of Hearing Loss**
SHHH Publications
7910 Woodmont Avenue
Bethesda, MD 20814-3572
301-657-2248
Fax: 301-913-9413
Offers editorials from the SHHH Journal that have shaped the past decade of self help with their focus on the plight and hopes and the aspirations of hard of hearing people everywhere.

4323 **Angels and Outcasts: An Anthology of Deaf Characters in Literature**
Gallaudet University
11030 S Langley Avenue
Chicago, IL 60628-3819
800-621-2736
Fax: 800-621-8476
TTY: 888-630-9347
www.gallaudet.edu
Collection of writings by and about deaf people revealing attitudes and prejudices common to western cultures.
375 pages

4324 **Approaching Equality**
TJ Publishers
817 Silver Spring Avenue
Silver Spring, MD 20910-4617
301-585-4440
800-999-1168
Fax: 301-585-5930
TTY: 301-585-4441
e-mail: tjpubinc@aol.com
Written by the former chair of the Commission on the Education of the deaf, this book reviews the dramatic developments in the education of deaf children.
112 pages Softcover
ISBN: 0-932666-39-6
Angela K Thames, President
Jerald A Murphy, VP

4325 **Assessment & Management of Mainstreamed Hearing-Impaired Children**
Pro-Ed, Inc.
8700 Shoal Creek Boulevard
Austin, TX 78757-6897
512-451-3246
800-897-3202
Fax: 800-397-7633
e-mail: info@proedin.com
www.proedinc.com
The theoretical and practical considerations of developing appropriate programming for hearing-impaired children who are being educated in mainstream educational settings are presented in this book.
415 pages Hardcover
ISBN: 0-890794-58-8
Lindy Jordaan, Marketing Coordinator

4326 **Assessment of Hearing Impaired People**
Gallaudet University
11030 S Langley Avenue
Chicago, IL 60628-3819
800-621-2736
Fax: 800-621-8476
TTY: 888-630-9347
www.gallaudet.edu
This is a comprehensive review of 62 tests used by educational institutions, rehabilitation agencies, and mental health centers.
128 pages Softcover

4327 **At Home Among Strangers**
Gallaudet University
11030 S Langley Avenue
Chicago, IL 60628-3819
800-621-2736
Fax: 800-621-8476
TTY: 888-630-9347
www.gallaudet.edu
Details the history and culture of the deaf community.
336 pages

4328 **Basic Course in Manual Communication**
National Association of the Deaf
8630 Fenton Street
Silver Spring, MD 20910-4500
301-587-1788
Fax: 301-587-1791
TTY: 301-587-1789
www.nad.org
Over 700 signs are grouped according to shape, location, and movement. Also includes dialogues for practice.
158 pages Paperback
Donna Morris, Publications Manager

4329 **Basic Sign Communication: Student Materials**
National Association of the Deaf
8630 Fenton Street
Silver Spring, MD 20910-4500
301-587-1788
Fax: 301-587-1791
TTY: 301-587-1789
www.nad.org
Includes study and reference materials for all three levels of Basic Sign Communication.
232 pages Paperback
ISBN: 0-913072-56-7
Donna Morris, Publications Manager

4330 **Basic Sign Communication: Vocabulary**
National Association of the Deaf
8630 Fenton Street
Silver Spring, MD 20910-4500
301-587-1788
Fax: 301-587-1791
TTY: 301-587-1789
www.nad.org
Features sections on Sign Vocabulary, Numbers, and Classifiers. Contains 1000 illustrated signs, organized alphabetically by gloss for quick reference.
162 pages Paperback
ISBN: 0-913072-55-9
Donna Morris, Publications Manager

4331 **Basic Vocabulary and Language Thesaurus for Hearing Impaired Children**
Alexander Graham Bell Association
3417 Volta Place NW
Washington, DC 20007-2737
202-337-5220
Fax: 202-337-8270
TTY: 202-337-5220

This simple thesaurus lists spontaneous vocabulary used by normally hearing children and lets patients and teachers check so that children with hearing losses have mastered these words.
1977 76 pages

4332 **Basic Vocabulary: American Sign Language for Parents and Children**
TJ Publishers
817 Silver Spring Avenue 301-585-4440
Silver Spring, MD 20910-4617 800-999-1168
Fax: 301-585-5930
TTY: 301-585-4441
e-mail: tjpubinc@aol.com
Carefully selected words and signs include those families use every day. Alphabetically organized vocabulary incorporates developmental lists helpful to both deaf and hearing children and over 1,000 clear sign language illustrations.
240 pages Softcover
ISBN: 0-932666-00-0
Angela K Thames, President
Jerald A Murphy, VP

4333 **Being in Touch**
Gallaudet University
11030 S Langley Avenue
Chicago, IL 60628-3819 800-621-2736
Fax: 800-621-8476
TTY: 888-630-9347
www.gallaudet.edu
Provides information on hearing and vision loss.
80 pages

4334 **Best Practices in Educational Interpreting**
Sign Enhancers
2625 SE Hawthorne Boulevard 503-304-4501
Portland, OR 97214-2941 Fax: 503-304-1063
TTY: 503-304-4501
e-mail: sign@signenhancers.com
www.signenhancers.com
Specific recommendations of best practices for working in preschool through graduate school. Case studies focus on real-life situations with suggested solutions and questions for further thought.
269 pages
ISBN: 0-205263-11-9

4335 **Between Friends**
Beltone Electronics Corporation
4201 W Victoria Street
Chicago, IL 60646-6772 773-583-3600
www.beltone.com
For hearing aid wearers: quizzes, jokes, health, recipes and financial items.
6 pages
Renee Rockoff, Editor

4336 **Black and Deaf in America**
TJ Publishers
817 Silver Spring Avenue 301-585-4440
Silver Spring, MD 20910-4617 800-999-1168
Fax: 301-585-5930
TTY: 301-585-4441
e-mail: tjpubinc@aol.com
An in depth look at some of the problems of the black deaf community, including undereducation and underemployment. This book includes an important chapter on signs used in the black community and presents interviews with prominent Black deaf individuals who share their joys, fears and hope for the future.
91 pages Softcover
ISBN: 0-932666-18-3
Angela K Thames, President
Jerald A Murphy, VP

4337 **Blueprint for Conversational Competence**
Alexander Graham Bell Association
3417 Volta Place NW 202-337-5220
Washington, DC 20007-2737 Fax: 202-337-8270
TTY: 202-337-5220
A book that develops conversational skills in children with hearing impairments.
175 pages

4338 **Book of Name Signs**
Gallaudet University
11030 S Langley Avenue
Chicago, IL 60628-3819 800-621-2736
Fax: 800-621-8476
TTY: 888-630-9347
www.gallaudet.edu
This text discusses the rules for ASL name sign formulation and their appropriate uses and presents a list of over 400 name signs.
112 pages

4339 **Broken Ears: Wounded Hearts**
Gallaudet University
11030 S Langley Avenue
Chicago, IL 60628-3819 800-621-2736
Fax: 800-621-8476
TTY: 888-630-9347
www.gallaudet.edu
An intimate journey into the lives of a deaf, multihandicapped child and her young hearing parents.
186 pages Hardcover

4340 **CUED Speech Resource Book for Parents of Deaf Children**
Alexander Graham Bell Association
3417 Volta Place NW 202-337-5220
Washington, DC 20007-2737 Fax: 202-337-8270
TTY: 202-337-5220
A comprehensive book describing cued speech, getting started, your child's rights in and out of school and families expectations with special attention on siblings and peer relationships.
832 pages Hardcover

4341 **Can't Your Child Hear?**
Gallaudet University
11030 S Langley Avenue
Chicago, IL 60628-3819 800-621-2736
Fax: 800-621-8476
TTY: 888-630-9347
www.gallaudet.edu
Is deafness a difference to be accepted or a defect to be corrected? This comprehensive reference will help parents, as well as educators and other professionals, recognize their options in understanding and handling a child who is deaf.
340 pages Softcover

4342 **Chelsea: The Story of a Signal Dog**
Gallaudet University
11030 S Langley Avenue
Chicago, IL 60628-3819 800-621-2736
Fax: 800-621-8476
TTY: 888-630-9347
www.gallaudet.edu
A story of a young deaf couple and their dog who acts as their ears.
169 pages

4343 **Choices in Deafness**
Woodbine House
6510 Bells Mill Road
Bethesda, MD 20817-1636 800-843-7323
Serving as an invaluable guide to the world of deaf education, this expanded edition covers a wide variety of communication options for children with hearing impairments. By providing medical, audiological, and educational information. It also contains numerous case studies. This indispensible book is an outstanding resource for parents.
1996 212 pages
ISBN: 0-933149-09-3

4344 **Chuck Baird**
Gallaudet University
11030 S Langley Avenue
Chicago, IL 60628-3819 800-621-2736
Fax: 800-621-8476
TTY: 888-630-9347
www.gallaudet.edu
Contains 35 full-color plates of the artwork of the deaf artist.
55 pages

4345 **Classroom Notetaker**
Alexander Graham Bell Association

3417 Volta Place NW
Washington, DC 20007-2737
202-337-5220
Fax: 202-337-8270
TTY: 202-337-5220

This detailed manual for instructors, administrators and staff note takers promotes classroom notetaking within long-term educational programs as vital for students who are deaf and hard of hearing from elementary school to college. This book will help readers to sell a notetaking program to schools and will give a good foundation for designing and implementing a notetaking program in a school or college.
1996 150 pages

4346 **Closer Look: The English Program at the Model Secondary School for the Deaf**
Gallaudet University
11030 S Langley Avenue
Chicago, IL 60628
800-621-2736
Fax: 800-621-8476
TTY: 888-630-9347
www.gallaudet.edu

Program highlighting student-centered activities using carefully selected novels and literature texts to enhance students' reading comprehension and writing abilities through interaction with real literature.
67 pages

4347 **Cochlear Implant Auditory Training Guidebook**
Alexander Graham Bell Association
3417 Volta Place NW
Washington, DC 20007-2737
202-337-5220
Fax: 202-337-8270
TTY: 202-337-5220

This guidebook full of reproducible masters was designed for parents and professionals working with children ages four and up who have cochlear implants. It includes an easy to follow hierarchy for listening goals and a quick placement test to help you find where to start.
236 pages

4348 **Cochlear Implantation for Infants and Children**
Alexander Graham Bell Association
3417 Volta Place NW
Washington, DC 20007-2737
202-337-5220
Fax: 202-337-8270
TTY: 202-337-5220

This comprehensive text presents the surgical, medical, audiological speech and language and habilitation aspects of cochlear implants in infants and children.
1997 263 pages

4349 **Cognition, Education and Deafness**
Gallaudet University
11030 S Langley Avenue
Chicago, IL 60628-3819
800-621-2736
Fax: 800-621-8476
TTY: 888-630-9347
www.gallaudet.edu

The work of 54 authors is gathered in this definitive collection of current research on deafness and cognition. The articles are grouped into seven sections: cognition, problem solving, thinking processes, language development, reading methodologies, measurement of potential and intervention programs.
260 pages Hardcover

4350 **Communicate with Me: Conversation Skills for Deaf Students**
Gallaudet University
11030 S Langley Avenue
Chicago, IL 60628-3819
800-621-2736
Fax: 800-621-8476
TTY: 888-630-9347
www.gallaudet.edu

Students learn how to begin and end conversations, choose appropriate topics and maintain subjects.
160 pages

4351 **Communication Access for Persons with Hearing Loss**
Mark Ross, author
Hearing Loss Association of America
7910 Woodmont Avenue
Bethesda, MD 20814-3079
301-657-2248
Fax: 301-913-9413
TTY: 301-657-2249
e-mail: info@hearingloss.org
www.hearingloss.org

Communication access for persons with hearing loss covers both visual and hearing techniques devoted to persons with hearingloss, ranging from mild to profound.
Jerry Portis, Executive Director
Brenda Battat, Assistant Executive Director

4352 **Communication Issues Among Deaf People**
Gallaudet University
11030 S Langley Avenue
Chicago, IL 60628-3819
800-621-2736
Fax: 800-621-8476
TTY: 888-630-9347
www.gallaudet.edu

Monograph discussing important aspects of communication including total communication and the value of ASL.
138 pages

4353 **Communication Issues Among Deaf People: Eyes, Hands and Voices**
National Association of the Deaf
8630 Fenton Street
Silver Spring, MD 20910-4500
301-587-1788
Fax: 301-587-1791
TTY: 301-587-1789
www.nad.org

Includes over thirty relevant articles reflecting a wide range of perceptions and attitutes on communication among deaf people.
145 pages
Donna Morris, Publications Manager

4354 **Communication Rules for Hard of Hearing People**
Hearing Loss Association of America
7910 Woodmont Avenue
Bethesda, MD 20814-3079
301-657-2248
Fax: 301-913-9413
TTY: 301-657-2249
e-mail: info@hearingloss.org
www.hearingloss.org

To open the world of communication to people with hearing loss through education, information, support and advocacy.
Jerry Portis, Executive Director
Brenda Battat, Assistant Executive Director

4355 **Communication and Adult Hearing Loss**
Alexander Graham Bell Association
3417 Volta Place NW
Washington, DC 20007-2737
202-337-5220
Fax: 202-337-8270
TTY: 202-337-5220

This informative book was written for anyone who wants to communicate more effectively with a person with adult hearing loss.
1993 136 pages

4356 **Comprehensive Signed English Dictionary**
Harris Communications
6541 City W Parkway
Eden Prairie, MN 55344-3248
612-906-1180
Fax: 612-946-0924

Complete dictionary offers 3100 signs, including signs reflecting contemporary vocabulary.
457 pages

4357 **Consumer Handbook on Dizziness and Vertigo**
Dennis Poe, MD, author
Hearing Loss Association of America
7910 Woodmont Avenue
Bethesda, MD 20814-3079
301-657-2248
Fax: 301-913-9413
TTY: 301-657-2249
e-mail: info@hearingloss.org
www.hearingloss.org

Learn the differences between dizziness and vertigo.
Hardcover
ISBN: 0-966182-64-2

4358 **Conversational Sign Language II: An Intermdiate Advanced Manual**
Harris Communications
6541 City W Parkway
Eden Prairie, MN 55344-3248
612-906-1180
Fax: 612-946-0924

This book presents English words and their American Sign Language equivalents.
218 pages

4359 **Dancing Without Music**
Gallaudet University
11030 S Langley Avenue
Chicago, IL 60628-3819
800-621-2736
Fax: 800-621-8476
TTY: 888-630-9347
www.gallaudet.edu
Investigates being deaf and its social ramifications.
320 pages

4360 **Deaf Children in Public Schools Placement, Context, and Consequences**
Gallaudet University
11030 S Langley Avenue
Chicago, IL 60628-3819
800-621-2736
Fax: 800-621-8476
TTY: 888-630-9347
www.gallaudet.edu
Assesses the progress of three second-grade deaf students to demonstrate the importance of placement, context, and language in their development.
August 1997 250 pages
ISBN: 1-563680-62-9

4361 **Deaf Culture, Our Way**
Gallaudet University
11030 S Langley Avenue
Chicago, IL 60628-3819
800-621-2736
Fax: 800-621-8476
TTY: 888-630-9347
www.gallaudet.edu
A revised edition of Silence is Golden, Sometimes, this new edition contains sections on Classic Humor, Bathroom Tales, Classic Hazards and New Technology.
115 pages

4362 **Deaf Empowerment, Emergence, Struggle and Rhetoric**
Gallaudet University
11030 S Langley Avenue
Chicago, IL 60628-3819
800-621-2736
Fax: 800-621-8476
TTY: 888-630-9347
www.gallaudet.edu
Examines the rhetorical foundation that motivated Deaf people to work for social change during the past two centuries. Assesses the goal of a multicultural society and offers suggestions for community building through a new humanitarianism.
July 1997 192 pages Hardcover
ISBN: 1-563680-61-0

4363 **Deaf Heritage: A Narrative History of Deaf America**
National Association of the Deaf
8630 Fenton Street
Silver Spring, MD 20910-4500
301-587-1788
Fax: 301-587-1791
TTY: 301-587-1789
www.nad.org
In-depth history of Deaf America contains pictures, vignettes, and biographical profiles.
483 pages Paperback
Donna Morris, Publications Manager

4364 **Deaf Heritage: Student Text and Workbook**
National Association of the Deaf
8630 Fenton Street
Silver Spring, MD 20910-4500
301-587-1788
Fax: 301-587-1791
TTY: 301-587-1789
www.nad.org
Each chapter is followed by a vocabulary section and workbook activities including questions and follow-up activities for students.
115 pages Paperback
Donna Morris, Publications Manager

4365 **Deaf History Unveiled: Interpretations from the New Scholarship**
Gallaudet University
11030 S Langley Avenue
Chicago, IL 60628-3819
800-621-2736
Fax: 800-621-8476
TTY: 888-630-9347
www.gallaudet.edu
Essays written by internationally renowned deaf studies scholars.
316 pages

4366 **Deaf Like Me**
Gallaudet University
11030 S Langley Avenue
Chicago, IL 60628-3819
800-621-2736
Fax: 800-621-8476
TTY: 888-630-9347
www.gallaudet.edu
Written by the uncle and father of a deaf girl, this is an account of parents coming to terms with deafness.
292 pages

4367 **Deaf President Now! The 1988 Revolution at Gallaudet University**
Gallaudet University
11030 S Langley Avenue
Chicago, IL 60628-3819
800-621-2736
Fax: 800-621-8476
TTY: 888-630-9347
www.gallaudet.edu
This book chronicles the events leading up to the revolution in which deaf people won social change for themselves and all disabled people.
240 pages

4368 **Deaf Sport: The Impact of Sports Within the Deaf Community**
Gallaudet University
11030 S Langley Avenue
Chicago, IL 60628-3819
800-621-2736
Fax: 800-621-8476
TTY: 888-630-9347
www.gallaudet.edu
Describes the full ramifications of athletics for deaf people.
224 pages

4369 **Deaf Students and the School-to-Work Transition**
Gallaudet University
11030 S Langley Avenue
Chicago, IL 60628-3819
800-621-2736
Fax: 800-621-8476
TTY: 888-630-9347
www.gallaudet.edu
Studies severely and profoundly hearing impaired students as they leave high school and enter the work force.
278 pages

4370 **Deaf Studies Curriculum Guide**
Gallaudet University
11030 S Langley Avenue
Chicago, IL 60628-3819
800-621-2736
Fax: 800-621-8476
TTY: 888-630-9347
www.gallaudet.edu
Designed to help students explore the history, language and culture of deaf people.
250 pages

4371 **Deaf Women: A Parade Through the Decades**
Gallaudet University
11030 S Langley Avenue
Chicago, IL 60628-3819
800-621-2736
Fax: 800-621-8476
TTY: 888-630-9347
www.gallaudet.edu
A compilation of information, history, anecdotes and research that showcases many deaf women from all walks of American life.
192 pages

4372 **Deaf and Hard of Hearing Individuals**
Mainstream
1030 5th Street NW
Washington, DC 20001-2504
202-898-1400

Mainstreaming deaf individuals into the workplace.
12 pages

4373 Deaf in America: Voices from a Culture
Gallaudet University
11030 S Langley Avenue
Chicago, IL 60628-3819
800-621-2736
Fax: 800-621-8476
TTY: 888-630-9347
www.gallaudet.edu

Written by authors who are themselves deaf.
134 pages

4374 Deafness and Child Development
Gallaudet University
11030 S Langley Avenue
Chicago, IL 60628-3819
800-621-2736
Fax: 800-621-8476
TTY: 888-630-9347
www.gallaudet.edu

Provides rational, informed and balanced approaches to the effects of deafness in child development.
236 pages

4375 Deafness: 1993-2013
National Association of the Deaf
8630 Fenton Street
Silver Spring, MD 20910
301-587-1788
Fax: 301-587-1791
TTY: 301-587-1789
www.nad.org

Over 30 articles cover such topics as magnet schools, deaf identity, technology, multicultural education, communication, leadership, and sign language research.
Paperback
Donna Morris, Publications Manager

4376 Deafness: A Personal Account
Faber & Faber
19 Union Square W
New York, NY 10003-3304
781-721-1427
e-mail: contact@faber.co.uk
www.faber.co.uk

Poet, critic and translator David Wright's enduring memoir (now with a substantial new introduction by the author) describes with humor and insight his early life, his development as a poet, and little-known history of deaf education.
202 pages

4377 Deafness: An Autobiography
Gallaudet University
11030 S Langley Avenue
Chicago, IL 60628-3819
800-621-2736
Fax: 800-621-8476
TTY: 888-630-9347
www.gallaudet.edu/~gupress

This book is intended to explore the author's own experiences with deafness, and satisfy the curiosity about the condition of deaf people.
238 pages

4378 Deafness: Historical Perspectives
National Association of the Deaf
8630 Fenton Street
Silver Spring, MD 20910
301-587-1788
Fax: 301-587-1791
TTY: 301-587-1789
www.nad.org

Focuses on the history of deaf people. Topics cover a spectrum from a history of deaf theaters, to a genealogy of our first deaf families, to a conversation with a ghost.
Paperback
Donna Morris, Publications Manager

4379 Deafness: Life and Culture II
National Association of the Deaf
8630 Fenton Street
Silver Spring, MD 20910
301-587-1788
Fax: 301-587-1791
TTY: 301-587-1789
www.nad.org

Continues to explore the variety and diversity of the deaf experience.
133 pages Paperback
ISBN: 0-913072-79-6
Donna Morris, Publications Manager

4380 Directory of Auditory-Oral Programs
Alexander Graham Bell Association
3417 Volta Place NW
Washington, DC 20007-2737
202-337-5220
Fax: 202-337-8270
TTY: 202-337-5220

This directory lists auditory/oral programs in public and private schools, auditory-oral programs in speech and hearing centers and therapists who offer private tutoring and auditory-oral therapy.
67 pages

4381 Discovering Sign Language
Gallaudet University
11030 S Langley Avenue
Chicago, IL 60628-3819
800-621-2736
Fax: 800-621-8476
TTY: 888-630-9347
www.gallaudet.edu/~gupress

Here is a book of information about deaf people and sign communication.
104 pages Softcover

4382 Douglas Tilden, the Man and His Legacy
Gallaudet University
11030 S Langley Avenue
Chicago, IL 60628-3819
800-621-2736
Fax: 800-621-8476
TTY: 888-630-9347
www.gallaudet.edu/~gupress

A beautiful tribute to the Deaf sculptor, Douglas Tilden.
216 pages

4383 Ear Book
Gallaudet University
11030 S Langley Avenue
Chicago, IL 60628-3819
800-621-2736
Fax: 800-621-8476
TTY: 888-630-9347
www.gallaudet.edu/~gupress

A how-to book on obtaining and using an otoscope, recognizing and managing common ear disorders, when to call the doctor and when your child needs ear tubes.
136 pages Softcover

4384 Ear Gear: A Student Workbook on Hearing and Hearing Aids
Gallaudet University
11030 S Langley Avenue
Chicago, IL 60628-3819
800-621-2736
Fax: 800-621-8476
TTY: 888-630-9347
www.gallaudet.edu/~gupress

Attractive workbook designed to teach elementary-age children about hearing loss and the use of hearing aids.
75 pages

4385 Educating Deaf Children Bilingually
Gallaudet University
11030 S Langley Avenue
Chicago, IL 60628-3819
800-621-2736
Fax: 800-621-8476
TTY: 888-630-9347
www.gallaudet.edu/~gupress

Discusses perspectives and practices of educating deaf children with goals of age-level achievement.
120 pages

4386 Educating the Deaf: Psychology, Principles and Practices
Gallaudet University
11030 S Langley Avenue
Chicago, IL 60628-3819
800-621-2736
Fax: 800-621-8476
TTY: 888-630-9347
www.gallaudet.edu/~gupress

Offers extensive coverage of the background and history of the education of the deaf, as well as specific information on working with multihandicapped students.
383 pages

4387 Education and Deafness
Longman Publishing Group
95 Church Street 914-993-5000
White Plains, NY 10601-1515
This comprehensive introduction to educating students with hearing impairments provides extensive coverage of the interrelated issues that affect the teaching of these students. It concentrates on the severely to profoundly hearing impaired but includes an entire chapter devoted to students whose impairments are less severe (hard-of-hearing students).
320 pages Paperback
ISBN: 0-801300-26-6

4388 Educational and Development Aspects of Deafness
Gallaudet University
11030 S Langley Avenue
Chicago, IL 60628-3819 800-621-2736
Fax: 800-621-8476
TTY: 888-630-9347
www.gallaudet.edu/~gupress
Book detailing the ongoing revolution in the education of deaf children.
415 pages

4389 Empowerment and Black Deaf Persons
Gallaudet University
11030 S Langley Avenue
Chicago, IL 60628-3819 800-621-2736
Fax: 800-621-8476
TTY: 888-630-9347
www.gallaudet.edu/~gupress
Conference proceedings focusing on the guidance and training of African American deaf individuals.
175 pages

4390 Encyclopedia of Deafness and Hearing Disorders
Facts on File
11 Penn Plaza 212-967-8800
New York, NY 10001 800-322-8755
Fax: 800-678-3633
A comprehensive guide to all aspects of hearing impairments.

4391 Eye-Centered: A Study of Spirituality of Deaf People
NCOD
814 Thayer Avenue 301-587-7992
Silver Spring, MD 20910-4500
The findings of the five-year De Sales Project conducted by The National Catholic Office for the Deaf.

4392 FM Auditory Trainers: A Winning Choice for Students, Teachers and Parents
Alexander Graham Bell Association
3417 Volta Place NW 202-337-5220
Washington, DC 20007-2737 Fax: 202-337-8270
TTY: 202-337-5220
A practical guide to the selection and use of FM trainers in class or at home.
67 pages

4393 For Teachers of the Hearing Impaired
Gallaudet University
11030 S Langley Avenue
Chicago, IL 60628-3819 800-621-2736
Fax: 800-621-8476
TTY: 888-630-9347
www.gallaudet.edu/~gupress
Contains practical articles by and for teachers of hearing impaired children.

4394 Foundations of Spoken Language for Hearing Impaired Children
Alexander Graham Bell Association
3417 Volta Place NW 202-337-5220
Washington, DC 20007-2737 Fax: 202-337-8270
TTY: 202-337-5220
This guide traces the individual progress of a child's speech development.
1978 87 pages

4395 Free Hand: Education of the Deaf
TJ Publishers
817 Silver Spring Avenue 301-585-4440
Silver Spring, MD 20910-4617 800-999-1168
Fax: 301-585-5930
TTY: 301-585-4441
e-mail: tjpubinc@aol.com
Based on the proceedings of a 1990 symposium on the educational uses of ASL, A Free Hand presents papers by prominent educators, researchers and linguists in the changing role of American sign language in the classroom.
204 pages Softcover
ISBN: 0-932666-40-X
Angela K Thames, President
Jerald A Murphy, VP

4396 GA and SK Etiquette
Gallaudet University
11030 S Langley Avenue
Chicago, IL 60628-3819 800-621-2736
Fax: 800-621-8476
TTY: 888-630-9347
www.gallaudet.edu/~gupress
This booklet presents guidelines for proper usage of the TDD.
53 pages

4397 Gallaudet Encyclopedia of Deaf People and Deafness
Gallaudet University
11030 S Langley Avenue
Chicago, IL 60628-3819 800-621-2736
Fax: 800-621-8476
TTY: 888-630-9347
www.gallaudet.edu/~gupress
Three-volume set of research and information on deaf people and deafness.
1400 pages

4398 Growing Together: Information for Parents of Deaf & Hard of Hearing Children
Gallaudet University
11030 S Langley Avenue
Chicago, IL 60628-3819 800-621-2736
Fax: 800-621-8476
TTY: 888-630-9347
www.gallaudet.edu/~gupress
This publication answers questions often asked by parents of children with a hearing loss.
92 pages

4399 Handtalk Zoo
Macmillan Publishing Company
866 3rd Avenue 212-702-2000
New York, NY 10022-6221 800-257-5755
www.mcp.com
Wonderful photographs are used to show children at the zoo communicating with sign language.
28 pages Hardcover
ISBN: 0-027008-01-0

4400 Hearing Aid Handbook
Gallaudet University
11030 S Langley Avenue
Chicago, IL 60628-3819 800-621-2736
Fax: 800-621-8476
TTY: 888-630-9347
www.gallaudet.edu/~gupress
A complete guide for wearers and clinicians for the use and maintenance of hearing aids.
172 pages Paperback

4401 Hearing Impaired Children and Youth and Developmental Disabilities
Gallaudet University

11030 S Langley Avenue
Chicago, IL 60628-3819 800-621-2736
Fax: 800-621-8476
TTY: 888-630-9347
www.gallaudet.edu/~gupress

Offers insights from 24 experts to help clarify relationships between hearing impairments and developmental difficulties.
416 pages

4402 Hearing Loss Help
Impact Publications
9104 Manassas Drive 703-361-7300
Manassas Park, VA 20111-5211 Fax: 703-335-9469
e-mail: info@impactpublications.com
www.impactpublications.com

Self-help guide provides factual information on how we hear, and on the causes and symptoms of hearing loss. Gives practical information on ways to improve everyday communication and create better listening conditions, and covers assistive listening devices.

4403 Hearing Loss and Hearing Aids: A Bridge to Healing
Richard Carmen, author
Hearing Loss Association of America
7910 Woodmont Avenue 301-657-2248
Bethesda, MD 20814-3079 Fax: 301-913-9413
TTY: 301-657-2249
e-mail: info@hearingloss.org
www.hearingloss.org

The Consumer Handbook on hearing loss and hearing aids.
Softcover
ISBN: 0-966182-61-8
Jerry Portis, Executive Director
Brenda Battat, Assistant Executive Director

4404 Hispanic Deaf
Gallaudet University
11030 S Langley Avenue
Chicago, IL 60628-3819 800-621-2736
Fax: 800-621-8476
TTY: 888-630-9347
www.gallaudet.edu/~gupress

Hispanic students now make up the largest minority in education for deaf students. This timely collection includes articles by many of the professionals most closely involved with the education of this very special population.
213 pages Hardcover

4405 History of Special Education: From Isolation to Integration
Gallaudet University
11030 S Langley Avenue
Chicago, IL 60628-3819 800-621-2736
Fax: 800-621-8476
TTY: 888-630-9347
www.gallaudet.edu/~gupress

Comprehensive volume examining the facts and events that shaped this field in Western Europe, United States and Canada.
464 pages

4406 Hollywood Speaks
Gallaudet University
11030 S Langley Avenue
Chicago, IL 60628-3819 800-621-2736
Fax: 800-621-8476
TTY: 888-630-9347
www.gallaudet.edu/~gupress

How deafness has been treated in movies and how it provides yet another window onto social history in addition to a fresh angle from which to view Hollywood.
167 pages Hardcover

4407 Hometown Heroes: Successful Deaf Youth in America
Gallaudet University
11030 S Langley Avenue
Chicago, IL 60628-3819 800-621-2736
Fax: 800-621-8476
TTY: 888-630-9347
www.gallaudet.edu/~gupress

A lively book showcasing more than 40 deaf and hard-of-hearing teenagers in the United States.
108 pages

4408 How Hearing Impacts Relationships
Richard Carmen, author
Hearing Loss Association of America
7910 Woodmont Avenue 301-657-2248
Bethesda, MD 20814-3079 Fax: 301-913-9413
TTY: 301-657-2249
e-mail: info@hearingloss.org
www.hearingloss.org

At last families of loved ones with untreated hearing loss can know they are not alone and what options are available.
Softcover
ISBN: 0-966182-63-4
Jerry Portis, Executive Director
Brenda Battat, Assistant Executive Director

4409 How the Student with Hearing Loss Can Succeed in College
Alexander Graham Bell Association
3417 Volta Place NW 202-337-5220
Washington, DC 20007-2737 Fax: 202-337-8270
TTY: 202-337-5220

This revised book details how students who are deaf or hard of hearing and professionals must work together for students in college to be successful.
1996 304 pages

4410 How to Survive a Hearing Loss
Gallaudet University
11030 S Langley Avenue
Chicago, IL 60628-3819 800-621-2736
Fax: 800-621-8476
TTY: 888-630-9347
www.gallaudet.edu/~gupress

This book presents the results of the author's intensive research about hearing and the ear.
241 pages

4411 Hug Just Isn't Enough
Gallaudet University
11030 S Langley Avenue
Chicago, IL 60628-3819 800-621-2736
Fax: 800-621-8476
TTY: 888-630-9347
www.gallaudet.edu/~gupress

Photos of deaf children and excerpts from interviews with parents of deaf youngsters.

4412 I Didn't Hear the Dragon Roar
Gallaudet University
11030 S Langley Avenue
Chicago, IL 60628-3819 800-621-2736
Fax: 800-621-8476
TTY: 888-630-9347
www.gallaudet.edu/~gupress

The remarkable true story of a deaf woman's journey from Hong Kong to Katmandu.
251 pages

4413 IDEA Advocacy for Children Who are Deaf or Hard of Hearing
Alexander Graham Bell Association
3417 Volta Place NW 202-337-5220
Washington, DC 20007-2737 Fax: 202-337-8270
TTY: 202-337-5220

This book offers up to date information about the 1997 Individuals with Disabilities Education Act which affects children who are deaf or hard of hearing.
1997 96 pages

4414 Implications and Complications for Deaf Students of Full Inclusion Movement
Gallaudet University
11030 S Langley Avenue
Chicago, IL 60628-3819 800-621-2736
Fax: 800-621-8476
TTY: 888-630-9347
www.gallaudet.edu/~gupress

A collection of papers discussing the full inclusion movement.
80 pages

4415 In Silence: Growing Up Hearing in a Deaf World
Gallaudet University

11030 S Langley Avenue
Chicago, IL 60628-3819 800-621-2736
Fax: 800-621-8476
TTY: 888-630-9347
www.gallaudet.edu/~gupress

Author's story of growing up as a hearing child of deaf parents.
335 pages

4416 In This Sign
Gallaudet University
11030 S Langley Avenue
Chicago, IL 60628-3819 800-621-2736
Fax: 800-621-8476
TTY: 888-630-9347
www.gallaudet.edu/~gupress

A modern classic following a family of deaf parents and their hearing impaired child through several decades of growth and pain, tragedy and triumph.
275 pages

4417 Inclusion?
Gallaudet University
11030 S Langley Avenue
Chicago, IL 60628-3819 800-621-2736
Fax: 800-621-8476
TTY: 888-630-9347
www.gallaudet.edu/~gupress

This book defines quality education for deaf and hard of hearing students.
213 pages

4418 International Directory of Periodicals Related to Deafness
Gallaudet University
11030 S Langley Avenue
Chicago, IL 60628-3819 800-621-2736
Fax: 800-621-8476
TTY: 888-630-9347
www.gallaudet.edu/~gupress

Offers information on more than 500 magazines and journals related to deafness.
150 pages

4419 International Telephone Directory for TDD Users
Gallaudet University
11030 S Langley Avenue
Chicago, IL 60628-3819 800-621-2736
Fax: 800-621-8476
TTY: 888-630-9347
www.gallaudet.edu/~gupress

Offers 12,000 TDD members and organizations serving deaf people.
190 pages

4420 Introduction to Communication
Gallaudet University
11030 S Langley Avenue
Chicago, IL 60628-3819 800-621-2736
Fax: 800-621-8476
TTY: 888-630-9347
www.gallaudet.edu/~gupress

Curriculum materials exploring the areas of sound, hearing and interpersonal communication.
100 pages

4421 Invisible Condition: The Human Side of Hearing Loss
Howard E Stone, author
Hearing Loss Association of America
7910 Woodmont Avenue 301-657-2248
Bethesda, MD 20814-3079 Fax: 301-913-9413
TTY: 301-657-2249
e-mail: info@hearingloss.org
www.hearingloss.org

A collection of 14 years of editorials by the author from the SHHH Journal. An inspiration book that transcends hearing loss.
1993
Jerry Portis, Executive Director
Brenda Battat, Assistant Executive Director

4422 Its Your Turn Now: Using Dialogue Journals with Deaf Students
Gallaudet University
11030 S Langley Avenue
Chicago, IL 60628-3819 800-621-2736
Fax: 800-621-8476
TTY: 888-630-9347
www.gallaudet.edu/~gupress

Based on years of experience, this book reviews teachers' questions and answers.
130 pages

4423 Journey Into the Deaf World
DawnSignPress
6130 Nancy Ridge Drive 858-625-0600
San Diego, CA 92121-3223 800-549-5350
Fax: 858-625-2336
TTY: 858-625-0600
e-mail: comments@dawnsign.com
www.dawnsign.com

Provides explanation about the nature and meaning of the deaf world. Comprehensive work discusses latest findings and theories for deaf studies students and professionals working with deaf people.
528 pages Paperback
ISBN: 0-915035-63-4
Barry Howland, Marketing Director

4424 Journey Out of Silence
Dora Tinglestad Weber, author
Hearing Loss Association of America
7910 Woodmont Avenue 301-657-2248
Bethesda, MD 20814-3079 Fax: 301-913-9413
TTY: 301-657-2249
e-mail: info@hearingloss.org
www.hearingloss.org

Dora Weber, who made a long and arduous journey out of silence, shares her experiences in an effort to encourage those who are hearing impaired and to increase the sensitivity of those who are not.
Softcover
ISBN: 1-890676-30-6
Jerry Portis, Executive Director
Brenda Battat, Assistant Executive Director

4425 Joy of Signing
Gospel Publishing House
1445 N Boonville Avenue 417-862-2781
Springfield, MO 65802-1894 Fax: 417-862-7566
e-mail: jclore@ag.org
www.GospelPublishing.com

Illustrated sign language text with descriptions of the origin of selected signs and examples of how each is used. Second edition.
352 pages
Judy Clore, Promotions Coordinator

4426 Kaleidoscope of Deaf America
Harris Communications
6541 City W Parkway 612-906-1180
Eden Prairie, MN 55344-3248 Fax: 612-946-0924

Puts you in touch with the trends, the events and the thinking that is shaping your future.
79 pages

4427 Kendall Demonstration Elementary School Curriculum Guides
Gallaudet University
11030 S Langley Avenue
Chicago, IL 60628-3819 800-621-2736
Fax: 800-621-8476
TTY: 888-630-9347
www.gallaudet.edu/~gupress

These guides provide detailed information to help teachers organize curriculum, structure classes and develop individualized education programs.
18 months+

4428 Kid-Friendly Parenting with Deaf and Hard of Hearing Children
Gallaudet University
11030 S Langley Avenue
Chicago, IL 60628-3819 800-621-2736
Fax: 800-621-8476
TTY: 888-630-9347
www.gallaudet.edu/~gupress

A step-by-step guide offering parents hundreds of ideas and play activities for children ages 3 to 12.
336 pages

4429 Learning to Hear Again
Alexander Graham Bell Association
3417 Volta Place NW
Washington, DC 20007-2737
202-337-5220
Fax: 202-337-8270
TTY: 202-337-5220

This audiologic rehabilitation curriculum guide is designed to help audiologists and speech language pathologist provide rehabilitation and education for adults with hearing losses. The authors are practicing audiologists and have used these methods successfully in individual and group sessions. This comprehensive manual comprises lesson plans, activities and materials ready to be duplicated and distributed to clients.
1996 224 pages

4430 Learning to See: American Sign Language as a Second Language
Gallaudet University
11030 S Langley Avenue
Chicago, IL 60628-3819
800-621-2736
Fax: 800-621-8476
TTY: 888-630-9347
www.gallaudet.edu/~gupress

Provides a comprehensive introduction to the history and structure of ASL to the deaf community.
134 pages

4431 Least Restrictive Environment: The Paradox of Inclusion
LRP Publications
PO Box 980
Horsham, PA 19044-0980
800-341-7874
Fax: 215-784-9639
e-mail: custserv@lrp.com
www.lrp.com

Analyzes relevant federal law and the inclusion reform movement, and discusses the premise that an effort to force one generic placement on all children will create more problems than thought imaginable.
Paperback

4432 Legal Rights for the Deaf and Hard of Hearing
Hearing Loss Association of America
7910 Woodmont Avenue
Bethesda, MD 20814-3079
301-657-2248
Fax: 301-913-9413
TTY: 301-657-2249
e-mail: info@hearingloss.org
www.hearingloss.org

A comprehensive analysis of recent laws passed to protect the rights of and guarantee equal access for people with hearing loss. The book explains in layman's terminology how legislation affects individuals with disabilities in everyday life.
2002 Softcover
Jerry Portis, Executive Director
Brenda Battat, Assistant Executive Director

4433 Legal Rights of Hearing-Impaired People
Gallaudet University
11030 S Langley Avenue
Chicago, IL 60628-3819
800-621-2736
Fax: 800-621-8476
TTY: 888-630-9347
www.gallaudet.edu/~gupress

Includes updated interpretations of legislation affecting hearing-impaired people, including chapters dealing with the ADA.
297 pages

4434 Lessons in Laughter: The Autobiography of a Deaf Actor
Gallaudet University
11030 S Langley Avenue
Chicago, IL 60628-3819
800-621-2736
Fax: 800-621-8476
TTY: 888-630-9347
www.gallaudet.edu/~gupress

Born deaf of deaf parents, Bernard Bragg dreamed of using sign language to act. This book recounts how he starred in his own television show.
237 pages

4435 Let's Learn About Deafness
Gallaudet University
11030 S Langley Avenue
Chicago, IL 60628-3819
800-621-2736
Fax: 800-621-8476
TTY: 888-630-9347
www.gallaudet.edu/~gupress

Hands-on school classroom activities for the deaf student.
82 pages

4436 Listen to Me: Auditory Exercises for Adults
Alexander Graham Bell Association
3417 Volta Place NW
Washington, DC 20007-2737
202-337-5220
Fax: 202-337-8270
TTY: 202-337-5220

Helps hard of hearing teenagers and adults to listen, lip read, pick up clues from conversations and remember what they have heard.
65 pages

4437 Listen with the Heart: Relationships and Hearing Loss
Hearing Loss Association of America
7910 Woodmont Avenue
Bethesda, MD 20814-3079
301-657-2248
Fax: 301-913-9413
TTY: 301-657-2249
e-mail: info@hearingloss.org
www.hearingloss.org

Written for family and friends as well as professionals. It is an excellent text for college and graduate level courses in psychology, mental health counseling, speech and hearing, special education, and deaf education.
Jerry Portis, Executive Director
Brenda Battat, Assistant Executive Director

4438 Listening
National Catholic Office for the Deaf
7201 Buchnan Street
Landover Hills, MD 20784-4500
301-577-1684
e-mail: nco@erols.com
www.ncod.org

Published as a pastoral service for the hearing impaired.

4439 Listening & Talking
Alexander Graham Bell Association
3417 Volta Place NW
Washington, DC 20007-2737
202-337-5220
Fax: 202-337-8270
TTY: 202-337-5220

This guide promotes spoken language in young hearing-impaired children.
191 pages

4440 Listening to Learn: A Handbook for Parents with Hearing-Impaired Children
Alexander Graham Bell Association
3417 Volta Place NW
Washington, DC 20007-2737
202-337-5220
Fax: 202-337-8270
TTY: 202-337-5220

Developed by teachers, this handbook provides parents with the essential steps necessary to develop effective spoken communication with their children.
98 pages

4441 Listening: Ways of Hearing in a Silent World
Hannah Merker, author
Hearing Loss Association of America
7910 Woodmont Avenue
Bethesda, MD 20814-3079
301-657-2248
Fax: 301-913-9413
TTY: 301-657-2249
e-mail: info@hearingloss.org
www.hearingloss.org

This book is about one woman's evocative account of her perceptions and rememberance of sound.
1999
Jerry Portis, Executive Director
Brenda Battat, Assistant Executive Director

4442 Literature Journal
Gallaudet University

11030 S Langley Avenue
Chicago, IL 60628-3819 800-621-2736
Fax: 800-621-8476
TTY: 888-630-9347
www.gallaudet.edu/~gupress

This book includes extensive examples of student and teacher entries taken from actual journals of deaf high school students.
44 pages

4443 Living with Hearing Loss
Marcia B Dugan, author
Hearing Loss Association of America
7910 Woodmont Avenue 301-657-2248
Bethesda, MD 20814-3079 Fax: 301-913-9413
TTY: 301-657-2249
e-mail: info@hearingloss.org
www.hearingloss.org

Living with Hearing Loss takes the reader from A to Z on the kinds and causes of hearing loss and its common early signs. Topics Include: Seeking Professional Evaluations, Hearing Aids, Assistive Technology, Speechreading, Communication Tips, Cochlear Implants, Dealing with Tinnitus, and resources.
2003
ISBN: 1-563681-34-0
Jerry Portis, Executive Director
Brenda Battat, Assistant Executive Director

4444 Looking Back: A Reader on the History of Deaf Communities & Sign Language
Gallaudet University
11030 S Langley Avenue
Chicago, IL 60628-3819 800-621-2736
Fax: 800-621-8476
TTY: 888-630-9347
www.gallaudet.edu/~gupress

Renowned researchers from around the world present provocative findings in six areas relating to the deaf culture.
558 pages

4445 Loss for Words
Gallaudet University
11030 S Langley Avenue
Chicago, IL 60628-3819 800-621-2736
Fax: 800-621-8476
TTY: 888-630-9347
www.gallaudet.edu/~gupress

The author's touching story of her life as an interpreter for her parents, head of her household by the age of eight and a teacher and helper to both of her deaf parents.
208 pages

4446 Mainstreaming Deaf and Hard of Hearing Students
Gallaudet University
800 Florida Avenue NE 202-651-5000
Washington, DC 20002-3695 800-621-2736
Fax: 800-621-8476
TTY: 888-630-9347
www.gallaudet.edu/~gupress

Gallaudet University is the world leader in liberal education and career development for deaf and hard-of-hearing undergraduate students.
40 pages

4447 Man Without Words
Gallaudet University
11030 S Langley Avenue
Chicago, IL 60628-3819 800-621-2736
Fax: 800-621-8476
TTY: 888-630-9347
www.gallaudet.edu/~gupress

Author relates her experiences teaching sign language to a 27 year old deaf Mexican man who had no education and no language.
203 pages

4448 Martimer
APSEA-RCHI
Box 308 902-667-3808
Amherst, NS, B4H 3Z6, Fax: 902-667-0893

Periodical describing programs and services provided by the APSEA Resource Center for the Hearing Impaired.
Phyllis Cameron, Editor

4449 Mask of Benevolence: Disabling the Deaf Community
Gallaudet University
11030 S Langley Avenue
Chicago, IL 60628-3819 800-621-2736
Fax: 800-621-8476
TTY: 888-630-9347
www.gallaudet.edu/~gupress

Written by a doctor who does not view deafness as a handicap but rather a different state of hearing.
310 pages

4450 Meeting Halfway in ASL
MSM Productions
PO Box 23380 716-442-6370
Rochester, NY 14692-3380 Fax: 716-442-6371
TTY: 716-442-6370
e-mail: Books@deaflife.com
www.deaflife.com

Illustrated photographic sign-language book containing 1,300 photos.

ISBN: 0-963401-67-
Matthew Moore, Publisher

4451 Meeting the Challenge: Hearing-Impaired Professionals in the Workplace
Gallaudet University
11030 S Langley Avenue
Chicago, IL 60628-3819 800-621-2736
Fax: 800-621-8476
TTY: 888-630-9347
www.gallaudet.edu/~gupress

Provides information on communication methods, educational backgrounds and job search tactics used by more than 1500 participants and their current employment conditions.
236 pages

4452 Mental Health Services for Deaf People
Gallaudet University
11030 S Langley Avenue
Chicago, IL 60628-3819 800-621-2736
Fax: 800-621-8476
TTY: 888-630-9347
www.gallaudet.edu/~gupress

Contains information on over 350 mental health programs and services for deaf people across the United States.
210 pages

4453 Missing Words: The Family Handbook on Adult Hearing Loss
Gallaudet University
11030 S Langley Avenue
Chicago, IL 60628-3819 800-621-2736
Fax: 800-621-8476
TTY: 888-630-9347
www.gallaudet.edu/~gupress

Written by a mother who lost her hearing and her daughter, learning to cope.
304 pages

4454 Mother Father Deaf: Living Between Sound and Silence
Harvard University Press
79 Garden Street 617-495-2480
Cambridge, MA 02138-1423 800-448-2242
Fax: 800-962-4983
www.hup.harvard.edu

Based on interviews with 150 adult hearing children of deaf parents who chart the sometimes difficult middle ground between spoken and signed language.

4455 Moving Toward the Standards
Gallaudet University
11030 S Langley Avenue
Chicago, IL 60628-3819 800-621-2736
Fax: 800-621-8476
TTY: 888-630-9347
www.gallaudet.edu/~gupress

A national action plan for mathematics education reform for the deaf.
55 pages

4456 Music in Motion
Modern Signs Press
PO Box 1181
Los Alamitos, CA 90720-1181
562-596-8548
800-572-7332
Fax: 562-795-6614
TTY: 562-493-4168
e-mail: modsigns@aol.com
www.modsigns.com
Includes guitar notes and glossary of sign descriptions for 325-word vocabulary.
109 pages
ISBN: 0-916708-07-1

4457 NAD Deaf Awareness Kit
National Association of the Deaf
8630 Fenton Street
Silver Spring, MD 20910
301-587-1788
Fax: 301-587-1791
TTY: 301-587-1789
www.nad.org
Includes information that can be used both during Deaf Awareness Week and year-round to recognize the accomplishments and heritage of the deaf community.
Donna Morris, Publications Manager

4458 Never the Twain Shall Meet: The Communications Debate
Gallaudet University
11030 S Langley Avenue
Chicago, IL 60628-3819
800-621-2736
Fax: 800-621-8476
TTY: 888-630-9347
www.gallaudet.edu/~gupress
Should sign language be used in the education of Deaf children or should they be forced to deal with a hearing, speaking world on its own terms?.
129 pages

4459 Next Step
Gallaudet University
11030 S Langley Avenue
Chicago, IL 60628-3819
800-621-2736
Fax: 800-621-8476
TTY: 888-630-9347
www.gallaudet.edu/~gupress
A national conference focusing on issues related to substance abuse in the deaf and hard of hearing population.
209 pages

4460 No Sound
Harris Communications
6541 City W Parkway
Eden Prairie, MN 55344-3248
612-906-1180
Fax: 612-946-0924
A moving, highly informative autobiography of Julius Wiggins, founder and president of the newspaper Silent News. Second edition.
211 pages

4461 No Walls of Stone: An Anthology of Literature by Deaf Writers
Gallaudet University
11030 S Langley Avenue
Chicago, IL 60628-3819
800-621-2736
Fax: 800-621-8476
TTY: 888-630-9347
www.gallaudet.edu/~gupress
Short fiction, essays, verse and drama written by the deaf and hard of hearing writer.
240 pages
Jill Jepson, Editor

4462 None So Deaf
Gallaudet University
11030 S Langley Avenue
Chicago, IL 60628-3819
800-621-2736
Fax: 800-621-8476
TTY: 888-630-9347
www.gallaudet.edu/~gupress
A student history of education of deaf people and the development of sign language.
51 pages Paperback

4463 Odyssey of Hearing Loss: Tales of Triumph
Michael A Harvey, PhD, author
Hearing Loss Association of America
7910 Woodmont Avenue
Bethesda, MD 20814-3079
301-657-2248
Fax: 301-913-9413
TTY: 301-657-2249
e-mail: info@hearingloss.org
www.hearingloss.org
A glimpse into the lives of 10 people; each showing how sharing insights about hearing loss helps people on the road to healing and a life well examined.
Jerry Portis, Executive Director
Brenda Battat, Assistant Executive Director

4464 Okada Hearing Ear Guide
RR 1 Box 640F
Fontana, WI 53125-9714
414-275-5226
Trains dogs to aid hearing-impaired persons.

4465 On My Own
Gallaudet University
11030 S Langley Avenue
Chicago, IL 60628-3819
800-621-2736
Fax: 800-621-8476
TTY: 888-630-9347
www.gallaudet.edu/~gupress
Book examining doorbell devices, alarm clocks, telephone amplifiers and other assistive devices for the deaf.
50 pages Teacher's Guide

4466 Oral Interpreting Selections from Papers from Kirsten Gonzales
Alexander Graham Bell Association
3417 Volta Place NW
Washington, DC 20007-2737
202-337-5220
Fax: 202-337-8270
TTY: 202-337-5220
These six easy to read articles discuss speech reading and oral interpreting. The articles answer questions that are frequently asked by professionals and the general public.
30 pages

4467 Other Side of Silence
Gallaudet University
11030 S Langley Avenue
Chicago, IL 60628-3819
800-621-2736
Fax: 800-621-8476
TTY: 888-630-9347
www.gallaudet.edu/~gupress
Explores the deaf community through interviews from across the country.
256 pages

4468 Our Forgotten Children: 3rd Edition
Alexander Graham Bell Association
3417 Volta Place NW
Washington, DC 20007-2737
202-337-5220
Fax: 202-337-8270
TTY: 202-337-5220
This simple book describes characteristics of hard-of-hearing children in the school and discusses their educational requirements, psychological and social needs and amplification options.
68 pages

4469 Our Forgotten Children: Hard of Hearing Pupils in the Schools
Julia M Davis, PhD, author
Hearing Loss Association of America
7910 Woodmont Avenue
Bethesda, MD 20814-3079
301-657-2248
Fax: 301-913-9413
TTY: 301-657-2249
e-mail: info@hearingloss.org
www.hearingloss.org
Important resource about the educational environment.
2001
Jerry Portis, Executive Director
Brenda Battat, Assistant Executive Director

4470 **Outsiders in a Hearing World**
Gallaudet University
11030 S Langley Avenue
Chicago, IL 60628-3819
800-621-2736
Fax: 800-621-8476
TTY: 888-630-9347
www.gallaudet.edu/~gupress
The author gives a sociologist's view of what it is like to be deaf.
240 pages

4471 **Parents and Teachers: Partners in Language Development**
Alexander Graham Bell Association
3417 Volta Place NW
Washington, DC 20007-2737
202-337-5220
Fax: 202-337-8270
TTY: 202-337-5220
Outlines the essential role of the teacher and parent in the development of language in the school aged child with hearing impairment.
386 pages

4472 **Perigee Visual Dictionary of Signing**
Harris Communications
6541 City W Parkway
Eden Prairie, MN 55344-3248
612-906-1180
Fax: 612-946-0924
An A-to-Z guide to American Sign Language vocabulary.
450 pages

4473 **Perspectives Folio: Mainstreaming**
Gallaudet University
11030 S Langley Avenue
Chicago, IL 60628-3819
800-621-2736
Fax: 800-621-8476
TTY: 888-630-9347
www.gallaudet.edu/~gupress
Presents 14 articles from Perspectives magazine that offer practical, experience-based advice on mainstreaming for parents and students themselves.
39 pages

4474 **Perspectives on Deafness**
National Association of the Deaf
8630 Fenton Street
Silver Spring, MD 20910
301-587-1788
Fax: 301-587-1791
TTY: 301-587-1789
www.nad.org
Focuses on the many perspectives which constitute diversity within the deaf community.
Paperback
Donna Morris, Publications Manager

4475 **Place of Their Own: Creating the Deaf Community in America**
Gallaudet University Press
11030 S Langley Avenue
Chicago, IL 60628-3819
800-621-2736
TTY: 888-630-9347
www.gallaudet.edu
Traces the history of deaf people and views deafness not from the perspective of a pathology, but of culture, not as a disease or disability to overcome or be cured, but as the distinguishing characteristic of a distinct community of individuals whose history and achievement are worthy of study.

4476 **Politics of Deafness**
Gallaudet University
11030 S Langley Avenue
Chicago, IL 60628
800-621-2736
Fax: 800-621-8476
TTY: 888-630-9347
www.gallaudet.edu/~gupress
Embarks upon a postmodern examination of the search for identity in deafness and its relationship to the prevalent Hearing culture that has marginalized Deaf people.
June 1997 304 pages Softcover
ISBN: 1-563680-58-0

4477 **Possible Dream: Mainstream Experiences of Hearing-Impaired Students**
Alexander Graham Bell Association
3417 Volta Place NW
Washington, DC 20007-2737
202-337-5220
Fax: 202-337-8270
TTY: 202-337-5220
This collection highlights the experiences of auditory-oral children who are Bell Association financial aid winners and their families.
66 pages
Mildred L Oberkotter, Editor

4478 **Post Milan**
Gallaudet University
11030 S Langley Avenue
Chicago, IL 60628-3819
800-621-2736
Fax: 800-621-8476
TDD: 800-621-8476
www.gallaudet.edu/~gupress
Timely issues covering trends in ASL and ASL/English literacy.
323 pages

4479 **PreReading Strategies**
Gallaudet University
11030 S Langley Avenue
Chicago, IL 60628-3819
800-621-2736
Fax: 800-621-8476
TTY: 888-630-9347
www.gallaudet.edu/~gupress
Here is a wealth of good advice for preparing students to understand what they read, building comprehension and enjoyment.
65 pages

4480 **Psychoeducational Assessment of Hearing-Impaired Students**
Pro-Ed, Inc.
8700 Shoal Creek Boulevard
Austin, TX 78757-6897
512-451-3246
Fax: 512-451-8542
e-mail: info@proedinc.com
www.proedinc.com
This book includes a comprehensive presentation of issues and procedures related to the assessment of hearing-impaired students.
251 pages Paperback
ISBN: 0-890794-55-3
Lindy Jordaan, Marketing Coordinator

4481 **Reading and Deafness**
Pro-Ed, Inc.
8700 Shoal Creek Boulevard
Austin, TX 78757-6897
512-451-3246
800-897-3202
Fax: 800-397-7633
e-mail: info@proedinc.com
www.proedinc.com
Three areas are looked at in this book: deaf children's prereading development of real-world knowledge; cognitive abilities and linguistic skills.
422 pages Hardcover
ISBN: 0-887441-07-6
Lindy Jordaan, Marketing Coordinator

4482 **Rebuilt: My Journey Back to the Hearing World**
Michael Chorost, author
Hearing Loss Association of America
7910 Woodmont Avenue
Bethesda, MD 20814-3079
301-657-2248
Fax: 301-913-9413
TTY: 301-657-2249
e-mail: info@hearingloss.org
www.hearingloss.org
Brimming with insight and written with charm and self-deprecating humor, Rebuilt unveils, in personal terms, the astounding possibilities of a new technological age.
240 pages Paperback
ISBN: 0-618717-60-9
Jerry Portis, Executive Director
Brenda Battat, Assistant Executive Director

4483 **Say That Again, Please**
Gallaudet University
11030 S Langley Avenue
Chicago, IL 60628-3819
800-621-2736
Fax: 800-621-8476
TTY: 888-630-9347
www.gallaudet.edu/~gupress

This book serves to enlighten those who are interested.
370 pages

4484 Schedules of Development for Hearing Impaired Infants and their Parents
Alexander Graham Bell Association
3417 Volta Place NW 202-337-5220
Washington, DC 20007-2737 Fax: 202-337-8270
TTY: 202-337-5220
Written for parents and teachers, this assessment record of verbal learning will help to evaluate each child's language development.
1977 14 pages

4485 Science of Sound
Gallaudet University
11030 S Langley Avenue
Chicago, IL 60628-3819 800-621-2736
Fax: 800-621-8476
TTY: 888-630-9347
www.gallaudet.edu/~gupress
This exciting book is carefully designed to help hearing-impaired students understand, use and enjoy the principles of sound.
32 pages

4486 Seeds of Disquiet: One Deaf Woman's Experience
Gallaudet University
11030 S Langley Avenue
Chicago, IL 60628-3819 800-621-2736
Fax: 800-621-8476
TTY: 888-630-9347
www.gallaudet.edu/~gupress
This book relates to the story of how Cheryl Heppner reacted to two severe losses in her hearing.
192 pages

4487 Seeing Voices: A Journey Into the World of the Deaf
Gallaudet University
11030 S Langley Avenue
Chicago, IL 60628-3819 800-621-2736
Fax: 800-621-8476
TTY: 888-630-9347
www.gallaudet.edu/~gupress
Dr. Sacks takes us into the world of deaf people.
180 pages

4488 Sign Communication: A Family Affair
Gallaudet University
11030 S Langley Avenue
Chicago, IL 60628-3819 800-621-2736
Fax: 800-621-8476
TTY: 888-630-9347
www.gallaudet.edu/~gupress
Book designed to help hearing parents communicate effectively with their deaf children on issues of good health and personal growth.
132 pages

4489 Sign Language Feelings
Gallaudet University
11030 S Langley Avenue
Chicago, IL 60628-3819 800-621-2736
Fax: 800-621-8476
TTY: 888-630-9347
www.gallaudet.edu/~gupress
Worksheets teach signs for happy, sad and all of the feelings in between.

4490 Sign Language Interpreters and Interpreting
Gallaudet University
11030 S Langley Avenue
Chicago, IL 60628-3819 800-621-2736
Fax: 800-621-8476
TTY: 888-630-9347
www.gallaudet.edu/~gupress
This monograph presents articles about personal characteristics and abilities of interpreters, the effects of lag time on interpreter errors, and the interpretation of register.
161 pages

4491 Sign Language Made Simple
Gospel Publishing House
1445 N Boonville Avenue 417-862-2781
Springfield, MO 65802-1894 Fax: 417-862-7566
e-mail: jclore@ag.org
www.GospelPublishing.com
Illustrated sign language text with descriptions of the origin of selected signs and examples of how each is used. Second edition.
240 pages
Judy Clore, Promotions Coordinator

4492 Sign Language Talk
Franklin Watts Grolier
90 Old Sherman Tpke 203-797-3500
Danbury, CT 06816-0001 800-843-3749
Fax: 203-797-3197
www.grolier.com
Using 300 easy-to-follow illustrations, this book introduces the structure of sign language, shows how sentences are formed and how signed conversations differ from spoken ones.
96 pages
ISBN: 0-531105-97-0

4493 Sign Language and the Deaf Community: Essays in Honor of William Stokoe
National Association of the Deaf
8630 Fenton Street 301-587-1788
Silver Spring, MD 20910 Fax: 301-587-1791
TTY: 301-587-1789
www.nad.org
Collection of essays, written by professionals in the field of sign language research and usage, describing how information has dramatically altered society's understanding of deaf people and their culture.
267 pages Paperback
Donna Morris, Publications Manager

4494 Signed English Starter
Harris Communications
6541 City W Parkway 612-906-1108
Eden Prairie, MN 55344-3248 Fax: 612-946-0924
The first book to use when learning Signed English.
208 pages

4495 Signing Exact English
Modern Signs Press
PO Box 1181 562-596-8548
Los Alamitos, CA 90720-1181 800-572-7332
Fax: 562-795-6614
TTY: 562-493-4168
e-mail: modsigns@aol.com
www.modsigns.com
A reference manual containing manual signs representing nearly 4,000 words, plus signs for letters, numbers, prefixes and suffixes.
1993 479 pages Softcover
ISBN: 0-196708-23-3

4496 Signing Illustrated
Gallaudet University
11030 S Langley Avenue
Chicago, IL 60628-3819 800-621-2736
Fax: 800-621-8476
TTY: 888-630-9347
www.gallaudet.edu/~gupress
A guide presenting illustrations of over 1,350 signs.
85 pages

4497 Signing Naturally: Teacher's Curriculum Guide-Level 1
DawnSignPress
6130 Nancy Ridge Drive 619-625-0600
San Diego, CA 92121-3223 800-549-5350
Fax: 619-625-2336
e-mail: DawnSign@aol.com
Guide and video.
336 pages 22 minutes
ISBN: 0-915035-07-3

4498 Signs Everywhere
Modern Signs Press

PO Box 1181 562-596-8548
Los Alamitos, CA 90720-1181 800-572-7332
Fax: 562-795-6614
TTY: 562-493-4168
e-mail: modsigns@aol.com
www.modsigns.com

Includes signs for cities, towns and states through United States, Canada and Mexico. Drawings and descriptions of the signs accompany maps showing locations of states and cities.
280 pages
ISBN: 0-916708-05-5

4499 Signs for Computing Terminology
National Association of the Deaf
8630 Fenton Street 301-587-1788
Silver Spring, MD 20910-4500 Fax: 301-587-1791
TTY: 301-587-1789
www.nad.org

Contains over 600 computer related sign illustrations used by deaf and hearing computer specialists.
182 pages Paperback
ISBN: 0-913072-63-X
Donna Morris, Publications Manager

4500 Silent Alarm: On the Edge with a Deaf EMT
Gallaudet University
11030 S Langley Avenue
Chicago, IL 60628-3819 800-621-2736
Fax: 800-621-8476
TTY: 888-630-9347
www.gallaudet.edu/~gupress

Silent Alarm tells the gripping story of survival and the good that the author did as a topnotch EMT.
160 pages

4501 Silent Garden: Raising Your Deaf Child
Gallaudet University
11030 S Langley Avenue
Chicago, IL 60628 800-621-2736
Fax: 800-621-8476
TTY: 888-630-9347
www.gallaudet.edu/~gupress

Provides parents with a firm foundation for making the difficult decisions necessary for their deaf child's future. Includes information on critical concerns, communication, technological alternative, and reassurance through case studies and interviews.
304 pages Softcover
ISBN: 1-563680-58-0

4502 Simultaneous Communication, ASL and Other Communication Modes
Gallaudet University
11030 S Langley Avenue
Chicago, IL 60628-3819 800-621-2736
Fax: 800-621-8476
TTY: 888-630-9347
www.gallaudet.edu/~gupress

This monograph presents four major articles that examine issues surrounding communications in an educational environment.
236 pages

4503 Sing Praise
Sunday School Board of the Southern Baptists
127 9th Avenue N
Nashville, TN 37234-0001 800-458-2772

For use by interpreters to the deaf.

4504 Sociolinguistics in Deaf Communities
Gallaudet University
11030 S Langley Avenue
Chicago, IL 60628-3819 800-621-2736
Fax: 800-621-8476
TTY: 888-630-9347
www.gallaudet.edu/~gupress

The first volume in a series offering assessments and up-to-date information on sign language linguistics.
280 pages

4505 Software to Go
Gallaudet University
11030 S Langley Avenue
Chicago, IL 60628-3819 800-621-2736
Fax: 800-621-8476
TTY: 888-630-9347
www.gallaudet.edu/~gupress

Lists and describes commercial software that may be borrowed by educators of hearing impaired students.
100 pages

4506 Sound and Sign, Childhood Deafness and Mental Health
Gallaudet University
11030 S Langley Avenue
Chicago, IL 60628-3819 800-621-2736
Fax: 800-621-8476
TTY: 888-630-9347
www.gallaudet.edu/~gupress

Presents research to support beliefs that deaf children should be educated using a combination manual and oral communication in residual hearing and speech.
265 pages

4507 Speak to Me
Gallaudet University
11030 S Langley Avenue
Chicago, IL 60628-3819 800-621-2736
Fax: 800-621-8476
TTY: 888-630-9347
www.gallaudet.edu/~gupress

A story of a single mother confronted with the deafness of her son.
160 pages

4508 Speech and the Hearing-Impaired Child
Alexander Graham Bell Association
3417 Volta Place NW 202-337-5220
Washington, DC 20007-2737 Fax: 202-337-8270
TTY: 202-337-5220

Provides a systematic approach to the teaching of speech and a challenge to all involved in the development of spoken language skills in hearing-impaired children.
402 pages

4509 Speechreading in Context
Gallaudet University
11030 S Langley Avenue
Chicago, IL 60628-3819 800-621-2736
Fax: 800-621-8476
TTY: 888-630-9347
www.gallaudet.edu/~gupress

This useful guide for teachers and therapists approaches speechreading instruction with the help of context cues.
32 pages

4510 Speechreading: A Way to Improve Understanding
Gallaudet University
11030 S Langley Avenue
Chicago, IL 60628-3819 800-621-2736
Fax: 800-621-8476
TTY: 888-630-9347
www.gallaudet.edu/~gupress

Designed for a wide audience, this book presents valuable information on the nature and process of speechreading and its benefits.
152 pages

4511 Speechreading: A Way to Improve Understand ing
Harriet Kaplan, author
Hearing Loss Association of America
7910 Woodmont Avenue 301-657-2248
Bethesda, MD 20814 Fax: 301-913-9413
TTY: 3016572249
e-mail: info@hearingloss.org
www.hearingloss.org

Discusses the nature and process of speechreading, its benefits, and its limitations. This useful book clarifies commonly-held misconceptions about speechreading. The beginning chapters address difficult communication situations and problems related to the speaker, the speechreader, and the environment It then offers strategies to manage them.
160 pages Paperback
Jerry Portis, Executive Director
Brenda Battat, Assistant Executive Director

4512 **Study of American Deaf Folklore**
Gallaudet University
11030 S Langley Avenue
Chicago, IL 60628-3819
800-621-2736
Fax: 800-621-8476
TTY: 888-630-9347
www.gallaudet.edu/~gupress

Presents a discussion of the different functions that folklore serves in the community.
156 pages

4513 **Substance Abuse and Recovery: Empowerment of Deaf Persons**
Gallaudet University
11030 S Langley Avenue
Chicago, IL 60628-3819
800-621-2736
Fax: 800-621-8476
TTY: 888-630-9347
www.gallaudet.edu/~gupress

Professionals in the field of substance abuse and deafness present their views on abuse.
217 pages

4514 **Talk with Me**
Alexander Graham Bell Association
3417 Volta Place NW
Washington, DC 20007-2737
202-337-5220
Fax: 202-337-8270
TTY: 202-337-5220

Written by a clinical psychologist and mother, this book educates parents and professionals about crucial early decisions that affect the speech, language, auditory, social and emotional development of children with hearing impairments.
222 pages

4515 **Teaching English to the Deaf as a Second Language**
Depart. of English, Gallaudet University
800 Florida Avenue NE
Washington, DC 20002
202-651-5000
e-mail: janice-johnson@gallaudet.edu
eli.gallaudet.edu/

Publishes articles of practical interest to classroom teachers of hearing impaired and second language students.

Kendall Green

4516 **There's a Hearing Impaired Child in my Class**
Gallaudet University
11030 S Langley Avenue
Chicago, IL 60628-3819
800-621-2736
Fax: 800-621-8476
TTY: 888-630-9347
www.gallaudet.edu/~gupress

This complete package provides basic facts about deafness, practical strategies for teaching hearing impaired children, and the question-and-answer information for all students.
44 pages

4517 **Thirteen Keys to A Successful High School Experience**
Alexander Graham Bell Association
3417 Volta Place NW
Washington, DC 20007-2737
202-337-5220
Fax: 202-337-8270
TTY: 202-337-5220

In this booklet, three students who have profound hearing losses share their mainstream education experiences. This booklet is great for teachers of any age child and many of the suggestions to make mainstreaming easier are practical and easy to implement.
1996 28 pages

4518 **Toward Effective Public School Programs for Deaf Students**
Thomas N. Kluwin, Donald F. Moores, Gonter Gaustad, author
Teachers College Press
1234 Amsterdam Avenue
New York, NY 10027
212-678-3929
Fax: 212-678-4149
e-mail: tcpress@tc.columbia.edu
www.teacherscollegepress.com

Examining various options for providing effective education-including the highly controversial practice of mainstreaming-the editors base their study on one of the largest and longest-running studies ever of public school programs for the deaf.
272 pages
ISBN: 0-807731-59-5
Martha Gonter Gaustad, Editors

4519 **Understanding Deafness Socially**
Gallaudet University
11030 S Langley Avenue
Chicago, IL 60628-3819
800-621-2736
Fax: 800-621-8476
TTY: 888-630-9347
www.gallaudet.edu/~gupress

Articles on the social dynamics of deafness.
196 pages

4520 **Understanding Ear Infections**
Alexander Graham Bell Association
3417 Volta Place NW
Washington, DC 20007-2737
202-337-5220
Fax: 202-337-8270
TTY: 202-337-5220

Based on medical research, this clinical aid for medical and hearing professionals explains ear infections and their complications to patients and their families. Sturdily designed of cardboard and spiral-bound, each page has photos and diagrams that explain each topic and answer commonly asked questions about ear infections.
1993 27 pages

4521 **Viewpoints on Deafness**
National Association of the Deaf
8630 Fenton Street
Silver Spring, MD 20910
301-587-1788
Fax: 301-587-1791
TTY: 301-587-1789
www.nad.org

Monograph presents a collection of viewpoints on deafness.
157 pages Paperback
Donna Morris, Publications Manager

4522 **Visible Speech**
SRC Software Research Corporation
Box 4277, Station A
Victoria, BC, V8X 3X8,
250-727-3744

Computerized speech culture, analysis and computer-based speech training.
6 pages
AE Wright, Publisher

4523 **Voyage to an Island**
Gallaudet University
11030 S Langley Avenue
Chicago, IL 60628-3819
800-621-2736
Fax: 800-621-8476
TTY: 888-630-9347
www.gallaudet.edu/~gupress

This book recounts the story of how the author, a deaf woman from Finland, adjusts to moving to the exotic island of St. Lucia.
248 pages

4524 **Week the World Heard Gallaudet**
Gallaudet University
11030 S Langley Avenue
Chicago, IL 60628-3819
800-621-2736
Fax: 800-621-8476
TTY: 888-630-9347
www.gallaudet.edu/~gupress

This book gives the readers a day-by-day description of the Deaf President Now movement as it unfolded from March 6 to 13, 1988.
176 pages Paperback

4525 **What is an Audiogram?**
Gallaudet University
11030 S Langley Avenue
Chicago, IL 60628-3819
800-621-2736
Fax: 800-621-8476
TTY: 888-630-9347
www.gallaudet.edu/~gupress

Here's a cheery friend to solve the mysteries of the audiogram.
16 pages

4526 **What's that Pig Outdoors? A Memoir of Deafness**
Henry Kisor, author
Pengiuin Group
375 Hudson Street
New York, NY 10014-3657 800-526-0275
Fax: 212-366-2952
e-mail: ecommerce@us.penguin.com
www.us.penguin.com
Life of a journalist who is deaf and lives in a hearing world lipreading. Discusses some of the technical advances which help the deaf.
288 pages Hardcover
ISBN: 0-140148-99-2

4527 **When Your Child is Deaf: A Guide for Parents**
Alexander Graham Bell Association
3417 Volta Place NW 202-337-5220
Washington, DC 20007-2737 Fax: 202-337-8270
TTY: 202-337-5220
This book gives encouragement and advice to parents on their essential roles in teaching speech to their child.
182 pages

4528 **When the Mind Hears**
Gallaudet University
11030 S Langley Avenue
Chicago, IL 60628-3819 800-621-2736
Fax: 800-621-8476
TTY: 888-630-9347
www.gallaudet.edu/~gupress
Told largely from the vantage point of Laurent Clerc.
460 pages

4529 **Who Speaks for the Deaf Community?**
National Association of the Deaf
8630 Fenton Street 301-587-1788
Silver Spring, MD 20910 Fax: 301-587-1791
TTY: 301-587-1789
www.nad.org
Paperback
Donna Morris, Publications Manager

4530 **Wired for Sound**
Gallaudet University
11030 S Langley Avenue
Chicago, IL 60628-3819 800-621-2736
Fax: 800-621-8476
TTY: 888-630-9347
www.gallaudet.edu/~gupress
Secondary school edition of Ear Gear, this attractive workbook is designed to give older students an in-depth understanding of hearing and hearing aids.
156 pages

4531 **Working with Deaf People: Accessibility and Accommodation in the Workplace**
2600 S 1st Street 217-789-8980
Springfield, IL 62704-4730 Fax: 217-789-9130
e-mail: books@ccthomas.com
www.ccthomas.com
Reveals the kinds of patterns of work adjustment problems that can surface among deaf employees, including the points of view of both supervisors an deaf people.
250 pages Paperback
ISBN: 0-398061-26-2
Charles C Thomas, Publisher

4532 **Working with Deaf Persons in Sunday School**
Sunday School Board of the Southern Baptists
127 9th Avenue N
Nashville, TN 37234-0001 800-458-2772
Provides guidance for organizing and conducting Sunday School classes/departments for deaf children, youth and adults.

4533 **Writer's Workshop**
Gallaudet University
11030 S Langley Avenue
Chicago, IL 60628-3819 800-621-2736
Fax: 800-621-8476
TTY: 888-630-9347
www.gallaudet.edu/~gupress
Offers suggestions to teachers who are interested in turning the classroom into an environment where students learn to express themselves in writing.
95 pages

4534 **You Just Don't Understand**
Deborah Tannen, author
Hearing Loss Association of America
7910 Woodmont Avenue 301-657-2248
Bethesda, MD 20814-3079 Fax: 301-913-9413
TTY: 301-657-2249
e-mail: info@hearingloss.org
www.hearingloss.org
Studded with lively and entertaining examples of real conversations, this book gives you the tools to understand what went wrong — and to find a common language in which to strengthen relationships at work and at home. A classic in the field of interpersonal relations, this book will change forever the way you approach conversations.
Softcover
ISBN: 0-060959-62-2
Jerry Portis, Executive Director
Brenda Battat, Assistant Executive Director

4535 **You and Your Deaf Child**
Gallaudet University
11030 S Langley Avenue
Chicago, IL 60628-3819 800-621-2736
Fax: 800-621-8476
TTY: 888-630-9347
www.gallaudet.edu/~gupress
This guide for parents explores how families interact to deal with the special impact of a child who is hearing impaired.
1997 224 pages 2nd edition

Children's Books

4536 **ABC's of Finger Spelling**
Modern Signs Press
PO Box 1181 562-596-8548
Los Alamitos, CA 90720-1181 800-572-7332
Fax: 562-795-6614
TTY: 562-493-4168
e-mail: modsigns@aol.com
www.modsigns.com
Helps teach upper and lower case letters of the alphabet. Includes printed letters and easy-to-follow drawings of the hand shapes.
60 pages
ISBN: 0-916708-13-6

4537 **Alphabet of Animal Signs**
Garlic Press
605 Powers Street 541-345-0063
Eugene, OR 97402-5337 Fax: 541-345-0063
e-mail: garlicpress@mindspring.com
www.garlicpress.com
Presents animal illustrations and associated signs for each letter of the alphabet.
16 pages Paperback
ISBN: 0-931993-65-2
SH Collins, Contact

4538 **Animal Signs: A First Book of Sign Language**
Gallaudet University
11030 S Langley Avenue
Chicago, IL 60628-3819 800-621-2736
Fax: 800-621-8476
TTY: 888-630-9347
www.gallaudet.edu/~gupress
Full-color photos of animals and their signs.
16 pages Ages 1-4

4539 **Another Handful of Stories**
Gallaudet University
11030 S Langley Avenue
Chicago, IL 60628-3819
800-621-2736
Fax: 800-621-8476
TTY: 888-630-9347
www.gallaudet.edu/~gupress
Second book contains a series of 37 stories told by deaf individuals.
124 pages

4540 **At Grandma's House**
Modern Signs Press
PO Box 1181
Los Alamitos, CA 90720-1181
562-596-8548
800-572-7332
Fax: 562-795-6614
TTY: 562-493-4168
e-mail: modsigns@aol.com
www.modsigns.com
Pictures, signs and printed words tell the tale of April, a cuddly little rabbit who loves to play with her beloved Grandma.
28 pages

4541 **Be Happy, Not Sad**
Modern Signs Press
PO Box 1181
Los Alamitos, CA 90720
562-596-8548
800-572-7332
Fax: 562-795-6614
TTY: 562-493-4168
e-mail: modsigns@aol.com
www.modsigns.com
These books help children understand hard to explain emotions through signing. Includes Be Happy Not Sad coloring workbook.
2 Book Set

4542 **Belonging**
Gallaudet University
11030 S Langley Avenue
Chicago, IL 60628-3819
800-621-2736
Fax: 800-621-8476
TTY: 888-630-9347
www.gallaudet.edu/~gupress
Gustie Blaine loses her hearing after an illness and must now learn to accept her loss and understand the changes it brings.
176 pages

4543 **Chris Gets Ear Tubes**
Gallaudet University
11030 S Langley Avenue
Chicago, IL 60628-3819
800-621-2736
Fax: 800-621-8476
TTY: 888-630-9347
www.gallaudet.edu/~gupress
A helpful book for parents and children to share concerning ear tubes and hospitals.
44 pages

4544 **Clerc: The Story of His Early Years**
Gallaudet University
11030 S Langley Avenue
Chicago, IL 60628-3819
800-621-2736
Fax: 800-621-8476
TTY: 888-630-9347
www.gallaudet.edu/~gupress
A novel by Laurent Clerc, a deaf teacher who helped Gallaudet establish schools to educate deaf Americans.
208 pages

4545 **Come Sign with Us: Sign Language Activities for Children**
Gallaudet University
11030 S Langley Avenue
Chicago, IL 60628-3819
800-621-2736
Fax: 800-621-8476
TTY: 888-630-9347
www.gallaudet.edu/~gupress
Revised version, offering more follow-up activities, including many in context, to teach children sign language. Features more than 300 line drawings of both adults and children signing familiar words, phrases, and sentences using ASL. Shows how to form each sign exactly and also presents the origins of ASL, facts about deafness, and the deaf community.
160 pages Softcover
ISBN: 1-563680-51-3

4546 **Day We Met Cindy**
Gallaudet University
11030 S Langley Avenue
Chicago, IL 60628-3819
800-621-2736
Fax: 800-621-8476
TTY: 888-630-9347
www.gallaudet.edu/~gupress
A picture storybook telling the story of Cindy, the hearing impaired aunt of one of the students of a first grade class.
32 pages

4547 **Finger Alphabet**
Gallaudet University
11030 S Langley Avenue
Chicago, IL 60628-3819
800-621-2736
Fax: 800-621-8476
TTY: 888-630-9347
www.gallaudet.edu/~gupress
Includes activities for improving fingerspelling.
30 pages

4548 **Flying Fingers Club**
Gallaudet University
11030 S Langley Avenue
Chicago, IL 60628-3819
800-621-2736
Fax: 800-621-8476
TTY: 888-630-9347
www.gallaudet.edu/~gupress
Three young friends, one deaf and two hearing find they can communicate secretly in sign language.
104 pages

4549 **Gift of the Girl Who Couldn't Hear**
Alexander Graham Bell Association
3417 Volta Place NW
Washington, DC 20007-2737
202-337-5220
Fax: 202-337-8270
TTY: 202-337-5220
This fictional novel for middle school readers introduces Eliza, a gifted singer and Lucy, her best friend who has been deaf since birth.
79 pages

4550 **Goldilocks and the Three Bears**
Gallaudet University
11030 S Langley Avenue
Chicago, IL 60628-3819
800-621-2736
Fax: 800-621-8476
TTY: 888-630-9347
www.gallaudet.edu/~gupress
Offers children ages 3-8 the classic story with new words and matching signs in Signed English.
48 pages Casebound
ISBN: 1-563680-57-2

4551 **Grandfather Moose**
Modern Signs Press
PO Box 1181
Los Alamitos, CA 90720-1181
562-596-8548
800-572-7332
Fax: 562-795-6614
TTY: 562-493-4168
e-mail: modsigns@aol.com
www.modsigns.com
Offers exciting and beautifully illustrated rhymes, games and chants in sign language.
32 pages

4552 **Handful of Stories**
Gallaudet University
11030 S Langley Avenue
Chicago, IL 60628-3819
800-621-2736
Fax: 800-621-8476
TTY: 888-630-9347
www.gallaudet.edu/~gupress

Sometimes incredible, moving and amusing, these stories are based on the personal experiences of deaf storytellers.
118 pages

4553 **Handmade Alphabet**
Gallaudet University
11030 S Langley Avenue
Chicago, IL 60628-3819
800-621-2736
Fax: 800-621-8476
TTY: 888-630-9347
www.gallaudet.edu/~gupress
This book presents 26 beautiful color drawings showing a hand forming a letter of the manual alphabet.
26 pages

4554 **Hasta Luego, San Diego**
Gallaudet University
11030 S Langley Avenue
Chicago, IL 60628-3819
800-621-2736
Fax: 800-621-8476
TTY: 888-630-9347
www.gallaudet.edu/~gupress
A Flying Fingers Club mystery.
104 pages

4555 **Hearing Loss**
Franklin Watts Grolier
90 Old Sherman Tpke
Danbury, CT 06816-0001
203-797-3500
800-621-1115
Fax: 203-797-3197
www.grolier.com
Offers a concise explanation of how and why hearing losses occur, how the ear works and how to protect your hearing.
144 pages Grades 7-12
ISBN: 0-531125-19-0

4556 **I Have a Sister, My Sister is Deaf**
TJ Publishers
817 Silver Spring Avenue
Silver Spring, MD 20910-4617
301-585-4440
800-999-1168
Fax: 301-585-5930
TTY: 301-585-4441
e-mail: tjpubinc@aol.com
An emphatic, affirmative look at the relationship between siblings, as a young deaf child is affectionately described by her older sister. This Coretta Scott King honor award winner helps young children develop an understanding that deaf children share the same interests as hearing children.
1977 32 pages Softcover
ISBN: 0-064430-59-6
Angela K Thames, President
Jerald A Murphy, VP

4557 **I Was So Mad!**
Modern Signs Press
PO Box 1181
Los Alamitos, CA 90720-1181
562-596-8548
800-572-7332
Fax: 562-795-6614
TTY: 562-493-4168
e-mail: modsigns@aol.com
www.modsigns.com
Includes manual alphabet and glossary of signs.
40 pages
ISBN: 0-916708-16-0

4558 **In Our House**
Modern Signs Press
PO Box 1181
Los Alamitos, CA 90720-1181
562-596-8548
800-572-7332
Fax: 562-795-6614
TTY: 562-493-4168
e-mail: modsigns@aol.com
www.modsigns.com
This colorful picturebook tells the story of Joy and Jason helping Mom and Dad around the house. Has a 140-word vocabulary listed in an alphabetical glossary.
32 pages
ISBN: 0-191670-81-1

4559 **Invisible Inc #4**
Alexander Graham Bell Association
3417 Volta Place NW
Washington, DC 20007-2737
202-337-5220
Fax: 202-337-8270
TTY: 202-337-5220
The intrepid trio accept an invitation to doom as they solve the mystery behind their school's haunted computer.
1996 42 pages

4560 **King Midas With Selected Sentences in ASL**
Gallaudet University
11030 S Langley Avenue
Chicago, IL 60628-3819
800-621-2736
Fax: 800-621-8476
TTY: 888-630-9347
www.gallaudet.edu/~gupress
Fairytale retold with full color illustrations and American Sign Language sentences.
72 pages Casebound
ISBN: 0-930323-75-0

4561 **Learning to Sign in my Neighborhood**
Gallaudet University
11030 S Langley Avenue
Chicago, IL 60628-3819
800-621-2736
Fax: 800-621-8476
TTY: 888-630-9347
www.gallaudet.edu/~gupress
Here are signs to learn and pictures to color, all in one friendly book.
32 pages

4562 **Little Green Monsters**
Modern Signs Press
PO Box 1181
Los Alamitos, CA 90720-1181
562-596-8548
800-572-7332
Fax: 562-795-6614
TTY: 310-493-4168
Forty-five word vocabulary in signs and printed words introduces concept of directionality. Includes manual alphabet and glossary of signs.
36 pages

4563 **Little Red Riding Hood**
Gallaudet University
11030 S Langley Avenue
Chicago, IL 60628-3819
800-621-2736
Fax: 800-621-8476
TTY: 888-630-9347
www.gallaudet.edu/~gupress
A beloved folktale that is told in American Sign Language format.
48 pages

4564 **Living with Deafness**
Franklin Watts Grolier
90 Old Sherman Tpke
Danbury, CT 06816-0001
203-797-3500
800-621-1115
Fax: 203-797-3197
www.grolier.com
Shows how deaf persons can overcome their disability and live happy, productive lives.
32 pages Grades 5-7
ISBN: 0-531108-42-2

4565 **Mandy**
Gallaudet University
11030 S Langley Avenue
Chicago, IL 60628-3819
800-621-2736
Fax: 800-621-8476
TTY: 888-630-9347
www.gallaudet.edu/~gupress
A beautiful story about a young deaf girl's relationship with her grandmother.
32 pages

4566 **Matthew Pinkowski's Special Summer**
Gallaudet University

11030 S Langley Avenue
Chicago, IL 60628-3819
800-621-2736
Fax: 800-621-8476
TTY: 888-630-9347
www.gallaudet.edu/~gupress

Matthew begins his special summer by moving to Minnesota, where he meets some special friends.
150 pages

4567 **Messy Monsters, Jungle Joggers and Bubble Baths**
Alexander Graham Bell Association
3417 Volta Place NW
Washington, DC 20007-2737
202-337-5220
Fax: 202-337-8270
TTY: 202-337-5220

This child's work book is filled with poems, stories and delightful drawings that make speaking lip reading and using residual hearing fun for the elementary school aged child.
97 pages

4568 **Mother Goose in Sign**
Garlic Press
605 Powers Street
Eugene, OR 97402-5337
541-345-0063
Fax: 541-345-0063
e-mail: garlicpress@mindspring.com
www.garlicpress.com

Fully illustrated Mother Goose nursery rhymes in sign language.
16 pages Paperback
ISBN: 0-931993-66-0
SH Collins, Contact

4569 **My ABC Signs of Animal Friends**
DawnSignPress
6130 Nancy Ridge Drive
San Diego, CA 92121-3223
619-625-0600
800-549-5350
Fax: 619-625-2336
e-mail: DawnSign@aol.com

Sign language primer for both hearing and deaf children from birth to age five.
32 pages
ISBN: 0-915035-31-6

4570 **My First Book of Sign**
Gallaudet University
11030 S Langley Avenue
Chicago, IL 60628-3819
800-621-2736
Fax: 800-621-8476
TTY: 888-630-9347
www.gallaudet.edu/~gupress

This book makes signing fun for children from three to eight.
76 pages

4571 **My Signing Book of Numbers**
Gallaudet University
11030 S Langley Avenue
Chicago, IL 60628-3819
800-621-2736
Fax: 800-621-8476
TTY: 888-630-9347
www.gallaudet.edu/~gupress

Picture book helps children learn their numbers in sign language.
56 pages

4572 **Nick's Mission**
Alexander Graham Bell Association
3417 Volta Place NW
Washington, DC 20007-2737
202-337-5220
Fax: 202-337-8270
TTY: 202-337-5220

Twelve-year-old Nick plans to spend his summer vacation at the lake, snorkeling and playing with Wags, his dog, not at speech therapy as his mother has planned. But the summer will embroil Nick and Wags in an exciting mystery that includes kidnapping, smuggling, stolen macaws and maybe even speech therapy.
1996 148 pages

4573 **Now I Understand**
Gallaudet University
11030 S Langley Avenue
Chicago, IL 60628-3819
800-621-2736
Fax: 800-621-8476
TTY: 888-630-9347
www.gallaudet.edu/~gupress

Explores what happens when a hard-of-hearing boy is mainstreamed.
56 pages

4574 **Number and Letter Games**
Gallaudet University
11030 S Langley Avenue
Chicago, IL 60628-3819
800-621-2736
Fax: 800-621-8476
TTY: 888-630-9347
www.gallaudet.edu/~gupress

A fascinating way to learning sign language with games, riddles and map skills for children and adults.
30 pages

4575 **Nursery Rhymes from Mother Goose**
Gallaudet University
11030 S Langley Avenue
Chicago, IL 60628-3819
800-621-2736
Fax: 800-621-8476
TTY: 888-630-9347
www.gallaudet.edu/~gupress

The complete nursery rhyme is presented in Signed English.
64 pages

4576 **Popsicles are Cold**
Modern Signs Press
PO Box 1181
Los Alamitos, CA 90720-1181
562-596-8548
800-572-7332
Fax: 562-795-6614
TTY: 562-493-4168
e-mail: modsigns@aol.com
www.modsigns.com

Colorful pictures and rhyming words highlight this storybook with a 33-word vocabulary in signs and printed words.
32 pages

4577 **Season of Change**
Gallaudet University
11030 S Langley Avenue
Chicago, IL 60628-3819
800-621-2736
Fax: 800-621-8476
TTY: 888-630-9347
www.gallaudet.edu/~gupress

A cheerful teenager tired of having people treat her as a problem just because she does not hear very well.
108 pages

4578 **Secret Signing: A Sign Language Activity Book**
Gallaudet University
11030 S Langley Avenue
Chicago, IL 60628-3819
800-621-2736
Fax: 800-621-8476
TTY: 888-630-9347
www.gallaudet.edu/~gupress

Children will enjoy this activity book with signs.
64 pages Level K-1

4579 **Secret in the Dorm Attic**
Gallaudet University
11030 S Langley Avenue
Chicago, IL 60628-3819
800-621-2736
Fax: 800-621-8476
TTY: 888-630-9347
www.gallaudet.edu/~gupress

Susan, Donald and Matt are back, as the Flying Fingers Club solving yet another mystery.
104 pages

4580 **Sesame Street Sign Language ABC**
Gallaudet University
11030 S Langley Avenue
Chicago, IL 60628-3819
800-621-2736
Fax: 800-621-8476
TTY: 888-630-9347
www.gallaudet.edu/~gupress

Muppets learn words and letters signed by Linda Bove.
30 pages

4581 **Sesame Street Sign Language Fun**
Gallaudet University

11030 S Langley Avenue
Chicago, IL 60628-3819 800-621-2736
Fax: 800-621-8476
TTY: 888-630-9347
www.gallaudet.edu/~gupress

This book uses the Muppets to explain concepts such as opposites, words and feelings.
62 pages

4582 **Sign Numbers**
Modern Signs Press
PO Box 1181 562-596-8548
Los Alamitos, CA 90720-1181 800-572-7332
Fax: 562-795-6614
TTY: 562-493-4168
e-mail: modsigns@aol.com
www.modsigns.com

A manual teaching sign language and written numbers that includes printed numbers and easy-to-follow drawings of the number hand shapes.
60 pages

4583 **Sign-Me-Fine**
Gallaudet University
11030 S Langley Avenue
Chicago, IL 60628-3819 800-621-2736
Fax: 800-621-8476
TTY: 888-630-9347
www.gallaudet.edu/~gupress

Written for young adults, this book introduces American Sign Language and how it differs from English.
120 pages

4584 **Signed Language Coloring Books**
Gallaudet University
11030 S Langley Avenue
Chicago, IL 60628-3819 800-621-2736
Fax: 800-621-8476
TTY: 888-630-9347
www.gallaudet.edu/~gupress

Six coloring books made up of easy-to-color pictures that include the printed, signed and fingerspelled words for each image.
16 pages

4585 **Signing for Kids**
Gallaudet University
11030 S Langley Avenue
Chicago, IL 60628-3819 800-621-2736
Fax: 800-621-8476
TTY: 888-630-9347
www.gallaudet.edu/~gupress

Contains 17 chapters dealing with special areas of interest to children like pets, family, friends and people.
142 pages

4586 **Signs for Me: Basic Vocabulary for Children, Parents and Teachers**
DawnSignPress
6130 Nancy Ridge Drive 619-625-0600
San Diego, CA 92121-3223 800-549-5350
Fax: 619-625-2336
e-mail: DawnSign@aol.com

ASL/English vocabulary primer filled with all the basics for preschoolers. The focus is on learning ASL signs and English words for better language development. Illustrates the meaning of the sign, the sign itself, and the English word in bold print.
112 pages
ISBN: 0-915035-27-8

4587 **Silent Dances**
Gallaudet University
11030 S Langley Avenue
Chicago, IL 60628-3819 800-621-2736
Fax: 800-621-8476
TTY: 888-630-9347
www.gallaudet.edu/~gupress

Space adventure story featuring a deaf graduate of Gallaudet University.
275 pages

4588 **Silent Garden: Raising Your Deaf Child**
Alexander Graham Bell Association
3417 Volta Place NW 202-337-5220
Washington, DC 20007-2737 Fax: 202-337-8270
TTY: 202-337-5220

This book provides parents of deaf children with crucial information on the possibilities afforded their children. Ogden, deaf since birth and a professor of deaf studies offers parents the foundation for making the difficult decisions necessary to start their children on the road to realizing their full potential.
1996 313 pages

4589 **Silent Observer**
Gallaudet University
11030 S Langley Avenue
Chicago, IL 60628-3819 800-621-2736
Fax: 800-621-8476
TTY: 888-630-9347
www.gallaudet.edu/~gupress

Lovely illustrations tell the story of an affectionate memoir of childhood presented through the eyes of a deaf girl.
48 pages

4590 **Simple Signs**
Gallaudet University
11030 S Langley Avenue
Chicago, IL 60628-3819 800-621-2736
Fax: 800-621-8476
TTY: 888-630-9347
www.gallaudet.edu/~gupress

Charming, full-color pictures and hints introducing ASL to children.
32 pages

4591 **Sleeping Beauty**
Gallaudet University
11030 S Langley Avenue
Chicago, IL 60628-3819 800-621-2736
Fax: 800-621-8476
TTY: 888-630-9347
www.gallaudet.edu/~gupress

Classic story with full-color illustrations and line drawings of more than 30 sentences rendered in ASL, offering new dimensions of imagination while also strengthening young readers' language skills.
64 pages
ISBN: 0-930323-97-1

4592 **Songs in Sign**
Gallaudet University
11030 S Langley Avenue
Chicago, IL 60628-3819 800-621-2736
Fax: 800-621-8476
TTY: 888-630-9347
www.gallaudet.edu/~gupress

Fully illustrated sign English.
30 pages

4593 **Very Special Sister**
Gallaudet University
11030 S Langley Avenue
Chicago, IL 60628-3819 800-621-2736
Fax: 800-621-8476
TTY: 888-630-9347
www.gallaudet.edu/~gupress

Tells the story of Laura who is deaf and her delight at the fact that she will soon have a brother.
36 pages

4594 **Where Is Spot?**
Gallaudet University
11030 S Langley Avenue
Chicago, IL 60628-3819 800-621-2736
Fax: 800-621-8476
TTY: 888-630-9347
www.gallaudet.edu/~gupress

A Signed English edition of a childhood favorite.
20 pages

4595 **Word Signs: A First Book of Sign Language**
Gallaudet University
11030 S Langley Avenue
Chicago, IL 60628-3819
800-621-2736
Fax: 800-621-8476
TTY: 888-630-9347
www.gallaudet.edu/~gupress
Full-color photos of basic words and their signs.
16 pages Ages 1-4

Magazines

4596 **American Annals of the Deaf**
Convention of American Instructors of the Deaf
800 Florida Avenue NE
Washington, DC 20002-3660
202-651-5530
Fax: 202-651-5860
TTY: 202-651-5530
e-mail: mary.carew@galludet.edu
gupress.gallaudet.edu/annals/
Scholarly journal at the forefront of research related to the education of deaf people. Annual reference Issue identifies programs and services for deaf people nationwide.
64 pages 5x Year
Donald Moores, Editor
Mary E Carew, Managing Editor

4597 **American Journal of Audiology**
American Speech-Language-Hearing Association
10801 Rockville Pike
Rockville, MD 20852-3226
301-897-5700
800-638-8255
e-mail: actioncenter@asha.org
www.asha.org
Russell L Malone PhD, Editor

4598 **American Journal of Speech-Language Pathology**
American Speech-Language-Hearing Association
10801 Rockville Pike
Rockville, MD 20852-3226
301-897-5700
800-638-8255
Russell L Malone PhD, Editor

4599 **Audiology Today**
1735 N Lynn Street
Arlington, VA 22209-2019
703-524-1923
Fax: 703-524-2303
Jerry Northern PhD, Editor

4600 **Auricle**
Auditory-Verbal International
2121 Eisenhower Avenue
Alexandria, VA 22314-4688
703-739-1049
Fax: 703-739-0395
TTY: 703-739-0874
e-mail: audiverb@aol.com
www.auditory-verbal.org
To provide the choice of listening and speaking as the way of life for children and adults who are deaf on hard of hearing.
Magazine
Sara Lake, Executive Director/CEO/Publisher
Mary Benson, Executive Assistant

4601 **Deaf Life**
MSM Productions
PO Box 23380
Rochester, NY 14692-3380
716-442-6370
Fax: 716-442-6371
www.deaflife.com
This magazine focuses on profiles, news, controversial issues, cultural topics and more relating to the Deaf community.
50 pages Monthly
Matthew Moore, Publisher

4602 **Deaf Sports Review**
American Athletic Association of the Deaf
3607 Washington Boulevard
Ogden, UT 84403-1737
801-393-8710
Fax: 801-393-2263
TTY: 801-393-7916
A magazine that describes deaf athletes and past and upcoming events.
Quarterly
Shirley Platt, Editor

4603 **Deaf USA**
Eye Festival Communications
6917B Woodley Avenue
Van Nuys, CA 91406-4844
818-902-9800
Fax: 818-902-9840
Provides news coverage on all activities and issues of interest to deaf and hard of hearing readers as well as professionals and associates within this specialized market.
Monthly
David Rosenbaum, Editor

4604 **Deaf-Blind American**
American Association of the Deaf-Blind
814 Thayer Avenue
Silver Spring, MD 20910-4500
800-735-2258
Fax: 301-588-8705
TTY: 301-588-6545
e-mail: aadb@erols.com
A journal of the American Association of the Deaf-Blind with articles on new technology, legislation news affecting deaf-blind Americans, success stories on deaf-blind, conference news, and many other topics of interest to deaf-blind people.
4x Year
Jamie McNamara, Editor

4605 **Hearing Health**
1050 17th Street NW
Washington, DC 20036
209-289-5850
e-mail: info@hearinghealthmag.com
A publication for deaf and hard-of-hearing people, as well as hearing health care professionals, libraries, agencies, schools and organizations.
BiMonthly
Paula Bartone-Bonillas, Editor

4606 **JADARA**
ADARA
PO Box 251554
Little Rock, AR 72225-1554
501-868-8850
Fax: 501-868-8812
A journal for professionals networking for excellence in service delivery with individuals who are deaf or hard of hearing. The journal is a vehicle for dissemination and exchange of information which has a large bearing on the quality of service delivery to the deaf and hearing impaired populations.
Quarterly
Gerry Walter, Editor

4607 **Journal of AAA**
American Academy of Audiology
1735 N Lynn Street
Arlington, VA 22209-2019
703-524-1923
800-222-2336
Fax: 703-524-2303
James Jerger, Editor

4608 **Journal of Speech-Language-Hearing Research**
American Speech-Language-Hearing Association
10801 Rockville Pike
Rockville, MD 20852-3226
301-897-5700
800-638-8255
Russell L Malone PhD, Editor

4609 **Language, Speech and Hearing Services in the Schools**
American Speech-Language-Hearing Association
10801 Rockville Pike
Rockville, MD 20852
301-897-5700
800-638-8255
Professional journal for clinicians, audiologists and speech-language pathologists.
Russell L Malone PhD, Editor

4610 **NADmag**
National Association of the Deaf
8630 Fenton Street
Silver Spring, MD 20910
301-587-1788
Fax: 301-587-1791
TTY: 301-587-1789
www.nad.org/nadmagadrates
Each NADmag focuses on a specific theme, such as technology and telecommunications, human services, deaf culture, education, and interpreting.
32 pages Bi-Monthly
Donna Morris, Publications Manager

4611 Perspectives in Education and Deafness
Gallaudet University
11030 S Langley Avenue
Chicago, IL 60628-3819
800-621-2736
Fax: 800-621-8476
TTY: 888-630-9347
www.gallaudet.edu/~gupress

A practical, reader-friendly magazine, offering help and advice in and beyond the classroom, tuned to the needs of today's students, teachers, and families.
5x Annually
Mary Abrams Perica, Editor

4612 SHHH Journal
Self Help For Hard of Hearing People
7910 Woodmont Avenue
Bethesda, MD 20814-3079
301-657-2248
Fax: 301-913-9413
TTY: 301-657-2249

An educational journal about hearing loss for hard-of-hearing people.
BiMonthly
Barbara G Harris, Editor

4613 Silent News
1425 Jefferson Road
Rochester, NY 14623-3139
716-272-4900
Fax: 716-272-4904
TTY: 716-272-4900

Covers news and events of interest to deaf and hard-of-hearing people all over the world.
Monthly
Tom Willard, Editor

4614 Silent News Job Bulletin
1425 Jefferson Road
Rochester, NY 14623-3139
716-272-4900
Fax: 716-272-4904
TTY: 716-272-4900

Lists current job openings and career opportunities working with deaf and hard-of-hearing people.
BiAnnually

4615 Tinnitus Today
American Tinnitus Association
PO Box 5
Portland, OR 97207-0005
503-248-9985
800-634-8978
Fax: 503-248-0024
www.ata.org

A quarterly magazine published by the American Tinnitus Association.
28 pages Quarterly
ISBN: 1-530656-9 -
David P. Fagerlie, Chief Executive Officer
Terri Baltus, Chief Development Officer

4616 USA Deaf Sports Federation
3607 Washington Boulevard
Ogden, UT 84403-1737
801-393-8710
Fax: 801-393-2263
TTY: 801-393-7916
e-mail: homeoffice@usadsf.org
www.usadsf.org

A glossy magazine called Deaf Sports Review featuring articles on all deaf sports and recreation.
Dr. Bobbie Beth Scoggins, President
Valerie Kinney, Adminstrative Assistant

4617 Volta Review
Alexander Graham Bell Association
3417 Volta Place NW
Washington, DC 20007-2737
202-337-5220
Fax: 202-337-8270
TTY: 202-337-5220

A professionally reviewed journal highlighting research and studies in the field of deafness.
5x Year
Michelle Vanderhoff, Managing Editor

4618 Volta Voices
Alexander Graham Bell Association
3417 Volta Place NW
Washington, DC 20007-2737
202-337-5220
Fax: 202-337-8270
TTY: 202-337-5220

A magazine highlighting inspirational stories from parents of children who are deaf, legislative news, technology update and stories pertaining to speech, speech reading, and the use of residual hearing.
BiMonthly
Michelle Vanderhoff, Managing Editor

4619 World Around You
Gallaudet University
11030 S Langley Avenue
Chicago, IL 60628-3819
800-621-2736
Fax: 800-621-8476
TTY: 888-630-9347
www.gallaudet.edu/~gupress

A current events magazine directed at keeping junior high and high school deaf and hard-of-hearing students informed about deaf people and the deaf community.
5x Year
Cathryn Carroll, Editor

Newsletters

4620 AAAD Bulletin
American Athletic Association of the Deaf
3607 Washington Boulevard
Ogden, UT 84403-1737
801-393-8710
Fax: 801-393-2263
TTY: 801-393-7916

A newsletter describing deaf athletes and upcoming events.
Quarterly
Shirley Platt, Editor

4621 ADARA Updated
ADARA
PO Box 251554
Little Rock, AR 72225-1554
501-868-8850
Fax: 501-868-8812

Updates readers on events, resources, legislation, information of national interest, conferences, workshops and employment opportunities. Information from and about local chapters, special interest sections, and national organizations is included in this publication.
Quarterly
Nanncy Long PhD, Editor

4622 ALDA News
Association of Late-Deafened Adults
1131 Lake Street
Oak Park, IL 60301
877-907-1738
Fax: 877-907-1738
TTY: 708-358-0135
www.alda.org

Marilyn Howe, Publisher

4623 Adult Bible Lessons for the Deaf
Sunday School Board of the Southern Baptists
127 9th Avenue N
Nashville, TN 37234-0001
800-458-2772

Bible study quarterly that relates to the needs of deaf and hearing impaired persons.
Quarterly

4624 Audiology Express
American Academy of Audiology
1735 N Lynn Street
Arlington, VA 22209-2019
703-524-1923
800-222-2336
Fax: 703-524-2303

4625 Better Hearing News
Better Hearing Institute
5021B Backlick Road
Annandale, VA 22003-6043
703-642-0580
800-327-9355
Fax: 703-750-9302

Quarterly
Jerry J Rizzo, Executive Director

4626 Canine Listener
Dogs for the Deaf
10175 Wheeler Road
Central Point, OR 97502-9360
541-826-9220

Offers information on various dogs for the deaf that are available, hotlines, support groups and articles on the newest technology for the hard of hearing person.
Quarterly
Robin Dickson, Executive Director

4627 **Caption Center News**
Caption Center
125 Western Avenue 617-429-9225
Boston, MA 02134-1008 Fax: 617-562-0590
Reports developments in closed captioning for persons with hearing impairments.

4628 **Deaf Artists of America**
302 Goodman Street N 716-244-3460
Rochester, NY 14607-1148 Fax: 716-244-3690
TTY: 716-244-3460
Tom Willard, Editor

4629 **Deaf Episcopalian**
Episcopal Conference of the Deaf
PO Box 27459 215-247-1059
Philadelphia, PA 19118-0459 e-mail: Bmose@aol.com
www.ecdeaf.com/
Rev. Virginia Nagel, Editor

4630 **Deaf Work**
Baptist Sunday School Board
127 9th Avenue N 615-251-2000
Nashville, TN 37234-0002
Offers information for religious workers and church educators who teach the handicapped.

4631 **Deafpride Advocate**
Deafpride
1350 Potomac Avenue SE 202-675-6700
Washington, DC 20003-4412

4632 **Endeavor**
American Society for Deaf Children
PO Box 3355 717-334-7922
Gettysburg, PA 17325-1373 800-942-2732
Fax: 717-334-8808
TTY: 717-334-7922
e-mail: asdc1@aol.com
www.deafchildren.org
Newsletter for parents of deaf children.
36 pages Quarterly
Linda Zumbrun, Operations Manager

4633 **Frat**
National Fraternal Society of the Deaf
1300 W NW Highway 847-392-9282
Mt Prospect, IL 60056-2217 Fax: 847-392-9298
TTY: 708-392-1409
Offers fraternal insurance information and news about members.
BiMonthly
Wayne D Shook, Editor

4634 **GA-SK Newsletter**
Telecommunications for the Deaf
8630 Fenton Street 301-589-3786
Silver Spring, MD 20910-3822 Fax: 301-589-3797
TTY: 301-589-3006
A newsletter focusing on issues for the deaf and hearing impaired person.
Quarterly
Barry Solomon, Editor
Alfred Sonnenstrahl, Manager

4635 **Gallaudet Today**
Galladet University
575 5th Avenue 212-599-0027
Washington, DC 20002 Fax: 212-599-0039
www.drf.org
A university publication with both general and special issues on deafness-related topics.
Quarterly
Vickie Walter, Editor

4636 **Hear**
Deafness Research Foundation
15 W 39th Street 212-768-1181
New York, NY 10018-3806
Offers information on the Foundation's activities and events, technical updates on assistive devices, legislative and medical information on the latest breakthroughs and laws for the hearing impaired, book reviews and resources.
Monte H Jacoby, Executive Director

4637 **NTID Focus**
National Technical Institute for the Deaf
52 Lomb Memorial Drive 716-475-6906
Rochester, NY 14623-5604 Fax: 716-475-5623
e-mail: ntidmc@rit.edu
www.rit.edu/ntid
A college publication featuring news and stories about NTID programs and community members.
TriAnnual
Kathryn Shwartz, Editor

4638 **Newsletter of American Hearing Research**
American Hearing Research Foundation
8 S Michigan Avenue 312-726-9670
Chicago, IL 60603-4539 Fax: 312-726-9695
e-mail: blederer@american-hearing.org
www.american-hearing.org
Concerned with hearing research and education.
6-8 pages 3 per year
William L Lederer, Executive Director
Sharon Parmet, Development/Communications Associate

4639 **Newsline**
Sertoma Foundation
1912 E Meyer Boulevard 816-333-8300
Kansas City, MO 64132-1141 Fax: 816-333-4320
e-mail: info@sertoma.org
www.sertoma.org
Reports on activities of the Sertoma Foundation in the field of speech and hearing impairments.

4640 **Otoscope**
EAR Foundation
1817 Patterson Street 615-329-7807
Nashville, TN 37203 800-545-4327
Fax: 615-329-7935
TTY: 615-329-7849
e-mail: ear@earfoundation.org
www.earfoundation.org
8-14 pages Quarterly
Amy Nielsen, Director Educational Progams

4641 **Research at Gallaudet**
Gallaudet University
11030 S Langley Avenue
Chicago, IL 60628-3819 800-621-2736
Fax: 800-621-8476
TTY: 888-630-9347
www.gallaudet.edu/~gupress
Newsletter reporting research and activities of the Institute.

4642 **Speech and Deafness Newsletter**
Hearing, Speech
1620 18th Avenue 206-323-5770
Seattle, WA 98122-2798
Agency newsletter for membership and community.
8 pages
Patty Tumberg, Editor

4643 **Tech Talk**
Caption Center
125 Western Avenue 617-492-9225
Boston, MA 02134-1008 Fax: 617-562-0590

4644 USA Deaf Sports Federation
3607 Washington Boulevard 801-393-8710
Ogden, UT 84403-1737 Fax: 801-393-2263
TTY: 801-393-7916
e-mail: homeoffice@usadsf.org
www.usadsf.org
A matte newsletter called USADSF Bulletin featuring articles on all deaf sports and recreation.
Dr. Bobbie Beth Scoggins, President
Valerie Kinney, Adminstrative Assistant

4645 World Federation of the Deaf News
Ilkantie 4, PO Box 65 358-058-0583
SF-00401 Helsinki Finland, Fax: 358-058-0377
The official magazine of the World Federation of the Deaf, features information on the work of the EFD, the latest news and interviews with people active in the Deaf communities throughout the world.
Quarterly
Antti Makipaa, Editor

Pamphlets

4646 25 Ways to Promote Spoken Language in Your Child with a Hearing Loss
Alexander Graham Bell Association
3417 Volta Place NW 202-337-5220
Washington, DC 20007-2737 Fax: 202-337-8270
TTY: 202-337-5220
This pamphlet teaches twenty-five golden rules about preparing your child to listen and to speak.
1995 62 pages

4647 Aging and Hearing Loss: Some Commonly Asked Questions
National Information Center on Deafness
800 Florida Avenue NE 202-651-5051
Washington, DC 20002-3660 Fax: 202-651-5054
TTY: 202-651-5052
Discusses the hearing evaulation, tests used to determine type and extent of hearing loss and what an audiogram tells us.

4648 Alerting and Communication Devices for Deaf and Hard of Hearing People
National Information Center on Deafness
800 Florida Avenue NE 202-651-5051
Washington, DC 20002 Fax: 202-651-5054
TTY: 202-651-5052
Describes general communication in everyday life.

4649 Alexander Graham Bell's Life
Alexander Graham Bell Association
3417 Volta Place NW 202-337-5220
Washington, DC 20007-2737 Fax: 202-337-8270
TTY: 202-337-5220
This pamphlet highlights Alexander Gram Bell's professional and personal involvement with deafness as a teacher of the deaf; a friend of many notable persons, including Helen Keller; a scientist interested in acoustics; the inventor of the telephone; and the founder of the Bell Association.
1996

4650 All About the New Generation of Hearing Aids
National Information Center on Deafness
800 Florida Avenue NE 202-651-5051
Washington, DC 20002-3660 Fax: 202-651-5054
TTY: 202-651-5052
Explains the terms digital hearing aid, and digitally controlled hearing aid.

4651 Assistive Devices Demonstration Centers
National Information Center on Deafness
800 Florida Avenue NE 202-651-5051
Washington, DC 20002-3660 Fax: 202-651-5054
TTY: 202-651-5052
A resource list identifying demonstration centers across the United States.

4652 Books for Parents of Deaf and Hard of Hearing Children
National Information Center on Deafness
800 Florida Avenue NE 202-651-5051
Washington, DC 20002 Fax: 202-651-5054
TTY: 202-651-5052
Identifies books written for parents and everday experiences of deaf and hard of hearing children.

4653 Care of the Ears and Hearing for Health
American Hearing Research Foundation
8 S Michigan Avenue 312-726-9670
Chicago, IL 60603-4539 Fax: 312-726-9695
e-mail: bledcrer@american-hearing.org
www.american-hearing.org
Offers information on ear infections relating to chronic progressive deafness.
William L Lederer, Executive Director
Sharon Parmet, Development/Communications Associate

4654 Consumer's Guide to Hearing Aids
Hearing Loss Association of America
7910 Woodmont Avenue 301-657-2248
Bethesda, MD 20814-3079 Fax: 301-913-9413
TTY: 301-657-2249
e-mail: info@hearingloss.org
www.hearingloss.org
Color booklet illustrating the different styles of hearing aids and comparing different models and features. Illustrates the technology pyramid and hearing aid pricing.
2006 24 pages
Jerry Portis, Executive Director
Brenda Battat, Assistant Executive Director

4655 Deaf Culture Videotapes
National Information Center on Deafness
800 Florida Avenue NE 202-651-5051
Washington, DC 20002-3660 Fax: 202-651-5054
TTY: 202-651-5052
This list identifies deaf culture and deaf history videotapes available from the Historic Film Collection of the National Association of the Deaf.

4656 Deaf Culture: Suggested Readings
National Information Center on Deafness
800 Florida Avenue NE 202-651-5051
Washington, DC 20002-3660 Fax: 202-651-5054
TTY: 202-651-5052
A selected reading list providing annotations for 62 books highlighting the community, and history of deaf people.

4657 Deafness: A Fact Sheet
National Information Center on Deafness
800 Florida Avenue NE 202-651-5051
Washington, DC 20002-3660 Fax: 202-651-5054
TTY: 202-651-5052

4658 Developing Cognition in Young Children Who are Deaf
Hope
55 E 100 N 435-752-9533
Logan, UT 84321-4648 Fax: 435-752-9533
Presents interesting, updated information on the importance of early cognition development in young children who are deaf. Contains many ideas for ways to promote early thinking skills, especially those that promote and enhance early communication and language development.

4659 Ear and Hearing
National Information Center on Deafness
800 Florida Avenue NE 202-651-5051
Washington, DC 20002-3660 Fax: 202-651-5054
TTY: 202-651-5052
An illustrated publication of the ear and what can go wrong with it.

4660 Educating Deaf Children: An Introduction
National Information Center on Deafness
800 Florida Avenue NE 202-651-5051
Washington, DC 20002-3660 Fax: 202-651-5054
TTY: 202-651-5052
Describes the different settings in which deaf children are currently educated.

4661 Facts About Hearing Aids
Alexander Graham Bell Association

3417 Volta Place NW 202-337-5220
Washington, DC 20007-2737 Fax: 202-337-8270
TTY: 202-337-5220

This brochure describes defferent types of hearing aids, factors to consider when choosing a hearing aid, the best way to go about purchasing a hearing aid. It also addresses cost and provides information on hearing conservation.

4662 Facts and Fancies About Hearing Aids
American Hearing Research Foundation
8 S Michigan Avenue 312-726-9670
Chicago, IL 60603-4539 Fax: 312-726-9695
e-mail: blederer@american-hearing.org
www.american-hearing.org

Offers information on types of hearing aids and hearing aid evaluations.

William L Lederer, Executive Director
Sharon Parmet, Development/Communications Associate

4663 Genetics and Deafness
National Information Center on Deafness
800 Florida Avenue NE 202-651-5051
Washington, DC 20002-3660 Fax: 202-651-5054
TTY: 202-651-5052

Written for deaf people and their families who wish to learn more about the relationship between heredity and deafness.

4664 Hearing Loss: Information for Professionals in the Aging Network
National Information Center on Deafness
800 Florida Avenue NE 202-651-5051
Washington, DC 20002-3660 Fax: 202-651-5054
TTY: 202-651-5052

Introduces professionals in the aging network to the realities of hearing loss.

4665 How Does Your Child Hear and Talk?
American Speech-Language-Hearing Association
10801 Rockville Pike 301-897-8682
Rockville, MD 20852-3226 800-638-8255
e-mail: actioncenter@asha.org
www.asha.org

Offers a chart to parents on children's growth pertaining to their hearing and speech.

4666 Late-Deafened Adults: A Selected Annotated Bibliography
National Information Center on Deafness
800 Florida Avenue NE 202-651-5051
Washington, DC 20002-3660 Fax: 202-651-5054
TTY: 202-651-5052

A selected reading list of books and articles for late-deafened people and their families.

4667 Leading National Publications of and for Deaf People
National Information Center on Deafness
800 Florida Avenue NE 202-651-5051
Washington, DC 20002 Fax: 202-651-5054
TTY: 202-651-5052

Identifies publications with national circulations to deaf audiences.

4668 Making New Friends
National Information Center on Deafness
800 Florida Avenue NE 202-651-5051
Washington, DC 20002-3660 Fax: 202-651-5054
TTY: 202-651-5052

Identifies resources that offer opportunities for deaf people.

4669 Meniere's Disease: Hearing Loss & Inner Ear Blood Flow
Self Help for Hard of H
7910 Woodmont Avenue 301-657-2248
Bethesda, MD 20814-3079 Fax: 301-913-9413
TTY: 301-657-2249
e-mail: national@shhh.org
www.shhh.org

Includes a personal narrative.

4670 National Information Center on Deafness Brochure
National Information Center on Deafness
800 Florida Avenue NE 202-651-5051
Washington, DC 20002 Fax: 202-651-5054
TTY: 202-651-5052

A description of services offered by NICD.

4671 Noise Can Be Harmful to Your Health
Deafness Research Foundation
15 W 39th Street 212-768-1181
New York, NY 10018-3806

Offers information, including a chart of noise levels, low to harmful, and the effects these noise levels have on your hearing.

4672 Otitis Media
Deafness Research Foundation
15 W 39th Street 212-768-1181
New York, NY 10018-3806

Offers information on Otitis Media, prevention, causes, treatments and symptoms.

4673 Perspectives Folio: Parent-Child
Gallaudet University
11030 S Langley Avenue
Chicago, IL 60628-3819 800-621-2736
Fax: 800-621-8476
TTY: 888-630-9347
www.gallaudet.edu/~gupress

Seven articles emphasizing family communication while providing important information for parents about deafness and the deaf culture.

29 pages

4674 Publications from the National Information Center on Deafness
National Information Center on Deafness
800 Florida Avenue NE 202-651-5051
Washington, DC 20002-3660 Fax: 202-651-5054
TTY: 202-651-5052

Order form and explanations of NICD publications.

4675 Questions and Answers About Employment of Deaf People
National Information Center on Deafness
800 Florida Avenue NE 202-651-5051
Washington, DC 20002-3660 Fax: 202-651-5054
TTY: 202-651-5052

4676 Questions and Answers on Hearing Loss
Self Help for Hard of H
7910 Woodmont Avenue 301-657-2248
Bethesda, MD 20814-3079 Fax: 301-913-9413
TTY: 301-657-2249
e-mail: national@shhh.org
www.shhh.org

4677 So You Have Had an Ear Operation...What Next?
American Hearing Research Foundation
8 S Washington Avenue 312-726-9670
Chicago, IL 60603-4539 Fax: 312-726-9695
e-mail: blederer@american-hearing.org
www.american-hearing.org

Offers information on ear infections and surgery.

William L Lederer, Executive Director
Sharon Parmet, Development/Communications Associate

4678 Statewide Services for Deaf and Hard of Hearing People
National Information Center on Deafness
800 Florida Avenue NE 202-651-5051
Washington, DC 20002 Fax: 202-651-5054
TTY: 202-651-5052

A resource list of states that have established commissions and other offices to serve deaf people.

4679 Travel Resources for Deaf and Hard of Hearing People
National Information Center on Deafness
800 Florida Avenue NE 202-651-5051
Washington, DC 20002 Fax: 202-651-5054
TTY: 202-651-5052

A publication list of travel industry resources for deaf and hard of hearing people.

4680 What are TTY's? TDDs? TTs?
National Information Center on Deafness

800 Florida Avenue NE | 202-651-5051
Washington, DC 20002-3660 | Fax: 202-651-5054
TTY: 202-651-5052

Discusses text telephones used by deaf people.

4681 World of Sound
International Hearing Society
16880 Middlebelt Road | 313-478-2610
Livonia, MI 48154-3367 | Fax: 313-478-4520

The purpose of this booklet is to provide basic information for those with questions about hearing loss, hearing aids and Hearing Instrument Specialists.

4682 You Don't Have to Hate Meetings: Try Computer-Assisted Notetaking Instead
Self Help for Hard of H
7910 Woodmont Avenue | 301-657-2248
Bethesda, MD 20814-3079 | Fax: 301-913-9413
TTY: 301-657-2249
e-mail: national@shhh.org
www.shhh.org

Audio & Video

4683 ASL Poetry: Selected Works of Clayton Valli
DawnSignPress
6130 Nancy Ridge Drive | 858-625-0600
San Diego, CA 92121-3223 | 800-549-5350
Fax: 858-625-2336
TTY: 858-625-0600
e-mail: comments@dawnsign.com
www.dawnsign.com

Twenty one original Valli poems recited by a diversity of native signers. Guided experience through the richness of poetry in another language.
105 minutes
ISBN: 0-915035-23-5
Barry Howland, Marketing Director

4684 Basic Course in American Sign Language Vid eotape Package
TJ Publishers
2544 Tarpley Road | 972-416-0800
Carrollton, TX 75006 | 800-999-1168
Fax: 972-416-0944
e-mail: customerservice@tjpublishers.com
www.tjpublishers.com/index.html

The A Basic Course in American Sign Language Vocabulary Videotape features four Deaf models signing each vocabulary word contained in all 22 lessons of the text plus the alphabet and numbers. The tape has captions and voice which can be turned off to sharpen visual acuity. It is ideal for classroom reinforcement and independent home study.
Angela K Thames, President
Jerald A Murphy, VP

4685 Beginning Reading and Sign Language Video
TJ Publishers
2544 Tarpley Road | 972-416-0800
Carrollton, TX 75006 | 800-999-1168
Fax: 972-416-0944
e-mail: customerservice@tjpublishers.com
www.tjpublishers.com/index.html

Learning sign improves reading, motor skills and visual perception and increases language acquisition abilities. For kids from 2 to 12, this video picture book features deaf actress Susan Bressler signing over a hundred words at the zoo, at home and around the community.
Video
Angela K Thames, President
Jerald A Murphy, VP

4686 Come Sign With Us
Gallaudet University
11030 S Langley Avenue
Chicago, IL 60628-3819 | 800-621-2736
Fax: 800-621-8476
TTY: 888-630-9347
www.gallaudet.edu/~gupress

Lessons including fingerspelling and signing are overviewed.
90 minutes
ISBN: 1-563680-50-5

4687 Deaf Children Signers
Harris Communications
15155 Technology Drive | 952-906-1180
Eden Prairie, MN 55344 | 800-825-6758
Fax: 952-906-1099
TTY: 800-825-9187
e-mail: info@harriscomm.com
www.harriscomm.com/

This 5-part collection of children signers is great for children, teachers, parents and interpreters.
Robert Harris Ph.D, Founder/President/CEO

4688 Deaf Culture Autobiographies
Harris Communications
15155 Technology Drive | 952-906-1180
Eden Prairie, MN 55344 | 800-825-6758
Fax: 952-906-1099
TTY: 800-825-9187
e-mail: info@harriscomm.com
www.harriscomm.com/

Inspiring videotapes offer encouragement and enlightenment to the hearing impaired. Total of eight videotapes.
Robert Harris Ph.D, Founder/President/CEO

4689 Deaf Culture Series
Harris Communications
15155 Technology Drive | 952-906-1180
Eden Prairie, MN 55344 | 800-825-6758
Fax: 952-906-1099
TTY: 800-825-9187
e-mail: info@harriscomm.com
www.harriscomm.com/

Each video in this 5-part series features a variety of Deaf talent. It is an excellent resource for Deaf studies programs, Interpreter Preparation programs and Sign Language programs.
Robert Harris Ph.D, Founder/President/CEO

4690 Deaf Mosaic Series
Harris Communications
15155 Technology Drive | 952-906-1180
Eden Prairie, MN 55344 | 800-825-6758
Fax: 952-906-1099
TTY: 800-825-9187
e-mail: info@harriscomm.com
www.harriscomm.com/

A national magazine show produced monthly by Gallaudet University, this show has been awarded nine Emmys. As the only nation-wide program about the Deaf community, these videotapes are the best of the best from the shows programs.
Robert Harris Ph.D, Founder/President/CEO

4691 Diagnosis and Treatment of Unilateral Hearing Loss
American Academy of Otolaryngology
1 Prince Street | 703-836-4444
Alexandria, VA 22314-3357 | Fax: 703-683-5100
www.entnet.org

This CD-ROM focuses on evaluation and treatment of unilateral hearing loss arising from skull base lesion.

4692 Do You Hear That?
Alexander Graham Bell Association
3417 Volta Place NW | 202-337-5220
Washington, DC 20007-2737 | Fax: 202-337-8270
TTY: 202-337-5220

This video documents auditory-verbal therapy as it is practiced at North York General Hospital in Toronto, Canada.
1992 35 minutes

4693 Fantastic Series
Gallaudet University Bookstore
800 Florida Avenue NE
Washington, DC 20002-3660 | 800-451-1073
Fax: 800-621-8476
TTY: 888-630-9347
www.gallaudet.edu/~gupress

Tapes designed to encourage both deaf and hearing children to use their imaginations.
Ages 6-10

4694 **Fingers that Tickle and Delight**
National Association of the Deaf
8630 Fenton Street
Silver Spring, MD 20910
301-587-1788
Fax: 301-587-1791
TTY: 301-587-1789
www.nad.org
One's woman's experiences from childhood, school, marriage, her career as a teacher and interpreter trainer, and her life as an entertainer. Closed captioned.
13+ 32 minutes
Bill Stark, Project Director
Donna Morris, Publications Manager

4695 **Fingerspelling and Numbers Software**
American Sign Language (ASL) Productions
c/o Harris Communications
Eden Prairie, MN 55344
952-906-1180
800-767-4461
Fax: 952-906-1099
TTY: 800-767-4461
e-mail: ASLProductions@harriscomm.com
www.americansignlanguageproductions.com
Fingerspelling practice partner that allows you to control the speed and vocabulary level. Requires Windows 3.1 or greater.
Robert Harris Ph.D, Founder/President-Harris Communications
Jenna Cassell, Founder ASL Productions

4696 **Getting in Touch**
Research Press
2612 N Mattis Avenue
Champaign, IL 61822-1053
217-352-3273
800-519-2707
Fax: 217-352-1221
e-mail: rp@researchpress.com
www.researchpress.com
Shows how to create an individualized communications system based on the abilities and needs of the child. Illustrates seven basic communication procedures that involve the use of touch cues and object cues.

4697 **Gospel of Luke**
Gallaudet University Bookstore
800 Florida Avenue NE
Washington, DC 20002-3660
800-451-0173
Fax: 800-621-8476
TTY: 888-630-9347
www.gallaudet.edu/~gupress
A set of five videotapes of the Gospel of Luke told in ASL.
Set of five

4698 **Granny Good's Sign of Christmas**
Gallaudet University Bookstore
800 Florida Avenue NE
Washington, DC 20002-3660
800-451-1073
Fax: 800-621-8476
TTY: 888-630-9347
www.gallaudet.edu/~gupress
Twas The Night Before Christmas told in American Sign Language.

4699 **Hearing Loss and Rehabilitation**
American Academy of Otolaryngology
1 Prince Street
Alexandria, VA 22314-3357
703-836-4444
Fax: 703-683-5100
www.entnet.org
Slides.

4700 **I Can Hear!**
Alexander Graham Bell Association
3417 Volta Place NW
Washington, DC 20007-2737
202-337-5220
Fax: 202-337-8270
TTY: 202-337-5220
This inspirational video describes the auditory-verbal approach for developing speech and language for hearing impaired children and adults.
1992 23 minutes

4701 **I Can Hear!: II**
Alexander Graham Bell Association
3417 Volta Place NW
Washington, DC 20007-2737
202-337-5220
Fax: 202-337-8270
TTY: 202-337-5220
An exciting videotape that gives more examples of auditory-verbal therapy and a variety of kids who have been taught to speak using this method.
1996 19 minute video

4702 **I See What You Say: Self Help Lip Reading Program**
Alexander Graham Bell Association
3417 Volta Place NW
Washington, DC 20007-2737
202-337-5220
Fax: 202-337-8270
TTY: 202-337-5220
Easy to follow videotape and manual for consumers teaches visual recognition of speech sounds in single words and phrases.
1995 54 minutes

4703 **Interpreters in Public Schools Kit**
Sign Media
4020 Blackburn Lane
Burtonsville, MD 20866-1167
301-421-0268
800-475-4756
Fax: 301-421-0270
TTY: 301-421-4460
e-mail: signmedia@aol.com
www.signmedia.com
Videotapes individually specialized for administrators, classroom teachers and for interpreters. Provides practical insights to some of the most crucial issues and problems facing mainstreamed programs. Contains reproducible printed material.
Three videos
Barbara Olmert, Director Marketing

4704 **Interview with Kirsten Gonzales**
Alexander Graham Bell Association
3417 Volta Place NW
Washington, DC 20007-2737
202-337-5220
Fax: 202-337-8270
TTY: 202-337-5220
Interviews a longtime user and trainer of oral interpreters who offers techniques in articulation and natural gestures.
20 minutes

4705 **It's Not Just Hearing AIDS: Deaf People and the Epidemic**
National Association of the Deaf
8630 Fenton Street
Silver Spring, MD 20910
301-587-1788
Fax: 301-587-1791
TTY: 301-587-1789
www.nad.org
Straightforward and factual information on how AIDS is transmitted, who gets AIDS, procedures for an HIV test, and an interview with a person who actually has the AIDS virus.
9 - 13+ Video
Bill Stark, Project Director
Donna Morris, Publications Manager

4706 **Joy of Signing**
Gallaudet University Bookstore
800 Florida Avenue NE
Washington, DC 20002-3660
800-451-1073
Fax: 800-621-8476
TTY: 888-630-9347
www.gallaudet.edu/~gupress
Three tapes full of useful information to help increase skill and comfort with sign.
1 Videotape

4707 **King Midas**
Gallaudet University
11030 S Langley Avenue
Chicago, IL 60628-3819
800-621-2736
Fax: 800-621-8476
TTY: 888-630-9347
www.gallaudet.edu/~gupress
30 minutes
ISBN: 0-930323-71-8

4708 **King Midas Videotape**
Gallaudet University Bookstore

800 Florida Avenue NE
Washington, DC 20002-3660 800-451-1073
Fax: 800-621-8476
TTY: 888-630-9347
www.gallaudet.edu/~gupress
Story of King Midas told in American Sign Language.

4709 **Learning to Communicate: The First Three Years Videotape**
Alexander Graham Bell Association
3417 Volta Place NW 202-337-5220
Washington, DC 20007-2737 Fax: 202-337-8270
TTY: 202-337-5220
This video shows normal communication development in young children under three years of age. It discusses factors which can affect speech and language development, including anatomy and environment. Closed captioned.
11 minutes

4710 **Let's Be Friends**
Britannica Film Company
345 4th Street 415-597-5555
San Francisco, CA 94107-1206
The teacher left the room and asked Shelly, a hearing impaired child to be the mother. Margaret, an emotionally disturbed child, became frightened and verbally attacked Shelly. The teacher worked to get them to become friends and understand each other's problems.
Films

4711 **Once Upon a Time - Children's Classics Ret old in American Sign Language**
Harris Communications
15155 Technology Drive 952-906-1180
Eden Prairie, MN 55344 800-825-6758
Fax: 952-906-1099
TTY: 800-825-9187
e-mail: info@harriscomm.com
www.harriscomm.com/
Children's classics come alive on videotapes.
Robert Harris Ph.D, Founder/President/CEO

4712 **Parent Sign Video Series**
TJ Publishers
2544 Tarpley Road 972-416-0800
Carrollton, TX 75006 800-999-1168
Fax: 972-416-0944
e-mail: customerservice@tjpublishers.com
www.tjpublishers.com/index.html
Ten instructional videotapes specifically designed for parents of deaf children, present frequently used vocabulary and phrases. The tapes are perfect for home use and as a compliment to sign language and educational programs. Deaf and hearing parents, each having a deaf and a hearing child, reflect common communication needs of all families.
Video
Angela K Thames, President
Jerald A Murphy, VP

4713 **People vs. Noise**
Better Hearing Institute
5021B Backlick Road 703-684-3391
Annandale, VA 22003-6043 e-mail: mail@betterhearing.org
www.betterhearing.org

4714 **Read My Lips**
Alexander Graham Bell Association
3417 Volta Place NW 202-337-5220
Washington, DC 20007-2737 Fax: 202-337-8270
TTY: 202-337-5220
A six videotape series that takes adults from lip reading to basic words to complex phrases and sentences in a variety of real life situations.

4715 **See What I'm Saying**
Thomas Kaufman, author
Fanlight Productions
4196 Washington Street 617-469-4999
Boston, MA 02131-1731 800-937-4113
Fax: 617-469-3379
e-mail: fanlight@fanlight.com
www.fanlight.com
Follows Patricia, a deaf child from a hearing, Spanish speaking family, through her first year of elementary school. Illustrates how the acquisition of communication skills enhances a child's self-esteem, confidence and family relationships. Open captioned.
1992 31 Minutes
ISBN: 1-572950-90-0

4716 **Seeing and Hearing Speech: Lessons in Lipreading and Listening**
Hearing Loss Association of America
7910 Woodmont Avenue 301-657-2248
Bethesda, MD 20814-3079 Fax: 301-913-9413
TTY: 301-657-2249
e-mail: info@hearingloss.org
www.hearingloss.org
This CD-Rom helps people with hearing loss learn to combine what they see with what they hear to understand speech better in difficult situations. This interactive CD-ROM contains carefully planned lessons to improve speech understanding through lipreading.
CD-ROM
Jerry Portis, Executive Director
Brenda Battat, Assistant Executive Director

4717 **Show & Tell: Explaining Hearing Loss to Teachers**
Alexander Graham Bell Association
3417 Volta Place NW 202-337-5220
Washington, DC 20007-2737 Fax: 202-337-8270
TTY: 202-337-5220
This video introduces mainstreamed teachers to the challenges that hearing impairments impose on normal communication.
20 minutes

4718 **Show 'N' Tell Stories**
Modern Signs Press
PO Box 1181 562-596-8548
Los Alamitos, CA 90720-1181 800-572-7332
Fax: 562-795-6614
TTY: 562-493-4168
e-mail: modsigns@aol.com
www.modsigns.com
A bilingual storytelling series for Deaf children and their families, featuring both Signing Exact English (SEE) and American Sign Language (ASL).
Videotape

4719 **Sign-Me-A-Story**
DawnSignPress
6130 Nancy Ridge Drive 858-625-0600
San Diego, CA 92121-3223 800-549-5350
Fax: 858-625-2336
TTY: 858-625-0600
e-mail: info@dawnsign.com
www.dawnsign.com/
Linda Bove, the deaf actress from Sesame Street, introduces children to American Sign Language. Teaches simple signs and then acts out fairy tales. Stories are voiced and closed captioned, accessible to all.
30 minutes
ISBN: 0-394892-32-1
Joe Dannis, Founder/Publisher/President

4720 **Sleeping Beauty Videotape**
Gallaudet University Bookstore
800 Florida Avenue NE
Washington, DC 20002-3660 800-451-1073
Fax: 800-621-8476
TTY: 888-630-9347
www.gallaudet.edu/~gupress
Presents the entire story of Sleeping Beauty told in American Sign Language.

4721 **Sleeping Beauty: With Selected Sentences in ASL**
Gallaudet University

11030 S Langley Avenue
Chicago, IL 60628-3819
800-621-2736
Fax: 800-621-8476
TTY: 888-630-9347
www.gallaudet.edu/~gupress

Features the full story in ASL and includes vocabulary and sentence structure focusing on adjectives, with a voice-over throughout.
30 minutes
ISBN: 0-930323-98-X

4722 **Sound Hearing**
Hearing Loss Association of America
7910 Woodmont Avenue
Bethesda, MD 20814-3079
301-657-2248
Fax: 301-913-9413
TTY: 301-657-2249
e-mail: info@hearingloss.org
www.hearingloss.org

Provides listening samples to illustrate sound, hearing, and hearing loss. Listeners will hear as people who have hearing loss might, listening to music, a story, etc.
CD-ROM, 26 mins
Jerry Portis, Executive Director
Brenda Battat, Assistant Executive Director

4723 **Telecoil: Plugging Into Sound**
Hearing Loss Association of America
7910 Woodmont Avenue
Bethesda, MD 20814-3079
301-657-2248
Fax: 301-913-9413
TTY: 301-657-2249
e-mail: info@hearingloss.org
www.hearingloss.org

In The Telecoil: Plugging Into Sound, members of SHHH give accounts of their experiences with using the telecoil, describing how the telecoil makes a noticeable difference in their social and professional lives.
Open Captioned
Jerry Portis, Executive Director
Brenda Battat, Assistant Executive Director

4724 **Telecoil: Plugging into Sound**
7910 Woodmont Avenue
Bethesda, MD 20814-3079
301-657-2248
Fax: 301-913-9413
TTY: 301-657-2249
e-mail: national@shhh.org
www.shhh.org

Guide for consumers concerning why they should include a telecoil in their hearing aid. SHHH members are featured, talking about their experiences. Includes 50 brochures. Open-captioned.
1996 10 minutes

4725 **Telling Stories**
Harris Communications
15155 Technology Drive
Eden Prairie, MN 55344
952-906-1180
800-825-6758
Fax: 952-906-1099
TTY: 800-825-9187
e-mail: info@harriscomm.com
www.harriscomm.com/

This international, award winning play, now on video, uses the symbols and myths drawn from the struggles between the world of the deaf and the world of the hearing.
Robert Harris Ph.D, Founder/President/CEO

4726 **Treasure**
Gallaudet University Bookstore
800 Florida Avenue NE
Washington, DC 20002-3660
773-568-1550
Fax: 800-621-8476
TTY: 888-630-9347
www.gallaudet.edu/~gupress

Ella Mae Lentz, a well-known deaf poet, signs some of her poems.

4727 **Unheard Voices**
Hearing Loss Association of America
7910 Woodmont Avenue
Bethesda, MD 20814-3079
301-657-2248
Fax: 301-913-9413
TTY: 301-657-2249
e-mail: info@hearingloss.org
www.hearingloss.org

Unheard Voices is a candid and compassionate portrayal of people coping with the life-changing impact of hearing loss. Open-captioned.
23 minutes
Jerry Portis, Executive Director
Brenda Battat, Assistant Executive Director

Web Sites

4728 **Alexander Graham Bell Association**
www.agbell.org

Information on pediatric hearing loss, and educational issues for hearing impaired children, promotes better public understanding of hearing loss in children and adults, provides scholarships and financial aid to families of children with hearing loss, and promotes early detection of hearing loss in infants.

4729 **American Academy of Audiology**
www.audiology.org

Provides professional development, education and research and provides increased public awareness of hearing disorders and audiologic services.

4730 **American Academy of Otolaryngology**
www.entnet.org

Advance the art and science of otalaryngology-head and neck surgury through state-of-the-art education, research, and learning; and to unite, serve, and represent the interests of its members and their patients to the public.

4731 **American Society for Deaf Children**
www.deafchildren.org

Provides support, encouragement, and current information about deafness to families with deaf and hard of hearing children.

4732 **American Tinnitus Association**
www.ata.org

Provides information about tinnitus and referrals to local contacts/support groups nationwide.

4733 **Auditory-Verbal International**
www.auditory-verbal.org

Promotes the Auditory-Verbal Therapy approach, which is based on the belief that the overwhelming majority of these children can hear and talk by using their residual hearing and hearing aids.

4734 **Better Hearing Institute**
www.betterhearing.org

Information programs on hearing loss and available medical, surgical, hearing aid, and rehabilitation assistance for millions with uncorrected hearing problems.

4735 **Council on Education of the Deaf**
www.deafed.net

Offers information and referral services to the hearing impaired.

4736 **Deafness Research Foundation**
www.drf.org

Committed to public awareness and support for basic and clinical research into deafness and hearing disabilities.

4737 **EAR Foundation**
www.earfoundation.org

Provides the general public support services promoting the integration of the hearing and balance impaired into mainstream society and to educate young people and adults about hearing preservation and early detection of hearing loss, enabling them to prevent at an early age hearing and balance disorders.

4738 **Healing Well**
www.healingwell.com

An online health resource guide to medical news, chat, information and articles, newsgroups and message boards, books, disease-related web sites, medical directories, and more for patients, friends, and family coping with disabling diseases, disorders, or chronic illnesses.

4739 **Health Finder**
www.healthfinder.gov

Searchable, carefully developed web site offering information on over 1000 topics. Developed by the US Department of Health and Human Services, the site can be used in both English and Spanish.

4740 Healthlink USA

www.healthlinkusa.com

Health information concerning treatment, cures, prevention, diagnosis, risk factors, research, support groups, email lists, personal stories and much more. Updated regularly.

4741 Hear Now

www.sotheworldmayhearnow.org

Committed to making technology accessible to deaf and hard of hearing individuals throughout the United States. Also raises funds to provide hearing aids, cochlear implants and related services to children and adults who have hearing losses but do not have financial resources to purchase their own devices.

4742 Hearing Education and Awareness for Rocker

www.hearnet.com

Educates the public about the real dangers of hearing loss resulting from repeated exposure to excessive noise levels.

4743 Helios Health

www.helioshealth.com

Online resource for your health information. Detailed information about specific health topics, access to expert advice from our Medical Advisory Board, and up-to-date health news.

4744 House Ear Institute

www.hei.org

A national non-profit otologic research and educational institute that provides information on hearing and balance disorders.

4745 John Tracy Clinic

www.johntracycyclinic.org

An educational facility for preschool age children who have hearing losses and their families. In addition to on-site services, worldwide correspondence courses in English and Spanish are offered to parents whose children are of preschool age and are hard of hearing, deaf, or deaf-blind.

4746 MedicineNet

www.medicinenet.com

An online resource for consumers providing easy-to-read, authoritative medical and health information.

4747 Medscape

www.mywebmd.com

Medscape offers specialists, primary care physicians, and other health professionals the Web's most robust and integrated medical information and educational tools.

4748 National Association of the Deaf

www.nad.org

Focus on advocacy, captioned media, deafness-related information/publications, legal assistance and more.

4749 National Captioning Institute

ncicap.org

Advocates captioned television for people who want to see, as well as hear, the dialogue of a television program. It not only enables deaf and hard-of-hearing people to understand all of a program's content, but it is also beneficial for new Americans learning English as a second language, as well as children learning to read.

4750 National Information Center on Deafness

www.gallaudet.edu

Provides information or referrals on questions about deafness, including general information, education, research, legislation, assistive devices and more. Offers a bibliography of readings available on 30 topics relating to deafness.

4751 National Information Clearinghouse on Children Who are Deaf-Blind

www.tr.wou.edu/dblink

Collects, organizes and disseminates information related to children and youth who are deaf-blind and connects consumers of deaf-blind information to sources of information about deaf-blindness, assistive technology and deaf-blind people.

4752 National Institute on Deafness and Other Communication Disorders

www.nih.gov/nidcd

A national resources center for information about hearing, balance, smell, taste, voice, speech and language.

4753 Registry of Interpreters for the Deaf

www.RID.org

Professional interpreters and translators, persons with deafness or hearing impairments and professionals in related fields.

4754 Self-Help for Hard of Hearing People

www.shhh.org/

Promotes awareness and information about hearing loss, communication, assistive devices, and alternative communication skills through publications, exhibits and presentations.

4755 USA Deaf Sports Federation

www.usadsf.org

Website published by a governing body for all deaf sports and recreation in the United States.

4756 WebMD

www.webmd.com

Information on deafness, including articles and resources.

Description

4757 # Heart Disease

There is a wide range of heart (cardiac) diseases that can be divided into several major categories: heart failure; problems in electrical conduction; heart rate and rhythm; and malfunction of the heart valves. Coronary disease relates to the arteries that supply oxygen to the heart muscle itself.

Heart failure is the general inability of the heart to function effectively as the pumping mechanism to distribute oxygenated blood and nutrients to the cells and tissues. As the heart's pumping action declines, blood does not get distributed properly and normal circulation gets disrupted. As a result, the fluid accumulates, or backs up, causing swelling (edema) in the body, often noticeable in the ankles, as well as within the lungs (pulmonary edema) causing difficulty in breathing. Numerous mechanisms are responsible for heart failure so treatment is aimed at the underlying causes, improving heart contractibility (and thus pump efficiency), and removal of excess fluid through the kidneys.

Problems in the electrical conduction that makes the heart contract result in irregular heart rate and rhythm, either slower, faster, or, in life-threatening situations, absence of heart beat or ineffective heart contractions. Specific medications and procedures are used in treatment, again depending on the underlying problem.

New diagnostic (angiography) and therapeutic catheter techniques have been developed to accurately identify the rhythm problem, and in some cases, cure it bydelivering radio frequency energy to the abnormal pathway.

Malfunctions of heart valves are also common, but surgical advances enable successful repair and replacement of defective or diseased valves.

The arteries that directly supply the heart (known as coronary arteries) can also be affected by disease processes. Deposits or fatty plaques may cause narrowing of the arteries, or the arteries can become blocked by a clot that originated somewhere else in the body. Either way, the heart may be deprived of oxygenated blood and the particular muscle that is fed by the artery is injured or dies. Angina is chest pain produced when the heart is not receiving enough oxygen but no direct damage occurs. A heart attack (or myocardial infarction) occurs when the heart is deprived of its blood for a significant amount of time. The outcome of a heart attack depends on the amount of damage sustained by the affected heart muscle and the speed with which treatment is started. Immediate medical intervention has a marked effect on long-term prognosis. Administration of agents that dissolve the clot (blood thinners, antithrombotics) significantly reduce heart atack deaths when given within 6 hours of the onset of chest pain. Catheter interventions (angioplasty) can include balloons and metallic stents that are placed in coronary arteries to push obstructions against the arterial walls thereby re-opening the vessel. The most recent advance is a stent that is coated with a drug that iscoated to prevent reformation of the clot.

The symptoms of heart disease are varied, but may include chest pain, difficulty breathing, fatigue, palpitations, dizziness and fainting. See also *Congenital Heart Disease*.

National Agencies & Associations

4758 **American Heart Association**
7272 Greenville Avenue
Dallas, TX 75231 800-242-8721
www.americanheart.org
Supports research education and community service programs with the objective of reducing premature death and disability from cardiovascular diseases and stroke; coordinates the efforts of health professionals and other engaged in the fight against heart disease.
M Cass Wheeler, CEO

4759 **Canadian Adult Congenital Heart Network**
6835 Century Avenue
Mississauga, Ontario, L5N-2L2 e-mail: jtherrien@cachnet.org
www.cachnet.org
Was created to pool the knowledge and experience of congenital heart disease professionals in Canada to help strengthen their skills and knowledge of the discipline, and to create a community of individuals committed to caring for adults with congenital heart disease and their families.

4760 **Children's Heart Society**
Box 52088 Garneau Postal Outlet 780-454-7665
Edmonton, Alberta, T6G-2T5 888-247-9404
Fax: 780-454-7665
e-mail: childrensheart@shaw.ca
www.childrensheart.org
Supports families of children with acquired and congenital heart disease.

4761 **National Heart, Lung and Blood Institute**
National Institutes of Health
31 Center Drive, Building 31 301-592-8573
Bethesda, MD 20892 Fax: 240-629-3246
TTY: 240-629-3255
e-mail: NHLBIinfo@nhlbi.nih.gov
www.nhlbi.nih.gov
Primary responsibility of this organization is the scientific investigation of heart, blood vessel, lung and blood disorders. Oversees research, demonstration, prevention, education, control and training activities in these fields and emphasizes the prevention and control of heart diseases.
Elizabeth G Nabel, MD, Director

4762 **Pulmonary Hypertension Association**
801 Roeder Road 301-565-3004
Silver Spring, MD 20910 800-748-7274
Fax: 301-565-3994
e-mail: pha@PHAssociation.org
www.PHAssociation.org
A nonprofit organization for pulmonary hypertension patients, families, caregivers and PH-treating medical professionals. The mission of the Pulmonary Hypertension Association (PHA) is to find ways to prevent and cure pulmonary hypertension, and to provide hope for the pulmonary hypertension community through support, education, advocacy and awareness.
Rino Aldrighetti, President

Research Centers

4763 Arizona Heart Institute
2632 N 20th Street
Phoenix, AZ 85006-1300
602-266-2200
800-345-4278
Fax: 602-604-5047
e-mail: information@azheart.com
www.azheart.com
Edward Diethrich, Medical Director and Founder

4764 Baylor College of Medicine: Debakey Heart Center
Texas Medical Center
1 Baylor Plaza
Houston, TX 77030-3411
713-798-1297
Fax: 713-798-6990
e-mail: research@bcm.edu
www.bcm.tmc.edu
Research activities have an emphasis on therapeutic intervention and prevention of heart disease.
Jeffrey R Steinbauer, Medical Director
Thomas J Riley, Vice President of Clinic & Hospital Oper

4765 Baylor College of Medicine: General Clinical Research Center Adults
Baylor College of Medicine
1 Baylor Plaza
Houston, TX 77030-3498
713-798-4945
Fax: 713-798-6990
e-mail: asander1@bcm.edu
www.bcm.tmc.edu
David J Tweardy M D, Chief of Infectious Diseases
Sarah Allen M D, Associate Professor

4766 Bees-Stealy Research Foundation
2001 4th Avenue
San Diego, CA 92101-2303
619-235-8744
Fax: 619-234-8190
Basic cardiac research.
HD Peabody Jr, Director

4767 Bockus Research Institute Graduate Hospital
Graduate Hospital
415 S 19th Street
Philadelphia, PA 19146-1464
215-893-2000
Offers research in cardiovascular diseases with emphasis on muscle tissue studies.
Dr Robert Cox, Director

4768 Boston University, Whitaker Cardiovascular Institute
80 E Concord Street
Boston, MA 02118-2307
617-638-7254
Fax: 617-638-8728
Offers basic and clinical care research relating to cardiovascular diseases.
Joseph Loscalzo MD, Director

4769 CHASER Congenital Heart Disease Anomalies Anomalies Support, Education & Resources
2112 N Wilkins Road
Swanton, OH 43558-9445
419-825-5575
Fax: 419-825-2880
e-mail: CHASER@compuserve.com
www.csun.edu
An organization established to meet the emotional and educational needs of parents and professionals who deal with congenital heart disease in children. Offers resource materials and support for parent to parent networking.

4770 Cardiovascular Research and Training Center University of Alabama
THT Room 311
Birmingham, AL 35294-6
205-934-3624
Fax: 205-345-96
Robert C Bueourge, Director

4771 Children's Heart Institute of Texas
PO Box 3966
Corpus Christi, TX 78463-3966
512-887-4505
Fax: 512-887-0539
Offers research and statistical information on pediatric cardiology.
Laura Berlanga, Director

4772 Cleveland Clinic Foundation Research Institute
9500 Euclid Avenue
Cleveland, OH 44195
216-444-3900
Fax: 216-444-3279
www.lerner.ccf.org
Research institute focusing on diseases of the cardiovascular system.
Amiya K Banerjee PhD, Head
Paul E DiCorleto PhD, Staff/ Institute Chairman

4773 Columbia University Irving Center for Clinical Research Adult Unit
Presbyterian Hospital
622 W 168th Street
New York, NY 10032-3784
212-305-2071
Fax: 212-053-13
www.columbia.edu
Research center focusing on pulmonary diseases.
Henry Ginsberg, Director

4774 Creighton University Cardiac Center
3006 Webster Street
Omaha, NE 68131-2137
402-280-4566
800-237-7828
thecardiaccenter.creighton.edu
Research into the clinical aspects of cardiology and heart disease.
Dennis J Esterbrooks MD, Chief of the Division of Cardiology
Michael G Del Core MD, Associate Professor of Medicine

4775 Duke University Pediatric Cardiac Catheterization Laboratory
7506 Hospital N
Durham, NC 27710-0001
919-220-4000
e-mail: john.rhodes@duke.edu
pediatrics.duke.edu
Research into pediatric cardiology.
Brenda E Armstrong MD, Director
John F Rhodes MD, Chief Clinical Cardiology

4776 Framingham Heart Study
73 Mount Wayte Avenue
Framingham, MA 01702-6334
508-935-3434
Fax: 508-626-1262
e-mail: levyD@nih.gov
www.framinghamheartstudy.org
Daniel Levy, Medical Director
Philip A Wolf, Principal Investigator

4777 General Clinical Research Center at Beth Israel Hospital
330 Brookline Avenue
Boston, MA 02215-5400
617-735-2151
Studies into cardiology pulmonary disorders and heart disease.
Lewis Landsb MD, Program Director

4778 General Clinical Research Center: University of California at LA
Center for Health Sciences
10833 Le Conte Avenue
Los Angeles, CA 90095
310-825-7177
Fax: 310-206-5012
e-mail: lshakerirwin@mednet.ucla.edu.
www.gcrc.medsch.ucla.edu
Cardiovascular and heart disease disorders and illness research.
Isidro Salus MD, Program Director
Gerald Levey, Principal Investigator

4779 Georgetown University Research Resources Facility
3800 Reservoir Road NW
Washington, DC 20007-2195
202-444-2000
www.georgetownuniversityhospital.org
Studies of medical sciences with particular emphasis on heart disease.
Linda Winger, Vice President of Professional Services
Joy Drass MD, President

4780 Hahnemann University Likoff Cardiovascular Institute
Broad & Vine Streets
Philadelpia, PA 19102
215-854-8100
Diseases of the heart and vessels.
William S Frankl MD, Director

4781 Harvard Throndike Laboratory Harvard Medical Center
Harvard Medical Center
330 Brookline Avenue
Boston, MA 02215-5400
617-735-3020
Fax: 617-735-4833
Dr James Morgan, Director

4782 Heart Disease Research Foundation
50 Court Street
Brooklyn, NY 11201-4801
718-649-6210
Robert A Teters, Director

4783 Heart Research Foundation of Sacramento
1007 39th Street 916-456-3365
Sacramento, CA 95816-5502 e-mail: rjfrink@pol.net
www.hrfsac.org
Dr Frink, Founder/Principal Investigator

4784 Hope Heart Institute
1710 E Jefferson Street 206-903-2001
Seattle, WA 98122 Fax: 206-903-2144
e-mail: info@hopeheart.org
www.hopeheart.org
Heart and blood vessel research.
Dr Lester Sauvage MD, Founder & Medical Director Emeritus
Mark Nudelman, President & CEO

4785 John L McClellan Memorial Veterans' Hospital Research Office
4300 W 7th Street 501-257-1000
Little Rock, AR 72205-5446 Fax: 501-671-2510
www2.va.gov
Karl David Straub MD, Chief Staff

4786 Krannert Institute of Cardiology
1801 N Senate Boulevard 317-962-0500
Indianapolis, IN 46202-4832 800-843-2786
Fax: 317-962-0501
medicine.iupui.edu/krannert
The cardiovascular program at the Indiana University School of Medicine is recognized throughout the world for its commitment to excellence in patient care research and education. While we're known for our experience and ability to take care of the most complex cardiovascular problems we are equally focused on prevention and early detection.
Peng-Sheng C MD, Division Chief

4787 Loyola University of Chicago Cardiac Transplant Program
2160 S 1st Avenue 708-216-4977
Maywood, IL 60153-3304 Fax: 708-216-4918
www.luhs.org
Loyola University Health System is committed to excellence in patient care and the education of health professionals. They believe that our Catholic heritage and Jesuit traditions of ethical behavior academic distinction and scientific research lead to new knowledge and advance our healing mission in the communities we serve.
Dr Maria Rosa Costanzo-Nordin, Director

4788 Miami Heart Institute
4701 N Meridian Avenue 305-672-1111
Miami Beach, FL 33140-2997 Fax: 305-743-09
www.msmc.com
General cardiovascular research.
Steven D Sonenreich, President & Chief Executive Officer

4789 Miami Heart Research Institute
4770 Biscayne Boulevard 305-674-3020
Miami, FL 33137 Fax: 305-535-3642
e-mail: pak@floridaheart.org
www.miamiheartresearch.org
General cardiovascular research.
Paul Kurlansky, Director Research
Maria Terris MD, Medical Director

4790 Oklahoma Medical Research Foundation: Cardiovascular Research Program
825 NE 13th Street 405-271-6673
Oklahoma City, OK 73104-5097 800-522-0211
Fax: 405-271-3980
www.omrf.ouhsc.edu
The Cardiovascular Biology Research Program investigates fundamental mechanisms involved in blood coagulation inflammation and atherogenesis with special emphasis on the regulation of theses processes.
William G Thurman MD, President
Rodger P McEver, Member and Program Chair

4791 Pennsylvania State University Artificial Heart Research Project
Milton S Hershey Medical Center
500 University Drive 717-531-8407
Hershey, PA 17033-2391 Fax: 717-531-5011
www.psu.edu
William S Pierce MD, Director

4792 Preventive Medicine Research Institute
900 Bridgeway 415-332-2525
Sausalito, CA 94965-2158 Fax: 415-325-30
e-mail: dean.ornish@pmri.org
www.pmri.org
Nonprofit organization focusing on prevention and treatment of heart disease through modification of diet exercise and relaxation techniques.
Dean Ornish MD, President
Anne Ornish, Vice President

4793 Purdue University William A Hillenbrand Biomedical Engineering Center
AA Potter Engineering Center
500 Central Drive 765-494-7015
W Lafayette, IN 47907 877-598-4233
Fax: 765-494-6628
engineering.purdue.edu/BME
Cardiology and heart disease research.
George R Wodicka, Professor and Head

4794 Rockefeller University Laboratory of Cardiac Physiology
1230 York Avenue 212-327-7458
New York, NY 10021-6399 Fax: 212-570-8996
Causes of cardiac arrhythmias and prevention of heart disease.
Paul F Cranefield, Head

4795 San Francisco Heart Institute
1900 Sullivan Avenue 650-991-6601
Daly City, CA 94015-2200 800-82H-EART
Fax: 650-755-7315
e-mail: webmaster@sfhi.com
www.sfhi.com
At Seton Medical Center we are committed to providing a full range of high quality services and state-of-the-art cardiovascular treatments for our patients. Our medical nursing and social services staff provide quality care and compassion as a coordinated team focusing on the medical emotional and spiritual needs of patients and their families.
Colman Ryan, Executive Director
Louis Manila RN BA, Manager of Research and Operations

4796 Specialized Center of Research in Ischemic Heart Disease
619 19th Street S 205-934-9999
Birmingham, AL 35294-0001 800-822-8816
www.health.uab.edu
Coronary artery disease.
Dr Marsha Sturdevant, Program Director
Becky Armstrong, Program Manager

4797 Texas Heart Institute St Lukes Episcopal Hospital
St Lukes Episcopal Hospital
6770 Bertner Avenue
Houston, TX 77225-0345 800-292-2221
Fax: 713-791-3089
e-mail: mmattsson@heart.thi.tmc.edu
www.texasheartinstitute.org
Marc C Mattsson, CEO
L Maximilian Buja MD, Chief Cardiovascular Pathology Research

4798 University of Alabama at Birmingham: Congenital Heart Disease Center
University Station 205-934-2344
Birmingham, AL 35294-0001 Fax: 205-934-7514
Dr. Albert Pacifico, Director

4799 University of California San Diego General Clinical Research Center
UCSD Medical Center
200 W Arbor Drive 619-543-6014
San Diego, CA 92103-1910 Fax: 619-435-36
gcrc.ucsd.edu
General clinical research.
Michael G Zieglor, Program Director
Melinda Richards, Administrative Manager

4800 University of California: Cardiovascular Research Laboratory
Center for Health Sciences
UCLA Medical Center 310-825-6824
Los Angeles, CA 90024 Fax: 310-206-5777
Cellular and subcellular cardiac conditions.
Dr Glenn Langer, Director

4801 University of Cincinnati Department of Pathology & Laboratory Medicine
231 Bethesda Avenue 513-558-4500
Cincinnati, OH 45267-1 Fax: 513-558-2289
e-mail: decourgm@ucmail.uc.edu
pathology.uc.edu
C Fenoglio Preiser, Director
Meifeng Xu PhD, Research Instructor

4802 University of Iowa: Iowa Cardiovascular Center
College of Medicine
616 MRC 319-335-8588
Iowa City, IA 52242 Fax: 319-335-6969
www.int-med.uiowa.edu
The purpose is to coordinate the cardiovascular programs of the College into a more cohesive unit to permit us to 1) utilize our cardiovascular resources optimally 2) intensify expand and integrate basic and clinical research programs in areas related to cardiovascular research and 3) evaluate the role of new measures for prevention diagnosis and treatment of cardiovascular disease.
Francois M Abboud, Director
Mark E Anderson MD PhD, Associate Director

4803 University of Michigan Pulmonary and Critical Care Division
University Hospital
1500 E Medical Center Drive 734-936-5383
Ann Arbor, MI 48109 888-287-1082
Fax: 734-763-7390
www2.med.umich.edu
Melvyn Rubenfire, Director

4804 University of Michigan: Division of Cardiology
1500 E Medical Center Drive 734-936-3236
Ann Arbor, MI 48109-0001
Focuses on the diagnosis, treatment and prevention of cardiovascular and heart diseases.
Dr. Bertram Pitt, Director

4805 University of Missouri Columbia Division of Cardiothoracic Surgery
School of Medicine
1 Hospital Drive 573-882-6955
Columbia, MO 65212 Fax: 573-884-0437
e-mail: sissonwhitem@health.missouri.edu
www.missouri.edu
Cardiac surgery research.
Brady J Deaton, Chancellor

4806 University of Pennsylvania Pennsylvania Muscle Institute
School of Medicine
3700 Hamilton Walk 215-898-4017
Philadelphia, PA 19104 Fax: 215-898-2653
e-mail: mafoster@mail.med.upenn.edu
www.med.upenn.edu
Studies in tissue science.
Yale E Goldman MD, Director
Michael Osta PhD, Associate Director

4807 University of Pittsburgh: Human Energy Research Laboratory
242 Trees Hall
Pittsburgh, PA 15261-0001 412-624-4387
www.pitt.edu
Focuses on exercise and cardiac rehabilitation.
Dr Robert Robertson, Director

4808 University of Rochester: Clinical Research Center
601 Elmwood Avenue 585-275-3676
Rochester, NY 14642-0001 Fax: 585-256-3805
e-mail: germaine_reinhardt@urmc.rochester.edu
www.urmc.rochester.edu
Studies of normal tissue functions pertaining to heart diseases.
John E Gerich MD, Director
David S Guzick MD, Principal Investigator

4809 University of Southern California: Coronary Care Research
1200 N State Street 213-226-7242
Los Angeles, CA 90033-1029
Dr. L Julian Haywood, Director

4810 University of Tennessee: Division of Cardiovascular Diseases
920 Madison Avenue 901-448-5750
Memphis, TN 38163-0001 Fax: 901-448-8084
www.utmem.edu\cardiology
Cardiovascular system disorders including heart disease prevention and treatment.
Karl T Weber MD, Director

4811 University of Texas Southwestern Medical Center at Dallas
University of Texas
5323 Harry Hines Boulevard 214-648-7500
Dallas, TX 75390-7208 Fax: 214-483-11
www.utsouthwestern.edu
Cardiology department research.
Kern Wildenthal PhD MD, President

4812 University of Utah: Artificial Heart Research Laboratory
803 N 300 W 801-581-6991
Salt Lake City, UT 84103-1414 Fax: 801-581-4044
healthsciences.utah.edu
Cardiac and blood vessel research.
Dr Don B Olsen, Director

4813 University of Utah: Cardiovascular Genetic Research Clinic
420 Chipeta Way 801-581-3888
Salt Lake City, UT 84108-0001 Fax: 801-581-6862
medicine.utah.edu
Cardiovascular genetics research.
Dr Roger Williams, Founder
Sara Frogley, Research Manager

4814 Urban Cardiology Research Center
2300 Garrison Boulevard 410-945-8600
Baltimore, MD 21216-2308
Causes diagnosis and treatment of cardiovascular diseases.
Arthur White MD, Director

4815 Warren Grant Magnuson Clinical Center
National Institute of Health
9000 Rockville Pike
Bethesda, MD 20892 800-411-1222
Fax: 301-480-9793
TTY: 866-411-1010
e-mail: prpl@mail.cc.nih.gov
www.clinicalcenter.nih.gov
Established in 1953 as the research hospital of the National Institutes of Health. Designed so that patient care facilities are close to research laboratories so new findings of basic and clinical scientists can be quickly applied to the treatment of patients. Upon referral by physicians, patients are admitted to NIH clinical studies.
John Gallin, Director
David Henderson, Deputy Director for Clinical Care

4816 Yeshiva University General Clinical Research Center
Eastchester Road & Morris Park Aven
Bronx, NY 10461 718-430-8514
www.yu.edu
Cardiovascular research.
Harriet S Gilbert MD, Program Director
William Arsenio, Research Training Director

Support Groups & Hotlines

4817 American Autoimmune Related Diseases Association
22100 Gratiot Avenue 586-776-3900
Eastpointe, MI 48021 800-598-4668
Fax: 586-776-3903
e-mail: aarda@aarda.org
www.aarda.org
Awareness, education, referrals for patients with any type of autoimmune disease.
Virginia T. Ladd, President/Executive Director

4818 Mended Hearts
7272 Greenville Avenue 214-706-1442
Dallas, TX 75231 888-432-7899
Fax: 214-706-5231
e-mail: dbonham@Heart.org
www.mendedhearts.org
Mutual support for persons who have heart disease, their families, friends, and other interested persons.

4819 Mitral Valve Prolapse Program of Cincinnati Support Group
10525 Montgomery Road 513-745-9911
Cincinnati, OH 45242 e-mail: kscordo@wright.edu
www.nursing.wright.edu
Brings together persons frightened by their symptoms in order to learn to better cope with MVP. Fosters use of non-drug therapies. Supervised exercise sessions, diagnostic evaluations and specialized testing. Information and referrals, conferences, literature, group meetings, MVP Hot Line, and assistance in starting groups.

4820 National Health Information Center
PO Box 1133 310-565-4167
Washington, DC 20013 800-336-4797
Fax: 301-984-4256
e-mail: info@nhic.org
www.health.gov/nhic
Offers a nationwide information referral service, produces directories and resource guides.

4821 National Society for MVP and Dysautonomia
880 Montclair Road 205-595-8229
Birmingham, AL 35213 866-595-8229
Fax: 205-595-8222
e-mail: nancysawyermd@bellsouth.net
Assists individuals suffering from mitral valve prolapse syndrome and dysautonomia to find support and understanding. Education on symptoms and treatment. Other areas of focus are Fibromyalgia and Sjogren's Syndrome.
Nancy Sawyer, MD

4822 Pulmonary Hypertension Association
850 Sligo Avenue 301-565-3004
Silver Spring, MD 20907 800-748-7274
Fax: 301-565-3994
e-mail: pha@phassociation.org
www.phassociation.org
A nonprofit organization funded and for pulmonary hypertension patients. Our mission is to seek a cure, provide hope, support, education and to promote awareness and advocate for the PH community.
Rind Alrrighetti, President

4823 Society of Mitral Valve Prolapse Syndrome
PO Box 431 630-250-9327
Itasca, IL 60143-0431 Fax: 630-773-0478
e-mail: bonnie0107@aol.com
www.mitralvalveprolapse.com/
Provides support and education to patients, families and friends about mitral valve prolapse syndrome.
Phillip C Watkins, Director MVP Center
Cheryl Durante, Editor

Books

4824 Advances in Cardiac and Pulmonary Rehabilitation
Haworth Press
10 Alice Street 607-722-5857
Binghamton, NY 13904-1580 800-429-6784
Fax: 607-722-0012
www.haworthpress.com
Enhance your rehabilitation program with this authoritative volume.
74 pages Hardcover
ISBN: 0-866569-86-0

4825 Congenital Heart Disease
Northwestern University Press
625 Colfax Street 847-491-5313
Evanston, IL 60208-4210 800-621-2736
www.nupress.nwu.edu
1993 300 pages
ISBN: 1-880416-82-4

4826 Dr. Dean Ornish's Program for Reversing Heart Disease
Random House Trade Books
400 Hahn Road
Westminster, MD 21157-4663 800-733-3000
Fax: 800-659-2436
ISBN: 0-804110-38-7

4827 Expert Guide to Beating Heart Disease: What You Absolutely Must Know
Dr. Harlan M. Krumholz, author
HarperCollins
10 E. 53rd Street 212-207-7000
New York, NY 10022-5299 e-mail: orders@harpercollins.com
www.harpercollins.com
Translates key medical data into clear guidelines capturing the highest treatment standards for heart disease. Profiles care alternatices from supplements to stress reduction as well as treatments on the horizon.
2005 288 pages
ISBN: 0-060578-34-3

4828 Heart Disease
Franklin Watts Grolier
90 Old Sherman Turnpike 203-797-3500
Danbury, CT 06816-0001 800-621-1115
Fax: 203-797-3197
www.grolier.com
Using diagrams, this book discusses strokes and other blood vessel disorders, as well as their treatment and prevention.
112 pages Grades 7-12
ISBN: 0-531108-84-8

4829 Heart of a Child: What Families Need to Know About Heart Disorders: 2nd Edition
Johnss Hopkins University Press
2715 N Charles Street 410-935-6900
Baltimore, MD 21218-4319 800-537-5487
Fax: 410-516-6998
www.press.jhu.edu
1993 352 pages Paperback
ISBN: 0-801866-36-7

4830 Living with Heart Disease
Franklin Watts Grolier
90 Old Sherman Turnpike 203-797-3500
Danbury, CT 06816-0001 800-621-1115
Fax: 203-797-3197
www.grolier.com
Shows how persons with heart disease can overcome their illness and lead productive lives.
32 pages Grades 5-7
ISBN: 0-531108-45-7

4831 Mitral Valve Prolapse Syndrome/Dysautonomia Survival Guide
Society of Mitral Valve Prolapse Syndrome
PO Box 431 630-250-9327
Itasca, IL 60143-0431 Fax: 630-773-0478
e-mail: bonnie0107@aol.com
www.mitralvalveprolapse.com
Provides support and education to patients, families and friends about mitral valve prolapse syndrome.
175 pages
ISBN: 1-572243-03-1
Bonnie Durante, Vice President
Cheryl Durante, Editor

4832 What Every Woman Must Know About Heart Disease
Warner Books

1271 Avenue of the Americas 212-484-2900
New York, NY 10020-1300 Fax: 818-507-5596
e-mail: nylandimmunojobs@boxter.com
www.twbookmark.com

1996
ISBN: 0-446519-86-3

4833 Women Take Heart
Putnam Publishing Group
200 Madison Avenue 212-951-8400
New York, NY 10016-3903
1993 224 pages
ISBN: 0-399138-88-9

4834 Women and Heart Disease
Random House Trade Books
400 Hahn Road
Westminster, MD 21157-4663 800-733-3000
Fax: 800-659-2436

ISBN: 0-345386-20-5

Children's Books

4835 Village by the Sea
Franklin Watts Grolier
90 Old Sherman Turnpike 203-797-3500
Danbury, CT 06816-0001 Fax: 203-797-3197
www.grolier.com
This story focuses on the relationship between Emma and her father as he prepares to undergo bypass surgery.
Grades 5-8

Newsletters

4836 American Heart Association News
American Heart Association
7272 Greenville Avenue 214-706-1162
Dallas, TX 75231-5129 Fax: 214-696-5211
News reports and journal reports on the latest information concerning heart disease.

4837 And the Beat Goes On
Society of Mitral Valve Prolapse Syndrome
PO Box 431 630-250-9327
Itasca, IL 60143-0431 Fax: 630-773-0478
e-mail: bonnie0107@aol.com
www.mitralvalveprolapse.com
Bi-monthly newsletter. Provides support and education to patients, families and friends about mitral valve prolapse syndrome.
6 pages
Bonnie Durante, Vice President
Cheryl Durante, Editor

4838 Heartstyle
American Heart Association
7272 Greenville Avenue 214-706-1162
Dallas, TX 75231-5129 Fax: 214-696-5211
Reports on heart and blood vessel diseases and stroke.
Quarterly

4839 MVPS & Anxiety
Society of Mitral Valve Prolapse Syndrome
PO Box 431 630-250-9327
Itasca, IL 60143-0431 Fax: 630-773-0478
e-mail: bonnie0107@aol.com
www.mitralvalveprolapse.com

6 pages
Bonnie Durante, Vice President
Cheryl Durante, Editor

Pamphlets

4840 About High Blood Pressure
American Heart Association
7272 Greenville Avenue 214-706-1162
Dallas, TX 75231-5129 Fax: 214-696-5211
Offers information on what blood pressure is, risk factors and at risk persons.

4841 American Heart Association Diet
American Heart Association
7272 Greenville Avenue 214-706-1162
Dallas, TX 75231-5129 Fax: 214-696-5211
An eating plan for healthy americans.

4842 Cholesterol and Your Heart
American Heart Association
7272 Greenville Avenue 214-706-1162
Dallas, TX 75231-5129 Fax: 214-696-5211
Offers information on lowering blood cholesterol levels.

4843 Congenital Heart Defects
March of Dimes
233 Park Avenue South 212-353-8353
New York, NY 10003 Fax: 212-254-3518
e-mail: NY639@marchofdimes.com
www.marchofdimes.com

4844 E is for Exercise
American Heart Association
7272 Greenville Avenue 214-706-1162
Dallas, TX 75231-5129 Fax: 214-696-5211
Offers information on what kinds of exercise are the best and how to exercise properly.

4845 Easy Food Tips for Heart Healthy Eating
American Heart Association
7272 Greenville Avenue 214-706-1162
Dallas, TX 75231-5129 Fax: 214-696-5211
Offers food selection hints for fat-controlled meals.

4846 Eat Well, But Wisely
American Heart Association
7272 Greenville Avenue 214-706-1162
Dallas, TX 75231-5129 Fax: 214-696-5211
Offers information on good nutrition to reduce the risks of heat attacks.

4847 Exercise and Your Heart
American Heart Association
7272 Greenville Avenue 214-706-1162
Dallas, TX 75231-5129 Fax: 214-696-5211
Offers information on how to get enough exercise from daily activities, what the benefits of exercise are and what the risks of exercising are.

4848 Heart Defects
Association of Birth Defect Children
5400 Diplomat Circle
Orlando, FL 32810-5603 800-922-9234
Informational sheet on the causes, symptoms and statistics of heart defects and heart disease in children.

4849 How to Have Your Cake and Eat It Too
American Heart Association
7272 Greenville Avenue 214-706-1162
Dallas, TX 75231-5129 Fax: 214-696-5211
A guide to low-fat, low-cholesterol eating.

Web Sites

4850 American Heart Association
www.americanheart.org
Supports research, education and community service programs with the objective of reducing premature death and disability from cardiovascular diseases and stroke; coordinates the efforts of health professionals, and other engaged in the fight against heart and circulatory disease.

4851 Healing Well
www.healingwell.com
An online health resource guide to medical news, chat, information and articles, newsgroups and message boards, books, disease-related web sites, medical directories, and more for patients, friends, and family coping with disabling diseases, disorders, or chronic illnesses.

4852 **Health Finder**

www.healthfinder.gov

Searchable, carefully developed web site offering information on over 1000 topics. Developed by the US Department of Health and Human Services, the site can be used in both English and Spanish.

4853 **Healthlink USA**

www.healthlinkusa.com

Health information concerning treatment, cures, prevention, diagnosis, risk factors, research, support groups, email lists, personal stories and much more. Updated regularly.

4854 **Helios Health**

www.helioshealth.com

Online resource for your health information. Detailed information about specific health topics, access to expert advice from our Medical Advisory Board, and up-to-date health news.

4855 **MedicineNet**

www.medicinenet.com

An online resource for consumers providing easy-to-read, authoritative medical and health information.

4856 **Medscape**

www.mywebmd.com

Medscape offers specialists, primary care physicians, and other health professionals the Web's most robust and integrated medical information and educational tools.

4857 **National Heart, Lung and Blood Institute**

www.nhlbi.nih.gov

Primary responsibility of this organization is the scientific investigation of heart, blood vessel, lung and blood disorders. Oversees research, demonstration, prevention, education, control and training activities in these fields and emphasizes the prevention and control of heart diseases.

4858 **WebMD**

www.webmd.com

Information on Heart disease, including articles and resources.

Description

4859 # Hemophilia

Hemophilia is a genetic disorder that disrupts the body's normal blood clotting function because there is a deficiency of specific proteins known as clotting factors—specifically, factor VIII and factor IX. About 20,000 Americans are affected with the disorder and, currently, there is no cure.

Hemophilia is linked to the X-chromosome because that is where both factor genes are located. As a result, hemophilia affects males almost exclusively, with females being carriers, whose sons have a 50 percent chance of having the disorder.

Hemophiliacs, like anyone else, will bleed if injured, but they will bleed longer and more profusely. They may also bleed in response to injuries that are inconsequential in other people. For instance, normal daily activities may cause bleeding within a joint, leading to severe pain and swelling, and over time destroying the joint.

The severity of hemophilia varies dramatically depending on the factor VIII and IX levels, thus, affecting a person's prognosis and need for therapy. Treatment is with transfusions of the appropriate factor, and usually has to be repeated frequently. Most hemophiliacs treated with plasma concentrate in the early 1980s are infected with HIV contracted from contaminated blood and transfusions. HIV is now responsible for over half of deaths among hemophiliacs.

Most hemophiliacs are now treated at comprehensive hemophilia centers, which offer not just factor replacement but multispecialty expertise, sophisticated laboratory testing, physical therapy and psychological support. New techniques allow for identification of carrier females in these families. This is important for genetic counseling and family planning.

National Agencies & Associations

4860 **American Red Cross Blood Services**
4333 Arlington Boulevard 202-303-5000
Arlington, VA 22203 800-733-2767
e-mail: lkeefe@arlingtonredcross.org
www.redcross.org
Distributes a wide variety of plasma therapeutics to benefit people with hemophilia A and B, immune disorders and hypoalbuminemia.
Lynne Kocik Keefe, CEO

4861 **Baxter Hyland Division**
One Baxter Parkway 847-948-4770
Deerfield, IL 60015-1900 800-422-9837
Fax: 847-948-3642
www.baxter.com
Government affairs office that monitors and selectively lobbies on issues relating to Medicare Medicaid Orphan Drugs and other subjects relating to hemophilia.
Pam Koo, Programs Manager

4862 **Canadian Hemophilia Society**
625, Avenue President Kennedy 514-848-0503
Montreal, Quebec, H3A-1K2 800-668-2686
Fax: 514-848-9661
e-mail: chs@hemophilia.ca
www.hemophilia.ca
Strives to improve the health and quality of life for all people with inherited bleeding disorders and to find a cure.
David Page, Executive Director
Wendy Wong, National Director Resource Development

4863 **Hemophilia Health Services**
201 Great Circle Road 615-352-2500
Nashville, TN 37228 800-800-6606
Fax: 615-261-6730
e-mail: info@hemophiliahealth.com
www.hemophiliahealth.com
Largest homecare company devoted solely to serving people with bleeding disorders.
Ken Trader, VP of Sales and Marketing

4864 **National Hemophilia Foundation**
116 W 32nd Street 212-328-3700
New York, NY 10001 800-424-2634
Fax: 212-328-3777
e-mail: info@hemophilia.org
www.hemophilia.org
Dedicated to the treatment and the cure of hemophilia, related bleeding disorders and complications of those disorders or their treatment, including HIV infection, as well as improving the quality of life of all those affected.
Val Bias, Chief Executive Officer
Howard A Balsam, COO

4865 **National Hemophilia Foundation's Information Center**
116 W 32nd Street 212-328-3700
New York, NY 10001 800-424-2634
Fax: 212-328-3777
e-mail: info@hemophilia.org
www.hemophilia.org
Offers various information articles resources books and more for the hemophilia and HIV/AIDS community.
Alan Kinnibu PhD, CEO
Paul Haas, President

4866 **World Federation of Hemophilia**
1425 Rene Levesque Boulevard W 514-875-7944
Montreal, Quebec, H3G-1T7 Fax: 514-875-8916
e-mail: wfh@wfh.org
www.wfh.org
An international not-for-profit organization to improving the lives of people with hemophilia and related bleeding disorders.
Miklos Fulop, CEO/Executive Director

State Agencies & Associations

Alabama

4867 **Alabama Chapter of the National Hemaphilia Foundation**
802 Midland Avenue 205-381-5925
Muscle Shoals, AL 35661-1640

Arkansas

4868 **Hemophilia Foundation of Arkansas**
351 Valley Oak Lane 501-941-3109
Austin, AR 72007 888-941-4366
e-mail: angieclark1315@sbcglobal.net
www.hemophilia.org

Angie Clark, President
John Little, VP

California

4869 Central California Chapter of the National Hemophilia Foundation
PO Box 163689 916-734-3461
Sacramento, CA 95816 Fax: 916-489-1569
e-mail: seanahubbert@yahoo.com
www.cchfsac.org
A very small and family-oriented chapter. Offers an active youth group, an annual summer camp, a men's and women's group and various family activities for persons living in the central California valley from its center in Sacramento to the borders of Nevada.
Sean Hubbert, President

4870 Hemophilia Association of San Diego County
3570 Camino Del Rio N 619-325-3570
San Diego, CA 92108 Fax: 619-325-4350
e-mail: info@hasdc.org
www.hasdc.org
Provides summer camp programs for young persons with hemophilia, sponsors educational programs for the general public, sponsors support groups for parents to help them deal with hemophilia, monitors legislation pertaining to hemophilia and related conditions.
Teresa Ramirez, Executive Director

4871 Hemophilia Foundation of Northern California
6400 Hollis Street 510-658-3324
Emeryville, CA 94608-3024 888-749-4362
Fax: 510-658-3384
e-mail: support@hemofoundation.org
www.hemofoundation.org
A volunteer, nonprofit organization serving the needs of people with hemophilia and other related bleeding disorders in 35 counties in Northern California. Provides hemophilia literature, scholarships, youth programs and annual summer camps.
Nancy Trunzo, Office Administrator
Merlin Wedepohl, Executive Director

4872 Hemophilia Foundation of Southern California
6720 Melrose Avenue 323-525-0440
Hollywood, CA 90038 800-371-4123
Fax: 323-525-0445
e-mail: hfsc@hemosocal.org
www.hemosocal.org
Helena Smith, Office Manager
Linda Corrente, Executive Director

Colorado

4873 Hemophilia Society of Colorado
1301 Ulysses Street 303-629-6990
Golden, CO 80203 888-687-CLOT
Fax: 303-629-7035
e-mail: hsc@cohemo.org
www.cohemo.org
Daniel Reilly, President
Diane Cadwell, Vice President

Florida

4874 Florida Chapter of the National Hemophilia Foundation
18001 Old Cutler Road 813-367-0050
Palmetto Bay, FL 33157 888-880-8330
Fax: 813-367-0051
e-mail: linda316@bellsouth.net
www.floridahemophilia.org
Debbi Adamkin, Executive Director
Linda Thomas, President

Georgia

4875 Hemophilia Foundation of Georgia
8800 Roswelll Road 770-518-8272
Atlanta, GA 30350 Fax: 770-518-3310
e-mail: mail.@hog.org
www.hog.org
Established to help Georgia residents with hemophilia lead normal and productive lives. Because this organization is comprised of patients, their friends and families, it is especially motivated to provide the best in personalized and comprehensive services.
Patricia Dominic, CEO
Dave Fronk, Vice Chief Governance Officer

Hawaii

4876 Hemophilia Foundation of Hawaii Kapiolani Medical Center
Kapiolani Medical Center
1164 Bishop Street 808-638-2910
Honolulu, HI 96813 Fax: 808-638-2910
e-mail: hemophiliafoundation@hawaii.rr.com
www.bleedingdisorders.org
Jeanine Keoh Kam, Executive Manager

Idaho

4877 Hemophilia Foundation of Idaho
PO Box 7622 208-344-4476
Boise, ID 83707-1622 e-mail: info@idahoblood.org
www.hemophilia.org
Janet Angell, Foundation Administrator

Illinois

4878 Hemophilia Foundation of Illinois
332 S Michigan Avenue 312-427-1495
Chicago, IL 60604-4305 Fax: 312-427-1602
e-mail: info@hfi-il.org
www.hemophiliaillinois.org
Serves as an information source referral service and advocate for persons with hemophilia and their families. The mission of this chapter is to provide counseling, educational information and support services to persons affected by hemophilia and related disorders.
Robert P Robinson, Executive Director
Lily Schwartz, Associate Director

Indiana

4879 Hemophilia Foundation of Indiana
5170 E 65th Street 317-570-0039
Indianapolis, IN 46220 800-241-2873
Fax: 317-570-0058
e-mail: cfeay@hoii.org
www.hemophiliaofindiana.org
Chad Feay, Executive Director
Debbie Ford, Office Manger

Kentucky

4880 Kentucky Hemophilia Foundation
1850 Taylor Avenue 502-456-3233
Louisville, KY 40213 800-582-2873
Fax: 502-456-3234
e-mail: info@kyhemo.org
www.kyhemo.org
Assists individuals with hemophilia and related inherited bleeding disorders through education, advocacy and support services. Services include quarterly newsletter, post secondary education scholarship, summer camp for children, seminars and support functions.
Quarterly
Ursela M Lacer, Executive Director

Louisiana

4881 Louisiana Chapter of the National Hemophilia Foundation
3636 S Sherwood Forest 225-291-1675
Baton Rouge, LA 70816-2285 800-749-1680
Fax: 225-291-1679
e-mail: lahemophilia@hipoint.net
www.louisianahemophilia.org
Lori Keels, Executive Director
Tres Major, President

Maryland

4882 **Hemophilia Foundation of Maryland**
13 Class Court 410-661-2307
Baltimore, MD 21234-2602 800-964-3131
Fax: 410-661-2308
www.hfmonline.org

The Hemophilia foundation of Maryland is a private not for profit organization which devotes its efforts to improving the quality of life for persons affected with bleeding disorders and their complications.

4883 **Maryland Chapter of the National Hemophilia Foundation**
PO Box 164 410-291-1675
Phoenix, MD 21131-0164 Fax: 410-285-3271

Massachusetts

4884 **New England Hemophilia Association**
347 Washington Street 781-326-7645
Dedham, MA 02026 Fax: 781-329-5122
e-mail: info@newenglandhemophilia.org
www.newenglandhemophilia.org

New England Hemophilia Association is dedicated to improving the quality of life for persons with bleeding disorders (hemophilia, von Willebrands, and other factor deficiencies) and their families through education, support and advocacy.

Kevin R Sorge, Executive Director
Jane Cavanau Smith, Director of Programs

Michigan

4885 **Hemophilia Foundation of Michigan**
1921 W Michigan Avenue 734-544-0015
Ypsilanti, MI 48197 800-482-3041
Fax: 734-544-0095
e-mail: hfm@hfmich.org
www.hfmich.org

Coordinates funding, professional education, and networking, with Hemophilia Treatment Centers in Michigan, Indiana, and Ohio. Provides educational services, including workshops, meetings, symposiums, and numerous publications.

Ivan C Harner, Executive Director
Tami Wood-Lively, Regional Coordinator

Minnesota

4886 **Hemophilia Foundation of Minnesota and the Dakotas**
750 S Plaza Drive 651-406-8655
Mendota Heights, MN 55120 Fax: 651-406-8656
e-mail: hemophiliafound@visi.com
www.hfmd.org

A nonprofit organization established to be a leader and a catalyst within the community to enable and inspire members to impact their own lives, with the ultimate aim of cures for both hemophilia and HIV/AIDS.

Aaron Reeves, President/Board of Directors
Bob Stone Jr, Vice President

Mississippi

4887 **Mississippi Hemophilia Foundation**
PO Box 13608 601-957-6483
Jackson, MS 39236 e-mail: haleyjones80@yahoo.com
www.hemophilia.org

Haley Jones, President
Patty Lyons, Treasurer

Missouri

4888 **Gateway Hemophilia Association**
4515 Olive Street 314-361-9500
Saint Louis, MO 63108 877-623-8300
Fax: 314-729-7033
e-mail: info@gatewayhemophilia.org
www.gatewayhemophilia.org

Daniel Kahmke, President
Bridget Tyrey, Vice-President

Nebraska

4889 **Nebraska Chapter of the National Hemophilia Foundation**
215 Centennial Mall S 402-742-5663
Lincoln, NE 68508 Fax: 402-742-5677
e-mail: office@nebraskanhf.org
www.nebraskanhf.org

The mission of this chapter is to provide support, education, communication and advocacy for men, women and children challenged by Hemophilia. Services provided include a toll free telephone hotline for persons seeking information on HIV and hemophilia.

Carl Clark, President
James Clarke, Vice-President

Nevada

4890 **Hemophilia Foundation of Nevada**
1850 Whitney Mesa 702-564-4368
Henderson, NV 89014 Fax: 702-446-8134
e-mail: Info@hfnv.org
www.hfnv.org

Ramona Alice RN, President Executive Committee
Greg Mireles, Vice President Executive Committee

New Mexico

4891 **Hemophilia Foundation of New Mexico**
1601 Valdez Drive NE 505-341-9321
Albuquerque, NM 87112 866-341-9321
Fax: 505-292-5818
e-mail: sangredeoro@comcast.net
www.hemophilia.org

Loretta Cordova, Executive Director
Johanna Chappelle, President

New York

4892 **Hemophilia Center of Western New York**
462 Grider Street 716-896-2470
Buffalo, NY 14215 800-669-2299
Fax: 716-898-5537
e-mail: info@hemophiliawny.com
www.hemophiliawny.com

Rosemary Holmberg, Executive Director
Thomas Long, President

4893 **Mary M Gooley Hemophilia Center: A Chapter of the NHF**
1415 Portland Avenue 585-922-5700
Rochester, NY 14621 Fax: 585-922-5775
e-mail: robert.fox@rochestergeneral.org
www.hemocenter.org

Robert Fox, CEO/ President
Peter Kouides, Medical & Research Director

North Carolina

4894 **Hemophilia Foundation of North Carolina**
PO Box 70 919-319-0014
Cary, NC 27512 800-990-5557
Fax: 919-319-0016
e-mail: info@hemophilia-nc.org
www.hemophilia-nc.org

A nonprofit organization that serves as an information source for the hemophilia community of North Carolina. Supply the most up-to-date information concerning hemophilia and hemophilia related HIV/AIDS.

Richard Atwood, President
Leonard Poe, Vice President & Advocacy Chair

Ohio

4895 **Central Ohio Chapter of the National Hemophilia Foundation**
834 W Third Avenue 614-429-2120
Columbus, OH 43212-0345 800-847-0345
Fax: 614-429-2122
e-mail: info@nhfcentralohio.org
www.nhfcentralohio.org

Jim Wasserstrom, President
Rob Alexander, Executive Director

4896 **Greater Cincinnati/Northern Kentucky Chapter of the NHF**
1008 Marshall Avenue 513-961-4366
Cincinnati, OH 45225 Fax: 513-961-1740
e-mail: hemophilia@fuse.net
tristatebleedingdisorderfoundation.org
Lisa Raterman, Executive Director
Brad Sanders, President

4897 **Northern Ohio Chapter of the National Hemophilia Foundation**
One Independence Place
4807 Rockside Road 216-834-0051
Independence, OH 44131 800-554-4366
Fax: 216-834-0055
e-mail: lynnecapretto@nohf.org
www.nohf.org
Lynne Capretto, Executive Director
Teresa Glass, President

4898 **Northwest Ohio Hemophilia Association**
241 N Superior Street 419-242-9587
Toledo, OH 43604 Fax: 419-242-4951
e-mail: hemo@uhs-toledo.org
www.uhs-toledo.org
Carla Wells, Executive Director
Scott Newsom, President

4899 **Southwestern Ohio Chapter of the National Hemophilia Foundation**
3131 S Dixie Drive 937-298-8000
Moraine, OH 45439 Fax: 937-298-8080
e-mail: info@swohiohemophilia.org
www.swohiohemophilia.org
This chapter serves persons with hemophilia and blood clotting disorders in an 11 county area. It is dedicated to offering people with hemophilia and related blood disorders and their families educational opportunities about the diseases.
Sharon DiLorenzo, Executive Director
Dena M Shepard, President

Oklahoma

4900 **Oklahoma Chapter of the National Hemophilia Foundation**
PO Box 30242 405-636-9831
Edmund, OK 73003 800-735-3855
e-mail: TAyers007@aol.com
www.okhemophilia.org
Tom Ayers, President
Genny Goodley, Secretary

Oregon

4901 **Hemophilia Foundation of Oregon**
5319 SW Westgate Drive 503-297-7207
Portland, OR 97221 Fax: 503-297-0127
e-mail: hfo@easystreet.com
www.hfo.info
Chris Leland, President
Alex Ell, Vice President

Pennsylvania

4902 **Delaware Valley Chapter of the National Hemophilia Foundation**
222 S Easton Road 215-885-6500
Glenside, PA 19038 Fax: 215-885-6074
e-mail: hemophilia@navpoint.com
www.hemophiliasupport.org
Ann Rogers, Executive Director
Clifford Cohn, President

4903 **Western Pennsylvania Chapter of the National Hemophilia Foundation**
532 S Aiken Avenue 412-683-2231
Pittsburgh, PA 15232 800-824-0016
Fax: 412-683-2568
e-mail: wpcnhf@earthlink.net
www.westpennhemophilia.org
Brings together and serves as a focal point for those segments of the community most concerned with hemophilia. They include medical and social service providers, people with hemophilia and their families educators and the general public.
Kerry Fatula, Executive Director
Ida McFarren, President

Rhode Island

4904 **Rhode Island Hemophilia Foundation**
160 Plainfield Street 401-944-6950
Providence, RI 02909

South Carolina

4905 **Hemophilia Association of South Carolina**
PO Box 2386
Irmo, SC 29063 888-829-4849
e-mail: Factoreight@aol.com

Tennessee

4906 **TN Hemo & Bleeding Disorders Foundation**
203 Jefferson Street 615-220-4868
Smyrna, TN 37167-5281 888-703-3269
Fax: 615-220-4889
e-mail: linda@thbdf.org
www.thbdf.org
Offers a hemophilia clinic social workers and consultants a state hemophilia program blood donor programs counseling programs genetic counseling literature and resources summer camp grants and more for the hemophilia and HIV/AIDS community.
Linda McClanahan, Executive Director
Sandy Jones, President

Texas

4907 **Lone Star Chapter of the National Hemophilia Foundation**
10500 NW Freeway 713-686-6100
Houston, TX 77092 888-LSC-NHF1
Fax: 713-686-6102
e-mail: Debbiedelariva@yahoo.com
www.lonestarhemophilia.org
Debbie De La Riva, Executive Director
Brian Compton, President

4908 **Texas Central Chapter of the National Hemophilia Foundation**
3530 Forest Lane 214-351-4595
Dallas, TX 75234 Fax: 214-654-9954
e-mail: mail@texcen.org
www.texcen.org
A group of volunteers seeking solutions to the various aspects of the hemophilia problem. Supports blood drives sponsors a summer camp for hemophiliac children, conducts educational member meetings, arranges for genetic counseling and sponsors group support meetings.
Shanna Garcia, President
Shelley Embry, Secretary and Executive Director

Utah

4909 **Utah Chapter of the National Hemophilia Foundation**
772 E 3300 S 801-484-0325
Salt Lake City, UT 84106 877-463-6893
Fax: 801-484-4177
www.hemophiliautah.org
Offers educational information, pamphlets, fundraising events and more for persons and families affected by hemophilia.
Scott Muir, Executive Director
David Ohlson, President

Virginia

4910 **Hemophilia Association of the Capital Area**
10560 Main Street 703-352-7641
Fairfax, VA 22030-1504 Fax: 703-352-2145
e-mail: hacacares@verizon.net
www.hacacares.org
A nonprofit organization serving persons with bleeding disorders and their families in northern Virginia Washington DC and Montgomery and Prince George's Counties in Maryland. This chapter's

mission is to improve the quality of life for persons with hemophelia.
Sandi Qualley, Executive Director
Kirstin Duggan, President

4911 United Virginia Chapter of the National Hemophilia Foundation
PO Box 188 804-748-7896
Midlothian, VA 23113-8824 800-266-8438
Fax: 804-740-8643
e-mail: vahemophiliaed@verizon.net
www.vahemophilia.org
Kelly Waters, Executive Director
Jeff Krecek, President

Washington

4912 Hemophilia Foundation of Washington
9659 Firdale Avenue 206-652-5789
Edmunds, WA 98020 Fax: 206-652-5790
e-mail: regina@bdfwa.org
www.bdfwa.org
Regina Timmons, Executive Director
Reid Morgan, President

4913 Inland Empire Bleeding Disorders
1010 Riverside Drive 509-967-7417
W Richland, WA 99353 866-710-4323
e-mail: iebd4u@verizon.net
www.hemophilia.org
Debbie Campeau, President
Jill McCary, President

Wisconsin

4914 Great Lakes Hemophilia Foundation
638 N 18th Street 414-257-0200
Milwaukee, WI 53233 888-797-4543
Fax: 414-257-1225
e-mail: info@glhf.org
www.glhf.org
The only Wisconsin organization that addresses the physical, emotional social and financial needs of individuals affected by hemophilia. This chapter supports high-quality cost-effective programs for patient care, education, research and public awareness.
Kathleen Roach, Executive Director
Beth Rodenhuis, President

Foundations

4915 National Hemophilia Foundation
116 West 32nd Street 212-328-3700
New York, NY 10001 800-42H-ANDI
Fax: 212-328-3777
e-mail: handi@hemophilia.org
www.hemophilia.org
The National Hemophilia Foundation is dedicated to finding better treatments and cures for bleeding and clotting disorders and to preventing the complications of these disorders through education, advocacy and research.
Alan Kinniburgh, PhD, Chief Executive Officer

Research Centers

4916 Albert Einstein Medical Center Hemophilia Program
5501 Old York Road 215-456-7890
Philadelphia, PA 19141 Fax: 215-456-6179
www.einstein.edu
With humanity humility and honor to heal by providing exceptionally intelligent and responsive healthcare and education for as many as we can reach
Mehdi K Kajani MD

4917 American Red Cross Hemophilia Center
4860 Sheboygan Avenue 608-227-1303
Madison, WI 53705-0905 Fax: 608-233-8318
www.redcross.org
Diane Nugent MD

4918 Boston Hemophilia Center Fegan 5 Children's Hospital
Fegan 5 Children's Hospital
300 Longwood Avenue 617-355-6101
Boston, MA 02115 Fax: 617-732-5706
www.childrenshospital.org
The program offers comprehensive care to people with hemophilia and their families. Our services range from medical treatment counseling and support to discounts on clotting-factor replacement and other products that people with hemophilia require.
Ellis Neufel MD PhD, Associate Chief Division of Hematology/
Estelle Thomas, Administrative Associate

4919 Bowman Grey School of Medicine: Hemophilia Diagnostic Center
Wake Forest University
Department of Pediatrics 919-716-4324
Winston Salem, NC 27157-0001 Fax: 910-716-7100
Christine A Johnson MD

4920 Children's Hospital Hemophilia Treatment Center
3333 Burnet Avenue 513-636-4200
Cincinnati, OH 45229 800-344-2462
Fax: 513-636-5599
TTY: 513-636-4900
www.cincinnatichildrens.org
Cincinnati Children's will improve child health and transform delivery of care through fully integrated globally recognized research education and innovation.
Ralph Gruppo MD, Director

4921 Childrens Hospital of Philadelphia Hemophilia Program
Division of Hematology
34th Street and Civic Center Boulev 215-590-1000
Philadelphia, PA 19104 Fax: 215-903-92
www.chop.edu
The Children's Hospital of Philadelphia the oldest hospital in the United States dedicated exclusively to pediatrics strives to be the world leader in the advancement of healthcare for children by integrating excellent patient care innovative research and quality professional education into all of its programs.
Alan R Cohen MD, Medical Director

4922 Comprehensive Hemophilia Diagnostic and Treatment Center
University of North Carolina
450 W Drive 919-966-3036
Chapel Hill, NC 27599-7016 Fax: 919-966-3036
e-mail: lccc@med.unc.edu
www.unchealthcare.org
Multidisciplinary clinics are dedicated to patients with hemophilia (through the Comprehensive Hemophilia Diagnostic and Treatment Center) sickle cell disease brain tumors late effects of anticancer therapy as well as general hematology/oncology.
Michelle Manning, Center Coordinator
Al Baldwin, Associate Director Basic Research

4923 Comprehensive Pediatric Hemophilia Center University of South Florida
University of South Florida
450 W Drive 813-974-2201
Tampa, FL 33612-4742
Sara Griggs RN

4924 Eastern Michigan Hemophilia Center St. Joseph Hospital
St. Joseph Hospital
302 Kensington Avenue 810-762-8656
Flint, MI 48503-2044
Leslie Kirschke

4925 Eau Claire Hemophilia Center
900 W Clairemont Avenue 715-839-4418
Eau Claire, WI 54701 Fax: 715-833-4976
Vicky Anders RN

4926 Fairview-University Hemophilia & Thrombosis Center
Harvard Street at E River Road 612-626-6455
Minneapolis, MN 55455 800-688-5252
Fax: 612-625-4955
Serves over 700 adults and children in Minnesota with inherited bleeding disorders. Offers access to current technologies and treatments. Special programs include patient support group family retreats and camps.
Linda Swanso RN, Program Manager

4927 Great Plains Regional Hemophilia Center University of Iowa Hospitals
University of Iowa Hospitals
200 Howkins Drive 319-384-8442
Iowa City, IA 52242 800-777-8442
Fax: 319-567-59
www.uiowa.edu
Donald E Macfarlane, Director

4928 Greater Grand Rapids Pediatric Hemophilia Program
DeVos at Spectrum Health Systems
100 Michigan NE 616-391-2033
Grand Rapids, MI 49503
James B Fahner MD

4929 Gulf States Hemophilia Diagnostic and Treatment Center
University of Texas Health Science Center Houston
6655 Travis Street 713-500-8360
Houston, TX 77030-3005 800-464-1440
Fax: 713-500-8364
www.livingwithhaemophilia.com
Marisela Trujillo, Financial Administer
W Hoots, Medical Director

4930 Gundersen Clinic Comprehensive Hemophilia Treatment Center
Gundersen Clinic
1900 S Avenue 608-782-7300
LaCrosse, WI 54601 800-362-9567
Fax: 608-775-6692
e-mail: info@GundLuth.org
www.gundluth.com
Jeff Thompson, Chief Executive Officer
Joan Curran, Chief Government Relations and External

4931 Hematology Treatment Center of the Great Lakes Hemophilia Foundation
8734 W Watertown Plank Road 414-257-2424
Wauwatosa, WI 53226-3548 Fax: 414-257-1225
Joan Gill MD

4932 Hemophilia Association of the Huntington Area
Marshall University School of Medicine
1600 Medical Center Drive 304-691-1384
Huntington, WV 25703-1518 877-691-1600
Fax: 304-691-1375
Andrew Tendleton, Medical Director

4933 Hemophilia Association of the Huntington A Marshall University School of Medicine
1600 Medical Center Drive 304-691-1384
Huntington, WV 25703 877-691-1600
Fax: 304-691-1375
Andrew Tendleton, Medical Director

4934 Hemophilia Center of Central Pennsylvania Penn State Milton S Hershey Medical Cent
Penn State Milton S Hershey Medical Center
500 University Drive 717-531-7468
Hershey, PA 17033 Fax: 717-310-47
M Elaine Eyster MD, Medical Director

4935 Hemophilia Center of Rhode Island Rhode Island Hospital
Rhode Island Hospital
593 Eddy Street 401-444-8250
Providence, RI 02903 Fax: 401-444-6104
Peter Smith MD

4936 Hemophilia Center of West Virginia University Health Sciences Center
University Health Sciences Center
Medical Center Drive 304-293-4229
Morgantown, WV 26506 Fax: 304-293-3793
John S Rogers II MD

4937 Hemophilia Center of Western New York Erie County Medical Center
Erie County Medical Center
462 Grider Street 716-896-2470
Buffalo, NY 14215-3021 Fax: 716-898-5537
www.hemophiliawny.com
The center provides a variety of services to the hemophilia and HIV/AIDS community. Included among these services are diagnostics registration outpatient treatment home care programs home visits school visits dental services and counseling services. Offers an adult unit and a pediatric unit.
Rosemary Holmberg, Executive Director
Thomas Long, President

4938 Hemophilia Center of the Huntington Hospital
100 W California Boulevard
Pasadena, CA 91105-3023 626-397-5000
www.huntingtonhospital.com
At Huntington our mission is to excel at the delivery of health care to our community.
Stephen Ralph, President and CEO
Bernadette Merlino, Vice President/Service Line and Ambulato

4939 Hemophilia Center of the New England Medical Center
Tufts New England Medical Center
800 Washington Street 617-636-5000
Boston, MA 02111-1526 Fax: 617-636-7738
www.tuftsmedicalcenter.org
Comprehensive care for pediatric and young adult individuals with bleeding and prothrombotic disorders.
Ellen Zane, President and Chief Executive Officer
David G Fairchild MD MP, Chief Medical Officer

4940 Hemophilia Clinic: Childrens' Rehabilitation Service
1870 Pleasant Avenue 334-479-8617
Mobile, AL 36617 800-879-8163
Nancy Woodall RN

4941 Hemophilia Treatment Center at Children's National Medical Center
Department of Hematology/Oncology
111 Michigan Avenue NW 202-884-3622
Washington, DC 20010 Fax: 202-884-2976
www.livingwithhaemophilia.com
Gordon L Bray MD

4942 Louisiana Comprehensive Hemophilia Care Center
1430 Tulane Avenue 504-988-5433
New Orleans, LA 70112-2699 Fax: 504-883-08
e-mail: cleissi@tulane.edu
tulane.edu
Cindy Leissinger, Director

4943 Maine Hemophilia Treatment Center
19 Bramhall Street 207-885-7683
Portland, ME 04102 Fax: 207-885-7565
Nancy Roy RN

4944 Mayo Comprehensive Hemophilia Center Mayo Clinic
Mayo Clinic
200 1st Street SW 507-284-2021
Rochester, MN 55905-1 800-344-7726
Fax: 507-284-8286
A World Federation of Hemophilia-designated International Hemophilia Training Center provides multidisciplinary assessment and care of persons with bleeding disorders. Offers consultation with hemotologists specializing in the care of pediatric and adult patients a special consultation laboratory testing center and more.
Harlan Langstraat, Director

4945 Miami Comprehensive Hemophilia Center Jackson Medical Towers
Jackson Medical Towers
1500 NW 305-243-4791
Miami, FL 33136-3609 Fax: 305-324-9785
Susan Schmal ARNP

4946 Michigan State University Hemophilia Comprehensive Care Clinic
Michigan State University
2900 Hannah Boulevard 517-353-9385
E Lansing, MI 48823 800-759-5595
Fax: 517-353-9421
John Penner MD, Head Physician

4947 Missouri Illinois Regional Hemophilia Comprehensive Treatment Center
3635 Vista Avenue & Grand Boulevard 314-268-5275
Saint Louis, MO 63104-1003 Fax: 314-268-5104
Kathleen P Gioia RN

4948 Mountain State Regional Hemophilia Center University of Arizona Health Sciences Ce
University of Arizona Health Sciences Center
1501 N Campbell Avenue 520-626-9688
Tucson, AZ 85724-0001 Fax: 520-626-9868
www.ahsc.arizona.edu
John J Hutter Jr

4949 Nadeene Brunini Comprehensive Hemophilia Care Center
St Michael s Medical Center
268 Martin Luther King Jr Boulevard 973-877-5340
Newark, NJ 07102-2011 Fax: 973-775-5466
e-mail: dominiquej@cathedralhealth.org
www.hanj.org
Hemophilia and other bleeding disorder treatment center.
Louis Greene, Director

4950 North Dakota Comprehensive Hemophilia Center
Roger Maris Cancer Center
820 4th Street N 701-234-7544
Fargo, ND 58122-0001 800-437-4010
Fax: 701-234-7592
A treatment center for diseases of hemotosis and thrombosis which includes a clinical research program in bleeding disorders. Hemotologists are available for consultation 24 hours a day.

4951 North Dakota Comprehensive Hemophilia and Thrombosis Treatment Center
Roger Maris Cancer Center
820 4th Street N 701-234-7544
Fargo, ND 58122-0001 800-437-4010
Fax: 701-234-7577
www.meritcare.com
A treatment center for diseases of hemotosis and thrombosis which includes a clinical research program in bleeding disorders. Hemotologists are available for consultation 24 hours a day.
Dr Nathan Kobrinsky MD, Hemophilia Treatment Director

4952 North Texas Comprehensive Adult Hemophilia Center
University of Texas Southwestern Medical Center
5323 Harry Hines Boulevard
Dallas, TX 75390-7208 214-648-3111
www.utsouthwestern.edu
Cynthia J Rutherford, Director

4953 North Texas Comprehensive Pediatric Hemophilia Center
1935 Motor Street 214-456-2382
Dallas, TX 75235-7701 Fax: 214-456-6133
www.hemophiliaregion6.org
Andrea Johns RN PNP

4954 Northwest Ohio Hemophilia Treatment Center
The Toledo Hospital
2142 N Cove Boulevard 419-471-2291
Toledo, OH 43606-3895 Fax: 412-916-01
www.toledochildrens.org
Barbara Steele, President
Ann Gilbert, Director

4955 Oklahoma Comprehensive Hemophilia Diagnostic Treatment Center
940 NE 13th Street 405-271-3661
Oklahoma City, OK 73126-0307 800-688-5288
Fax: 405-271-3756
Beverly Stev RN

4956 Orthopaedic Hospital's Hemophilia Treatment Center
2400 S Flower Street 213-742-1402
Los Angeles, CA 90007-2629 Fax: 213-742-1103
e-mail: info@laoh.ucla.edu
www.orthohospital.org
Carol K Kasper, Hematology

4957 Puget Sound Blood Center
921 Terry Avenue 206-292-6500
Seattle, WA 98104-1256 e-mail: keithw@psbc.org
www.psbc.org
Arthur R Thompson, Director

4958 Regional Comprehensive Center for Hemophilia and VonWillebrand Disease
47 New Scotland Avenue 518-262-5827
Albany, NY 12208-3479 800-773-7080
Fax: 518-262-6320
e-mail: albanyhtc@mail.amc.edu
www.amc.edu
Providing excellence in medical education biomedical research and patient care.ÿ
Joanne Porter, Medical Director
Christine Coonrad, Billing/ Grant Support

4959 Regional Hemophilia Treatment Center Children's Hospital of Michigan
Children's Hospital of Michigan
3901 Beaubien Street 313-745-5437
Detroit, MI 48201-2196 Fax: 313-745-5237
www.hfmich.org
Jeanne M Lusher MD

4960 Richland Memorial Comprehensive Pediatric Hemophilia Center
Children's Hospital for Cancer & Blood Disorders
7 Richland Medical Park Drive 803-434-3533
Columbia, SC 29203 Fax: 803-434-4598
Robert S Etinger MD

4961 Riley Hemophilia & Hemophilia Center Riley Hospital for Children
Riley Hospital for Children
702 Barnhill Drive 317-274-2060
Indianapolis, IN 46202-5200 800-248-1199
Fax: 317-278-0616
e-mail: mheiny@iupui.edu
rileychildrenshospital.com
Elaine South RN PNP, Nurse Coordinator

4962 South Texas Comprehensive Hemophilia Center: Santa Rosa Health Corporation
Children's Hospital
333 N Santa Rosa Street 210-704-2011
San Antonio, TX 78207-3108 Fax: 210-704-2396
www.christussantarosa.org
John Drake RN

4963 Southern Tier Hemophilia Center United Health Services-Wilson Hospital
United Health Services-Wilson Hospital
33-57 Harrison Street 607-763-6436
Johnson City, NY 13790 Fax: 607-763-5514
Doris Michal RN

4964 St. Joseph's Hemophilia Center
2927 N 7th Avenue 602-406-3770
Phoenix, AZ 85013-4102
Rachel Stuar RN

4965 Ted R Montoya Hemophilia Program University of New Mexico
University of New Mexico
2211 Lomas Boulevard NE 505-272-4461
Albuquerque, NM 87131-0001 Fax: 505-272-6845
www.unm.edu
Prasad Mathe MD, Director

4966 Thomas Jefferson University: Cardenza Foundation for Hematologic Research
833 Chesnut E Street 215-955-4730
Philadelphia, PA 19107-5005 Fax: 215-955-2342
www.jefferson.edu
Sandor Shapi MD, Director

4967 UCD Northern Central California Hemophilia Program
PO Box 163689 916-734-3461
Sacramento, CA 95816-2208 Fax: 916-489-1569
www.cchfsac.org

An all-volunteer nonprofit organization dedicated to helping people with bleeding disorders.
Charles F Abildgaard MD

4968 UCSD Comprehensive Hemophilia Treatment Center
200 W Arbor Drive 619-471-0336
San Diego, CA 92103 Fax: 858-822-6288
e-mail: kdherbst@ucsd.edu
hem-onc.ucsd.edu
George Davig MD
Kenneth D Herbst, Medical Director

4969 University Medical Center Hemophilia Program
1800 W Charleston Boulevard
Las Vegas, NV 89102-2329 702-383-2000
www.umcsn.com
Jack Lazerso MD

4970 University Treatment Center of University Hospitals of Cleveland
11100 Euclid Avenue 216-844-3345
Cleveland, OH 44106 Fax: 216-844-5431
www.uhhospitals.org
Susan B Shurin MD
Alex Y Huang, Director

4971 University of Cincinnati Adult Hemophilia Treatment Program
231 Bethesda Avenue 513-558-4233
Cincinnati, OH 45267-0001 Fax: 513-558-3878
Kathleen E Palascak MD

4972 University of Michigan Hemophilia Center
1500 E Medical Center Drive 734-647-5705
Ann Arbor, MI 48109 Fax: 734-635-15
www.umich.edu
Mary Sue Coleman, President

4973 University of Tennessee Hemophilia Clinic
920 Madison Avenue 901-448-1751
Memphis, TN 38103-0001 Fax: 901-488-7929
www.thbdf.org
Marion Dugda MD

4974 Vanderbilt Comprehensive Hemophilia Center
2220 Pierce Avenue 615-936-1765
Nashville, TN 37232-6310 866-372-5663
Fax: 615-936-1767
www.mc.vanderbilt.edu/vhtc
The mission of the Vanderbilt Hemostasis-Thrombosis Clinic is to provide the highest quality compassionate care for individuals with inherited disorders of bleeding or clotting. The team emphasizes the empowerment of patients in their own care while also providing opportunities to participate in scientific advances in the diagnosis and treatment of bleeding and clotting disorders.
Dr Robert L Janco, Director Hematologist
Dr Anne Neff, Co-Director Hematologist

4975 Vermont Regional Hemophilia Center
108 Cherry Street 802-651-1550
Burlington, VT 05402 Fax: 802-651-1573
e-mail: vtadap@vdh.state.vt.us
healthvermont.gov
Provides care to persons with types of bleeding disorders. We see people from Vermont and upstate New York.
Miriam Huste RN, Hemophilia Nurse Coordinator
Donald R Swartz, Medical Director

4976 West Central Ohio Hemophilia Center Childens Medical Center
Childens Medical Center
1 Childrens Plaza 937-641-3111
Dayton, OH 45404-1815 800-228-4055
Fax: 937-641-5878
www.childrensdayton.org
The center provides complete care for individuals and families with hemophilia and related bleeding disorders. Some of the services offered include a comprehensive clinic emergency treatment network consultations diagnostic coagulation laboratory home infusion programs HIV/AIDS education and counseling and more.
James French II, Medical Director
Emmett Broxson, Director Hemothology

Support Groups & Hotlines

4977 National Health Information Center
PO Box 1133 310-565-4167
Washington, DC 20013 800-336-4797
Fax: 301-984-4256
e-mail: info@nhic.org
www.health.gov/nhic
Offers a nationwide information referral service, produces directories and resource guides.

Books

4978 Avoiding Indecision and Hesitation with Hemophilia-Related Emergencies
American Health Consultants
3525 Piedmont Road NE
Atlanta, GA 30305 800-688-2421
Provides detailed information necessary for physicians, and ED staff to deal effectively and expeditiously with hemophilia emergencies.
12 pages

4979 Federal Medicaid Drug Program
1730 E Street NW 202-628-9292
Washington, DC 20006-5300
Discusses changes in government reimbursement and its effect on plasma derived products distributed by the American Red Cross. Includes law information, individual state billing procedures and Medicaid program coverage for the hemophilia community.

4980 Guide to Insurance Coverage for People with Hemophilia
Armour Pharmaceutical Company
500 Arcola Road 215-454-3720
Collegeville, PA 19426-3930
An educational guide designed to assist with health insurance concerns.

4981 Hemophilia Camp Directory
National Hemophilia Foundation
116 W 32nd Street 212-219-8180
New York, NY 10001-3212 800-424-2634
Fax: 212-328-3777
www.hemophilia.org
Lists camps in the United States for children with hemophilia and other coagulation disorders.
16 pages
Alan Kinniburgh, PhD, CEO

4982 Procedure Coding for Hemophilia Treatment
Armour Pharmaceutical Company
500 Arcola Road 215-454-3720
Collegeville, PA 19426-3930
Educational guide designed to facilitate the appropriate use of CPT codes for the hemophilia community.

Children's Books

4983 Adventures of Maxx
Nova Factor
1620 Century Centery Parkway 901-348-8129
Memphis, TN 38137 800-424-2634
Fax: 901-385-3778
An activity book for children with hemophilia, this publication is intended to be both educational and entertaining.
15 pages

4984 Children's Hemophilia Book
Porton Products Limited
30401 Agoura Road 818-879-2200
Agoura Hills, CA 91301-2006
Coloring book that discusses what hemophilia is, bleeding episodes and treatment from a child's point of view.
25 pages

4985 Harold Talks About How He Inherited Hemophilia
Kentucky Hemophilia Foundation

982 Eastern Parkway
Louisville, KY 40217-1571
502-634-8161
800-582-2873
Fax: 502-634-9995
e-mail: info@kyhemo.org
www.kyhemo.org

Children's brochure explaining hemophilia causes, symptoms and living a regular life.
Ursela M Lacer, Executive Director

4986 Harold's Secret: A Boy with Hemophilia
Bayer
400 Morgan Lane
West Haven, CT 06516-4175
203-937-2765

A comic book for youngsters pertaining to children with hemophilia and understanding of the illness among school friends.
16 pages

4987 Understanding Hemophilia: A Young Person's Guide
Armour Pharmaceuticals Company
500 Arcola Road
Collegeville, PA 19426-3930
800-424-2634

This publication is designed for young persons with hemophilia. Presented in very basic and accessible language, this text with colored illustrations points out what hemophilia is, how to cope and more.
91 pages

Magazines

4988 HEMALOG
Maleria Medica
101 W 23rd Street PMB 2246
New York, NY 10011-2490
212-725-5151
Fax: 212-725-2794
e-mail: hemalog@hotmail.com

The purpose of Hemalog is to serve as a national forum for the hemophilia community, providing current news, information, opinion and contact with others in the community. The material contained in this journal reflects the experience and opinion of a wide range of people connected with hemophilia and encourages story and art contributions.
36 pages Quarterly
Barbara Robin Slonevsky, Publisher
Janet Spencer-King, Editor-in-Chief

4989 HemAware
National Hemophilia Foundation
116 W 32nd Street
New York, NY 10001-3212
888-463-6643
800-424-2634
Fax: 212-328-3777
www.hemophilia.org

NHF magazine that offers treatment news about bleeding disorders and provides comprehensive articles on the latest developments in treatment and research as well as highlighting new programs and new resources in the field.
Bi-Monthly
Alan Kinniburgh, PhD, CEO

4990 Human Factor
Hemophilia Health Services
6820 Charlotte Pike
Nashville, TN 37209-4206
800-800-6606

This journal is provided as a free service for the purpose of informing, educating and empowering the hemophilia community.
Quarterly

Newsletters

4991 Artery
Hemophilia Foundation of Michigan
230 1 Platt Road
Ann Arbor, MI 48103-2973
734-761-2535
800-482-3041
Fax: 734-975-2889
www.hfmich.org

Offers information on the chapter's activities and events, support groups and hotlines, technical and medical updates pertaining to the hemophilia and HIV/AIDS community.
Quarterly
Susan Lerch, Editor

4992 Big Red Factor
National Hemophilia Foundation: Nebraska
215 Centennial Mall South
Lincoln, NE 68508
402-742-5663
Fax: 402-742-5677
e-mail: office@nebraskanhf.org
www.nebraskanhf.org/chapter/

Chapter newsletter offering legislative and medical updates, technology, resources, assistive devices and more for persons affected by hemophilia and other blood disorders.

4993 Bloodlines
Hemophilia Association of San Diego County
3570 Camoni del Rio N
San Diego, CA 92108
619-325-3570
Fax: 619-325-4350
www.hasdc.org

Updates membership on the newest techniques and technologies on the treatment of hemophilia.
Quarterly
Jessica Swann, Executive Director
Teresa Ramirez, Coordinator Member Services

4994 Concentrate
Hemophilia of North Carolina
2 Centerview Drive
Greensboro, NC 27407-3708
919-852-4788

Offers information on summer camps, resources, book reviews, parent information and articles pertaining to hemophilia.
Monthly

4995 Factor Nine News
Coalition for Hemophilia B
225 W 34th Street
New York, NY 10122
212-628-3445
Fax: 212-554-6906
e-mail: cfb@web-depot.com
www.boygenius.com/cfb

Offers information on FDA approvals, annual meetings and the latest in technology and information regarding hemophilia.
Kimberly Phelan, VP

4996 Hemophilia NewsBriefs
Great Lakes Hemophilia Foundation
638 North 18th Street
Milwaukee, WI 53233
414-257-0200
Fax: 414-257-1225
e-mail: info@glhf.org
www.glhf.org

4997 Infusion
Kentuckian Hemophilia Foundation
982 Eastern Parkway
Louisville, KY 40217-1571
510-634-8161
800-582-CURE
Fax: 510-568-6111
e-mail: officeinfo@HFNonline.org
www.hfnconline.org

Offers information on summer camps, association activities and events, national projects touching on hemophilia and HIV related disorders and articles on the newest breakthroughs and technology for fighting bleeding disorders.
Quarterly

4998 Initiatives
Quantum Health Resources
790 The City Drive S
Orange, CA 92868-4941
714-750-1610

Aimed at keeping patients and other interested individuals informed on important economic trends, legislation and medical issues.
Quarterly
Lynne Brightman

4999 Linking Factor
National Hemophila Foundation: Utah Chapter
340 E 400 S
Salt Lake City, UT 84111-2909
800-800-6606

A newsletter offering chapter association news and information.
BiMonthly
Charles Hand, Executive Director
Linda Aagard, Editor

5000 New England Hemophilia Association Newsletter
180 Rustcraft Road 781-326-7645
Dedham, MA 02026-4558 800-228-6342
e-mail: neha@world.std.com
www.newenglandhemophilia.org
New England Hemophilia Association is dedicated to improving the quality of life for persons with bleeding disorders (hemophilia, von Williebrands, and other factor deficiencies) and their families through education, support and advocacy. NEHA is a chapter of the National Hemophilia Foundation.
Quarterly
Catherine I Cornell, Executive Director

5001 Ways & Means
Quantum Health Resources
790 The City Drive S 714-750-1610
Orange, CA 92868-4941
Features pertinent health care information for hemophilia patients and their families.
Quarterly
Lynne Brightman

5002 Infusion
Northern California Chapter of the NHF
7700 Edgewater Drive 650-568-NCHF
Oakland, CA 94621-3023
Informs members of medical, dental and orthopedic treatment advances and the latest research in the field. Helps to keep people with hemophilia and their families aware of relevant local and national meetings and includes important updates regarding research and treatment.
BiMonthly

Pamphlets

5003 Anyone Can Have a Bleeding Problem
Hemophilia Foundation of Michigan
411 Huronview Boulevard 734-761-2535
Ann Arbor, MI 48103-2973 800-482-3041
Offers information on Hemophilia and Von Willebrand's Disease. How persons can get it, prevention and causes of the illnesses.

5004 Article Reprint Exchange
HANDI-The National Hemophilia Foundation
116 W 32nd Street 212-219-8180
New York, NY 10001-3212 800-424-2634
Fax: 212-328-3777
Offers various reprinted articles concerning hemophilia and the newest medical technology.

5005 Basics of HIV Disease: Questions and Answers
National Hemophilia Foundation
116 W 32nd Street 888-463-6643
New York, NY 10001-3212 800-424-2634
Fax: 212-328-3777
www.hemophilia.org
This publication contains basic information about hemophilia and HIV disease.
1992 28 pages
Alan Kinniburgh, PhD, CEO

5006 Clotting Agents Are Lifesavers
Hemophilia Foundation of Michigan
411 Huronview Boulevard 734-761-2535
Ann Arbor, MI 48103-2973
Offers information on what hemophilia is, treatments, occurances, heredity, Von Willebrand's Disease, patient services and direct services for hemophiliacs and HIV/AIDS patients.

5007 Comprehensive Care
National Hemophilia Foundation
116 W 32nd Street 888-463-6643
New York, NY 10001-3212 800-424-2634
Fax: 212-328-3777
www.hemophilia.org
Discusses the nature of comprehensive care and its functions and defines the care team. Also touches upon essential resources, HIV, and the benefits of comprehensive care.
1991 12 pages
Alan Kinniburgh, PhD, CEO

5008 Comprehensive Services for Persons with Hemophilia
Hemophilia Foundation of Minnesota/Dakotas
2304 Park Avenue 612-871-3340
Minneapolis, MN 55404-3712 Fax: 612-871-1359
Offers information on what hemophilia is and information and resources for persons with hemophilia and other bleeding disorders.

5009 Consumer Bill of Rights and Responsibilities for Healthcare Service
National Hemophilia Foundation
116 W 32nd Street 888-463-6643
New York, NY 10001-3212 800-424-2634
Fax: 212-328-3777
www.hemophilia.org
Serves as a set of goals for both the provider and consumer in seeking, providing, and receiving high quality health care within a setting of honesty and respect.
1994
Alan Kinniburgh, PhD, CEO

5010 Countdown to a Cure
Louisiana Hemophilia Foundation
3636 S Sherwood Forest Boulevard 225-291-1675
Baton Rouge, LA 70816-2285 Fax: 225-291-1679
e-mail: lahemophilia@hipoint.net
www.louisianahemophilia.org/
Offers information on chapter resources and services for hemophiliacs and their families. Offers information and services to families/patients affected by bleeding disorders.
Lori Keels, Executive Director

5011 Fight Hemophilia with Facts Not Fiction
Great Lakes Hemophilia Foundation
638 North 18th Street 414-257-0200
Milwaukee, WI 53233 Fax: 414-257-1225
www.glhf.org
Offers information on what hemophilia is, research information and treatments.

5012 Get Real and Be Safe!
National Hemophilia Foundation
116 W 32nd Street 888-463-6643
New York, NY 10001-3212 800-424-2634
Fax: 212-328-3777
www.hemophilia.org
Comic book style, this pamphlet offers information to young adults on the hazards and precautions of sex. Offers an Ask The Doctor question and answer section to books and resources for young adults on safer sex and HIV/AIDS.
1991 14 pages
Alan Kinniburgh, PhD, CEO

5013 Guidelines for Finding Childcare
National Hemophilia Foundation
116 W 32nd Street 888-463-6643
New York, NY 10001-3212 800-424-2634
Fax: 212-328-3777
www.hemophilia.org
Information for parents on how to hire a good babysitter, information on daycare centers, how to tell daycare staff about hemophilia, cooperative childcare and suggested reading for parents.
1987 10 pages
Alan Kinniburgh, PhD, CEO

5014 HIV Disease in People with Hemophilia: Your Questions Answered
National Hemophilia Foundation

116 W 32nd Street 888-463-6643
New York, NY 10001-3212 800-424-2634
Fax: 212-328-3777
www.hemophilia.org
Discusses hemophilia and HIV disease, AIDS, management of HIV disease, risks to sexual partners, and issues for children with hemophilia.
1991 48 pages
Alan Kinniburgh, PhD, CEO

5015 **HIV Infection and Hemophilia**
Hemophilia Foundation of Illinois
332 S Michigan Avenue 312-427-1495
Chicago, IL 60604-4434
Offers information on HIV/AIDS relating to persons with hemophilia.

5016 **Hemophilia: Current Medical Management**
National Hemophilia Foundation
116 W 32nd Street 888-463-6643
New York, NY 10001-3212 800-424-2634
Fax: 212-328-3777
www.hemophilia.org
Provides an overview of all aspects of hemophilia treatment, including prophylaxis, home therapy, inhibitors, orthopedic solutions, surgery, and dental care.
1994 30 pages
Alan Kinniburgh, PhD, CEO

5017 **How to Control Bleeds: Inspired by Vince, an 8-year-old Boy with Hemophilia**
Bayer
400 Morgan Lane 203-937-2765
West Haven, CT 06516-4175
An educational comic book story by Vince about hemophilia and treatment for bleeds.
26 pages

5018 **Living with HIV: Talking with Your Child**
Bobbie Steinhart, author
National Hemophilia Foundation
116 W 32nd Street 888-463-6643
New York, NY 10001-3212 800-424-2634
Fax: 212-328-3777
www.hemophilia.org
A pamphlet directed at caregivers of young children living with hemophilia and HIV disease.
1990 8 pages
Alan Kinniburgh, PhD, CEO

5019 **Mild Hemophilia**
National Hemophilia Foundation
116 W 32nd Street 888-463-6643
New York, NY 10001-3212 800-424-2634
Fax: 212-328-3777
www.hemophilia.org
Defines mild hemophilia and details its discovery, diagnosis, inheritance, symptoms, treatment, and activity limitations.
1994 25 pages
Alan Kinniburgh, PhD, CEO

5020 **Participating in a Clinical Trial: Your Life, Your Choice**
National Hemophilia Foundation
116 W 32nd Street 888-463-6643
New York, NY 10001-3212 800-424-2634
Fax: 212-328-3777
www.hemophilia.org
This brochure explains what clinical trials are and what they are like for patients, describes what kinds of HIV therapies are being tested in clinical trials, and lists questions to ask before joining a trial. This publication is ideal for patients, their families, and/or healthcare personnel who counsel HIV-positive patients.
1994 6 pages
Alan Kinniburgh, PhD, CEO

5021 **Physical Therapy in Hemophilia**
Nationa Hemophilia Foundation
110 Greene Street 212-328-3700
New York, NY 10012-3832 800-424-2634
Fax: 212-328-3777
www.hemophilia.org
Targeted at physical therapy students or new therapists at comprehensive hemophilia care clinics. Also provides basic treatment care information for persons with hemophilia and their families.
1986 13 pages

5022 **Simple & Complex: A Hemophilia Primer**
Western Pennsylvania Chapter of the NHF
580 S Aiken Avenue 412-685-2231
Pittsburgh, PA 15232-1531 Fax: 412-683-2568
Offers information on what hemophilia is, explains AIDS and HIV infection, offers information on the treatments for hemophilia and what hemophilia care costs.

5023 **Student with Hemophilia: A Resource for the Educator**
National Hemophilia Foundation
116 W 32nd Street 888-463-6643
New York, NY 10001-3212 800-424-2634
Fax: 212-328-3777
www.hemophilia.org
Written for teachers, nurses, and other school personnel, this booklet aims to dispel the myths and fears surrounding hemophilia.
1995 16 pages
Alan Kinniburgh, PhD, CEO

5024 **Treatment of Hemophilia: Current Orthopedic Management**
Marvin Gilbert, Jerome Wiedel, author
National Hemophilia Foundation
116 W 32nd Street 888-463-6643
New York, NY 10001-3212 800-424-2634
Fax: 212-328-3777
www.hemophilia.org
Covers a wide range of orthopedic treatment issues, including hemophilic arthropathy, clinical considerations, diagnostic imaging, surgical and nonsurgical treatments, hemophilic synovitis, soft-tissue bleeding, the hemophilia pseudotumor, fracture care, other musculoskelatal problems, and HIV infections.
1995 25 pages
Alan Kinnibrugh, PhD, CEO

5025 **Understanding Hepatitis**
Leonard Seeff, Maribel Johnson, author
National Hemophilia Foundation
116 W 32nd Street 888-463-6643
New York, NY 10001-3212 800-424-2634
Fax: 212-328-3777
www.hemophilia.org
Provides comprehensive information about viral hepatitis for people with bleeding disorders, their caregivers, and families. Discusses the different hepatitis viruses, viral transmissions, how the liver is affected by hepatitis, blood product concerns, prevention, diagnosis, treatment, and psychosocial issues.
1997 24 pages
Alan Kinniburgh, PhD, CEO

5026 **Von Willebrand Disease: A Guide for Patients and Families**
Hemophilia Health Services
6820 Charlotte Pike
Nashville, TN 37209-4206 800-800-6606
Offers information on this disease, explains the causes, treatments, prevention and offers resources and books.

5027 **What Is Hemophilia?**
Hemophilia Foundation of Georgia
8800 Roswell Road 770-518-8272
Atlanta, GA 30328-1689 800-866-4366
Fax: 770-518-3310
e-mail: hog@america.net
www.hog.org
Offers information on what hemophilia is, common factors in hemophilia, the cost and treatments offered to hemophiliacs and more.

5028 **What Women Should Know About HIV Infection AIDS and Hemophilia**
Hemophilia Foundation of Illinois

332 S Michigan Avenue 312-427-1495
Chicago, IL 60604-4434
For spouses/partners of men with hemophilia and women with bleeding disorders. Provides information about HIV/AIDS and how it affects women in the hemophilia community.
25 pages

5029 What You Should Know About Hemophilia
National Hemophilia Foundation
116 W 32nd Street 888-463-6643
New York, NY 10001-3212 800-424-2634
Fax: 212-328-3777
www.hemophilia.org
Defines hemophilia, explains its effects, and provides a historical overview of treatment and treatment complications.
1991 13 pages
Alan Kinniburgh, PhD, CEO

5030 Who Will Tell Them of Your Special Needs?
MedicAlert
2323 Colorado Avenue
Turlock, CA 95382-2018 800-432-5378
Offers information on MedicAlert bracelets, personal identification medical information needed for treatment in case of emergency.

Audio & Video

5031 Song of Superman
National Hemophilia Foundation
116 W 32nd Street 888-463-6643
New York, NY 10001-3212 800-424-2634
Fax: 212-328-3777
www.hemophilia.org
Designed to help young people with bleeding disorders come to terms with their HIV status, sexuality, and living with HIV. The video explores issues of disclosure in relationships and safer sex through dramatic scenes and frank testimonials by young people living with hemophilia and/or HIV. The companion workbook contains group exercises that follow each of the main topics of the video and serve as a bridge to discussion.
1993 49 pages
Alan Kinnibrugh, PhD, CEO

5032 Treat Yourself to a Brighter Future - It's Time to Hit the Freedom Trail
c/o Hemophilia Association of the Capital Area
10560 Main Street 703-352-7641
Fairfax, VA 22030-7182 Fax: 703-352-2145
e-mail: info@hacacares.org
www.hacacares.org/ed_publist.html
A booklet and videotape published by the American Red Cross providing a list of required supplies and equipment for self-infusion concentrates for persons with hemophilia A. It is an instructional piece for home self-infusion and concise text and illustrations depict seven steps for self-infusion.
20 pages Video & Booklet
Keith Bushey, President
Cliff Krug Jr, Vice President

Web Sites

5033 American Red Cross Blood Services
www.redcross.org/services/biomed
Distributes a wide variety of plasma therapeutics to benefit people with hemophilia A and B, immune disorders and hypoalbuminemia.

5034 Healing Well
www.healingwell.com
An online health resource guide to medical news, chat, information and articles, newsgroups and message boards, books, disease-related web sites, medical directories, and more for patients, friends, and family coping with disabling diseases, disorders, or chronic illnesses.

5035 Health Finder
www.healthfinder.gov
Searchable, carefully developed web site offering information on over 1000 topics. Developed by the US Department of Health and Human Services, the site can be used in both English and Spanish.

5036 Healthlink USA
www.healthlinkusa.com
Health information concerning treatment, cures, prevention, diagnosis, risk factors, research, support groups, email lists, personal stories and much more. Updated regularly.

5037 Helios Health
www.helioshealth.com
Online resource for your health information. Detailed information about specific health topics, access to expert advice from our Medical Advisory Board, and up-to-date health news.

5038 MedicineNet
www.medicinenet.com
An online resource for consumers providing easy-to-read, authoritative medical and health information.

5039 Medscape
www.mywebmd.com
Medscape offers specialists, primary care physicians, and other health professionals the Web's most robust and integrated medical information and educational tools.

5040 National Hemophilia Foundation
www.hemophilia.org
Information on the treatment and the cure of hemophilia, related bleeding disorders and complications of those disorders or their treatment, including HIV infection, as well as improving the quality of life of all those affected.

5041 WebMD
www.webmd.com
Information on Hemophilia, including articles and resources.

Description

5042 **Hepatitis**

Hepatitis, or inflammation of the liver, has multiple causes and several stages. Hepatitis is usually caused by viruses or by excess alcohol consumption. Less common causes include prescription medications, accidental poisoning, and auto-immune diseases in which the body attacks its own liver.

The severity of the disease is highly variable. At an early stage, hepatitis may cause no symptoms, vague mild symptoms, or overwhelming disease. Early symptoms include vague abdominal pain, jaundice, fever, loss of appetite and nausea. If the disease becomes chronic, it may lead to irreversible scarring, or cirrhosis, which causes weakness, fatigue and weight loss. Late stage disease includes fluid accumulation in the abdominal cavity, gastrointestinal bleeding and mental changes. Abdominal pain and liver enlargement are generally present. Advanced cirrhosis is a risk factor for cancer of the liver.

There are four major kinds of viral hepatitis. Type A is very common world-wide, is spread by contaminated food and water, and generally causes a mild to moderately severe illness that runs its course over several weeks and disappears without further damage. Type B is also very common, and is spread by bodily fluids, generally through blood transfusion, sexual intercourse, sharing of needles or contaminated items like shaving razors and tattoo needles. The disease may resolve without further consequences, but frequently becomes chronic and may lead to cirrhosis as well as chronic infections. Hepatitis C is also spread through blood transfusion and needle sharing. Although it is not usually severe at onset, it can lead to the same serious consequences as type B. Finally, there is a type D, which is spread by blood products, and only infects people who already have Type B. Type D is associated with a more severe course.

Prevention of any of these forms of viral hepatitis depends on avoiding the usual routes of transmission. In addition, there is an effective vaccine available for hepatitis B. Close family contacts of persons with this disease should receive the vaccine if they have not yet received it as part of routine childhood immunization.

Treatment of hepatitis is largely supportive, but antiviral drugs and interferon are used in certain stages of Type B and Type C infection. End-stage or overwhelming infection may necessitate liver transplantation. See also *Liver Disease*.

National Agencies & Associations

5043 **American Hepatitis Association**
133 E 58th Street 212-753-8068
New York, NY 10022
Conducts educational and prevention programs concerning hepatitis provides screening and vaccines and offers support groups for individuals with hepatitis.

5044 **Centers for Disease Control and Prevention Hepatitis Branch**
1600 Clifton Road 404-639-2709
Atlanta, GA 30333 800-232-4636
www.cdc.gov/ncidod/diseases/hepatitis
Monitors the rates of viral hepatitis in the United States; provides epidemiologic assistance for outbreaks of viral hepatitis; coordinates and implements epidemiologic studies to define the risk factors for acute and chronic viral hepatitis; provides viral hepatitis reference/diagnostic services; serves as the World Health Organization Collaborating Center for Reference and Research on Viral Hepatitis.
Julie Louise Gerberding, MD, Director

5045 **HIV/Hepatitis C in Prison (HIP) Committee**
California Prison Focus 510-665-1935
San Francisco, CA 94103 e-mail: contact@prisons.org
www.prisons.org/hivin
The HIV/HCV in Prison Committee of California Prison Focus works on behalf of prisoners to fight for consistent access to quality medical care including access of all new HIV and hepatitis C medications, diagnostic testing and combination therapies.
Michelle Foy, Contact
Judy Greenspan, Contact

5046 **Hepatitis B Coalition**
1573 Selby Avenue 651-647-9009
Saint Paul, MN 55104 Fax: 651-647-9131
e-mail: admin@immunize.org
www.immunize.org
Works to prevent transmission of hepatitis B in high-risk groups; to promote HBsAG screening for all pregnant women; to achieve vaccination of all infants children and adolescents; and to promote education and treatment for the person who is chronically ill.
Deborah L Wexler MD, Executive Director
Diane C Peterson, Associate Director for Immunization

5047 **Hepatitis Foundation International**
504 Blick Drive 301-622-4200
Silver Spring, MD 20904-2901 800-891-0707
Fax: 301-622-4702
e-mail: hfi@comcast.net
www.hepfi.org
Grassroots support network for persons with viral hepatitis. Provides education about the prevention diagnosis and treatment of viral hepatitis as well as phone network support and various literature.
Thelma King Thiel, Chief Executive Officer
Karen Wirth MBA, Vice Chairwoman

5048 **Immunization Action Coalition**
1573 Selby Avenue 651-647-9009
Saint Paul, MN 55104 Fax: 651-647-9131
e-mail: admin@immunize.org
www.immunize.org
The mission of the Immunization Action Coalition is to boost immunization rates and prevent disease. The coalition promotes physician, community and family awareness of and responsibility for appropriate immunization of all children and adults against all diseases.
Deborah L Wexler MD, Executive Director
Diane C Peterson, Associate Director for Immunization

5049 **Living Positive Resource Centre**
#101-266 Lawrence Avenue 250-862-2437
Kelowna, BC, V1Y-6L3 800-616-2437
Fax: 260-868-8662
e-mail: info@iprc.ca
www.iprc.ca
Through partnerships and collaboration, will work to reduce the incidence of new HIV/AIDS/HEP C and other blood borne pathogens and to improve the quality of life for those infected and affected.
Daryle Roberts, Executive Director
Sheila Karr, Prevention Coordinator

5050 **National Hepatitis C Coalition**
PO Box 5058 951-766-8238
Hemet, CA 92544 e-mail: mail@nationalhepatitis-c.org
www.nationalhepatitis-c.org

The National Hepatitis C Coalition is a 501(c) (3) tax exempt organization that relies on private donations from good folks like you in order to continue helping others with hepatitis C.
Patty Krueger, Co-Founder/Board Chair/President

Foundations

5051 Hepatitis B Foundation
3805 Old Easton Road — 215-489-4900
Doylestown, PA 18902 — Fax: 215-489-4313
e-mail: info@hepb.org
www.hepb.org

We are dedicated to finding a cure and improving the quality of life for those affected by hepatitis B worldwide. Our commitment includes funding focused research, promoting disease awareness, supporting immunization and treatment initiatives, and serving as the primary source of information for patients and their families, the medical and scientific community, and the general public.

Molli Conti, Chair
Timothy Block, PhD, Founder/President

Libraries & Resource Centers

5052 Hepatitis Education Project
4603 Aurora Avenue N — 206-732-0311
Seattle, WA 98103 — Fax: 206-732-0312
e-mail: hep@scn.org
www.scn.org/hepatitis

The mission of the Hepatitis Education Project is to help raise awareness among patients, medical personnel and the public of the facts concerning hepatitis patients and the resources available to help those who live with the disease.
Steve Graham, President
Michael Ninburg, Executive Director

Support Groups & Hotlines

5053 Christ Hospital Hepatitis C Support Group
Christ Hospital
176 Palisade Avenue — 201-795-1230
Jersey City, NJ 07306 — e-mail: dkatz@65717@aol.com

For anyone interested in becoming advocates for increasing awareness of this illness.

5054 Hepatitis Education Project
The Maritime Building — 206-732-0311
Seattle, WA 98104 — e-mail: hepinfo@hepeducation.org
www.hepeducation.org

Helps raise awareness among patients, medical personeel and the public of the facts concerning hepatitis patients and the resources available to help those who live with the disease
Steve Graham, President
Michael Ninburg, Executive Director

5055 National Health Information Center
PO Box 1133 — 310-565-4167
Washington, DC 20013 — 800-336-4797
Fax: 301-984-4256
e-mail: info@nhic.org
www.health.gov/nhic

Offers a nationwide information referral service, produces directories and resource guides.

Books

5056 Hepatitis B Prevention: A Resource Guide
National Digestive Diseases Info. Clearinghouse
2 Information Way — 301-654-3810
Bethesda, MD 20824 — 800-891-5389
Fax: 301-907-8906
e-mail: nddic@info.niddk.uih.goc
www.niddk.nih.gov

Designed to assist health care and other professionals who work in planning or administering hepatitis B prevention programs.
252 pages

5057 Understanding Hepatitis
James L Achord, MD, author
University Press of Mississippi
3825 Ridgewood Road — 601-432-6205
Jackson, MS 39211-6492 — Fax: 601-432-6217
e-mail: kburgess@ihl.state.ms.us
www.upress.state.ms.us

For general readers a comprehensive discussion of the causes and of the treatments of hepatitis.
2002 152 pages Paperback
ISBN: 1-578064-36-8
Kathy Burgess, Advertising/Marketing Services Manager

5058 Viral Hepatitis: Scientific Basis and Clinical Management
Churchill Livingstone
PO Box 3188 — 201-319-9800
Secaucus, NJ 07096-3188 — 800-553-5426
Fax: 201-319-9659
www.harcourt-international.com/cl/

1997 800 pages Hardcover
ISBN: 0-443057-97-4

Magazines

5059 Hepatitis Magazine
Quality Publishing Services
523 N Sam Houston Parkway E — 281-272-2744
Houston, TX 77060 — 800-310-7047
Fax: 281-847-5440
e-mail: info@hepatitismag.com
www.hepatitismag.com

Magazine for those with hepatitis. Price listed is for a one year subscription.
Quarterly
Barbara Veres, Publisher
Geoff Drushel, Editor

Newsletters

5060 American Liver Foundation: Progress Newsletter
75 Maiden Lane — 212-668-1000
New York, NY 10038-4826 — 800-465-4837
Fax: 212-483-8179
e-mail: info@liverfoundation.org
www.liverfoundation.org

The American Liver Foundation is the nation's leading nonprofit organization promoting liver health and disease prevention. ALF provides research education and sdvocacy for those affected by liver-related diseases, including hepatitis
8 pages 2 per year
Sarah Wilson Brown, Manager Marketing/Communications

5061 B Connected
3805 Old Easton Road — 215-489-4900
Doylestown, PA 18902 — Fax: 215-489-4313
e-mail: info@hepb.org
www.hepb.org

Features practical health tips, frequently asked questions, and other useful information for patients and families to live well with chronic hepatitis B. Available in both print and online versions.
3x/year
Molli Conti, Chair
Timothy Block, PhD, Founder/President

5062 B-Informed Newsletter
Hepatitis B Foundation
3805 Old Easton Road — 215-489-4900
Doylestown, PA 18902 — Fax: 215-489-4920
e-mail: info@hepb.org
www.hepb.org

Includes a "Drug Watch" of approved and experimental therapies for Hepatitis B, reasearch updates, Foundation news and events, and feature articles on special topics. Available in print and online.
Molli C. Conti, Executive Director

5063 Hepatitis Alert
Hepatitis Foundation International (HFI)
30 Sunrise Terrace 973-239-1035
Cedar Grove, NJ 07009-1423 800-891-0707
Fax: 973-875-5044
e-mail: hfi@intac.com
www.hepfi.org
Provides information for the public, patients, educators, and medical professionals about the diagnosis, treatment, and prevention of viral hepatitis.

5064 Hepatitis B Coalition News
Hepatitis B Coalition
1573 Selby Avenue 651-647-9009
Saint Paul, MN 55104-6328 Fax: 651-647-9131
e-mail: admin@inmunize.org
Newsletter with brochures, articles, videotapes, audio-cassette tapes and manuals for different ethnic populations.

5065 NEEDLE TIPS & the Hepatitis B Coalition News
Hepatitis B Coalition
1573 Selby Avenue 651-647-9009
St. Paul, MN 55104-6328 Fax: 651-647-9131
e-mail: admin@immunize.org
www.immunize.org
Information on immunization for health professionals.
28 pages 2x Year
Deborah L Wexler

5066 VACCINATE ADULTS! Coalition News
Hepatitis B Coalition
1573 Selby Avenue 651-647-9009
St. Paul, MN 55104-6328 Fax: 651-647-9131
e-mail: admin@immunize.org
www.immunize.org
Information on immunization: adult medicine specialist.
12 pages 2x Year
Deborah L Wexler MD

Pamphlets

5067 Advice to Parents of Children with HBV
Hepatitis B Foundation
3805 Old Easton Road 215-489-4900
Doylestown, PA 18902 Fax: 215-489-4920
e-mail: info@hepb.org
www.hepb.org
Provides information to people affected by hepatitis B and their loved ones. Current HBV research, telephone numbers, and a medical glossary.
Molli C. Conti, Executive Director

5068 Caring for Your Liver
Hepatitis Foundation International (HFI)
30 Sunrise Terrace 973-239-1035
Cedar Grove, NJ 07009-1423 800-891-0707
Fax: 973-875-5044
e-mail: hfi@intac.com
www.hepfi.org
Information for the person with hepatitis.

5069 Caution! Treating Children with Acetaminophen
Hepatitis Foundation International (HFI)
30 Sunrise Terrace 973-239-1035
Cedar Grove, NJ 07009-1423 800-891-0707
Fax: 973-875-5044
e-mail: hfi@intac.com
www.hepfi.org
Information on hepatitis.

5070 Chronic Viral Hepatitis Backgrounder
Schering Corporation
Kenilworth, NJ 07033
908-298-4000
www.sch-plough.com
Offers information and statistics on viral hepatitis.

5071 Cirrhosis: Many Causes
American Liver Foundation
1425 Pompton Avenue
Cedar Grove, NJ 07009-1000 800-223-0179
Fax: 973-256-3214
e-mail: info@liverfoundation.org
www.liverfoundation.org
Gives basic facts about cirrhosis including causes, signs, symptoms and treatments.
Rick Smith, President & CEO
Rebecca Frank, Chief Development Officer

5072 Diagnosis and Treatment
Hepatitis Foundation International (HFI)
30 Sunrise Terrace 973-239-1035
Cedar Grove, NJ 07009-1423 800-891-0707
Fax: 973-875-5044
e-mail: hfi@intac.com
www.hepfi.org
Information for the person with hepatitis.

5073 Health Insurance
Hepatitis Foundation International (HFI)
30 Sunrise Terrace 973-239-1035
Cedar Grove, NJ 07009-1423 800-891-0707
Fax: 973-875-5044
e-mail: hfi@intac.com
www.hepfi.org
Information on hepatitis and health insurance.

5074 Helpful Tips for Carriers of HBV
Hepatitis Foundation International (HFI)
30 Sunrise Terrace 973-239-1035
Cedar Grove, NJ 07009-1423 800-891-0707
Fax: 973-875-5044
e-mail: hfi@intac.com
www.hepfi.org
Information for people with Hepatitis B.

5075 Hepatitis
National Institute of Allergy & Infectious Disease
31 Center Drive
Bethesda, MD 20892-0001 301-496-4000
www.niaid.nih.gov/default.htm
A pamphlet discussing the cause, symptoms, transmission, diagnosis, tests, prevention and the latest research on Hepatitis.

5076 Hepatitis A and B Vaccination
Hepatitis Foundation International (HFI)
30 Sunrise Terrace 973-239-1035
Cedar Grove, NJ 07009-1423 800-891-0707
Fax: 973-875-5044
e-mail: hfi@intac.com
www.hepfi.org
Information on hepatitis vaccination.

5077 Hepatitis A, B & C
Hepatitis Foundation International (HFI)
30 Sunrise Terrace 973-239-1035
Cedar Grove, NJ 07009-1423 800-891-0707
Fax: 973-875-5044
e-mail: hfi@intac.com
www.hepfi.org
Information for the person with hepatitis.

5078 Hepatitis A, B & C: Liver Disease You Should Know About
American Liver Foundation
1425 Pompton Avenue
Cedar Grove, NJ 07009 800-465-4837
Fax: 973-256-3214
e-mail: info@liverfoundation.org
www.liverfoundation.org
Explains viral hepatitis, transmission, symptoms, testing and acute chronic hepatitis.
Rick Smith, President & CEO
Rebecca Frank, Chief Development Officer

5079 **Hepatitis B Prevention**
National Center For Infectious Diseases
Hepatitis Branch 404-332-4555
Atlanta, GA 30333
Explains what hepatitis B is, what behaviors are risky and how to protect oneself against it.

5080 **Hepatitis Fact Sheet**
www.cdc.gov/ncidod/diseases/hepatitis/c
Offers information on the causes, symptoms, prevention and treatments for hepatitis.

5081 **How Many Times a Day Do You Risk Being Infected with Hepatitis B?**
American Liver Foundation
1425 Pompton Avenue
Cedar Grove, NJ 07009 800-465-4837
Fax: 973-256-3214
e-mail: info@liverfoundation.org
www.liverfoundation.org
A flyer emphasizing the importance of vaccination against hepatitis B.
Rick Smith, President & CEO
Rebecca Frank, Chief Development Officer

5082 **Is Your Liver Giving You the Silent Treatment?**
Hepatitis Foundation International (HFI)
30 Sunrise Terrace 973-239-1035
Cedar Grove, NJ 07009-1423 800-891-0707
Fax: 973-875-5044
e-mail: hfi@intac.com
www.hepfi.org
Provides information for patients with hepatitis.

5083 **Living with Hepatitis C: Self Help Tips**
Hepatitis Foundation International (HFI)
30 Sunrise Terrace 973-239-1035
Cedar Grove, NJ 07009-1423 800-891-0707
Fax: 973-875-5044
e-mail: hfi@intac.com
www.hepfi.org
Information for people with Hepatitis C.

5084 **Protect Yourself and Those You Love Against HBV**
Hepatitis B Foundation
3805 Old Easton Road 215-489-4900
Doylestown, PA 18902 Fax: 215-489-4920
e-mail: info@hepb.org
www.hepb.org
Provides information to people affected by hepatitis B and their loved ones.
Molli C. Conti, Executive Director

5085 **Q and A: Hepatitis B Prevention**
SmithKline Beecham Pharmaceuticals
1 Franklin Plaza 215-751-4000
Philadelphia, PA 19102-1282
Informational booklet written for healthcare personnel by the manufacturer of Engerix-B vaccine, reviews hepatitis B prevention.

5086 **Someone You Know Has Hepatitis B**
Hepatitis B Foundation
3805 Old Easton Road 215-489-4900
Doylestown, PA 18902 Fax: 215-489-4920
e-mail: info@hepb.org
www.hepb.org
Provides information to people affected by hepatitis B and their loved ones.
Molli C. Conti, Executive Director

5087 **Tips on Coping with Chronic Hepatitis**
Hepatitis Foundation International (HFI)
30 Sunrise Terrace 973-239-1035
Cedar Grove, NJ 07009-1423 800-891-0707
Fax: 973-875-5044
e-mail: hfi@intac.com
www.hepfi.org
Information for people with hepatitis.

5088 **Viral Hepatitis: Everybody's Problem?**
American Liver Foundation
1425 Pompton Avenue
Cedar Grove, NJ 07009-1000 800-223-0179
Fax: 973-256-3214
e-mail: info@liverfoundation.org
www.liverfoundation.org
Covering a broad range of topics including: a definition of the disease, descriptions of types of infections, transmission, symptoms, treatment options and prevention of hepatitis.
Rick Smith, President & CEO
Rebecca Frank, Chief Development Officer

5089 **What Health Care Workers Should Know About Hepatitis B**
Channing L Bete Company
200 State Road
South Deerfield, MA 01373 800-628-7733
Presents information in easy-to-read, simple English for health care workers about hepatitis B.
15 pages

Audio & Video

5090 **Hepatitis B Video**
Hepatitis B Foundation
3805 Old Easton Road 215-489-4900
Doylestown, PA 18902 Fax: 215-489-4920
e-mail: info@hepb.org
www.hepb.org
Provides information to people affected by hepatitis B and their loved ones.
Molli C. Conti, Executive Director

5091 **Hepatitis C: A Viral Mystery**
Terry Strauss, Stephen Steady, author
Fanlight Productions
4196 Washington Street 617-469-4999
Boston, MA 02131-1731 800-937-4113
Fax: 617-469-3379
e-mail: fanlight@fanlight.com
www.fanlight.com
This timely video is about living with a serious, chronic illness. In addition to discussing the medical treatments available, the video also explores alternatives which appear to help some people.
2000 30 Minutes
ISBN: 1-572953-08-X

Web Sites

5092 **HIV/Hepatitis C in Prison (HIP) Committee**
www.prisons.org/hivin.htm
Fighting for consistent access to quality medical care including access to all new HIV and Hepatitis C medications, diagnostic testing and combination therapies.

5093 **Healing Well**
www.healingwell.com
An online health resource guide to medical news, chat, information and articles, newsgroups and message boards, books, disease-related web sites, medical directories, and more for patients, friends, and family coping with disabling diseases, disorders, or chronic illnesses.

5094 **Health Finder**
www.healthfinder.gov
Searchable, carefully developed web site offering information on over 1000 topics. Developed by the US Department of Health and Human Services, the site can be used in both English and Spanish.

5095 **Healthlink USA**
www.healthlinkusa.com
Health information concerning treatment, cures, prevention, diagnosis, risk factors, research, support groups, email lists, personal stories and much more. Updated regularly.

5096 **Healthy Lives**
www.healthylives.com/hepatitis

5097 **Helios Health**
www.helioshealth.com

Online resource for your health information. Detailed information about specific health topics, access to expert advice from our Medical Advisory Board, and up-to-date health news.

5098 Hepatitis B Coalition

www.immunize.org

Works to prevent transmission of hepatitis B in high-risk groups; to promote HBsAG screening for all pregnant women; to achieve vaccination of all infants, children, and adolescents; and to promote education and treatment for the person who is chronically infected with hepatitis B.

5099 Hepatitis Information Network

www.hepnet.com

5100 MedicineNet

www.medicinenet.com

An online resource for consumers providing easy-to-read, authoritative medical and health information.

5101 Medscape

www.mywebmd.com

Medscape offers specialists, primary care physicians, and other health professionals the Web's most robust and integrated medical information and educational tools.

5102 WebMD

www.webmd.com

Information on hepatitis, including articles and resources.

Description

5103 **Hydrocephalus**

The normal brain and spinal cord are surrounded with a watery substance called cerebro-spinal fluid, CSF, which collects within the brain in several larger pools called ventricles, connected to one another through tiny channels. The CSF is formed in some of these ventricles, circulates widely and is eventually reabsorbed. If CFS production exceeds reabsorption, or if the fluid is blocked from circulating and it may build up pressure that expands the ventricles and presses on the normal brain tissue, causing hydrocephalus, or water on the brain.

Hydrocephalus can cause change in behavior, headache, visual loss, vomiting and weakness. Hydrocephalus may be congenital, that is, present from birth. If it occurs in a child whose skull bones have not yet fused together, it may cause the head to enlarge.

In adults whose brains are encased in the rigid skull, there is no room to expand and pressure builds up in the brain. Excess CSF may be in response to infection such as meningitis or to blockage of CSF movement by tumor. Treatment and outlook depend on the underlying cause. Medical therapy may cause limited temporary improvement. Surgical treatment may be able to correct the underlying cause. If it cannot, the surgeon may still give substantial relief by placing a shunt which allows extra CSF to drain from the ventricles to some other part of the body.

National Agencies & Associations

5104 **Association of Hydrocephalus Education Advocacy & Discussion (AHEAD)**
1730 Autumn Leaf Lane 215-355-4728
Huntingdon Valley, PA 19006-1515
Organized by young adults with hydrocephalus for the purpose of providing telephone support nationwide.
Lane Borden, NE Regional Contact

5105 **Guardians of Hydrocephalus Research Foundation**
2640 E 28 Street 718-743-9650
Brooklyn, NY 11235-2023 Fax: 718-743-9650
e-mail: ghrf2618@aol.com
ghrf.homestead.com/ghrf.html
Non-profit organization made up of concerned parents and dedicated volunteers. The goal is to wipe out this top ranking birth defect.
Michael Fischetti, Founder
Jamie Fischetti, Secretary

5106 **Hydrocephalus Association Hydrocephalus Association**
Hydrocephalus Association
870 Market Street 415-732-7040
San Francisco, CA 94102 888-598-3789
Fax: 415-732-7044
e-mail: info@hydroassoc.org
www.hydroassoc.org
The association provides support education and advocacy for families and professionals. The goal is to insure that families and individuals dealing with the complexities of hydrocephalus receive personal support, comprehensive educational materials and outreach.
Dory Kranz, Director of Research
Pip Marks, Director of Support & Education

5107 **Hydrocephalus Foundation**
910 Rear Broadway 781-942-1161
Saugus, MA 01906 e-mail: HyFII@netscape.net
www.hydrocephalus.org
Dedicated to providing support educational resources and networking opportunities to patients and families affected by hydrocephalus. The Foundation also promotes related research and facilitates the training of healthcare professionals to improve patient care.
Greg A Tocco MIR, Founder/Executive Director
Donna H West, Board of Directors Member

5108 **Kidney Foundation**
300-5165 Sherbrooke Street W 514-369-4806
Montreal, QC, H4A-1T6 800-361-7494
Fax: 514-369-2472
e-mail: webmaster@kidney.ca
www.kidney.ca
A national volunteer organization committed to reducing the burden of kidney disease through: funding and stimulating innovative research; providing education and support; promoting access to high quality healthcare; and increasing public awareness and commitment to advancing kidney health and organ donation.

5109 **National Hydrocephalus Foundation**
12413 Centralia Road 562-924-6666
Lakewood, CA 90715 888-857-3434
Fax: 562-924-6666
e-mail: nhf@earthlink.net
www.nhfonline.org
The foundation is a national organization with almost 30 years of history. We provide information and education along with peer-to-peer support a physician referral sheet along with patient and family comments and several different types of help sheets.
Debbi Fields, Executive Director
Michael Fields, President/Treasurer

5110 **Spina Bifida & Hydrocephalus Association of Nova Scotia**
PO Box 341 902-679-1124
Coldbrook, Nova Scotia, B4R-1B6 800-304-0450
Fax: 902-679-1433
e-mail: spina.bifida@ns.sympatico.ca
www3.ns.sympatico.ca
It is a non-profit, registered charitable organization affiliated with the Spina Bifida and Hydrocephalus Association of Canada, and currently has one chapter in Cape Breton.

5111 **Spina Bifida & Hydrocephalus Association o f Ontario**
PO Box 341 902-679-1124
Coldbrook Nova Scotia, B4R 1-3B1 800-304-0450
Fax: 902-679-1433
e-mail: spina.bifida@ns.sympatico.ca
www.sbhans.ca
It is a non-profit registered charitable organization affiliated with the Spina Bifida and Hydrocephalus Association of Canada and currently has one chapter in Cape Breton.

5112 **World Hypertension League**
Medical University of Ohio 419-383-5270
Toledo, OH 43614-5809 Fax: 419-383-3120
e-mail: gmonhollen@meduohio.edu
hsc.utoledo.edu
Devoted to the advancement of hypertension prevention and control through joint efforts of all national leagues and societies.
Lloyd A Jacobs MD, President

State Agencies & Associations

California

5113 **Hydrocephalus Support Group of Southern California**
870 Market Street 415-732-7040
San Francisco, CA 94102 888-598-3789
Fax: 415-732-7044
e-mail: info@hydroassoc.org
www.hydroassoc.org

Founded in 1976 this group was formed as a group of concerned families and patients with hydrocephalus to share information and experiences in dealing with this disease locally and nationwide.
Rick Smith, Interim Executive Director
Karima Roumi MPH, Outreach Coordinator

Michigan

5114 **Hydrocephalus Support Group of Michigan Children's Hospital of Michigan**
Children's Hospital of Michigan
3901 Beaubien 313-745-5437
Detroit, MI 48201 Fax: 313-993-8744
Founded in 1992 this group provides information to families and gives them support.
Mary Smellie RN MSN, Clinical Nurse Specialist

Pennsylvania

5115 **Hydrocephalus Association of Philadelphia**
PO Box 2099 610-497-0375
Boothwyn, PA 19061-8099 Fax: 610-497-2836
Founded in 1992 the Association provides support information advocacy and telephone support to families in Pennsylvania New Jersey and Delaware.

Rhode Island

5116 **Hydrocephalus Association of Rhode Island**
PO Box 343 401-723-6065
Valley Falls, RI 02864-0343
Founded in 1993 the mission of this Association is to provide information support and advocacy for individuals with hydrocephalus and for friends and family members.
Gabriella Halmi, Director

Texas

5117 **Hydrocephalus Association of North Texas**
PO Box 670552 972-690-4342
Dallas, TX 75367-0552
Founded in 1987 the mission is to provide information and support to parents of children with hydrocephalus in the state of Texas and neighboring states.
Beverly Pike, President

Washington

5118 **Hydrocephalus Support Group of Seattle**
PO Box 1611 425-482-0479
Woodinville, WA 98072 e-mail: lpoliski@hydrosupport.org
www.hydrosupport.org
Founded in 1993 the group of Seattle provides support to individuals with hydrocephalus.
Diana Pozzi

Libraries & Resource Centers

5119 **LINK Program**
Emily Fudge, author
Hydrocephalus Association
870 Market Street 415-732-7040
San Francisco, CA 94102-2912 888-598-3789
Fax: 415-732-7044
e-mail: info@hydroassoc.org
www.hydroassoc.org
National network of 1300 individuals and families listed in directory format, giving our members direct access to others in similar circumstances.
Dory Kranz, Executive Director
Pip Marks, Director Outreach Services

Support Groups & Hotlines

5120 **Cerebrospinal Fluid Shunt Systems for the Management of Hydrocephalus**
Hydrocephalus Association
870 Market Street 415-732-7040
San Francisco, CA 94102-2912 888-598-3789
Fax: 415-732-7044
e-mail: info@hydroassoc.org
www.hydroassoc.org
Nonprofit organization that provides support, education and advocacy for all families, individuals and professionals affected by hydrocephalus.
Pip Marks, Director Outreach Services

5121 **Hydrocephalus Parents Support Group**
1325 Louis Street 908-722-4691
Manville, NJ 08835
Founded in 1993, the group provides support for parents of children with hydrocephalus.
Andrea Liptak, Founder

5122 **National Health Information Center**
PO Box 1133 310-565-4167
Washington, DC 20013 800-336-4797
Fax: 301-984-4256
e-mail: info@nhic.org
www.health.gov/nhic
Offers a nationwide information referral service, produces directories and resource guides.

Books

5123 **Hydrocephalus: A Guide for Patients, Families, and Friends**
O'Reilly and Associates
101 Morris Street
Sebastopol, CA 95472 800-998-9938
Fax: 707-829-0104
e-mail: order@oreilly.com
www.oreilly.com
Hydrocephalus: A Guide for Patients, Families, and Friends provides individuals and families with the guidance, information and support needed to make the right decisions at the right time.
350 pages Paperback
ISBN: 1-565924-10-X

5124 **Spina Bifida Association of America: Insights into Spina Bifida**
Spina Bifida Association of America
4590 MacArthur Boulevard NW 202-944-3285
Washington, DC 20007-4226 800-621-3141
Fax: 202-944-3295
e-mail: sbaa@sbaa.org
www.sbaa.org
News on medical, legislative and education topics relevant to individuals with spina bifida.
bi-monthly
Marybeth Leamyini, Communications Director

Children's Books

5125 **Loving Ben**
Delacorte
1540 Broadway 212-354-6500
New York, NY 10036-4039
This is a moving story of a sister who cares for her baby brother and tries to help him learn despite his birth defects and deteriorating health.
Grades 7-10

Newsletters

5126 **Alliance of Genetic Support Groups**
35 Wisconsin Circle 202-331-0942
Chevy Chase, MD 20815 800-336-4363

A coalition of voluntary genetic support groups, consumers and professionals addressing the needs of individuals and families affected by genetic disorders from a national perspective.

5127 **Hydrocephalus Association Newsletter**
Hydrocephalus Association
870 Market Street
San Francisco, CA 94102-2912
415-732-7040
888-598-3789
Fax: 415-732-7044
e-mail: info@hydroassoc.org
www.hydroassoc.org
Offers information on association news, conference articles, meetings, support and educational groups.
12 pages Quarterly
Dory Kranz, Executive Director
Pip Marks, Director Outreach Services

5128 **Hydrocephalus Parents Support Group Newsletter**
1325 Louis Street
Manville, NJ 08835
908-722-4691
Founded in 1993, the group provides support for parents of children with hydrocephalus.
Andrea Liptak, Founder

5129 **Hydrocephalus Support Group Newsletter**
PO Box 4236
Chesterfield, MO 63005-4236
636-532-8228
Fax: 314-995-4108
e-mail: hydrodb@earthlink.net
Founded in 1986, this group provides information, education and support to anyone dealing with hydrocephalus.
Debby Buffa, Founder/Chairman

5130 **National Hydrocephalus Foundation Newsletter**
12413 Centrailia Road
Lakewood, CA 90715-1623
562-402-3523
888-857-3434
Fax: 562-924-6666
e-mail: hydrobrat@earthlink.net
nhfonline.org
Founded in 1979, the foundation is a national organization whose purpose is to provide information and education, along with peer support newsletter quarterly. Group meeting quarterly in Long Beach, CA. $35 a year.
Quarterly
Debbie Fields, Executive Director

5131 **New York University Medical Center Auxiliary of Tisch Hospital**
560 1st Avenue
New York, NY 10016
212-263-5040
www.nyukidshealth.org
Conducts national symposiums on hydrocephalus.
Doris Farrelly, Contact

Pamphlets

5132 **About Hydrocephalus: A Book for Families**
Hydrocephalus Association
870 Market Street
San Francisco, CA 94102-2912
415-732-7040
888-598-3789
Fax: 415-732-7044
e-mail: info@hydroassoc.org
www.hydroassoc.org
A booklet in either English or Spanish, detailing all aspects of hydrocephalus from diagnosis and treatment to complications and follow-up care.
36 pages Paperback
Dory Kranz, Executive Director
Pip Marks, Director Outreach Services

5133 **About Normal Pressure Hydrocephalus: A Book for Adults & Their Families**
Hydrocephalus Association
870 Market Street
San Francisco, CA 94102-2912
415-732-7040
888-598-3789
Fax: 415-732-7044
e-mail: info@hydroassoc.org
www.hydroassoc.org
Booklet discusses the diagnosis and treatment of adult-onset normal pressure hydrocephalus.
24 pages Paperback
Dory Kranz, Executive Director
Pip Marks, Director Outreach Services

5134 **Directory of Neurosurgeons Who Treat Adults**
Hydrocephalus Association
870 Market Street
San Francisco, CA 94102-2912
415-732-7040
888-598-3789
Fax: 415-732-7044
e-mail: info@hydroassoc.org
www.hydroassoc.org
Names and addresses of neurosurgeons who treat adult-onset normal pressure hydrocephalus and adult-acquired hydrocephalus, listed alphabetically and geographically.
Dory Kranz, Executive Director
Pip Marks, Director Outreach Services

5135 **Directory of Pediatric Neurosurgeons**
Hydrocephalus Association
870 Market Street
San Francisco, CA 94102-2912
415-732-7040
888-598-3789
Fax: 415-732-7044
e-mail: info@hydroassoc.org
www.hydroassoc.org
Names and addresses of more than 200 neurosurgeons who specialize in pediatrics, listed alphabetically and geographically.
Dory Kranz, Executive Director
Pip Marks, Director Outreach Services

5136 **Endoscopic Third Ventriculotomy**
Hydrocephalus Association
870 Market Street
San Francisco, CA 94102-2912
415-732-7040
888-598-3789
Fax: 415-732-7044
e-mail: info@hydroassoc.org
www.hydroassoc.org
Series includes information on primary care, learning disabilities, eye problems, social skills development, headaches, endoscopic third ventriculostomy, shunts and more.
Dory Kranz, Executive Director
Pip Marks, Director Outreach Services

5137 **Eye Problems Associated with Hydrocephalus in Children**
Hydrocephalus Association
870 Market Street
San Francisco, CA 94102-2912
415-732-7040
888-598-3789
Fax: 415-732-7044
e-mail: info@hydroassoc.org
www.hydroassoc.org
Series includes information on primary care, learning disabilities, eye problems, social skills development, headaches, endoscopic third ventriculostomy, shunts and more.
Dory Kranz, Executive Director
Pip Marks, Director Outreach Services

5138 **Fact Sheet: Hydrocephalus**
Hydrocephalus Association
870 Market Street
San Francisco, CA 94102-2912
415-732-7040
888-598-3789
Fax: 415-732-7044
e-mail: info@hydroassoc.org
www.hydroassoc.org
Available in Spanish.
Dory Kranz, Executive Director
Pip Marks, Director Outreach Services

5139 **Headaches and Hydrocephalus**
Hydrocephalus Association
870 Market Street
San Francisco, CA 94102-2912
415-732-7040
888-598-3789
Fax: 415-732-7044
e-mail: info@hydroassoc.org
www.hydroassoc.org
Series includes information on primary care, learning disabilities, eye problems, social skills development, headaches, endoscopic third ventriculostomy, shunts and more.
Dory Kranz, Executive Director
Pip Marks, Director Outreach Services

5140 **Hospitalization Tips**
Hydrocephalus Association
870 Market Street
San Francisco, CA 94102-2912
415-732-7040
888-598-3789
Fax: 415-732-7044
e-mail: info@hydroassoc.org
www.hydroassoc.org

1997
Dory Kranz, Executive Director
Pip Marks, Director Outreach Services

5141 **How to Be an Assertive Parent on the Treatment Team**
Hydrocephalus Association
870 Market Street
San Francisco, CA 94102-2912
415-732-7040
888-598-3789
Fax: 415-732-7044
e-mail: info@hydroassoc.org
www.hydroassoc.org

Dory Kranz, Executive Director
Pip Marks, Director Outreach Services

5142 **ID Card for Third Ventriculostomy Patients**
Hydrocephalus Association
870 Market Street
San Francisco, CA 94102-2912
415-732-7040
888-598-3789
Fax: 415-732-7044
e-mail: info@hydroassoc.org
www.hydroassoc.org

Dory Kranz, Executive Director
Pip Marks, Director Outreach Services

5143 **LINK Directory Information**
Hydrocephalus Association
870 Market Street
San Francisco, CA 94102-2912
415-732-7040
888-598-3789
Fax: 415-732-7044
e-mail: info@hydroassoc.org
www.hydroassoc.org

A nationwide network of individuals listed in directory format giving members direct access to others in similar circumstances.
Dory Kranz, Executive Director
Pip Marks, Director Outreach Services

5144 **Learning Disabilities in Children with Hydrocephalus**
Hydrocephalus Association
870 Market Street
San Francisco, CA 94102-2912
415-732-7040
888-598-3789
Fax: 415-732-7044
e-mail: info@hydroassoc.org
www.hydroassoc.org

Available in Spanish.
Dory Kranz, Executive Director
Pip Marks, Director Outreach Services

5145 **Nonverbal Learning Disorder Syndrome**
Hydrocephalus Association
870 Market Street
San Francisco, CA 94102-2912
415-732-7040
888-598-3789
Fax: 415-732-7044
e-mail: info@hydroassoc.org
www.hydroassoc.org

1998
Dory Kranz, Executive Director
Pip Marks, Director Outreach Services

5146 **Prenatal Hydrocephalus: A Book for Parents**
Hydrocephalus Association
870 Market Street
San Francisco, CA 94102-2912
415-732-7040
888-598-3789
Fax: 415-732-7044
e-mail: info@hydroassoc.org
www.hydroassoc.org

Dory Kranz, Executive Director
Pip Marks, Director Outreach Services

5147 **Resource Guide**
Hydrocephalus Association
870 Market Street
San Francisco, CA 94102-2912
415-732-7040
888-598-3789
Fax: 415-732-7044
e-mail: info@hydroassoc.org
www.hydroassoc.org

A comprehensive listing of 450 articles on all aspects of hydrocephalus. Articles may be ordered from the association for a small fee.
Dory Kranz, Executive Director
Pip Marks, Director Outreach Services

5148 **Resource Guide: Normal Pressure Hydrocephalus/Adult Onset**
Hydrocephalus Association
870 Market Street
San Francisco, CA 94102-2912
415-732-7040
888-598-3789
Fax: 415-732-7044
e-mail: info@hydroassoc.org
www.hydroassoc.org

Dory Kranz, Executive Director
Pip Marks, Director Outreach Services

5149 **Social Skills Development in Children with Hydrocephalus**
Hydrocephalus Association
870 Market Street
San Francisco, CA 94102-2912
415-732-7040
888-598-3789
Fax: 415-732-7044
e-mail: info@hydroassoc.org
www.hydroassoc.org

Dory Kranz, Executive Director
Pip Marks, Director Outreach Services

5150 **Survival Skills for the Family Unit**
Hydrocephalus Association
870 Market Street
San Francisco, CA 94102-2912
415-732-7040
888-598-3789
Fax: 415-732-7044
e-mail: info@hydroassoc.org
www.hydroassoc.org

Dory Kranz, Executive Director
Pip Marks, Director Outreach Services

5151 **Understanding Your Child's Education Needs/Individualized Education Program**
Hydrocephalus Association
870 Market Street
San Francisco, CA 94102-2912
415-732-7040
888-598-3789
Fax: 415-732-7044
e-mail: info@hydroassoc.org
www.hydroassoc.org

Dory Kranz, Executive Director
Pip Marks, Director Outreach Services

Audio & Video

5152 **Hydrocephalus: A Neglected Disease**
Guardians of Hydrocephalus Research Foundation
2618 Avenue Z
Brooklyn, NY 11235-2023
718-743-4473
Fax: 718-743-1171
e-mail: ghrf2618@aol.com
www.homestead.com/ghrf.html

Marie Fischetti, Founder

Web Sites

5153 **Healing Well**
www.healingwell.com

An online health resource guide to medical news, chat, information and articles, newsgroups and message boards, books, disease-related web sites, medical directories, and more for patients, friends, and family coping with disabling diseases, disorders, or chronic illnesses.

5154 **Health Finder**
www.healthfinder.gov

Searchable, carefully developed web site offering information on over 1000 topics. Developed by the US Department of Health and Human Services, the site can be used in both English and Spanish.

5155 **Healthlink USA**

www.healthlinkusa.com

Health information concerning treatment, cures, prevention, diagnosis, risk factors, research, support groups, email lists, personal stories and much more. Updated regularly.

5156 **Helios Health**

www.helioshealth.com

Online resource for your health information. Detailed information about specific health topics, access to expert advice from our Medical Advisory Board, and up-to-date health news.

5157 **Hydrocephalus Association**

www.hydroassoc.org

Provides support, education and advocacy for families and professionals. The goal is to insure that families and individuals dealing with the complexities of hydrocephalus receive personal support, comprehensive educational materials and on-going medical care.

5158 **Hydrocephalus Center**

www.patientcenters.com/hydrocephalus

An online reference that was created especially as a resource for those with hydrocephalus and their families.

5159 **MedicineNet**

www.medicinenet.com

An online resource for consumers providing easy-to-read, authoritative medical and health information.

5160 **Medscape**

www.mywebmd.com

Medscape offers specialists, primary care physicians, and other health professionals the Web's most robust and integrated medical information and educational tools.

5161 **Neurology Channel**

www.neurologychannel.com

Find clearly explained, medically accurate information regarding conditions, including an overview, symptoms, causes, diagnostic procedures and treatment options. On this site it is possible to ask questions and get information from a neurologist and connect to people who have similar health interests.

5162 **WebMD**

www.webmd.com

Information on hydrocephalus, including articles and resources.

Description

5163 **Hypertension**

Hypertension is an abnormal elevation of blood pressure. Blood pressure is noted as a top number (systolic) over a bottom number (diastolic) with a reading of 120/80 being recognized as normal. Hypertension is defined as a systolic pressure greater than 140 and/or a diastolic pressure greater than 90. It is a common disorder that affects about 20 percent of the population. Primary, or essential, hypertension is the most common form, and it has no known cause. It is more prevalent in African-Americans, males, and those with a family history of high blood pressure. Other risk factors include obesity, diabetes, high levels of fat and cholesterol, smoking, sedentary lifestyle and psychological stress. It is a significant risk factor for coronary heart disease, heart failure, stroke, and kidney failure.

Patients with hypertension generally have no symptoms. Diagnosis is made by simple measurement with a blood pressure cuff. Several measurements are necessary at different times to establish the diagnosis.

Treatment of hypertension is done in a step-wise fashion beginning with lifestyle modifications (weight reduction, regular exercise, smoking cessation, a low salt, fat and cholesterol diet and improved stress reduction.) If medications are necessary, doctors can choose from a wide variety of effective and usually well-tolerated drugs. Therapy generally must be lifelong.

Occasionally the blood pressure may be refractory, or difficult to control with medicines. In this instance, screening is needed for unusual causes of hypertension, such as renovascular disease (narrowing of the arteries feeding the kidneys), hyperaldosteronism (a tumor or overgrowth of the adrenal gland which secretes hormones that raise the blood pressure), or aortic coarctation (a congenital malformation of the major blood vessels near the heart.) If no specifically treatable cause is identified, the patient will require combination therapy with high doses of drugs. Given a commitment to doing so, it is almost always possible to control the pressure.

National Agencies & Associations

5164 **American Society of Hypertension**
148 Madison Avenue 212-696-9099
New York, NY 10016 Fax: 212-696-0711
e-mail: ash@ash-us.org
www.ash-us.org

To organize and conduct educational seminars, materials and products in all aspects of hypertension and other cardiovascular diseases.
Torry Mark Sansone, Executive Director
Mary Trifault, Executive Associate

5165 **Lifeclinic.Com**
4032 Blackburn Lane 301-476-9888
Burtonsville, MD 20866 Fax: 301-476-9388
e-mail: salesteam@lifeclinic.com
www.lifeclinic.com

The lifeclinic.com web site was developed to provide an in-depth resource for information about prevalent, long-term health conditions and an online service to track your health over time. It also provides the information, resources and tools that can help patients and their families.
David Read, SVP
Shane Knee, VP-Business Development

5166 **National Heart, Lung & Blood Institute**
PO Box 30105 301-592-8573
Bethesda, MD 20824-0105 Fax: 240-629-3246
TTY: 240-629-3255
e-mail: nhlbiinfo@nhlbi.nih.gov
www.nhlbi.nih.gov

Primary responsibility of this organization is the scientific investigation of heart, blood vessel, lung and blood disorders. Oversee research, demonstration, prevention, education and training activities in these fields and emphasizes the control of stroke.
Elizabeth G Nabel, MD, Director

5167 **National Hypertension Association**
324 E 30th Street 212-889-3557
New York, NY 10016 Fax: 212-447-7032
e-mail: nathypertension@aol.com
www.nathypertension.org

Conducts research on the cause of hypertension through basic laboratory and clinical studies sponsors seminars and symposia to keep the medical profession and public abreast of services and advances in the treatment of hypertension.
William M Manger MD PhD, Chairman

5168 **National Stroke Association**
9707 E Easter Lane 303-649-9299
Centennial, CO 80112-3747 800-787-6537
Fax: 303-649-1328
e-mail: Info@stroke.org
www.stroke.org

A national organization whose sole purpose is to reduce the incidence and impact of stroke through prevention treatment rehabilitation and research and support for stroke survivors and their families. NSA produces a variety of education materials and other support services.
James Baranski, Chief Executive Officer
Mike Stefanski, Controller

5169 **Pulmonary Hypertension Association**
801 Roeder Road 301-565-3004
Silver Spring, MD 20910 800-748-7274
Fax: 301-565-3994
e-mail: pha@PHAssociation.org
www.PHAssociation.org

A nonprofit organization for pulmonary hypertension patients families caregivers and PH-treating medical professionals. The mission of the Pulmonary Hypertension Association (PHA) is to find ways to prevent and cure pulmonary hypertension.
Rino Aldrighetti, President
Carl Hicks, Chair

Research Centers

5170 **Creighton University Midwest Hypertension Research Center**
601 N 30th Street 402-280-4507
Omaha, NE 68131-2137 Fax: 402-280-4101
Dr William Pettinger, Director

5171 **Hahnemann University: Division of Surgical Research**
Broad & Vine Streets 215-762-7000
Philadelphia, PA 19102 Fax: 215-762-8109
www.hahnemannhospital.com

Studies hypertension and management of stress ulcers.
Teuro Matsum PhD, Director

5172 **Henry Ford Hospital: Hypertension and Vascular Research Division**
2799 W Grand Boulevard 313-972-1693
Detroit, MI 48202-2689 Fax: 313-876-1479
e-mail: ocarret1@hfhs.org
www.hypertensionresearch.org

Basic biomedical research seeks to understand: The role of vasoconstrictors and vasodilators (angiotensin II bradykinin nitric oxide natriuretic peptides) in the regulation of blood pressure development of hypertension and development of target organ damage (myocardial infarction heart failure vascular injury and renal disease); The generation of reactive oxygen species by blood vessels and kidney cells and how this contributes to target organ damage; and The mechanisms by which therape
Dr Oscar Carretero, Division Head
William H Beierwaltes, Scientist

5173 **Indiana University: Hypertension Research Center**
541 Clinical Drive 317-274-8153
Indianapolis, IN 46202-0001 800-274-4862
Fax: 317-278-0673
www.indiana.edu/medical
The mission of the Center is to conduct research in the causes diagnosis treatment and prevention of high blood pressure and its complications.
Dr Myron Weinberger, Director

5174 **New York University General Clinical Research Center**
NYU Medical Center
550 First Avenue 212-263-7900
New York, NY 10016 Fax: 212-263-8501
www.med.nyu.edu
Focuses in the areas of hypertension and studies into endocrinology.
Dr William Rom MPH, Director
Eric Schips, Divisional Administrator

5175 **University of Michigan: Division of Hypertension**
1500 E Medical Center 734-936-4000
Ann Arbor, MI 48109 800-914-8561
www.med.umich.edu
Excellence in medical education patient care and research.
Douglas L Strong, Director
Robert P Kelch, Executive Vice President for Medical Aff

5176 **University of Minnesota: Hypertensive Research Group**
611 Beacon Street SE 612-624-1438
Minneapolis, MN 55455
Research pertaining to hypertension and stress disorders.
Jack Stoulil, Study Coordinator

5177 **University of Southern California: Division of Nephrology**
2025 Zonal Avenue 213-226-7307
Los Angeles, CA 90033-1034 Fax: 213-226-3958
Research into hypertension and sleep disorders.
Dr. Shaul G Massry, Head

5178 **University of Virginia: Hypertension and Atherosclerosis Unit**
Medical Center 804-924-8470
Charlottesville, VA 22908-0001 Fax: 804-924-2581
Dr Carlos Ayers, Director

5179 **Wake Forest University: Arteriosclerosis Research Center**
Department of Comparative Medicine
300 S Hawthorne Road 336-764-3600
Winston-Salem, NC 27103-2732 Fax: 336-764-5818
Hypertension research.
Thomas Clark DVM, Director

Support Groups & Hotlines

5180 **National Health Information Center**
PO Box 1133 310-565-4167
Washington, DC 20013 800-336-4797
Fax: 301-984-4256
e-mail: info@nhic.org
www.health.gov/nhic
Offers a nationwide information referral service, produces directories and resource guides.

Books

5181 **Courage: Poems & Positive Thoughts for Stroke Survivors**
National Stroke Association
9707 E Easter Lane 303-649-9299
Englewood, CO 80112-3747 800-787-6537
Fax: 303-649-1328
www.stroke.org
Words of inspiration from survivors and caregivers.
83 pages
Colette Lafosse, Director Rehabilitation/Recovery Program

5182 **Discovery Circles**
National Stroke Association
9707 E Easter Lane 303-649-9299
Englewood, CO 80112-3747 800-787-6537
Fax: 303-649-1328
www.stroke.org
NSA's guide to organizing and facilitating stroke support groups. This detailed manual describes the support group structure and the facilitator's role.
213 pages
Colette Lafosse, Director Rehabilitation/Recovery Program

5183 **Magic of Humor in Caregiving**
National Stroke Association
9707 E Easter Lane 303-649-9299
Englewood, CO 80112-3747 800-787-6537
Fax: 303-649-1328
www.stroke.org
A dynamic researching tool focusing on the necessity of humor in daily caregiving interaction.
Colette Lafosse, Director Rehabilitation/Recovery Program

5184 **Management of Hypertension**
EMIS Medical Publishers
PO Box 1607 580-924-0643
Durant, OK 74702-1607 800-225-0694
Fax: 580-924-9414

ISBN: 0-929240-62-6

5185 **November Days**
National Stroke Association
9707 E Easter Lane 303-649-9299
Englewood, CO 80112-3747 800-787-6537
Fax: 303-649-1328
www.stroke.org
A caregiver's story of her struggle with a loved one's stroke.
225 pages

5186 **Ted's Stroke: The Caregiver's Story**
National Stroke Association
9707 E Easter Lane 303-649-9299
Englewood, CO 80112-3747 800-787-6537
Fax: 303-649-1328
www.stroke.org
Personal experiences, guidance and tips for caregivers.
175 pages
ISBN: 0-962487-61-9

5187 **Women in Your Life: Protect Yourself, Protect Your Family**
National Stroke Association
9707 E Easter Lane 303-649-9299
Englewood, CO 80112-3747 800-787-6537
Fax: 303-649-1328
www.stroke.org
Valuable information about the unique toll stroke takes on women.
Colette Lafosse, Director Rehabilitation/Recovery Program

Magazines

5188 **American Journal of Hypertension**
American Society of Hypertension
515 Madison Avenue 212-644-0650
New York, NY 10022 Fax: 212-644-0658
e-mail: ash@ash-us.org
www.ash-us.org

5189 **Ethnicity & Disease**
International Society on Hypertension in Blacks

2045 Manchester Street NE 404-875-6263
Atlanta, GA 30324-4110 Fax: 404-875-6334
e-mail: member@ishib.org
www.ishib.org

International journal on ethnic minority population differences in diease patterns. Provides a comprehensive source of information on the causal relationships in the etiology of common illnesses through the study of ethnic patterns of disease.
Quarterly
Christopher T Fitzpatrick, CEO
Melanie T Cockfield, Director Administration

5190 **Ethnicity Disease**
International Society on Hypertension in Blacks
2045 Manchester Street NE 404-875-6263
Atlanta, GA 30324-4110 Fax: 404-875-6334
e-mail: member@ishib.org
www.ishib.org

Determined to accomplish the overall mission to improving the health and life expectancy of ethnic minority populations around the world. Publishes a quarterly journal and holds an annual conference.
150 pages Quarterly
Christopher T Fitzpatrick, CEO
Melanie T Cockfield, Director Administration

5191 **Magazine of the National Institute of Hypertension Studies**
13217 Livernois Avenue 313-931-3427
Detroit, MI 48238-3162
Association news.

Newsletters

5192 **News Report**
National Hypertension Association
324 E 30th Street 212-889-3557
New York, NY 10016-8329 Fax: 212-447-7032
e-mail: nathypertension@aol.com
www.nathypertension.org

Offers information and medical updates regarding hypertension. Recent book publication: 100 Questions and Answers about Hypertension by WM Manger, MD, PhD, and RW Gifford, Jr, MT available throught National Hypertension Association.
W.M. Manger MD, PhD, Chairman

Pamphlets

5193 **African-Americans and Stroke**
National Stroke Association
9707 E Easter Lane 303-649-9299
Englewood, CO 80112-3747 800-787-6537
Fax: 303-649-1328
www.stroke.org
Colette Lafosse, Director Rehabilitation/Recovery Program

5194 **Aneurysm Answers**
National Stroke Association
9707 E Easter Lane 303-649-9299
Englewood, CO 80112-3747 800-787-6537
Fax: 303-649-1328
www.stroke.org
Colette Lafosse, Director Rehabilitation/Recovery Program

5195 **Check Your Pulse, America: Atrial Fibrillation**
National Stroke Association
9707 E Easter Lane 303-649-9299
Englewood, CO 80112-3747 800-787-6537
Fax: 303-649-1328
www.stroke.org
Colette Lafosse, Director Rehabilitation/Recovery Program

5196 **Cholesterol and Stroke**
National Stroke Association
9707 E Easter Lane 303-649-9299
Englewood, CO 80112-3747 800-787-6537
Fax: 303-649-1328
www.stroke.org
Colette Lafosse, Director Rehabilitation/Recovery Program

5197 **High Blood Pressure and Stroke**
National Stroke Association
9707 E Easter Lane 303-649-9299
Englewood, CO 80112-3747 800-787-6537
Fax: 303-649-1328
www.stroke.org
Colette Lafosse, Director Rehabilitation/Recovery Program

5198 **Mobility: Issues Facing Stroke Survivors and Their Families**
National Stroke Association
9707 E Easter Lane 303-649-9299
Englewood, CO 80112-3747 800-787-6537
Fax: 303-649-1328
www.stroke.org
Colette Lafosse, Director Rehabilitation/Recovery Program

5199 **Recurrent Stroke**
National Stroke Association
9707 E Easter Lane 303-649-9299
Englewood, CO 80112-3747 800-787-6537
Fax: 303-649-1328
www.stroke.org
Colette Lafosse, Director Rehabilitation/Recovery Program

5200 **Smoking Cessation: Be Smoke Free in 3 Minutes**
National Stroke Association
9707 E Easter Lane 303-649-9299
Englewood, CO 80112-3747 800-787-6537
Fax: 303-649-1328
www.stroke.org
Colette Lafosse, Director Rehabilitation/Recovery Program

5201 **Transient Ischemic Attack**
National Stroke Association
9707 E Easter Lane 303-649-9299
Englewood, CO 80112-3747 800-787-6537
Fax: 303-649-1328
www.stroke.org
Colette Lafosse, Director Rehabilitation/Recovery Program

Audio & Video

5202 **Stroke: Touching the Soul of Your Family**
National Stroke Association
9707 E Easter Lane 303-649-9299
Englewood, CO 80112-3747 800-787-6537
Fax: 303-649-1328
www.stroke.org

Fifteen minute video chronicling three stroke survivors and their courageous struggle to overcome daily challenges and educate others about stroke.
Colette Lafosse, Director Rehabilitation/Recovery Program

Web Sites

5203 **American Society of Hypertension**
www.ash-us.org

To organize and conduct educational seminars, materials, and products in all aspects of hypertension and other cardiovascular diseases.

5204 **Healing Well**
www.healingwell.com

An online health resource guide to medical news, chat, information and articles, newsgroups and message boards, books, disease-related web sites, medical directories, and more for patients, friends, and family coping with disabling diseases, disorders, or chronic illnesses.

5205 **Health Finder**
www.healthfinder.gov

Searchable, carefully developed web site offering information on over 1000 topics. Developed by the US Department of Health and Human Services, the site can be used in both English and Spanish.

5206 **Healthlink USA**
www.healthlinkusa.com

Links to websites which may include treatment, cures, diagnosis, prevention, support groups, email lists, messageboards, personal stories, risk factors, statistics, research and more.

5207 **Helios Health**

www.helioshealth.com

Online resource for your health information. Detailed information about specific health topics, access to expert advice from our Medical Advisory Board, and up-to-date health news.

5208 **Hypertension: Journal of the American Heart Association**

hyper.ahajournals.org

Lists current issues of journals about hypertension and the American Heart Association.

5209 **Inter-American Society of Hypertension**

www.iashonline.org

Website hosted by IASH, a non-profit professional organization devoted to the understanding, prevention and control of hypertension and vascular diseases in the American population. Members from 20 different countries in the Americas as well as Europe, Australia and Asia. Stimulates research and the exchange of ideas in hypertension and vascular diseases amoung physicians and scientists. Promotes the detection, control and prevention of hypertension and other cardiovascular risk factors.

5210 **Lifeclinic.Com**

www.lifeclinic.com

Online information about blood pressure, hypertension, diabetes, cholesterol, stroke, heart failure and more. Maintains current, up-to-date and accurate information for patients to help them manage their conditions better and to improve communications between them and their doctors.

5211 **Mayo Clinic Health Oasis**

www.mayohealth.org

Mission is to empower people to manage their health, by providing useful and up-to-date information and tools that reflect the expertise and standard of excellence of the Mayo Clinic.

5212 **MedicineNet**

www.medicinenet.com

An online resource for consumers providing easy-to-read, authoritative medical and health information.

5213 **Medscape**

www.mywebmd.com

Medscape offers specialists, primary care physicians, and other health professionals the Web's most robust and integrated medical information and educational tools.

5214 **National Heart, Lung & Blood Institute**

www.nhlbi.nih.gov

Information on the scientific investigation of heart, blood vessel, lung and blood disorders. Oversee research, demonstration, prevention, education and training activities in these fields and emphasizes the control of stroke.

5215 **WebMD**

www.webmd.com

Information on hypertension, including articles and resources.

Description

5216 **Impotence**

Impotence, also called erectile dysfunction (ED), is defined as the inability of a male to achieve and maintain an erection of sufficient quality to allow sexual intercourse. ED is very common, affecting millions of American males. Although it may occur at any age, it becomes dramatically more common with advancing age. Impotence may be caused by diabetes, circulatory disturbance, genital injury, hormonal disorders, medication side effects, depression, surgery (for instance, prostate removal) and many less well-characterized physical and psychological states. Impotence may be situational, that is, involving place, time, partner and degree of self-esteem.

Few cases of impotence are completely cured, but several kinds of effective treatment exist, including correction, if possible, of underlying causes. Oral medications that increase blood flow to the penis have been effective in many instances. Psychological factors that accompany ED should be considered in every case, including behavioral therapy and counseling, as needed.

National Agencies & Associations

5217 **Impotence Institute of America**
119 S Ruth Street 865-379-2154
Maryville, TN 37803 800-669-1603
e-mail: iwatenn@aol.com
A non-profit organization dedicated to education about impotence. The IIA is a division of the Impotence World Association. Provides information on the causes, impact and treatments on this topic. Also publishes a quarterly newsletter on impotence topics.

5218 **Impotence Resource Center of the Geddings Osbon Sr Foundation**
PO Box 1593
Augusta, GA 30903 800-433-4215
Fax: 706-821-2782
e-mail: impotence@afud.org
www.impotence.org
Offers a free medical discussion where the consumer can obtain accurate unblessed information in a confidential understanding and thoughtful manner.

5219 **National Kidney and Urologic Diseases Information Clearinghouse**
Center Drive MSC 2560 301-654-4415
Bethesda, MD 20892-2560 800-891-5390
Fax: 301-907-8906
e-mail: nkudic@info.niddk.nih.gov
www.niddk.nih.gov
Provides information about diseases of the kidneys and urologic system to people with such afflictions and to their families, health care professionals and the public. Answers inquiries; develops, reviews and distributes publications.
Griffin P Rodgers, Director

5220 **Sexual Function Health Council American Foundation for Urologic Disease**
American Foundation for Urologic Disease
1000 Corporate Boulevard 410-689-3700
Linthicum, MD 21090 866-746-4282
Fax: 410-689-3800
e-mail: auafoundation@auafoundation.org
www.auafoundation.org
The American Foundation for Urologic Disease Inc. is a charitable organization established to raise funds for research lay education and patient advocacy for the prevention detection management and cure of urologic disease.
John M Barry, President
Sandra Vassos, Executive Director

Research Centers

5221 **CNY Male Sexual Dysfunction Center**
357 Genesee Street 315-363-8862
Oneida, NY 13421 888-269-6732
Fax: 315-363-5477
www.cnymsdc.com

5222 **Male Sexual Dysfunction Clinic**
3401 N Central Avenue 800-788-2873
Chicago, IL 60634 800-788-2873
Fax: 847-231-4130
e-mail: info@msdclinic.com
www.msdclinic.com
Helping men overcome male sexual dysfunctions such as impotence since 1981.
Sheldon O Burman, Director

5223 **New York Male Reproductive Center: Sexual Dysfunction Unit**
161 Fort Washington Avenue 212-305-0123
New York, NY 10032 Fax: 212-305-0126
e-mail: rshabsigh@urology.columbia.edu
The New York Male Reproductive Center at Columbia-Presbyterian Medical Center offers state-of-the-art diagnosis and treatment for impotence. Treatments include surgical and non-surgical procedures.
Ridwan Shabs MD, Director

Support Groups & Hotlines

5224 **Impotence Information Center**
PO Box 9
Minneapolis, MN 55440 800-843-4315

5225 **Impotents Anonymous**
8630 Fenton Street 301-588-5777
Silver Spring, MD 20910-3803
Serves as an educational organization providing concerned individuals with information regarding impotence.
Bruce MacKenzie, Founder

5226 **National Health Information Center**
PO Box 1133 310-565-4167
Washington, DC 20013 800-336-4797
Fax: 301-984-4256
e-mail: info@nhic.org
www.health.gov/nhic
Offers a nationwide information referral service, produces directories and resource guides.

Books

5227 **Impotence: How to Overcome It**
HealthProInk Publishing
562 Wind Drift Lane 313-355-3686
Spring Lake, MI 49456-2168

5228 **It's Not All in Your Head**
Impotence Institute of America
8201 Corporate Drive 301-577-0650
Landover, MD 20785-2230
A couple's guide to overcoming impotence.

Newsletters

5229 **Impotence Worldwide**
8201 Corporate Drive 301-577-0650
Landover, MD 20785-2230
Provides information from professionals and lay persons concerning impotence plus manufactured product information.
Monthly

5230 Your Sexuality & Health
Impotence Resource Center
PO Box 1593
Augusta, GA 30903-1593
800-433-4215
e-mail: info@gdo.org
www.impotence.org

Quarterly newsletter that features articles by medical experts and highlights current research and tidbits of healthy living advice.
Quarterly

Pamphlets

5231 Answers to the Most Asked Questions About Impotence
Impotence World Services
8201 Corporate Drive
Landover, MD 20785-2230
301-577-0650

5232 Impotence Causes and Treatments
American Medical Systems
10700 Bren Road E
Minnetonka, MN 55343
952-933-4666
800-843-4315
Fax: 952-930-6157
www.visitams.com

Offers information on what impotence is, physical and emotional causes, treatments, questions and answers.

5233 Male Treatment Guide
Impotence Resource Center
PO Box 1593
Augusta, GA 30903-1593
800-433-4215
e-mail: info@gdo.org
www.impotence.org

Explains impotence - what it is, what causes it and how it is treated.
Free

5234 Woman's Perspective
Impotence Resource Center
PO Box 1593
Augusta, GA 30903-1593
800-433-4215
e-mail: info@gdo.org
www.impotence.org

Talking with your partner about impotence and choosing a treatment together.
Free

Audio & Video

5235 Impotence Treatment Options
Impotence Resource Center
PO Box 1593
Augusta, GA 30903-1593
800-433-4215
e-mail: info@gdo.org
www.impotence.org

Actual taping of a men's sexual health seminar - presented by Gary Leach, MD.

5236 Male Treatment Guide
Impotence Resource Center
PO Box 1593
Augusta, GA 30903-1593
800-433-4215
e-mail: info@gdo.org
www.impotence.org

Explains impotence - what it is, what causes it and how it is treated.
Audio Tape

5237 Medical Management of Impotence
Impotence Resource Center
PO Box 1593
Augusta, GA 30903-1593
800-433-4215
e-mail: info@gdo.org
www.impotence.org

5238 Woman's Perspective
Impotence Resource Center
PO Box 1593
Augusta, GA 30903-1593
800-433-4215
e-mail: info@gdo.org
www.impotence.org

Talking with your partner about impotence and choosing a treatment together.
Audio Tape

Web Sites

5239 American Foundation for Urologic Disease
www.impotence.org

Online information about impotence, provided by the Sexual Function Health Council of the American Foundation for Urologic Disease.

5240 Family Meds
www.familymeds.com

A site providing information on impotence and its various treatments, including over the counter, natural, and prescription medication choices.

5241 Healing Well
www.healingwell.com

An online health resource guide to medical news, chat, information and articles, newsgroups and message boards, books, disease-related web sites, medical directories, and more for patients, friends, and family coping with disabling diseases, disorders, or chronic illnesses.

5242 Health Finder
www.healthfinder.gov

Searchable, carefully developed web site offering information on over 1000 topics. Developed by the US Department of Health and Human Services, the site can be used in both English and Spanish.

5243 Healthlink USA
www.healthlinkusa.com

Health information concerning treatment, cures, prevention, diagnosis, risk factors, research, support groups, email lists, personal stories and much more. Updated regularly.

5244 Helios Health
www.helioshealth.com

Online resource for your health information. Detailed information about specific health topics, access to expert advice from our Medical Advisory Board, and up-to-date health news.

5245 Impotence Resource Center of the Geddings Osbon Sr Foundation
www.impotence.org

Offers a free medical discussion service where the consumer can obtain accurate, unblassed information in a confidential, understanding and thoughtful manner.

5246 Impotence Specialists.com
www.impotencespecialists.com

Offers information on physicians in your area, treatment options, online resources and more. A guide to the nation's impotence specialists.

5247 Impotence World Association
www.impotence.com

Informs and educates the public on the subject of impotence and its causes and treatments. Serving the impotence industry since 1983 by bringing total care to the treatment of impotence.

5248 MedicineNet
www.medicinenet.com

An online resource for consumers providing easy-to-read, authoritative medical and health information.

5249 Medscape
www.mywebmd.com

Medscape offers specialists, primary care physicians, and other health professionals the Web's most robust and integrated medical information and educational tools.

5250 WebMD
www.webmd.com

Information on impotence, including articles and resources.

Description

5251 **Incontinence**

Urinary incontinence is the involuntary leakage of urine, whether during waking or sleeping hours. One common type is urge incontinence, resulting from involuntary bladder contractions. The person feels a sudden urge to urinate, so intense that it may not be controlled long enough to reach the toilet. Common causes of urge incontinence are urinary tract infections, spinal cord injury, and kidney stones. Stress incontinence is the instantaneous leakage of urine without bladder contractions. It manifests as loss of urine during stress events, such as coughing, sneezing, laughing, or lifting. This may occur in women due to weak bladder tone from multiple pregnancies. In men, stress incontinence can occur after prostate removal or trauma to the bladder. Overflow incontinence, in which the bladder cannot control urine output, can be caused by nerve injury, alcoholism, and some diseases. Symptoms incude urgency, and having to urinate more often (frequency) and at night (nocturia).

Treatment of incontinence focuses on therapy for the underlying causes. Infections are treated with the appropriate antibiotics. Stress incontinence in women can be treated with exercises to strengthen the bladder muscles. Other therapies include biofeedback and electrical stimulation. Severe cases may require surgical repair. Urinary incontinence remains largely a neglected problem, despite the fact that it can often be successfully treated.

National Agencies & Associations

5252 **American Urological Association**
1000 Corporate Boulevard 410-689-3700
Linthicum, MD 21090 866-746-4282
Fax: 410-689-3800
e-mail: auafoundation@auafoundation.org
www.urologyhealth.org
A charitable organization whose mission is the prevention and cure of urologic diseases through the expansion of research education and public awareness.
Sandra Vasso MPA, Executive Director
John M Barry MD, President

5253 **International Foundation for Functional Gastrointestinal Disorders (IFFGD)**
PO Box 170864 414-964-1799
Milwaukee, WI 53217-8076 888-964-2001
Fax: 414-964-7176
e-mail: iffgd@iffgd.org
www.iffgd.org
Nonprofit education, support and research organization devoted to increasing awareness and understanding of functional gastrointestinal disorders including irritable bowel syndrome (IBS), constipation, diarrhea, pain and incontinence.
Nancy J Norton, President

5254 **Intestinal Disease Foundation**
100 W Station Square Drive 412-261-5888
Pittsburgh, PA 15219-1122 877-587-9606
Fax: 412-471-2722
www.intestinalfoundation.org
Provides one-on-one telephone support, educational programs and materials and self-help groups for people with irritable bowel syndrome (IBS), diverticular disease, inflammatory bowel diseases and short bowel syndrome; sponsors educational seminars; provides educational materials.
Harriet Gibb LPN, Client Services Manager

5255 **National Association for Continence**
PO Box 1019 843-377-0900
Charleston, SC 29402-1019 800-252-3337
Fax: 843-377-0905
e-mail: memberservices@nafc.org
www.nafc.org
Founded as Help for Incontinent People, NAFC is the foremost consumer advocacy organization dedicated to helping people who struggle with incontinence and related voiding dysfunction. Its mission is focused on public education, awareness and collaboration.
Nancy Muller, Executive Director
Pam Knox, Communications and Public Relations

5256 **National Council on Aging**
1901 L Street NW 202-479-1200
Washington, DC 20036 Fax: 202-479-0735
TTY: 202-479-6674
TDD: 202-479-6674
e-mail: info@ncoa.org
www.ncoa.org
Organizations and professionals promoting the dignity self-determination and well-being of older persons.
James P Firman EdD, President/CEO

5257 **Simon Foundation for Continence**
PO Box 815 847-864-3913
Wilmette, IL 60091 800-237-4666
Fax: 847-864-9758
e-mail: cbgartley@simonfoundation.org
www.simonfoundation.org
Seeks to bring the topic of incontinence out of the closet and remove the associated stigma; provides educational materials to patients their families and the health care professionals who provide patient care.
Cheryle B Gartley, President/Founder
Anita Saltmarche, Vice President

Support Groups & Hotlines

5258 **Greater New York Pull-Thru Network**
62 Edgewood Avenue 201-891-5977
Wyckoff, NJ 07481
National support network providing emotional support and information to patients and families of children who have had or will have a pull-thru type surgery to correct an imperforate anus or associated malformation, Hirschsprung's or other fecal incontinence problems. Support group meetings held quarterly.

5259 **National Health Information Center**
PO Box 1133 310-565-4167
Washington, DC 20013 800-336-4797
Fax: 301-984-4256
e-mail: info@nhic.org
www.health.gov/nhic
Offers a nationwide information referral service, produces directories and resource guides.

5260 **Simon Foundation Helpline for Incontinence Information**
Simon Foundation for Continence
PO Box 815 847-864-3913
Wilmette, IL 60091 800-237-4666
Fax: 847-864-9758
e-mail: cbgartley@simonfoundation.org
www.simonfoundation.org
Offers information and help to persons with incontinence problems and professionals who work with them.
Cheryle Gartley, Founder/President
Jasmine Schmidt, Director of Education

5261 **University of California at San Francisco Women's Continence Center**
2356 Sutter Street 415-885-7788
San Francisco, CA 94115 877-366-8325
coe.ucsf.edu/wcc

Offers a comprehensive array of clinical services for women with incontinence, urethal or bladder dysfuntion and pelvic support problems.
Jeanette S Brown MD, Director

Books

5262 Managing Incontinence: a Guide to Living with Loss of Bladder Control
Simon Foundation for Incontinence
PO Box 815
Wilmette, IL 60091
847-864-3913
800-237-4666
Fax: 847-864-9768
e-mail: simoninfo@simonfoundation.org
www.simonfoundation.org
Seeks to bring the topic of incontinence out of the closet and remove the associated stigma; provides information to patients, their families and the health care professionals who provide patient care.
Quarterly
Cheryle B Gartley, President

5263 Pocket Guide for Continence Care
National Association for Continence
PO Box 1019
Charleston, SC 29402
843-377-0900
800-252-3337
Fax: 843-377-0905
e-mail: memberservices@nafc.org
www.nafc.org
Condensed version of the Blueprint for Continence Care, this guide is designed for a first line supervisor or any health care professional in any eldercare environment to help address any issues related to bladder health. The guide is perfect for a quick referral because it can actually fit in the healthcare professional's pocket.
Nancy Muller, Executive Director
Caryn Antos, Publicity/Publications Associate

5264 Resource Guide: Products and Services for Incontinence
National Association for Continence
PO Box 1019
Charleston, SC 29402
843-377-0900
800-252-3337
Fax: 843-377-0905
e-mail: memberservices@nafc.org
www.nafc.org
Complete directory of products and services available. Categories include disposable products, reusable products, skin care products, deodorizing products, pelvic organ support devices, medications to treat incontinence and others. Also includes a listing of distributors and mail/phone order companies.
Nancy Muller, Executive Director
Caryn Antos, Publicity/Publications Associate

5265 Your Personal Guide to Bladder Health
National Association for Continence
PO Box 1019
Charleston, SC 29402
843-377-0900
800-252-3337
Fax: 843-377-0905
e-mail: memberservices@nafc.org
www.nafc.org
Designed for residents of assisted living environments, other older individuals living independently and their involved family members. It encompasses a wide variety of informative topics, including diet and daily habits, pelvic muscle exercises odor control and more.
48 pages
Nancy Muller, Executive Director
Caryn Antos, Publicity/Publications Associate

Magazines

5266 Digestive Health Matters
Intl. Foundation for Gastrointestinal Disorders
PO Box 170864
Milwaukee, WI 53217-0864
414-964-1799
888-964-2001
Fax: 414-964-7176
e-mail: iffgd@iffgd.org
www.iffgd.org
Quarterly journal focuses on upper and lower gastrointestinal disorders in adults and children. Educational pamphlets and factsheets are available. Patient and professional membership.

Newsletters

5267 Discoveries
National Association for Continence
PO Box 1019
Charleston, SC 29402
843-377-0900
800-252-3337
Fax: 843-377-0905
e-mail: memberservices@nafc.org
www.nafc.org
Compendium comprised of the most recently released incontinence products and newly approved protocol. Includes editorial sections, authored by leading clinicians and researchers, describing new product technology and research in other medical advances related to continence care.
32 pages BiAnnual
Nancy Muller, Executive Director
Caryn Antos, Publicity/Publications Associate

5268 Informer
Simon Foundation for Incontinence
PO Box 815
Wilmette, IL 60091
847-864-3913
800-237-4666
Fax: 847-864-9768
e-mail: simoninfo@simonfoundation.org
www.simonfoundation.org
Seeks to bring the topic of incontinence out of the closet and remove the associated stigma; provides information to patients, their families, and the health care professionals who provide patient care.
Quarterly
Cheryle B Gartley, President

5269 Intestinal Fortitude
Intestinal Disease Foundation
One Station Square, Suite 525
Pittsburgh, PA 15219
412-261-5888
Fax: 412-471-2722
www.intestinalfoundation.org
Newsletter, brochures and books for Intestinal Disease Foundation members.

5270 Participate
IFFGD
PO Box 17864
Milwaukee, WI 53217-0864
414-964-1799
888-964-2001
Fax: 414-964-7176
e-mail: iffgd@iffgd.org
www.aboutincontinence.org
Provides information for people affected by the various forms of functional bowel disorders, including irritable bowel syndrome, constipation, diarrhea, pain and incontinence.
Quarterly

5271 Pull-Thru Network News
Greater New York Pull-Thru Network
62 Edgewood Avenue
Wyckoff, NJ 07481-3456
201-891-5977
www.pullthrough.org/ptnn.html
Quarterly newsletter for patients and families who have had or will have a pull-thru type surgery to correct an imperforate anus or associated malformation, Hirschsprung's or other fecal incontinence problem.

5272 Quality Care
National Association for Continence
PO Box 1019
Charleston, SC 29402
843-377-0900
800-252-3337
Fax: 843-377-0905
e-mail: memberservices@nafc.org
www.nafc.org
Quarterly newsletter addressing causes, symptoms, management and treatment options for incontinence and related disorders.
Quarterly
Nancy Muller, Executive Director
Caryn Antos, Publicity/Publications Associate

Pamphlets

5273 Bladder Control for Women
National Kidney and Urologic Diseases Information
3 Information Way
Bethesda, MD 20892-3580
800-891-5390
Fax: 301-907-8906
e-mail: nkudic@info.nidkk.nih.gov
Comprehensive introduction to the causes, symptoms, and treatments for bladder control problems in women.

5274 Exercising Your Pelvic Muscles
National Kidney and Urologic Diseases Information
3 Information Way
Bethesda, MD 20892-3580
800-891-5390
Fax: 301-907-8906
e-mail: nkudic@info.nidkk.nih.gov
A description of exercises for the pelvic floor muscles, called Kegel exercises, and how they can help to restore or maintain bladder control.

5275 Menopause and Bladder Control
National Kidney and Urologic Diseases Information
3 Information Way
Bethesda, MD 20892-3580
800-891-5390
Fax: 301-907-8906
e-mail: nkudic@info.nidkk.nih.gov
An introduction to the changes to your body that occur during menopause, how these changes can result in loss of bladder control, and how your health care team can help you restore or maintain bladder control.

5276 NAFC Fact Sheets
National Association for Continence
PO Box 1019
Charleston, SC 29402
843-377-0900
800-252-3337
Fax: 843-377-0905
e-mail: memberservices@nafc.org
www.nafc.org
Offering helpful tips and information on a variety of topics, the sheets provide consumers and professionals with the necessary information on managing incontinence. Some titles include medications, diet and daily habits, odor control, prostatectomy and many more.
Nancy Muller, Executive Director
Caryn Antos, Publicity/Publications Associate

5277 Pregnancy, Childbirth, and Bladder Control
National Kidney and Urologic Diseases Information
3 Information Way
Bethesda, MD 20892-3580
800-891-5390
Fax: 301-907-8906
e-mail: nkudic@info.nidkk.nih.gov
A look at the effects that pregnancy and childbearing can have on bladder control and ways you can counter those effects.

5278 Talking to Your Health Care Team About Bladder Control
National Kidney and Urologic Diseases Information
3 Information Way
Bethesda, MD 20892-3580
800-891-5390
Fax: 301-907-8906
e-mail: nkudic@info.nidkk.nih.gov
Tips for giving your health care provider the information needed to diagnose and treat your bladder control problem. Includes a questionnaire for you to fill out and take to your first appointment.

5279 Urinary Incontinence in Women
National Kidney and Urologic Diseases Information
3 Information Way
Bethesda, MD 20892-3580
800-891-5390
Fax: 301-907-8906
e-mail: nkudic@info.nidkk.nih.gov
An overview of the types, diagnosis, and treatment of urinary incontinence in women.

5280 What Your Female Patients Want to Know About Bladder Control
National Kidney and Urologic Diseases Information
3 Information Way
Bethesda, MD 20892-3580
800-891-5390
Fax: 301-907-8906
e-mail: nkudic@info.nidkk.nih.gov
Fact sheet with tips for health care providers on raising the issue of incontinence with female patients who may be reluctant to talk about their problem.

5281 Your Body's Design for Bladder Control
National Kidney and Urologic Diseases Information
3 Information Way
Bethesda, MD 20892-3580
800-891-5390
Fax: 301-907-8906
e-mail: nkudic@info.nidkk.nih.gov
An introduction to the female urinary system. Includes diagrams of the bladder and pelvic floor muscles.

5282 Your Daily Bladder Diary
National Kidney and Urologic Diseases Information
3 Information Way
Bethesda, MD 20892-3580
800-891-5390
Fax: 301-907-8906
e-mail: nkudic@info.nidkk.nih.gov
An easy-to-use form for patients to note liquid intake, trips to the bathroom, urine leaks, and other details that may help explain your incontinence.

5283 Your Medicines and Bladder Control
National Kidney and Urologic Diseases Information
3 Information Way
Bethesda, MD 20892-3580
800-891-5390
Fax: 301-907-8906
e-mail: nkudic@info.nidkk.nih.gov
Booklet describing the effects that your medications could have on bladder control, with a recommendation for discussing all your medicines with your doctor.

Audio & Video

5284 Solution Starts with You
Simon Foundation for Continence
PO Box 815
Wilmette, IL 60091
847-864-3913
800-237-4666
Fax: 847-864-9758
e-mail: cbgartley@simonfoundation.org
www.simonfoundation.org
Seeks to bring the topic of incontinence out of the closet and remove the associated stigma; provides information to patients, their families, and the health care professionals who provide patient care.
Quarterly
Cheryle Gartley, Founder/President
Jasmine Schmidt, Director of Education

Web Sites

5285 American Foundation for Urologic Disease
www.incontinence.org
Large website detailing information on incontinence, ranging from various treatment options to links and resources.

5286 Healing Well
www.healingwell.com
An online health resource guide to medical news, chat, information and articles, newsgroups and message boards, books, disease-related web sites, medical directories, and more for patients, friends, and family coping with disabling diseases, disorders, or chronic illnesses.

5287 Health Finder
www.healthfinder.gov
Searchable, carefully developed web site offering information on over 1000 topics. Developed by the US Department of Health and Human Services, the site can be used in both English and Spanish.

5288 Healthlink USA
www.healthlinkusa.com

Health information concerning treatment, cures, prevention, diagnosis, risk factors, research, support groups, email lists, personal stories and much more. Updated regularly.

5289 **Helios Health**

www.helioshealth.com

Online resource for your health information. Detailed information about specific health topics, access to expert advice from our Medical Advisory Board, and up-to-date health news.

5290 **MedicineNet**

www.medicinenet.com

An online resource for consumers providing easy-to-read, authoritative medical and health information.

5291 **Medscape**

www.mywebmd.com

Medscape offers specialists, primary care physicians, and other health professionals the Web's most robust and integrated medical information and educational tools.

5292 **National Association for Continence**

www.nafc.org

Interactive website packed with useful information about diagnosis, treatment options and management solutions for incontinence. The site currentlyfeatures a specialist search engine of healthcare providers who have recieved specific training in the diagnosis and treatment of incontinence to assist consumers in locating a specialist in their area. Other features include archived Quality Care articles, a message board, online database of active support groups and much more.

5293 **Simon Foundation for Continence**

www.simonfoundation.org

Seeks to bring the topic of incontinence out of the closet and remove the associated stigma; provides educational materials to patients, their families, and the health care professionals who provide patient care.

5294 **WebMD**

www.webmd.com

Information on incontinence, including articles and resources.

Description

5295 **Infertility**

Infertility is defined as the failure to achieve conception by couples who have not used contraception for at least one year, and affects 1 in 5 couples in the United States.

Female causes of infertility include dysfunction of the ovaries (20 percent of couples), blockage of the tubes connecting the ovaries to the uterus (30 percent), and abnormal secretions (5 percent). Infertility in males is mostly related to sperm disorders (35 percent of couples), either insufficient production of sperm, ineffective sperm, or defective delivery of sperm. Unidentified factors account for the remaining 10 percent of couples.

A variety of tests are needed to determine the exact cause of infertility and then identify the appropriate treatment options. Failure to conceive can be both an emotional and financial burden on couples. Counseling and psychologic support are important parts of treatment.

National Agencies & Associations

5296 **Adopt-A-Special-Kid America**
8201 Edgewater Drive 510-553-1748
Oakland, CA 94621 888-680-7349
Fax: 510-553-1747
e-mail: info@aask.org
www.adoptaspecialkid.org
Adopt-A-Special-Kid provides information on adoption of children with special needs.
Amirah Revels-Bey, President/Board of Directors
Vali Ebert, Executive Director

5297 **American Fertility Association**
666 5th Avenue
New York, NY 10103-0004 888-917-3777
Fax: 718-601-7722
e-mail: info@theafa.org
www.theafa.org
Purpose is to educate the public about reproductive disease and support families during struggles with infertility and adoption. Exists to serve the unique needs of men and women confronting infertility issues.
Ken Mosesian, Executive Director
Stuart Miller, Co-Chair of the Board

5298 **American Society for Reproductive Medicine**
1209 Montgomery Highway 205-978-5000
Birmingham, AL 35216-2809 Fax: 205-978-5005
e-mail: asrm@asrm.org
www.asrm.com
Purpose is to educate the public about reproductive disease and support families during struggles with infertility and adoption. Exists to serve the unique needs of men and women confronting infertility issues.
Robert W Rebar MD, Executive Director
Andrew LaBar PhD, Scientific Director

5299 **Hysterectomy Educational Resources & Services (HERS) Foundation**
422 Bryn Mawr Avenue 610-667-7757
Bala Cynwyd, PA 19004 888-750-4377
Fax: 610-677-8096
e-mail: hersfdn@earthlink.net
www.hersfoundation.com
A nonprofit foundation which provides information about the alternatives to hysterectomy the risks of the alternatives and the consequences of the surgery. HERS provides telephone counseling by appointment.

5300 **International Council on Infertility Information Dissemination**
PO Box 6836 703-379-9178
Arlington, VA 22206 Fax: 703-379-1593
e-mail: INCIIDinfo@inciid.org
www.inciid.org
Provides information on infertility pregnancy loss adoption high risk pregnancy and parenting after the above.
Gary S Berger MD FACOG, Member of Advisory Board
Mike Berkley LAc DA, Member of Advisory Board

5301 **RESOLVE: The National Infertility**
7910 Woodmont Avenue 301-652-8585
Bethesda, MD 20814 Fax: 301-652-9375
e-mail: info@resolve.org
www.resolve.org
A nationwide nonprofit consumer organization serving the unique needs of those striving to build a family. Provides compassionate and informed help to people who are experiencing the infertility crisis and strives to increase the visibility of infertility in the community.
Joseph C Isaacs CAE, President/CEO
Barbara Collura, Executive Director

State Agencies & Associations

Alabama

5302 **RESOLVE of Alabama**
1760 Old Meadow Road 703-556-7172
McLean, VA 22102 888-623-0744
Fax: 703-506-3266
e-mail: bcollura@resolve.org
www.resolve.org
Barbara Collura, Executive Director
Dawn Gannon, Professional Outreach Manager

Arizona

5303 **RESOLVE of Valley of the Sun**
PO Box 36252 602-995-3933
Phoenix, AZ 85067-6252 e-mail: resolveaz@hotmail.com
www.resolveaz.org
Tina Nelson, President
Denny Ceizyk, VP

Arkansas

5304 **RESOLVE Affiliate of Northwest Arkansas**
2230 Country Way 501-521-3763
Fayetteville, AR 72703-4215

California

5305 **RESOLVE of Greater Los Angeles**
PO Box 12529 310-326-2630
Newport Beach, CA 92658 866-888-7452
e-mail: socalresolve@gmail.com
www.southwest.resolve.org
Jennifer Munro, Los Angeles Local Area Affiliate Chair
Kirsten Hanson-Press, Adoption

5306 **RESOLVE of Greater San Diego**
PO Box 12529 310-326-2630
Newport Beach, CA 92658-7385 866-888-7452
e-mail: mariwaldron@yahoo.com
www.southwest.resolve.org
Mari Waldron, San Diego Chair
Jennifer Bolger, Speaker Coordinator

5307 **RESOLVE of Northern California**
312 Sutter Street 415-788-6772
San Francisco, CA 94108 Fax: 415-788-6774
e-mail: info@YourOpenPath.org
www.resolvenc.org
Volunteer-based organization that provides infertility education adoption information advocacy and support.
Roberta Rodriguez-Ha, Executive Director
Renee Cullinan, President

5308 **RESOLVE of Orange County**
PO Box 12529
Newport Beach, CA 92658-0693
949-451-8437
866-888-7452
e-mail: pennyjf@sbcglobal.net
www.southwest.resolve.org
Penny Joss Fletcher, Local Area Affiliate Chair
Cathy Cochrane, Education Coordinator

Colorado

5309 **RESOLVE of Colorado**
PO Box 260725
Littleton, CO 80163-0725
303-469-5261
866-469-5261
www.resolvecolorado.org

Connecticut

5310 **RESOLVE of Fairfield County**
PO Box 930
S Norwalk, CT 06856-0930
914-686-1490
Fax: 203-255-2561
e-mail: anncrane4@aol.com
northeast.resolve.org
Joan Gill, Volunteer Coordinator

5311 **RESOLVE of Greater Hartford**
PO Box 290964
Wetherfield, CT 06129-0964
860-523-8337
e-mail: info@resolveofgreaterhartford.org
www.resolveofgreaterhartford.org
Janice Falk, President
Gwen Hamil, Treasurer

District of Columbia

5312 **RESOLVE of the Washington Metro Area**
PO Box 3423
Merrifield, VA 22116-3423
202-362-5555
e-mail: mary.stern@erols.com
www.resolvedc.org
Mary Stern, Adoption Resource

Florida

5313 **RESOLVE Affiliate of Central Florida**
1050 W Morse Boulevard
Winter Park, FL 32789
407-637-0142
e-mail: admin@resolveofcentralflorida.org
www.resolveofcentralflorida.org

5314 **RESOLVE of North Florida**
1929 Logging Lane
Jacksonville, FL 32221-2071
904-737-0140
rushservices.com/resolve

5315 **RESOLVE of South Florida**
3342 SW 51 Street
Ft Lauderdale, FL 33312
954-749-9500
e-mail: elinder33134@gmail.com
southeast.resolve.org
Elise Linder, Cooordinator

Georgia

5316 **RESOLVE of Georgia**
3904 N Druid Hills Road
Decatur, GA 30333
404-233-8443
e-mail: Katie9924@hotmail.com
southeast.resolve.org
Kate Badey, Coordinator
Renee Whitley, Advocacy Chair

Hawaii

5317 **RESOLVE of Hawaii**
PO Box 29193
Honolulu, HI 96820
808-528-8559
e-mail: info@resolveofhawaii.org
www.resolveofhawaii.org

Illinois

5318 **RESOLVE of Illinois**
PO Box 56
Hinsdale, IL 60521
773-743-1623
e-mail: info@resolveofillinios.org
greatlakes.resolve.org

Indiana

5319 **RESOLVE of Indiana**
5155 Sandy Court
Pittsboro, IN 46167-9129
317-329-9519
e-mail: resolveofindiana@hotmail.com
greatlakes.resolve.org
Robin Scott, President

Iowa

5320 **RESOLVE Affiliate of Iowa**
1348 Atlantic
Dunuque, IA 52001
319-557-2763

Kentucky

5321 **RESOLVE of Kentucky**
851 Van Dyke Mill Road
Taylorsville, KY 40071-9502
502-834-7568
e-mail: jannetteburns@msn.com
greatlakes.resolve.org

Louisiana

5322 **RESOLVE of Louisiana**
PO Box 55693
Metairie, LA 70055-5693
504-454-6987

Maryland

5323 **RESOLVE of Maryland**
PO Box 3423
Merrifield, VA 22116
202-362-5555
888-362-4414
e-mail: info@resolve.org
www.resolve.org
Holly Kortright, Support Services Coordinator
Jane Castanias, Co-Chair

5324 **RESOLVE of West Virginia**
PO Box 3423
Merrifield, VA 22116
202-362-5555
888-362-4414
e-mail: info@resolve.org
www.resolve.org
Joanne MacMillan, Co-Chair
Joann Mirgon, Professional Relations Coordinator

Massachusetts

5325 **RESOLVE of the Bay State**
395 Totten Pond Road
Waltham, MA 02451-1553
781-890-2225
Fax: 781-890-2249
e-mail: admin@resolveofthebaystate.org
www.resolveofthebaystate.org
Information on the Massachusetts chapter of a national, nonprofit consumer based infertility support organization. Information and a variety of services to answer your questions about infertility, treatments, coping techniquesand insurance issues.
1,000 Homes
Rebecca Lubens, Executive Director
Lisa Rothstein, Programming Coordinator

Michigan

5326 **RESOLVE of Michigan**
3601 W Thirteen Mile Road
Royal Oak, MI 48068-9998
248-975-8866
888-255-1399
e-mail: info@greatlakes.resolve.org
www.greatlakes.resolve.org
Kathy Rollinger, President
Heather Hall, Vice President

Minnesota

5327 **RESOLVE: Minnesota Chapter**
1161 E Wayzata Boulevard
Wayzata, MN 55391
651-659-0333
888-959-0333
e-mail: info@midwest.resolve.org
www.resolve.org

Missouri

5328 **RESOLVE of St. Louis, Missouri**
PO Box 411072 314-567-8788
Saint Louis, MO 63141-3072 e-mail: info@resolvestl.org
www.resolvestl.org
Jan DeMasters, MD, Media Contact

Nevada

5329 **RESOLVE of Nevada Barbara Greenspun Women's Care Center**
Barbara Greenspun Women's Care Center
8280 W Warm Springs Road 702-616-4900
Las Vegas, NV 89074 877-203-7778
e-mail: rpbooklover@cox.net
www.southwest.resolve.org
Robyn Isaacson, Local Area Affiliate Chair\Help Line
Suzanne Allen, Office Liaison/New Member Coordinator

New Hampshire

5330 **RESOLVE of New Hampshire**
131 Daniel Webster Highway 603-303-9144
Nashua, NH 03060-5224

New Jersey

5331 **RESOLVE of New Jersey**
1830 Front Street 908-322-9180
Scotch Plains, NJ 07076-0335 888-RNJ-2810
e-mail: info@resolvenj.org
www.resolvenj.org
Dr Lidia Abrams, Executive Director
Daria Venezia, Secretary

New Mexico

5332 **RESOLVE of New Mexico**
PO Box 93386 505-291-5066
Albuquerque, NM 87199 888-895-6055
e-mail: info@southcentral.resolve.org
www.resolve.org

New York

5333 **RESOLVE of Long Island**
PO Box 303 631-385-5026
Long Island, NY 11714-0303 e-mail: racchair@northeast.resolve.org
www.northeast.resolve.org
Arelys Soto-Lugo, President Advocacy Chair
April R Simanoff, VP Outreach Coordinator

5334 **RESOLVE of New York City**
178 Columbus Avenue 212-799-7400
New York, NY 10023 888-765-2810
e-mail: info@resolve.org
www.northeast.resolve.org

5335 **RESOLVE of the Capital District**
PO Box 14591 518-242-3848
Albany, NY 12212-4591

North Carolina

5336 **RESOLVE of North Carolina**
101 Gettysburg Drive 919-380-8497
Cary, NC 27513

Ohio

5337 **RESOLVE of Ohio**
3000 NW Boulevard 614-340-0905
Columbus, OH 43221 800-414-6446
Fax: 614-340-0916
e-mail: info@greatlakes.resolve.org
www.resolveofohio.org
Carole White, President
Kris Henniger, Secretary

Oklahoma

5338 **RESOLVE of Oklahoma**
PO Box 18151 405-949-8857
Oklahoma City, OK 73154-0151 888-895-6055
e-mail: info@southcentral.resolve.org
www.resolve.org

Oregon

5339 **RESOLVE of Oregon**
PO Box 175 503-762-0449
Scappoose, OR 97056 e-mail: resolve_oregon@yahoo.com
www.northpacific.resolve.org

Pennsylvania

5340 **RESOLVE of Philadelphia**
PO Box 2456 215-849-3920
Southeastern, PA 19399-2456 888-765-2810
e-mail: info@resolve.org
www.northeast.resolve.org
Marge McKeone, President and Conference Co-Chair
Jennifer Kaczur, Recording Secretary

5341 **RESOLVE of Pittsburgh**
PO Box 11203 703-861-2910
Pittsburgh, PA 15238-0203 888-255-1399
e-mail: CantrellMVHS@hotmail.com
www.greatlakes.resolve.org

5342 **RESOLVE of Southcentral Pennsylvania**
PO Box 402 717-234-8583
Camp Hill, PA 17001-0402

Rhode Island

5343 **RESOLVE of the Ocean State**
PO Box 28201 401-421-4695
Providence, RI 02908-0201

South Carolina

5344 **RESOLVE of South Carolina**
204 Fernbrook Circle 864-542-9092
Spartanburg, SC 29307-2966 888-867-7970
www.resolve.org

Tennessee

5345 **RESOLVE of Tennessee**
4770 Riverdale Road 615-244-5582
Memphis, TN 38141-8529 888-867-7970
www.resolve.org

Texas

5346 **RESOLVE of Central Texas**
PO Box 49783 512-453-2171
Austin, TX 78765 e-mail: resolvecentraltexas@gmail.com
www.resolvecentraltexas.org
Renaye Thornborrow

5347 **RESOLVE of Dallas/Fort Worth**
434 N Manus Drive
Dallas, TX 77244 888-563-6376

5348 **RESOLVE of Houston**
PO Box 441212 713-975-5324
Houston, TX 77244-1212 888-814-1119
e-mail: info@southcentral.resolve.org
www.southcentral.resolve.org

5349 **RESOLVE of South Texas**
PO Box 782061 210-967-6771
San Antonio, TX 78278 e-mail: info@southcentral.resolve.org
www.southcentral.resolve.org
Christie Goo APR, Contact

Utah

5350 **RESOLVE of Utah**
PO Box 57531
Salt Lake City, UT 84157-0531
801-483-4024
888-592-4449
e-mail: info@resolve.org
www.mountain.resolve.org

Vermont

5351 **RESOLVE of Vermont**
PO Box 1094
Williston, VT 05495-1094
802-657-2542

Washington

5352 **RESOLVE of Washington State**
1760 Old Meadow Road
McLean, VA 22102-1231
703-556-7172
888-591-6663
Fax: 703-506-3266
e-mail: WAinfo@northpacific.resolve.org
www.resolvewa.org

Wisconsin

5353 **RESOLVE of Wisconsin**
PO Box 13842
Wauwatosa, WI 53213-0842
262-521-4590
e-mail: info@resolvewi.org
www.resolvewi.org

Gary Dalton, Web Site Contact

5354 **Society for the Study of Reproduction**
1619 Monroe Street
Madison, WI 53711-2063
608-256-2777
Fax: 608-256-4610
e-mail: ssr@ssr.org
www.ssr.org
International scientific society promotes the study of reproductive biology by fostering interdisciplinary communication within the science by holding conferences and by publishing meritorious studies.
2,400 members
Judith Jansen, Executive Director
Asgerally T Fazleabas, President

Foundations

5355 **Fertility Research Foundation**
877 Park Avenue
New York, NY 10021
212-744-5500
Fax: 212-744-6536
e-mail: info@frfbaby.com
www.frfbaby.com
Offers information on treatment and the latest research on male and female infertility.
Masood Khatamee MD, Executive Director

Libraries & Resource Centers

5356 **National Women's Health Resource Center**
157 Broad Street, Suite 106
Red Bank, NJ 07701
877-986-9472
Fax: 732-530-3347
e-mail: info@healthywomen.org
www.healthywomen.org
NWHRC provides the most current women's health care information through website articles, online mini-courses, a monthly electronic newsletter, and periodic news releases.
Elizabeth Battaglino Cahill, RN, Executive Director
Maria Bushee, Director of Marketing & Communications

Research Centers

5357 **Fertility Clinic at the Shepherd Spinal Center**
Shepherd Spinal Center
2020 Peachtree Road NW
Atlanta, GA 30309-1465
404-352-2020
www.shepherd.org
This clinic makes it possible for paralyzed men to father children.
Gary Ulicny, Chief Executive Officer

5358 **Fertility and Women's Health Care Center**
130 Maple Street
Springfield, MA 01103-2202
413-781-8220
Fax: 413-732-9088
Conducts basic and clinical studies of male and female infertility.
Ronald K Burke MD, Head

5359 **Melpomene Institute for Women's Health Research**
550 Rice Street
Saint Paul, MN 55103
651-789-0140
Fax: 651-292-9417
e-mail: shawne@melpomene.org
www.melpomene.org
Focuses on women's health including fertility issues.
Judy Mahle Lutter, President

5360 **Tufts University: Baystate Medical Center**
759 Chestnut Street
Springfield, MA 01199-1001
413-784-5252
www.tufts.edu
Dr Donald Higby, Director

5361 **University of California: UCLA Population Research Center**
1124 W Carson Street
Torrance, CA 90502-2006
310-212-1867
Fax: 310-320-6515
Clinical investigations of overpopulation and infertility.
Dr Ronald Swerdloff, Director

5362 **University of Michigan Reproductive Sciences Program**
1301 E Catherine Street
Ann Arbor, MI 48109
734-764-0445
Fax: 734-368-20
e-mail: jenic@umich.edu
www.med.umich.edu
Research done into reproductive medicine and infertility treatments.
Larry Warren, Chief Executive Director
Jeffrey B Halter, Director

5363 **Vand erbilt University: Center for Fertili**
C-1100 MCN
Nashville, TN 37232
615-322-6576
Fax: 615-343-4902
Reproductive biology and fertility research.

5364 **Vanderbilt University: Center for Fertility and Reproductive Research**
C-1100 MCN
Nashville, TN 37232-0001
615-322-6576
Fax: 615-343-4902
Reproductive biology and fertility research.

5365 **Wayne State University**
4707 St Antoine
Detroit, MI 48201
313-993-2666
Fax: 313-745-0203
wsupg.med.wayne.edu
Reproductive endocrine infertility and gynecologic surgery research. The research spans the woman's life cycle. Reseach projects include: endometriosis polycystic ovary syndrome sexual dysfunction fibroids and menopause.
Michael Diam MD, Director

5366 **Wayne State University: University Women's Care**
26400 W 12 Mile Road
Southfield, MI 48034
248-352-8200
Fax: 248-356-8224
wayne.edu
Reproductive endocrine infertility and gynecologic surgery research. The research spans the woman's life cycle. Research projects include: endometriosis polycystic ovary syndrome sexual dysfunction fibroids and menopause. Additional studies pertaining to women's health and male infertility.
Elizabeth Pu MD, Associate Professor
Nancy Angel RN, Research Nurse Coordinator

Support Groups & Hotlines

5367 **National Health Information Center**
PO Box 1133
Washington, DC 20013
310-565-4167
800-336-4797
Fax: 301-984-4256
e-mail: info@nhic.org
www.health.gov/nhic

Offers a nationwide information referral service, produces directories and resource guides.

5368 **National Infertility Network Exchange**
PO Box 204 516-794-5772
East Meadow, NY 11554 Fax: 516-794-0008
e-mail: info@nine-infertility.org
www.nine-infertility.org/
The National Infertility Network Exchange (NINE) is a national, notfor profit organization for persons and couples with impaired fertility. NINE supportes the decision of legal and medical means to build families as well as the decision to remain childfree.

Books

5369 **Adopt the Baby You Want**
Simon & Schuster
1230 Avenue of the Americas 212-698-7000
New York, NY 10020-1586 800-223-2348
A how-to adoption book written by an attorney specializing in all areas of adoption.
272 pages

5370 **Adopting After Infertility: The Decision, the Commitment, the Experience**
American Society for Reproductive Medicine
1209 Montgomery Highway 205-978-5000
Birmingham, AL 35216-2809 Fax: 205-978-5018
Emphasizes the importance of communication between partners and offers several guidelines for maintaining a healthy relationship during such a stressful process.
318 pages

5371 **Adoption Directory**
American Society for Reproductive Medicine
1209 Montgomery Highway 205-978-5000
Birmingham, AL 35216-2809 Fax: 205-978-5018
An extensive reference text covering such specifics as state statutes, adoption agencies, exchanges and agencies.
515 pages

5372 **Adoption Fact Book**
American Society for Reproductive Medicine
1209 Montgomery Highway 205-978-5000
Birmingham, AL 35216-2809 Fax: 205-978-5018
A comprehensive source of statistics, regulations and facts on adoption.
277 pages

5373 **Adoption Resource Book**
Harper Collins
10 E 53rd Street 212-207-7000
New York, NY 10022-5299 800-242-7737
Explores and describes all types and styles of adoption and provides excellent resources for each path taken.
421 pages Third edition

5374 **Baby of Your Own: New Ways to Overcome Infertility**
Taylor Publishing Company
1550 W Mockingbird Lane 214-637-2800
Dallas, TX 75235-5007
Provides current information regarding the psychological aspects of infertility.
244 pages

5375 **Conquering Infertility: A Guide for Couples**
Prentice Hall Press
15 Columbus Circle 212-373-8000
New York, NY 10023-7707
Covers various aspects of infertility.

5376 **Consumer's Guide to Insurance**
American Society for Reproductive Medicine
1209 Montgomery Highway 205-978-5000
Birmingham, AL 35216-2809 Fax: 205-978-5018
A how-to book for infertile couples who are experiencing difficulty with insurance reimbursement.
106 pages

5377 **Consumer's Legal Guide to Today's Health Care**
American Society for Reproductive Medicine
1209 Montgomery Highway 205-978-5000
Birmingham, AL 35216-2809 Fax: 205-978-5018
Provides accurate and up-to-date information concerning patient rights and medical care.
384 pages

5378 **Designs on Life**
American Society for Reproductive Medicine
1209 Montgomery Highway 205-978-5000
Birmingham, AL 35216-2809 Fax: 205-978-5018
Provides real life stories regarding assisted reproductive technology.
276 pages

5379 **Family Bonds: Adoption and the Politics of Parenting**
American Society for Reproductive Medicine
1209 Montgomery Highway 205-978-5000
Birmingham, AL 35216-2809 Fax: 205-978-5050
A well organized book is written for people struggling with some of the issues encountered in their journey through infertility and ultimately adoption.
1993 273 pages

5380 **Fertility and Pregnancy Guide for DES Daughters and Sons**
American Society for Reproductive Medicine
1209 Montgomery Highway 205-978-5000
Birmingham, AL 35216-2809 Fax: 205-978-5018
Guide offering information related to the reproductive potential of individuals who have been exposed to DES in utero.
48 pages

5381 **For Want of a Child: A Psychologist and His Wife Explore Infertility**
Continuum Publishing Corporation
370 Lexington Avenue 212-532-3650
New York, NY 10017-6503
A psychologist and his wife go through the emotional effects and challenges of infertility.

5382 **Getting Pregnant When You Thought You Couldn't**
Warner Books
1271 Avenue of the Americas
New York, NY 10020 www.twbookmark.com
A concise guide to understanding infertility that covers issues from diagnosis to treatment and is useful for couples at any stage of infertility treatment.
1993 512 pages

5383 **Guide for the Childless Couple**
American Society for Reproductive Medicine
1209 Montgomery Highway 205-978-5000
Birmingham, AL 35216-2809 Fax: 205-978-5018
A short text which focuses on the emotional aspects of infertility, including its effects on marriage and self-esteem.
201 pages

5384 **Guide to In Vitro Fertilization & Other Assisted Reproduction Methods**
Pharos Books
200 Park Avenue 212-692-3700
New York, NY 10166-0005 800-221-4816
This book discusses assisted reproductive technologies from a laboratory and a patient's perspective.

5385 **Having Your Baby By Donor Insemination**
Houghton Mifflin Company
222 Berkeley Street
Boston, MA 02116 617-351-5000
www.hmco.com
A resource guide to donor insemination which discusses the experience, traditions and techniques of donor insemination, sperm freezing, and known vs. anonymous donors.
352 pages

5386 **Healing the Infertile Family**
University of California Press

1445 Lower Ferry Road
Ewing, NJ 08618
205-978-5000
800-777-4726
Fax: 800-999-1958
e-mail: orders@cpfs.pupress.princeton.edu
This well-written book is dedicated to the psychological concerns of the infertile couple.
335 pages
ISBN: 0-520211-80-4

5387 **Hormones**
American Society for Reproductive Medicine
1209 Montgomery Highway 205-978-5000
Birmingham, AL 35216-2809 Fax: 205-978-5018
Highly recommended text for patients who are suffering from reproductive disorders.
216 pages

5388 **How Can I Help?: A Handbook for Practical Suggestions for Infertility**
American Society for Reproductive Medicine
1209 Montgomery Highway 205-978-5000
Birmingham, AL 35216-2809 Fax: 205-978-5018
Designed to provide greater understanding of the infertility experience.
18 pages

5389 **How to Be a Successful Fertility Patient**
American Society for Reproductive Medicine
1209 Montgomery Highway 205-978-5000
Birmingham, AL 35216-2809 Fax: 205-978-5018
Offers extensive interviews with dozens of male and female infertility patients.
1993 447 pages

5390 **In Pursuit of Fertility**
American Society for Reproductive Medicine
1209 Montgomery Highway 205-978-5000
Birmingham, AL 35216-2809 Fax: 205-978-5018
A comprehensive text which can be used as a tool for couples who want to achieve an understanding of their problem as well as treatment options.
348 pages

5391 **In Vitro Fertilization**
Facts on File
11 Penn Plaza 212-967-8800
New York, NY 10001 800-322-8755
Fax: 800-678-3633
The A.R.T. of making babies. (Assisted Reproductive Technology) A complete and caring overview of the options available to infertile couples.
208 pages Hardcover
ISBN: 0-816032-69-6

5392 **Infertility Book: A Comprehensive Medical & Emotional Guide**
American Society for Reproductive Medicine
1209 Montgomery Highway 205-978-5000
Birmingham, AL 35216-2809 Fax: 205-978-5018
Enables the infertile couple to learn how to take control and educate themselves about the trials and tribulations of infertility treatment.
420 pages Softcover

5393 **Infertility: A Comprehensive Text**
Appleton & Lange
11 W 19th Street 203-838-4400
New York, NY 10011-4209 800-423-1359
A medical reference book.

5394 **Issues in Reproductive Management**
Thieme Med Publishers
381 Park Avenue S 212-683-5088
New York, NY 10016-8806 Fax: 212-779-9020
1993
ISBN: 0-865775-05-2

5395 **Lethal Secrets: The Psychology of Donor Insemination**
Warner Books
1271 Avenue of the Americas
New York, NY 10020 www.twbookmark.com
An interview of a cross-section of people who participated in donor insemination.
1993 277 pages
ISBN: 1-567430-20-1

5396 **Lifeline: The Action Guide to Adoption Search**
American Society for Reproductive Medicine
1209 Montgomery Highway 205-978-5000
Birmingham, AL 35216-2809 Fax: 205-978-5018
A very interesting text describing how an adoptee or adoptive parent may track down birth parents.
384 pages

5397 **Long-Awaited Stork: A Guide to Parenting After Infertility**
Jossey-Bass
350 Sansome Street 415-433-1740
San Francisco, CA 94104 Fax: 415-433-0499
e-mail: webperson@jbp.com
www.josseybass.com
An excellent resource for couples who are moving from being patients to being parents.
300 pages
ISBN: 0-787940-53-4

5398 **Love Cycles: The Science of Intimacy**
Random House
1540 Broadway 212-782-9000
New York, NY 10036 Fax: 212-302-7985
Book providing patients with refreshing, scientific concepts of rhythms and relationships between the sexes.
330 pages

5399 **Loving Journeys Guide to Adoption**
American Society for Reproductive Medicine
1209 Montgomery Highway 205-978-5000
Birmingham, AL 35216-2809 Fax: 205-978-5018
Describes the basic prerequisits agencies and social workers expectations of prospective adoptive parents. Part two offers a directory of state-by-state listings of public and private adoption agencies and adoption attorneys.
394 pages

5400 **Male Body**
Firestone Touchstone Paperbacks/Simon & Schuster
200 Old Tappan Road
Old Tappan, NJ 07675-7005 800-999-5479
An informative and reassuring reference written to meet increasing interest in male health issues. This book discusses varied aspects of health such as infections and injuries, vasectomies, the emotional aspects of sexual difficulties and preventive measures that can be taken against AIDS and other sexually transmitted diseases.
208 pages
ISBN: 0-671864-26-2

5401 **Men, Women and Infertility**
American Society for Reproductive Medicine
1209 Montgomery Highway 205-978-5000
Birmingham, AL 35216-2809 Fax: 205-978-5018
A helpful book offering suggestions for a positive self-image and high self-esteem through the trauma of infertility.
1993 256 pages

5402 **Miscarriage Women: Sharing from the Heart**
American Society for Reproductive Medicine
1209 Montgomery Highway 205-978-5000
Birmingham, AL 35216-2809 Fax: 205-978-5018
A well organized book offering help and information to benefit patients who have experienced pregnancy loss as well as professionals working with these couples.
1993 258 pages

5403 **Missed Conceptions: Overcoming Infertility**
McGraw-Hill
1221 Avenue of the Americas 212-512-2000
New York, NY 10020
Book about infertility and the emotional agony that goes along with it. Addresses all aspects surrounding infertility care and of-

fers in-depth discussions of the many fertility options now available.
377 pages

5404 Motherhood: A Feminist Perspective
American Society for Reproductive Medicine
1209 Montgomery Highway 205-978-5000
Birmingham, AL 35216-2809 Fax: 205-978-5018
A compilation of papers from conference proceedings designed to define motherhood. Offers information on infertility, emotional and financial difficulties and daily living.
234 pages

5405 Mothers of Thyme: Customs and Rituals of Infertility and Miscarriage
Lida Rose Press
PO Box 5076
Ann Arbor, MI 48106
An interesting book that offers details on rituals and misconceptions concerning infertility and miscarriage.
128 pages
ISBN: 0-962595-75-6

5406 Never to Be a Mother
Harper Collins Publishers
10 E 53rd Street 212-207-7000
New York, NY 10022-5299 800-242-7737
Offers childless women a plan for confronting their grief, anger and guilt, as well as offering alternative ways to mother and live.

5407 No-Hysterectomy Option
American Society for Reproductive Medicine
1209 Montgomery Highway 205-978-5000
Birmingham, AL 35216-2809 Fax: 205-978-5018
An excellent reference for women faced with decisions regarding hysterectomy.
265 pages

5408 One Women's Passionate Quest to Complete Her Family
Viking Penguin
375 Hudson Street 212-366-2000
New York, NY 10014-3658
The author presents a highly emotional account of the years of anguish, disappointment, and finally the joy she achieved in trying to complete her family.

5409 Overcoming Infertility
Doubleday
666 5th Avenue 212-765-6500
New York, NY 10103-0001 800-223-6834
Paints a clear picture of the medical and emotional aspects of infertility.

5410 Preventing Miscarriage: The Good News
American Society for Reproductive Medicine
1209 Montgomery Highway 205-978-5000
Birmingham, AL 35216-2809 Fax: 205-978-5018
Provides information on possible causes of miscarriages with information on infections, abnormalities and more.
240 pages Softcover

5411 Reproductive Hazards in the Workplace: Mending Jobs, Managing Pregnancies
Regina H Kenen, PhD, author
Haworth Press
10 Alice Street 607-722-5857
Binghamton, NY 13904-1580 800-429-6784
Fax: 607-722-0012
www.haworthpress.com
Offers information on the history and present of potential reproductive hazards. Includes pregnancy hazard hotlines, specific contact points where women can get information on working environments and more.
286 pages Hardcover
ISBN: 1-560241-54-3

5412 Resolving Infertility
RESOLVE: National Infertility Association
1310 Broadway 617-623-1156
Somerville, MA 02144-1779 888-623-0744
Fax: 617-623-0252
e-mail: info@resolve.org
www.resolve.org
Understanding the options and choosing solutions when you want to have a baby is a definitive resource to help you sort out the options and negative through the experience with confidence. This book tells you everything you need to know about infertility treatment and exploring other family building options.
370 pages
ISBN: 0-062735-22-5
Bonny Gilbert, Executive Director

5413 Science and Babies: Private Decisions, Public Dilemmas
American Society for Reproductive Medicine
1209 Montgomery Highway 205-978-5000
Birmingham, AL 35216-2809 Fax: 205-978-5018
Offers a superb summary of key reproductive issues ranging from conception to contraception.
250 pages

5414 Silent Sorrow
Delta-Dell Publishers
666 5th Avenue 212-765-6500
New York, NY 10103-0001 800-223-6834
A book dealing with the emotional and psychological aspects of losing a child.

5415 Surrogate Motherhood: The Legal and Human Issues
Harvard University Press
79 Garden Street 617-495-2600
Cambridge, MA 02138-1423
A discussion of the psychological, legal and policy questions raised by surrogacy.

5416 Surviving Infertility
Tapestry Books
PO Box 359 908-806-6695
Ringoes, NJ 08551-0359 800-765-2367
Fax: 732-288-2999
A valuable source of support and practical advice for coping with the many intense feelings associated with being infertile.
389 pages

5417 Surviving Pregnancy Loss: A Complete Sourcebook for Women & Their Families
American Society for Reproductive Medicine
1209 Montgomery Highway 205-978-5000
Birmingham, AL 35216-2809 Fax: 205-978-5018
Contains practical approaches to coping with the emotional and psychological problems associated with pregnancy loss.
298 pages

5418 Sweet Grapes: How to Stop Being Infertile and Living Again
American Society for Reproductive Medicine
1209 Montgomery Highway 205-978-5000
Birmingham, AL 35216-2809 Fax: 205-978-5018
Recommended for couples nearing the end of their options or for those who are unsure if they wish to pursue infertility therapy.

5419 To Love a Child
Addison Wesley Publishing
Route 128 781-944-3700
Reading, MA 01867 800-447-2226
A thoughtful and informative overview of alternatives to bio/genetic parenting.

5420 Understanding and Infertility
Tapestry Books
PO Box 359 908-806-6695
Ringoes, NJ 08551-0359 800-765-2367
Fax: 732-288-2999
Provides specific advice to the family on how to be supportive of members and/or friends who suffer from infertility.
28 pages

5421 WHO Laboratory Manual
American Society for Reproductive Medicine

1209 Montgomery Highway 205-978-5000
Birmingham, AL 35216-2809 Fax: 205-978-5018
Third edition

5422 Waiting: A Diary of Loss and Hope in Pregnancy
American Society for Reproductive Medicine
1209 Montgomery Highway 205-978-5000
Birmingham, AL 35216-2809 Fax: 205-978-5018
Provides clear insight into coping with the trials and tribulations of infertility.
121 pages

5423 Without Child
American Society for Reproductive Medicine
1209 Montgomery Highway 205-978-5000
Birmingham, AL 35216-2809 Fax: 205-978-5018
Covers topics including the doctor-patient relationship, religion and infertility, living child-free and the adoption process for persons without children investigating their options.
226 pages

5424 Women Without Children
Pharos Books
200 Park Avenue 212-692-3700
New York, NY 10166-0005 800-221-4816
Offers women without children support through their struggle and decision making.

Children's Books

5425 Mommy, Did I Grow in Your Tummy? Where Some Babies Come From
American Society for Reproductive Medicine
1209 Montgomery Highway 205-978-5000
Birmingham, AL 35216-2809 Fax: 205-978-5018
Illustrated book that helps parents explain the different ways children can come into the world, including IVF, surrogacy, game donation and adoption.
28 pages Ages 4-8

Magazines

5426 American Society for Reproductive Medicine: Clinic Specific Annual Report
1209 Montgomery Highway 205-978-5000
Birmingham, AL 35216-2809 Fax: 205-978-5005
e-mail: asrm@asrm.com
www.asrm.com
Gives the success rates of treatment for fertility centers around the country.

5427 Biology of Reproduction
1603 Monroe Street 608-256-2777
Madison, WI 53711-2021 Fax: 608-256-4610
e-mail: bor@ssr.org
www.biolreprod.org
A monthly, peer-reviewed journal.
250 pages Monthly

5428 Family Building Magazine
RESOLVE: National Infertility Association
1310 Broadway 617-623-1156
Somerville, MA 02144-1779 888-623-0744
Fax: 617-623-0252
e-mail: info@resolve.org
www.resolve.org
Offers various information on the newest technology and advances in infertility treatments, support groups, helplines, centers and in depth articles written by professionals in the field.
15-18 pages Quarterly
Bonny Gilbert, Executive Director

5429 Infertility and Adoption
RESOLVE: National Infertility Association
1310 Broadway 617-623-1156
Somerville, MA 02144-1779 888-623-0744
Fax: 617-623-0252
e-mail: info@resolve.org
www.resolve.org
Published by RESOLVE: The National Infertility Association.
Bonny Gilbert, Executive Director

5430 Journal of Occupational & Environmental Medicine
Williams & Wilkins
351 W Camden Street 301-528-4000
Baltimore, MD 21201-7912 800-638-0672

Newsletters

5431 Hers Newsletter
Hysterectomy Educational Resources & Services
422 Bryn Mawr Avenue 610-667-7757
Bala Cynwyd, PA 19004-2708 800-777-4377
Fax: 610-667-8096
e-mail: hersfdn@aol.com
www.hersfoundation.com
Offers information and support for women who have had or are going through hysterectomies.
Quarterly
Nora W Coffey, President

5432 RESOLVE of the Bay State
PO Box 541553 781-647-1614
Waltham, MA 02454-1553 Fax: 781-899-7207
e-mail: admin@resolveofthebaystate.org
www.resolveofthebaystate.org
Information on the Massachusetts chapter of a national, nonprofit, consumer based infertility support organization. Information on a variety of services to answer your questions about infertility, treatments, coping techniques, insurance issues and family building options.

Pamphlets

5433 ART-Assisted Reproductive Technologies
Serono Symposia USA
100 Longwater Circle
Norwell, MA 02061-1616 800-283-8088

5434 Abnormal Uterine Bleeding
American Society for Reproductive Medicine
1209 Montgomery Highway 205-978-5000
Birmingham, AL 35216-2809 Fax: 205-978-5018
e-mail: asrm@asrm.com
1996

5435 Adoption
American Society for Reproductive Medicine
1209 Montgomery Highway 205-978-5000
Birmingham, AL 35216-2809 Fax: 205-978-5018
e-mail: asrm@asrm.com
1990

5436 Affording Your Infertility
Serono Symposia USA
100 Longwater Circle
Norwell, MA 02061-1616 800-283-8088

5437 Age and Fertility
American Society for Reproductive Medicine
1209 Montgomery Highway 205-978-5000
Birmingham, AL 35216-2809 Fax: 205-978-5018
e-mail: asrm@asrm.com
1996

5438 Bibliography
RESOLVE: National Infertility Association
1310 Broadway 617-623-1156
Somerville, MA 02144-1779 888-623-0744
Fax: 617-623-0252
e-mail: info@resolve.org
www.resolve.org

Annotated guide to books and articles on medical and emotional aspects of infertility.
Bonny Gilbert, Executive Director

5439 Birth Defects of the Female Reproductive System
American Society for Reproductive Medicine
1209 Montgomery Highway 205-978-5000
Birmingham, AL 35216-2809 Fax: 205-978-5018
e-mail: asrm@asrm.com
1993

5440 Coping with the Holidays
RESOLVE
1310 Broadway 781-643-0744
Somerville, MA 02144-1779

5441 Donor Insemination
American Society for Reproductive Medicine
1209 Montgomery Highway 205-978-5000
Birmingham, AL 35216-2809 Fax: 205-978-5018
e-mail: asrm@asrm.com
1995

5442 Early Menopause (Premature Ovarian Failure)
American Society for Reproductive Medicine
1209 Montgomery Highway 205-978-5000
Birmingham, AL 35216-2809 Fax: 205-978-5018
e-mail: asrm@asrm.com
1996

5443 Ectopic Pregnancy
American Society for Reproductive Medicine
1209 Montgomery Highway 205-978-5000
Birmingham, AL 35216-2809 Fax: 205-978-5018
e-mail: asrm@asrm.com
1996

5444 Emotional Aspects of Infertility
RESOLVE: National Infertility Association
1310 Broadway 617-623-1156
Somerville, MA 02144-1779 888-623-0744
Fax: 617-623-0252
e-mail: info@resolve.org
www.resolve.org
Published by RESOLVE: The National Infertility Association.
Bonny Gilbert, Executive Director

5445 Ending Infertility Treatment
RESOLVE: National Infertility Association
1310 Broadway 617-623-1156
Somerville, MA 02144-1779 888-623-0744
Fax: 617-623-0252
e-mail: info@resolve.org
www.resolve.org
Published by RESOLVE: The National Infertility Association.
Bonny Gilbert, Executive Director

5446 Endometriosis
American Society for Reproductive Medicine
1209 Montgomery Highway 205-978-5000
Birmingham, AL 35216-2809 Fax: 205-978-5018
e-mail: asrm@asrm.com
Available in Spanish.
1994

5447 Environmental Toxins and Fertility
RESOLVE: National Infertility Association
1310 Broadway 617-623-1156
Somerville, MA 02144-1779 888-623-0744
Fax: 617-623-0252
e-mail: info@resolve.org
www.resolve.org
Published by the National Infertility Association (RESOLVE).
Bonny Gilbert, Executive Director

5448 Fertility After Cancer Treatment
American Society for Reproductive Medicine
1209 Montgomery Highway 205-978-5000
Birmingham, AL 35216-2809 Fax: 205-978-5018
e-mail: asrm@asrm.com
1995

5449 Getting Started: How Do I Know If I'm Infertile?
RESOLVE
1310 Broadway 781-643-0744
Somerville, MA 02144-1779

5450 Hirsutism and Polycystic Ovarian Syndrome
American Society for Reproductive Medicine
1209 Montgomery Highway 205-978-5000
Birmingham, AL 35216-2809 Fax: 205-978-5018
e-mail: asrm@asrm.com
1995

5451 Husband Insemination
American Society for Reproductive Medicine
1209 Montgomery Highway 205-978-5000
Birmingham, AL 35216-2809 Fax: 205-978-5018
e-mail: asrm@asrm.com
1995

5452 IVF & GIFT: A Guide to Assisted Reproductive Technologies
American Society for Reproductive Medicine
1209 Montgomery Highway 205-978-5000
Birmingham, AL 35216-2809 Fax: 205-978-5018
e-mail: asrm@asrm.com
Available in Spanish.
1995

5453 If You are Having Trouble Conceiving
American Society for Reproductive Medicine
1209 Montgomery Highway 205-978-5000
Birmingham, AL 35216-2809 Fax: 205-978-5018

5454 Infertility Insurance
Serono Symposia USA
100 Longwater Circle
Norwell, MA 02061-1616 800-283-8088

5455 Infertility: An Overview
American Society for Reproductive Medicine
1209 Montgomery Highway 205-978-5000
Birmingham, AL 35216-2809 Fax: 205-978-5018
e-mail: asrm@asrm.com
Available in Spanish.
1994

5456 Infertility: Causes and Treatment
American College/Obstetricians and Gynecologists
409 12th Street SW
Washington, DC 20024 www.acog.com
To obtain a free copy of this publication, please send a self-addressed stamped #10 envelope and request by title. (#AP002)

5457 Infertility: Coping and Decision Making
American Society for Reproductive Medicine
1209 Montgomery Highway 205-978-5000
Birmingham, AL 35216-2809 Fax: 205-978-5018
e-mail: asrm@asrm.com
1995

5458 Infertility: The Emotional Roller Coaster
Serono Symposia USA
100 Longwater Circle
Norwell, MA 02061-1616 800-283-8088

5459 Insights Into Infertility
Serono Symposia USA
100 Longwater Circle
Norwell, MA 02061-1616 800-283-8088

5460 Introduction to Infertility: The First Steps
RESOLVE: National Infertility Association
1310 Broadway 617-623-1156
Somerville, MA 02144-1779 888-623-0744
Fax: 617-623-0252
e-mail: info@resolve.org
www.resolve.org
Published by RESOLVE: The National Infertility Association.
Bonny Gilbert, Executive Director

5461 Laparoscopy and Hysteroscopy
American Society for Reproductive Medicine

1209 Montgomery Highway
Birmingham, AL 35216-2809
205-978-5000
Fax: 205-978-5018
e-mail: asrm@asrm.com

1995

5462 **Male Infertility**
Serono Symposia USA
100 Longwater Circle
Norwell, MA 02061-1616
800-283-8088

5463 **Male Infertility and Vasectomy Reversal**
American Society for Reproductive Medicine
1209 Montgomery Highway
Birmingham, AL 35216-2809
205-978-5000
Fax: 205-978-5018
e-mail: asrm@asrm.com

1995

5464 **Managing Family & Friends**
RESOLVE
1310 Broadway
Somerville, MA 02144-1779
781-643-0744

5465 **Miscarriage**
American Society for Reproductive Medicine
1209 Montgomery Highway
Birmingham, AL 35216-2809
205-978-5000
Fax: 205-978-5018
e-mail: asrm@asrm.com

1995

5466 **Myths & Facts**
RESOLVE
1310 Broadway
Somerville, MA 02144-1779
781-643-0744

5467 **Ovulation Detection**
American Society for Reproductive Medicine
1209 Montgomery Highway
Birmingham, AL 35216-2809
205-978-5000
Fax: 205-978-5018
e-mail: asrm@asrm.com

1995

5468 **Ovulation Drugs**
American Society for Reproductive Medicine
1209 Montgomery Highway
Birmingham, AL 35216-2809
205-978-5000
Fax: 205-978-5018
e-mail: asrm@asrm.com

1995

5469 **Patient Information Series Publications**
American Society for Reproductive Medicine
1209 Montgomery Highway
Birmingham, AL 35216-2809
205-978-5000
Fax: 205-978-5018
e-mail: asrm@asrm.com

Offers a set of 20 various brochures ranging from artificial insemination to male infertility problems.

5470 **Pelvic Pain**
American Society for Reproductive Medicine
1209 Montgomery Highway
Birmingham, AL 35216-2809
205-978-5000
Fax: 205-978-5018
e-mail: asrm@asrm.com

1997

5471 **Pregnancy After Infertility**
American Society for Reproductive Medicine
1209 Montgomery Highway
Birmingham, AL 35216-2809
205-978-5000
Fax: 205-978-5018
e-mail: asrm@asrm.com

1997

5472 **Premenstrual Syndrome (PMS)**
American Society for Reproductive Medicine
1209 Montgomery Highway
Birmingham, AL 35216-2809
205-978-5000
Fax: 205-978-5018
e-mail: asrm@asrm.com

1997

5473 **Third Party Reproduction (Donor Eggs, Donor Sperm, Donor Embryos, & Surrogacy)**
American Society for Reproductive Medicine
1209 Montgomery Highway
Birmingham, AL 35216-2809
205-978-5000
Fax: 205-978-5018
e-mail: asrm@asrm.com

1996

5474 **Tubal Factor Infertility**
American Society for Reproductive Medicine
1209 Montgomery Highway
Birmingham, AL 35216-2809
205-978-5000
Fax: 205-978-5018
e-mail: asrm@asrm.com

1995

5475 **Understanding: A Guide to Impaired Fertility for Family and Friends**
American Society for Reproductive Medicine
1209 Montgomery Highway
Birmingham, AL 35216-2809
205-978-5000
Fax: 205-978-5018

A pamphlet designed for families of patients with infertility and for distribution to individuals who may want to become involved in the counseling and support of these couples.
28 pages

5476 **Unexplained Infertility**
American Society for Reproductive Medicine
1209 Montgomery Highway
Birmingham, AL 35216-2809
205-978-5000
Fax: 205-978-5018
e-mail: asrm@asrm.com

1997

5477 **Uterine Fibroids**
American Society for Reproductive Medicine
1209 Montgomery Highway
Birmingham, AL 35216-2809
205-978-5000
Fax: 205-978-5018
e-mail: asrm@asrm.com

1997

Audio & Video

5478 **Candid Talk About Loss in Adoption**
Mary Martin Mason
4505 York Avenue S
Minneapolis, MN 55410-1422
612-922-1136

Discusses losses incurred by the adopted persons and adoptive persons issues for children adopted into different race families.
Videotape

5479 **Coping with Infertility**
Distributed By UC Video
425 Ontario Street SE
Minneapolis, MN 55414-3002
612-627-4444

Features five couples talking about their infertility experiences.
Odessa Flores

5480 **Infertility: Exploring the Male Factor**
American Society for Reproductive Medicine
1209 Montgomery Highway
Birmingham, AL 35216-2809
205-978-5000
Fax: 205-978-5018

A well-orchestrated video discussing male factor infertility, including the infertility workup, physical exam, semen analysis, and surgical options available.
1993 47 minutes

5481 **One, Two, Three, Zero: Infertility**
Filmmaker's Library
133 E 58th Street
New York, NY 10022-1236
212-355-6545

Videotape

5482 **Six Phases of Infertility Treatment: Medical & Emotional Aspects**
RESOLVE of Maryland
PO Box 19049
Baltimore, MD 21284-9049
410-243-0235

Gives an overview of infertility treatment, addressing the medical and emotional aspects.
Videotape

5483 **So You're Going to Adopt**
Mary Martin Mason
4505 York Avenue S
Minneapolis, MN 55410-1422
612-922-1136

This video prepares adoptive parents for pre and post adoption issues.
Videotape

Web Sites

5484 Adopt-A-Special-Kid America
www.adoptaspecialkid.org
Adopt-A-Special-Kid provides information on adoption of children with special needs.

5485 American Society for Reproductive Medicine
www.asrm.com
Devoted to advancing the knowledge, understanding and expertise in all phases of reproductive medicine and biology. Offers patient education brochures, recommended readings and support.

5486 Center for Disease Control
www.cdc.gov
Reproductive health information source. Also a resource for the Society of Reproductive Technology. Invitro fertilization data reports and men's reproductive health. Interesting well balanced site.

5487 Fertilethoughts.com
www.fertilethoughts.com
A support sytem concerned with helping reach a goal of finding the perfect doctor, the diagnosis, as well as the treatment.

5488 Healing Well
www.healingwell.com
An online health resource guide to medical news, chat, information and articles, newsgroups and message boards, books, disease-related web sites, medical directories, and more for patients, friends, and family coping with disabling diseases, disorders, or chronic illnesses.

5489 Health Finder
www.healthfinder.gov
Searchable, carefully developed web site offering information on over 1000 topics. Developed by the US Department of Health and Human Services, the site can be used in both English and Spanish.

5490 Healthlink USA
www.healthlinkusa.com
Health information concerning treatment, cures, prevention, diagnosis, risk factors, research, support groups, email lists, personal stories and much more. Updated regularly.

5491 Helios Health
www.helioshealth.com
Online resource for your health information. Detailed information about specific health topics, access to expert advice from our Medical Advisory Board, and up-to-date health news.

5492 Infertility Books
www.infertilitybooks.com
Nonprofit site includes book titles regarding infertility and a short explanation of each book and how to get it.

5493 International Council on Infertility Information Dissemination
www.inciid.org
A nonprofit organization that helps individuals and couples explore their family-building options.

5494 Internet Health Resources
www.ihr.com/infertility
This web site provides extensive information about IVF, ICSI, infertility clinics, donor egg and surrogacy services, sperm banks, pharmacies, infertility books and videotapes, sperm testing, infertility newsgroups and support organizations, and drugs and medications.

5495 Ivf.com
www.ivf.com
Goal is to provide the latest women's healthcare innovations to address infertility, polycystic ovaries, endometriosis, and pelvic pain treatment.

5496 MedicineNet
www.medicinenet.com
An online resource for consumers providing easy-to-read, authoritative medical and health information.

5497 Medscape
www.mywebmd.com
Medscape offers specialists, primary care physicians, and other health professionals the Web's most robust and integrated medical information and educational tools.

5498 National Institutes of Health
www.medlineplus.gov
Information regarding all aspects of infertility. Some of the topics include: Latest news, overview of anatomy and physiology, clinical trails, diagnoses and symptoms, treatment, genetics, plus lots of links to other sites. Type infertility into the search engine.

5499 RESOLVE
www.resolve.org
Provides help to people who are experiencing the infertility crisis and strives to increase the visibility of infertility issues via concerted advocacy and public education.

5500 Uterine Artery Embolization
www.uterinearteryembolization.com
Provides information on Uterine Artery Embolization, or Uterine Fibroid Embolization as an alternative to hysterectomy or myomectomy as a treatment for uterine fibroids.

5501 WebMD
www.webmd.com
Information on infertility, including articles and resources.

Description

5502 **Kidney Disease**

The diseases that affect the kidney can be divided into diseases of the kidney itself, such as nephritis, polycystic kidney disease, kidney infections and stones, and diseases of other body systems that cause damage to the kidneys, such as diabetes, high blood pressure and lupus. In either instance, disruption of kidney function results in failure to remove excess fluids and wastes from the blood. This may lead to end stage kidney, or renal, failure.

Symptoms of kidney disease and their severity, depend on the underlying cause. If there is damage or disease in the urinary tract, there can be pain when urinating, blood in the urine, or changes in frequency and urgency of urination. If excess fluid cannot be removed, there may be swelling around the eyes and ankles. When the kidney is damaged directly, back or flank tenderness may be present. In many cases, kidney disease causes no symptoms until the advanced stages, although it may be detected much earlier through tests of blood or urine.

Treatment is directed to the cause, and may include antibiotics for infections, removal of kidney stones by surgery or ultrasound waves, management of the systemic disease such as diabetes, dietary modification, especially of salt and protein intake, and close monitoring and correction of fluids and electrolytes. Treatment may also include control of high blood pressure, which can be caused by kidney disease and further damage the kidney. The most severe cases of kidney failure require either dialysis, in which the blood's toxins are mechanically filtered and removed, or a kidney transplant.

National Agencies & Associations

5503 **American Association of Kidney Patients**
3505 East Frontage Road 813-636-8100
Tampa, FL 33607-1796 800-749-2257
Fax: 813-636-8122
e-mail: info@aakp.org
www.aakp.org
Serves the needs and interests of all kidney patients and their families. Founded in 1969 by kidney patients, for kidney patients, the purpose of this association is to help patients and their families cope with the emotional, physical and social impact of kidney disease.
Kim Buettner, Executive Director

5504 **American Kidney Fund**
6110 Executive Boulevard 301-881-3052
Rockville, MD 20852 800-638-8299
Fax: 301-881-0898
e-mail: helpline@kidneyfund.org
www.akfinc.org
A nonprofit national health organization providing direct financial assistance to thousands of Americans who suffer from kidney disease.
Mike Hartness, Council Chair
Robert J Burnstein, Council Treasurer

5505 **National Institute of Diabetes & Digestive & Kidney Diseases**
National Institutes of Health
31 Center Drive MSC 2560 301-496-4000
Bethesda, MD 20892-2560 e-mail: NIHInfo@OD.NIH.GOV
www.diabetes.niddk.nih.gov
Conducts and supports research on many of the most serious diseases affecting public health. The Institute supports much of the clinical research on the diseases of internal medicine and related subspecialty fields as well as many basic science disciplines.
Dr Griffin Rodgers, Acting Director

5506 **National Kidney Foundation**
30 E 33rd Street 212-889-2210
New York, NY 10016 800-622-9010
Fax: 212-689-9261
e-mail: info@kidney.org
www.kidney.org
A major voluntary health organization dedicated to preventing kidney and urinary tract diseases improving the health and well-being of individuals and families affected by these diseases and increasing the availability of all organs for transplantation.
Allan J Collins MD, Immediate Past President
Bryan N Becker, President

5507 **National Kidney and Urologic Diseases Information Clearinghouse**
31 Center Drive MSC 2560 301-496-3583
Bethesda, MD 20892-3580 800-891-5390
Fax: 301-907-8906
e-mail: nkudic@info.niddk.nih.gov
www.niddk.nih.gov
Strives to increase knowledge and understanding about diseases of the kidneys and urologic system among people with these conditions their families health care professionals and the general public.
Griffin P Rodgers, Director

State Agencies & Associations

Alabama

5508 **Alabama Chapter of the American Association of Kidney Patients**
3404 Sheffield Drive 205-967-4307
Birmingham, AL 35223-2238
Lynn Royale

5509 **National Kidney Foundation of Alabama**
4150 Carmichael Court 334-396-9870
Montgomery, AL 36106 888-533-1981
Fax: 334-396-9872
e-mail: nkfal@kidney.org
www.nkfalabama.org
Barbara A Jackson, Regional Vice President
Renae White, Division Special Events Manager

Arizona

5510 **Arizona Kidney Foundation**
4203 E Indian School Road 602-840-1644
Phoenix, AZ 85018 Fax: 602-840-2360
www.azkidney.org
Jeffrey D Neff, Chief Executive Officer
Samuel H Rogers Jr, Chairman

5511 **Central Arizona Chapter of the American Association of Kidney Patients**
4401 W Hatcher Road 602-939-7248
Glendale, AZ 85302-3821
Dale A Ester, President

Arkansas

5512 **National Kidney Foundation of Arkansas**
1818 N Taylor Street 501-664-4343
Little Rock, AR 72207 800-282-0190
Fax: 816-221-7984
e-mail: nkfar@kidney.org
www.kidney.org
Nonprofit health organization. Our mission is to prevent kidney and urinary tract disease improve the health and well being of indi-

viduals and families affected by these diseases and increase the availability of all organs for transplantation.
R D Todd Baur, Member of the Board of Directors
Derek E Bruce, Member of the Board of Directors

California

5513 Harbor-South Bay Orange County Chapter of the American Assoc. of Kidney Patients
PO Box 8 — 714-527-8009
Seal Beach, CA 90740 — e-mail: delrita@aol.com
www.aakp.org
Rita McQuire, President

5514 Los Angeles Chapter of the American Association of Kidney Patients
9854 National Boulevard — 310-364-1807
Los Angeles, CA 90034 — e-mail: aakpla@yahoo.com
www.aakp.org
Robin Siegal, President

5515 National Kidney Foundation of Northern California
131 Steuart Street — 415-543-3303
San Francisco, CA 94105 — Fax: 415-543-3331
e-mail: info@kidneynca.org
www.kidneynca.org
Work with kidney patients both pre ESRD dialysis and transplant. Financial assistance educational workshops scholarships children's and family camps transplant games information and referral.
Brad J Price, President
Pamela Evans, Vice President

5516 National Kidney Foundation of Southern California
15490 Ventura Boulevard — 818-783-8153
Sherman Oaks, CA 91403 — 800-747-5527
Fax: 818-783-8160
e-mail: info@kidneysocal.org
www.kidneysocal.org
Linda D Small, Division President
Connie M Nieri, Division Director of Finance/Operations

5517 Redding Chapter of the American Association of Kidney Patients
790 Pioneer Drive — 530-241-6451
Redding, CA 96001-0258 — e-mail: teamward@c-zone.net
www.aakp.org

5518 Sacramento Valley Chapter of the American Association of Kidney Patients
565 Morrison Avenue — 916-924-1996
Sacramento, CA 95838
Patricia Jones

Colorado

5519 Colorado Chapter of the American Association of Kidney Patients
PO Box 8442 — 303-758-8610
Denver, CO 80201
Lew Gaiter

5520 National Kidney Foundation of Colorado: Idaho, Montana, and Wyoming
30 East 33rd Street — 720-748-9991
New York, NY 10016 — 800-263-4005
Fax: 720-748-1273
www.kidney.org

5521 Western Slope Chapter of the American Association of Kidney Patients
1539 Ptarmigan Ridge — 970-244-9196
Grand Junction, CO 81056
Vicki Ladd

Connecticut

5522 National Kidney Foundation of Connecticut
2139 Silas Deane Highway — 860-257-3770
Rocky Hill, CT 06067 — 800-441-1280
Fax: 860-257-3429
e-mail: info@kidneyct.org
www.kidneyct.org
Kimberly Hathaway, CEO
Donna Sciacca, Director of Patient Programs/Services

District of Columbia

5523 Georgetown University Center for Hypertension and Renal Disease Research
3800 Reservoir Road NW — 202-687-9183
Washington, DC 20007 — Fax: 202-687-7893
e-mail: wilcoxch@qunet.georgetown.edu
www.georgetown.edu/research/hrdrc
International institute for basic and clinical investigation education and clinical practice in hypertension and renal disease.
Christopher MD PhD, Chief

5524 National Kidney Foundation of the National Capital Area
5335 Wisconsin Avenue NW — 202-244-7900
Washington, DC 20015-2030 — Fax: 202-244-7405
e-mail: info@kidneywdc.org
www.kidneywdc.org
Preston A Englert, Jr. CAE, President/CEO

5525 National Kidney Foundation of the Texas
5335 Wisconsin Avenue NW — 202-244-7900
Washington, DC 20015 — Fax: 202-244-7405
e-mail: ncdc@kidney.org
www.kidneywdc.org
Preston A Englert, Division President/Government Relations
Lisa Taylor, Division Development Director

Florida

5526 National Kidney Foundation of Florida
1040 Woodcock Road — 407-894-7325
Orlando, FL 32803 — 800-927-9659
Fax: 407-895-0051
e-mail: nkf@kidneyfla.org
www.kidneyfla.org
Stephanie Hutchinson, CEO
Richard Salick, Community Relations Director

5527 Palm Beach Chapter of the American Association of Kidney Patients
6801 Lake Worth Road — 561-434-4559
Lake Worth, FL 33467 — e-mail: jansym@bellsouth.net
www.aakp.org
Jan Symonette, President

5528 South Florida Chapter of the American Association of Kidney Patients
2375 NE 173rd Street — 305-324-1727
N Miami Beach, FL 33160 — e-mail: diazgray@aol.com
www.aakp.org
Robert Kirby, President

5529 Sunshine Chapter of the American Association of Kidney Patients
PO Box 4716 — 305-821-4827
Hialeah, FL 33014-0716
Elaine Kamsler

Georgia

5530 Atlanta Georgia Chapter of the American Association of Kidney Patients
6409 Lakeview Drive — 404-932-1100
Buford, GA 30518
Pamela Printup

5531 **National Kidney Foundation of Georgia**
2951 Flowers Road S
Atlanta, GA 30341
770-452-1539
800-633-2339
Fax: 770-452-7564
e-mail: nkfga@kidney.org
www.kidneyga.org
Barbara Sachs, Division President
Tracy Jenny, Division Program Director

5532 **Rome Georgia Chapter of the American Association of Kidney Patients**
118 Woodcrest Drive
Rome, GA 30161
706-232-8989
Hazel McDowell, President

Hawaii

5533 **National Kidney Foundation of Hawaii**
1314 S King Street
Honolulu, HI 96814
808-593-1515
800-488-2277
Fax: 808-589-5993
e-mail: Glen@kidneyhi.org
www.kidneyhi.org
Hawaii's leading voluntary health agency to the education prevention and treatment of kidney and urinary tract diseases and increase the availability of all organs for transplantation in Hawaii.
Glen Hayashida, Chief Executive Officer
Diana Pinard, Director of Organization Planning

Idaho

5534 **National Kidney Foundation of Colorado, Idaho, Montana, and Wyoming**
3545 South Tamarac Drive
Denver, CO 80237
303-713-1523
800-263-4005
Fax: 303-713-0989
www.kidney.org
ML Hanson, CEO

Illinois

5535 **Chicagoland Chapter of the American Association of Kidney Patients**
70 Lincoln Oaks Drive
Chicago, IL 60514
708-325-3475
Gloria Combs, President

5536 **National Kidney Foundation of Illinois**
215 W Illinois
Chicago, IL 60610
312-321-1500
Fax: 312-321-1505
e-mail: kidney@nkfi.org
www.nkfi.org
Willa Iglitz Lang, Chief Executive Officer
Kate Grubbs O'Connor, Chief Operating Officer

Indiana

5537 **National Kidney Foundation of Indiana**
911 E 86th Street
Indianapolis, IN 46240-1840
317-722-5640
800-382-9971
Fax: 317-722-5650
e-mail: nkfi@kidneyindiana.org
www.kidneyindiana.org
The mission of the NKFI is to prevent kidney and urinary tract disease improve the health and well-being of individuals and family affected by these disease and increase the availability of all organs for transplantation.
Margie Fort, CEO
Marilyn Winn, Programs Director

Iowa

5538 **Mississippi Valley, Iowa Chapter of the Association of Kidney Patients**
2203 75th Place
Davenport, IA 52806-1107
319-391-1194
Dave King

5539 **National Kidney Foundation of Iowa NKFI Mercy Medical Center**
NKFI Mercy Medical Center
PO Box 1364
Cedar Rapids, IA 52406-1364
319-369-4474
800-369-3619
Fax: 800-724-8314
e-mail: info@kidneyia.org
www.kidneyia.org
Diane Hagarty, Executive Director
Lori Donald, Accounting Coordinator

Kansas

5540 **National Kidney Foundation of Kansas and Western Missouri**
6405 Metcalf Avenue
Overland Park, KS 66202
913-262-1551
800-444-8113
Fax: 913-722-4841
e-mail: nkfkswmo@kidney.org
www.kidneyksmo.org
Randy K Williams, Regional Vice President
Holly Hagman, Division Program Manager

Kentucky

5541 **National Kidney Foundation of Kentucky**
250 E Liberty Street
Louisville, KY 40202
502-585-5433
800-737-5433
Fax: 502-585-1445
e-mail: lallgood@nkfk.org
www.nkfk.org
Lisa Allgood, Program Director
Leann Wiley, Bookkeeper/Office Manager

Louisiana

5542 **Bayou Area Chapter of the American Association of Kidney Patients**
PO Box 400
Lockport, LA 70374
504-532-3542
Louisiana Barrios

5543 **National Kidney Foundation of Louisiana**
8200 Hampson Street
New Orleans, LA 70118
504-861-4500
800-462-3694
Fax: 504-861-1976
e-mail: info@kidneyla.org
www.kidneyla.org
Torie Kranze, Chief Executive Officer
Tracey Eldridge, Director of Special Events

Maine

5544 **National Kidney Foundation of Maine**
470 Forest Avenue
Portland, ME 04101
207-772-7270
800-639-7220
Fax: 207-772-4202
e-mail: nkfme@kidney.org
www.kidneyme.org
Tammy Atwood, Regional Vice President
Jaime Hanks, Regional Programs Assistant

Maryland

5545 **National Kidney Foundation of Maryland**
1107 Kenilworth Drive
Baltimore, MD 21204-2136
410-494-8545
800-671-5369
Fax: 410-494-8549
e-mail: rmcguire@kidneymd.org
www.kidneymd.org
Also covers the Harrisburg area of Pennsylvania and portions of Virginia and West Virginia.
Raquel McGuire, Executive Director
Brenda Falcone, Director of Community/Patient Services

Massachusetts

5546 **National Kidney Foundation of MA/RI/NH/VT**
11 Vanderbilt Avenue 781-278-0222
Norwood, MA 02062 800-542-4001
Fax: 781-278-0333
e-mail: asavisky@kidneyhealth.org
www.kidneyhealth.org
Andrea Savisky RN CNN, Director Patient Services

Michigan

5547 **National Kidney Foundation of Michigan**
1169 Oak Valley Drive 734-222-9800
Ann Arbor, MI 48108 800-482-1455
Fax: 734-222-9801
e-mail: info@nkfm.org
www.nkfm.org
Dan Carney, President and Chief Executive Officer
Maurie Ferriter, Director of Programs and Services

Minnesota

5548 **National Kidney Foundation of Minnesota**
1970 Oakcrest Avenue 651-636-7300
Saint Paul, MN 55113 800-596-7943
Fax: 651-636-9700
e-mail: nkfmndk@kidney.org
www.nkfmn.org
Also covers North Dakota and South Dakota.
Jill Evenocheck, Division President
Julie Iverson, Regional Vice President

Mississippi

5549 **National Kidney Foundation of Mississippi**
3000 Old Canton Road 601-981-3611
Jackson, MS 39216 800-232-1592
Fax: 601-981-3612
www.kidneyms.org
Gail G Sweat, Executive Director
Lynda Richards, Director of Patient Services

Missouri

5550 **National Kidney Foundation of Eastern Missouri and Metro East**
10803 Olive Boulevard 314-961-2828
Saint Louis, MO 63141 800-489-9585
Fax: 314-961-0888
e-mail: nkfemo@kidney.org
www.kidneyemo.org
Steve Engel, Division President
Anne Carpenter, Director of Program Services

Montana

5551 **National Kidney Foundation of Colorado/Idaho/Montana/Wyoming**
3151 South Vaughn Way 720-748-9991
Aurora, CO 80014 800-263-4005
Fax: 720-748-1273
www.kidneycimw.org

5552 **National Kidney Foundation of Colorado,**
3151 S Vaughn Way 720-748-9991
Aurora, CO 80014 Fax: 720-748-1273
e-mail: jnorman@kidneycimw.org
www.kidneycimw.org
Judy Norman, Executive Director
Tracey Nilson, Director of Development

Nebraska

5553 **National Kidney Foundation of Nebraska**
11725 Arbor Street 402-932-7200
Omaha, NE 68144-2116 800-642-1255
Fax: 402-933-0087
e-mail: nkfnoffice@kidneyne.org
www.kidneyne.org
Support research and training continuing education of health care professionals expanding of patient services and community resources educating he public fund raising...all the mission of the National Kidney Foundation to prevent kidney and urinary tract infections.
Tim Neal, Chief Executive Officer
Sherri Petersen, Development Director

Nevada

5554 **National Kidney Foundation of Nevada**
2550 E Desert Inn Road 702-735-9222
Las Vegas, NV 89121-3611 800-282-0190
Fax: 816-221-7984
e-mail: info@nkfnv.org
www.kidney.org

New Hampshire

5555 **National Kidney Foundation of MA/RI/NH/VT**
11 Vanderbilt Avenue 781-278-0222
Norwood, MA 02062 800-542-4001
Fax: 781-278-0333
e-mail: asavisky@kidneyhealth.org
www.kidneyhealth.org
Andrea Savisky RN CNN, Director Patient Services

New Jersey

5556 **Garrett Mountain Chapter of the American Association of Kidney Patients**
PO Box 8496 973-523-3959
Haledon, NJ 07538

5557 **Meadowlands Chapter of the American Association of Kidney Patients**
PO Box 3032 201-471-5674
Clifton, NJ 07012-3032
Howard Hurwitz, President

5558 **Northern New Jersey Chapter of the American Association of Kidney Patients**
1095 Stone Street 732-382-1092
Rahway, NJ 07065-1913

New Mexico

5559 **National Kidney Foundation of New Mexico**
3167 San Mateo Boulevard NE 505-830-3542
Albuquerque, NM 87110 800-282-0190
Fax: 816-221-7984
e-mail: nkfnm@kidney.org
www.kidney.org
Connie Burnett

New York

5560 **Kidney & Urology Foundation of America**
152 Madison Avenue 212-629-9770
New York, NY 10016 800-633-6628
Fax: 212-629-5652
e-mail: info@kidneyurology.org
www.kidneyurology.org
Sam Giarrusso, President
Shirley Baer, Executive Director

5561 **Long Island Chapter of the American Association of Kidney Patients**
2 Maplewood Avenue 516-756-9126
Farmingdale, NY 11735
Margie Ng Gencarelli, President

5562 **National Kidney Foundation of Central New York**
731 James Street 315-476-0311
Syracuse, NY 13203 877-8KI-DNEY
Fax: 315-476-3707
e-mail: info@cnykidney.org
www.cnykidney.org
Marion E Makhuli, Chief Executive Officer
Laura Squadrito, Director of Programs and Services

5563 **National Kidney Foundation of Northeast New York**
99 Troy Road
E Greenbush, NY 12061
518-458-9697
800-999-9697
Fax: 518-458-9690
e-mail: info@nkfneny.org
www.nkfneny.org
Carol LaFleur, Executive Director
Alicia Jacobs, Director of Special Events

5564 **National Kidney Foundation of Upstate New York**
15 Prince Street
Rochester, NY 14607
585-697-0874
800-724-9421
Fax: 585-697-0895
e-mail: infoupny@kidney.org
www.kidneynyup.org
Jan Miller MS Ed CFRE, Executive Director
Mary Jones, Division Development Director

5565 **National Kidney Foundation of Western New York**
3871 Harlem Road
Buffalo, NY 14215
716-835-1323
Fax: 716-835-2281
e-mail: nkfofwny@hotmail.com
www.nkfwny.org
Nonprofit health organization.
Victoria Keidel, CEO
E Timothy Danahy III, Board President

5566 **New York Chapter of the American Association of Kidney Patients**
450 Clarkson Avenue
Brooklyn, NY 11203
718-270-1548
e-mail: linda.cohen@downstate.edu
www.aakp.org
Linda Cohen, President

North Carolina

5567 **National Kidney Foundation of North Carolina**
5950 Fairview Road
Charlotte, NC 28210
704-552-1351
800-356-5362
Fax: 704-552-7870
www.nkfnc.org
Kenya Welch, Kidney Early Evaluation Program Contact

5568 **National Kidney Foundation of North Texas**
5950 Fairview Road
Charlotte, NC 28210
704-552-1351
Fax: 704-552-7870
e-mail: info@nkfnc.org
www.nkfnc.org
Kenya Welch, Kidney Early Evaluation Program Contact

Ohio

5569 **Miami Valley Ohio Chapter of the American Association of Kidney Patients**
4511 W State Route
W Milton, OH 45383
513-698-5847
Bob Felter, President

5570 **National Kidney Foundation of Ohio**
1373 Grandview Avenue
Columbus, OH 43212-2804
614-481-4030
800-242-2133
Fax: 614-481-4038
e-mail: patti.gold@kidney.org
www.nkfofohio.org
Patti V B Gold, Division President
Danielle Estep, Division Program Director

Oklahoma

5571 **American Association of Kidney Patients**
911 N Woodland Drive
Sand Springs, OK 74063
918-241-3969
800-749-2257
e-mail: jasonmikles@hotmail.com
Jason Mikles, President

5572 **American Association of Kidney Patients: Tulsa Chapter**
911 North Woodland Drive
Sand Springs, OK 74063
918-241-3969
800-749-2257
e-mail: jasonmikles@hotmail.com
Jason Mikles, President

5573 **National Kidney Foundation of Oklahoma**
10600 S Pennsylvania Avenue
Oklahoma City, OK 73170
816-221-9559
800-282-0190
Fax: 816-221-7984
e-mail: nkfok@kidney.org
www.kidneyok.org
Jeff Tallent, CEO

Oregon

5574 **National Kidney Foundation of Oregon and Washington**
465 NE 181st Avenue
Portland, OR 97230
503-963-5364
888-354-3639
Fax: 503-238-1754
e-mail: nkforwa@kidney.org
www.kidney.org
Prevention treatment and cures for kidney diseases! Provides public education health screenings research funding and dialysis and transplant patient services. Increases awareness for organ donation.
Susan Baumgardner, CEO
Glenda McClure, Operations Manager

Pennsylvania

5575 **Lehigh Valley Chapter of the American Association of Kidney Patients**
1242 N 19th Street
Allentown, PA 18104-3058
610-776-1091
e-mail: info@aakp.org
www.aakp.org
Jill Davis, President

5576 **National Kidney Foundation of Delaware Valley**
111 S Independence Mall E
Philadelphia, PA 19106
215-923-8611
800-697-7007
Fax: 215-923-2199
e-mail: nkfdv@kidney.org
www.nkfdv.org
Also covers Delaware and Southern New Jersey.
Joanne Spink, Division President
Mary Reilly, Development Director

5577 **National Kidney Foundation of Western Pennsylvania**
700 5th Avenue
Pittsburgh, PA 15219
412-261-4115
800-261-4115
Fax: 412-261-1405
e-mail: nkfalg@kidney.org
www.kidneyall.org
Also covers Northern West Virginia.
Mary Grace Diana, Regional Program Director
Deborah A Hartman CFRE, Regional Vice President

Rhode Island

5578 **National Kidney Foundation of MA/RI/NH/VT**
85 Astor Avenue
Norwood, MA 02062
781-278-0222
800-542-4001
Fax: 781-278-0333
e-mail: nkfmarinhvt@kidney.org
www.kidneyhealth.org
Andrea Savis RN CNN, Division Program Director
Linda Plazonja, Division President

South Carolina

5579 **National Kidney Foundation of South Carolina**
500 Taylor Street
Columbia, SC 29201
803-798-3870
800-488-2277
e-mail: info@kidney-sc.org
www.kidney-sc.org
Beth Irick, CEO
Sheilah Derrick, Office Manager

South Dakota

5580 **National Kidney Foundation of South Dakota**
1000 East 21st Street
Sioux Falls, SD 57105
605-322-7025
Fax: 605-322-7029
Kori Baade, Executive Director

5581 **National Kidney Foundation of Southeast**
2601 S Minnesota Avenue 605-321-1668
Sioux Falls, SD 57105 Fax: 651-636-9700
e-mail: nkfmndk@kidney.org
www.nkfdak.org

Jill Evenocheck, Division President
Julie Iverson, Regional Vice President

Tennessee

5582 **National Kidney Foundation of East Tennessee**
4450 Walker Boulevard 865-688-5481
Knoxville, TN 37917-1523 Fax: 865-688-5495
e-mail: nkfetn@kidney.org
www.kidneyetn.org

The National Kidney Foundation of East Tennessee works to prevent kidney and urinary tract diseases improve the health and well-being of individuals and family members affected by these diseases and increase the availability of all organs for transplantation.
Helen Harb, President
Judy Roitman, Senior Program Manager

5583 **National Kidney Foundation of Middle Tennessee**
2120 Crestmoor Road 615-383-3887
Nashville, TN 37215-2613 800-380-3887
Fax: 615-383-2647
e-mail: nkfmdtn@bellsouth.net
www.nkfmdtn.org

Teresa Davidson, Executive Director
Leah Engle, Administrative Assistant

5584 **National Kidney Foundation of West Tennessee**
849 Mount Moriah Road 901-683-6185
Memphis, TN 38117 800-273-3869
Fax: 901-683-6189
e-mail: nkf@bellsouth.net
www.kidney.org

5585 **National Kidney Foundation of West Texas**
857 Mount Moriah Road 901-683-6185
Memphis, TN 38117 Fax: 901-683-6189
e-mail: info@nkfwtn.org
www.nkfwtn.org

Texas

5586 **American Association of Kidney Patients**
PO Box 1012 903-537-7031
Mount Vernon, TX 75457 800-749-2257
e-mail: edwinhargraves@webtv.net
www.aakp.org

Edwin Hargraves, President

5587 **American Association of Kidney Patients: Piney Woods Chapter**
PO Box 1012 903-537-7031
Mount Vernon, TX 75457 800-749-2257
e-mail: edwinhargraves@webtv.net

Edwin Hargraves, President

5588 **Lone Star Chapter of the American Association of Kidney Patients**
10042 Sugarloaf Drive
San Antonio, TX 78245 210-523-1605
www.aakp.org

Robert Wager, President

5589 **National Kidney Foundation of North Texas**
5429 Lyndon B Johnson Freeway 214-351-2393
Dallas, TX 75240 877-543-6397
Fax: 214-351-3797
e-mail: nkfntx@kidney.org
www.nkft.org

Public and professional education about kidney and urinary tract diseases. Peer mentoring medical emergency identification jewelry kidney early evaluation program Camp Reynal transplant games.
Mary Van Eaton, CEO
Cameron Hernholm, Director of Development

5590 **National Kidney Foundation of South Texas**
1919 Oakwell Farms Parkway 210-829-1299
San Antonio, TX 78218-1777 888-829-1299
Fax: 210-829-1248
e-mail: nkfsctx@kidney.org
www.kidneytx.org

5591 **National Kidney Foundation of Southeast Texas**
2400 Augusta Drive 713-952-5499
Houston, TX 77057 800-961-5683
Fax: 713-952-5497
e-mail: customerservice@nkfset.org
www.nkfset.org

Provides services for people who suffer with kidney and urinary tract diseases.

5592 **National Kidney Foundation of West Texas**
4601 50th Street 806-799-7753
Lubbock, TX 79414 Fax: 806-799-0277
e-mail: nkfwtx@kidney.org
www.nkfwt.org

Amy Garms, Regional Vice President
Jennifer Ray, Regional Administrative Assistant

5593 **National Kidney Foundation of the Texas Coastal Bend**
PO Box 9172 361-884-5892
Corpus Christi, TX 78469 Fax: 361-884-2332
e-mail: info@coastalbendkidneyfoundation.org
www.coastalbendkidneyfoundation.org

Bess Stone, President
William Alle MD, Vice President

Utah

5594 **National Kidney Foundation of Utah**
3707 N Canyon Road 801-226-5111
Provo, UT 84604-4585 800-869-5277
Fax: 801-226-8278
e-mail: NKFU@KidneyUT.org
www.kidneyut.org

Serving kidney dialysis and transplant patients through out Utah providing patient service and support programs medical research and public and patient education regarding kidney disease and its treatment and prevention and the promotion of organ donations.
David C Trimble, President
Dean Vetterli, CEO

Vermont

5595 **National Kidney Foundation of MA/RI/NH/VT**
85 Astor Avenue 781-278-0222
Norwood, MA 02062 800-542-4001
Fax: 781-278-0333
e-mail: nkfmarinhvt@kidney.org
www.kidneyhealth.org

Andrea Savis RN CNN, Division Program Director
Linda Plazonja, Division President

Virginia

5596 **National Kidney Foundation of Virginia**
1742 E Parham Road 804-288-8342
Richmond, VA 23228 800-543-6398
Fax: 804-282-7835
e-mail: welcome@kidneyva.org
www.kidneyva.org

An affiliate of the National Kidney Foundation it serves kidney patients and their families in Virginia and portions of West Virginia. Mission includes professional and public education prevention and working to increase the availability of all organs for donation.
Lou Markwith, CEO
Betty Sloan, Executive Assistant

Washington

5597 National Kidney Foundation of Oregon and Washington
2142 NW Overton
Portland, OR 97210
503-963-5364
Fax: 503-238-1754
e-mail: help@kidneyorwa.org
www.kidneyorwa.org+R16

Susan Baumgardner, CEO
Glenda McClure, Operations Manager

Wisconsin

5598 National Kidney Foundation of Wisconsin
16655 W Bluemound Road
Brookfield, WI 53005-5935
262-821-0705
800-543-6393
Fax: 262-821-5641
e-mail: nkfw@kidneywi.org
www.kidneywi.org

Offers prevention detection and education programs for those at risk for kidney disease. The National Kidney Foundation of Wisconsin is making life's better through its programs and services. Brochures are offered at no charge.
Cindy Huberÿ, Chief Executive Officer
Kimberly Mueller, Director of Special Events

Wyoming

5599 National Kidney Foundation of Colorado/Idaho/Montana/Wyoming
3151 South Vaughn Way
Aurora, CO 80014
720-748-9991
800-263-4005
Fax: 720-748-1273
www.kidneycimw.org

5600 National Kidney Foundation of Colorado,
3151 S Vaughn Way
Aurora, CO 80014
720-748-9991
Fax: 720-748-1273
e-mail: jnorman@kidneycimw.org
www.kidneycimw.org

Judy Norman, Executive Director
Tracey Nilson, Director of Development

Research Centers

5601 Associates in Nephrology
210 S Desplaines Street
Chicago, IL 60611
312-654-2720
Fax: 312-654-0118
e-mail: charlotte.chapple@ainmd.com
www.associatesinnephrology.com

A medical group practicing nephrology in the Chicago metropolitan area and it suburbs. Includes 21 nephrologists with expertise in many areas in the field of nephrology including hypertension chronic and acute renal failure hemodialysis and peritoneal dialysis glomerulonephritis acid base disturbances fluid and electrolytes management. Provides personal high quality care to patients with kidney diseases.
Eduardo Cremer, Physician
Paul Crawford, Physician

5602 Kantor Nephrology Consultants
1750 E Desert Inn Road
Las Vegas, NV 89169
702-732-2438
Fax: 702-737-5043
www.kncvegas.com

Specializes in nephrology hypertension evaluation and treatment osteoporosis evaluation and treatment chronic in-center hemodialysis home dialysis programs transplantation nephrology nutritional support and more.
Gary L Kantor MD, Founder

5603 Kidney Disease Institute Wadsworth Center for Laboratories and Re
Wadsworth Center for Laboratories and Research
Empire State Plaza
Albany, NY 12201
518-474-7354
Fax: 518-737-71
www.nyhealth.gov

An information and referral organization for polycystic kidney disease autoimmune kidney disease and transplantation.
Lorraine Fla MD, Director

5604 Kidney Disease Program of the University of Louisville
615 S Preston Street
Louisville, KY 40202-0001
502-852-7350
Fax: 502-852-7643
e-mail: cbrown@kdp.louisville.edu
kdpnet.kdp.louisville.edu

Educates residents and patients regarding kidney diseases and offers a dialysis clinic for people afflicted with kidney disease.
George R Aronoff MD, Chief
Cynthia Brown, Program Coordinator

5605 Lovelace Medical Foundation
2425 Ridgecrest Drive SE
Albuquerque, NM 87108-5127
505-348-9400
Fax: 505-348-8541
e-mail: info@lrri.org
www.lrri.org

David J Ottensmeyer, President

5606 PKD Foundation Polycystic Kidney Disease Foundation
Polycystic Kidney Disease Foundation
9221 Ward Parkway
Kansas City, MO 64114-3367
816-931-2600
800-PKD-CURE
Fax: 816-931-8655
e-mail: pkdcure@pkdcure.org
www.pkdcure.org

The foundation exists to win the war with PKD. Their mission is to promote research into the treatment and cure of polycystic kidney disease by raising financial support for peer approved biomedical research projects and fostering public awareness among medical professionals patients and the general public.
Dave Switzer, National Director, Educational Programs

5607 University of Kansas Kidney and Urology Research Center
3901 Rainbow Boulevard
Kansas City, KS 66160
913-588-5000
Fax: 913-588-3995
TTY: 913-588-7963
www.kumc.edu

Jared J Grantham, Director
Tomas L Griebling, Vice Chair

5608 University of Michigan Nephrology Division
University of Michigan Health System
1500 E Medical Center Drive
Ann Arbor, MI 48109
734-936-5645
Fax: 734-763-4151
www.med.umich.edu/intmed/nephrology

Focuses on kidney research.
Frank Brosius, Chief
Joseph Messana, Professor/ Service Chief

5609 University of Rochester: Nephrology Research Program
601 Elmwood Avenue
Rochester, NY 14642-0001
585-275-3660
Fax: 716-442-9201
www.urmc.rochester.edu

Focuses on kidney disorders.
Rebeca Monk, Fellowship Director
Marilyn C Miran, Fellowship Coordinator

5610 Warren Grant Magnuson Clinical Center
National Institute of Health
9000 Rockville Pike
Bethesda, MD 20892
800-411-1222
Fax: 301-480-9793
TTY: 866-411-1010
e-mail: prpl@mail.cc.nih.gov
www.clinicalcenter.nih.gov

Established in 1953 as the research hospital of the National Institutes of Health. Designed so that patient care facilities are close to research laboratories so new findings of basic and clinical scientists can be quickly applied to the treatment of patients. Upon referral by physicians, patients are admitted to NIH clinical studies.
John Gallin, Director
David Henderson, Deputy Director for Clinical Care

5611 Washington University Chromalloy American Kidney Center
One Barnes-Jewish Hospital Plaza
Saint Louis, MO 63110-1036
314-362-7209
Fax: 314-747-3743
renal.wustl.edu

Offers a dialysis unit for people afflicted with kidney disease.
Dr Eduardo Slatopolsky, Director

Support Groups & Hotlines

5612 **Kidneeds**
Greater Cedar Rapids Community Foundation
200 First Street Southwest 319-366-2862
Cedar Rapids, IA 52404 Fax: 319-386-0431
e-mail: kidneedsmpgn@yahoo.com
www.medicine.uiowa.edu/kidneeds/
Primary mission of kidneeds is to fund research on membranoproliferative giomerulonephritis type 2 (MPON type 2, aka, dense deposit disease). Phone support and annual newsletter availiable. No computerized version availiable. No mailing list availble.
Lynne Lanning RN/JD, President Board of Directors
Sean Tully, Vice President Board of Directors

5613 **National Health Information Center**
PO Box 1133 310-565-4167
Washington, DC 20013 800-336-4797
Fax: 301-984-4256
e-mail: info@nhic.org
www.health.gov/nhic
Offers a nationwide information referral service, produces directories and resource guides.

Books

5614 **Family and ADPKD: A Guide for Children and Parents**
Polycystic Kidney Disease Foundation
9221 Ward Parkway 816-931-2600
Kansas City, MO 64114 800-753-2873
Fax: 816-931-8655
e-mail: pkdcure@pkdcure.org
www.pkdcure.org
This book focuses on the questions most commonly asked by children and parents about ADPKD. It is divided into two sections: one for children and one for parents.
48 pages
ISBN: 0-961456-75-2
Dave Switzer, National Director, Educational Programs

5615 **Kidney Beginnings: A Patient's Guide to Li ving with Reduced Kidney Function**
American Association of Kidney Patients
3505 E Frantage Road 813-636-8100
Tampa, FL 33607 800-749-2257
Fax: 813-636-8122
e-mail: info@aakp.org
www.aakp.org
Provides patients with the information they need to take control of their healthcare and do what is necessary to preserve and protect their kidney function. The book addresses concerns of those at risk for kidney disease and their family members; featuring information about the workings of the kidneys, common medications, hypertention, testing, and answers to health, diet and lifestyle questions.
62 pages
Kim Buettner, Executive Director

5616 **Kidney Cooking**
National Kidney Foundation of Georgia
1639 Tullie Circle NE 404-248-1315
Atlanta, GA 30329-2304
A unique cookbook with over one hundred recipes that have been analyzed for sodium, potassium and protein content.

5617 **Nutrition & the Kidney**
Little Brown & Company
34 Beacon Street 617-227-0730
Boston, MA 02108-1415 Fax: 617-227-4633
1993 480 pages
ISBN: 0-316575-00-3

5618 **PKD Patient's Manual**
Polycystic Kidney Disease Foundation
9221 Ward Parkway 816-931-2600
Kansas City, MO 64114 800-753-2873
Fax: 816-931-8655
e-mail: pkdcure@pkdcure.org
www.pkdcure.org
Covers everything from cysts to how persons can be active if they have ARPKD.
Dave Switzer, National Director, Educational Programs

5619 **Q&A on PKD**
Polycystic Kidney Disease Foundation
9221 Ward Parkway 816-931-2600
Kansas City, MO 64114 800-753-2873
Fax: 816-931-8655
e-mail: pkdcure@pkdcure.org
www.pkdcure.org
A goldmine of information for the PKD patient and physician. Includes 88 pages of PKD questions and answers by the scientific advisers of the PKR Foundation.
88 pages Paperback
ISBN: 0-961456-72-8
Dave Switzer, National Director, Educational Programs

5620 **Real Lifestyles Manual**
R&D Laboratories
4204 Glencoe Avenue
Marina Del Rey, CA 90292-5612 800-338-9066
A complete renal guide including diets for hemodialysis and CAPD patients. Delicious menus, ADA exchange lists, gourmet recipes with nutritional analysis for renal patients and exercises.

5621 **Your Child, Your Family & ARPKD**
Polycystic Kidney Disease Foundation
9221 Ward Parkway 816-931-2600
Kansas City, MO 64114 800-753-2873
Fax: 816-931-8655
e-mail: pkdcure@pkdcure.org
www.pkdcure.org
This second edition book focuses on the questions most commonly asked about ARPKD in order to help families understand more about the disease.
Dave Switzer, National Director, Educational Programs

5622 **Your Child, Your Family and Autosomal Recessive Polycystic Kidney Disease**
Polycystic Kidney Disease Foundation
9221 Ward Parkway 816-931-2600
Kansas City, MO 64114 800-753-2873
Fax: 816-931-8655
e-mail: pkdcure@pkdcure.org
www.pkdcure.org
This secong edition book focuses on the questions most commonly asked about autosomal recessive PKD in order to help families understand more about the disease.
26 pages Paperback
Dave Switzer, National Director, Educational Programs

Magazines

5623 **Kindey Beginnings: The Magazine**
American Association of Kidney Patients
3505 E Frantage Road 813-636-8100
Tampa, FL 33607 800-749-2257
Fax: 813-636-8122
e-mail: info@aakp.org
www.aakp.org
This quarterly member magazine provides articles, news items and information of interest to those at risk or recently diagnosed with kidney disease, their famliy, and healthcare professionals.
Kmi Buettner, Executive Director

5624 **aakpRENALIFE**
American Association of Kidney Patients
35052 E Frantage Road 813-636-8100
Tampa, FL 33607 800-749-2257
Fax: 813-636-8122
e-mail: info@aakp.org
www.aakp.org

The official publication for AAKP members, offering articles, news and health care information for kidney patients,and health care professionals.
BiMonthly
Kim Buettner, Executive Director

Newsletters

5625 **Family Focus**
National Kidney Foundation
30 E 33rd Street 212-889-2210
New York, NY 10016-5337 800-622-9010
Fax: 212-689-9261
www.kidney.org
A patient and family newspaper targeted toward dialysis populations.
Quarterly

5626 **PKD Progress**
PKD Foundation
4901 Main Street 816-931-2600
Kansas City, MO 64112-2634 800-753-2873
Fax: 816-931-8655
e-mail: pkdcure@pkdcure.org
www.pkdcure.org
Offers information and updated medical news for persons and professionals with an interest in kidney disorders.
Monthly
Dave Switzer, Marketing/Public Relations Director

5627 **Renal Recipes Quarterly**
R&D Laboratories
4204 Glencoe Avenue
Marina Del Rey, CA 90292-5612 800-338-9066
Features timely holiday and ethnic food menus and recipes, shopping and food tips, analysis of nutrients and calculation of food exchanges.
Quarterly

5628 **Transplant Chronicles**
National Kidney Foundation
30 E 33rd Street 212-889-2210
New York, NY 10016 800-622-9010
Fax: 212-689-9261
www.kidney.org
A patient and family newsletter targeted towards transplant recipients.
Quarterly

Pamphlets

5629 **About Kidney Stones**
National Kidney Foundation
30 E 33rd Street 212-889-2210
New York, NY 10016 800-622-9010
Fax: 212-689-9261
www.kidney.org
Discusses causes, treatment and prevention of kidney stones.

5630 **Advance Directives: A Guide for Patients and Their Families**
National Kidney Foundation
30 E 33rd Street 212-889-2210
New York, NY 10016-5337 800-622-9010
Fax: 212-689-9261
www.kidney.org
Everyone has the right to make an advance directive, which is a legal document stating how you want decisions made concerning your medical care when your no longer able to make them yourself. This booklet describes the different types of advance directives and the medical decisions they cover.
12 pages Package

5631 **American Kidney Fund Helps When Nobody Else Will**
American Kidney Fund
6110 Executive Boulevard 301-881-3052
Rockville, MD 20852-3915 800-638-8299
Fax: 301-881-0898
e-mail: helpline@AFINC.org
www.kidneyfund.org
Focuses on the services and programs offered by the American Kidney Fund.

5632 **At Home with AAKP**
American Association of Kidney Patients
3505 E Frantage Road 813-636-8100
Tampa, FL 33607 800-749-2257
Fax: 813-636-8122
e-mail: info@aakp.org
www.aakp.org
A free publication, this was developed to address the growing need for information about home dialysis treatment options.
Kim Buettner, Executive Director

5633 **Children and Kidney Disease**
American Kidney Fund
6110 Executive Boulevard 301-881-3052
Rockville, MD 20852-3915 800-638-8299
Fax: 301-881-0898
www.arbon.com/kidney/

5634 **Choosing a Treatment for Kidney Failure**
National Kidney Foundation
30 E 33rd Street 212-889-2210
New York, NY 10016 800-622-9010
Fax: 212-689-9261
www.kidney.org
Introduces treatment options for kidney failure and explains the pros and cons of each.
16 pages

5635 **Diabetes and Kidney Disease**
National Kidney Foundation
30 E 33rd Street 212-889-2210
New York, NY 10016-5337 800-622-9010
Fax: 212-689-9261
www.kidney.org
Explains the connection between diabetes and kidney disease covering prevention, recognition and treatments.
12 pages Pkg. of 100

5636 **Dialysis Patient: An Informative Guide for the Dentist**
American Kidney Fund
6110 Executive Boulevard 301-881-3052
Rockville, MD 20852-3915 800-638-8299
Fax: 301-881-0898
www.arbon.com/kidney/

5637 **Diet Guide for the CAPD Patient**
American Kidney Fund
6110 Executive Boulevard 301-881-3052
Rockville, MD 20852-3915 800-638-8299
Fax: 301-881-0898
www.arbon.com/kidney/

5638 **Diet Guide for the Hemodialysis Patient**
American Kidney Fund
6110 Executive Boulevard 301-881-3052
Rockville, MD 20852-3915 800-638-8299
Fax: 301-881-0898
www.arbon.com/kidney/

5639 **Facts About Kidney Diseases and Their Treatment**
American Kidney Fund
6110 Executive Boulevard 301-881-3052
Rockville, MD 20852-3915 800-638-8299
Fax: 301-881-0898
www.arbon.com/kidney/
Offers information about what kidneys are and their functions, diagnosis and treatment of kidney disease.

5640 **Facts About Kidney Stones**
American Kidney Fund

6110 Executive Boulevard 301-881-3052
Rockville, MD 20852-3915 800-638-8299
Fax: 301-881-0898
www.arbon.com/kidney/

5641 **Glomerulonephritis**
National Kidney Foundation
30 E 33rd Street 212-889-2210
New York, NY 10016-5337 800-622-9010
Fax: 212-689-9261
www.kidney.org
Defines the types of Glomerulonephritis, signs, causes and symptoms.
8 pages Pkg. of 100

5642 **Hemodialysis**
National Kidney Foundation
30 E 33rd Street 212-889-2210
New York, NY 10016 800-622-9010
Fax: 212-689-9261
www.kidney.org
Introduces and explains the hemodialysis treatment process.
12 pages Pkg. of 100

5643 **High Blood Pressure and Your Kidneys**
National Kidney Foundation
30 E 33rd Street 212-889-2210
New York, NY 10016-5337 800-622-9010
Fax: 212-689-9261
www.kidney.org
Offers a description of hypertension, including symptoms, detection, causes and effects. Also available in Spanish.
8 pages Pkg. of 100

5644 **High Blood Pressure and its Effects on the Kidneys**
American Kidney Fund
6110 Executive Boulevard 301-881-3052
Rockville, MD 20852 800-638-8299
Fax: 301-881-0898
www.arbon.com/kidney/

5645 **Kid**
American Kidney Fund
6110 Executive Boulevard 301-881-3052
Rockville, MD 20852-3915 800-638-8299
Fax: 301-881-0898
www.arbon.com/kidney/

5646 **Kidney Disease: A Guide for Patients and Their Families**
American Kidney Fund
6110 Executive Boulevard 301-881-3052
Rockville, MD 20852 800-638-8299
Fax: 301-881-0898
www.arbon.com/kidney/
Offers information on how the kidneys work, symptoms of kidney disease, kidney failure and treatment alternatives.

5647 **Kidney Transplant: A New Lease on Life**
National Kidney Foundation
30 E 33rd Street 212-889-2210
New York, NY 10016 800-622-9010
Fax: 212-689-9261
www.kidney.org
A brochure that answers common questions about transplants, such as patient expectations, drug therapy, complications including rejection and recovery.
10 pages Pkg. of 100

5648 **Kidneys for Kids**
American Kidney Fund
6110 Executive Boulevard 301-881-3052
Rockville, MD 20852-3915 800-638-8299
Fax: 301-881-0898
www.arbon.com/kidney/

5649 **Nutrition and Changing Kidney Function**
National Kidney Foundation
30 E 33rd Street 212-889-2210
New York, NY 10016-5337 800-622-9010
Fax: 212-689-9261
www.kidney.org
Explains how to slow the progression of kidney disease by controlling the intake of vitamins, minerals, fluids, calories and proteins.
12 pages Pkg. of 100

5650 **Organ Donor Program**
National Kidney Foundation
30 E 33rd Street 212-889-2210
New York, NY 10016-5337 800-622-9010
Fax: 212-689-9261
www.kidney.org
A comprehensive description of the organ donor program that explains organ and tissue donation, brain death, routine inquiry and becoming an organ donor.
12 pages Pkg. of 100

5651 **Peritoneal Dialysis**
National Kidney Foundation
30 E 33rd Street 212-889-2210
New York, NY 10016 800-622-9010
Fax: 212-689-9261
www.kidney.org
Introduces and explains the peritoneal dialysis treatment process
8 pages

5652 **Understanding Nephrotic Syndrome**
American Kidney Fund
6110 Executive Boulevard 301-881-3052
Rockville, MD 20852-3915 800-638-8299
Fax: 301-881-0898
www.arbon.com/kidney/

5653 **Urinary Tract Infections**
National Kidney Foundation
30 E 33rd Street 212-889-2210
New York, NY 10016-5337 800-622-9010
Fax: 212-689-9261
www.kidney.org
Defines urinary tract infections, its symptoms, causes and treatments.
10 pages Pkg. of 100

5654 **Warning Signs of Kidney Disease**
National Kidney Foundation
30 E 33rd Street 212-889-2210
New York, NY 10016-5337 800-622-9010
Fax: 212-689-9261
www.kidney.org
A one-panel leaflet that numbers and lists the six early warning signs of kidney disease.
Pkg. of 100

5655 **Winning the Fight Against Silent Killers**
National Kidney Foundation
30 E 33rd Street 212-889-2210
New York, NY 10016-5337 800-622-9010
Fax: 212-689-9261
www.kidney.org
Written for the African-American community, this brochure discusses the increased risk of high blood pressure and diabetes in this population.
12 pages Pkg. of 100

5656 **Your Kidneys: Master Chemists of the Body**
National Kidney Foundation
30 E 33rd Street 212-889-2210
New York, NY 10016-5337 800-622-9010
Fax: 212-689-9261
www.kidney.org
Offers an overview of kidneys and urinary system, describing the kidneys' filtering system, hereditary, congenital and acquired kidney diseases.
12 pages Pkg. of 100

Audio & Video

5657 **It's Just Part of My Life**
National Kidney Foundation

30 E 33rd Street
New York, NY 10016-5337
212-889-2210
800-622-9010
Fax: 212-689-9261
www.kidney.org

A 15-minute program for adolescent dialysis patients and their families.

5658 People Like Us
National Kidney Foundation
30 E 33rd Street
New York, NY 10016-5337
212-889-2210
800-622-9010
Fax: 212-689-9261
www.kidney.org

A seven-part video series targeted toward the newly-diagnosed chronic kidney disease patient.

Web Sites

5659 American Association of Kidney Patients
www.aakp.org

Serves the needs and interests of kidney patients, for kidney patients, the purpose of this Association is to help patients and their families cope with the emotional, physical and social impact of kidney disease.

5660 American Kidney Fund
www.akfinc.org/

A nonprofit, national health organization providing direct financial assistance to thousands of Americans who suffer from kidney disease.

5661 Healing Well
www.healingwell.com

An online health resource guide to medical news, chat, information and articles, newsgroups and message boards, books, disease-related web sites, medical directories, and more for patients, friends, and family coping with disabling diseases, disorders, or chronic illnesses.

5662 Health Finder
www.healthfinder.gov

Searchable, carefully developed web site offering information on over 1000 topics. Developed by the US Department of Health and Human Services, the site can be used in both English and Spanish.

5663 Healthlink USA
www.healthlinkusa.com

Links to websites which may include treatment, cures, diagnosis, prevention, support groups, email lists, messageboards, personal stories, risk factors, statistics, research and more.

5664 Helios Health
www.helioshealth.com

Online resource for your health information. Detailed information about specific health topics, access to expert advice from our Medical Advisory Board, and up-to-date health news.

5665 MedicineNet
www.medicinenet.com

An online resource for consumers providing easy-to-read, authoritative medical and health information.

5666 Medscape
www.mywebmd.com

Medscape offers specialists, primary care physicians, and other health professionals the Web's most robust and integrated medical information and educational tools.

5667 Polycystic Kidney Research Foundation
www.pkdcure.org

Provide information on research into the cause, treatment, and cure of polycystic kidney disease by raising financial support for peer approved biomedical research projects and fostering public awareness among medical professionals, patients and the general public.

5668 WebMD
www.webmd.com

Information on kidney disease, including articles and resources.

Description

5669 # Liver Disease

Liver disease covers a wide range of disorders that can result in chronic liver damage, such as scarring (fibrosis) or the development of cirrhosis. An estimated 43,000 Americans die each year from liver disease.

Specific liver diseases that damage the liver include infection (e.g., viral hepatitis), chronic alcoholism or drug abuse, medications and certain systemic illnesses. Severe disease can permanently damage the liver, causing it to fail totally.

Common signs of liver damage are fatigue, loss of appetite, nausea and tea-colored urine. Yellowing of the skin and the whites of the eye (jaundice) is seen in 50 percent of cases. Other symptoms include liver enlargement and tenderness, and fluid collection in the abdominal cavity. A shriveling liver indicates more chronic and severe damage.

Treatment for liver disease depends on the underlying cause. In less severe injury, due to its remarkable capacity to heal itself, the liver can completely recover. Liver transplantation is accepted as appropriate treatment for end-stage liver dysfunction. See also *Hepatitis*.

National Agencies & Associations

5670 **(AASLD) American Association for the Study of Liver Diseases**
1729 King Street 703-299-9766
Alexandria, VA 22314 Fax: 703-299-9622
e-mail: aasld@aasld.org
www.aasld.org
Physicians, researchers, and allied hepatology health professionals.
Sherrie H. Cathcart, Executive Director

5671 **American Liver Foundation**
75 Maiden Lane 212-668-1000
New York, NY 10038 800-465-4837
Fax: 212-483-8179
e-mail: info@liverfoundation.org
www.liverfoundation.org
National, nonprofit organization dedicated to the prevention treatment and cure of hepatitis and other liver diseases through research and advocacy. The ALF offers information, physician referrals, a 24-hour, 7 day-a-week national helpline and support groups.
Rick Smith, President/CEO
Newton Guerin, COO

State Agencies & Associations

Arizona

5672 **American Liver Foundation Arizona Chapter**
4545 E Shea Boulevard 602-953-1800
Phoenix, AZ 85028 866-953-1800
Fax: 602-953-1806
e-mail: arizona@liverfoundation.org
www.liverfoundation.org
Melissa McCracken, Executive Director
Pamela White, Events Manager

California

5673 **American Liver Foundation Greater Los Angeles Chapter**
5777 Century Boulevard 310-670-4624
Los Angeles, CA 90045 Fax: 310-670-4672
e-mail: sfranklin@liverfoundation.org
www.liverfoundation.org
Taly Fantini, Executive Director
Jessica Goltermann, Event Coordinator

5674 **American Liver Foundation Northern CA Chapter**
870 Market Street 415-248-1060
San Francisco, CA 94102 800-292-9099
Fax: 415-248-1066
e-mail: northernca@liverfoundation.org
www.liverfoundation.org
Linden Young, Division Vice President
Michelle Flatley, Special Events Manager

5675 **American Liver Foundation San Diego Chapte r**
2515 Camino del Rio S 619-291-5483
San Diego, CA 92108 800-749-2630
Fax: 619-295-7181
e-mail: KFurrow@liverfoundation.org
www.liverfoundation.org
Kristina Furrow, Executive Director
Lisa A Haile JD PhD, President of the Board

Colorado

5676 **American Liver Foundation Rocky Mountain Chapter**
2100 S Corona Street 303-988-4388
Denver, CO 80210 Fax: 303-988-4398
e-mail: rminfo@liverfoundation.org
www.liverfoundation.org
Regina Musyl, Executive Director
Brooke Fritz, Community Events Manager

Connecticut

5677 **American Liver Foundation: Connecticut Chapter**
127 Washington Avenue 203-234-2022
N Haven, CT 06473 Fax: 203-234-1386
e-mail: info@ctalf.org
www.ctalf.org
Offers support for patients and families provides educational meetings and conferences raising vital liver research dollars; encouraging the beautifully unselfish gift of organ donation and the medical miracle of organ transplantation.
12 pages Quarterly
JoAnn Thompson, Executive Director
Marla Hannah Sadler, Event Coordinator

Florida

5678 **American Liver Foundation Gulf Coast Chapter**
202 S 22nd Street 813-248-3337
Ybor City, FL 33605 Fax: 813-248-3340
e-mail: jbourgeois@liverfoundation.org
www.liverfoundation.org
Jennifer Bourgeois, Executive Director

Hawaii

5679 **American Liver Foundation Hawaii Chapter**
3660 Waialae Avenue 808-737-0400
Honolulu, HI 96816 Fax: 808-737-3230
e-mail: alfhawaii@liverfoundation.org
www.liverfoundation.org
Janice M Nillias, Executive Director

Illinois

5680 **American Liver Foundation Illinois Chapter**
180 N Michigan Avenue 312-377-9030
Chicago, IL 60601 Fax: 312-377-9035
e-mail: info@illinois-liver.org
www.illinois-liver.org
Kevin Gianotto, Executive Director
Emily Nuzzo MA LSW, Program Manager

Indiana

5681 **American Liver Foundation Indiana Chapter**
921 E 86th Street 317-635-5074
Indianapolis, IN 46240 877-548-3730
Fax: 317-635-5075
e-mail: dsparksunsworth@liverfoundation.org
www.liverfoundation.org
Natalie Sutton, Executive Director
Kristin Gray, Development Coordinator

Massachusetts

5682 **American Liver Foundation New England Chapter**
88 Winchester Street 617-527-5600
Newton, MA 02461 800-298-6766
Fax: 617-527-5636
e-mail: info@liverfoundation.org
www.liverfoundation.org
Kelly Leigh Beckett, Executive Director
Laura Dempsey, Director of Campaigns

Michigan

5683 **American Liver Foundation Michigan Chapter**
21886 Farmington Road 248-615-5768
Farmington, MI 48336 888-MYL-IVER
Fax: 248-615-5778
e-mail: michigan@liverfoundation.org
www.liverfoundation.org
Jennifer L Dale, Executive Director

Minnesota

5684 **American Liver Foundation Minnesota Chapte r**
2626 E 82nd Street 952-854-6181
Bloomington, MN 55425 Fax: 952-854-6956
e-mail: dstibbe@liverfoundation.org
www.liverfoundation.org
David Stibbe, Executive Director
Meghan Likes, Community Events Coordinator

Missouri

5685 **American Liver Foundation Greater Kansas Greater kC Chapter**
Greater kC Chapter
309 NE 88th Terrace 816-420-9446
Kansas City, MO 64155 Fax: 612-892-8442
e-mail: kcchapal@amail.com
Stan Adkins, Chapter Director

New York

5686 **American Liver Foundation Greater New York Chapter**
75 Maiden Lane 212-943-1059
New York, NY 10004 877-307-7507
Fax: 212-943-1314
e-mail: greaterny@liverfoundation.org
www.liverfoundation.org
Gina Parziale, Executive Director
Tracy Merlau, Programs Manager

5687 **American Liver Foundation Western New York Chapter**
25 Canterbury Road 585-271-2859
Rochester, NY 14607 Fax: 585-271-8642
e-mail: nkoris@liverfoundation.org
www.liverfoundation.org
Nancy Koris, Executive Director

Ohio

5688 **American Liver Foundation Ohio Chapter**
5755 Granger Road 216-635-2780
Independence, OH 44131-1455 Fax: 216-635-2781
e-mail: ohio@liverfoundation.org
www.liverfoundation.org
Susan S Rodwa MNO, Executive Director

Pennsylvania

5689 **American Liver Foundation Delaware Valley Chapter**
111 Presidential Boulevard 610-668-0152
Bala Cynwyd, PA 19004 Fax: 610-668-0155
e-mail: emurphy@liverfoundation.org
www.liverfoundation.org
Elizabeth Murphy, Executive Director

5690 **American Liver Foundation Western Pennsylv ania**
100 W Station Square Drive 412-434-7044
Pittsburgh, PA 15219 Fax: 412-434-7040
e-mail: spmasartis@liverfoundation.org
www.liverfoundation.org
Suzanna Masartis, Division Vice-President
Kara Hartner, Event Manager

Tennessee

5691 **American Liver Foundation Midsouth Chapter**
5050 Poplar Avenue 901-766-7668
Memphis, TN 38157 866-756-7668
Fax: 901-766-2061
e-mail: midsouth@liverfoundation.org
www.liverfoundation.org
Karen Viotti, Executive Director
Deri Whittaker, Community Events Coordinator

Texas

5692 **American Liver Foundation South Texas Chap ter**
2425 W Loop S 713-622-1318
Houston, TX 77027 Fax: 713-622-1376
e-mail: texas@liverfoundation.org
www.liverfoundation.org
Patricia Wittlif, Executive Director

Virginia

5693 **American Liver Foundation National Capital**
127 S Peyton Street 703-535-8880
Alexandria, VA 22314 Fax: 703-535-8890
e-mail: jjacobs@liverfoundation.org
www.liverfoundation.org
Jodie Campbe Jacobs, Community Events Coordinator

Washington

5694 **American Liver Foundation Pacific Northwest Chapter**
2033 6th Avenue 206-443-3805
Seattle, WA 98121 800-465-4837
Fax: 206-443-1511
www.liverfoundation.org
David de la Fuente, Executive Director
Molly Scott, Community Events Manager

Wisconsin

5695 **American Liver Foundation Wisconsin Chapter**
4927 N Lydell Avenue 414-961-4936
Glendale, WI 53217 Fax: 414-961-7288
e-mail: infowi@liverfoundation.org
www.liverfoundation.org
Dee Girard, Executive Director
Samantha Chartrau, Event/Program Coordinator

Research Centers

5696 **Clinical Research Center: Pediatrics Children's Hospital Research Foundation**
Children's Hospital Research Foundation
Elland & Bethesda Avenues 513-559-4412
Cincinnati, OH 45229 Fax: 513-559-7431
Studies of pediatric acquired diseases including liver disease and Reye's Syndrome.
Dr James Heubi, Director

5697 **University of California Liver Research Unit**
7601 E Imperial Highway 562-940-8961
Downey, CA 90242 Fax: 562-940-6628
Dr Allan G Redeker, Co-director

5698 **University of Texas Southwestern Medical Center**
5323 Harry Hines Boulevard
Dallas, TX 75390-9151 214-648-8311
www.utsouthwestern.edu
William M Lee MD Facp, Professor InteRNal Medicine / Director

5699 **University of Texas Southwestern Medical**
5323 Harry Hines Boulevard 214-648-3404
Dallas, TX 75235 Fax: 214-648-9119
e-mail: news@utsouthwestern.edu
www.utsouthwestern.edu
William M Lee MD Facp, Professor Internal Medicine / Director

5700 **Yeshiva University Marion Bessin Liver Research Center**
Albert Einstein College of Medicine
1300 Morris Park Avenue 718-430-2000
Bronx, NY 10461-1975 Fax: 718-918-0857
www.aecom.yu.edu
Liver disease research and therapy.
Dr David Shafritz, Director

Support Groups & Hotlines

5701 **Children's Liver Association for Support S ervices**
27023 McBean Parkway 661-263-9099
Valencia, CA 91355 877-679-8256
Fax: 661-263-9099
e-mail: Support Srv@aol.com
www.classkids.org
Dedicated to addressing the emotional, educational, and financial needs of families with children with liver disease or liver transplantation. Telephone hotline, newsletter, parent matching, literature and financial assistance. supports research and educates public about organ donations.
Diane Summer, President Board of Directors
Ann Whitehead RN/JD, Vice President Board of Directors

5702 **National Gaucher Foundation (NGF)**
2227 Idlewood Road
Tucker, GA 30084 800-504-3189
Fax: 770-934-2911
e-mail: rhonda@gaucherdisease.org
www.gaucherdisease.org/
The National Gaucher Foundation (NGF), established in 1984, supports and promotes research into the causes of, and a cure for Gaucher Disease. NGF provides information and assistance for those affected by Gaucher disease in addition to education and outreach to increase public awareness. NGF operates the Gaucher Disease Family Support Network.
Robin A Ely MD, President/Medical Director
Rhonda P Buyers, CEO/Executive Director

5703 **National Health Information Center**
PO Box 1133 310-565-4167
Washington, DC 20013 800-336-4797
Fax: 301-984-4256
e-mail: info@nhic.org
www.health.gov/nhic
Offers a nationwide information referral service, produces directories and resource guides.

5704 **National Reye's Syndrome Foundation**
PO Box 829 419-636-2679
Bryan, OH 43506 800-233-7393
Fax: 419-636-9897
e-mail: nrsf@reyesyndrome.org
www.reyessyndrome.org
Devoted to conquering Reye's syndrome, primarily a children's disease affecting the liver and brain, but can affect all ages. Provides support, information and referrals. Encourages research.
John Freudenberger, President
Larry Lasky, Vice President

5705 **Wilson's Disease Association**
1802 Brookside Drive 330-264-1450
Wooster, OH 44691 888-264-1450
Fax: 330-264-0974
e-mail: info@wilsonsdisease.org
www.wilsonsdisease.org
Serves as a communications support network for individuals affected by Wilson's disease; distributes information to professionals and the public; makes referrals; and holds meetings.
8 pages
Kimberly Symonds, Executive Director

Books

5706 **Liver Cancer**
Churchill Livingstone
PO Box 3188 201-319-9800
Secaucus, NJ 07096-3188 800-553-5426
Fax: 201-319-9659
www.churchillmed.com
1997 640 pages Hardcover
ISBN: 0-443054-81-9

5707 **Liver Disease in Children**
Mosby Year Book
11830 Westline Industrial Drive 314-872-8370
Saint Louis, MO 63146-3313 800-325-4177
1993 800 pages
ISBN: 1-556443-77-2

Magazines

5708 **American Association for the Study of Liver Diseases**
1729 King Street 703-299-9766
Alexandria, VA 22314 Fax: 703-299-9622
e-mail: aasld@aasld.org
www.aasld.org
Information for professionals interested in disease of the liver and biliary tract.
Sherrie H Cathcart, Executive Director

5709 **Hepatology**
American Assoc. for the Study of Liver Disease
1729 King Street 703-299-9766
Alexandria, VA 22314 Fax: 703-299-9622
e-mail: aasld@aasld.org
www.aasld.org
Information for professionals interested in disease of the liver and biliary tract.
Sherrie H Cathcart, Executive Director

Newsletters

5710 **Liver Update**
American Liver Foundation
1425 Pompton Avenue
Cedar Grove, NJ 07009-1000 800-465-4837
Fax: 973-256-3214
e-mail: info@liverfoundation.org
www.liverfoundation.org
Clinical newsletter for physicians.
BiAnnually
Rick Smith, President & CEO
Rebecca Frank, Chief Development Officer

5711 **LiverLink**
Alagille Syndrome Alliance
10630 SW Garden Park Place 503-639-6217
Tigard, OR 97223-3832
Newsletter for Alagille Syndrome.

5712 **Progress**
American Liver Foundation

1425 Pompton Avenue
Cedar Grove, NJ 07009-1000
800-465-4837
Fax: 973-256-3214
e-mail: info@liverfoundation.org
www.liverfoundation.org

Newsletter about liver disease and ALF.
TriAnnually
Rick Smith, President & CEO
Rebecca Frank, Chief Development Officer

Pamphlets

5713 **Alcohol and the Liver: Myth vs. Facts**
American Liver Foundation
1425 Pompton Avenue
Cedar Grove, NJ 07009-1000
973-256-2550
800-223-0179
e-mail: info@liverfoudation.org
www.liverfoundation.org

Rick Smith, President & CEO
Rebecca Frank, Chief Development Officer

5714 **Biliary Atresia**
American Liver Foundation
1425 Pompton Avenue
Cedar Grove, NJ 07009-1000
973-857-2626
800-223-0179
e-mail: info@liverfoundation.org
www.liverfoundation.org

Rick Smith, President & CEO
Rebecca Frank, Chief Development Officer

5715 **Diet and Your Liver**
American Liver Foundation
1425 Pompton Avenue
Cedar Grove, NJ 07009-1000
800-223-0179
Fax: 973-256-3214
e-mail: info@liverfoundation.org
www.liverfoundation.org

Rick Smith, President & CEO
Rebecca Frank, Chief Development Officer

5716 **Facts on Liver Transplantation**
American Liver Foundation
1425 Pompton Avenue
Cedar Grove, NJ 07009-1000
800-223-0179
Fax: 973-256-3214
e-mail: info@liverfoundation.org
www.liverfoundation.org

Rick Smith, President & CEO
Rebecca Frank, Chief Development Officer

5717 **Fatty Liver**
American Liver Foundation
1425 Pompton Avenue
Cedar Grove, NJ 07009-1000
800-223-0179
Fax: 987-256-3214
e-mail: info@liverfoundation.org
www.liverfoundation.org

Rick Smith, President & CEO
Rebecca Frank, Chief Development Officer

5718 **Gallstones**
American Liver Foundation
1425 Pompton Avenue
Cedar Grove, NJ 07009-1000
800-223-0179
Fax: 973-256-3214
e-mail: info@liverfoundation.org
www.liverfoundation.org

Rick Smith, President & CEO
Rebecca Frank, Chief Development Officer

5719 **Getting Help to Hepatitis**
American Liver Foundation
1425 Pompton Avenue
Cedar Grove, NJ 07009-1000
800-223-0179
Fax: 973-256-3214
e-mail: info@liverfoundation.org
www.liverfoundation.org

Rick Smith, President & CEO

5720 **Hemochromatosis**
American Liver Foundation
1425 Pompton Avenue
Cedar Grove, NJ 07009-1000
800-223-0179
Fax: 973-256-3214
e-mail: info@liverfoundation.org
www.liverfoundation.org

Rick Smith, President & CEO

5721 **Hepatitis A, B & C**
American Liver Foundation
1425 Pompton Avenue
Cedar Grove, NJ 07009-1000
800-223-0179
Fax: 973-256-3214
e-mail: info@liverfoundation.org
www.liverfoundation.org

Rick Smith, President & CEO

5722 **Hepatitis B: Your Child at Risk**
American Liver Foundation
1425 Pompton Avenue
Cedar Grove, NJ 07009-1000
800-223-0179
Fax: 973-256-3214
e-mail: info@liverfoundation.org
www.liverfoundation.org

Rick Smith, President & CEO

5723 **How Can You Love Me**
American Liver Foundation
1425 Pompton Avenue
Cedar Grove, NJ 07009-1000
973-857-2626
800-223-0179
Fax: 973-256-3214
e-mail: info@liverfoundation.org
www.liverfoundation.org

Rick Smith, President & CEO

5724 **Liver Function Tests**
American Liver Foundation
1425 Pompton Avenue
Cedar Grove, NJ 07009-1000
973-256-2550
800-223-0179
Fax: 973-256-3214
e-mail: info@liverfoundation.org
www.liverfoundation.org

Rick Smith, President & CEO

5725 **Liver Transplant Fund**
American Liver Foundation
1425 Pompton Avenue
Cedar Grove, NJ 07009-1000
973-256-2550
800-223-0179
Fax: 973-256-3214
e-mail: info@liverfoundation.org
www.liverfoundation.org

Rick Smith, President & CEO

5726 **Liver Transplantation**
American Liver Foundation
1425 Pompton Avenue
Cedar Grove, NJ 07009-1000
973-857-2626
800-223-0179
Fax: 973-256-3214
e-mail: info@liverfoundation.org
www.liverfoundation.org

Rick Smith, President & CEO

5727 **Viral Hepatitis**
American Liver Foundation
1425 Pompton Avenue
Cedar Grove, NJ 07009-1000
973-256-2550
800-223-0179
Fax: 973-256-3214
e-mail: info@liverfoundation.org
www.liverfoundation.org

Rick Smith, President & CEO

5728 **Your Liver Lets You Live**
American Liver Foundation
1425 Pompton Avenue
Cedar Grove, NJ 07009-1000
973-256-2550
800-223-0179
Fax: 973-256-3214
e-mail: info@liverfoundation.org
www.liverfoundation.org

Rick Smith, President & CEO

Web Sites

5729 **American Association for the Study of Liver Diseases**
www.aasld.org/
Conducts symposia and educational courses for professionals interested in disease of the liver and biliary tract. The leading organization for advancing the science and practice of hepatology.

5730 **Children's Liver Alliance**
www.liverkids.org.au/
Empowering the hearts and minds of children with liver disease, their families and the medical professionals who care for them.

5731 **Healing Well**
www.healingwell.com
An online health resource guide to medical news, chat, information and articles, newsgroups and message boards, books, disease-related web sites, medical directories, and more for patients, friends, and family coping with disabling diseases, disorders, or chronic illnesses.

5732 **Health Finder**
www.healthfinder.gov
Searchable, carefully developed web site offering information on over 1000 topics. Developed by the US Department of Health and Human Services, the site can be used in both English and Spanish.

5733 **Healthlink USA**
www.healthlinkusa.com
Health information concerning treatment, cures, prevention, diagnosis, risk factors, research, support groups, email lists, personal stories and much more. Updated regularly.

5734 **Helios Health**
www.helioshealth.com
Online resource for your health information. Detailed information about specific health topics, access to expert advice from our Medical Advisory Board, and up-to-date health news.

5735 **Liver Support**
www.liversupport.com
Information about the world's safest, most powerful liver-protecting supplement, milk thistle. Specifically facts about the safe, yet highly potent, Phytosome form.

5736 **MedicineNet**
www.medicinenet.com
An online resource for consumers providing easy-to-read, authoritative medical and health information.

5737 **Medscape**
www.mywebmd.com
Medscape offers specialists, primary care physicians, and other health professionals the Web's most robust and integrated medical information and educational tools.

5738 **WebMD**
www.webmd.com
Information on liver disease, including articles and resources.

Description

5739 **Lung Disease**

The lungs are in intimate contact with a person's environment, so they may be damaged by scores of agents, including dusts, gases and micro-organisms. The majority of lung, or pulmonary, diseases are related to exposure to external irritants, such as cigarette smoke, asbestos, bacteria and viruses. The most common chronic lung diseases of this type are emphysema and chronic bronchitis; both are part of the class of diseases called Chronic Obstructive Pulmonary Disease, or COPD. Most cases are associated with tobacco usage. High-risk occupations for lung disease include mining, farming, building construction and certain types of manufacturing. Lung cancer may be primary (originating in the lung) or secondary (spread, or metastasized, from another area). Bronchogenic cancer accounts for more than 90 percent of all lung tumors; cigarette smoking is the principal cause. Lung cancer is usually seen in people with COPD, because the two conditions have similar causes. Other lung disorders are secondary to clots originating from other sites in the body, systemic illness, and skeletal abnormalities that interfere with chest expansion during breathing.

Symptoms of lung disease may include coughing, sputum production, breathlessness, and sometimes fever or chest pain. In advanced cases, breathlessness is constant, and cyanosis (a bluish discoloration of the lips and fingernails) may occur.

Diagnosis of pulmonary disorders depends on a very careful history, physical examination, chest x-ray and pulmonary function testing, or spirometry. These measures are also important in following disease progression and response to treatment. Other chest imaging techniques, such as computed tomography (CT) scans and MRIs, and examination of fluid in the lung and lung tissue help establish a diagnosis. Recent research indicates that PET (positron emission tomography) scans may be helpful in the earlier diagnosis and treatment of lung cancer. Treatment of lung disease depends on the underlying cause. Management of COPD includes avoiding tobacco or other environmental exposure, antibiotics to control heavy sputum production and drugs to open up the narrowed airways. In advanced cases, breathing oxygen directly by nasal prongs improves quality of life and survival. Lung transplantation has occasionally been attempted, usually when COPD is due to a genetic disorder. Early screening for lung cancer has been disappointing; quitting smoking early is the only meaningful way of reducing one's risk of dying of the disease. Treatment may include surgery, radiation, or chemotherapy; success depends on the stage of the tumor and its precise type as determined by tissue biopsy.

Severe Acute Respiratory Syndrome, known as SARS, is an infectious disease that first appeared in China in 2002. SARS is caused by a corona-virus, which is related to the virus behind the common cold. The symptoms of SARS are a fever, greater than 100.4 degrees, fatigue, headache and chills. It is also accompanied by a dry cough and difficulty breathing, owing to the inflamed lungs. Until effective treatment or a vaccine is developed, prevention in SARS-infected areas includes isolating patients, wearing protective surgical masks, and restricting travel.

National Agencies & Associations

5740 **American Association for Respiratory Care**
9425 N MacArthur Boulevard
Irving, TX 75063-4706
972-243-2272
Fax: 972-484-2720
e-mail: info@aarc.org
www.aarc.org

Committed to enhancing professionalism as a respiratory care practitioner improving your performance on the job and helping to broaden the scope essential for success.
Sam Giordano, Executive Director
Tim Goldsbury, Sales Director

5741 **American Lung Association**
1301 Pennsylvania Avenue NW
Washington, DC 20004
212-315-8700
800-LUN-GUSA
www.lungusa.org

The mission of the American Lung Association is to prevent lung disease and promote lung health. Founded in 1904 to fight tuberculosis the American Lung Association today fights disease in all its forms with special emphasis on asthma and tobacco control.
H James Gooden, Secretary
Stephen J Nolan, Chair

5742 **Coalition for Pulmonary Fibrosis**
1659 Branham Lane
San Jose, CA 95118
888-222-8541
Fax: 408-266-3289
e-mail: info@coalitionforpf.org
www.coalitionforpf.org

Founded to further education patient support and research efforts for pulmonary fibrosis specifically idiopathic pulmonary fibrosis.
Marvin Schwa MD, Chairman

5743 **Lung Association**
1750 Courtwood Crescent
Ottawa, K2C 2-2B5
613-569-6411
888-566-5864
Fax: 613-569-8860
e-mail: info@lung.ca
www.lung.ca

At the national provincial and community levels to improve and promote lung health.
Nora Sobolov, President/CEO
Mary-Pat Shaw, VP National Programs & Operations

5744 **National Jewish Medical and Research Center**
1400 Jackson Street
Denver, CO 80206
303-388-4461
800-222-5864
e-mail: allstetterw@njhealth.orgÿ
www.nationaljewish.org

Offers comprehensive diagnosis treatment and rehabilitation of people with chronic obstructive pulmonary disease asthma allergies and other respiratory and immune diseases.
William Allstetter, Media Contact
Pamela Meister, Patient Representative Office

5745 **Public Information Center US Environmental Protection Agency**
US Environmental Protection Agency
1200 Pennsylvania Avenue NW
Washington, DC 20460
202-272-0167
800-368-5888
TTY: 202-272-0165
www.epa.gov

Provides information on handling asbestos and explanation of legislation.
Lisa Jackson, Administrator

5746 **Pulmonary Fibrosis Association**
1332 N Halstead Street 312-587-9272
Chicago, IL 60642-0004 Fax: 312-587-9273
e-mail: pulmonaryfibrosisinfo@yahoo.com
www.pulmonaryfibrosis.org
Dedicated to finding a cure for and raising awareness of pulmonary fibrosis an often fatal lung disease.
Michael Rose PhD, President/CEO
Leanne Storch, Executive Director

5747 **Pulmonary Fibrosis Foundation**
1332 N Halsted Street 312-587-9272
Chicago, IL 60642 Fax: 312-587-9273
e-mail: pulmonaryfibrosisinfo@yahoo.com
www.pulmonaryfibrosis.org
A non-profitý corporation founded in the state of Colorado in 2000 by Albert Rose and Michael Rosenzweig, both of whom were diagnosed with Pulmonary Fibrosis (IPF).
Mike Rosenzweig, President/CEO
Leanne Storch, Executive Director

5748 **Pulmonary Hypertension Association**
801 Roeder Road 301-565-3004
Silver Spring, MD 20910 800-748-7274
Fax: 301-565-3994
e-mail: pha@PHAssociation.org
www.PHAssociation.org
A nonprofit organization for pulmonary hypertension patients, families, caregivers and PH-treating medical professionals. The mission of the Pulmonary Hypertension Association (PHA) is to find ways to prevent and cure pulmonary hypertension.
Rino Aldrighetti, President
Carl Hicks, Chair

5749 **US Environmental Protection Agency: Indoor Environments Division**
1200 Pennsylvania Avenue NW 202-343-9370
Washington, DC 20460 Fax: 202-343-2392
e-mail: iaqinfo@aol.com
www.epa.gov/iaq
Responsible for implementing EPA's Indoor Environments Program, a voluntary (non-regulatory) program to address indoor air pollution.

5750 **White Lung Association**
PO Box 1483 410-243-5864
Baltimore, MD 21203-1483 e-mail: jfite@whitelung.org
www.whitelung.org
A national nonprofit organization dedicated to the education of the public to the hazards of asbestos exposure. The association developed programs of public education and consults with victims of asbestos exposure, school boards, building owners and government representatives.
Jim Fite, Contact

State Agencies & Associations

Alabama

5751 **American Lung Association of Alabama**
3125 Independence Drive 205-933-8821
Birmingham, AL 35209 e-mail: kperry@alabamalung.org
www.alabamalung.org
Kim Perry, Director of Development

Alaska

5752 **American Lung Association of Alaska**
500 W International Airport Road 907-276-5864
Anchorage, AK 99518-1105 800-LUN-GUSA
Fax: 907-565-5587
e-mail: mlarson@aklung.org
www.aklung.org
Marge Larson, Steering Committee Member
Michelle Ferreira, Asthma Coalition Coordinator

Arizona

5753 **American Lung Association of Arizona**
102 W McDowell Road 602-258-7505
Phoenix, AZ 85003-1299 800-LUN-GUSA
Fax: 602-258-7507
e-mail: bpfeifer@lungaz.org
www.lungarizona.org
Through research education and advocacy the American Lung Association of Arizona works to prevent lung disease and promote lung health. Our areas of focus are asthma air quality and tobacco control.
Bill J Pfeifer, President/CEO

Arkansas

5754 **American Lung Association of Arkansas**
211 Natural Resources Drive 501-224-5864
Little Rock, AR 72205-1539 800-880-5864
Fax: 501-224-5654
e-mail: klackey@lungark.org
www.lungark.org
Karen S Lackey, CEO
Melinda Rogers, Data Entry Coordinator

California

5755 **American Lung Association of California**
424 Pendleton Way 510-638-5864
Oakland, CA 94621-2189 Fax: 510-638-8984
e-mail: contact@californialung.org
www.californialung.org
Ben Abate, President/CEO
Sylvia Goodin, Secretary

Colorado

5756 **American Lung Association of Colorado**
5600 Greenwood Plaza Boulevard 303-388-4327
Greenwood Village, CO 80111 800-LUN-GUSA
Fax: 303-377-1102
e-mail: chuber@lungcolorado.org
www.alacolo.org
Curt Huber, Executive Director
Connor Michael, Communications Manager

Connecticut

5757 **American Lung Association of Connecticut**
45 Ash Street 860-289-5401
E Hartford, CT 06108-3272 800-586-4872
Fax: 860-289-5405
e-mail: bcase@alact.org
www.alact.org
Part of the American Lung Association the oldest voluntary health agency dedicated to fighting a single disease. Highest priorities are asthma tobacco control and clean air.
Lisa Blumetti, Director Development/Special Events

Delaware

5758 **American Lung Association of Delaware**
1021 Gilpin Avenue 302-655-7258
Wilmington, DE 19806-3280 800-LUN-GUSA
Fax: 302-655-8546
e-mail: dbrown@aladc.org
www.lunginfo.org
Deborah Brown, VP Community Outreach
Susan DeNardo, Development Director

District of Columbia

5759 **American Lung Association of the District of Columbia**
1725 K Street N.W. 202-466-5864
Washington, DC 20001-2617 e-mail: info@aladc.org
www.aladc.org
Resource for information and programs in the area of lung health, including asthma, tobacco control, air quality, sarcoidosis, and turberculosis.

5760 **American Lung Association of the Northern**
530 7th Street SE
Washington, DC 20003
202-546-5864
Fax: 202-546-5607
e-mail: info@aladc.org
www.aladc.org

Resource for information and programs in the area of lung health, including asthma, tobacco control, air quality, sarcoidosis, and tuberculosis.

David A McWilliams Sr, Chairman
Henry Yeager Jr MD, Vice Chairman

Florida

5761 **American Lung Association of Florida**
6852 Belfort Oaks Place
Jacksonville, FL 32216-5216
904-743-2933
800-940-2933
Fax: 904-743-2916
e-mail: alaf@lungfla.org
www.lungfla.org

Works for the prevention and control of lung disease through education, advocacy and research.

Denise Grimsley, President

5762 **Goodwill Industries-Suncoast**
Goodwill Industries-Suncoast
10596 Gandy Boulevard
St. Petersburg, FL 33702
727-523-1512
888-279-1988
Fax: 727-563-9300
e-mail: gw.marketing@goodwill-suncoast.com
www.goodwill-suncoast.org

A non-profit community based organization whose purpose is to improve the quality of life for people who are disabled, disadvantaged and/or aged. This mission is accomplished through a staff of over 1,200 employees providing independent living skills, affordable housing, career assessment and planning, job skills, training, placement, and job retention assistance with useful employment. Annually, Goodwill Industries-Suncoast serves over 30,000 people in Citrus, Hernando, Levy, Marion and more.

R Lee Waits, CEO
Martin W Gladysz, Chair

Georgia

5763 **American Lung Association of Georgia**
2452 Spring Road
Smyrna, GA 30080-3862
770-434-5864
Fax: 770-319-0349
e-mail: aburger@alase.org
www.alaga.org

Charles J White, Chief Executive Officer
June Deen, Vice President of Public Affairs

Hawaii

5764 **American Lung Association of Hawaii**
680 Iwilei Road
Honolulu, HI 96817
808-537-5966
Fax: 808-537-5971
e-mail: lung@ala-hawaii.org
www.ala-hawaii.org

Jean Evans, Executive Director
Karen J Lee, President

Idaho

5765 **American Lung Association of Idaho**
8030 Emerald Street
Boise, ID 83704
208-345-5864
800-LUN-GUSA
Fax: 208-345-5896
www.lungidaho.org

Illinois

5766 **American Lung Association of Illinois**
3000 Kelly Lane
Springfield, IL 62711
217-787-5864
800-LUN-GUSA
Fax: 217-787-5916
e-mail: info@lungil.org
www.lungil.org

Harold Wimmer, CEO
Kim Streib, Vice President Finance

Indiana

5767 **American Lung Association of Indiana**
115 W Washington Street
Indianapolis, IN 46204-1470
317-819-1181
800-LUN-GUSA
Fax: 317-819-1187
e-mail: info@lungin.org
www.lungin.org

Chris Brooks, Director Program Services
Melissa Henderson, Director Operations

Iowa

5768 **American Lung Association of Iowa**
2530 73rd Street
Des Moines, IA 50322-1800
515-278-5864
800-LUN-GUSA
Fax: 515-334-9564
e-mail: info@lungia.org
www.lungia.org

Harold Wimmer, President & CEO
Kim Streib, Manager/Controller

Kansas

5769 **American Lung Association of Kansas**
4300 SW Drury Lane
Topeka, KS 66604-2419
785-272-9290
800-LUN-GUSA
Fax: 785-272-9297
e-mail: jkeller@kslung.org
www.kslung.org

Judy Keller, Executive Officer
Kris Scothorn, Office Manager

Kentucky

5770 **American Lung Association of Kentucky**
4100 Churchman Avenue
Louisville, KY 40209-0067
502-363-2652
800-LUN-GUSA
Fax: 502-363-0222
e-mail: info@kylung.org
www.kylung.org

Ann Evans, Regional Director
Barry Gottschalk, Senior VP Operations

Louisiana

5771 **American Lung Association of Louisiana**
2325 Severn Avenue
Metairie, LA 70001-6918
504-828-5864
800-586-4872
Fax: 504-828-5867
e-mail: info@louisianalung.org
www.louisianalung.org

Aline Palmisano-Vita, Deputy Executive Director
Thomas P Lotz RRT MEd, Chief Executive Officer

Maine

5772 **American Lung Association of Maine**
122 State Street
Augusta, ME 04330
207-622-6394
888-241-6566
Fax: 207-626-2919
e-mail: info@lungme.org
www.lungme.org

Edward Miller, Executive Director
Norman Anderson, Regional Research Director

Maryland

5773 **American Lung Association of Maryland**
11350 McCormick Road
Hunt Valley, MD 21031
410-560-2120
800-LUN-GUSA
Fax: 410-560-0829
e-mail: info@marylandlung.org
www.marylandlung.org

Stephen J Nolan Esq, Chairman of the Board
Melina Davis-Martin, President and CEO

Massachusetts

5774 **American Lung Association of Massachusetts**
5 Mountain Road
Burlington, MA 01903
781-272-2866

Michigan

5775 **American Lung Association of Michigan**
25900 Greenfield Road
Oak Park, MI 48237
248-784-2000
800-543-LUNG
Fax: 248-784-2008
e-mail: alam@alam.org
www.alam.org

Rose Adams, CEO
Nicole Crumpton, Executive Office Manager

Minnesota

5776 **American Lung Association of Minnesota**
490 Concordia Avenue
Saint Paul, MN 55103-2441
651-227-8014
800-LUN-GUSA
Fax: 651-227-5459
e-mail: info@alamn.org
www.alamn.org

Jerry Orr, CEO

Mississippi

5777 **American Lung Association of Mississippi**
PO Box 2178
Ridgeland, MS 39157
601-206-5810

5778 **American Lung Association of Missouri**
731 Pear Orchard Road
Ridgeland, MS 39157
601-206-5810
Fax: 601-206-5813
www.alams.org

Greg Wynne, Chairman
Tara Pierre Ellis, Vice-Chairman

Missouri

5779 **American Lung Association of Eastern Missouri**
1118 Hampton Avenue
Saint Louis, MO 63139-3196
314-645-5505
Fax: 314-645-7128
www.lungusa2.org/missouri/index.html

5780 **American Lung Association: Kansas City Office**
2400 Troost
Kansas City, MO 64108
816-842-5242
Fax: 816-842-5470
e-mail: qnimrod@breathehealthy.org
www.lungusa.org

National health association dedicated to promoting lung health and preventing lung disease.

Montana

5781 **American Lung Association of Northern Rockies**
825 Helena Avenue
Helena, MT 59601-3459
406-442-6556
Fax: 406-442-2346
e-mail: ala-nr@ala-nr.org
www.lungusa.org

Nebraska

5782 **American Lung Association of Nebraska**
7101 Newport Avenue
Omaha, NE 68152
402-572-3030
800-LUN-GUSA
e-mail: ala@lungnebraska.org
www.lungnebraska.org

Nevada

5783 **American Lung Association of Nevada**
PO Box 7056
Reno, NV 89510
775-829-5864
800-LUN-GUSA
Fax: 775-829-5850
e-mail: dszabo@lungs.org
www.lungusa.org

New Hampshire

5784 **American Lung Association of New Hampshire**
9 Cedarwood Drive
Bedford, NH 03110
603-669-2411
800-83L-UNGS
Fax: 603-645-6220
e-mail: dfortin@nhlung.org
www.nhlung.org

Dan Fortin, President/CEO
Lois McKenna, Office Manager

New Jersey

5785 **American Lung Association of New Jersey**
1600 Route 22 E
Union, NJ 07083-3410
908-687-9340
Fax: 908-851-2625
e-mail: info@alanewjersey.org
www.alanewjersey.org

John A Rutkowski MBA RRT, President
Howard Hellman, First Vice President

New Mexico

5786 **American Lung Association of New Mexico**
7001 Menaul Boulevard NE
Albuquerque, NM 87110
505-265-0732
800-LUN-GUSA
Fax: 505-260-1739
e-mail: jdemaria@LungNewMexico.org
www.lungnewmexico.org

Support group for adults with lung disease. Also offers lung health education.

JoAnna DeMaria, Lung Health Coordinator
Lorrie Loomis, Office Coordinator

New York

5787 **American Lung Association of New York State**
155 Washington Avenue
Albany, NY 12210-2804
518-465-2013
Fax: 518-465-2926
e-mail: info@alany.org
www.alany.org

Deborah Carioto, President
Michael Seilback, Vice President of Public Policy

North Carolina

5788 **American Lung Association of North Carolina**
3801 Lake Boone Trail
Raleigh, NC 27607
919-832-8326
800-586-4872
Fax: 919-856-8530
e-mail: info@lungnc.org
www.lungnc.org

Better breathing clubs for chronic lung disease patients.

Deborah Bryan, CEO
Susan King Cope, VP Programs/Advocacy

North Dakota

5789 **American Lung Association of North Dakota**
PO Box 5004
Bismarck, ND 58501
701-223-5613
800-252-6325
Fax: 701-223-5727
e-mail: lungnd@gcentral.com

A voluntary health agency whose objective is the conquest of lung disease and the promotion of lung health. We sponsor Super Asthma Saturday and open airways for schools events to educate asthmatics and their families and Dakota Superkids Asthma Camp for kids 8-15 with asthma. Smoking cessation classes for adults and youth.

Ohio

5790 **American Lung Association of Ohio**
1950 Arlingate Lane
Columbus, OH 43228-4102
614-279-1700
800-LUN-GUSA
Fax: 614-279-4940
www.ohiolung.org

Tracy Ross, President/CEO

Oklahoma

5791 American Lung Association of Oklahoma
11212 N May Avenue
Oklahoma City, OK 73120
405-748-4674
800-LUN-GUSA
Fax: 405-748-6274
e-mail: ktodd@oklung.org
www.oklung.org

Kay Todd PhD CAE, CEO
Jimmy Beth, Member

Oregon

5792 American Lung Association of Oregon
7420 SW Bridgeport Road
Tigard, OR 97224-7790
503-924-4094
800-LUN-GUSA
Fax: 503-924-4120
e-mail: info@lungoregon.org
www.lungoregon.org

Dana Kaye, Executive Director
Jennifer Baldwin, Director of Development

Pennsylvania

5793 American Lung Association of Pennsylvania
3001 Old Gettysburg Road
Camp Hill, PA 17011
717-541-5864
800-932-0903
Fax: 717-541-8828
e-mail: info@lunginfo.org
www.lungusa.org

Provide education, research and information on lung disease and lung health, including asthma, tobacco prevention and cessation, chronic obstructive pulmonary disease, indoor and outdoor air quality, children's summer camps, support groups and specialty programs.

5794 American Respiratory Alliance of Western Pennsylvania
201 Smith Drive
Cranberry Township, PA 16066
724-772-1750
800-220-1990
Fax: 724-772-1180
www.healthylungs.org

Dedicated to the prevention and control of lung disease through education training, direct services, research funding and advocacy since 1904.

Christine R Weaver, Executive Director
George B Miller, President

Rhode Island

5795 American Lung Association of Rhode Island
260 W Exchange Street
Providence, RI 02903-3700
401-421-6487
800-586-4872
Fax: 401-331-5266
e-mail: ALARI@lungri.org
www.lungne.org

Lucille Cavan, Director
Robert Petix, Chair/Executive Committee

South Carolina

5796 American Lung Association of South Carolina
1212 West Elkhorn Street
Columbia, SC 29201-2344
803-779-5864
800-849-5864
Fax: 803-254-2711
www.lungsc.org

South Dakota

5797 American Lung Association of South Dakota
1212 West Elkhorn
Sioux Falls, SD 57104-0233
605-336-7222
800-873-5864
Fax: 605-336-7227
e-mail: lung@americanlungsd.org

Linda Redder, Coordinator

Tennessee

5798 American Lung Association of Tennessee
1 Vantage Way
Nashville, TN 37228
615-329-1151
800-LUN-GUSA
Fax: 615-329-1723
e-mail: alastaff@alatn.org
www.lungtn.org

A statewide organization the oldest national health agency in the US. Our mission is to prevent lung disease and to promote lung health. Our program priorities include environmental health asthma education tobacco control for children and finding a cure.

Texas

5799 American Lung Association of Texas
5926 Balcones Drive
Austin, TX 78731
512-467-6753
800-252-LUNG
Fax: 512-467-7621
e-mail: info@texaslung.org
www.texaslung.org

Lewis Brown MD, Chairman
Ted Balistreri, Member

Utah

5800 American Lung Association of Utah
1930 S 1100 E
Salt Lake City, UT 84106-2317
801-484-4456
800-548-8252
Fax: 801-484-5461
e-mail: info@utahlung.org
www.lungutah.org

Craig Cutright, Executive Director
Don Hooper, Development Director

Virginia

5801 American Lung Association of Virginia
9221 Forest Hill Avenue
Richmond, VA 23235
804-267-1900
800-345-5864
Fax: 804-267-5634
e-mail: info@lungac.org
www.lungva.org

Washington

5802 American Lung Association of Washington
2625 3rd Avenue
Seattle, WA 98121
206-441-5100
800-732-9339
Fax: 206-441-3277
e-mail: alaw@alaw.org
www.alaw.org

Marina Cofer-Wildsmi, CEO
Darlene Madenwald, President

West Virginia

5803 American Lung Association of West Virginia
415 Dickinson Street
Charleston, WV 25301
304-342-6600
800-LUN-GUSA
Fax: 304-342-6096
e-mail: sara@alawv.org
www.alawv.org

Sarah Crickenberger, Executive Director
Chantal Fields, Assistant Executive Director

Wisconsin

5804 American Lung Association of Wisconsin
13100 W Lisbon Road
Brookfield, WI 53005-2508
262-703-4200
800-LUN-GUSA
Fax: 262-781-5180
e-mail: amlung@lungwisconsin.org
www.lungwi.org

Susan Gloede Swan, Executive Director
Dona Wininsky, Director of Public Policy

Research Centers

5805 **Enzymology Research Laboratory Dept. of Veterans Affairs Medical Center**
Dept. of Veterans Affairs Medical Center
150 Muir Road 925-228-6800
Martinez, CA 94553
Studies affecting emphysema in mankind.
Michael C Geokas MD, Chief

5806 **National Jewish Center for Immunology**
1400 Jackson Street
Denver, CO 80206 303-388-4461
www.nationaljewish.org
Offers basic and clinical research into the causes and treatments of various lung diseases and respiratory problems.
Lynn Gaussig, President

5807 **University of Utah Rocky Mountain Center for Occupational & Environmental Health**
University of Utah
391 Chipeta Way 801-581-4800
Salt Lake City, UT 84108 Fax: 801-817-24
e-mail: rmoser@rmcoeh.utah.edu
www.rmcoeh.utah.edu
Provides graduate and continuing education programs in occupational medicine occupational health nursing ergonomics and safety industrial hygiene and hazardous materials. Additionally provides clinical evaluations and consultations in the listed areas.
Royce Moser Jr MD, Deputy Director
Kurt Hedmann, Director

5808 **Warren Grant Magnuson Clinical Center**
National Institute of Health
9000 Rockville Pike
Bethesda, MD 20892 800-411-1222
Fax: 301-480-9793
TTY: 866-411-1010
e-mail: prpl@mail.cc.nih.gov
www.clinicalcenter.nih.gov
Established in 1953 as the research hospital of the National Institutes of Health. Designed so that patient care facilities are close to research laboratories so new findings of basic and clinical scientists can be quickly applied to the treatment of patients. Upon referral by physicians, patients are admitted to NIH clinical studies.
John Gallin, Director
David Henderson, Deputy Director for Clinical Care

Support Groups & Hotlines

5809 **American Lung Association Help Line**
American Lung Association
3000 Kelly Lane 217-787-5864
Springfield, IL 62711 800-586-4872
Fax: 217-787-5916
www.helpline.org
Provides information for the lung association of the state in which you make the call. Offers support group referrals.
Michael Mark, Lung Help Line Director

5810 **Lung Facts**
National Jewish Center for Immunology
1400 Jackson Street 303-388-4461
Denver, CO 80206 800-222-5864
Fax: 303-270-2220
e-mail: allstetterw@njc.org
www.njc.org/
An automated information service with recorded health messages developed by Lung Line Information Service. The information provided on this system offers help and support, as well as medical updates for persons suffering from lung diseases.
Michael Salem MD, President/CEO
William Allstetter, Public Affairs/Media

5811 **National Health Information Center**
PO Box 1133 310-565-4167
Washington, DC 20013 800-336-4797
Fax: 301-984-4256
e-mail: info@nhic.org
www.health.gov/nhic
Offers a nationwide information referral service, produces directories and resource guides.

Books

5812 **American Lung Association Family Guide to Asthma and Allergies**
American Lung Association
1740 Broadway 212-315-8700
New York, NY 10019-4315 e-mail: info@lungusa.org
www.lungusa.org

5813 **Health Consequences of Smoking: Cancer & Chronic Lung Disease in the Workplace**
DIANE Publishing Company
330 Pusey Avenue, Unit #3 Rear 610-461-6200
Darby, PA 19023 800-782-3833
Fax: 610-461-6130
e-mail: dianepublishing@gmail.com
www.dianepublishing.net
Examines the relationship between cigarette smoking and occupational exposures. Establishes that in order to protect the workers fully, forces of labor, management, insurers and government must become as engaged in attempts to reduce the prevalence of cigarette smoking as they are in occupational exposure. Tables and figure. Extensive bibliography, index.
542 pages Paperback
ISBN: 0-788123-11-4
Herman Baron, Publisher

5814 **Management of Acute Exacerbations of Chronic Obstructive Pulmonary Disease**
DIANE Publishing Company
330 Pusey Avenue, Unit #3 Rear 610-461-6200
Darby, PA 19023 800-782-3833
Fax: 610-461-6130
e-mail: dianepublishing@gmail.com
www.dianepublishing.net
This report describes evidence about the clinical assessment and management of patients presenting with acute exacerbation of chronic obstructive pulmonary disease, a frequent cause of health care utilization, morality and decreased quality of life.
256 pages Paperback
ISBN: 0-756721-99-7
Herman Baron, Publisher

5815 **Seven Steps to a Smoke-Free Life**
American Lung Association
1740 Broadway 212-315-8700
New York, NY 10019-4315 e-mail: info@lungusa.org
www.lungusa.org

Pamphlets

5816 **Around the Clock with COPD**
American Lung Association
1740 Broadway 212-315-8700
New York, NY 10019-4315 800-586-4872
e-mail: info@lungusa.org
www.lungusa.org
A booklet with non-medical helpful hints written by persons living with a chronic lung disease for others.

5817 **Asbestos in Your Home**
American Lung Association
1740 Broadway 212-315-8700
New York, NY 10019-4315 800-586-4872
Offers information on asbestos.

5818 **Black Lung**
National Jewish Center for Immunology

1400 Jackson Street 303-388-4461
Denver, CO 80206-2762 800-222-5864
Offers information on black lung and the respiratory system.

5819 **Emphysema**
American Lung Association of Connecticut
45 Ash Street 860-289-5401
East Hartford, CT 06108-3294 800-586-4872
Fax: 860-289-5405
www.alact.org
Offers information on who gets emphysema, how it attacks, causes, effects, prevention and treatment.
John E Zinn, President/CEO

5820 **Exercise Guidelines for the Person with Lung Disease**
American Lung Association of Connecticut
45 Ash Street 860-289-5401
East Hartford, CT 06108-3294 800-586-4872
Fax: 860-289-5405
www.alact.org
Offers exercise information and illustrations for persons with lung disease.
John E Zinn, President/CEO

5821 **Facts About AAT Deficiency-Related Emphysema**
American Lung Association
1740 Broadway 212-315-8700
New York, NY 10019-4315
Offers information on this type of emphysema, risk factors, development, symptoms and early detection.

5822 **Facts About Asbestos**
American Lung Association
1740 Broadway 212-315-8700
New York, NY 10019-4315
Offers information on lung hazards on the job and what employers can do to protect themselves and the people that work for them.

5823 **Facts About Asthma**
American Lung Association
1740 Broadway 212-315-8700
New York, NY 10019-4315 800-586-4872

5824 **Steps to a Better Understanding of Lung Cancer: A Patient and Family Guide**
American Lung Association
1740 Broadway 212-315-8700
New York, NY 10019-4315 800-586-4872
e-mail: info@lungusa.org
www.lungusa.org
A booklet with non-medical helpful hints written by persons living with a chronic lung disease for others.

5825 **Understanding Emphysema**
National Jewish Center for Immunology
1400 Jackson Street 303-388-4461
Denver, CO 80206-2762 800-222-5864
Offers information on emphysema, causes, treatments, symptoms and prevention.

Audio & Video

5826 **Keeping the Balance**
Fanlight Productions
4196 Washington Street 617-469-4999
Boston, MA 02131-1731 800-937-4113
Fax: 617-469-3379
e-mail: fanlight@fanlight.com
www.fanlight.com
Siblings of children with serious lung disease share their experiences of being the normal child, exploring the frequent conflict between their feelings of love and concern and their resentment over the attention denied to them because of the sibling's illness. Offers advice on how parents can keep the balance between the needs of all of their children.
1993 23 Minutes
ISBN: 1-572950-89-7

5827 **Sickle Cell Disease: Faces of Our Children**
Fanlight Productions
4196 Washington Street 617-469-4999
Boston, MA 02131-1731 800-937-4113
Fax: 617-469-3379
e-mail: fanlight@fanlight.com
www.fanlight.com
This program examines the devastating impact of sickle cell disease on these young people and their families and caregivers. It will be an important tool for increasing awareness in the community and among healthcare and social service providers in community clinics, hospitals, and other settings.
1999 14 Minutes
ISBN: 1-572953-05-5

Web Sites

5828 **American Lung Association**
www.lungusa.org
Offers research, medical updates, fund-raising, educational materials and public awareness campaigns relating to lung disease causes.

5829 **Healing Well**
www.healingwell.com
An online health resource guide to medical news, chat, information and articles, newsgroups and message boards, books, disease-related web sites, medical directories, and more for patients, friends, and family coping with disabling diseases, disorders, or chronic illnesses.

5830 **Health Central**
www.healthcenter.com
Provides support group and diagnostic information regarding lung disease.

5831 **Health Finder**
www.healthfinder.gov
Searchable, carefully developed web site offering information on over 1000 topics. Developed by the US Department of Health and Human Services, the site can be used in both English and Spanish.

5832 **Healthlink USA**
www.healthlinkusa.com
Health information concerning treatment, cures, prevention, diagnosis, risk factors, research, support groups, email lists, personal stories and much more. Updated regularly.

5833 **Helios Health**
www.helioshealth.com
Online resource for your health information. Detailed information about specific health topics, access to expert advice from our Medical Advisory Board, and up-to-date health news.

5834 **Lung Disease**
www.lungusa.org
The American Lung Association's website, including information on diseases A to Z, living with lung disease, tobacco control, air quality, data, statistics, research, and more.

5835 **MedicineNet**
www.medicinenet.com
An online resource for consumers providing easy-to-read, authoritative medical and health information.

5836 **Medscape**
www.mywebmd.com
Medscape offers specialists, primary care physicians, and other health professionals the Web's most robust and integrated medical information and educational tools.

5837 **National Heart, Lung & Blood Institute**
www.nhlbi.nih.gov
A website maintained by the National Institute of Health offering general information regarding the heart, lungs, and blood.

5838 **WebMD**
www.webmd.com
Information on lung disease, including articles and resources.

Description

5839 Lupus Erythematosus

Lupus erythematosus refers to two distinct but overlapping conditions. Systemic lupus erythematosus, SLE, is a chronic multi-organ inflammatory illness that may involve the brain, skin, kidneys, joints, bowel, and eyes. Discoid lupus erythematosus, DLE, is a much less serious disease that is limited to the skin. In DLE, patches of skin may turn red and develop white scales, followed by thinning and scarring. About 10 percent of patients with DLE will go on to develop SLE; roughly 25 percent of patients with SLE also have the manifestations of DLE.

Of SLE cases, 90 percent are women, and the disease usually begins during the child-bearing years. Although the cause is unclear, SLE causes its damage through auto-immune mechanisms. The body's own immune system, designed to fight off invasion from micro-organisms, turns against its own tissues, evidence of which can be measured in the blood. Almost any organ system can be affected, and symptoms include fatigue, fever, loss of appetite, skin rash, sensitivity to light (photophobia), joint pain, headaches, personality change, eye irritation, and inflammation of the kidney.

In general, the course of SLE is chronic and relapsing, often with long periods (years) of remission. It may only be mild or progress towards more serious illness and death from infection, kidney failure, or neurologic damage. Survival has improved markedly in the past two decades because, for most patients with SLE, the disease can be controlled with large, prolonged doses of steroids, and other drugs that affect the immune system. Some of these therapies may be associated with long-term complications.

National Agencies & Associations

5840 **American Juvenile Arthritis Organization (AJAO)**
1330 West Peachtree Street 404-872-7100
Atlanta, GA 30309 800-283-7800
Fax: 440-872-9559
e-mail: help@arthritis.org
www.arthritis.org
A council of the Arthritis Foundation devoted to serving the special needs of children, teens and young adults with childhood rheumatic diseases (including systemic lupus erythematosus) and their families. Provides support groups, information, advocacy, research updates, and conferences.
Janet S Austin, PhD

5841 **American Juvenile Arthritis Organization**
1330 W Peachtree Street 404-872-7100
Atlanta, GA 30309 800-283-7800
Fax: 440-872-9559
e-mail: help@arthritis.org
www.arthritis.org
A council of the Arthritis Foundation devoted to serving the special needs of children teens and young adults with childhood rheumatic diseases (including systemic lupus erythematosus) and their families. Provides support groups, information and advocacy.
John H Klippel, President/CEO
Roberta K Byrum, Assistant Secretary

5842 **Autoimmune Diseases Association**
22100 Gratiot Avenue 586-776-3900
E Detroit, MI 48021 Fax: 586-776-3903
e-mail: aarda@aarda.org
www.aarda.org
Provides mutual support and education for patients with any type of autoimmune disease. Support includes advocacy referral to support groups literature and conferences.
Stanley M Finger PhD, Chairman of the Board
Noel R Rose MD PhD, Chairman Emeritus

5843 **Lupus Foundation of America**
2000 L Street NW 202-349-1155
Washington, DC 20036 800-558-0121
Fax: 202-349-1156
e-mail: info@lupus.org
www.lupus.org
The Lupus Foundation of America is the nation's leading non-profit voluntary health organization dedicated to finding the causes and cure for lupus. Our mission is to improve the diagnosis and treatment of lupus and support individuals and families affected by this disease.
Karen B Evans, Chair
Sandra C Raymond, President & CEO

5844 **Lupus Network**
230 Ranch Drive 203-372-5795
Bridgeport, CT 06606
Seeks to foster better understanding of the disease among patients and the general public educators and professionals through the distribution of educational materials.

State Agencies & Associations

Alabama

5845 **Lupus Foundation of America: Alabama Chapter**
4 Office Park Circle 205-870-0504
Birmingham, AL 35223

Alaska

5846 **Lupus Foundation of America: Alaska Chapter**
PO Box 240628 907-338-6332
Anchorage, AK 99524 800-307-5878
e-mail: LFA_Alaska@hotmail.com
www.geocities.com/lfa_alaska
Anna Tillman, Executive Director
Judy Powell, President

Arizona

5847 **Lupus Foundation of America: Greater Arizona Chapter**
2001 West Camelback Road 602-242-2213
Phoenix, AZ 85015-4908 e-mail: LupusAZ@aol.com
www.lupusarizona.org
Catherine Lamphier

5848 **Lupus Foundation of America: Southern Arizona Chapter**
2583 North 1st Avenue 520-622-9006
Tucson, AZ 85719
Sharon Smiley, Office Manager

Arkansas

5849 **Lupus Foundation of America: Arkansas Chapter**
220 Mockingbird 501-525-9380
Hot Springs, AR 71913 800-294-8878
e-mail: lupusarkhs@direclynx.net
www.lupus-arkansas.com

California

5850 **Bay Area LE Foundation**
2635 N 1st Street 408-954-8600
San Jose, CA 95134 800-523-3363
Chapter of the Lupus Foundation of America.

5851 **Lupus Foundation of America: San Diego/Imperial County Chapter**
PO Box 837 760-579-7744
El Cajon, CA 92022-0837

5852 **Lupus Foundation of America: Northern California Chapter**
2775 Cottage Way 916-973-0776
Sacramento, CA 95825 877-225-8787
Fax: 916-973-8124
e-mail: Saclupus@excite.com
www.saclupus.org

Cynthia L Holton, Executive Director Team
Stephanie Pringle-Fox, Executive Director Team

5853 **Lupus Foundation of America: Sacramento Chapter**
4200 Prospect Drive 916-973-0776
Carmichael, CA 95608-1941

5854 **Lupus Foundation of America: Southern California Chapter**
17985 Sky Park Circle 714-833-2121
Irvine, CA 92614 800-426-6026

Colorado

5855 **Lupus Foundation of Colorado**
1211 S Parker Road 303-597-4050
Denver, CO 80231 800-858-1292
Fax: 303-597-4054
e-mail: info@lupuscolorado.org
www.lupuscolorado.org

Chapter of the Lupus Foundation of America.
Skip Schlenk, CEO
Debbie Lynch, Director of Development

Connecticut

5856 **Lupus Foundation of America: Connecticut Chapter**
97 S Street 860-953-0387
W Hartford, CT 06110-2402 800-699-6967
e-mail: CTLFA@sbcglobal.net
www.lupusct.org

A non-profit organization and a National Health Agency established for the purpose of enlightening the public by focusing professional and public attention on Lupus Erythematosus promotes research by providing financial assistance and serves as the support bond for patients and their families.
Marilyn Sousa, Founder
Lisa Voglesong, President

Delaware

5857 **Lupus Foundation of America: Delaware Chapter**
PO Box 6391 302-622-8700
Wilmington, DE 19804 800-880-8686

Florida

5858 **Lupus Foundation of America: Northeast Florida Chapter**
PO Box 10486 904-645-8398
Jacksonville, FL 32247-0486 800-853-8398

5859 **Lupus Foundation of America: Northwest Florida Chapter**
PO Box 17841 904-444-7070
Pensacola, FL 32522-7841 800-458-8211
e-mail: info@lupus.pensacola.com
www.lupus.pensacola.com

Brenda Lee, President
Jon Kagan, Vice President

5860 **Lupus Foundation of America: Southeast Florida Chapter**
75 NE 6th Avenue 561-279-8606
Delray Beach, FL 33483 800-339-0586
Fax: 561-279-9772
e-mail: info@lupusfl.org
www.lupusfl.com

Claudia Kirk Barto, Executive Director
Kathleen Laca, Director of Operations

5861 **Lupus Foundation of America: Suncoast Chapter**
3637 4th Street N 727-447-7075
St Petersburg, FL 33704-7485 800-684-9276
Fax: 727-447-8925
e-mail: info@lupusflorida.org
www.lupusfl.com

Michael J Keefer, President/CEO
Maggi McQueen, Chairman

5862 **Lupus Foundation of America: Tampa Area Chapter**
Dibbs Plaza
4119-20A Gunn Highway 813-960-3992
Tampa, FL 33624 800-330-3992
www.milupus.org/southeast.htm

5863 **Lupus Foundation of Florida**
4406 Urban Court 727-447-7075
Orlando, FL 32810 800-684-9276
Fax: 727-447-7075

Chapter of the Lupus Foundation of America.

Georgia

5864 **Lupus Foundation of America: Columbus Chapter**
233 12th Street
Columbus, GA 31901 706-571-8950
www.milupus.org/southeast.htm

5865 **Lupus Foundation of America: Greater Atlanta Chapter**
340 Interstate North Parkway NW 404-952-3891
Atlanta, GA 30339-2203 800-800-4532

Hawaii

5866 **Hawaii Lupus Foundation**
1200 College Walk 808-538-1522
Honolulu, HI 96817 800-201-1522
Chapter of the Lupus Foundation of America.

Idaho

5867 **Lupus Foundation of America: Idaho Chapter**
4696 Overland Road
Boise, ID 83705-2864 208-343-4907
www.lupuswest.topcities.com

Illinois

5868 **Lupus Foundation of America: Illinois Chapter**
740 N Rush Street 312-542-0002
Chicago, IL 60611 800-258-7872
Fax: 312-255-8020
e-mail: Paul@lupusil.org
www.lupusil.org

Paul Sakol, Interim President & CEO
Mary Dollear, Vice President of Health Promotion

Indiana

5869 **Lupus Foundation of America: Northeast Indiana Chapter**
5401 Keystone Drive 219-482-8205
Fort Wayne, IN 46825

5870 **Lupus Foundation of America: Northwest Indiana Lupus Chapter**
PO Box 2763 219-762-6575
Portage, IN 46368 800-948-8806
e-mail: lupusnwichapter@aol.com
www.lupusnwichapter.org

Tammie Largent, Director

5871 **Lupus Foundation of Indiana**
PO Box 51066
Indianapolis, IN 46251 317-858-9133
www.milupus.org/midwest.htm

Chapter of the Lupus Foundation of America.

Iowa

5872 **Lupus Foundation of America: Iowa Chapter**
PO Box 13174
Des Moines, IA 50310-1044
515-279-3048
888-279-3048
e-mail: info@lupusia.org
www.lupusia.org

Barb Hildebrandt, Executive Director
Braxton Pulley, Chair

Kansas

5873 **Lupus Foundation of America: Kansas Chapter**
PO Box 16094
Wichita, KS 67216
316-262-6180
e-mail: lupus@kansaslupus.org
www.kansaslupus.org

James Logue, President
Marilyn Rumsey, Treasurer

5874 **Lupus Foundation of America: Kansas City**
PO Box 12204
Wichita, KS 67277
316-262-6180
e-mail: lupus@kansaslupus.org
www.kansaslupus.org

Ruth Busch, President
Sandy Blaylock, Recording Secretary

Kentucky

5875 **Lupus Foundation of Kentuckiana**
1939 Goldsmith Lane
Louisville, KY 40218
502-456-5265
800-277-9681
www.milupus.org/southeast.htm
Chapter of the Lupus Foundation of America.

Louisiana

5876 **Louisiana Lupus Foundation**
7732 Goodwood Boulevard
Baton Rouge, LA 70806
225-927-8052
800-355-7473
www.milupus.org/southwest.htm
Chapter of the Lupus Foundation of America.

5877 **Lupus Foundation of America: Cenla Chapter**
PO Box 12565
Alexandria, LA 71315-2565
318-473-0125
www.lupus.org

5878 **Lupus Foundation of America: Northeast Louisiana**
102 Susan Drive
West Monroe, LA 71291
318-396-1333

5879 **Lupus Foundation of America: Shreveport Chapter**
6321 W Canal Boulevard
Shreveport, LA 71108
318-631-6531
www.lupus.org

Maine

5880 **Lupus Group of Maine**
PO Box 8168
Portland, ME 04104
207-878-8104
www.milupus.org/northeast.htm
Chapter of the Lupus Foundation of America.

Maryland

5881 **Maryland Lupus Foundation**
7400 York Road
Baltimore, MD 21204
410-337-9000
800-777-0934
Fax: 410-337-7406
e-mail: dwatson@lupusmd.org
www.lupusmd.org

Chapter of the Lupus Foundation of America.
Dick Watson, Executive Director
Jessica Gilbart, Health Education Coordinator

Massachusetts

5882 **Lupus Foundation of America: Massachusetts Chapter**
425 Watertown Street
Newton, MA 02158
617-332-9014
e-mail: info@lupusne.org
www.lupusmass.org

Elyse Smith, President
Lee McGraw, Board of Trustees Chair

Michigan

5883 **Lupus Foundation of America: Michigan Lupus Foundation**
26507 Harper Avenue
Saint Clair Shores, MI 48081
586-775-8310
800-705-6677
Fax: 586-775-8494
e-mail: info@milupus.org
www.milupus.org

Minnesota

5884 **Lupus Foundation of America: Minnesota Chapter**
2626 E 82nd Street
Bloomington, MN 55425
952-746-5151
800-645-1131
e-mail: info@lupusmn.org
www.lupusmn.org

Lynn Clarey, Chair
Chris McPartland, Chair Elect

Mississippi

5885 **Lupus Foundation of America: Mississippi Chapter**
PO Box 24292
Jackson, MS 39225-4292
601-366-5655
800-866-9606
www.milupus.org/southeast.htm

Missouri

5886 **Lupus Foundation of America: Kansas City Chapter**
6700 Troost
Kansas City, MO 64131
816-761-0850
866-761-0850
Fax: 816-361-0446
e-mail: info@lifewithlupus.org
www.lifewithlupus.org

5887 **Lupus Foundation of America: Missouri Chapter**
5701 Columbia Avenue
Saint Louis, MO 63139
314-644-2222
800-9LU-PUS6
e-mail: adminlupus@sbcglobal.net
www.lupusmo.org

Gina Banks, Chair
Necole Powell, Vice-Chair

5888 **Lupus Foundation of America: Ozarks Chapter**
3150 W Marty Street
Springfield, MO 65807
417-887-1560
www.lupus.org

Montana

5889 **Lupus Foundation of America: Montana Chapter**
29 1/2 Alderson
Billings, MT 59102
406-254-2082
www.lupus.org

Nebraska

5890 **Lupus Foundation of America: Omaha Chapter**
Community Health Plaza
7101 Newport Avenue
Omaha, NE 68152
402-572-3150
www.milupus.org/midwest.htm

5891 **Lupus Foundation of America: Western Nebraska Chapter**
HCR 72 Box 58
Sutherland, NE 69165
308-764-2474

Nevada

5892 **Lupus Foundation of America: Las Vegas Chapter**
1555 E Flamingo Suite 439
Las Vegas, NV 89119
702-369-0474
www.lupus.org

5893 **Lupus Foundation of America: Northern Nevada Chapter**
1755 Vassar Street
Reno, NV 89502
702-323-2444
www.lupus.org

New Hampshire

5894 **New Hampshire Lupus Foundation**
PO Box 444
Nashua, NH 03061-0444
603-424-0111
www.milupus.org

Chapter of the Lupus Foundation of America.

New Jersey

5895 **Lupus Foundation of America: New Jersey Chapter**
150 Morris Avenue Suite 102
Springfield, NJ 07081
973-379-3226
800-322-5816
Fax: 973-379-1053
e-mail: info@lupusnj.org
www.lupusnj.org

Dianna Beck-Clemens, Interim President and CEO
Adam Gold, Development Associate

5896 **Lupus Foundation of America: South Jersey Chapter**
One Greentree Center
Marlton, NJ 08053
856-988-5444
Fax: 856-596-8359
e-mail: lupusinfo@sjlupus.org
www.sjlupus.org

New Mexico

5897 **Lupus Foundation of America: New Mexico Chapter**
6001 Marble Avenue NE
Albuquerque, NM 87110
505-881-9081
800-843-9081
e-mail: info@lupusnm.org
www.lfanm.org

New York

5898 **Lupus Foundation of America: Long Island/Queens Chapter**
2255 Centre Avenue
Bellmore, NY 11710
516-783-3370
888-57L-UPUS
Fax: 516-826-2058
e-mail: LupusLiQueens@aol.com
www.lupusliqueens.org

Jo Ann Quinn, Executive Director
Nancy Beder, Director of Resources

5899 **Lupus Foundation of America: Bronx Chapter**
PO Box 1117
Bronx, NY 10462
718-822-6542
www.milupus.org/northeast.htm

5900 **Lupus Foundation of America: Central New York Chapter**
Pickard Office Building
5858 E Molloy Road
Syracuse, NY 13211
315-454-9886
e-mail: cnylupus@dreamscape.com
www.milupus.org/northeast.htm

5901 **Lupus Foundation of America: Genessee Valley Chapter**
500 Helendale Road
Rochester, NY 14609
585-288-2910
Fax: 585-288-1608
e-mail: lupusgvc@frontiernet.net
www.lupusgvc.org

Eileen M Aman, President/CEO
Bob Stewart, Chairperson

5902 **Lupus Foundation of America: Marguerite Curri Chapter**
PO Box 139
Utica, NY 13503
315-829-4272
866-2LU-PUS4
Fax: 315-829-4272
e-mail: lupusmidny@aol.com
www.nolupus.org

Kathleen A Arntsen, President/CEO
James E Mitchell Jr, Vice President

5903 **Lupus Foundation of America: New York Southern Tier Chapter**
PO Box 139
Utica, NY 13503
315-829-4272
866-2LU-PUS4
Fax: 315-829-4272
e-mail: lupusmidny@aol.com
www.nolupus.org

Kathleen A Arntsen, President/CEO
James E Mitchell Jr, Vice President

5904 **Lupus Foundation of America: Northeastern New York Chapter**
1300 Piccard Drive
Rockville, MD 20850-4303
301-670-9292
800-558-0121
Fax: 301-670-9486
e-mail: nenylfa@aol.com
nenylfa.tripod.com

5905 **Lupus Foundation of America: Westchester**
100 S Bedford Road
Mt Kisco, NY 10549
914-948-1032
888-57L-UPUS
e-mail: pguidice@stellarishealth.org
www.lupushudsonvalley.org

5906 **Lupus Foundation of America: Western New York Chapter**
3871 Harlem Road
Cheektowaga, NY 14215
716-835-7161
800-300-4198
Fax: 716-835-7251
e-mail: info@lupusupstateny.org
www.lupusupstateny.org

5907 **SLE Foundation**
330 Seventh Avenue
New York, NY 10001
212-685-4118
800-74L-UPUS
Fax: 212-545-1843
e-mail: lupus@lupusny.org
www.lupusny.org

Chapter of the Lupus Foundation of America.
Richard D DeScherer, President
Margaret G Dowd, Executive Director

North Carolina

5908 **Lupus Foundation of America: Winston-Triad Lupus Chapter NCLF**
2841 Foxwood Lane
Winston Salem, NC 27103
910-768-1493
Ruth Banbury, President

5909 **Lupus Foundation of America: Charlotte Chapter**
2540 Plantation Center Drive
Matthews, NC 28105
704-849-8271
877-849-8271
Fax: 704-849-8272
e-mail: info@lupuslinks.org
www.lupuslinks.org

Christine M John, President/CEO
Ginger Dickerson, Chairman of the Board

5910 **Lupus Foundation of America: Raleigh Chapter**
5409 Belsay Drive
Raleigh, NC 27612
919-783-8288
www.milupus.org/southeast.htm

Ohio

5911 **Lupus Foundation of America: Akron Area Chapter**
2769 Front Street
Cuyahoga Falls, OH 44221
330-945-6767
877-635-8787
Fax: 330-945-5703
www.lupus.org

Sharon Combs

5912 Lupus Foundation of America: Columbus
6119 E Main Street 614-755-5077
Columbus, OH 43213 Fax: 614-755-5066
e-mail: lupusoff@aol.com
www.lupusohio.org
Janice Washington, President
Melvyn Little, Chair of Public Relations

5913 Lupus Foundation of America: Columbus, Marcy Zitron Chapter
6161 Busch Boulevard 614-221-0811
Columbus, OH 43229

5914 Lupus Foundation of America: Greater Cleveland Chapter
12930 Chippewa Road 440-717-0183
Brecksville, OH 44141 Fax: 440-717-0186
e-mail: info@lupuscleveland.org
www.lupuscleveland.org
Suzanne Tierney, Executive Director
David Wonsetler, Counselor

5915 Lupus Foundation of America: North Texas
1800 N Blanchard Street 419-423-9313
Findlay, OH 45840 Fax: 419-423-5959
e-mail: info@lupusnwoh.org
www.lupus.org
Bob Scherger, President/CEO
Jackie Urbanski, VP Education & Volunteer Programs

5916 Lupus Foundation of America: Northwest Ohio Lupus Chapter
1710 Manor Hill Road 419-423-9313
Findlay, OH 45840 888-33L-UPUS
Fax: 419-423-5959
e-mail: info@lupusnwoh.org
www.lupusnwoh.org

Oklahoma

5917 Oklahoma Lupus Association
4100 N Lincoln Boulevard 405-427-8787
Oklahoma City, OK 73105 Fax: 405-427-8778
e-mail: oklupus@flash.net
www.oklupus.com
Chapter of the Lupus Foundation of America.
Katherine Scheirman, Vice Chairman
Janna D Hall, Chairman

Pennsylvania

5918 Lupus Foundation of America: Central Pennsylvania Chapter
Old Liberty Square
4813 Jonestown Road 717-671-9515
Harrisburg, PA 17109 e-mail: cplclfa@aol.com

5919 Lupus Foundation of America: Delaware Valley Chapter
25 Washington Lane 215-517-5070
Wyncote, PA 19095 866-517-5070
Fax: 215-517-8483
e-mail: info@lupustristate.org
www.lupustristate.org
Eileen Harmo Council, President
Cheri M Perron, Secretary

5920 Lupus Foundation of America: Northeast Pennsylvania Chapter
615 Jefferson Avenue 570-558-2008
Scranton, PA 18510 888-995-8787
Fax: 570-558-2009
e-mail: neinfo@lupuspa.org
www.lupuspa.org
Beth Rundell MS, Branch Director
Cathy Wilcox, Patient Services Director

5921 Lupus Foundation of America: Northwestern Pennsylvania Chapter
PO Box 885 724-962-0368
Erie, PA 16512-0885 866-292-1472
Fax: 724-962-0368
e-mail: ericinfo@lupuspa.org
www.lupuspa.org
Jane Lippinc RN, Patient Services Consultant
Bill Trainor, Events Coordinator

5922 Lupus Foundation of America: West Texas Landmarks Building
100 W Station Square Drive 412-261-5886
Pittsburgh, PA 15219 Fax: 412-261-5365
e-mail: info@lupuspa.org
www.lupuspa.org
Deborah Nigro, Executive Director
Marian Belotti, Patient Services Director

5923 Lupus Foundation of America: Western Pennsylvania Chapter
Landmarks Building
100 West Station Square Drive 412-261-5886
Pittsburgh, PA 15219 800-800-5776
Fax: 412-261-5365
e-mail: info@lupuspa.org
www.lupuspa.org
Deborah Nigro, Executive Director
Barbara Hastings, RN, Patient Services Director

5924 Lupus Foundation of Philadelphia
5415 Claridge Street 215-877-9061
Philadelphia, PA 19124
Chapter of the Lupus Foundation of America.

Rhode Island

5925 Lupus Foundation of America: Rhode Island Chapter
#8 Fallon Avenue
Providence, RI 02908 401-421-7227
www.milupus.org

South Carolina

5926 Lupus Foundation of America: South Carolina Chapter
L.E. Support Club
8039 Nova Court 843-764-1769
Charleston, SC 29420-8934 e-mail: hmeisic@awod.com
www.galaxymall.com/commerce/lupus

Tennessee

5927 Lupus Foundation of America: East Tennessee Chapter
5612 Kingston Pike 615-584-5215
Knoxville, TN 37919 e-mail: lupustn@aol.com
www.lupus.org/chapters/southeastern.html

5928 Lupus Foundation of America: Memphis Area Chapter
3181 Poplar Avenue 901-458-5302
Memphis, TN 38111 e-mail: MemphisLFA@yahoo.com
www.memphislfa.com
Acquanetta Thomas, President/CEO
John J Davis, Vice President/Chair of Board

5929 Lupus Foundation of America: Mid-South Area Chapter
4004 Hillsboro Road 615-298-2273
Nashville, TN 37215 877-865-8787
Fax: 615-292-0520
e-mail: info@lupusmidsouth.org
www.lupustennessee.org
Sherry Hammond, Executive Director
Renee Levay Stewart, President

Texas

5930 Lupus Foundation of America: North Texas Chapter
15441 Knoll Trail 469-374-0590
Dallas, TX 75248 800-285-2369
Fax: 469-374-0794
e-mail: info@lupus-northtexas.org
www.lupus-northtexas.org
Tessie Holloway, President/CEO
Lisa Christensen, Development Director

5931 Lupus Foundation of America: South Central Texas Chapter
9330 Corporate Drive 210-651-9480
Selma, TX 78154 800-809-3953
e-mail: salupus@texas.net
www.milupus.org/southwest.htm

5932 **Lupus Foundation of America: Texas Gulf Coast Chapter**
3730 Kirby Drive
Houston, TX 77098
713-529-0126
800-458-7870
Fax: 713-529-0780
e-mail: info@lupustexas.org
www.lupustexas.org

Janice Gipson, President
Christine Smith, Vice President

5933 **Lupus Foundation of America: West Texas Chapter**
1717 Avenue K
Lubbock, TX 79401
806-744-6666
800-580-5878
e-mail: lfawesttx@juno.com
www.milupus.org/southwest.htm

Utah

5934 **Lupus Foundation of America Utah Chapter**
455 E 500 S
Salt Lake City, UT 84111
801-364-0366
800-657-6398
e-mail: info@utahlupus.org
www.utahlupus.org

Noelle Reymond, Executive Director
Katie Fillnow, President

Vermont

5935 **Lupus Foundation of America: Vermont Chapter**
57 S Main Street
Waterbury, VT 05676
802-244-5988
877-735-8787
e-mail: lupusvermont@myfairpoint.net
www.central-vt.com/web/lupus

Virginia

5936 **Lupus Foundation of America: Central Virginia Chapter**
PO Box 25418
Richmond, VA 23260-5418
804-262-9622

5937 **Lupus Foundation of America: Eastern Virginia Chapter**
Pembroke One
281 Independence Boulevard
Virginia Beach, VA 23462
757-490-2793
www.lupus.org

5938 **Lupus Foundation of Greater Washington**
2000 L Street NW
Washington, DC 20036
202-349-1167
888-349-1167
Fax: 202-223-1970
e-mail: info@lupusgw.org
www.lupusgw.org

Penelope C Fletcher, President
Sarah Guy, Executive Assistant

Washington

5939 **Lupus Foundation of America: Pacific Northwest Chapter**
1207 N 200th Street
Shoreline, WA 98133
206-546-6785
Fax: 206-546-8946
e-mail: lupus@lupuspnw.org
www.lupuspnw.org

Kathy Casey, Executive Director
Tonita Webb, President

Wisconsin

5940 **Lupus Foundation of America: Wisconsin Chapter**
1109 N Mayfair Road
Milwaukee, WI 53226
414-443-6400
866-LUP-USWI
Fax: 414-443-6400
e-mail: lupuswi@lupuswi.org
www.lupuswi.org

Sandra Hofstetter, Executive Director
Angela K Nelson, Chairman

Foundations

5941 **SLE Lupus Foundation**
330 Seventh Avenue
New York, NY 10001
212-685-4118
Fax: 212-545-1843
e-mail: lupus@lupusny.org
www.lupusny.org

The Foundation helps people with lupus, as well as their families and friends, cope with the anxieties and frustrations that often accompany daily living with a chronic illness. Sharing information and networking among patients and their families further helps dispel myths and provides daily support to those learning to live with lupus.
Richard K DeScherer, President
Margaret G Dowd, Executive Director

Research Centers

5942 **Alliance for Lupus Research**
28 W 44th Street
New York, NY 10036
212-218-2840
800-867-1743
e-mail: info@lupusresearch.org
www.lupusresearch.org

Research foundation dedicated to providing information about lupus.

5943 **Hahnemann University Lupus Study Center Hahnemann University Medical Center**
Hahnemann University Medical Center
Broad and Vine Street
Philadelphia, PA 19102
215-762-7000
Fax: 215-762-8109
www.hahnemannhospital.com

Raphael J Dehoratius, Director

5944 **Terri Gotthelf Lupus Research Institute**
3 Duke Place
S Norwalk, CT 06854
800-828-87
Fax: 203-852-9720

Founded to help millions of lupus victims in the world and to encourage coordinate and direct future progress in the etiology diagnosis and treatment of this disease.
Theodore Gotthelf, President

Support Groups & Hotlines

5945 **National Health Information Center**
PO Box 1133
Washington, DC 20013
310-565-4167
800-336-4797
Fax: 301-984-4256
e-mail: info@nhic.org
www.health.gov/nhic

Offers a nationwide information referral service, produces directories and resource guides.

Books

5946 **Coping with Lupus**
Lupus Foundation of America
1300 Piccard Drive
Rockville, MD 20850-4303
301-670-9292
800-558-0121
www.lupus.org

A practicing psychologist offers sound, meaningful and compassionate advice to individuals who must deal with lupus.
276 pages Paperback
ISBN: 0-895294-75-3

5947 **Disability Workbook for Social Security Disability Applicants**
Lupus Foundation of America
1300 Piccard Drive
Rockville, MD 20850-4303
301-670-9292
800-558-0121
www.lupus.org

Helps people get their disability benefits promptly, without unnecessary appeals. Tells what you have to prove and how to prove it.
137 pages

5948 **Get to Sleep! How to Sleep Well...Despite Lupus**
Lupus Foundation of America

1300 Piccard Drive 301-670-9292
Rockville, MD 20850-4303 800-558-0121
Written in a simple, straightforward style, this easy-to-follow action guide teaches you the most effective strategies for enabling you to get the sleep you want and need!
17 pages

5949 Lupus Book
Lupus Foundation of America
1300 Piccard Drive 301-670-9292
Rockville, MD 20850-4303 800-558-0121
Packed with useful, easy-to-understand information and practical guidance for people with lupus, their family members, friends and physicians. This hardcover book explains virtually every aspect of the disease and will help people better manage their day-to-day fight with lupus.

ISBN: 0-195084-43-8

5950 Lupus Erythematosus: A Handbook for Physicians, Patients & Families
Lupus Foundation of America
1300 Piccard Drive 301-670-9292
Rockville, MD 20850-4303 800-558-0121
www.lupus.org
Written for physicians, people with lupus, their families and friends, this is LFA's most popular publication. The handbook provides a brief, but detailed, overview of the disease and guide for living well with lupus.
60 pages

5951 Lupus: Everything You Need to Know
Lupus Foundation of America
1300 Piccard Drive 301-670-9292
Rockville, MD 20850-4303 800-558-0121
e-mail: lupusinfo@aol.com
www.lupus.org
Resource written for patients that want to learn more about lupus than what their doctors may or may not tell them.
236 pages

5952 Sick and Tired of Feeling Sick and Tired
Lupus Foundation of America
1300 Piccard Drive 301-670-9292
Rockville, MD 20850-4303 800-558-0121
www.lupus.org
Written in simple terms, the authors offer all readers- people with invisible chronic illness (ICI's), spouses, friends, family members, employers or health care providers, both understanding and practical guidance. This is a very useful resource for all those who live with ICI's and those who care for and about them.
288 pages

5953 We Are Not Alone: Learning to Live with Chronic Illness
Lupus Foundation of America
1300 Piccard Drive 301-670-9292
Rockville, MD 20850-4303 800-558-0121
www.lupus.org
Complete and comprehensive, this book is about redesigning your life... about how to live better, not just differently.
335 pages

Children's Books

5954 Embracing the Wolf: A Lupus Victim and Her Family Learn to Live
Cherokee Publishing Company
PO Box 1730 770-438-7366
Marietta, GA 30061-1730 800-653-3952
This book gives a very detailed account of the effects of the disease that include emotions and moods for the victim and the way in which these attributes affect loved ones.
192 pages Hardcover
ISBN: 0-877971-66-8
Kenneth W Boyd, Publisher

5955 In Search of the Sun: A Woman's Courageous Victory Over Lupus
Scribner
866 3rd Avenue 212-702-2000
New York, NY 10022-6221 800-257-5755
This book is a revision of Henrietta Aladjem's book, The Sun Is My Enemy. In this book, with Peter Schur she discusses her fight with this deadly and widespread disease.
Grades 10-12

5956 When Mom Gets Sick
Lupus Foundation of America
1300 Piccard Drive 301-670-9292
Rockville, MD 20850-4303 800-558-0121
www.lupus.org
Written and illustrated by a 9-year-old, this is a compelling story based on the experiences of a sensitive and insightful young girl who makes the best from what could be a devastating situation.
27 pages

Newsletters

5957 Heliogram
Lupus Network
230 Ranch Drive 203-372-5795
Bridgeport, CT 06606-1747
Includes book reviews, medical abstracts and resource listings of physicians.
Quarterly
ISBN: 0-887168-0 -
Linda Rosinsky, Editor

5958 Informer
Simon Foundation
PO Box 815 847-864-3913
Wilmette, IL 60091-0815 Fax: 847-864-9758
Offers information and the latest updates concerning incontinence treatments, cures, medical aspects, resources and more.
Quarterly

5959 Lupus News
Lupus Foundation of America
1300 Piccard Drive 301-670-9292
Rockville, MD 20850-4303 800-558-0121
Provides detailed news for physicians, patients, their families and friends on lupus.
Quarterly

5960 The Loop
SLE Lupus Foundation
330 Seventh Avenue 212-685-4118
New York, NY 10001 Fax: 212-545-1843
e-mail: lupus@lupusny.org
www.lupusny.org

Richard K DeScherer, President
Margaret G Dowd, Executive Director

Pamphlets

5961 Control Your Pain!
Lupus Foundation of America
1300 Piccard Drive 301-670-9292
Rockville, MD 20850-4303 800-558-0121
www.lupus.org
This easy to read booklet offers 144 concrete strategies for reducing and managing the pain of lupus.
48 pages

5962 Facts About Lupus
Lupus Foundation of America
1300 Piccard Drive 301-670-9292
Rockville, MD 20850-4303 800-558-0121
A series of brochures on a wide range of lupus-related topics including lab tests, medications, joint and muscle involvement, skin involvement, lupus and the kidneys, central nervous system involvement, lupus in men, pregnancy, well/coping, etc.
21 Brochures

5963 Handout on Health: Systemic Lupus Erythematosus
NAMSIC/National Institutes of Health

1 AMS Circle
Bethesda, MD 20892-0001
301-495-4484
877-226-4267
Fax: 301-718-6366
TTY: 301-565-2966
e-mail: niamsinfo@mail.nih.gov
www.nih.gov/niams

5964 **Living Well, Despite Lupus!**
Lupus Foundation of America
1300 Piccard Drive
Rockville, MD 20850
301-670-9292
800-558-0121
This booklet offers 204 sure-fire strategies for taking charge of your life to enable you to live well.
1996 50 pages
ISBN: 0-895294-75-3

5965 **Lupus Eritematoso (Spanish Booklet)**
Lupus Foundation of America
1300 Piccard Drive
Rockville, MD 20850-4303
301-670-9292
800-558-0121
www.lupus.org
Written for physicians, people with lupus, their families and friends, this is LFA's most popular publication. The handbook provides a brief, but detailed, overview of the disease and guide for living well with lupus.

5966 **Lupus Erythematosus**
Lupus Foundation of America
1300 Piccard Drive
Rockville, MD 20850-4303
301-670-9292
800-558-0121
www.lupus.org/lupus
This booklet is intended to help patients understand what lupus is, how it may affect their lives and what they can do to help themselves and their physician in the management of the illness.

5967 **Lupus Information Package**
NAMSIC/National Institutes of Health
1 AMS Circle
Bethesda, MD 20892-0001
301-495-4484
877-226-4267
Fax: 301-718-6366
TTY: 301-565-2966
e-mail: niamsinfo@mail.nih.gov
www.nih.gov/niams

5968 **Many Shades of Lupus: Information for Multicultural Communities**
NAMSIC/National Institutes of Health
1 AMS Circle
Bethesda, MD 20892-0001
301-495-4484
877-226-4267
Fax: 301-587-4352
TTY: 301-565-2966
e-mail: niamsinfo@mail.nih.gov
www.nih.gov/niams

Audio & Video

5969 **For Life: More Stories of Lupus**
Marcia Urbin Raymond, author
Fanlight Productions
4196 Washington Street
Boston, MA 02131
617-469-4999
800-937-4113
Fax: 617-469-3349
e-mail: fanlight@fanlight.com
www.fanlight.com
Three years after 'Stories of Lupus', the filmmaker revisits five people from the earlier film, to explore the day-to-day challenges and gifts that come to people living with a chronic illness as it evolves over time.
2002 53 Minutes
ISBN: 1-572954-17-5
Nicole Johnson, Publicity Coordinator

5970 **Stories of Lupus**
Fanlight Productions
4196 Washington Street
Boston, MA 02131
617-469-4999
800-937-4113
Fax: 617-469-3379
e-mail: fanlight@fanlight.com
www.fanlight.com
Recently diagnosed with lupus, the filmmakers go on the road to interview others enduring the precarious roller coaster of symptoms, treatment, flare-ups and recoveries which characterize this complex, mysterious, and often life-threatening disease.
1999 27 Minutes
ISBN: 1-572954-16-7
Nicole Johnson, Publicity Coordinator

Web Sites

5971 **Healing Well**
www.healingwell.com
An online health resource guide to medical news, chat, information and articles, newsgroups and message boards, books, disease-related web sites, medical directories, and more for patients, friends, and family coping with disabling diseases, disorders, or chronic illnesses.

5972 **Health Finder**
www.healthfinder.gov
Searchable, carefully developed web site offering information on over 1000 topics. Developed by the US Department of Health and Human Services, the site can be used in both English and Spanish.

5973 **Healthlink USA**
www.healthlinkusa.com
Health information concerning treatment, cures, prevention, diagnosis, risk factors, research, support groups, email lists, personal stories and much more. Updated regularly.

5974 **Helios Health**
www.helioshealth.com
Online resource for your health information. Detailed information about specific health topics, access to expert advice from our Medical Advisory Board, and up-to-date health news.

5975 **Lupus Foundation of America**
www.lupus.org
The LFA mission is to assist local chapters in their efforts to provide supportive services to individuals living with lupus, educate the public about lupus, and supports research into the cause and cure of lupus.

5976 **MedicineNet**
www.medicinenet.com
An online resource for consumers providing easy-to-read, authoritative medical and health information.

5977 **Medscape**
www.mywebmd.com
Medscape offers specialists, primary care physicians, and other health professionals the Web's most robust and integrated medical information and educational tools.

5978 **WebMD**
www.webmd.com
Information on Lupus Erythematosus, including articles and resources.

Description

5979 **Mental Illness/General**

Mental illness includes disorders of mood, thinking and behavior, with psychiatry being the branch of medicine responsible for their study, diagnosis, treatment, and prevention. Mental illness may be determined by genetic, physical, chemical, psychologic, and social factors. Mental or emotional illness includes such conditions as major depression, schizophrenia, bipolar disorder (i.e., manic depression), panic and other anxiety disorders, substance abuse and dependence, and dementia and other cognitive disorders.

Psychiatric diagnoses generally are based on criteria outlined in *Diagnostic and Statistical Manual of Mental Disorders* (DSM-IV), published by the American Psychiatric Association. Depending on the specific diagnosis, treatment can include medication, counseling, behavior modification, psychotherapy, and modification of the patient's environment. See also *Mental Illness/Depression* and *Mental Illness/Schizophrenia*.

National Agencies & Associations

5980 **Action Autonomie**
1260 Ste-Cataherine E #208 514-525-5060
Montreal, Quebec, H2L-2H2 Fax: 514-525-5580
e-mail: lecollectif@actionautonomie.qc.ca
www.actionautonomie.qc.ca
Community organization set up by people living or having lived with mental health problems who believed in the necessity of uniting their efforts collectively in order to defend their rights.

5981 **American Academy of Child & Adolescent Psychiatry**
3615 Wisconsin Avenue NW 202-966-7300
Washington, DC 20016 Fax: 202-966-2891
e-mail: communications@aacap.org
www.aacap.org
A professional organization that represents 7 500 child and adolescent psychiatrists that actively research diagnose and treat psychiatric and mental illness disorders in children and adolescents.
Robert Hendren, President

5982 **American Association of Children's Residential Centers**
11700 W Lake Park Drive 877-332-2272
Milwaukee, WI 53224 Fax: 877-36A-ACRC
e-mail: info@aacrc-dc.org
www.aacrc-dc.org
Brings professionals together to advance the frontiers of knowledge pertaining to the spectrum of therapeutic living environments for adolescents with behavioral health disorders.
Steven Elson, President
Richard Altman, Secretary

5983 **American Association on Mental Retardation**
444 N Capitol Street NW 202-387-1968
Washington, DC 20001-1512 800-424-3688
Fax: 202-387-2193
www.aamr.org
Promotes progressive policies sound research effective practices and universal human rights for people with intellectual and developmental disabilities.
Steve M Eidelman, President
Doreen M Croser, Executive Director

5984 **American Psychiatric Association**
1000 Wilson Boulevard 703-907-7300
Arlington, VA 22209-3901 888-357-7924
e-mail: apa@psych.org
www.psych.org
Works to promote the best interest of patients and those actually or potentially making use of psychiatric services.

5985 **American Psychological Association**
750 1st Street NE 202-336-5500
Washington, DC 20002-4242 800-374-2721
TTY: 202-336-6123
e-mail: practice@apa.org
www.apa.org
A scientific and professional organization the represents psychology in the United States. The largest association of psychologists worldwide.
James H Bray, President

5986 **Calgary Association of Self Help**
1019-7th Avenue SW 403-266-8711
Calgary, Alberta, T2P-1A8 Fax: 403-266-2478
e-mail: calgaryselfhelp@shaw.ca
www.calgaryselfhelp.com
Calgary Association of Self Help have been assisting people with a mental illness to live full lives within our community since 1973.
Marion McGrath, CEO
Anneisa Lauchlan, COO

5987 **Canadian Federation of Mental Health Nurse s**
1185 Eglinton Avenue E 416-426-7029
Toronto, Ontario, M3C-3C6 Fax: 416-426-7280
e-mail: info@cfmhn.ca
www.cfmhn.ca
A national voice for psychiatric and mental health (PMH) nursing.
Chris Davis, President

5988 **Canadian Mental Health Association**
180 Dundas Street W 416-484-7750
Toronto, Ontario, M5G-1Z8 Fax: 416-484-4617
e-mail: info@cmha.ca
www.cmha.ca
Promotes the mental health of all and supports the resilience and recovery of people experiencing mental illness.
Glenn Thompson, CEO
Christine Saracino, Director Finance

5989 **Center for Mental Health Services: Knowledge Exchange Network**
PO Box 42557
Washington, DC 20015 800-789-2647
Fax: 240-221-4295
TTY: 866-889-2647
TDD: 866-889-2647
e-mail: ken@mentalhealth.org
www.mentalhealth.org
Goal is to provide the treatment and support services needed by adults with mental disorders and children with serious emotional problems.
A Kathryn Power MEd, Director
Jeffrey A Buck PhD, Branch Chief

5990 **Coalition of Voluntary Mental Health Agencies**
90 Broad Street 212-742-1600
New York, NY 10014 Fax: 212-742-2080
e-mail: mailbox@cvmha.org
www.coalitionny.org
An umbrella advocacy organization of New York's mental health community representing over 100 non-profit community health agencies that serve more than 300 000 clients in the five boroughs of New York City and its environs.
Peter Campan PsyD, Past President
Donna Colonna, Vice President

5991 **Community Access**
666 Broadway 212-780-1400
New York, NY 10012 Fax: 212-780-1412
e-mail: info@communityaccess.org
www.cairn.org
A nonprofit agency providing housing and advocacy for people with psychiatric disabilities.
Stephen Chase, President
Karen Roth, Vice President

5992 Federation of Families for Children's Mental Health
1101 King Street
Alexandria, VA 22314
703-684-7710
Fax: 703-836-1040
e-mail: ffcmh@ffchm.org
www.ffcmh.org
Provides leadership to develop and sustain a nationwide network of family-run organizations.
Sandra Spencer, Executive Director
Marion Mealing, Administrative Assistant

5993 Mental Health America
2000 N Beauregard Street
Alexandria, VA 22311
703-684-7722
800-969-6642
Fax: 703-684-5968
TTY: 800-433-5959
e-mail: infoctr@mentalhealthamerica.net
www.mentalhealthamerica.net
Mental Health America (formerly National Mental Health Association) is dedicated to helping all people live mentally healthier lives. With our more than 320 affiliates nationwide, we represent a growing movement of Americans who promote mental health.
340+ Members
David L Shern PhD, President/CEO
Eileen Sexton, Vice President Communications

5994 Mental Health America (formerly NMHA) Resource Center
2000 North Beauregard Street
Alexandria, VA 22311
703-684-7722
800-969-6642
Fax: 703-684-5968
TTY: 800-433-5959
e-mail: www.mentalhealthamerica.net/help/index.c
www.nmha.org
The NMHA publishes pamphlets and booklets on many aspects of mental health and mental illnesses. Topics include children and families, recovery, doctor/patient communication, mental health policy, culturally competent services, teen suicide, coping, schizphrenia, stress, depression and many others.
340+ Members

5995 National Alliance for the Mentally Ill
Colonial Place Three
2107 Wilson Boulevard
Arlington, VA 22201-3042
703-524-7600
800-950-6264
Fax: 703-524-9094
TDD: 703-516-7227
e-mail: bbc@naimi.org
www.nami.org
The leading self-help organization for families and friends of those suffering from serious mental illnesses and those persons themselves. Over 900 affiliate groups nationwide offer support to members, advocate better lives for their loved ones, support research efforts and educate the public to reduce the stigma attached to serious mental illnesses.
Bob Carolla, Director Communications

5996 National Association of State Mental Health Program Directors
66 Canal Center Plaza
Alexandria, VA 22314
703-739-9333
Fax: 703-548-9517
e-mail: webmaster@nasmhpd.org
www.nasmhpd.org
Offers referrals to state mental health programs services and physicians for persons with mental illness.
Virginia Tro Betts, President
James S Reinhard, Vice President

5997 National Association of Therapeutic Wilderness Camps
437 William Avenue Suite 5
Davis, WV 26260
e-mail: natwc@gcol.net
www.natwc.org
Represents nearly fifty therapeutic wilderness camps located all over the US. We believe therapeutic wilderness camps represent the most effective method to help troubled young people change the way they deal with their parents, school and other authorities.
Rick McClintock, Executive Director

5998 National Council for Community Behavior Healthcare
12300 Twinbrook Parkway
Rockville, MD 20852
301-984-6200
Fax: 301-881-7159
e-mail: lindar@thenationalcouncil.org
www.thenationalcouncil.org
Represents community mental health centers working on Capitol Hill to ensure funding for community mental health services. Offers technical support and guidance and serves as a liaison with state organizations and other mental health related organizations.
Linda Rosenb MSW CSW, President/ CEO
Jeannie Campbell, Executive Vice President

5999 National Hispanic Coalition of Health and Human Service Organizations
1501 16th Street NW
Washington, DC 20036
202-387-5000
Fax: 202-265-8027
e-mail: alliance@hispanichealth.org
www.hispanichealth.org
Members are Spanish-speaking mental health professionals and patients and those interested in the special emotional needs of Hispanics.
Jane L Delgado PhD, President
Adolph Falcon, Vice President for Science and Policy

6000 National Institute of Mental Health
6001 Executive Boulevard
Bethesda, MD 20892-9663
301-443-4513
866-615-6464
Fax: 301-443-4279
TTY: 301-443-8431
e-mail: nimhinfo@nih.gov
www.nimh.nih.gov
A federal agency that supports research nationwide on mental illness and mental health. The Institute provides research, demonstrations and technical assistance concerning the housing and service needs of the homeless mentally ill population.
Thomas R Insel MD, Director
Aleisha S James, Grants Management Specialist (AFP)

6001 National Mental Health Services Knowledge Exchange Network
PO Box 42557
Washington, DC 20015
800-789-2647
Fax: 240-747-5470
TTY: 866-889-2647
TDD: 866-889-2647
e-mail: nmhic-info@samhsa.hhs.gov
www.mentalhealth.org
The National Mental Health Information Center was developed for users of mental health services and their families, the general public, policy makers, providers and the media.
A Kathryn Power MEd, Director
Edward B Searle, Deputy Director

6002 National Network for Mental Health (NNMH) s
55 King Street
St. Catharines, Ontario, L2R-3H5
905-682-2423
888-406-4663
Fax: 905-682-7469
e-mail: info@nnmh.ca
www.nnmh.ca
Network with Canadian consumer/survivors and family and friends of consumer/survivors to provide opportunities for resource sharing, information distribution and education on mental health issues.
Roy Muise, President
Joan Edwards-Karmazyn, VP

6003 Obsessive Compulsive Information Center Dean Foundation
Dean Foundation
7617 Mineral Point Road
Madison, WI 53717-1914
608-827-2470
Fax: 608-827-2479
e-mail: mim@miminc.org
www.miminc.org
Provides access to published literature on obsessive compulsive disorder certain obsessive compulsive spectrum disorders and their treatments.

6004 Option Istitute Learning and Training Center
2080 S. Undermountain Road
Sheffield, MA 01257
413-229-2100
800-714-2779
Fax: 413-229-8931
e-mail: happiness@option.org
www.option.org
As the worldwide teaching center for the Option Process(R). The Option Institute offers empowering personal growth programs and seminars using life-changing experiential learning techniques that help people overcome adversity, maximize their success and hap-

piness and greatly improve their health, career, relationships and quality of life.
Zoe

6005 Texas Mining and Reclamation Association
100 Congress Avenue 512-236-2325
Austin, TX 78701 Fax: 512-236-2002
e-mail: information@tmra.com
www.tmra.com
Serves as a unified voice for mental health patients in consumer social and political affairs. Helps members to live outside a hospital setting by providing assistance in the areas of resocialization, employment and housing.
Mark Pelizza, Chairman
Mike Kezar, Vice Chair

6006 World Federation for Mental Health
12940 Harbor Drive 703-494-6515
Woodbridge, VA 22192 Fax: 703-494-6518
e-mail: info@wfmh.com
www.wfmh.com
WFMH is an international membership organization founded in 1948 to advance among all peoples and nations the prevention of mental and emotional disorders the proper treatment and care of those with such disorders and the promotion of mental health.
John Copeland, President
Preston J Garrison, Secretary-General/CEO

State Agencies & Associations

Alabama

6007 National Alliance on Mental Illness of Alabama
4122 Wall Street 334-396-4797
Montgomery, AL 36106-1902 800-626-4199
Fax: 334-396-4794
e-mail: Terri@NAMIAlabama.org
www.namialabama.org
Greg Carlson, President
Terri Beasley, Executive Director

Alaska

6008 National Alliance on Mental Illness of Alaska
144 W 15th Avenue 907-277-1300
Anchorage, AK 99501-5106 Fax: 907-277-1400
e-mail: trishmcd@nami.org
www.nami.org/sites/alaska
Trish McDonald, Program/Education Director
Beth LaCrosse, Treasurer

Arizona

6009 Mentally Ill Kids In Distress
2642 E Thomas Road 602-253-1240
Phoenix, AZ 85016-2723 800-35M-IKID
Fax: 602-253-1250
e-mail: Phoenix@MIKID.org
www.mikid.org
Vicki Johnso MA, Executive Director
Steve Carter, President

6010 Mentally Ill Kids in Distress Sue Gilbertson
Sue Gilbertson
2642 E Thomas Road 602-253-1240
Phoenix, AZ 85016 800-35M-IKID
Fax: 602-253-1250
e-mail: Phoenix@MIKID.org
www.mikid.org
Vicki Johnso MA, Executive Director
Steve Carter, President

6011 National Alliance on Mental Illness of Arizona
2210 N 7th Street 602-244-8166
Phoenix, AZ 85006-1604 Fax: 602-244-9264
e-mail: namiaz@namiaz.org
www.namiaz.org
Provides emotional support education and advocacy to persons of all ages who are affected by serious mental illnesses. Supports research to find a cure.
Robert Hess, Executive Director
Cheryl Fanning, President

6012 Navaho Nation K'E Project: Tuba City Children & Families Advocacy Corp
PO Box 3937 520-283-5415
Tuba City, AZ 86045 Fax: 520-283-5413
Rueben McCabe

6013 Navaho Nation K'E Project: Winslow Children & Families Advocacy Corp
HC 63 Box E 520-657-3234
Winslow, AZ 86047 Fax: 520-657-3207
Jayne Clark

Arkansas

6014 Arkansas FFCMH Jane Burgan
Jane Burgan
PO Box 56667 501-374-7218
Little Rock, AR 72215-4023 Fax: 501-374-2711
e-mail: pammarshall7218@sbcglobal.net
www.ffcmh.org

6015 NAMI Arkansas
1012 Autumn Road 501-661-1548
Little Rock, AR 72211-2222 800-844-0381
Fax: 501-312-7540
e-mail: karnold@nami.org
www.nami.org
Grassroots organization that focuses on improving mental health services. The mission is three prong: Support, Education, and Advocacy. Support Group meetings are held at 11 locations across the state.
Rick Owen, President
Kim Arnold, Executive Director

California

6016 NAMI California
1010 Hurley Way 916-567-0163
Sacramento, CA 95825-3218 Fax: 916-567-1757
e-mail: support@namicalifornia.org
www.namicalifornia.org
Brenda Scott, First Vice President
Karen H Henry, President

6017 United Advocates for Children of California
2035 Hurley Way 916-643-1530
Sacramento, CA 95825 866-643-1530
Fax: 916-643-1592
e-mail: sduval@uacf4hope.org
www.uacf4hope.org
Oscar Wright, Chief Executive Officer
Poppy Johal, Chief Officer of Strategic Planning

Colorado

6018 Colorado FFCMH
2950 Tennyson Street 303-572-0302
Denver, CO 80212 888-569-7500
Fax: 303-433-1605
e-mail: tdillingham@coloradofederation.org
www.coloradofederation.org
Tom Dillingham, Executive Director
Margie Grimsley, Technical Assistance Coordinator

6019 FFCMH: Denver/Aurora Chapter
12485 E 13th Avenue 303-343-1019
Aurora, CO 80011 Fax: 720-859-9367
e-mail: **ffcmhda@comcast.net
Carmen Held
Debra White

6020 National Alliance for the Mentally Ill of Colorado
1100 Fillmore Street
Denver, CO 80206-3334
303-321-3104
888-566-6264
Fax: 303-321-0912
e-mail: nami-co@nami.org
www.namicolorado.org

The National Alliance for the Mentally Ill Of Colorado is a statewide, grassroots, nonprofit organization whose mission is; To give strength and hope to individuals with mental illness and their families.

Henry Mohr, President
Carol Reynolds, Executive Director

6021 No. Colorado FFCMH
1400 White Peak Court
Fort Collins, CO 80525
970-223-3036
Fax: 303-377-0245
e-mail: thefeds@attbi.com
www.ffcmh.org

Connecticut

6022 Families United For CMH, Inc.
PO Box 151
New London, CT 06320
860-537-6125
Fax: 860-537-6130
e-mail: **ctfamiliesunited@sbcglobal.net
www.familiesunited.org

Morgan Meltz

6023 National Alliance for the Mentally Ill of Connecticut
30 Jordan Lane
Wethersfield, CT 06109
860-882-0236
800-215-3021
Fax: 860-882-0240
e-mail: namicted@namict.org
www.namict.org

Robert Correll, President
Sheila King, Executive Director

Delaware

6024 Alliance for the Mentally Ill in Delaware (AMID)
2400 W 4th Street
Wilmington, DE 19805-3306
302-427-0787
888-427-2643
Fax: 302-427-2075
e-mail: namide@namide.org
www.namide.org

Julius Meisel, President
Ken Singleton, Executive Director

6025 Delaware FFMCH
19 Baltusrol Court
Dover, DE 19904
302-730-0325
866-994-0000
Fax: 302-730-8952
e-mail: marags1@aol.com
www.ffcmh.org

Earline Jackson, Executive Director

6026 Mental Health Association of Delaware
100 W 10th Street
Wilmington, DE 19801
302-654-6833
800-287-6423
Fax: 302-654-6838
e-mail: information@mhainde.org
www.mhainde.org

Laurie McArthur, Director Development/Communications

District of Columbia

6027 DC Threshold Alliance for the Mentally Ill
422 8th Street SE
Washington, DC 20003-2832
202-546-0646
Fax: 202-546-6817
e-mail: namidc@juno.com
www.nami.org

Adrian Green, President

6028 Family Advocacy and Support Association
PO Box 74884
Washington, DC 20056
202-234-2325
Fax: 202-576-7154

Lynne M Smilth

Florida

6029 Career Assessment & Planning Services Goodwill Industries-Suncoast
Goodwill Industries-Suncoast
10596 Gandy Boulevard
St Petersburg, FL 33702
727-523-1512
888-279-1988
Fax: 727-579-0850
e-mail: gw.marketing@goodwill-suncoast.com
www.goodwill-suncoast.org

Provides a comprehensive assessment, which can predict current and future employment and potential adjustment factors for physically, emotionally or developmentally disabled persons who may be unemployed or underemployed.

Martin W Gladysz, Chair
R Lee Waits, President

6030 Florida Alliance for the Mentally Ill
316 E Park Avenue
Tallahassee, FL 32301-2646
850-671-4445
877-626-4352
Fax: 850-671-5272
e-mail: namifl@namifl.org
www.nami.org

Marcia Mathes, President
Judith Evans, Executive Director

6031 Florida FFCMH: Tampa Chapter
13301 Bruce B Downs Boulevard
Tampa, FL 33612
813-974-7930
Fax: 813-974-7712
e-mail: ffcmh@earthlink.net
www.federationoffamilies.org

Linda M Callejas, Board of Director
Albert J Duchnowski, Board of Director

6032 Suncoast Residential Training Center/Developmental Services Program
Goodwill Industries-Suncoast
10596 Gandy Boulevard
St. Petersburg, FL 33733
727-523-1512
888-279-1988
Fax: 727-577-2749
e-mail: gw.marketing@goodwill-suncoast.com
www.goodwill-suncoast.org

A large group home which serves individuals diagnosed as mentally retarded with a secondary diagnosed of psychiatric difficulties as evidenced by problem behavior. Providing residential, behavioral and instructional support and services that will promote the development of adaptive, socially appropriate behavior, each individual is assessed to determine strecths and needs in such skill areas as self-care, daily living, human growth and development, socialization, basic academics and recreation.

Martin W Gladysz, Chair
R Lee Waits, President/CEO

Georgia

6033 Georgia Alliance for the Mentally Ill
3050 Presidential Drive
Atlanta, GA 30340-3916
770-234-0855
800-728-1052
Fax: 770-234-0237
e-mail: nami-ga@nami.org
www.namiga.org

Nora Haynes, President
Eric Spencer, Executive Director

Hawaii

6034 NAMI: The Local Affiliate of the National Alliance for the Mentally Ill
85-175 Farrington Highway
Waianae, HI 96792-2025
808-591-1297
Fax: 808-591-2058
e-mail: namihawaii@hawaiiantel.net
namihawaii.org

Members include consumers families health professionals and interested persons/organizations. Programs include advocacy support and education and are free and open to the public. Office has lending library of books and videos. Newsletter is published.

6 pages Quarterly
Marion Poirier, Executive Director
Mike Durant, President

Idaho

6035 FFCMH: Idaho Chapter
1509 S Robert Street
Boise, ID 83705
208-433-8845
800-905-3436
Fax: 208-433-8337
e-mail: info@idahofederation.org
www.idahofederation.org
Courtney Lester, Administrative Director
Lacey Sinn, Development Director

6036 Idaho Alliance for the Mentally Ill
362 W Street
Albion, ID 83311-0068
208-673-6672
800-572-9940
Fax: 208-673-6685
e-mail: namiid@atcnet.ne
www.nami.org
President, President
Lee Woodland, Executive Director

Illinois

6037 Illinois Alliance for the Mentally Ill
218 W Lawrence Avenue
Springfield, IL 62704-2612
217-522-1403
800-346-4572
Fax: 217-522-3598
e-mail: namiil@sbcglobal.net
il.nami.org
Doug Call, President
Lora Thomas, Executive Director

6038 Illinois Federation of Families
PO Box 413
McHenry, IL 60051
847-265-0500
800-871-8400
Fax: 847-265-0501
e-mail: iffcmh@msn.com
www.iffcmh.net
Cynthia Sheppard, Executive Director

Indiana

6039 FFCMH: Indiana Chapter
2205 Costello Drive
Anderson, IN 46011
765-643-4357
Fax: 765-643-4357
e-mail: Indianafedfam@insightbb.com
www.ffcmh.org
Brenda Hamilton

6040 Family Action Network
214 W 2nd Street
Anderson, IN 46016-2206
765-643-4357
Brenda Hamilton

6041 NAMI Indiana
PO Box 22697
Indianapolis, IN 46222-0697
317-925-9399
800-677-6442
Fax: 317-925-9398
e-mail: NAMI-IN@nami.org
www.nami.org
Grass roots advocacy support and educational group for families affected by severe and persistent mental illnesses.
Pamela McConey, Executive Director
Teresa Hatten, President

Iowa

6042 FFCMH: Iowa Chapter
106 S Booth
Anamosa, IA 52205
319-462-2187
888-400-6302
Fax: 319-462-6789
e-mail: help@iffcmh.org
www.iffcmh.org
Lori Reynolds

6043 NAMI Iowa: Alliance for the Mentally Ill of Iowa
5911 Meredith Drive
Des Moines, IA 50322-1903
515-254-0417
800-417-0417
Fax: 515-254-1103
e-mail: info@namiiowa.com
www.namiiowa.com
Bruce Sielen MD, President
Margaret Stout, Executive Director

Kansas

6044 Keys for Networking: Kansas FFCMH
211 W 33rd Street
Topeka, KS 66611
785-233-8732
800-499-8732
Fax: 785-235-8732
e-mail: jadams@keys.org
www.keys.org
Jane Adams

6045 NAMI Kansas: Kansas' Voice on Mental Illness
112 SW 6th Avenue
Topeka, KS 66601-0675
785-233-0755
800-539-2660
Fax: 785-233-4804
e-mail: namikansas@nami.org
www.nami.org
Sharon Manson, President
Richard Cagan, Executive Director

Kentucky

6046 KY Partnership For Families and Children
207 Holmes Street
Frankfort, KY 40601
502-875-1320
Fax: 502-875-1399
e-mail: kpfc@kypartnership.org
www.kypartnership.org
Carol W Cecil, Executive Director
Kate Tilton, Program Coordinator

6047 Kentucky Alliance for the Mentally Ill
10510 Lagrange Road
Louisville, KY 40223-1277
502-245-5284
800-257-5081
Fax: 502-245-6390
e-mail: namiky@nami.org
www.nami.org
Bob McFadden, President
Carol Carrithers, Executive Director

Louisiana

6048 Louisiana Alliance for the Mentally Ill
5700 Florida Boulevard
Baton Rouge, LA 70806-2398
225-926-8770
866-851-6264
Fax: 225-926-8773
e-mail: namilouisiana@bellsouth.net
www.namilouisiana.org
Roselynn Nobles, President
Jennifer N Jantz, Executive Director

Maine

6049 Maine Alliance for the Mentally Ill
1 Bangor Street
Augusta, ME 04330-4701
207-622-5767
800-464-5767
Fax: 207-621-8430
e-mail: info@namimaine.org
www.nami.org
Julie O'Brien, President
Carol Carothers, Executive Director

6050 United Families for Children's Mental Health
PO Box 2107
Augusta, ME 04338-2107
207-622-3309
Fax: 207-622-1661
Pat Hunt

Maryland

6051 **National Alliance for the Mentally Ill: Maryland**
804 Landmark Drive 410-863-0470
Glen Burnie, MD 21061-4486 800-467-0075
Fax: 410-863-0474
e-mail: amimd@aol.com
md.nami.org
Barbara Bellack, Executive Director
Dana Lefko

6052 **Parents Supporting Parents of MD**
PO Box 30
Kensington, MD 20895-0030 800-498-5551
e-mail: Marge_Samels@umail.umd.edu
Marge Samels, Executive Director

Massachusetts

6053 **Massachusetts Alliance for the Mentally Ill**
400 W Cummings Park 781-938-4048
Woburn, MA 01801-6528 800-370-9085
Fax: 781-938-4069
e-mail: helpline@namimass.org
www.namimass.org
Rita Sagalyn, President
Toby Fisher, Director of Public Policy

Michigan

6054 **Association for Children's Mental Health**
6017 W Street Joseph Highway 517-372-4016
Lansing, MI 48917 888-226-4543
Fax: 517-372-4032
e-mail: ajwinans@aol.com
www.acmh-mi.org
Amy J Winans, Executive Director
Mary Porter, Business Manager

6055 **JIMHO Affiliated Centers (Justice in Mental Health Organization)**
421 Seymour Street 517-371-2266
Lansing, MI 48933 800-831-8035
Fax: 517-371-5770
e-mail: brwellwood@aol.com
members.aol.com/jimhofw/
JIMHO advocates for the rights and dignity that all people suffering from mental or emotional illness deserve.

6056 **Michigan Alliance for the Mentally Ill**
921 N Washington Avenue 517-485-4049
Lansing, MI 48906-5137 800-331-4264
Fax: 517-485-2333
e-mail: namimichigan@acd.net
mi.nami.org
Hubert Huebl, President
Sharon Solomon, Executive Director

Minnesota

6057 **Minnesota Alliance for the Mentally Ill**
800 Transfer Road 651-645-2948
Saint Paul, MN 55114-1146 888-NAM-IHEL
Fax: 651-645-7379
e-mail: nami-mn@nami.org
www.namihelps.org
Karen Lloyd, President
Sue Abderholden, Executive Director

6058 **Minnesota Association for Children's Mental Health**
165 Western Avenue 651-644-7333
Saint Paul, MN 55102 800-528-4511
Fax: 651-644-7391
e-mail: dsaxhaug@macmh.org
www.macmh.org
Deborah Saxhaug, Executive Director
Michele Willert, President

Mississippi

6059 **Mississippi Alliance for the Mentally Ill**
411 Briarwood Drive 601-899-9058
Jackson, MS 39206-3058 800-357-0388
Fax: 601-956-6380
e-mail: namimiss1@aol.com
www.nami.org
Annette Giessner, President
Wendy Mahoney, Executive Director

6060 **Mississippi Families as Allies**
5166 Keele Street 601-981-1618
Jackson, MS 39206 800-833-9671
Fax: 601-981-1696
e-mail: info@msfaacmh.org
www.msfaacmh.org
Tessie Bruni LMSW, Executive Director
Tressa Knuts LMSW, Family Support Coordinator

Missouri

6061 **MO-SPAN**
440 Rue Saint Francois 314-972-0600
Florissant, MO 63031 Fax: 314-972-0606
www.mo-span.org
Donna Dittrich, Executive Director
Tina VarVera, Administrative Assistant

6062 **Missouri Coalition Alliance for the Mentally Ill**
230 W Dunklin Street 573-634-7727
Jefferson City, MO 65101-3260 800-374-2138
Fax: 573-761-5636
e-mail: Keele@aol.com

6063 **NAMI of Missouri**
1001 SW Boulevard 573-634-7727
Jefferson City, MO 65109-2501 800-374-2138
Fax: 573-761-5636
e-mail: namimosjf@yahoo.com
mo.nami.org
A nonprofit education adudcacy, referal and support organization serving people with mental illness and their families.
12 pages newsletter
Cindi Keele, Executive Director
Karren Jones, President

Montana

6064 **Family Support Network**
1002 10th Street W 406-256-7783
Billings, MT 59102 877-376-4850
Fax: 406-256-9879
e-mail: admin@mtfamilysupport.org
www.mtfamilysupport.org
Barbara Sample, Executive Director

6065 **Montana Alliance for the Mentally Ill Mihelish's Residence**
Mihelish's Residence
616 Helena Avenue 406-443-7871
Helena, MT 59624-6946 888-280-6264
Fax: 406-862-6352
e-mail: mattkuntz@msn.com
www.namimt.org
Gary Milhelish, President
Matt Kuntz, Executive Director

Nebraska

6066 **National Alliance for the Mentally Ill: Nebraska (NAMI)**
1941 South 42nd Street 402-345-8101
Omaha, NE 68105-2986 877-463-6264
Fax: 402-346-4070
e-mail: nami.nebraska@nami.org
www.nami.org/sites/ne
NAMI is a nonprofit organization dedicated to providing support, education and advocacy to and for anyone whose life has been touched by a mental illness.
Colleen Wuebben, Executive Director
Carole Denton, President

Nevada

6067 **Nevada Alliance for the Mentally Ill**
2251 N Rampart Boulevard 702-310-5764
Las Vegas, NV 89128 Fax: 775-329-1618
e-mail: joetyler@sdi.net
www.nami-nevada.org
Joe Tyler, President
Mark Burchell, Vice President

New Hampshire

6068 **Granite State FFCMH**
940 Mammoth Road 603-296-0692
Manchester, NH 03104 e-mail: gsffcmh@aol.com
www.ffcmh.org
Kathleen Abate

6069 **National Alliance for the Mentally Ill**
15 Green Street 603-225-5359
Concord, NH 03301 800-242-6264
Fax: 603-228-8848
e-mail: info@naminh.org
www.naminh.org
Family support and advocacy for consumers and family members.
Michael Cohen, Executive Director
Win Saltmarsh, Development Director

6070 **National Alliance for the Mentally Ill: New Hampshire**
15 Green Street 603-225-5359
Concord, NH 03301-4020 800-242-6264
Fax: 603-228-8848
e-mail: naminh@naminh.org
www.naminh.org
Family support and advocacy for consumers and family members.
Michael Cohen, Executive Director
Mary Ann Aldrich, President

New Jersey

6071 **Association for Advancement of Mental Health**
Information
819 Alexander Road 609-452-2088
Princeton, NJ 08540 Fax: 609-452-0627
e-mail: info@aamh.org
www.aamh.org
This organization was founded to create a permanent community support system for mentally ill and developmentally disabled adults and their families living in the Greater Mercer County area of New Jersey.
Lisa Lynch, Director of Development
Marc Helberg, President

6072 **Community Mental Health Foundation**
610 Industrial Avenue 201-986-5070
Paramus, NJ 07652 Fax: 201-265-3543
e-mail: staff@cmhf.org
www.cmhf.org

6073 **New Jersey Alliance for the Mentally Ill**
1562 US Highway 130 732-940-0991
N Brunswick, NJ 08902-3004 Fax: 732-940-0355
e-mail: info@naminj.org
www.naminj.org
Mark Perrin, President
Sylvia Axelrod, Executive Director

New Mexico

6074 **Navaho Nation K'E Project Children and Families Advocacy Corp**
PO Box 309 505-733-2474
Tohatchi, NM 87325 Fax: 505-733-2444
Vera Kieyoomia

6075 **Navajo Nation K'E Project: Shiprock Children & Families Advocacy Corp**
PO Box 1240 505-368-4479
Shiprock, NM 87420 Fax: 505-368-5582
Evelyn Balwin

6076 **New Mexico Alliance for the Mentally Ill**
6001 Marble NE Suite 8 505-260-0154
Albuquerque, NM 87190-3086 Fax: 505-260-0342
e-mail: naminm@aol.com
www.nami.org
Becky Beckett, President
Elaine Jones, Executive Director

New York

6077 **Children's Mental Health Coalition of WNY, Inc.**
814 Kenmore Avenue 716-871-8997
Buffalo, NY 14216 Fax: 716-871-8656
e-mail: mtskorupa@aol.com
www.raisingminds.org
Mary Skorupa, Executive Director

6078 **Families Together in New York State**
737 Madison Avenue 518-432-0333
Albany, NY 12208 888-326-8644
Fax: 518-434-6478
e-mail: info@ftnys.org
www.ftnys.org
Paige Pierce, Executive Director
Joan Cullen, Program Director/Family Specialist

6079 **New York Alliance for the Mentally Ill**
260 Washington Avenue 518-462-2000
Albany, NY 12210 800-950-3228
Fax: 518-462-3811
e-mail: info@naminys.org
www.naminys.org
Trix Niernberger, Executive Director
Jeff Keller, Deputy Director

6080 **Parents United Network: Parsons Child Family Center**
60 Academy Road 518-426-2600
Albany, NY 12208 Fax: 518-447-5234
e-mail: info@parsonscenter.org
www.parsonscenter.org
Rose Mary Bailly, Executive Director
Thomas Luzzi, Chief Financial Officer

North Dakota

6081 **North Dakota Alliance for the Mentally Ill**
PO Box 3215 701-852-8202
Minot, ND 58702-6016 Fax: 701-725-4334
e-mail: naminwnd@min.midco.net
www.nami.org
Janet Sabol, President

6082 **North Dakota FFCMH**
PO Box 3061 701-222-1223
Bismarck, ND 58502-3061 Fax: 701-250-8835
e-mail: carlottamccleary@bis.midco.nrt
www.ffcmh.org

Ohio

6083 **1st Capital FFCMH**
394 Chestnut Street 740-775-2674
Chillicothe, OH 45601 Fax: 740-775-7834
e-mail: rmh1@adelphia.net
Rosemary Hill

6084 **Ohio Alliance for the Mentally Ill**
747 E Broad Street 614-224-2700
Columbus, OH 43205 800-686-2646
Fax: 614-224-5400
TTY: 866-924-1478
e-mail: amiohio@amiohio.org
www.namiohio.org
Harvey Snider, President
Jim Mauro, Executive Director

Oklahoma

6085 **Oklahoma Alliance for the Mentally Ill**
500 N Broadway Avenue
Oklahoma City, OK 73102-6200
405-230-1900
800-583-1264
Fax: 405-230-1903
e-mail: nami-OK@swbell.net
www.nami.org

Barney Allen, President
Karina Forrest, Executive Director

6086 **Tulsa Unified FFCMH**
1022 N Howard
Tulsa, OK 74115
918-838-8033
e-mail: sherryscoobydoo@aol.com
www.ffcmh.org

Sherry Hamby

Oregon

6087 **NAMI-Oregon**
3550 SE Woodward Street
Portland, OR 97202-1552
503-230-8009
800-343-6264
Fax: 503-230-2751
e-mail: namioregon@qwest.net
www.nami.org

Providing support education and advocacy for people with biological mental illness and their families. The in-state 800 phone number is Oregon's NAMI-Line. Callers to this line are provided with information about mental illnesses and referrals to support and treatment services.
Molly Gorger, Education Program Director
Cora Palazzolo, Communications Coordinator

6088 **Oregon Family Support Network**
PO Box 324
Marylhurst, OR 97036
503-675-2294
800-323-8521
Fax: 503-675-6932
e-mail: ofsn@ofsn.org
www.ofsn.org

Jammie Farish, Executive Director
Sandy Bumpus, President

Pennsylvania

6089 **Parents Involved Network**
1211 Chestnut Street
Philadelphia, PA 19107
215-751-1800
800-688-4226
e-mail: pin@pinofpa.org
www.pinofpa.org

Janet Lonsdale

6090 **Pennsylvania Alliance for the Mentally Ill**
2149 N 2nd Street
Harrisburg, PA 17110-1005
717-238-1514
800-223-0500
Fax: 717-238-4390
TTY: 800-890-6093
e-mail: nami-pa@nami.org
namipa.nami.org

James W Jordan Jr, Executive Director
Jyoti Shah, President

Rhode Island

6091 **National Alliance for the Mentally Ill**
154 Waterman Street
Providence, RI 02906
401-331-3060
800-749-3197
Fax: 401-274-3020
e-mail: chaznami@cox.net
www.namirhodeisland.org

Fred Sneesby, President
Charles Gross, Executive Director

6092 **National Alliance for the Mentally Ill of Rhode Island (NAMI)**
82 Pitman Street
Providence, RI 02906-4312
401-331-3060
800-749-3197
Fax: 401-274-3020
e-mail: nicknami@aol.com
www.namiri.org

Henry Saccoccia, President
Nicki Sahlin, Executive Director

South Carolina

6093 **South Carolina Alliance for the Mentally Ill**
PO BOX 1267
Columbia, SC 29202-1267
803-733-9592
800-788-5131
Fax: 803-733-9593
e-mail: namisc@namisc.org
www.namisc.org

Kennard Howell, President
David Almeida, Executive Director

South Dakota

6094 **NAMI South Dakota**
3920 S Western Avenue
Sioux Falls, SD 57109-1204
605-271-1871
800-551-2531
Fax: 605-271-1871
e-mail: namisd@midconetwork.com
www.nami.org/sites/NAMISouthDakota

Shelly Fuller, President
Robin Deming

Tennessee

6095 **Tennessee Alliance for the Mentally Ill**
1101 Kermit Drive
Nashville, TN 37217-2126
615-361-6608
800-467-3589
Fax: 615-361-6698
e-mail: sdiehl@namitn.org
www.namitn.org

Tod Jablonski, President
Sita Diehl, Executive Director

Texas

6096 **Central Texas FFCMH**
6814 Orange Blossom
Austin, TX 78744
512-282-7126
Fax: 512-282-5817
e-mail: mattie_dixon@hotmail.com

Mattie Dixon

6097 **North Texas FFCMH**
722 E Summitt
Sherman, TX 75090
e-mail: patoadv@msn.com
Pat Owens

6098 **San Antonio Bexar County FFCMH**
2516 Bandara
San Antonio, TX 78238
210-523-2351
Fax: 210-523-2352
e-mail: ideasjn@aol.com

Joseph Nazaroff

6099 **Texas Alliance for the Mentally Ill**
Foundtain Park Plaza III
Austin, TX 78704
512-693-2000
800-633-3760
Fax: 512-693-8000
e-mail: rpeyson@namitexas.org
www.namitexas.org

Robin Peyson, Executive Director
Donna Fisher, President

6100 **Texas FFCMH**
7800 Shoal Creek Road
Austin, TX 78752
512-407-8844
866-893-3264
Fax: 512-407-8266
e-mail: PattiDerr@txffcmh.org
www.txffcmh.org

Patti Derr, Executive Director

Utah

6101 **Utah Alliance for the Mentally Ill**
450 S 900 E
Salt Lake City, UT 84102-1701
801-323-9900
Fax: 801-323-9799
e-mail: Education@namiut.org
www.namiut.org

Don Muller, President
Sherri Wittwer, Executive Director

Vermont

6102 **Vermont Alliance for the Mentally Ill**
162 S Main Street
Waterbury, VT 05676-1519
802-244-1396
800-639-6480
Fax: 802-244-1405
e-mail: info@namivt.org
www.nami.org
Fran Levine, President
Larry Lewack, Executive Director

6103 **Vermont FFCMH**
95 Main Street
Waterbury, VT 05676-0607
802-244-1955
800-639-6071
Fax: 802-329-2135
e-mail: vffcmh@vffcmh.org
www.vffcmh.org
Kathy Holsopple, Executive Director
Ted Tighe, President

Virginia

6104 **Virginia Alliance for the Mentally Ill**
PO Box 8260
Richmond, VA 23226-1903
804-225-8264
888-486-8264
Fax: 80 -85 -464
e-mail: namiva@comcast.net
www.nami.org
Bill Farrington, President
Mira Signer, Executive Director

Washington

6105 **NAMI Washington (National Alliance for the Mentally Ill of Washington)**
4305 Lacey Boulevard SE
Lacey, WA 98503-5580
360-584-9622
800-782-9264
e-mail: office@namiwa.comcastbiz.net
www.nami.org
Advocacy, support and education for the mentally ill, their families and friends.
Barbara Bate, President
Bill Waters, Vice President

6106 **Washington FFCMH**
801 E 141 Street
Tacoma, WA 98445-2768
253-537-2145
Fax: 253-537-2162
e-mail: acvmarge@comcast.net
www.ffcmh.org/
Marge Critchlow

West Virginia

6107 **Mountain State/Parents/Children/ Adolescents Network**
1201 Garfield Street
McMechen, WV 26040
304-233-5399
800-CHI-LD35
Fax: 304-233-3847
e-mail: ttoothman@mcpcan.org
www.mspcan.org
Hope Coleman, President
Terrie Isaly, Fast Track Program Director

6108 **NAMI West Virginia**
PO Box 2706
Charleston, WV 25330-2706
304-342-0497
800-598-5653
Fax: 304-342-0499
e-mail: namiwv@aol.com
www.namiwv.org
Educational advocacy and support for families consumers and friends of people with mental illnesses.
Randal Johnson, President
Michael W Ross, Executive Director

Wisconsin

6109 **Wisconsin Alliance for the Mentally Ill**
4233 W Beltline Highway
Madison, WI 53711-3814
608-268-6000
800-236-2988
Fax: 608-268-6004
e-mail: namiwisc@choiceonemail.com
www.namiwisconsin.org
Pat Rutkowski, Co-President
Terence Schnapp, Interim Executive Director

6110 **Wisconsin Family Ties**
16 N Carroll Street
Madison, WI 53703
608-267-6888
800-422-7145
Fax: 608-267-6801
e-mail: info@wifamilyties.org
www.wifamilyties.org
Hugh Davis, Executive Director
Ginger Fobart, Statewide Family Network Coordinator

Wyoming

6111 **Wyoming Alliance for the Mentally Ill**
133 W 6th Street
Casper, WY 82601-3124
307-265-2573
888-882-4968
Fax: 307-234-0440
e-mail: nami-wyo@qwestoffice.net
www.nami.org/sites/namiwyoming
Jane Johnson, President
Deion Hagemeister, Vice-President

Libraries & Resource Centers

6112 **Alta Bates Summit Medical Center**
2001 Dwight Way
Berkeley, CA 94704-2608
510-204-4444
www.altabatesherrick.org
Alta Bates Summit Medical Center has made community healthcare a priority. We are proud of our many areas of clinical excellence including cardiovascular, behavioral health, women and infants, orthopedics, rehabilitation, and oncology care.
Carolyn Kemp, Director Public Relations

6113 **Central Louisiana State Hospital Medical and Professional Library**
242 West Shamrock Street
Pineville, LA 71360
318-484-6363
Fax: 318-484-6284
e-mail: bentonmcgee@hotmail.com
www.clmlc.org
The Consortium was established to increase and better utilize the health information resources of Central Louisiana. Information offered on psychiatry, psychology and mental health.
Carol McGee, Medical Librarian

6114 **National Mental Health Consumer's Self-Help Clearinghouse**
1211 Chestnut Street
Philadelphia, PA 19107
215-751-1810
800-553-4539
Fax: 215-735-0275
e-mail: info@mhselfhelp.org
www.mhselfhelp.org
The National Mental Health Consumers' Self-Help Clearinghouse, the nation's first national consumer technical assistance center, has played a major role in the development of the mental health consumer movement. The consumer movement strives for dignity, respect, and opportunity for those with mental illnesses.
Joseph Rogers, Director

6115 **National Mental Health Consumers' Self- Help Clearinghouse**
1211 Chestnut Street
Philadelphia, PA 19107
215-751-1810
800-553-4539
Fax: 215-636-6312
e-mail: info@mhselfhelp.org
www.mhselfhelp.org
The National Mental Health Consumers' Self-Help Clearinghouse, the nation's first national consumer technical assistance center, has played a major role in the development of the mental health consumer movement. The consumer movement strives for dignity, respect, and opportunity for those with mental illnesses. Consumers—those who receive or have received mental health

services—continue to reject the label of 'those who cannot help themselves.'
Joseph Rogers, Director

Research Centers

6116 Anxiety Disorders Center University of Wisconsin
University of Wisconsin
Department of Psychiatry 608-263-1530
Madison, WI 53792-0001
Provides evaluation and treatment for individuals suffering from anxiety disorders as well as training and education for clinicians.

6117 Institute of Psychiatry and Human Behavior: University of Maryland
701 Weat Pratt Street 410-328-6735
Baltimore, MD 21201-1542 Fax: 410-328-3693
e-mail: alehman@psych.umaryland.edu
www.medschool.umaryland.edu
Studies in psychiatric disorders.
Anthony Lehm MD, Director

6118 Langley Porter Psychiatric Institute University of California
University of California
401 Parnassus Avenue
San Francisco, CA 94143-9911 415-476-7365
www.universityofcalifornia.edu
Conducts clinical studies of psychiatric disorders.
Samuel Barno MD, Director
Craig Vantyke, Chief Executive Officer

6119 Medical College of Pennsylvania: Eastern Psychiatric Institute
3200 Henry Avenue 215-842-6990
Philadelphia, PA 19129-1137
Offers research into all aspects of mental illness.
Michael Faucher, Director

6120 Menninger Clinic: Department of Research
PO Box 829 785-350-5000
Topeka, KS 66601-0829 Fax: 785-350-5392
Focuses research on mental illness and mental health issues.
Dr Herbert Spohn, Director

6121 Mental Illness Research and Education Institute
Eastern State Hospital
PO Box 800 509-299-3121
Medical Lake, WA 99022-800 Fax: 509-997-15
Governmental organization focusing on mental illness research.
Harold Wilson, Director

6122 State University of New York At Stony Brook: Mental Health Research
450 Clarkson Avenue 718-270-1270
Brooklyn, NY 11203-2056
Oliver David, Director

6123 Thresholds Psychiatric Rehabilitation
2700 N Ravenswood Avenue 773-281-3800
Chicago, IL 60614-1894 Fax: 773-818-90
e-mail: thresholds@thresholds.org
www.luc.edu
A psychosocial rehabilitation agency serving persons with severe and persistent mental illness.
Tom Kinley, Director
Ellen Rodman, Assistant Director

6124 University of California Los Angeles Program on Psychosocial Adaptation
Neuropsychiatric Institute
760 Westwood Plaza 310-825-0511
Los Angeles, CA 90024 800-825-9989
www.semel.ucla.edu
Studies behavior disorders and psychosocial adaptation and the future.
Roderic GoRN MD, Director
Peter Whybrow, Director

6125 University of Michigan: Mental Health Research Institute
205 Washtenaw Place 734-763-2462
Ann Arbor, MI 48109 e-mail: UMresearch@umich.edu
www.umich.edu
Focuses on the diagnosis treatment and prevention of mental illnesses and disorders.
Dr Bernard Agranoff, Director

6126 University of Minnesota Department of Psychiatry
420 Delaware Street SE 612-624-2430
Minneapolis, MN 55455-374 Fax: 612-265-91
www.umn.edu
Behavior and mental illness research.
S Charles Schulz, Chair of Psychiatry

6127 University of Missouri: Columbia Missouri Institute of Mental Health
5247 Fyler Avenue 573-634-8787
Saint Louis, MO 63139-1300 Fax: 314-644-8834
Mental health policy and ethics studies.
Danny Weddin PhD, Director

6128 University of Pittsburgh: Western Psychiatric Institute & Clinic
3811 Ohara Street 412-246-6356
Pittsburgh, PA 15213-2593 Fax: 412-246-6350
e-mail: reitzpm@msx.upmc.edu
www.pitt.edu
Advancement of basic and clinical knowledge in mental health and psychiatric care.
Thomas Detre MD, Director

6129 Vanderbilt University John F Kennedy Center for Research/Human Development
Vanderbilt University
230 Appleton Place 615-322-8240
Nashville, TN 37203-5701 Fax: 615-228-36
e-mail: kc@vanderbilt.edu
www.kc.vanderbilt.edu
Mental health research.
Stephen Camarata, Acting Director

6130 Veterans Medical Center: Mental Health Clinical Research Center
3801 Miranda Avenue
Palo Alto, CA 94304-1207 650-858-3941
www.va.gov
Jerome Yesavage, Director Advanced Psychiatry
Ruth O'Hara, Co-Director Advanced Psychology

6131 Warren Grant Magnuson Clinical Center National Institute of Health
National Institute of Health
9000 Rockville Pike 301-496-4000
Bethesda, MD 20892 800-411-1222
Fax: 301-480-9793
TTY: 866-411-1010
e-mail: prpl@mail.cc.nih.gov
www.cc.nih.gov
Established in 1953 as the research hospital of the National Institutes of Health. Designed so that patient care facilities are close to research laboratories so new findings of basic and clinical scientists can be quickly applied to the treatment of patients. Upon referral by physicians patients are admitted to NIH clinical studies.
John I Gallin, Director
David Henderson, Deputy Director for Clinical Care

6132 Yeshiva University: Soundview-Throgs Neck Community Mental Health Center
2527 Glebe Avenue 718-904-4400
Bronx, NY 10461-3109 Fax: 718-931-7307
Mental health mental illness and recovery from mental illness research.
Dr Itamar Salamon, Director

Support Groups & Hotlines

6133 National Health Information Center
PO Box 1133
Washington, DC 20013
310-565-4167
800-336-4797
Fax: 301-984-4256
e-mail: info@nhic.org
www.health.gov/nhic
Offers a nationwide information referral service, produces directories and resource guides.

Alabama

6134 Alabama Education of Homeless Children and Youth Program
Alabama State Department of Education
5348 Gordon Persons Building
Montgomery, AL 36130-3901
334-242-8199
Fax: 334-420-9633
e-mail: mrivers@alsde.edu
www.alsde.edu/html/home.asp
The major responsibilities of the Federal Programs Section are to administer all federally funded education programs and to provide technical assistance to local education agencies and schools. These responsibilities include promoting, supervising, and coordinating statewide educational programs with federal programs in addition to assisting schools in developing, revising, and implementing their school wide plans.
Maggie Rivers, Federal Program Coordinator

Alaska

6135 National Alliance for the Mentally Ill (NA MI) Alaska
144 West 15th Avenue
Anchorage, AK 99501-5106
907-227-1300
800-478-4462
Fax: 907-227-1400
e-mail: info@nami-alaska.org
www.nami.org/sites/alaska
NAMI Alaska is a grassroots, 501(c)(3) nonprofit, support, educational and advocacy organization of consumers, families, and friends of people with severe brain disorders such as schizophrenia, schizo-affective disorder, bipolar disorder, major depressive disorder, obsessive-compulsive disorder, panic and anxiety disorders, and attention deficit/hyperactivity disorder. In addition, NAMI provides information and referral services and works with local media on stories about mental illness.
Trish McDonald, Program/Education Director
Augusta Reimer, Leadership Project Coordinator

Arizona

6136 Navajo Nation Office Special Education & R ehabilitation Services
IHS PO Box 1337
Gallup, NM 87301
505-722-1454
Fax: 505-722-1554
e-mail: osers@navajo.org
www.osers.navajo.org/
Navajo OSERS is a program within the Division of DINE Education, which offers vocational rehabilitation to people with disabilities. Vocational Rehabilitation includes an array of services, which are funded by a grant to the Navajo Nation from the U.S. Department of Education. The goal of vocational rehabilitation is to assist people with disabilities to obtain or maintain employment.
Rosemary Smith, Parent Training Coordinator

6137 Navajo Nation Office of Special Education & Rehabilitation Services (OSERS)
PO Box 1420
Window Rock, AZ 86515
928-871-6338
866-341-9918
Fax: 928-871-7865
e-mail: osers@navajo.org
www.osers.navajo.org/
Navajo OSERS is a program within the Division of DINE Education, which offers vocational rehabilitation to people with disabilities. Vocational Rehabilitation includes an array of services, which are funded by a grant to the Navajo Nation from the U.S. Department of Education. The goal of vocational rehabilitation is to assist people with disabilities to obtain or maintain employment.
Treva M Roanhorse, Director
Paula S Seanez, Assistant Director

Colorado

6138 Laradon Services for Children and Adults w ith Developmental Disabilities
5100 Lincoln Street
Denver, CO 80216
303-296-2400
Fax: 303-296-4012
TDD: 7209746821
www.laradon.org/Index.shtml#
Laradon specializes in services to children and adults with developmental disabilities, operating 15 programs that are designed to help each individual develop to his or her fullest potential and maximize self-sufficiency.
Annie Green, Deputy Director

Florida

6139 Florida Institute for Family Involvement (FIFI)
3927 Spring Creek Highway
Crawfordville, FL 32327
305-293-7626
877-926-3514
Fax: 863-582-9358
e-mail: HewFLMOM@aol.com
www.fifionline.org
Florida Institute for Family Involvement (FIFI), an affiliate of Federation of Families for Children's Mental Health (FFCMH), enhances, facilitates, and supports family and consumer involvement in the development of responsive, family centered, and community based systems of care. FIFI works in collaboration with state, federal, and private programs to develop a resource and training information center to enable individuals to advocate for appropriate services and make wise service choices.
Connie Wells, Executive Director
Lindsay Phillips, Business Manager

6140 Parent Education Network (PEN) Project Health
Family Network on Disabilities of Florida
2735 Whitney Road
Clearwater, FL 33760
727-523-1130
800-825-5736
Fax: 727-523-8687
e-mail: wilbur@fndfl.org
www.fndfl.org/PEN/index.htm
The PEN Project provides: information on specific disabilities; individual assistance by telephone, email, and in-person; referrals to local, state, and national resources; opportunities for youths with disabilities to be involved in training to parents and students; and, collaboration with Family Network on Disabilities Heart and Hope annual statewide conference for families.
Wilbur Hawke, Co-Director
Tara Bremer, Co-Director

Georgia

6141 Georgia Parent Support Network (GPSN)
1381 Metropolitan Parkway
Atlanta, GA 30310
404-758-4500
Fax: 404-758-6833
e-mail: rheba.smith@gpsn.org
www.gpsn.org/
Georgia Parent Support Network (GPNS) provides support, education, and advocacy for children and youth with mental illness, emotional disturbances, and behavioral differences and their families.
Sue L Smith, Co-Chief Executive Officer
Anna M McLaughlin, Co-Chief Executive Officer

Hawaii

6142 Hawaii Families As Allies (HFAA)
99-209 Moanalua Road
Aiea, HI 96701
808-487-8785
866-361-8825
Fax: 808-487-0514
e-mail: hfaa@hfaa.net
www.hfaa.net/
Hawaii Families as Allies (HFAA) is a statewide parent-controlled family network organization that provides support, services and information for families of children and adolescents with emotional and/or behavioral challenges. HFAA is the Hawaii state chapter of the Federation of Families for Children's Mental Health, a national organization that advocates for service system change so that families are valued and treated as true partners.
Susan Cooper, Executive Director
Shanelle Lum, Public Policy Information Specialist

Illinois

6143 CANDU Parent Group
24W 681 Woodcrest Drive 630-983-9027
Naperville, IL 60540
Cathy Bozett

6144 KALEIDOSCOPE
1279 N Milwaukee Avenue 773-278-7200
Chicago, IL 60622
Fax: 773-278-5663
TTY: 773-292-4086
e-mail: information@kaleidoscope4kids.org
www.kaleidoscope4kids.org
Karl Dennis

6145 Parents Information Network FFCMH
1926 1700th Avenue 217-735-1662
Lincoln, IL 62656
Bridget Schneider

Indiana

6146 Bloomington: NAMI Bloomington
NAMI Indiana
PO Box 22697 812-334-8117
Indianapolis, IN 46222-0697 800-677-6442
Fax: 317-925-9398
e-mail: lev@bloomington.in.us
www.namiindiana.org
Meets on the first and third Thursday at 7:00 p.m., at the First United Methodist Church on 219 E 4th Street, room 307.
Paul Van Gogh, President

6147 Elkhart: NAMI Elkhart County
NAMI Indiana
PO Box 22697
Indianapolis, IN 46222-0697 800-677-6442
Fax: 317-925-9398
e-mail: hsgjan@aol.com
www.namiindiana.org
Meets on the second and fourth Thursday at 7:30 p.m., at the St. Paul Methodist Church.
Harold Grieb, President

6148 Evansville NAMI Evansville
NAMI Indiana
PO Box 22697 317-925-9399
Indianapolis, IN 46222-697 800-677-6442
Fax: 317-925-9398
e-mail: daRNeson4051@insightbb.com
www.namiindiana.org
Meets on the second and fourth Tuesday, 6:45 p.m., at Southwestern Indiana CMHC.
Diane Arneson, President
Jo Vanable, President Nami Indiana

6149 Fort Wayne: NAMI Fort Wayne
NAMI Indiana
PO Box 22697 260-447-8990
Indianapolis, IN 46222-0697 800-677-6442
Fax: 317-925-9398
e-mail: tahat10@aol.com
www.namiindiana.org
Meets every Tuesday, 6:45 p.m., at Carriage House, 3327 Lake Avenue.
Teresa Hatten, President

6150 Indianapolis: NAMI Indianapolis
NAMI Indiana
PO Box 22697 317-767-7653
Indianapolis, IN 46222-0697 800-677-6442
Fax: 317-925-9398
www.namiindiana.org
For information please call our voice mail information line (317-767-7653) or write P.O. Box 40866, Indianapolis, IN 46240-0866. We have central, east, north, south and west support groups.
Don Fearrin, President

6151 Jeffersonville: NAMI Sunnyside
NAMI Indiana
PO Box 22697 812-282-6494
Indianapolis, IN 46222-0697 800-677-6442
Fax: 317-925-9398
www.namiindiana.org
Consumers meet on the second Monday of each month, 6:00 p.m., and family members meet on the second Tuesday of each month at 7:00 p.m. at Clark Memorial Hospital. Please call for directions.
Charlotte Davis, Contact Person

6152 Kendallville NAMI Northeast
NAMI Indiana
PO Box 22697 260-347-2291
Indianapolis, IN 46222-697 800-677-6442
Fax: 317-925-9398
www.namiindiana.org
Meets on the first Thursday of each month, 7:00 p.m., at the Kendallville Public Library.
Mary Smith, President

6153 Kokomo NAMI Kokomo
NAMI Indiana
128 Grant 765-628-7920
Green town, IN 46936-697 800-677-6442
Fax: 317-925-9398
e-mail: vkharris1010@aol.com
www.namiindiana.org
Meets on the first Tuesday of every month, 7:00 p.m., at the First Christian Church.
Alice Harris, President
Verl Harris, Treasurer

6154 Lafayette: NAMI West Central
NAMI Indiana
PO Box 22697 765-423-6939
Indianapolis, IN 46222-0697 800-677-6442
Fax: 317-925-9398
www.namiindiana.org
Meets on the second and fourth Monday of each month, at St. Elizabeth School of Nursing, room 4-901.
Cecilia Weber, Executive Director

6155 Lake County: NAMI Lake County
NAMI Indiana
PO Box 22697 219-374-5408
Indianapolis, IN 46222-0697 800-677-6442
Fax: 317-925-9398
www.namiindiana.org
Meets on the second and fourth Friday, 7:00 p.m., at the Southlake Mental Health Center.
Debbie Ganns, President

6156 Lawrenceburg: NAMI Southeast
NAMI Indiana
PO Box 22697 812-926-0199
Indianapolis, IN 46222-0697 800-677-6442
Fax: 317-925-9398
www.namiindiana.org
Meets on the first Tuesday of each month at the Dearborn County Mental Health Clinic, Dearborn Shopping Plaza. Call for meeting time.
Nancy McDaniel, President

6157 Logansport: NAMI Cass County
NAMI Indiana
PO Box 22697 574-753-6667
Indianapolis, IN 46222-0697 800-677-6442
Fax: 317-925-9398
www.namiindiana.org
Meets on the second Monday, 6:00 p.m., at the Four County Counseling Center. Call for more information.
Karen Menzie, President

6158 Marion NAMI Grant Blackford Counties
NAMI Indiana
PO Box 22697 765-664-0227
Indianapolis, IN 46222-697 800-677-6442
Fax: 317-925-9398
www.namiindiana.org
Meets on the first Wednesday, 7:00 p.m. Please call details.
Sandy Westafer, President

6159 Muncie: NAMI Delaware County
NAMI Indiana
PO Box 22697
Indianapolis, IN 46222-0697
800-677-6442
Fax: 317-925-9398
www.namiindiana.org

Please call the state office for details.

6160 NAMI Highland
NAMI
PO Box 22697
Indianapolis, IN 46222-697
317-925-9399
800-677-6442
Fax: 317-925-9398
e-mail: namiin@nami.org
www.namiindiana.org

Pamela Mcconey, Executive Director
Leslie Gay, Office Coordinator

6161 NAMI Indiana - National Alliance on Mental Illness
PO Box 22697
Indianapolis, IN 46222-0697
317-925-9399
800-677-6442
Fax: 317-925-9398
e-mail: nami-in@nami.org
www.namiindiana.org

NAMI Indiana is a non-profit grassroots organization dedicated to improving the lives of people afflicted by serious and persistent mental illness. NAMI Indiana consists of families, consumers, and professionals that are dedicated to helping families through a network of support, education, advocacy, and promotion of research. NAMI Indiana is affiliated with the National Alliance on Mental Illness (NAMI), which is located in Arlington, Virginia.
Pamela McConey, Executive Director
B Kellie Meyer, Development Director

6162 NAMI South Central Indiana
National Alliance for the Mentally Ill
1916 Central Avenue
Columbus, IN 47201
812-376-0020
Fax: 317-925-9398
e-mail: dweeks@scidata.com OR nami-in@nami.org
www.namiindiana.org

NAMI Indiana is a non-profit grassroots organization dedicated to improving the lives of people afflicted by serious and persistent mental illness. NAMI Indiana consists of families, consumers, and professionals that are dedicated to helping families through a network of support, education, advocacy, and promotion of research. NAMI Indiana is affiliated with the National Alliance on Mental Illness (NAMI), which is located in Arlington, Virginia.
Dee Weeks, Executive Director

6163 Richmond: NAMI East Central
NAMI Indiana
PO Box 22697
Indianapolis, IN 46222-0697
765-458-6758
800-677-6442
Fax: 317-925-9398
e-mail: nami@dunncenter.org
www.namiindiana.org

Meets on the first Tuesday of each month, 7:00 p.m., at 831 Dillon Drive, room 231.
Bernice Issac, Contact Person

6164 South Bend: NAMI St. Joseph County
NAMI Indiana
PO Box 22697
Indianapolis, IN 46222-0697
574-272-8580
800-677-6442
Fax: 317-925-9398
e-mail: Gary.E.Herr.1@nd.edu
www.namiindiana.org

Please call for our schedule.
Patricia Herr, President

6165 Terre Haute: NAMI Wabash Valley
NAMI Indiana
PO Box 22697
Indianapolis, IN 46222-0697
812-877-9950
800-677-6442
Fax: 317-925-9398
www.namiindiana.org

Currently meeting on the second Wednesday of each month, 7:00 p.m., at the Hamilton Center. Please call for directions and more information.
Betty Porter, Contact Person

6166 Warsaw NAMI Warsaw
NAMI Indiana
NAMI Indiana
Indianapolis, IN 46222-697
317-925-9399
800-677-6442
Fax: 317-925-9398
e-mail: toddataeq@earthlink.com
www.namiindiana.org

Meets every Tuesday from 7:00 to 9:00 p.m. at the First United Methodist Church.
Todd Biller, President
Joseph Vanable, President Nami Indiana

Iowa

6167 Iowa Federaion of Families for Children's Mental Health (FFCMH)
106 South Boothtreet
Anamosa, IA 52205
319-462-2187
888-400-6302
Fax: 319-462-6789
e-mail: lori@iffcmh.org
www.iffcmh.org

The mission of Iowa Federation of Families for Children's Mental Health is to link families to community, county and state partners for needed supports and services; and to promote systems change that will enable families to live in a safe, stable and respectful environment.
Lori Reynolds, Executive Director

Kentucky

6168 Kentucky IMPACT
275 E Main Street
Frankfort, KY 40621
502-564-7610
Sandra Noble Canon

Massachusetts

6169 Parent Professional Advocacy League
59 Temple Place
Boston, MA 2111
617-542-7860
866-815-8122
Fax: 617-542-7832
e-mail: info@ppal.net
www.ppal.net

Donna Welles, Executive Director

6170 Windhorse Associates
Windhorse Associates
31 Trumbull Road
Northampton, MA 01060-2328
413-586-0207
Fax: 413-585-1521
e-mail: info@windhorseassociates.org
www.windhorseassociates.org

Creating therapeutic environments to promote recovery from mental illness.
Molly Fortuna, Director Nursing/Admissions

Minnesota

6171 Emotional Health Anonymous
PO Box 4245
St Paul, MN 55104-0245
651-647-9712
Fax: 651-647-1593
e-mail: infodf3498fjsd@enotionsanonymous.org
www.emotionsanonymous.org

A twelve-step organization, similar to Alcoholics Anonymous. Compsed of people who come together in weekly meetings for the purpose of working toward recovery from emotional difficulties.

6172 PACER Center
8161 Normandale Boulevard
Minneapolis, MN 55437-1044
952-838-9000
800-537-2237
Fax: 952-838-0199
TTY: 952-838-0190
e-mail: pacer@pacer.org
www.pacer.org

Dixie Jordan, Advocate
Paula Goldberg, Executive Director

Missouri

6173 MO-SPAN Southwest Region
210 W Vine Street
Butler, MO 64730
660-679-5767
Eldonna Carroll

6174 MOSPAN Northwest Region
440 Rue Street François
Jefferson City, MO 63031
314-972-0600
Fax: 314-720-06
e-mail: mospan2@fid.net.com
www.mospan.org
Donna Dittrich, Executive Director
Tina Vervara, Administrative Assistant

Nevada

6175 Nevada PEP
2355 Red Rock Street
Las Vegas, NV 89146
702-388-8899
800-216-5188
Fax: 702-388-2966
e-mail: pepinfo@nvpep.org
www.nvpep.org
A statewide non-profit helping families who have children with disabilities, and the professionals who work with them. Support groups, training, workshops, lending resource library. Services are provided at no cost.
Karen Taycher, Executive Director

New Hampshire

6176 National Alliance for the Mentally Ill: New Hampshire
15 Green Street
Concord, NH 03301
603-225-5359
800-242-6264
Fax: 603-228-8848
e-mail: info@naminh.org
www.naminh.org
Family support and advocacy for consumers and family members.
Michael Cohen, Executive Director

New York

6177 Family Ties of Orange County
Mental Health Association of Orange County
20 Walker Street
Goshen, NY 10924-1906
845-294-7411
800-832-1200
Fax: 845-294-7348
e-mail: mha@mhaorangeny.com
www.mhaorangeny.com/
Mental Health Association of Orange County/MHA is a private, not-for-profit organization seeking to promote the mental health and emotional well being of Orange County residents. Under the leadership of a volunteer Board of Directors, MHA's staff members, consultants and volunteers provide free mental health services to thousands of Orange County residents each year. Several volunteers answer several hotlines, provide companionship, public education, direct services and assist with fundraisers.
Nadia Allen, Executive Director

6178 Mental Health Association in Dutchess Coun ty
510 Haight Avenue
Poughkeepsie, NY 12603
845-473-2500
Fax: 845-473-4870
e-mail: mhadc@hvc.rr.com
www.mhadc.com/
The Mental Health Association in Dutchess County promotes mental well-being and advances the recovery from mental illness, provides rehabilitation programs and support services for adults with a history of mental illness and their families.
Jacki Brownstein MPS, Executive Director
Emily Robisch, Director Finance and Operations

North Dakota

6179 ND FFCMH Region II
PO Box 3061
Bismarck, ND 58502-3061
701-222-1223
Fax: 701-250-8835
e-mail: carlottamccleary@bis.midco.nrt
www.ffcmh.org
Carlotta McCleary

6180 ND Region V FFCMH Chapter-Federation of Fa milies for Children's Mental Health
1104 2nd Avenue South
Fargo, ND 58103
701-235-9923
Fax: 701-235-9923
e-mail: ndffrgv@nbinternet.com
www.ffcmh.org/who_chapters.php
The FFCMH, a national family-run organization serves to: provide advocacy at the national level for the rights of children and youth with emotional, behavioral and mental health challenges and their families; provide leadership and technical assistance to a nation-wide network of family run organizations; and, collaborate with family run and other child serving organizations to transform mental health care in America.
Deborah Jendro, Executive Director

6181 ND Region VII FFCMH-Federation of Families for Children's Mental Health
2252 La Corte Loop
Bismarck, ND 58503
701-258-1628
Fax: 701-258-1628
e-mail: ndffrg7@btinet.net
www.ffcmh.org/who_chapters.php
The FFCMH, a national family-run organization serves to: provide advocacy at the national level for the rights of children and youth with emotional, behavioral and mental health challenges and their families; provide leadership and technical assistance to a nation-wide network of family run organizations; and, collaborate with family run and other child serving organizations to transform mental health care in America.
Becky Sevart, Executive Director

Ohio

6182 Child & Adolescent Service Center (CASC)
919 2nd Street NE
Canton, OH 44704
330-454-7917
Fax: 330-454-1476
e-mail: bsnyder@casrv.org
www.casrv.org/
The Child and Adolescent Service Center (CASC) was founded and incorporated in 1976 by a standing committee of the Stark County Mental Health Foundation. CASC provides dynamic leadership through innovative service, training and evaluation and is committed to providing culturally-sensitive programs and services throughout the community.
Bobbi L Beale Psy.D, Group Programs Director
David J Coleman Ph.D, Director of Psychological Services

6183 First Ohio Chapter: FFCMH
4505 Quaker Court
Canfield, OH 44406-9131
330-726-9570
Fax: 330-726-9031
e-mail: xuparents@aol.com OR ffcmh@ffcmh.org
www.ffcmh.org/who_chapters.php
The Federation of Families for Children's Mental Health (FFCMH) is a national organization dedicated exclusively to helping children with mental health needs and their families achieve a better quality of life.
Chrysanne Mitzel, Director First Ohio Chapter
Sandra Spencer, Executive Director Corporate Office (MD)

Rhode Island

6184 Parent Support Network
400 Warwick Avenue Suite 12
Warwick, RI 2888
401-467-6855
800-483-8844
Fax: 401-467-6903
e-mail: psnosri@aol.com
www.psnri.org
Cathy Cianon, Executive Director
Brenda Alego, Assistant Director

6185 Parent Support Network of Rhode Island
400 Warwick Avenue
Warwick, RI 2888
401-467-6855
800-483-8844
Fax: 401-467-6903
e-mail: psnori@aol.com
www.psnori.org
Family-run organization whose mission is to provide support, education and advocacy to parents of children at risk for or who have emotional, behavioral, and/or mental health challenges.
Cathy Cianon, Executive Director

South Carolina

6186 **FFCMH: South Carolina Chapter**
PO Box 1266 803-779-0402
Columbia, SC 29201 866-779-0402
Fax: 803-779-0450
e-mail: diane.flashnick@fedfamsc.org
www.fedfamsc.org/
The Federation of Families of South Carolina (FFCMH) is a non-profit organization established to serve the families of children with any degree of emotional, behavioral or psychiatric disorder. Through support networks, educational materials, publications, conferences/workshops and other activities, the Federation provides many avenues of support for families of children with emotional, behavioral or psychiatric disorders.
Dianne Flashnick, Executive Director
Phoebe Malloy, Board of Directors President

6187 **Family Support Network/SC AMI**
PO Box 2538 803-779-7849
Columbia, SC 29202 800-788-5131
Fax: 803-779-2655
Diane Flashnick

6188 **Federation of Families of South Carolina**
PO Box 1266 803-779-0402
Columbia, SC 29202-2344 866-779-0402
Fax: 803-779-0450
e-mail: FedFamSC@yahoo.com
www.midnet.sc.edu/ffsc
Cookie Cloyd

Tennessee

6189 **Tennessee Voices for Children**
1315 8th Avenue S 615-269-7751
Nashville, TN 37203 800-670-9882
Fax: 615-269-8914
e-mail: tvc@tnvoices.org
www.tnvoices.org
Charlotte Bryson, Director

Texas

6190 **Harris County FFCMH**
431 Breeze Park Drive 713-455-8962
Houston, TX 77015 e-mail: annn@flash.net
Elizabeth Neimeyer

Utah

6191 **Allies with Families**
450 East 1000 801-292-2515
North Salt Lake, UT 84054-2979 877-477-0764
Fax: 801-292-2680
e-mail: Allies@AlliesWithFamilies.org
www.allieswithfamilies.org
Allies with Families was created in 1991 to offer practical support and resources for parents and their children and youth who face serious emotional, behavioral and mental health challenges. It was created to support all families in the state of Utah.
Lori Cerar, Executive Director
Karen Greenwell, Community Education Coordinator

Vermont

6192 **Vermont FFCMH**
PO Box 607 802-434-6757
Montpelier, VT 05676-0507 800-639-6071
Fax: 802-434-6741
e-mail: vffcmh@together.net OR ffcmh@ffcmh.org
www.ffcmh.org/who_chapters.php
The Federation of Families for Children's Mental Health (FFCMH) is a national organization dedicated exclusively to helping children with mental health needs and their families achieve a better quality of life,
Kathleen Holsopple, Executive Director
Sandra Spencer, Executive Director Corporate Office (MD)

Virginia

6193 **PACCT**
8032 Mechanicsville Turnpike 804-559-6833
Mechancsville, VA 23111 Fax: 804-559-6835
Joyce Kube

6194 **PACCT of Roanoke Valley**
PO Box 21112 703-989-5042
Roanoke, VA 24018 Fax: 703-989-5675
e-mail: scheibe.p@worldnet.att.net
Sue Scheibe

Washington

6195 **Common Voice for Pierce County Parents**
801 East 141st Street 253-537-2145
Tacoma, WA 98445-2768 Fax: 253-537-2162
e-mail: acvmarge@comcast.net OR ffcmh@ffcmh.org
www.ffcmh.org/who_chapters.php
A Common Voice for Pierce County Parents is affiliated with the Federation of Families for Children's Mental Health (FFCMH), a national organization dedicated exclusively to helping children with mental health needs and their families achieve a better quality of life.
Marge Critchlow, Director
Sandra Spencer, Executive Director Corporate Office (MD)

Wisconsin

6196 **We Are the Children's Hope/Support Group**
First Love Outreach Ministries
PO Box 06204 414-263-1323
Milwaukee, WI 53206 Fax: 414-263-1148
e-mail: zelodius@aol.com
www.firstlovelifecoaching.com
Pr Zelodius Morton, CEO

Wyoming

6197 **Concerned Parent Coalition**
1125 Sioux Avenue 307-682-6684
Gillette, WY 82718-6529
Michelle Gerlosky

6198 **Uplift**
200 W 17th Street 307-778-8686
Cheyenne, WY 82003 888-875-4383
Fax: 307-778-8681
e-mail: uplift@upliftwy.org
www.upliftwy.org
Peggy Nikkel, Executive Director
Carla Schroeder, Deputy Director

Books

6199 **Anatomy of a Psychiatric Illness**
American Psychiatric Press
1400 K Street NW 202-682-6268
Washington, DC 20005-2403 Fax: 202-789-2648
Answers questions, provides clinical anecdotes, explains what medical science does and does not know about mental illnesses and discusses compassion and hard scientific facts surrounding the psychiatric profession.
230 pages
ISBN: 0-880485-21-3

6200 **Assessing Psychopathology and Behavior Problems: Mentally Ill Persons**
National Clearinghouse for Alcohol and Drug Abuse
PO Box 2345
Rockville, MD 20857-0001 800-729-6686
www.health.org
239 pages

6201 **Caring for People with Severe Mental Disorders: A National Plan**
Superintendent of Documents
PO Box 371954 202-512-2250
Pittsburgh, PA 15250-7954

This report offers, from three panels of expert consultants, recommendations for strengthening both services research and research resources that should lead to improvement of the standard and provision of care for persons who have severe mental disorders.
80 pages

6202 Complete Mental Health Directory
Grey House Publishing
4919 Route 22 518-789-8700
Amenia, NY 12501 800-562-2139
Fax: 518-789-0545
e-mail: books@greyhouse.com
www.greyhouse.com
Offers critical and comprehensive information on disorders, support groups, clinical management, government agencies, professional conferences, research centers and training.
687 pages
ISBN: 1-930956-06-1
Leslie Mackenzie, Publisher

6203 Creating New Options
Bazelon Center for Mental Health Law
1101 15th Street NW 202-467-5730
Washington, DC 20005-5002 Fax: 202-223-0409
TDD: 202-467-4342
e-mail: pubs@bazelon.org
www.bazelon.org
Training for corrections administrators and staff on access to federal benefits for people with mental illnesses who are leacing jail or prison. Available as a manual ($7.50),a PowerPoint presentation on CD ($5), or both ($11).
2008
Lee Carly, Communications Director

6204 Creating a Circle of Learning: The Church and the Mentally Ill
National Alliance for the Mentally Ill
PO Box 753 301-524-7600
Waldorf, MD 20604-0753 Fax: 301-843-0159
www.NAMI.org
A curriculum designed to sensitize adults in the church to the plight of people with severe mental illnesses and their families. Leaders can teach the study as 12 one-hour lessons or six two-hour lessons. The teaching sessions build on a Biblical-based theological reflection calling congregations to minister to their brothers and sisters with mental illnesses.
1997

6205 Culture and the Restructuring of Community Mental Health
William A Vega, author
Greenwood Publishing Group, Inc.
PO Box 6926
Portsmouth, NH 03802-6926 800-225-5800
Fax: 877-231-6980
e-mail: service@greenwood.com
www.greenwood.com
Examines treatment, organizational planning and research issues and offers a critique of the theoretical and programmatic aspects of providing mental health services to traditionally undeserved populations.
168 pages
ISBN: 0-313268-87-8

6206 Dealing with Mental Incapacity
Center for Public Representation
PO Box 260049 608-251-4008
Madison, WI 53726-0049 800-369-0388
Fax: 608-251-1263
This manual contains a comprehensive introduction to the problem of guardianship as well as chapters of financial and health care planning tools, guardianship under Wisconsin law, protective placement and Watts reviews.
Training Manual

6207 Design of Rehabilitation Services in Psychiatric Hospital Settings
American Occupational Therapy Association
PO Box 1725 301-948-9626
Rockville, MD 20849-1725 800-729-2082
Presents a design for constructing a rehabilitation system that will ensure the delivery of quality services to patients in a psychiatric hospital setting.
130 pages
Jeanette Bair, Executive Director

6208 Dimensions of State Mental Health Policy
Greenwood Publishing Group, Inc/Praeger Publishers
PO Box 6926
Portsmouth, NH 03802-6926 800-225-5800
Fax: 877-231-6980
e-mail: service@greenwood.com
www.greenwood.com
Introduces students to the emerging field of state mental health policy.
320 pages
ISBN: 0-275932-52-4

6209 Dual Diagnosis of Major Mental Illness and Substance Disorder
National Alliance for the Mentally Ill
PO Box 753 703-524-7600
Waldorf, MD 20604-0753 Fax: 703-524-9094
www.NAMI.org
Written for professionals, readable for families including descriptions of model programs.

6210 Educating Patients and Families About Mental Illness: A Practical Guide
Aspen Publishers
7201 McKinney Circle
Frederick, MD 21704-8356 800-638-8437
Introducing the manual to specifically address educating your patients and their families about mental illness.
496 pages

6211 Elderly with Chronic Mental Illness
Springer Publishing Company
536 Broadway 212-431-4370
New York, NY 10012-3955 877-687-7476
Fax: 212-941-7842
e-mail: marketing@springerpub.com
www.springerpub.com
384 pages Hardcover
ISBN: 0-826172-80-6
Annette Imperati, Marketing Director

6212 Elders Assert Their Rights
Bazelon Center for Mental Health Law
1101 15th Street NW 202-467-5730
Washington, DC 20005-5002 Fax: 202-223-0409
TDD: 202-467-4342
e-mail: pubs@bazelon.org
www.bazelon.org
A guide for residents, family members and advocates to the legal rights of elderly people with mental disabilities in nursing homes.
Paperback
Lee Carly, Communications Director

6213 Encyclopedia of Mental Health
Facts on File
11 Penn Plaza 212-967-8800
New York, NY 10001 800-322-8755
Fax: 800-678-3633
Here, readers will find inciseve definitions of theories, syndromes, symptons, treatments, and contemporary issues in easy-to-understand language.
480 pages Hardcover

6214 Encyclopedia of Phobias, Fears, and Anxieties
Facts on File
11 Penn Plaza 212-967-8800
New York, NY 10001 800-322-8755
Fax: 800-678-3633
500 pages Hardcover

6215 Evaluation and Treatment of the Psychogeriatric Patient
Diane Gibson, MS, author
Haworth Press

10 Alice Street
Binghamton, NY 13904-1580
607-722-5857
800-429-6784
Fax: 607-722-0012
www.haworthpress.com

This pertinent book assists occupational therapists and other health care providers in developing up-to-date psychogeriatric programs.
111 pages Hardcover
ISBN: 1-560240-52-1

6216 **Family Caregiving in Mental Illness**
National Alliance for the Mentally Ill
PO Box 753
Waldorf, MD 20604-0753
301-524-7600
Fax: 301-843-0159
www.NAMI.org

Examines patients' rights and treatment needs from the point of view of all those involved. Focuses on family burden and research and theoretical perspectives that influence mental health professionals.
1996

6217 **Federal Law of the Mentally Handicapped**
William Hein & Company
1285 Main Street
Buffalo, NY 14209-1987
716-882-2600

Chronological compilation of all relevant federal laws dealing with the mentally handicapped along with supporting documentation necessary to create a complete legislative history.
42 volumes/set

6218 **Focal Group Psychotherapy for Mental Health Professionals**
New Harbinger Publications
5674 Shattuck Avenue
Oakland, CA 94609-1662
800-748-6273
Fax: 510-652-5472
www.newharbinger.com

Definitive guide to leading brief, theme-based groups. This book offers an extensive week-by-week description of the basic concepts and interventions for 14 theme or focal groups.
544 pages

6219 **Handbook of Mental Health and Mental Disor der Among Black Americans**
Greenwood Publishing Group, Inc.
PO Box 6926
Portsmouth, NH 03802-6926
800-225-5800
Fax: 877-231-6980
e-mail: service@greenwood.com
www.greenwood.com

In addition to providing a wealth of new data on the mental health status of black communities, this handbook presents analyses of specific social, structural, and cultural conditions that affect the lives of individual black Americans.
352 pages
ISBN: 0-313263-30-2

6220 **How to Live with a Mentally Ill Person: A Handbook of Day-to-Day Strategies**
National Alliance for the Mentally Ill
PO Box 753
Waldorf, MD 20604-0753
301-524-7600
Fax: 301-843-0159
www.NAMI.org

Offers self-help-styled advice to caregivers. Includes personal experiences, education, stigma, coping, and the mental health system.
1996

6221 **Last in Line**
Bazelon Center for Mental Health Law
1101 15th Street NW
Washington, DC 20005-5002
202-467-5730
Fax: 202-223-0409
TDD: 202-467-4342
e-mail: pubs@bazelon.org
www.bazelon.org

discusses barriers to community integration of older adults with mental illnesses, and recommendations for change.
2006 72 pages
Lee Carly, Communications Director

6222 **Living with Mental Handicaps**
Jessica Kingsley Publishers
118 Pentonville Road
London, England,
071-833-2307
Fax: 071-837-2917

The focus of this book lies in its insistence that mentally handicapped people make transitions like the rest of us from youth to old age.
176 pages

6223 **Madness in the Streets**
Free Press
866 3rd Avenue
New York, NY 10022-6221
800-323-7445
Fax: 800-943-9831
www.simonsays.com

How psychiatry and the law abandoned the mentally ill.
436 pages
ISBN: 0-029153-80-8

6224 **Making Child Welfare Work**
Bazelon Center for Mental Health Law
1101 15th Street NW
Washington, DC 20005-5002
202-467-5730
Fax: 202-223-0409
TDD: 202-467-4342
e-mail: pubs@bazelon.org
www.bazelon.org

How the RC lawsuit forged new partnership to protect children and sustain families. The story of systems reform from the bottom up and the rededication of a burocracy to focus on the children and families it is meant to serve.
1998 126 pages
Lee Carly, Communications Director

6225 **Managed Mental Health Care**
American Psychiatric Press
1400 K Street NW
Washington, DC 20005-2403
202-682-6268
Fax: 202-789-2648

This text presents the collective wisdom of 40 experts experienced in clinical and managerial issues in managed care.
425 pages Hardcover
ISBN: 0-880483-55-5

6226 **Managing Managed Care: A Mental Health Practitioner's Survival Guide**
American Psychiatric Press
1400 K Street NW
Washington, DC 20005-2403
202-682-6268
Fax: 202-789-2648

Provides an easy-to-learn system for communicating with external reviewers and documenting quality of care.
200 pages Hardcover
ISBN: 0-880483-69-5

6227 **Manic Depressive Illness**
National Alliance for the Mentally Ill
PO Box 753
Waldorf, MD 20604-0753
703-524-7600
Fax: 703-524-9094
www.NAMI.org

A definitive overview of bipolar disorder.

6228 **Medicare Rx Consumer Workbook**
Mental Health America
2000 North Beauragard Street
Alexandria, VA 22311
703-684-7722
800-969-6642
Fax: 703-684-5968
TTY: 800-433-5959
www.mentalhealthamerica.net

This workbook is designed to help you as a mental health consumer to get educated about and get enrolled in the new Medicare prescription drug program. Designed as a pocket folder, the workbook includes basic language explanations, tips for enrollment preparation, questions you should ask regarding plan options, worksheets, and definitions.

6229 **Membership Directory**
Natl. Council for Community Behavioral Healthcare
12300 Twinbrook Parkway
Rockville, MD 20852
301-984-6200

6230 **Mental Disability Law: A Primer**
Commission on The Mentally Disabled

1800 M Street NW
Washington, DC 20036-5802
202-331-2240
An updated and expanded version of the 1984 edition. Addresses the considerations involved in representing clients with mental disabilities.

6231 Mental Health Care in Prisons and Jails
Vance Bibliographies
PO Box 229
Monticello, IL 61856-0229
217-762-3831
A bibliography regarding health care in prisons.
30 pages
ISBN: 0-792006-94-1

6232 Mental Health Concepts and Techniques for the Occupational Therapy Assistant
Raven Press
1185 Avenue of the Americas
New York, NY 10036-2601
212-930-9500
800-777-2295
This text offers clear and easily understood explanations of the various theoretical and practice health models. Second edition.
344 pages
ISBN: 0-781700-74-4

6233 Mental Health Law Reporter
Business Publishers, Inc.
PO Box 17592
Baltimore, MD 21297
800-274-6737
e-mail: custserv@bpinews.com
www.bpinews.com
Brings you the most timely, focused and thorough information on the legal issues that concern you in mental health litigation.
monthly
Leonard Eiserer, Publisher

6234 Mental Health: Counseling Services
Vance Bibliographies
PO Box 229
Monticello, IL 61856-0229
217-762-3831
Selected annotated bibliography on counseling services for the mentally handicapped from a black perspective.
23 pages
ISBN: 1-555903-76-2

6235 Mental Illness-Opposing Viewpoints Series
Greenhaven Press
Thomson Gale
Farmington Hills, MI 48333-9187
800-877-4253
Fax: 800-414-5043
e-mail: gale.customerservice@thomson.com
www.gale.com/greenhaven
In-depth overview of the topic written for upper elementary and junior/senior high school students.
2006
ISBN: 1-560061-68-5

6236 Mental and Physical Disability Law Report
American Bar Association
1800 M Street NW
Washington, DC 20036-5802
202-331-2240
Covers case law, legislative and regulatory developments that affect persons with mental or physical disabilities.

6237 Mentally Ill Individuals
Mainstream
1030 5th Street NW
Washington, DC 20001-2504
202-898-1400
Mainstreaming mentally ill individuals into the workplace.
12 pages

6238 Mood Apart: Depression, Mania, and Other Afflictions of the Self
National Alliance for the Mentally Ill
PO Box 753
Waldorf, MD 20604-0753
301-524-7600
Fax: 301-843-0159
www.NAMI.org
Discussion of depression and mania includes the symptoms, human costs, biological underpinnings, and therapies. Uses case histories, appendices, and historical references.
1997

6239 National Plan for Research on Child and Adolescent Mental Disorders
Superintendent of Documents
PO Box 371954
Pittsburgh, PA 15250-7954
202-512-2250
Summarizes the current knowledge about the prevalence and causes of mental disorders among children, identifies the possible treatments and prevention strategies and notes promising areas of research.
64 pages

6240 Occupational Therapy Practice Guidelines for Adults with Mood Disorders
American Occupational Therapy Association
4720 Montgomery Lane
Bethesda, MD 20824-1220
301-652-2682
Fax: 301-652-7711
TDD: 800-377-8555
www.aota.org
27 pages
ISBN: 1-569001-10-3

6241 Playing Cure
Jason Aronson
PO Box 15100
York, PA 17405-7100
800-782-0015
www.aronson.com
400 pages Hardcover
ISBN: 0-765700-21-2

6242 Protection and Advocacy Program for the Mentally Ill
US Department of Health and Human Services
5600 Fishers Lane
Rockville, MD 20857-0001
301-443-3667
Federal formula grant program to protect and advocate the rights of people with mental illnesses who are in residential facilities and to investigate abuse and neglect in such facilities.
Natalie Reatia, Chief

6243 Somatization Disorder in the Medical Setting
Superintendent of Documents
PO Box 371954
Pittsburgh, PA 15250-7954
202-512-2250
Somatization is a process in which psychological distress is expressed in multiple physical symptoms that have no discernible medical cause.
98 pages

6244 Strengthening the Role of Families in States' Early Intervention Systems
CEC, Department K00757
Herdon, VA 22091
703-471-9543
Policy guide for procedural safeguards for infants and toddlers under Part H of the Individuals with Disabilities Education Act.
213 pages Report

6245 Surviving Mental Illness
National Alliance for the Mentally Ill
PO Box 753
Waldorf, MD 20604-0753
703-524-7600
Fax: 703-524-9094
www.NAMI.org
The subjective experiences of people with multiple diagnoses including schizophrenia, bipolar disorder and manic depression.

6246 Teaching Adults with Mental Handicaps
Sunday School Board of the Southern Baptists
127 9th Avenue N
Nashville, TN 37234-0001
800-458-BSSB
Offers guidelines in methods of teaching adults with mental handicaps, their needs, outreach ideas, curriculum resources, adaptation procedures, and ministry suggestions.

6247 Troubled Journey
National Alliance for the Mentally Ill
PO Box 753
Waldorf, MD 20604-0753
301-524-7600
Fax: 301-843-0159
www.NAMI.org
Long associated with NAMI's former Siblings and Adult Children Network, the authors use their years of listening to stories - plus Marsh's professional experience - to provide a book that offers support to siblings and a caring and heartfelt approach to healing.
1997

6248 **Turning Point**
American Psychiatric Press
1400 K Street NW 202-682-6268
Washington, DC 20005-2403 Fax: 202-789-2648
The first comprehensive chronicle of the contributions made by conscientious objectors who volunteered for service in America's mental hospitals and state institutions for the developmentally disabled.
314 pages Hardcover
ISBN: 0-880485-60-4

6249 **Understanding Depression**
Patricia Ainsworth, MD, author
University Press of Mississippi
3825 Ridgewood Road 601-432-6205
Jackson, MS 39211-6492 Fax: 601-432-6217
e-mail: kburgess@ihl.state.ms.us
www.upress.state.ms.us
A clear explanation for those who know the illness personally and for those who want to understand them.
2000 120 pages Paperback
ISBN: 1-578061-69-5
Kathy Burgess, Advertising/Marketing Services Manager

6250 **Understanding Mental Retardation**
Patricia Ainsworth, MD; Pamela C Baker, PhD, author
University Press of Mississippi
3825 Ridgewood Road 601-432-6205
Jackson, MS 39211-6492 Fax: 601-432-6217
e-mail: kburgess@ihl.state.ms.us
www.upress.state.ms.us
A resource for parents, caregivers, and counselors.
2004 192 pages Paperback
ISBN: 1-578066-47-6
Kathy Burgess, Advertising/Marketing Services Manager

6251 **Understanding Panic and Other Anxiety Disorders**
Benjamin Root, MD, author
University Press of Mississippi
3825 Ridgewood Road 601-432-6205
Jackson, MS 39211-6492 Fax: 601-432-6217
e-mail: kburgess@ihl.state.ms.us
www.upress.state.ms.us
A patients guide to panic disorders, panic attacks, and other stress-related maladies.
2000 128 pages Paperback
ISBN: 1-578062-45-4
Kathy Burgess, Advertising/Marketing Services Manager

6252 **Victims of Dementia**
Haworth Press
10 Alice Street 607-722-5857
Binghamton, NY 13904-1580 800-429-6784
Fax: 607-722-0012
www.haworthpress.com
Provides an in-depth look at the concept, construction and operation of Wesley Hall, a special living area at the Chelsea United Methodist retirement home in Michigan.
1993 155 pages Hardcover
ISBN: 1-560242-64-0

6253 **Way to Go: School Success for Children wit h Mental Health Care Needs**
Bazelon Center for Mental Health Law
1101 15th Street NW 202-467-5730
Washington, DC 20005-5002 Fax: 202-223-0409
TDD: 202-467-4342
e-mail: pubs@bazelon.org
www.bazelon.org
A report and fact sheets that document how states and school districts have successfully combined school-wide positive behavior support (PBS) with effective mental health services to foster a school environment that is conducive to learning, and improves children's lives. Order book and fact sheets sheets seperately or together. Pricing according to volume begins at $25 per book, $10 per fact sheet, or $29 for the combination.
1998
Lee Carly, Communications Director

6255 **What Fair Housing Means for People with Disabilities**
Bazelon Center for Mental Health Law
1101 15th Street NW 202-467-5730
Washington, DC 20005-5002 Fax: 202-223-0409
TDD: 202-467-4342
e-mail: pubs@bazelon.org
www.bazelon.org
Explains in plain language how three federal laws protect the housing rights of people with mental or physical disabilities. 2003 edition available as pdf download.
2006 56 pages
Lee Carly, Communications Director

6256 **When Madness Comes Home**
National Alliance for the Mentally Ill
PO Box 753 301-524-7600
Waldorf, MD 20604-0753 Fax: 301-843-0159
www.NAMI.org
Personal accounts offer first-hand, day-to-day experiences with mental illness of a sibling (mostly) and partner/spouse (briefly) and discuss the effects of growing up in a family whose energies are focused on an ill family member.
1997

6257 **When Someone You Love Has a Mental Illness**
National Alliance for the Mentally Ill
PO Box 753 703-524-7600
Waldorf, MD 20604-0753 Fax: 703-524-9094
www.NAMI.org
Excellent for families recently stricken with severe mental illness.

Children's Books

6258 **Compassion Books**
7036 State Highway 80 S 828-675-5909
Burnsville, NC 28714-7569 800-970-4220
Fax: 828-675-9687
e-mail: heal2grow@aol.com
www.compassionbooks.com
Hand picked resources to help people through loss, grief and changes of all kinds. Carry over 400 books and videos on death and dying, bereavement and change, comfort and healing, hope and much more.
Bruce Greene, VP

Magazines

6259 **AJMR**
American Association on Mental Retardation
444 N Capitol Street NW 202-387-1968
Washington, DC 20001-1508 800-424-3688
Fax: 202-387-2193
e-mail: AAMR@access.digex.net
www.aamr.org
Provides information on the latest program advances, current research, and information on products and services in the developmental disabilities field.
BiMonthly

6260 **American Journal of Psychiatry**
American Psychiatric Association
1400 K Street NW 202-682-6220
Washington, DC 20005-2492
Professional papers on topics in psychiatry.
Monthly
Public Affairs, Division

6261 **American Psychologist**
American Psychological Association
750 First Street NE 202-336-5510
Washington, DC 20002-4242 800-374-2721
Fax: 202-336-5502
TDD: 202-336-6123
e-mail: books@apa.org
www.apa.org

Articles on current issues in psychology as well as empirical, theoretical and practical articles on broad aspects of psychology.
9x a year

6262 **Journal of Clinical Psychology**
Clinical Psychology Publishing Company
4 Conant Square 802-247-6877
Brandon, VT 05733-1018
Scholarly research reports in the field of psychology.

6263 **Mental Retardation**
American Association on Mental Retardation
444 N Capitol Street NW 202-387-1968
Washington, DC 20001-1508 800-424-3688
Fax: 202-387-2193
e-mail: AAMR@access.digex.net
www.aamr.org
Provides information on the latest program advances, current research, and information on products and services in the developmental disabilities field.
BiMonthly

6264 **Psychopharmacology Bulletin**
Superintendent of Documents/NIMH Journal
PO Box 371954 202-512-2250
Pittsburgh, PA 15250-7954
Emphasizes rapid, informal dissemination of recent research findings that have not previously appeared in the more formal literature.
Quarterly

6265 **Psychosocial Rehabilitation Journal**
Int'l Assoc. of Psychosocial Rehab. Services
730 Commonwealth Avenue 617-353-3549
Boston, MA 02215-1209
Discusses issues, programs and research on psychiatric rehabilitation.

Newsletters

6266 **ACMH Newsletter**
Association for Children's Mental Health
1705 Coolidge Road 517-336-7222
East Lansing, MI 48823-1735 800-782-0883
Offers the latest information, including unmet needs and notices of relevant agency and legislative activities, hearings, public meetings and other opportunities for promoting children's mental health.
Quarterly
Gail Allen, Director
Marla Holle, Parent Advocate

6267 **Advocate**
National Alliance for the Mentally Ill
200 N Glebe Road 703-524-7600
Arlington, VA 22203-3754 Fax: 703-524-9094
Offers reviews of books, medical information, legislative information and Alliance activities for persons with mental illness, their families and professionals who work with them.
Quarterly

6268 **Mental Health Law News**
Interwood Publications
PO Box 20241 513-221-3715
Cincinnati, OH 45220-0241
Mental health case law summaries.
6 pages Monthly
ISBN: 0-889017-0 -
Frank J Bardack, Editor

6269 **News & Notes**
American Association on Mental Retardation
444 N Capitol Street NW 202-387-1968
Washington, DC 20001-1508 800-424-3688
Fax: 202-387-2193
e-mail: AAMR@access.digex.net
www.aamr.org
Covers legislative, program, and research developments of interest to the field, as well as international news, Association activities, job ads and other classifieds, and upcoming events.
BiMonthly

Pamphlets

6270 **14 Worst Myths About Recovered Mental Patients**
National Institutes of Health
5600 Fishers Lane 301-496-4000
Rockville, MD 20857-0001 e-mail: NIHInfo@nih.gov
www.nih.gov
Refutes false beliefs that stigmatize recovered mental patients and suggests ways that the public can help advance the truth.

6271 **Bipolar Disorder**
National Institutes of Health
5600 Fishers Lane 301-443-3706
Rockville, MD 20857-0001 Fax: 301-443-6349
A short booklet offering a concise description of this disorder, which is also called manic-depressive illness.

6272 **Coping with Mental Illness in the Family**
National Alliance for the Mentally Ill
PO Box 753 703-524-7600
Waldorf, MD 20604-0753 Fax: 703-524-9094
www.NAMI.org
A handbook for families.

6273 **Dual Diagnosis: Substance Abuse and Mental Illness**
National Alliance for the Mentally Ill
PO Box 753 703-524-7600
Waldorf, MD 20604-0753 Fax: 703-524-9094
www.NAMI.org
A booklet for families and consumers.

6274 **Helping Families Understand PTSD**
National Veterans Services Fund
PO Box 2465 203-656-0003
Darien, CT 06820-0465 Fax: 203-656-1957
e-mail: NatVetSvc@aol.com
Pamphlet

6275 **Let's Talk Facts About Childhood Disorders**
American Psychiatric Association
1400 K Street NW 202-682-6220
Washington, DC 20005-2492
Offers information on depression and depressive disorders including the causes, symptoms, treatments, anxiety, and various other phobias.
Public Affairs, Division

6276 **Mental Health Problems of Vietnam Veterans**
National Veterans Services Fund
PO Box 2465 203-656-0003
Darien, CT 06820-0465 Fax: 203-656-1957
e-mail: NatVetSvc@aol.com
Pamphlet

6277 **Minority Advocacy Notebook**
Bazelon Center for Mental Health Law
1101 15th Street NW 202-467-5730
Washington, DC 20005-5002 Fax: 202-223-0409
TDD: 202-467-4342
e-mail: pubs@bazelon.org
www.bazelon.org
Selected materials and models from our manual on outreach and advocacy for African Americans and Latinos with mental disabilities; includes "Impediments to Services and Advocacy for Black and Hispanic People with Mental Illness".
1998
Lee Carly, Communications Director

6278 **New Challenge: Responding to Families**
Federation for Children with Special Needs
95 Berkeley Street 617-482-2915
Boston, MA 02116-6230 800-331-0688
Addresses the needs of children with emotional, behavioral and mental disorders and their families.

6279 **PTSD and the Family: Secondary Traumatization**
National Veterans Services Fund
PO Box 2465 203-656-0003
Darien, CT 06820-0465 Fax: 203-656-1957
e-mail: NatVetSvc@aol.com
Pamphlet

6280 **Plain Talk About...Dealing with the Angry Child**
Superintendent of Documents
PO Box 371954 202-512-2250
Pittsburgh, PA 15250-7954
A flyer that offers suggestions for helping children cope with their anger in a healthy and constructive way.

6281 **Plain Talk About...Handling Stress**
Superintendent of Documents
PO Box 371954 202-512-2250
Pittsburgh, PA 15250-7954
Information on stress and how you can make it work for you rather than against you.

6282 **Psychotherapy with Traumatized Vietnam Combatants**
National Veterans Services Fund
PO Box 2465 203-656-0003
Darien, CT 06820-0465 Fax: 203-656-1957
e-mail: NatVetSvc@aol.com
Pamphlet

6283 **Triumph Over Fear**
National Alliance for the Mentally Ill
PO Box 753 703-524-7600
Waldorf, MD 20604-0753 Fax: 703-524-9094
www.NAMI.org
Step-by-step treatment plans for the many faces of phobias, panic disorder, obsessive-compulsive disorder, and post-traumatic stress. Includes case histories.
1994 Softcover

Audio & Video

6284 **And After Tomorrow**
G. Allan Roeher Institute
4700 Keele Street 416-661-9611
Downsview, ON, M3J 1P3,
A film about lives of people with a mental handicap and their families, in which parents and friends speak candidly about their personal experiences.
Films

6285 **With a Little Help from My Friends**
L'institut Roeher Institute
York University, 4700 Keele Street 416-661-9611
North York, ON, M3J 1P3, Fax: 416-661-5701
This three-part video provides insight into inclusive education for people with mental handicaps.

Web Sites

6286 **American Psychological Association**
www.apa.org
Mission is to advance psychology as a science and professional organization that represents psychology in the United States.

6287 **Coalition of Voluntary Mental Health Agencies**
www.cvmha.org/
An umbrella advocacy organization of New York's mental health community, representing over 100 non-profit community based mental health agencies that serve more than 300,000 clients in the five boroughs of New York City and its environs.

6288 **Community Access**
www.cairn.org/
A nonprofit agency providing housing and advocacy for people with psychiatric disabilities.

6289 **Federation of Families for Children's Mental Health**
www.ffcmh.org/
Providing leadership to develop and sustain a nationwide network of family-run organizations.

6290 **Healing Well**
www.healingwell.com
An online health resource guide to medical news, chat, information and articles, newsgroups and message boards, books, disease-related web sites, medical directories, and more for patients, friends, and family coping with disabling diseases, disorders, or chronic illnesses.

6291 **Health Finder**
www.healthfinder.gov
Searchable, carefully developed web site offering information on over 1000 topics. Developed by the US Department of Health and Human Services, the site can be used in both English and Spanish.

6292 **Healthlink USA**
www.healthlinkusa.com
Health information concerning treatment, cures, prevention, diagnosis, risk factors, research, support groups, email lists, personal stories and much more. Updated regularly.

6293 **Helios Health**
www.helioshealth.com
Online resource for your health information. Detailed information about specific health topics, access to expert advice from our Medical Advisory Board, and up-to-date health news.

6294 **Internet Mental Health**
www.mentalhealth.com
A site whose goal is to improve understanding, diagnosis, and treatment of mental illness throughout the world. Includes information on specific disorders, medications, diagnosis, research, news, and other internet links.

6295 **MedicineNet**
www.medicinenet.com
An online resource for consumers providing easy-to-read, authoritative medical and health information.

6296 **Medscape**
www.mywebmd.com
Medscape offers specialists, primary care physicians, and other health professionals the Web's most robust and integrated medical information and educational tools.

6297 **Mental Health America (formerly NMHA) Information Center**
www.mentalhealthamerica.net
Provides informational materials, lobbies for Federal mental health legislation, stimulates funding of research on the causes and treatment of mental illnesses.

6298 **National Alliance for the Mentally Ill**
www.nami.org
Over 900 affiliate groups nationwide offer support to members, advocate better lives for their loved ones, support research efforts and educate the public to reduce the stigma attached to serious mental illnesses.

6299 **National Mental Health Services Knowledge Exchange Network**
www.mentalhealth.org
Leading the national system that delivers mental health services. Provides the treatment and support services neede by adults with mental disorders and children with serious emotional problems.

6300 **WebMD**
www.webmd.com
Information on mental illness, including articles and resources.

6301 **World Federation for Mental Health**
www.wfmh.com
Mission is to promote, among all people and nations, the highest possible level of mental health in its broadest biological, medical, educational, and social aspects.

Description

6302 **Mental Illness/Depression**

Depression is a mood disorder that can cause marked impairment of physical and social function and work capacity. It differs from normal grief which occurs in response to a significant separation or loss. It affects twice as many women as men and is more common in people with a family history of depression.

Research is gathering evidence of the relationship between depression and chemical imbalances in the brain. Clinical depression can also be associated with medication or other physical illnesses.

Common symptoms associated with depression include irritability, sleeping problems, changes in appetite, sadness, apathy, loss of interest in previously enjoyed activities and anxiety. Depression frequently disrupts a person's relationship with friends, family members and colleagues. It is also associated with alcohol and substance abuse. Suicide is the cause of death in approximately 15 percent of untreated patients.

Treatment must be tailored to the individual and can include talk therapy and/or medication. Newer groups of antidepressant medications have markedly improved the success of treatment. Patient and family education can play a crucial role. See also *Mental Illness/General and Mental Illness/Schizophrenia.*

National Agencies & Associations

6303 **American Counseling Association**
5999 Stevenson Avenue
Alexandria, VA 22304
800-347-6647
Fax: 800-473-2329
www.counseling.org

The American Counseling Association is a non-profit professional and educational organization that is dedicated to the growth and enhancement of the counseling profession. Founded in 1952 ACA is the world's largest such association.
Colleen R Logan, President
Richard Yep, Executive Director

6304 **American Psychiatric Association**
1000 Wilson Boulevard
Arlington, VA 22209-3901
703-907-7300
888-357-7924
e-mail: apa@psych.org
www.psych.org

The American Psychiatric Association is a medical specialty society recognized world wide. Its over 35,000 U.S. and international member physicians work together to ensure humane care and effective treatment for all persons with mental disorders.

6305 **Anxiety Disorders Association of America**
8730 Georgia Avenue
Silver Spring, MD 20910
240-485-1001
Fax: 240-485-1035
e-mail: information@adaa.org
www.adaa.org

The Anxiety Disorders Association (ADAA) is a non profit organization whose mission is to promote the prevention treatment and cure of anxiety disorders and to improve the lives of all people who suffer from them.
Abby J Fyer, Treasurer
Jerilyn Ross, President & CEO

6306 **NARSAD: Mental Health Research Association**
60 Cutter Miller Road
Great Neck, NY 11021-3104
516-829-0091
800-829-8289
Fax: 516-487-6930
e-mail: info@narsad.org
www.narsad.org

NARSAD Information and helpline staff is available to answer basic questions about the symptoms, causes and treatments of psychiatric illnesses. Information on support groups and other mental health organizations can also be provided.
Joel Gurin, Acting President
Louis Innamorato, Vice President Finance/CFO

6307 **National Alliance for the Mentally Ill**
2107 Wilson Boulevard
Arlington, VA 22201
703-524-7600
800-950-6264
Fax: 703-524-9097
TDD: 703-516-7227
www.nami.org

Membership organization with over 858 affiliates in 50 states, offers newsletters, a mail-order bookstore and many programs, conferences, symposia and groups meetings for family members and patients.
Liz Smith, Regional Director

6308 **National Anxiety Foundation**
3135 Custer Drive
Lexington, KY 40517-4001
606-272-7166
www.lexington-on-line.com/naf.html

Offers information and help to persons with panic disorders manic and depressive disorders and mental illness.
Stephen Cox, President & Medical Director
Linda Vermon Blair, Vice President

6309 **National Foundation for Depressive Illness**
PO Box 2257
New York, NY 10116-2257
800-239-1265
www.depression.org

Founded in 1983 to correct the myths and misconceptions surrounding the illness and help reverse the devastating effects depression has on the individual and our society. NAFDI's purpose is to educate the public and primary health care providers.
Jim Estepp, President/CEO
Joe Conoscenti, Vice President of Global Customers

6310 **National Mental Health Association**
2000 N Beauregard Street
Alexandria, VA 22311
703-684-7722
800-969-6642
Fax: 703-684-5968
TTY: 800-433-5959
e-mail: infoctr@nmha.org
www.mentalhealthamerica.net

Serves over 700 affiliates nationally providing information publications and other services.
David L Shern PhD, President & CEO
Eileen Sexton, Vice President Communications

6311 **National Mental Health Information Center**
PO Box 42557
Washington, DC 20015
800-789-2647
Fax: 240-747-5470
TTY: 866-889-2647
TDD: 866-889-2647
e-mail: nmhic-info@samhsa.hhs.gov
www.mentalhealth.samhsa.gov

The Center for Mental Health Services (CMHS) is charged with leading the national system that delivers mental health services. The goal of this system is to provide the treatment and support services needed by adults and children with mental disorders.
A Kathryn Power, Director
Edward B Searle, Deputy Director

6312 **Option Institute**
2080 S Undermountain Road
Sheffield, MA 01257
413-229-2100
800-714-2779
Fax: 413-229-8931
e-mail: participantsupport@option.org
www.option.org

Self-defeating beliefs, along with attitudes and judgments can lead to depression and a host of physical and psychological challenges.

The Option Institute offers programs designed to help uproot self-defeating beliefs and remove roadblocks to happiness.
Barry Kaufman, Co-Founder
Samahria Lyt Kaufman, Co-Founder

6313 **Screening For Mental Health**
Screening For Mental Health
One Washington Street 781-239-0071
Wellesley Hills, MA 02481 Fax: 781-431-7447
e-mail: smhinfo@mentalhealthscreening.org
www.mentalhealthscreening.org
Screening for Mental Health (SHM) is the non-profit organization that first introduced the concept of large-scale mental health screenings with its flagship program National Depression Screening Day in 1991. SHM programs now include both in-person and online.
Douglas G Jacobs, President/CEO
James Henry Scully Jr, Medical Director

Research Centers

6314 **University of Pennsylvania: Depression Research Unit**
School of Medicine
Department of Psychiatry 215-662-3462
Philadelphia, PA 19104 Fax: 215-662-6443
Focuses on mental health and depression.
Jay D Amsterdam MD, Director

6315 **University of Texas Mental Health Clinical Research Center**
University of Texas
5323 Harry Hines Boulevard 214-648-5555
Dallas, TX 75390 Fax: 214-485-99
e-mail: news@utsouthwester.edu
www.utsouthwesteRN.edu
Research activity of major and atypical depression.
Eric Nestler MD, Chairman
Alex Cabrera, Clinic Manager

6316 **Yale University: Behavioral Medicine Clinic**
Yale School of Medicine
333 Cedar Street 203-785-4184
New Haven, CT 06510
Focuses on mental disorders including schizophrenia and depression.
Hoyle Leigh MD, Director

6317 **Yale University: Ribicoff Research Facilities/CT Mental Health Center**
34 Park Street 203-789-7300
New Haven, CT 06511 Fax: 203-562-7079
Clinical research in the areas of schizophrenia depression and mental disorders.
George Henin MD, Director

Support Groups & Hotlines

6318 **National Depressive and Manic Depressive Association**
730 N Franklin Street 312-642-0049
Chicago, IL 60610 800-826-3632
Fax: 312-642-7243
www.dbsalliance.org
Consists of 250 patient groups providing support and direct services to persons with clinical depression.
Lydia Lewis, President

6319 **National Health Information Center**
PO Box 1133 310-565-4167
Washington, DC 20013 800-336-4797
Fax: 301-984-4256
e-mail: info@nhic.org
www.health.gov/nhic
Offers a nationwide information referral service, produces directories and resource guides.

Books

6320 **Columbia University Complete Home Guide to Mental Health**
Henry Holt & Company
115 W 18th Street 212-886-9200
New York, NY 10011-4113 Fax: 212-633-0748
A compendium of information on all aspects of mental health; written primarily for the lay reader.
476 pages

6321 **Coping with Depression and Mood Disorders**
Rosen Publishing Group
29 E 21st Street 212-777-3017
New York, NY 10010 800-237-9932
Fax: 888-436-4643
e-mail: customerservice@rosenpub.com
www.rosenpublishing.com
With an emphasis on life's myriad difficulties, the authors help teens find practical ways to cope with depression.

ISBN: 0-823929-73-6
Lawrence Clayton PhD, Author
Sharon Carter, Author

6322 **Depression Sourcebook**
Brian P. Quinn, author
McGraw-Hill Companies
Returns Department
Dubuque, IA 52002 877-833-5524
Fax: 614-759-3749
e-mail: pbg.ecommerce_custserv@mcgrw-hill.com
www.mcgraw-hill.com
Everything anyone afflicted with a depressive disorder - or the people who care about them - need to know about unipolar and bipolar depression.
2000 288 pages
ISBN: 0-737303-79-4

6323 **Depression and its Treatment**
Warner Books
1271 Avenue of the Americas 212-522-7200
New York, NY 10020-1300
A layman's guide to help one understand and cope with America's #1 mental health problem.
157 pages

6324 **Depressive Illnesses: Treatments Bring New Hope**
Superintendent of Documents
PO Box 371954 202-512-2250
Pittsburgh, PA 15250-7954
Offers the general public an overview of the various depressive illnesses. Topics include causes, symptoms and types of depression, clinical evaluation and treatment, helpful suggestions for family and friends, and other sources of information.
28 pages

6325 **Encyclopedia of Depression**
Facts on File
11 Penn Plaza 212-967-8800
New York, NY 10001 800-322-8755
Fax: 800-678-3633
This volume defines and explains all terms and topics relating to depression.
170 pages Hardcover

6326 **Essential Guide to Psychiatric Drugs**
St. Martin's Press
175 5th Avenue 212-674-5151
New York, NY 10010-7848 800-221-7945
Fax: 212-420-9314
Basic information on 123 drugs used for depression, anxiety and bipolar illness.

6327 **Everything You Need to Know About Depression**
Rosen Publishing Group

29 E 21st Street
New York, NY 10010
212-777-3017
800-237-9932
Fax: 888-436-4643
e-mail: customerservice@rosenpub.com
www.rosenpublishing.com

An important resource for teens who are looking for help with depression.

Grades 7-12

ISBN: 0-823934-39-X

Elanor H Ayer, Author

6328 **Inside Manic Depression**
Sunnyside Press
PO Box 1717
San Marcos, CA 92079-1717
619-424-3348

The true story of one victim's triumph over despair. A first person account.

176 pages

6329 **Medical Management of Depression**
EMIS Medical Publishers
PO Box 1607
Durant, OK 74702-1607
580-924-0643
800-225-0694
Fax: 580-924-9414

ISBN: 0-929240-62-6

6330 **Mood Apart**
Basic Books
10 E 53rd Street
New York, NY 10022-5244
212-207-7057

An overview of the depression and manic depression and the available treatments for them.

363 pages

6331 **Overcoming Depression**
Harper & Row
10 E 53rd Street
New York, NY 10022-5299
212-207-7000

318 pages Paperback

6332 **Panic Disorder in the Medical Setting**
Superintendent of Documents
PO Box 371954
Pittsburgh, PA 15250-7954
202-512-2250

This book serves the primary care physicians as a helpful guide in recognizing and treating panic disorder in patients and in identifying those who need psychiatric consultation or rerferrals.

1993 135 pages

6333 **Pastoral Care of Depression**
The Haworth Press
10 Alice Street
Binghamton, NY 13904-1580
607-722-5857
800-429-6784
Fax: 607-895-0582
e-mail: getinfo@haworth.com
www.haworth.com

Helps caregivers by overcoming the simplistic myths about depressive disorders and probing the real issues.

Paperback

ISBN: 0-789002-65-5

6334 **Prozac Nation: Young & Depressed in America: A Memoir**
Houghton Mifflin Company
Wayside Road
Burlington, MA 01803
800-225-3362

Struck with depression at 11, now 27, Wurtzel chronicles her struggle with the illness. Witty, terrifying and sometimes funny, it tells the story of a young life almost destroyed by depression.

317 pages

6335 **Psychotherapy of Severe and Mild Depression**
Jason Aronson
PO Box 15100
York, PA 17405-7100
800-782-0015
Fax: 201-840-7242
www.aronson.com

464 pages Softcover

ISBN: 1-568211-46-5

6336 **Questions & Answers About Depression & Its Treatment**

Ivan K Goldberg, MD, author

Charles Press Publishers
PO Box 15715
Philadelphia, PA 19103-0715
215-561-2786
Fax: 215-561-0191
e-mail: mailbox@charlespresspub.com
www.charlespresspub.com

All the questions you'd like to ask, asked and answered.

139 pages

ISBN: 0-914783-68-8

6337 **Report of the Secretary's Task Force on Youth Suicide, Volume 1**
Superintendent of Documents
PO Box 371954
Pittsburgh, PA 15250-7954
202-512-2250

A comprehensive review of information about youth suicide. The task force recommendations are presented in Volume 1.

110 pages

6338 **Touched with Fire:- Manic Depressive Illness & the Artistic Temperment**
Free Press
866 3rd Avenue
New York, NY 10022-6221
Fax: 800-943-9831
www.simonsays.com

Describing and discussing the markedly increased rates of severe mood disorders and suicides among the artistically creative and the reasons why.

370 pages

6339 **Winter Blues**

Norman E Rosenthal, author

Guilford Press
72 Spring Street
New York, NY 10012-4019
800-265-7006
Fax: 212-966-6708
e-mail: info@guilford.com
www.guilford.com

Complete information about Seasonal Affective Disorder and its treatment.

2005

ISBN: 1-593852-14-2

6340 **Women and Depression**
Springer Publishing Company
536 Broadway
New York, NY 10012-3955
212-431-4370
877-687-7476
Fax: 212-941-7842
e-mail: marketing@springerpub.com
www.springerpub.com

This volume examines depression in women within a developmental context. It ranges from issues in childhood and adolescence through premenstrual syndrome and postpartum depression to issues of menopause and aging.

328 pages Hardcover

ISBN: 0-826151-40-X

Annette Imperati, Marketing Director

6341 **Yesterday's Tomorrow**
Hazelden
15251 Pleasant Valley Road
Center City, MN 55012-9640
651-257-4010
800-328-9000
Fax: 651-213-4426
www.hazelden.org

A meditation book that shows why and how recovery works, from the author's own experiences.

432 pages Paperback

ISBN: 1-568381-60-3

Children's Books

6342 **Compassion Books**
7036 State Highway 80 S
Burnsville, NC 28714-7569
828-675-5909
800-970-4220
Fax: 828-675-9687
e-mail: heal2grow@aol.com
www.compassionbooks.com

Hand picked resources to help people through loss, grief and changes of all kinds. Carry over 400 books and videos on death and dying, bereavement and change, comfort and healing, hope and much more.
Bruce Greene, VP

Newsletters

6343 NFDI Newsletter
National Foundation for Depressive Illness
PO Box 2257 212-268-4260
New York, NY 10116-2257 800-248-4344
Fax: 212-268-4434
e-mail: pross@att.net
www.depression.org
To correct the myths and misconceptions surrounding the illness and help reverse the devastating effects depression has on the individual and our society and to inform the public, primary health care providers, other healthcare professionals and corporations about depression and manic depression and to provide the information about correct diagnosis and treatment and the availability of qualified doctors and support groups.
4 pages Quarterly

Pamphlets

6344 Depression is a Treatable Illness: A Patients Guide
Department of Health & Human Services
2101 E Jefferson Street 301-217-1245
Rockville, MD 20852-4908
Tells about major depressive disorder, which is only one form of depressive illness. This booklet answers important questions regarding this disorder and gives information on where to go for more help.

6345 If You're Over 65 and Feeling Depressed...
National Institutes on Mental Health
5600 Fishers Lane 301-443-3706
Rockville, MD 20857-0001 Fax: 301-443-6349
Many older people believe that their age alone is responsible for feelings of exhaustion, helplessness and worthlessness. This brochure discusses the causes of depression in the older years, symptoms, types of treatment and where to go for help.
12 pages

6346 Let's Talk About Depression
Superintendent of Documents
PO Box 371954 202-512-2250
Pittsburgh, PA 15250-7954
Targeted especially for inner-city youth. The colorful design will capture attention and focus on depression in a way that young people will understand and identify with.

6347 Lithium and Manic Depression
Lithium Info. Center-Dean Foundation for Health
8000 Excelsior Drive 608-836-8070
Madison, WI 53717-1972
A guidebook about lithium and its effects on bipolar affective disorders and manic depression.
1992 32 pages

6348 Living Without Depression & Manic Depression: A Workbook
National Alliance for the Mentally Ill
PO Box 753
Waldorf, MD 20604-0753 703-524-7600
www.NAMI.org
Workbook offering checklists and helpful advice targeted for individuals whose depressive illness is stabilized.
1994

6349 Panic Disorder
National Institutes of Health
5600 Fishers Lane 301-443-3706
Rockville, MD 20857-0001 Fax: 301-443-6349
Written for the lay public, this pamphlet contains a description of panic disorder, gives the symptoms, describes treatment methods, and encourages the person who has the symptoms to seek treatment.

6350 Plain Talk About Depression
Superintendent of Documents
PO Box 371954 202-512-2250
Pittsburgh, PA 15250-7954
A flyer discussing types of depression, major depression, symptoms and causes.

6351 Understanding Panic Disorder
National Institutes of Health
5600 Fishers Lane 301-443-3706
Rockville, MD 20857-0001 Fax: 301-443-6349
Offers information on what an panic disorder is, symptoms, causes, treatment, medications and therapy.

6352 Useful Information on Phobias and Panic
Superintendent of Documents
PO Box 371954 202-512-2250
Pittsburgh, PA 15250-7954
This booklet provides information on both phobias and panic. Symptoms, causes and treatments of these disorders are referred to. If you know someone who is excessively fearful, this booklet will be of great help to them in understanding their problem.
40 pages 50 copies

6353 What to Do When a Friend is Depressed: Guide for Students
Superintendent of Documents
PO Box 371954 202-512-2250
Pittsburgh, PA 15250-7954
Offers information on depression and its symptoms and suggests things a young person can do to guide a depressed friend in finding help.

6354 What to Do When an Employee is Depressed: A Guide for Supervisors
Superintendent of Documents
PO Box 371954 202-512-2250
Pittsburgh, PA 15250-7954
A D/ART program brochure that will enable an employer to recognize the symptoms of depression in an employee and offers suggestions on what to say to the employee to encourage him or her to seek help.

Audio & Video

6355 Four Lives: A Portrait of Manic Depression
Fanlight Productions
4196 Washington Street 617-469-4999
Boston, MA 02131-1731 800-937-4113
Fax: 617-469-3379
e-mail: fanlight@fanlight.com
www.fanlight.com
Four patients, families and psychiatrists share their perspectives on living with manic depression.
1987 60 Minutes
ISBN: 1-572950-29-3

6356 Taking Control of Depression

800-228-2495
Dramatic program offering new hope in the understanding and treatment of depression, with actor Ed Asner and Alan Xenakis, M.D.

6357 When Someone You Love Suffers from Depression
Medcom/Trainex

800-320-1444
Helping family and friends identify depression in a loved one - offers ways to help stop the suffering and get appropriate treatment.

Web Sites

6358 Healing Well
www.healingwell.com
An online health resource guide to medical news, chat, information and articles, newsgroups and message boards, books, disease-related web sites, medical directories, and more for patients, friends,

and family coping with disabling diseases, disorders, or chronic illnesses.

6359 Health Finder

www.healthfinder.gov

Searchable, carefully developed web site offering information on over 1000 topics. Developed by the US Department of Health and Human Services, the site can be used in both English and Spanish.

6360 Healthlink USA

www.healthlinkusa.com

Health information concerning treatment, cures, prevention, diagnosis, risk factors, research, support groups, email lists, personal stories and much more. Updated regularly.

6361 Helios Health

www.helioshealth.com

Online resource for your health information. Detailed information about specific health topics, access to expert advice from our Medical Advisory Board, and up-to-date health news.

6362 MedicineNet

www.medicinenet.com

An online resource for consumers providing easy-to-read, authoritative medical and health information.

6363 Medscape

www.mywebmd.com

Medscape offers specialists, primary care physicians, and other health professionals the Web's most robust and integrated medical information and educational tools.

6364 National Anxiety Foundation

www.lexington-on-line.com/naf.html

Offers information and help to persons with panic disorders, manic and depressive disorders and mental illness.

6365 National Foundation for Depressive Illness

www.depression.org

Provide the information about correct diagnosis and treatment and the availability of qualified doctors and support groups.

6366 WebMD

www.webmd.com

Information on depression, including articles and resources.

Description

6367 **Mental Illness/Schizophrenia**

Schizophrenia is a chronic mental illness that is characterized by disturbances of thinking, feeling, and behavior. It usually begins in late adolescence or early adult life, with a lifetime prevalance between 0.2 to 1 percent. Despite its literal translation of split mind, schizophrenia is not the same as split personality. Although its specific cause is unknown, most cases of schizophrenia are believed to result from a complex interaction between biologic, inherited and environmental factors.

Symptoms of schizophrenia vary in type and severity and may include delusions and auditory hallucinations (hearing voices), incoherent thought patterns, catatonic behavior, and a flat or grossly inappropriate emotional state.

Drug treatment is the cornerstone of managing schizophrenia. When treated early, patients tend to respond quickly and more fully. Effective drugs have been available for several decades, and have revolutionized treatment of the disease. However, these drug treatments may be limited by side effects (especially movement disorders resembling Parkinsons disease) and by the patient's failure or refusal to stay on treatment. Patient non-compliance is sometimes addressed with long-acting injectable medications. A new class of drugs, lacking the Parkinson-like side effects, and sometimes dramatically more effective than previously used drugs, became available during the 1990s. Their use is limited by high costs and the threat of serious blood-related side effects. Treatment includes counseling, social support, rehabilitation, and skills retraining. Poor outcome frequently leads to extensive and long-term disability. Psychological and educational interventions can reduce the rate of relapse. People close to persons with schizophrenia are often very affected by the disease and can be helped by support and advocacy groups. See also *Mental Illness/General and Mental Illness/Depression.*

National Agencies & Associations

6368 **International Society for the Study of Dissociation**
8400 Westpark Drive 703-610-9037
McLean, VA 22102 Fax: 703-610-0234
e-mail: info@isst-d.org
www.issd.org

A nonprofit professional association that promotes research and training in the identification of treatment of multiple personality, provides professional and public education about multiple personality and initiates international communication among clinicians.
Kathy Steele, President
Paul F Dell PhD, President-Elect

6369 **NARSAD: Mental Health Research Association**
60 Cutter Miller Road 516-829-0091
Great Neck, NY 11021-3104 800-829-8289
Fax: 516-487-6930
e-mail: info@narsad.org
www.narsad.org

NARSAD Information and helpline staff is available to answer basic questions about the symptoms, causes and treatments of psychiatric illnesses. Information on support groups and other mental health organizations can also be provided.
Joel Gurin, Acting President
Louis Innamorato, Vice President Finance/CFO

6370 **National Alliance for the Mentally Ill**
Colonial Place Three
2107 Wilson Boulevard 703-524-7600
Arlington, VA 22201-3042 800-950-6264
Fax: 703-524-9094
TDD: 703-516-7227
e-mail: membership@naminyc.org
www.nami-nyc-metro.org

Nonprofit, self-help, volunteer organization that offers practical support, useful education, advocacy, comfort and understanding to those in the greater New York area who suffer or have family members suffering from mental illnesses. Chapter of the National Alliance for the Mentally Ill and the New York State Alliance for the Mentally Ill.
Charolette Moses Fischman, President
Karen Gormandy, Vice President

Research Centers

6371 **Huxley Insititute-American Schizophrenic Association**
86-B Dorchester Drive
Lakewood, NJ 08701 www.schizohprenia.org

The ASA works to bring effective, low-cost treatment to patients woth schizophrenia and help them in a cooperative effort to cope with the disorder.
Abram Hoffer, MD PhD, President
Elizabeth Plante, Director, Huxley Institute

6372 **Maryland Psychiatric Research Center**
Box 21247 410-402-7666
Baltimore, MD 21228 Fax: 410-788-3837
www.umaryland.edu/mprc

Providing treatment to patients with schizophrenia and related disorders educating professionals and consumers about schizophrenia and conducting basic and translational research into the manifestations causes and treatment of schizophrenia.
Dr William Carpenter Jr, Director
Vito J Seskunas, Deputy Director for Administration

6373 **National Alliance for Research on Schizophrenia and Depression**
Grants Office
60 Cutter Mill Road 516-829-0091
Great Neck, NY 11021 800-829-8289
Fax: 516-487-6930
e-mail: info@narsad.org
www.narsad.org

Research focusing on varieties of mental illness and mental disorders.
Steve Lieber, Chairman of the Board & Treasurer
Joel Gurin, Acting President

6374 **Schizophrenia Research Branch: Division of Clinical and Treatment Research**
5600 Fisher Lane, Parklawn Building 301-443-4707
Rockville, MD 20857 Fax: 301-443-6000

Plans, supports, and conducts programs of research, research training, and resource development of schizophrenia and related disorders. Reviews and evaluates research developments in the field and recommends new program directors. Collaborates with organizations in and outside of the National Institue of Mental Health (NIMH) to stimulate work in the field through conferences and workshops.

6375 **Schizophrenia Research Branch: Division of**
5600 Fisher Lane Parklawn Building 301-443-4707
Rockville, MD 20857 Fax: 301-443-6000

Plans supports and conducts programs of research research training and resource development of schizophrenia and related disorders. Reviews and evaluates research developments in the field and recommends new program directors. Collaborates with organizations in and outside of the National Institute of Mental Health (NIMH) to stimulate work in the field through conferences and workshops.

6376 Tennessee Neuropsychiatric Institute Middle Tennessee Mental Health Institute
Middle Tennessee Mental Health Institute
221 Stewarts Ferry Pike 615-902-7535
Nashville, TN 37217
Michael Eber MD, Director

6377 University of Iowa Mental Health Clinical Research Center
University of Iowa Hospitals & Clinics
200 Hawkins Drive 319-356-1553
Iowa City, IA 52242 877-575-2864
Fax: 319-353-8300
www.iowa-mhcrc.psychiatry.uiowa.edu
Schizophrenia studies and other cognitive disorder research.
Nancy C Andreassen MD, Director

Support Groups & Hotlines

6378 National Health Information Center
PO Box 1133 310-565-4167
Washington, DC 20013 800-336-4797
Fax: 301-984-4256
e-mail: info@nhic.org
www.health.gov/nhic
Offers a nationwide information referral service, produces directories and resource guides.

Books

6379 Encyclopedia of Schizophrenia and the Psychotic Disorders
Facts on File
11 Penn Plaza 212-967-8800
New York, NY 10001 800-322-8755
Fax: 800-678-3633
This volume details recent theories and research findings on schizophrenia and psychotic disorders, together with a complete overview of the field's history.
368 pages Hardcover

6380 Experiences of Schizophrenia
Guilford Press
72 Spring Street
New York, NY 10012 800-365-7006
Fax: 212-966-6708
e-mail: info@guilford.com
www.guilford.com
This authoritative book presents new information on seasonal affective disorder. It includes remedies such as recent advances in light box therapy,research on the effectiveness of antidepressants, and new recipes to counterbalance unhealthy winter food cravings. This book also helps distinguish various degrees of the disorder ranging from winter blues to full blown SAD, and provides a self test that readers can use to evalutate their own seasonal mood changes.
2005 372 pages
ISBN: 1-593852-14-2

6381 Occupational Therapy Practice Guidelines for Adults with Schizophrenia
American Occupational Therapy Association
4720 Montgomery Lane 301-652-2682
Bethesda, MD 20824-1220 Fax: 301-652-7711
TDD: 800-377-8555
www.aota.org
24 pages
ISBN: 1-569001-53-7

6382 Return from Madness
Jason Aronson
PO Box 15100
York, PA 17405-7100 800-783-0015
www.aronson.com
256 pages Hardcover
ISBN: 1-568216-25-4

6383 Schizophrenia and Primitive Mental States
Jason Aronson
PO Box 15100
York, PA 17405-7100 800-782-0015
Fax: 201-840-7242
www.aronson.com
288 pages Softcover
ISBN: 0-765700-27-1

6384 Schizophrenia: From Mind to Molecule
American Psychiatric Press
1400 K Street NW 202-682-6268
Washington, DC 20005-2403 Fax: 202-789-2648
Presents a change in the scientific understanding and outlook regarding the devastating disorder of schizophrenia. It provides a thorough, up-to-date look at schizophrenia that includes neural behavioral studies, technologies and medical treatments.
274 pages Hardcover
ISBN: 0-880489-50-2

Children's Books

6385 Year it Rained
MacMillan Publishing Company
866 3rd Avenue
New York, NY 10022-6221 212-702-2000
www.mcp.com
The story of a girl traumatized by an alcoholic father and her desire to commit suicide. Hospitalized for schizophrenia, Elizabeth reaches a catharsis and, with the help of a poet, discovers that her talent and therapy may be in writing.
Grades 7-10

Magazines

6386 Dissociation
ISSMP&D
5700 Old Orchard Road 847-966-4322
Skokie, IL 60077-1036 Fax: 847-966-9418
A professional journal offering the latest information about the issues and research into multiple personalities and related disorders.

6387 Schizophrenia Bulletin
Superintendent of Documents/NIMH Journal
PO Box 371954 202-512-2250
Pittsburgh, PA 15250-7954
Serves as a forum for multidisciplinary exchange of information about schizophrenia and is exclusively devoted to the exploration of this severe disorder.
Quarterly

Newsletters

6388 ISSD News
Int'l Society for the Study of Dissociation
60 Revere Drive 847-480-0899
Northbrook, IL 60062 Fax: 847-480-9282
e-mail: issd@issd.org
www.issd.org
Includes current news from other onzations of interest to members, information about recent articles and books, news from US and international affiliates and the latest issues concerning multiple personality/dissociative states.
17 pages 6 times a year
Julie A Theander, Administrative Director
Richard Koepke, Executive Director

Pamphlets

6389 Schizophrenia
National Alliance for the Mentally Ill
200 N Glebe Road 703-524-7600
Arlington, VA 22203-3754 Fax: 703-524-9094
Part of the NAMI medical information series offering information on the causes, symptoms and treatments of Schizophrenia.

Web Sites

6390 **Healing Well**

www.healingwell.com

An online health resource guide to medical news, chat, information and articles, newsgroups and message boards, books, disease-related web sites, medical directories, and more for patients, friends, and family coping with disabling diseases, disorders, or chronic illnesses.

6391 **Health Finder**

www.healthfinder.gov

Searchable, carefully developed web site offering information on over 1000 topics. Developed by the US Department of Health and Human Services, the site can be used in both English and Spanish.

6392 **Healthlink USA**

www.healthlinkusa.com

Health information concerning treatment, cures, prevention, diagnosis, risk factors, research, support groups, email lists, personal stories and much more. Updated regularly.

6393 **Helios Health**

www.helioshealth.com

Online resource for your health information. Detailed information about specific health topics, access to expert advice from our Medical Advisory Board, and up-to-date health news.

6394 **International Society for the Study of Dissociation**

www.issd.org

Association that promotes research and training in the identification of treatment of multiple personality.

6395 **MedicineNet**

www.medicinenet.com

An online resource for consumers providing easy-to-read, authoritative medical and health information.

6396 **Medscape**

www.mywebmd.com

Medscape offers specialists, primary care physicians, and other health professionals the Web's most robust and integrated medical information and educational tools.

6397 **National Alliance for the Mentally Ill**

www.nami-nyc-metro.org

Organization that offers practical support, useful education, advocacy, comfort, and understanding to those in the greater New York area who suffer or have family members suffering from neurobiologically based disorders.

6398 **Schizophrenia Therapy Online Resource Center**

www.schizophreniatherapy.com

A website which provides effective and lasting alternatives to traditional treatment for individuals suffering with schizophrenia. Offers an effective and full continium of services ranging from psychopharmacology to individual and group psychotherapy to social rehabilitation, supported work experience, assertive community training and supported housing.

6399 **WebMD**

www.webmd.com

Information on schizophrenia, including articles and resources.

Description

6400 **Migraine**

Roughly 45 million Americans suffer from chronic headaches, the most disabling of which is migraine. Classified as a vascular headache, migraine headaches are caused by intracranial vasospasm, that is, alternating swelling and constricting of blood vessels on the surface of the brain. The swelling phase brings on intense pain and nausea, while the constricting phase may cause neurologic symptoms such as focal loss of vision or numbness involving one side of the body. Another theory is that migraines are due to a different dysfunction of the neurovascular system that results in the release of a substance that leads to migraine. More than 50 percent of patients have a family history of migraine. They also appear to have a hormonal component, being more common in women and often affected by menstrual cycles or pregnancy.

Management of migraine begins with careful observation for triggering agents like foods, alcohol, or irregular sleep patterns. Acute treatment to stop a migraine involves a class of drugs which antagonize the action of the 5-HT that aggravates the migraine process. They block inflammation and can abort migraine in about 70 percent of patients. Sumatriptan, the prototype, is available in oral and subcutaneous injection forms. Ergot drugs, also available in oral and injectable forms, work by helping the swollen blood vessels constrict down to normal size. If headaches become very frequent, doctors may recommend preventive therapy, which requires daily drug administration. Drugs used in this way include beta-blockers and calcium-channel blockers, which were originally developed for hypertension and heart disease, and certain medicines ordinarily used for depression or seizures.

Pain medication should be used sparingly. Nonsteroidal anti-inflammatory drugs, such as ibuprofen are best for mild to moderate headaches. Narcotic medications should be avoided except under special circumstances and with strict guidelines. Most migraine sufferers can be satisfactorily managed by their primary care physician or a neurologist, but in refractory cases a multi-disciplinary headache center may be of help.

Tension is the other common cause of disabling headaches. They are not migraine and are not considered vascular headache, but are mentioned here because they are so common. Some of the resources listed in this section may be helpful for persons with tension headache.

National Agencies & Associations

6401 **American Academy of Neurology**
1080 Montreal Avenue
Saint Paul, MN 55116-2311
651-695-2717
800-879-1960
Fax: 651-695-2791
e-mail: memberservices@aan.com
www.aan.com

A professional organization representing neurologists worldwide.
Catherine Rydell, Executive Director & CEO
Stephen M Sergay, President

6402 **American Council for Headache Education**
19 Mantua Road
Mount Royal, NJ 08061
856-423-0258
800-255-2243
Fax: 856-423-0082
e-mail: achehq@talley.com
www.achenet.org

A not-for-profit alliance of headache sufferers and physicians who are working together to improve the quality of care and the quality of information available to people with chronic or severe headache conditions.
Jan Lewis Brandes MD, President

6403 **American Headache Society**
19 Mantua Road
Mount Royal, NJ 08061
856-423-0043
Fax: 856-423-0082
e-mail: ahshq@talley.com
www.ahsnet.org

Professional society of health care providers who study and treat headache and face pain. AHS brings physicians from various fields and specialties together to share concepts and developments about headache and related conditions.
Linda McGillicuddy, Executive Director
Fred Sheftell, President

6404 **Help for Headaches**
515 Richmond Street
London, Ontario, N6A-5M3
519-434-0008
e-mail: brent@helpforheadaches.org
www.headache-help.org

A non-profit organization, and a registered Canadian charity that is committed to educational services for those suffering from and treating headaches.
G Brent Lucas BA, Director

6405 **Migraine Association of Canada**
356 Bloor Street E
Toronto Ontario, M4W
416-920-4916
800-663-3557
Fax: 416-920-3677
www.migraine.ca

A registered charity funded through memberships. Activities include a 24 hour telephone information access line the development of materials and assistance for those who start community self-help groups, workplace seminars and awareness programs.

6406 **Migraine Awareness Group: A National Understanding for Migraineurs**
100 N Union Street
Alexandria, VA 22314
703-349-1929
Fax: 703-739-2432
e-mail: comments@migraines.org
www.migraines.org

Works to bring public awareness utilizing the electronic print and artistic mediums to the fact that migraine is a true organic neurological disease.
Michael J Coleman, President
Terri Miller Burchfield, Exec VP & Legislative Director

6407 **National Headache Foundation**
820 N Orleans
Chicago, IL 60610-3132
312-640-5399
888-643-5552
Fax: 312-640-9049
e-mail: nhf1970@headaches.org
www.headaches.org

A nonprofit organization established in 1970 dedicated to serve as an information resource to headache sufferers, their families and the healthcare providers who treat them. Promotes research into potential headache causes and treatments.
Arthur HE Elkind MD, President
Roger K Cady M D, Vice President

Research Centers

6408 **Baltimore Headache Institute**
11 E Chase Street
Baltimore, MD 21202
410-547-0200
Brian E Mondell MD, Medical Director

6409 San Francisco Clinical Research Center
909 Hyde Street 415-673-4600
San Francisco, CA 94109 Fax: 415-673-9352
e-mail: SFHACLIN@aol.com
www.sfcrc.com
This research center also specializes in diagnosis of Alzheimer's related dementia in addition to migraine headaches.
Jerome Goldstein, Director

Support Groups & Hotlines

6410 National Health Information Center
PO Box 1133 310-565-4167
Washington, DC 20013 800-336-4797
Fax: 301-984-4256
e-mail: info@nhic.org
www.health.gov/nhic
Offers a nationwide information referral service, produces directories and resource guides.

Books

6411 Conquering Headache
Alan Rapoport, MD, author
B.C Decker, Inc.
50 King Street E, Floor 2 PO Box620 905-522-7017
Ontario, Canada L8N 3K7, 800-568-7281
Fax: 905-522-7839
e-mail: info@bcdecker.com
www.bcdecker.com
2003 128 pages Paperback
ISBN: 1-550092-33-2

6412 Freedom from Headaches
Simon & Schuster Order Department
200 Old Tappan Road
Old Tappan, NJ 07675-7095 800-999-5479
ISBN: 0-671254-04-9

6413 Handbook of Headache Disorders
Essential Medical Information Systems
PO Box 1607 580-924-0643
Durant, OK 74702-1607 800-225-0694
Fax: 580-924-9414
1993 Paperback
ISBN: 0-929240-62-6

6414 Handbook of Headache Management: A Practic al Guide to Diagnosis & Treatment
Williams & Wilkins
351 W Camden Street 301-528-4000
Baltimore, MD 21201-7912 800-638-0672
www.wwilkins.com
1993 224 pages
ISBN: 0-683058-01-0

6415 Migraine and Other Headaches: Vascular Mechanisms
Raven Press
1185 Avenue of the Americas 212-930-9500
New York, NY 10036-2601 800-777-2295
www.raven.com
Leading international experts present new concepts on the mechanisms of migraine and other vascular headaches and detail the latest strategies for diagnosis and treatment of migraine with and without aura, tension-type headaches, cluster headaches and other vascular disorders.
368 pages
ISBN: 0-881677-95-7

6416 Migraine: The Complete Guide
American Council for Headache Education
19 Mantua Road 856-423-0258
Mount Royal, NJ 08061 800-255-2243
Fax: 856-423-0082
e-mail: achehq@talley.com
www.achenet.org
A comprehensive resource book for people with migraine, their families and physicians (updated in 1999) by Lynne M Constantine, Suzanne Scott and ACHE.

6417 Overcoming Headaches & Migraines
Longmeadow Press
PO Box 10218 203-352-2110
Stamford, CT 06904-1469
1993 128 pages Paperback
ISBN: 0-681417-92-7

6418 Understanding Migrain and Other Headaches
Stewart J Tepper, MD, author
University Press of Mississippi
3825 Ridgewood Road 601-432-6205
Jackson, MS 39211-6492 Fax: 601-432-6217
e-mail: kburgess@ihl.state.ms.us
www.upress.state.ms.us
A comprehensive overview of causes, diagnoses, and treatments.
2004 112 pages Paperback
ISBN: 1-578065-92-5
Kathy Burgess, Advertising/Marketing Services Manager

6419 Wolff's Headaches & Other Head Pain
Oxford University Press
2001 Evans Road 212-726-6000
Cary, NC 27513-2010 800-451-7556
Fax: 919-677-1303
www.oup-usa.org
1993
ISBN: 0-195082-50-8

Newsletters

6420 Headache
American Council for Headache Education
19 Mantua Road 856-423-0258
Mount Royal, NJ 08061 800-255-2243
Fax: 856-423-0082
e-mail: achehq@talley.com
www.achenet.org
The ACHE 12 page quarterly newsletter provides valuable and current information on new treatments, as well as time proven headache management strategies. All articles are written or reviewed by headache experts from the American Headache Society (AHS). Recent issues have included articles by headache experts on drug and nondrug treatment options and information on new treatments and research is regularly included.
Quarterly

6421 NHF Head Lines
National Headache Foundation
820 N Orleans 312-640-5399
Chicago, IL 60610-3132 888-643-5552
Fax: 312-640-9049
e-mail: nhf1970@headaches.org
www.headaches.org
Offers the latest information on headaches, causes and treatments. Contains news on drugs and medical forums, in depth discussions of headaches and preventions and a question and answer section in which physicians respond to reader inquiries and support group information.
16 pages Quarterly

Pamphlets

6422 52 Proven Stress Reducers
National Headache Foundation
820 N Orleans
Chicago, IL 60610 888-643-5552
Fax: 312-640-9049
e-mail: nhf1970@headaches.org
www.headaches.org
Members only.
Suzanne Simons, Executive Director

6423 About Headaches
National Headache Foundation
820 N Orleans
Chicago, IL 60610
888-643-5552
Fax: 312-640-9049
e-mail: nhf1970@headaches.org
www.headaches.org
Contains an in depth look at headaches, tips on when to seek medical advice, methods of treatment and more.
16 pages
Suzanne Simons, Executive Director

6424 Analgesic Rebound Headaches: Fact Sheet
National Headache Foundation
820 N Orleans
Chicago, IL 60610
888-643-5552
Fax: 312-640-9049
e-mail: nhf1970@headaches.org
www.headaches.org
Offers information on analgesic agents or drugs used to control pain including migraine and other types of headaches.
Suzanne Simons, Executive Director

6425 Cluster Headache: Fact Sheet
National Headache Foundation
820 N Orleans
Chicago, IL 60610
888-643-5552
Fax: 312-640-9049
e-mail: nhf1970@headaches.org
www.headaches.org
Offers information on cluster headaches and the treatment available for them. This information sheet can be downloaded from the web site.
Suzanne Simons, Executive Director

6426 Diet and Headache: Fact Sheet
National Headache Foundation
820 N Orleans
Chicago, IL 60610
888-643-5552
Fax: 312-640-9049
e-mail: nhf1970@headaches.org
www.headaches.org
Offers information on what foods should be avoided and what foods trigger headaches in all migraine sufferers. This information sheet can be dowloaded from the web site.
Suzanne Simons, Executive Director

6427 Headache Facts: What Everyone Should Know
American Council for Headache Education
19 Mantua Road
Mount Royal, NJ 08061
856-423-0258
800-255-2243
Fax: 856-423-0082
e-mail: achehq@talley.com
www.achenet.org

6428 Headache Handbook
National Headache Foundation
820 N Orleans
Chicago, IL 60610
888-643-5552
Fax: 312-640-9049
e-mail: nhf1970@headaches.org
www.headaches.org
Gives information on causes and types of headaches as well as treatments available.
8 pages

6429 Headache in Children: Fact Sheet
National Headache Foundation
820 N Orleans
Chicago, IL 60610
888-643-5552
Fax: 312-640-9049
e-mail: nhf1970@headaches.org
www.headaches.org
Offers information on vascular headaches, tension-type headaches, traction and inflammatory headaches and treatment. This information sheet can be downloaded from the web site.
Suzanne Simons, Executive Director

6430 Hormones and Migraines: Fact Sheet
National Headache Foundation
820 N Orleans
Chicago, IL 60610
888-643-5552
Fax: 312-640-9049
e-mail: nhf1970@headaches.org
www.headaches.org
Offers information on the link between hormones and migraines.
Suzanne Simons, Executive Director

6431 How to Talk to Your Doctor About Headaches
National Headache Foundation
820 N Orleans
Chicago, IL 60610
888-643-5552
Fax: 312-640-9049
e-mail: nhf1970@headaches.org
www.headaches.org
Learn how to keep a headache diary to pinpoint symptoms and effective diagnosis.
Suzanne Simons, Executive Director

6432 Impact of Migraine: A Disabling and Costly Condition
American Council for Headache Education
19 Mantua Road
Mount Royal, NJ 08061
856-423-0258
800-255-2243
Fax: 856-423-0082
e-mail: achehq@talley.com
www.achenet.org

6433 Migraine and Coexisting Conditions: Other Illnesses That May Affect Migraine
American Council for Headache Education
19 Mantua Road
Mount Royal, NJ 08061
856-423-0258
800-255-2243
Fax: 856-423-0082
e-mail: achehq@talley.com
www.achenet.org

6434 Migraine: Fact Sheet
National Headache Foundation
820 N Orleans
Chicago, IL 60610
888-643-5552
Fax: 312-640-9049
e-mail: nhf1970@headaches.org
www.headaches.org
Offers information on migraines and treatments.
Suzanne Simons, Executive Director

6435 Tap the Best Resource
National Headache Foundation
820 N Orleans
Chicago, IL 60610
888-643-5552
Fax: 312-640-9049
e-mail: nhf1970@headaches.org
www.headaches.org
Informational brochure offering facts and statistics on headaches. Everything from muscle contraction, vascular headaches, sinus headaches, TMJ and much more.
Suzanne Simons, Executive Director

6436 Tension-Type Headache: Fact Sheet
National Headache Foundation
820 N Orleans
Chicago, IL 60610
888-643-5552
Fax: 312-640-9049
e-mail: nhf1970@headaches.org
www.headaches.org
Offers information on the least known type of headache, chronic tension-type headaches. This information sheet can be downloaded from the web site.

6437 What's the Best Medicine for My Headaches?
American Council for Headache Education
19 Mantua Road
Mount Royal, NJ 08061
856-423-0258
800-255-2243
Fax: 856-423-0082
e-mail: achehq@talley.com
www.achenet.org

Audio & Video

6438 **Relaxation Tape**
National Headache Foundation
820 N Orleans
Chicago, IL 60610
888-643-5552
Fax: 312-640-9049
e-mail: nhf1970@headaches.org
www.headaches.org
Contains techniques to assist the listener in experiencing greater self control and relaxation.
Audio Tape
Suzanne Simons, Executive Director

6439 **Stretch and Relax Tape**
National Headache Foundation
820 N Orleans
Chicago, IL 60610
888-643-5552
Fax: 312-640-9049
e-mail: nhf1970@headaches.org
www.headaches.org
Based on a series of progressive relaxation techniques which involve the tightening and relaxing of specific muscle groups.
Audio Tape
Suzanne Simons, Executive Director

Web Sites

6440 **American Academy of Neurology**
www.aan.com/
A professional organization representing neurologists worldwide.

6441 **American Council for Headache Education (ACHE)**
www.achenet.org
The ACHE website offers an extensive library of headache information, including a searchable database of past articles from our newsletter, discussion forums that provide virtual contact with leading headache specialists and fellow headache sufferers, a searchable database of physicians to find a specialist in your area and more.

6442 **American Headache Society**
www.ahsnet.org
The AHS website offers clinically oriented information on headache, as well as information on AHS programs and activities.

6443 **American Medical Association**
Journal of the American Medical Association
www.ama-assn.org/
An organized web site focusing on treatment options, education and support available to those suffering from migraine headaches.

6444 **Cluster Headaches**
www.clusterheadaches.com
A web site devoted completely and exclusively to those that suffer from cluster headaches.

6445 **Healing Well**
www.healingwell.com
An online health resource guide to medical news, chat, information and articles, newsgroups and message boards, books, disease-related web sites, medical directories, and more for patients, friends, and family coping with disabling diseases, disorders, or chronic illnesses.

6446 **Health Finder**
www.healthfinder.gov
Searchable, carefully developed web site offering information on over 1000 topics. Developed by the US Department of Health and Human Services, the site can be used in both English and Spanish.

6447 **Healthlink USA**
www.healthlinkusa.com
Health information concerning treatment, cures, prevention, diagnosis, risk factors, research, support groups, email lists, personal stories and much more. Updated regularly.

6448 **Helios Health**
www.helioshealth.com
Online resource for your health information. Detailed information about specific health topics, access to expert advice from our Medical Advisory Board, and up-to-date health news.

6449 **MedicineNet**
www.medicinenet.com
An online resource for consumers providing easy-to-read, authoritative medical and health information.

6450 **Medscape**
www.mywebmd.com
Medscape offers specialists, primary care physicians, and other health professionals the Web's most robust and integrated medical information and educational tools.

6451 **Medsupport**
www.medsupport.com
An up-to-date website dedicated towards giving the headache sufferer some important insights through the eyes of those who treat headache disorders.

6452 **Migraine Awareness Group: A National Understanding for Migraineurs**
www.migraines.org/
Works to bring public awareness, utilizing the electronic, print, and artistic mediums, to the fact that migraine is a true organic neurological disease.

6453 **National Headache Foundation**
www.headaches.org
Information for headache sufferers, their families, and the physicians who treat them.

6454 **Neurology Channel**
www.neurologychannel.com
Find clearly explained, medically accurate information regarding conditions, including an overview, symptoms, causes, diagnostic procedures and treatment options. On this site it is possible to ask questions and get information from a neurologist and connect to people who have similar health interests.

6455 **WebMD**
www.webmd.com
Information on migraine, including articles and resources.

Description

6456 # Multiple Sclerosis

Multiple sclerosis, MS, is a chronic disease that affects the central nervous system and impairs many of its functions. Over 300,000 Americans have MS. Although its cause is unknown, an immunologic abnormality is suspected. There also appear to be both genetic and environmental factors involved. Interestingly, the incidence of MS increases the further one lives from the equator.

Age of onset is typically between 20 and 40 years, and women are affected somewhat more than men. MS destroys the protective myelin sheath that surrounds nerve fibers. This special sheath normally allows passage of electrical signals through the brain, spinal cord, and nerves of the body. The disease is characterized by remissions and recurring exacerbations. The clinical signs vary depending on the area of demyelination and can include: generalized or focal weakness; difficulty walking; clumsiness; slurred speech; easy fatigability; numbness and tingling; visual loss; incontinence (loss of bladder and bowel control); loss of sexual function; and problems with short-term memory, judgment, or reason.

Significant strides are being made in both treating and understanding MS. Currently there is no curative treatment, but corticosteroids, interferon and other new medications may shorten or prevent relapses.

Supportive treatment includes medications to control muscle spasticity, fatigue and pain. Maintaining a normal lifestyle is recommended, avoiding fatigue and exposure to excessive heat. Physical therapy may also be helpful. Because of the debilitating nature of MS, counseling, psychiatric support, and antidepressant medication may be warranted.

National Agencies & Associations

6457 **Multiple Sclerosis Association of America**
706 Haddonfield Road
Cherry Hill, NJ 08002-2652
856-488-4500
800-532-7667
Fax: 856-661-9797
e-mail: webmaster@msaa.com
www.msassociation.org

A national nonprofit organization dedicated to enhancing the quality of life for those affected. Mission is to ease day-to-day challenges of individuals with MS, their families and their care partners.
Douglas Franklin, President & CEO
Bruce Makous, Vice President for Development

6458 **Multiple Sclerosis Foundation**
6350 N Andrews Avenue
Fort Lauderdale, FL 33309
954-776-6805
888-MSF-OCUS
Fax: 954-938-8708
e-mail: admin@msfocus.org
www.msfocus.org

Dedicated to helping create a brighter tomorrow for those with MS the foundation offers a wide array of free services including: national toll-free support, educational programs, homecare, support groups, assistive technology and publications.
Toni Somma, Public Relations Coordinator

6459 **National Institute of Neurological Disorders and Stroke**
Neurology Institute
31 Center Drive, Msc 2540
Bethesda, MD 20892-0001
301-496-5751
800-352-9424
Fax: 301-402-2186
www.ninds.nih.gov

America's focal point for support of research on brain and nervous system disorders.
Story Landis, Director

6460 **National Multiple Sclerosis Society**
733 3rd Avenue
New York, NY 10017-3288
212-986-3240
800-344-4867
Fax: 212-986-7981
e-mail: nat@nmss.org
www.nmss.org

Serves persons with MS, their families, health professionals and the interested public. The Society provides funding for research, public and professional education, advocacy and the design of rehabilitative and psychosocial programs. Direct services to MS persons are provided through local chapters and branches. Among the services offered are counseling, referral, equipment loan and other support activities.
Joyce Nelson, President & CEO

6461 **Toronto Parents of Multiple Births Associa tion**
790 Bay Street
Toronto, Ontario, M5G-1N9
416-760-3944
e-mail: info@tpomba.org
www.tpomba.org

A not-for-profit self-help and support organization in Canada for parents of twins, triplets, and more.
Laura Dallal, President

State Agencies & Associations

Alabama

6462 **National Multiple Sclerosis Society: Alabama Chapter**
3840 Ridgeway Drive
Birmingham, AL 35209
205-879-8881
800-FIG-HTMS
e-mail: alc@nmss.org
www.nationalmssociety.org/alc

Dedicated to serving people with MS and their families by providing programs and services designed to enhance quality of life.
Melissa Daniel, Chapter President
Taylor Lander, Development Manager

6463 **National Mutiple Sclerosis Society: Alabama Chapter**
3840 Ridgeway Drive
Birmingham, AL 35209
205-879-8881
800-344-4867
Fax: 205-879-8869
e-mail: alc@nmss.org
www.nationalmssociety.org

Serving people with MS and their families through education and emotional support.
Melissa Dani Patterson, Chapter President
Hillary Ball Ryan, Development Manager

Alaska

6464 **National Multiple Sclerosis Society: Alaska Chapter**
511 W 41st Avenue
Anchorage, AK 99503-6643
907-563-1115
800-344-4867
Fax: 907-562-6673
e-mail: aka@nmss.org
www.nationalmssociety.org/aka

Nonprofit organization providing equipment loan, information and referral, leading library, self-help groups, advocacy, education, training, newsletter, educational programs, volunteer opportunities, exercise/aquatics, newly diagnosed support and educational material.
Gary Wells, Regional Development Manager
Pam McElrath, President, All American Chapter

Arizona

6465 **Desert Southwest Chapter 1 National Multiple Sclerosis Society**
National Multiple Sclerosis Society

315 S 48th Street 602-968-2488
Tempe, AZ 85281-2343 Fax: 602-966-4049
e-mail: info@dsw.nmss.org
www.dsw.nmss.org

Serves Central and Northern Arizona.

6466 **Desert Southwest Chapter 2 National Multiple Sclerosis Society**
National Multiple Sclerosis Society
3003 S Country Club Road 520-322-6601
Tucson, AZ 85713 Fax: 520-322-6739
Serves Southern Arizona.

Arkansas

6467 **National Multiple Sclerosis Society: Arkansas Chapter**
Evergreen Place
1100 N University Avenue 501-663-6767
Little Rock, AR 72207-6367 Fax: 501-666-4355
e-mail: arr@nmss.org
www.nationalmssociety.org/arr

Rick Selig, Division Manager

California

6468 **Central California Chapter National Multiple Sclerosis Society**
National Multiple Sclerosis Society
334 Shaw Avenue 209-325-9293
Clovis, CA 93612-3839 Fax: 209-325-9295
Dan Dietrich, Development Director
Karen Nunn, Service Director

6469 **National Multiple Sclerosis Society: Southern California Chapter**
2440 S Sepulveda Boulevard 310-479-4456
Los Angeles, CA 90064 800-344-4867
Fax: 310-479-4436
e-mail: cal@nmss.org
www.cal.nmss.org

Leon A LeBuffe, President

6470 **National Multiple Sclerosis Society Channel Islands Chapter**
14 W Valerio Street 805-682-8783
Santa Barbara, CA 93101 Fax: 805-563-1489
e-mail: cat@nmss.org
nationalmssociety.org

Joan Young, Chapter President

6471 **National Multiple Sclerosis Society: Silicon Valley Chapter**
2589 Scott Boulevard 408-988-7557
Santa Clara, CA 95050-2508 800-344-4867
Fax: 408-988-1816
e-mail: cau@nmss.org
www.nmss.org

Funds, researches and supports people with MS and their families to end the devastating effects of multiple sclerosis.
Carla Hines, Chapter President
Michelle Spam-Allen, Program Director

6472 **Northern California Chapter National Multiple Sclerosis Society**
National Multiple Sclerosis Society
1700 Owens Street 415-230-6678
San Francisco, CA 94158 800-344-4867
Fax: 510-268-0575
e-mail: info@msconnection.org
www.nationalmssociety.org

David Hartman, Chapter President
Denise Casey, Director of Chapter Programs

6473 **Orange County Chapter National Multiple Sclerosis Society**
National Multiple Sclerosis Society
5950 La Place Court 760-448-8400
Carlsbad, CA 92008-5677 800-344-4867
Fax: 949-833-3104
e-mail: msinfo@mspacific.org
www.nmssoc.org

Richard V Israel, Chapter President
Karen Hooper, Vice President Programs & Services

6474 **San Diego Area Chapter National Multiple Sclerosis Society**
National Multiple Sclerosis Society
8840 Complex Drive 619-974-8640
San Diego, CA 92123-1498 Fax: 619-974-8646
e-mail: mswalksd@aol.com
www.nmssoc.org

Allan Shaw, Chapter President
Karen Barton, Service Director

Colorado

6475 **National MS Society: Colorado Chapter**
900 S Broadway 303-698-7400
Denver, CO 80209-3442 800-344-4867
Fax: 303-698-7421
e-mail: COCRECEPTIONIST@NMSS.ORG
www.nationalmssociety.org/chapters/COC/i

Carrie Nolan, President
Mary Ann Peters, Executive Assistant

Connecticut

6476 **National MS Society: Greater Connecticut Chapter**
659 Tower Avenue 860-714-2300
Hartford, CT 06112 Fax: 860-714-2301
e-mail: info@ctfightsMS.org
www.nationalmssociety.org/chapters/CTN/i
Lisa Gerrol, President and Chief Professional Officer
Cheryl Donati, Executive Vice President

6477 **National MS Society: Western Connecticut Chapter**
1 Selleck Street 203-831-2971
Norwalk, CT 06855-1120 Fax: 203-831-2973
www.nationalmssociety.org/chapters/CTN/i

Delaware

6478 **National MS Society: Delaware Chapter**
2 Mill Road 302-655-5610
Wilmington, DE 19806-2175 Fax: 302-655-0993
e-mail: KATE.COWPERTHWAIT@DED.NMSS.ORG
www.nationalmssociety.org/chapters/DED/i
Provides the encouragement, materials and skills needed to achieve and maintain a productive lifestyle with multiple sclerosis. The organization is a voluntary, nonprofit entity.
1100 members
Kate Cowperthwait, Chapter President
Helen Serbu, Director of Finance

District of Columbia

6479 **National MS Society: National Capital Chapter**
1800 M Street 202-296-5363
Washington, DC 20036-1003 Fax: 202-296-3425
e-mail: INFORMATION@MSandYOU.ORG
www.nationalmssociety.org/chapters/DCW/i
J Christophe Broullire, Chapter President
Kevin Dougherty, Vice President Programs and Services

Florida

6480 **Central Florida Chapter**
2701 Maitland Center Parkway 407-478-8880
Orlando, FL 32751-6726 Fax: 407-478-8893
e-mail: INFO@FLC.NMSS.ORG
www.nationalmssociety.org/chapters/FLC/i

Tami Caesar, President
Ryan Bumgardner, Bike MS Manager

6481 **Florida Gulf Coast Chapter National Multiple Sclerosis Society**
National Multiple Sclerosis Society
4919 Memorial Highway 813-889-8303
Tampa, FL 33634-3540 800-344-4867
Fax: 813-889-8313
www.nationalmssociety.org/chapters/FLC/i
Judy Wilkinson, Service Director
Tim Hanke, Chairman

6482 **Goodwill Industries-Suncoast**
Goodwill Industries-Suncoast

10596 Gandy Boulevard
St. Petersburg, FL 33733
727-523-1512
Fax: 727-577-2749
www.goodwill-suncoast.org

A nonprofit community based organization whose purpose is to improve the quality of life for people who are disabled, disadvantaged and/or aged. This mission is accomplished through a staff of over 1,200 employees providing independent living skills, affordable housing, career assessment and planning, job skills, training, placement, and job retention assistance with useful employment. Annually, Goodwill Industries-Suncoast serves over 30,000 people in Citrus, Hernando, Levy, Marion and more.
Jay Mc Cloe, Director Resource Development

6483 **Mid Florida Chapter National Multiple Sclerosis Society**
National Multiple Sclerosis Society
733 Third Avenue
New York, NY 10017
212-463-7787
Fax: 212-986-7981
e-mail: INFO@MSNYC.ORG
www.nationalmssociety.org/chapters/NYN/i
Ruth Brenner, President
Robin Einbinder, Executive Vice President Programs

6484 **National Multiple Sclerosis Society: North Florida Chapter**
9550 Regency Square Boulevard
Jacksonville, FL 32225-8171
904-725-6800
800-344-4867
Fax: 904-725-0500
TDD: 800-955-8770
e-mail: msnorfla@fln.nmss.org
www.nationalmssociety.org/fln
Jennifer Lee, Chapter President
Sabrah Witkamp, Client Program Director

6485 **South Florida Chapter National Multiple Sclerosis Society**
National Multiple Sclerosis Society
3201 W Commercial Boulevard
Fort Lauderdale, FL 33309-6350
954-731-4224
800-344-4867
Fax: 954-739-1398
e-mail: fls@nmss.org
fls.nationalmssociety.org
Karen Dresbach, Chapter President
Fred Zuckerman, Chairman

Georgia

6486 **National MS Society: Georgia Chapter**
1117 Perimeter Center W
Atlanta, GA 30338-3097
678-672-1000
800-822-3379
Fax: 678-672-1015
e-mail: mailbox@nmssga.org
www.nationalmssociety.org/chapters/GAA/i
Roy A Rangel, Chapter President
Nicole Hill, Director of Finance & Administrative

Hawaii

6487 **National MS Society: Hawaii Chapter**
418 Kuwili Street
Honolulu, HI 96817
808-532-0806
Fax: 808-532-0814
e-mail: HIH@NMSS.ORG
www.nationalmssociety.org/chapters/HIH/i
Jeffrey D Peier, Chairman
Pam McElrath, President

Idaho

6488 **National MS Society: Idaho Division**
6901 W Emerald Street
Boise, ID 83704
208-388-4253
800-344-4867
Fax: 208-388-1907
e-mail: idi@nmss.org
www.nationalmssociety.org/chapters/IDI/i
Pam McElrath, Chapter President
Suzanne Bland, Executive Vice President

Illinois

6489 **National MS Society: Chicago, Greater Illinois Chapter**
600 S Federal Street
Chicago, IL 60605-3814
312-922-8000
Fax: 312-922-2752

The Greater Illnois Chapter is comprised of all the Illinoisans whohave chosen to fight MS and the work that they do through the National Multiple Sclerosis Society Volunteers, staff, healthcare workers, researchers, donors, advocated, and partners together represent the Greater Illinoisans Chapter, and all the many ways it's possible to join the fight against multiple sclerosis.
Steven Pratapous, Chapter President

Indiana

6490 **National MS Society: Indiana State Chapter**
7301 Georgetown Road
Indianapolis, IN 46268
317-870-2500
800-344-4867
Fax: 317-870-2520
e-mail: Indiana@nmss.org
www.nationalmssociety.org/chapters/INI/i
Tiffany Bogard, Chapter President
Lisa Coffman, Director of Chapter Programs

Iowa

6491 **National MS Society: Iowa Chapter**
8187 University Boulevard
Clive, IA 50325
515-270-6337
800-798-6677
Fax: 515-270-0337
e-mail: mark.davis@nmss.org
www.nationalmssociety.org/chapters/NTH/a
Brett Ridge, Chapter President
Mark Davis, Area Director

Kansas

6492 **National MS Society: Mid-America Chapter**
7611 State Line
Kansas City, KS 64114-2915
913-432-3926
800-745-3148
Fax: 913-432-6912
e-mail: info@nmsskc.org
www.nationalmssociety.org/chapters/KSG/i

The National Multiple Sclerosis Society is a not-for-profit organization serving people with MS in every state. The Mid-America Chapter serves the 25,000 people who are affected by MS in eastern Kansas and western Missouri.
Kay Julian, Chapter President
Amy Goldstein, Program Director

6493 **National MS Society: South Central & West Kansas Division**
9415 E Harry Street
Wichita, KS 67211-1515
316-264-7043
800-344-4867
Fax: 316-264-5436
e-mail: KSS@NMSS.ORG
www.nationalmssociety.org/chapters/KSS/i
Cammy Mathews, Donor Relations Coordinator
Becky Kimbell, Regional Programs and Services Manager

Kentucky

6494 **National MS Society: Kentucky Chapter**
11700 Commonwealth Drive
Louisville, KY 40299
502-451-0014
e-mail: KYW@NMSS.ORG
www.nationalmssociety.org
Jeff Hamilton, Chairman
Stacy Funk, Chapter President

Louisiana

6495 **National Multiple Sclerosis Society**
4613 Fairfield Street
Metairie, LA 70006
504-832-4013
800-344-4867
Fax: 504-831-7188
e-mail: louisianachapter@lam.nmss.org
www.nationalmssociety.org/chapters/LAM/i
Brian Berrigon, Chapter President
Crystal Smith, Director of Programs and Services

6496 **National Multiple Sclerosis Society: Louisiana Chapter 3**
3616 S I 10 Service Road W 504-832-4013
Metairie, LA 70001-1874 800-344-4867
Fax: 504-831-7188
e-mail: louisianachapter@lam.nmss.org
www.nationalmssociety.org
Brian Berrigon, Chapter President
Crystal Smith, Director Chapter Programs

Maine

6497 **National MS Society: Maine Chapter**
170 US Route One 800-344-4867
Falmouth, ME 04105 Fax: 207-781-7961
e-mail: info@msmaine.org
www.nationalmssociety.org/chapters/MEM/i
The National Multiple Sclerosis Societ is dedicated to enind the devastating the devastating effects of multiple sciersis, a chronic, disease of the central nervous system often diagnosed in young adults
Robin Doughty, Director of Finance & Operations
Denise Clavette, Chapter President

Maryland

6498 **National MS Society: Maryland Chapter Hunt Valley Business Center**
Hunt Valley Business Center
11403 Cronhill Drive 443-641-1200
Owings Mills, MD 21117 Fax: 443-641-1201
e-mail: INFO@NMSS-MD.ORG
www.nationalmssociety.org/chapters/MDM/i
Mark Roeder, Chapter President
Nicole Weedon, Executive Assistant/Office Manager

Massachusetts

6499 **National MS Society: Central New England Chapter**
101A 1st Avenue 781-890-4990
Waltham, MA 02451-1160 800-493-9255
Fax: 781-890-2089
e-mail: COMMUNICATIONS@MAM.NMSS.ORG
www.nationalmssociety.org/chapters/MAM/i
Linda Guiod, Executive Vice President
Arlyn White, Chapter President & CEO

6500 **National MS Society: Massachusetts Chapter**
101A 1st Avenue 781-890-4990
Waltham, MA 02451-1160 Fax: 781-890-2089
e-mail: COMMUNICATIONS@MAM.NMSS.ORG
www.nationalmssociety.org/chapters/MAM/i
Linda Guiod, Executive Vice President
Arlyn White, Chapter President & CEO

Michigan

6501 **National MS Society: Michigan Chapter**
21311 Civic Center Drive 248-350-0020
Southfield, MI 48076-3911 Fax: 248-350-0029
e-mail: info@mig.nmss.org
www.nationalmssociety.org/chapters/MIG/i
Elana Sullivan, Chapter President
Melissa Ryan, Executive Administrative Assistant

Minnesota

6502 **National MS Society: Minnesota Chapter**
200 12th Avenue S 612-335-7900
Minneapolis, MN 55415 800-582-5296
Fax: 612-335-7997
e-mail: INFO@MSSOCIETY.ORG
www.nationalmssociety.org/chapters/MNM/i

Mississippi

6503 **National MS Society: Mississippi Chapter**
145 Executive Drive 601-856-5831
Madison, MS 39110-9198 800-344-4867
Fax: 601-856-7173
e-mail: MSM@NMSS.ORG
www.nationalmssociety.org/chapters/MSM/i
Rebecca Traweek, Donor Relations
Andi Agnew, Programs and Services Coordinator

Missouri

6504 **National MS Society: Gateway Area Chapter**
1867 Lackland Hill Parkway 314-781-9020
Saint Louis, MO 63146-3545 800-344-4867
Fax: 314-781-1440
e-mail: info@mos.nmss.org
www.nationalmssociety.org/chapters/MOS/i
Sponsors research and offers educational programs, counseling, lending library, referral services, independent living aids, legislative advocacy and therapeutic recreation for people with MS.
Phyllis Robsham, Chapter President
Kathi Taylor, Executive Assistant

Montana

6505 **National MS Society: Montana Division**
1629 Avenue D 406-252-5927
Billings, MT 59102 800-344-4867
Fax: 406-252-5956
e-mail: MTT@NMSS.ORG
www.nationalmssociety.org/chapters/MTT/i
Rebecca Wiehe, Regional Programs and Services Manager
Heather Ohs, Regional DevelopmentÿManager

Nebraska

6506 **National MS Society: Midlands Chapter Community Health Plaza**
Community Health Plaza
328 S 72nd Street 402-505-4000
Omaha, NE 68114-2153 Fax: 402-572-3002
e-mail: NEN@NMSS.ORG
www.nationalmssociety.org/chapters/NEN/i
Lisa Brink, Chapter President
Milton Trabal, Director of Finance

Nevada

6507 **Desert Southwest Chapter 3 National Multiple Sclerosis Society**
National Multiple Sclerosis Society
6000 S Eastern Avenue 702-736-1478
Las Vegas, NV 89119-3157 800-344-4867
Fax: 702-736-2487
e-mail: NVL@NMSS.ORG
www.nationalmssociety.org/chapters/NVL/i
Serves southern Nevada & northwest Arizona.
Nicole Rainey, Development Coordinator Special Events
Linda Nowell, Programs and Services Coordinator

6508 **National MS Society: Great Basin Sierra Chapter**
4600 Keitzke Lane 702-329-7180
Reno, NV 89502 800-344-4867
Fax: 775-827-3167
e-mail: nvn@nvn.nmss.org
www.nationalmssociety.org/chapters/NVN/i
Linda Lott, Regional Development Manager
Danielle Lutzow, Programs and Services Coordinator

New Hampshire

6509 **National MS Society: Central New England Chapter**
101A First Avenue 781-890-4990
Waltham, MA 02451-1115 800-493-9255
Fax: 781-490-2089
e-mail: COMMUNICATIONS@MAM.NMSS.ORG
www.msnewengland.org

Serving people with MS in Massachusetts and New Hampshire.
Judy Cotton, Director Chapter Services
Arlyn White, Chapter President & CEO

New Jersey

6510 **National MS Society: Greater North Jersey Chapter**
1 Kalisa Way
Paramus, NJ 07652-3550
201-967-5599
Fax: 201-967-7085
e-mail: INFO@NJM.NMSS.ORG
www.nationalmssociety.org/chapters/NJM/i
Michael Elkow, Chapter President
Marianne Maddocks, Vice President of Operations

6511 **National MS Society: Mid-Jersey Chapter**
246 Monmouth Road
Oakhurst, NJ 07755
732-660-1005
800-344-4867
Fax: 732-660-1388
e-mail: INFO@NJM.NMSS.ORG
www.nationalmssociety.org/chapters/NJM/i
The National Multiple Sclerosis Society is the only voluntary health agency that supports an international program of scientific research designed to cure, prevent and treat MS.
Michael Elkow, Chapter President
Marianne Maddocks, Vice President of Operations

New Mexico

6512 **National MS Society: Rio Grande Division**
4125-A Carlisle Boulevard NE
Albuquerque, NM 87107
505-243-2792
800-344-4867
Fax: 505-244-0629
e-mail: NMX@NMSS.ORG
www.nationalmssociety.org/chapters/NMX/i
Maggie Schold, Development Coordinator Special Events
Sheri Wharton, Programs and Services Coordinator

New York

6513 **National MS Society: Long Island Chapter**
40 Marcus Drive
Melville, NY 11747
631-864-8337
Fax: 631-864-8342
e-mail: PMASTROTA@NMSSLI.ORG
www.nationalmssociety.org/chapters/NYH/i
The National Multiple Sclerosis Society, Long Island Chapter, is dedicated to helping people with MS and their families live useful and fulfilling lives by opening their minds to opportunities and providing the tools to live with dignity.
Pamela Jones Mastrota, President & CEO
Barbara Travis, Vice President of Donor Development

6514 **National MS Society: New York City Chapter**
733 Third Avenue
New York, NY 10017-2098
212-463-7787
800-344-4867
Fax: 212-989-4362
e-mail: INFO@MSNYC.ORG
www.nationalmssociety.org/chapters/NYN/i
Committed to providing comprehensive support services to help people with MS and their families cope with the consequences of the disease. The goal is to empower people with MS and their loved ones so that they can better control their lives.
Ruth Brenner, Chapter President
Robin Einbinder, Executive Vice President Programs

6515 **National MS Society: Northeastern New York Chapter**
421 New Karner Road
Albany, NY 12205-5156
518-464-0630
800-344-4867
Fax: 518-464-1232
e-mail: chapter@msupstateny.org
www.nationalmssociety.org/chapters/NYR/i
Barbara R Milano, Chapter President
Elliey Kiale-Ingalsb, Chapter Chair

6516 **National MS Society: Southern New York Chapter**
2 Gannett Drive
White Plains, NY 10604-2145
914-694-1655
800-344-4867
Fax: 914-345-3504
e-mail: NYV@NMSS.ORG
www.nationalmssociety.org/chapters/NYV/i
The mission of the National MS Society is to end the devastating effects of multiple sclerosis. The Southern NY Chapter is committed to helping people with MS to live independently.
Andrea Maloney, Interim Chapter President
Christina Szeliga, Administrative Coordinator

6517 **National MS Society: Upstate New York Chapter**
457 State Street
Binghamton, NY 13901-2341
607-724-5464
800-344-4867
Fax: 607-722-1485
e-mail: chapter@msupstateny.org
www.nationalmssociety.org/chapters/NYR/i
James Ahearn, Chapter President
Jonathan Smith, Program Coordinator

6518 **National MS Society: Western New York/ Northwestern Pennsylvania Chapter**
4245 Union Road
Buffalo, NY 14225-5040
716-634-2261
800-344-4867
Fax: 716-634-2979
e-mail: chapter@msupstateny.org
www.nationalmssociety.org/chapters/NYR/i
Arthur V Cardella, Chapter President
Betsy Farkas, Director Chapter Programs

6519 **National Multiple Sclerosis: Upstate New York Chapter**
National Multiple Sclerosis Society
1650 S Avenue
Rochester, NY 14620-3901
716-271-0801
877-869-6677
Fax: 716-442-2817
e-mail: CHAPTER@MSUPSTATENY.ORG
www.nationalmssociety.org/chapters/NYR/i
Randal A Simonetti, Presidentÿ& CEO
Stephanie Mincer, Senior Vice President of Programs

North Carolina

6520 **National MS Society: Central North Carolina Chapter**
2211 W Meadowview Road
Greensboro, NC 27407-3400
336-299-4136
Fax: 336-855-3039
e-mail: NCC@NMSS.ORG
www.nationalmssociety.org/chapters/NCC/i
Elizabeth Green, Chapter President
Davishia Baldwin, Volunteer Coordinator

6521 **National MS Society: Eastern North Carolina Chapter**
3101 Industrial Drive
Raleigh, NC 27609-7577
919-781-0676
Fax: 919-781-1042
e-mail: NCT@NMSS.ORG
www.nationalmssociety.org/chapters/NCT/i
Craig Robertson, Interim Chapter President
Debbie Hoffman, Vice President Operations

6522 **National Multiple Sclerosis Society**
9801-I Southern Pine Boulevard
Charlotte, NC 28273-5561
704-525-2955
Fax: 704-527-0406
e-mail: NCP@NMSS.ORG
www.nationalmssociety.org/chapters/NCP/i
The Mid-Atlantic chapter of the National Multiple Sclerosis helps people learn to manage and understand MS and to achieve maximum independence.
Lori Hurd, Chapter President
Susan Jordan, VP of Chapter Programs

North Dakota

6523 **National MS Society: Dakota Chapter**
5990 14th Street S
Fargo, ND 58104
701-235-2678
Fax: 701-235-6358
www.nationalmssociety.org/chapters/NTH/i
Kelly Boeddeker, Senior Development Manager
Amanda Noce, Programs Manager

Ohio

6524 **Columbus Center of the National Multiple Sclerosis Society**
National Multiple Sclerosis Society

651 G Lakeview Plaza Boulevard 614-880-2290
Worthington, OH 43229-3626 800-667-7131
Fax: 614-880-2296
www.nationalmssociety.org
Stacey Wilko LSW, Program Coordinator
Tony Bernard LSW, Program Coordinator

6525 **National MS Soceity: Western Ohio Chapter The Woolpert Building**
The Woolpert Building
409 E Monument Avenue 937-461-5232
Dayton, OH 45402-1261 800-344-4867
Fax: 937-461-3500
e-mail: donnasimpson@ohm.nmss.org
www.nationalmssociety.org
Providing accurate, up-to-date information to individuals with MS, their families and healthcare providers is central to our mission.
12 pages
Karen Joseph, Program Director
Judy LaMusga, Chapter Chair

6526 **National MS Society: Southwestern Ohio/Northern Kentucky**
4460 Lake Forest Drive 513-281-5200
Cincinnati, OH 45242-3755 Fax: 513-769-6019
Tena Bunnell, Chapter President
Becky Wiehe, Service Director

6527 **National MS Society: Northeast Ohio Chapter**
The Hanna Building
6155 Rockside Road 216-696-8220
Independence, OH 44131-1901 800-667-7131
Fax: 216-696-2817
e-mail: WEBMASTER@NMSSOHA.ORG
www.nationalmssociety.org
Janet Kramer, Chapter President
Greg Kovach, Director of Services

6528 **National MS Society: Northwest Ohio Chapter**
401 Tomahawk Drive 419-897-9533
Maumee, OH 43537-1633 800-368-7459
Fax: 419-897-9733
e-mail: NWOHIO@AMPLEX.NET
www.nationalmssociety.org/chapters/OHO/i
Jacque Pratt, Chapter Program Coordinator
Tonya Scherf, Program Director

Oklahoma

6529 **National MS Society: Oklahoma Chapter**
4604 E 67th Street 918-488-0882
Tulsa, OK 74136-4946 800-777-7814
Fax: 918-488-0913
e-mail: LISA.GRAY@OKE.NMSS.ORG
www.nationalmssociety.org/chapters/OKE/i
Paula Cortner, Chapter President
Denise Allenÿÿÿÿÿÿÿÿ, Finance/HR Managerÿÿÿÿ

Oregon

6530 **National MS Society: Oregon Chapter**
104 SW Clay Street 503-223-9511
Portland, OR 97201 800-344-4867
Fax: 503-223-2912
e-mail: INFO@DEFEATMS.COM
www.nationalmssociety.org/chapters/ORC/i
The Pregon Chapter is aggressively pursuing the mission to end the devastating effects of MS by providing programs designed to enhance the families throughout Oregon and Clark County, Washington.
Wendy Allison, Office Coordinator
Sally Alworth, Director of Financeÿ

Pennsylvania

6531 **National MS Society: Central Pennsylvania Chapter**
2040 Linglestown Road 717-652-2108
Harrisburg, PA 17110-1095 Fax: 717-652-2590
e-mail: PAC@NMSS.ORG
www.nationalmssociety.org/chapters/PAC/i
Margie Adelmann, President
Debbie Rios, Executive Vice President

6532 **National MS Society: Greater Delaware Valley Chapter**
1 Reed Street 215-271-1500
Philadelphia, PA 19147-5519 800-548-4611
Fax: 215-271-6122
e-mail: PAE@NMSS.ORG
www.nationalmssociety.org/chapters/PAE/i
John H Scott, President
Randee Forstein, VP Programs & Community Outreach

Rhode Island

6533 **National MS Society: Rhode Island Chapter**
205 Hallene Road 401-738-8383
Warwick, RI 02886-2452 800-344-4867
Fax: 401-738-8469
e-mail: CATIE.DUSSAULT@RIR.NMSS.ORG
www.nationalmssociety.org/chapters/RIR/i
Provides local programs and services to people with MS and their families. These services include information and referral, equipment loans, purchase assistance, programs for the newly diagnosed and education and support groups.
3M Members
Kathy Mechnig, Chapter President
Catie Dussault, Director of Special Events

South Carolina

6534 **National MS Society: South Carolina Branch**
2711 Middleburg Drive 803-799-7848
Columbia, SC 29204-2413 800-922-7591
www.nationalmssociety.org/chapters/NCP/i

Tennessee

6535 **National MS Society: Sutheast Tennessee/North Georgia Chapter**
5720 Uptain Road 423-954-9700
Chattanooga, TN 37411-5642 Fax: 423-855-9667
e-mail: questions@msmidsouth.org
www.nationalmssociety.org
Jeanne Brice, Services Manager

6536 **National MS Society: Mid-South Chapter**
3100 Walnut Grove Road 901-324-9610
Memphis, TN 38111-3530 Fax: 901-324-9668
The mission of the National Multiple Sclerosis Society is to end the devastating effects of MS.
Dee Blake, Chapter President
Sherree Wilson, Services Director

6537 **National MS Society: Mid-South Chapter, Nashville Office**
4219 Hillsboro Road 615-269-9055
Nashville, TN 37215-3332 800-269-9055
Fax: 615-269-9470
e-mail: TNS@NMSS.ORG
www.nationalmssociety.org/chapters/TNS/i
Jim Ward, Chapter President
Beth Smith, Vice President of Client Programs

Texas

6538 **National MS Society: North Central Texas Chapter**
4086 Sandshell Drive 817-306-7003
Fort Worth, TX 76137 Fax: 817-877-1205
www.nationalmssociety.org/chapters/TXH/i
Educational programs, self-help groups, and information and referral for persons and families diagnosed with multiple sclerosis.
12 pages Quarterly
Justin Martin, Coordinator Development
Lynette Jarvis-Barre, Senior Manager Programs & Services

6539 **National MS Society: Panhandle Chapter**
6222 Canyon Drive 806-468-8005
Amarillo, TX 79109-6730 800-344-4867
Fax: 806-468-8022
e-mail: TXP@NMSS.ORG
www.nationalmssociety.org/chapters/TXP/i
Gail Lindsey, Programs and Services Coordinator
April Brownlee, Development Coordinator Special Events

6540 **National MS Society: Southern Texas**
8111 N Stadium Drive 713-526-8967
Houston, TX 77054 Fax: 713-394-7422
e-mail: TXH@NMSS.ORG
www.nationalmssociety.org/chapters/TXH/i
Mark Neagli, Chapter President
Deborah Pope, VP - Operations

6541 **National MS Society: West Texas Division**
1031 Andrews Highway 432-522-2143
Midland, TX 79701-4636 Fax: 432-694-7970
e-mail: TXQ@NMSS.ORG
www.nationalmssociety.org/chapters/TXQ/i
Sharon Rader, Regional Development Manager
Rona Bowerman, Regional Programs and Services Manager

6542 **National MS Socisty: Southeast Texas Chapter**
8111 N Stadium Drive 713-526-8967
Houston, TX 77054-4051 Fax: 281-526-4049
www.nationalmssociety.org
Mark Neagli, Chapter President
Jim Tidwell, Chairman

Utah

6543 **National MS Society: Utah State Chapter**
6364 S Highland Drive 801-493-0113
Salt Lake City, UT 84121-3537 800-527-8116
Fax: 801-493-0122
e-mail: infoutah@nmss.org
www.fightmsutah.org
Our mission is to end the devastating effects of MS. Serving individuals with MS and their families through programs, research, awareness and education.
Annette Royleÿÿÿÿÿÿÿ, Chapter President
Dee Dee Fox, Director of Client Programs and Services

Vermont

6544 **National MS Society: Vermont Division**
75 Talcott Road 802-864-6356
Williston, VT 05495 800-344-4867
Fax: 802-864-6509
e-mail: VTN@NMSS.ORG
www.nationalmssociety.org/chapters/VTN/i
Committed to ending the devastating effects of MS.
Christine Newberr, Programs and Services Coordinator
Lindsay Going, Development Coordinator Special Events

Virginia

6545 **National MS Society: Blue Ridge Chapter**
One Morton Drive 804-971-8010
Charlottesville, VA 22903 Fax: 804-979-4475
e-mail: VAB@NMSS.ORG
www.nationalmssociety.org/chapters/VAB/i
Faith Painter, Chapter President
Delton Hanson, Operations Director

6546 **National MS Society: Central Virginia Chapter**
2112 W Laburnum Avenue 804-353-5008
Richmond, VA 23227 Fax: 804-353-5595
e-mail: JUDY.GRIFFIN@NMSS.ORG
www.nationalmssociety.org/chapters/VAR/i
Sherri Ellis, Chapter President
Andy Page, Director of Community Development

6547 **National MS Society: Hampton Roads Chapter**
760 Lynnhaven Parkway 757-490-9627
Virginia Beach, VA 23452-6311 Fax: 757-490-1617
e-mail: info@fightms.com
www.nationalmssociety.org/chapters/VAX/i
Sharon Grossman, Chapter President
Michelle Derr, Vice President Finance/Administration

Washington

6548 **National MS Society: Greater Washington Chapter**
192 Nickerson Street 206-284-4236
Seattle, WA 98109 800-800-7047
Fax: 206-284-4972
e-mail: GREATERWAINFO@NMSSWAS.ORG
www.nationalmssociety.org/chapters/WAS/i
Patricia Shepherd-Ba, Chapter President
Erin Poznanski, Vice President Chapter Programs

6549 **National MS Society: Inland Northwest Chapter**
818 E Sharp Avenue 509-482-2022
Spokane, WA 99202-1935 Fax: 509-483-1077
e-mail: WAI@NMSS.ORG
www.nationalmssociety.org/chapters/WAI/i
Robert Hansen, Chapter President
Patty Mathias, Office Manager

West Virginia

6550 **National MS Society: West Virginia Chapter**
1 Morton Drive 434-971-8010
Charlottesville, VA 22903 800-344-4867
Fax: 434-979-4475
e-mail: VAB@NMSS.ORG
www.nationalmssociety.org/chapters/VAB/i
The National MS Society is committed to building a movement by and for people with MS that will move us closer to a world free of this disease.
Fay Painter, Chapter President
Delton Hanson, Operations Director

Wisconsin

6551 **National MS Society: Wisconsin Chapter**
1120 James Drive 262-369-4400
Hartland, WI 53029 Fax: 262-369-4410
e-mail: info@wisms.org
www.nationalmssociety.org/chapters/WIG/i
Colleen Kalt, President & CEO
Melissa Palfery, Executive Assistant

Wyoming

6552 **National MS Society: Wyoming Chapter**
525 Randall Avenue 307-433-9590
Cheyenne, WY 82001-1627 Fax: 307-433-8657
e-mail: WYY@NMSS.ORG
www.nationalmssociety.org/chapters/WYY/i
Cheryl Seaberg, Programs and Services Coordinator
Stephanie Batson, Development Coordinator Special Events

Libraries & Resource Centers

6553 **Information Resource Center and Library**
National Multiple Sclerosis Society
733 Third Avenue
New York, NY 10017 800-344-4867
www.nationalmssociety.org
The primary venue for educating the community about multiple sclerosis.Offers the latest information about MS information and provides referrals to local MS care centers, physicians and service providers.
Weyman T Johnson, Jr, Chairman
Joyce M Nelson, President/CEO

6554 **St. Agnes Hospital Medical: Health Science Library**
305 North Street 914-681-4500
White Plains, NY 10605 Fax: 914-328-6408
Labe C Scheinberg MD, Director

Research Centers

6555 **Brigham and Women's Hospital: Center for Neurologic Diseases**
LMRC Building
75 Francis Street 617-732-5500
Boston, MA 02115 800-294-9999
TTY: 617-732-6458
www.brighamandwomens.org
Offers research relating to Multiple Sclerosis and other autoimmune diseases.
Dr Howard Weiner, Coordinator

6556 **Center for Neuroimmunology: University of Alabama at Birmingham**
1720 7th Ave S 205-934-0683
Birmingham, AL 35294 Fax: 205-996-4039
www.main.uab.edu/neurology
Evaluate and treat acute and chronic neurological and neuromuscular diseases which are caused by autoimmune mechanisms or linked to presumed abnormalities affecting the immune system.
Khurram Bashir, Director

6557 **Jimmie Heuga Center**
27 Main Street 970-926-1290
Edwards, CO 81632 800-367-3101
Fax: 970-926-1295
e-mail: Info@heuga.org
www.heuga.org
Conducts research and studies on multiple sclerosis patients.
Kim Lennox Sharkey, Chief Executive Officer
Carrie Van Beek, Office Coordinator

6558 **Neuromuscular Treatment Center: Univ. of Texas Southwestern Medical Center**
Department of Neurology
Dallas, TX 75390 214-648-3111
www.utsouthwestern.edu
Basic and clinical studies of myasthenia gravis.
Dr Ralph Greenlee, Director

6559 **Rush University Multiple Sclerosis Center**
1725 W Harrison Street 312-942-8011
Chicago, IL 60612 888-352-RUSH
TTY: 312-942-2207
e-mail: contact_rush@rush.edu
www.rush.edu
The Multiple Sclerosis Center combines comprehensive treatment with clinical and laboratory research to provide the highest quality patient care.
Floyd A Davis, Director

Support Groups & Hotlines

6560 **MS Toll-Free Information Line**
National Multiple Sclerosis Society
733 3rd Avenue
New York, NY 10017-3288 800-344-4867
Offers public and professional information, brochures and referrals to MS patients, their families and health care professionals.

6561 **MSWorld**
1943 Morrill Street 415-701-1117
Sarasota, FL 34236 877-710-0302
e-mail: msworld@msworld.org
www.msworld.org/
MSWorld is for people with multiple sclerosis their families and friends, offer support via chat, e-mail, message boards, magazines.
Kathleen Wilson, Founder/President

6562 **Multiple Sclerosis Action Group**
National Multiple Sclerosis Society
733 3rd Avenue 409-883-2282
New York, NY 10017 800-344-4867
e-mail: msag@erasems.com
www.nmss.org
Richard J Mengel, Treasurer
Fred J Lublin, Director

6563 **National Health Information Center**
PO Box 1133 310-565-4167
Washington, DC 20013 800-336-4797
Fax: 301-984-4256
e-mail: info@nhic.org
www.health.gov/nhic
Offers a nationwide information referral service, produces directories and resource guides.

6564 **Traditional Tibetan Healing**
13 Harrison Street 617-666-8635
Sommerville, MA 2143-6504 866-628-6504
e-mail: Kelob@gte.net
www.tibetanherbalhealing.com/
To rid mankind from chronic illnesses using alternative methods.
Keyzon Bhutti, Chief Physician

Books

6565 **300 Tips for Making Life with Multiple Sclerosis Easier**
Demos Medical Publishing
386 Park Avenue S 212-683-0072
New York, NY 10016 Fax: 212-683-0118
e-mail: orderdept@demospub.com
www.demosmedpub.com
Techniques for better living.
109 pages
ISBN: 1-888799-23-4
Dr. Diana M Schneider

6566 **Alternative Medicine and Multiple Sclerosis**
Demos Medical Publishing
386 Park Avenue S 212-683-0072
New York, NY 10016 Fax: 212-683-0118
e-mail: orderdept@demospub.com
www.demosmedpub.com
272 pages
ISBN: 1-888799-52-8
Dr. Diana M Schneider

6567 **Fall Down Seven Times Get Up Eight**
Miramar Communications
PO Box 8987
Malibu, CA 90265-8987 800-543-4116
The second in Dr. Wolf's series on MS management: including chapters on stress and fatigue, planning for serious disability and lots more.
211 pages

6568 **Living with Multiple Sclerosis**
Demos Medical Publishing
386 Park Avenue S 212-683-0072
New York, NY 10016 Fax: 212-683-0118
e-mail: orderdept@demospub.com
www.demosmedpub.com
ISBN: 1-888799-26-9
Dr. Diana M Schneider

6569 **Living with Multiple Sclerosis: A Wellness Approach**
Demos Vermande
386 Park Avenue S 212-683-0072
New York, NY 10016-8804 800-532-8663
112 pages
ISBN: 1-888799-00-5

6570 **Meeting the Challenge of Progressive Multiple Sclerosis**
Demos Medical Publishing

386 Park Avenue S
New York, NY 10016
212-683-0072
Fax: 212-683-0118
e-mail: orderdept@demospub.com
www.demosmedpub.com

128 pages
ISBN: 1-888799-46-3
Dr. Diana M Schneider

6571 **Multiple Sclerosis**
Demos Medical Publishing
386 Park Avenue S
New York, NY 10016
212-683-0072
800-532-8663
Fax: 212-683-0118
e-mail: orderdept@demospub.com
www.demosmedpub.com

A consistent bestseller in multiple sclerosis management.
224 pages
ISBN: 1-888799-54-4
Dr. Diana M Schneider

6572 **Multiple Sclerosis, The Questions you Have Answers You Need**
Demos Medical Publishing
386 Park Avenue S
New York, NY 10016
212-683-0072
Fax: 212-683-0118
e-mail: orderdept@demospub.com
www.demosmedpub.com

592 pages
ISBN: 1-888799-43-9
Dr. Diana M Schneider

6573 **Multiple Sclerosis: A Guide for Families**
Demos Medical Publishing
386 Park Avenue S
New York, NY 10016-8804
212-683-0072
800-532-8663
Fax: 212-683-0118
e-mail: orderdept@demospub.com
www.demosmedpub.com

With its complex and unpredictable course, MS affects every area of family life. This book covers a broad range of medical, psychological, social, vocational, economic and legal problems.
1997 207 pages Paperback
ISBN: 1-888799-14-5
Dr. Diana M Schneider, President

6574 **Multiple Sclerosis: A Guide for Patients and Their Families**
Raven Press
1185 Avenue of the Americas
New York, NY 10036-2601
212-930-9500
800-777-2295

Second edition.
288 pages Paperback
ISBN: 0-881672-55-6

6575 **Multiple Sclerosis: A Personal Exploration**
Demos Vermande
386 Park Avenue S
New York, NY 10016-8804
212-683-0072
800-532-8663
Fax: 212-683-0118

1993 192 pages
ISBN: 0-285650-18-1

6576 **Multiple Sclerosis: Your Legal Rights**
Demos Medical Publishing
386 Park Avenue S
New York, NY 10016
212-683-0072
Fax: 212-683-0118
e-mail: orderdept@demospub.com
www.demosmedpub.com

156 pages
ISBN: 1-888799-31-5
Dr. Diana M Schneider

6577 **The Comfort of Home Multiple Sclerosis Edi tion: A Guide for Caregivers**
Marie M. Meyer and Paula Derr, RN, author
CareTrust Publications
PO Box 10283
Portland, OR 97296-0283
800-565-1533
Fax: 415-673-2005
e-mail: sales@comfortofhome.com
www.comfortofhome.com

Reviews caregiving options and discusses the financial and legal decisions you may encounterr. Readers will learn how to set up a safe and comfortable home for the person whose needs are changing and abilities declining. Comfort offers guidance through every caregiving stage and most decisions one will face in daily living, as well as in avoiding caregiver burnout. Valuable for the caregiver and the patient.
324 pages
ISBN: 0-966476-76-X

6578 **Understanding Multiple Sclerosis**
Melissa Stauffer, author
University Press of Mississippi
3825 Ridgewood Road
Jackson, MS 39211-6492
601-432-6205
Fax: 601-432-6217
e-mail: kburgess@ihl.state.ms.us
www.upress.state.ms.us

For patients and companions, an overview of all aspects of MS.
2006 144 pages Paperback
ISBN: 1-578068-03-7
Kathy Burgess, Advertising/Marketing Services Manager

Magazines

6579 **Inside MS**
National Multiple Sclerosis Society
733 3rd Avenue
New York, NY 10017-3288
212-986-3240
800-344-4867
Fax: 212-986-7981
www.nmss.org

Full color quarterly magazine on living well with mutiple sclerosis. Articles by people with MS; daily living, achievments, news, treatments, research, advocacy, humor, travel, helpful resources, large type. The magazine is a benefit of membership.
64 pages 4x Year

Newsletters

6580 **Inside MS Bulletin**
National Multiple Sclerosis Society
733 3rd Avenue
New York, NY 10017-3288
212-986-3240
800-344-4867
Fax: 212-986-7981

Newsletter offering information on the organization activities. Profiles of donors, and reports on MS research programs.

6581 **MS Connection**
National MS Society: Oregon Chapter
104 SW Clay Street
Portland, OR 97201
503-223-9511
800-344-4867
Fax: 503-223-2912
e-mail: info@defeatms.com
www.defeatms.com

Available to members of the National MS Society in Oregon and Southwest Washington.
Virginia Silvey, President
Ann Balzell, Program Director

6582 **Motivator**
Multiple Sclerosis Foundation
6350 N Andrews Avenue
Fort Lauderdale, FL 33309-2130
954-776-6805
800-441-7055
e-mail: msfacts@icanect.net
www.msfacts.org

Reports on the latest advancements regarding medical treatments/therapies for MS, inspirational feature stories, coping skills, correspondence from readers, and ongoing MSAA programs, services, and activities.
BiMonthly

6583 **Multiple Sclerosis Quarterly Report**
Demos Vermande
386 Park Avenue S
New York, NY 10016-8804
212-683-0072
800-532-8663
Fax: 212-683-0118

This is the definitive newsletter for everyone who has MS, with feature articles, research updates, book reviews, and more. It is de-

veloped with the sponsorship of the Eastern Paralyzed Veterans of America and the National Multiple Sclerosis Society. The MSQR will keep you informed of new developments in the management of MS and strategies for living successfully with the disease.
1997 Quarterly

6584 **National Multiple Sclerosis Society: Allegheny District Chapter**
1040 5th Avenue 412-261-6347
Pittsburgh, PA 15219-6220 800-544-5250
Fax: 412-232-1461
e-mail: pa@nmss.org
www.nmss-pgh.org
12 pages 4 per year
Colleen McGuire, Chapter President

Pamphlets

6585 **ADA and People with MS**
National Multiple Sclerosis Society
733 3rd Avenue 212-986-3240
New York, NY 10017-3288 800-344-4867
Fax: 212-986-7981
What the Americans with Disabilities Act means in employment, public accommodations, transportation, and telecommunications.
24 pages

6586 **At Home with MS: Adapting Your Environment**
National Multiple Sclerosis Society
733 3rd Avenue 212-986-3240
New York, NY 10017-3288 800-344-4867
Fax: 212-986-7981
Modify a house or apartment to save energy, compensate for reduced vision or mobility, and live comfortably. Many do-it-yourself changes.
28 pages

6587 **At Our House**
National Multiple Sclerosis Society
733 3rd Avenue 212-986-3240
New York, NY 10017-3288 800-344-4867
Fax: 212-986-7981
A coloring book for children, ages 5-8, about a Mama Bear with MS. contains some very basic facts with an afterword for parents on how to talk to young children about MS.
20 pages

6588 **Chapter Services at a Glance**
National Multiple Sclerosis Society
733 3rd Avenue 212-986-3240
New York, NY 10017-3288 800-344-4867
Fax: 212-986-7981
A summary of services offerred by local chapters. Contains membership form.

6589 **Check Your Multiple Sclerosis Facts**
National Multiple Sclerosis Society
733 3rd Avenue 212-986-3240
New York, NY 10017-3288 800-344-4867
Fax: 212-986-7981
A brief checklist of MS basics - definition, symptoms, and outlook.

6590 **Choosing a Pharmacy Service**
National Multiple Sclerosis Society
733 3rd Avenue 212-986-3240
New York, NY 10017-3288 800-344-4867
Fax: 212-986-7981
What to look for when choosing a prescription drug provider.
20 pages

6591 **Clear Thinking About Alternative Therapies**
National Multiple Sclerosis Society
733 3rd Avenue 212-986-3240
New York, NY 10017-3288 800-344-4867
Fax: 212-986-7981
Highlights facts and common misconceptions, compares alternative and conventional medicine, and suggests ways to evaluate benefits and risks.

6592 **Controlling Spasticity**
National Multiple Sclerosis Society
733 3rd Avenue 212-986-3240
New York, NY 10017-3288 800-344-4867
Fax: 212-986-7981
An overview of ways to control this common and sometimes disabling MS symtpom. Includes roles of self-help, medications, physical therapists, nurses, and physicians.

6593 **Food for Thought: MS and Nutrition**
National Multiple Sclerosis Society
733 3rd Avenue 212-986-3240
New York, NY 10017-3288 800-344-4867
Fax: 212-986-7981
A guide to healthy eating and coping with symptoms that may affect eating habits.
20 pages

6594 **Getting a Grip on Gait**
National Multiple Sclerosis Society
733 3rd Avenue 212-986-3240
New York, NY 10017-3288 800-344-4867
Fax: 212-986-7981
Walking problems and how they can be addressed.

6595 **Hiring Help at Home?**
National Multiple Sclerosis Society
733 3rd Avenue 212-986-3240
New York, NY 10017-3288 800-344-4867
Fax: 212-986-7981
Checklists and worksheets for people who need help at home. Forms for needs assessment, job description, and employment contract.

6596 **Insight Into Eyesight**
National Multiple Sclerosis Society
733 3rd Avenue 212-986-3240
New York, NY 10017-3288 800-344-4867
Fax: 212-986-7981
Current therapy for MS-related eye disorders. Discusses low-vision aids.

6597 **Living with MS**
National Multiple Sclerosis Society
733 3rd Avenue 212-986-3240
New York, NY 10017-3288 800-344-4867
Fax: 212-986-7981
Answers to 28 questions most often asked when the diagnosis is MS - from possible causes to advice on coping.
20 pages

6598 **Moving with Multiple Sclerosis**
National Multiple Sclerosis Society
733 3rd Avenue 212-986-3240
New York, NY 10017-3288 800-344-4867
Fax: 212-986-7981
Step-by-step illustrations of passive and active stretching, balance, and conditioning exercises.
30 pages

6599 **Multiple Sclerosis and Your Emotions**
National Multiple Sclerosis Society
733 3rd Avenue 212-986-3240
New York, NY 10017-3288 800-344-4867
Fax: 212-986-7981
How to manage some of the emotional challenges created by MS.
32 pages

6600 **On the Question of Pregnancy**
National Multiple Sclerosis Society
733 3rd Avenue 212-986-3240
New York, NY 10017-3288 800-344-4867
Fax: 212-986-7981
Reassuring answers on pregnancy, delivery, and nursing.

6601 **On: Alternative Therapies**
National Multiple Sclerosis Society
733 3rd Avenue 212-986-3240
New York, NY 10017-3288 800-344-4867
Fax: 212-986-7981
Checklist for people who are considering an alternative treatment.

6602 On: Diagnosis...Putting the Pieces Together
National Multiple Sclerosis Society
733 3rd Avenue
New York, NY 10017-3288
212-986-3240
800-344-4867
Fax: 212-986-7981
Explains usual steps and tests. Includes how to prepare for an MRI.

6603 On: Energy Management
National Multiple Sclerosis Society
733 3rd Avenue
New York, NY 10017-3288
212-986-3240
800-344-4867
Fax: 212-986-7981
Guidelines for budgeting your energy when it's limited by fatigue through prioritizing, delegating, and simplifying tasks.

6604 On: Fatigue
National Multiple Sclerosis Society
733 3rd Avenue
New York, NY 10017-3288
212-986-3240
800-344-4867
Fax: 212-986-7981
The mystery of MS fatigue, practical tips for coping, and the medications sometimes prescribed.

6605 On: Genes
National Multiple Sclerosis Society
733 3rd Avenue
New York, NY 10017-3288
212-986-3240
800-344-4867
Fax: 212-986-7981
Recent information on MS and heredity.

6606 On: Pain
National Multiple Sclerosis Society
733 3rd Avenue
New York, NY 10017-3288
212-986-3240
800-344-4867
Fax: 212-986-7981
Myths and facts about MS pain. Covers types of pain and possible treatment.

6607 Plaintalk: A Booklet About MS for Families
National Multiple Sclerosis Society
733 3rd Avenue
New York, NY 10017-3288
212-986-3240
800-344-4867
Fax: 212-986-7981
Discusses some of the more difficult physical and emotional problems families may face.
32 pages

6608 Rehab Outlook
National Multiple Sclerosis Society
733 3rd Avenue
New York, NY 10017-3288
212-986-3240
800-344-4867
Fax: 212-986-7981
What rehabilitation can do for mobility, fatigue, driving, speech, memory, bowel or bladder problems, sexuality, and more.
24 pages

6609 Research Directions in Multiple Sclerosis
National Multiple Sclerosis Society
733 3rd Avenue
New York, NY 10017-3288
212-986-3240
800-344-4867
Fax: 212-986-7981
An overview of current research on key areas of immunology, genetics, virology, and cell biology explained for nonscientists.
16 pages

6610 Sexual Problems Your Doctor Didn't Mention
National Multiple Sclerosis Society
733 3rd Avenue
New York, NY 10017-3288
212-986-3240
800-344-4867
Fax: 212-986-7981
How MS may affect sexuality and what can be done.

6611 Solving Cognitive Problems
National Multiple Sclerosis Society
733 3rd Avenue
New York, NY 10017-3288
212-986-3240
800-344-4867
Fax: 212-986-7981
Mental functions most likely to be affected by MS. Suggestions for self-help and information about cognitive rehabiitation.
20 pages

6612 Someone You Know Has MS: A Book for Families
National Multiple Sclerosis Society
733 3rd Avenue
New York, NY 10017-3288
212-986-3240
800-344-4867
Fax: 212-986-7981
For children ages 6-12 who have a parent with MS. Provides facts and explores children's fears and concerns.
32 pages

6613 Taking Care: A Guide for Well Partners
National Multiple Sclerosis Society
733 3rd Avenue
New York, NY 10017-3288
212-986-3240
800-344-4867
Fax: 212-986-7981
Introduces the concept of carepartnering to balance both partners' needs. Includes practical suggestions about getting and giving help.
16 pages

6614 Taming Stress in Multiple Sclerosis
National Multiple Sclerosis Society
733 3rd Avenue
New York, NY 10017-3288
212-986-3240
800-344-4867
Fax: 212-986-7981
Stress and depression, and how both relate to MS. Tips on simplifying daily life. Instructions on muscle relaxation, deep breathing, and visualization relaxation.
36 pages

6615 Things I Wish Someone Had Told Me
National Multiple Sclerosis Society
733 3rd Avenue
New York, NY 10017-3288
212-986-3240
800-344-4867
Fax: 212-986-7981
First-person story. A positive and practical approach to adjusting to life with MS.
20 pages

6616 Understanding Bladder Problems in Multiple Sclerosis
National Multiple Sclerosis Society
733 3rd Avenue
New York, NY 10017-3288
212-986-3240
800-344-4867
Fax: 212-986-7981
The three main types of bladder dysfunction explained. Guidelines for management.
12 pages

6617 Understanding Bowel Problems in MS
National Multiple Sclerosis Society
733 3rd Avenue
New York, NY 10017-3288
212-986-3240
800-344-4867
Fax: 212-986-7981
An exploration of ways to manage bowel problems in MS.
24 pages

6618 What Everyone Should Know About Multiple Sclerosis
National Multiple Sclerosis Society
733 3rd Avenue
New York, NY 10017-3288
212-986-3240
800-344-4867
Fax: 212-986-7981
Overview of MS, suitable for the whole family.
16 pages

6619 What Is Multiple Sclerosis?
National Multiple Sclerosis Society
733 3rd Avenue
New York, NY 10017-3288
212-986-3240
800-344-4867
Fax: 212-986-7981
For the newly diagnosed and others who need an overview of symptoms, disease patterns, diagnosis, prognosis, treatment, and research efforts.

6620 When a Parent Has MS: A Teenager's Guide
National Multiple Sclerosis Society
733 3rd Avenue
New York, NY 10017-3288
212-986-3240
800-344-4867
Fax: 212-986-7981
For older children and teenagers who have a parent with MS. Discusses issues brought up by real kids.
24 pages

6621 Win-Win Approach to Reasonable Accommodations
National Multiple Sclerosis Society
733 3rd Avenue 212-986-3240
New York, NY 10017-3288 800-344-4867
Fax: 212-986-7981

A practical guide to obtaining workplace accommodations.
20 pages

Audio & Video

6622 Aqua Exercises for Multiple Sclerosis
National Multiple Sclerosis Society
733 3rd Avenue 212-986-3240
New York, NY 10017-3288 800-344-4867
Fax: 212-986-7981

A workout that cools and supports the body, with exercises to reduce spasticity, build muscles, and improve posture. With waterproof chart.
20 minutes

6623 Clinical Trials in Multiple Sclerosis: Searching for New Therapies
National Multiple Sclerosis Society
733 3rd Avenue 212-986-3240
New York, NY 10017 800-344-4867
Fax: 212-986-7981

Describes studies to determine the safety and efficacy of new drugs to treat MS. Why studies are essential, how they are conducted, and the role of participants.
20 minutes

6624 Now, More Than Ever: Progress in Multiple Sclerosis Research
National Multiple Sclerosis Society
733 3rd Avenue 212-986-3240
New York, NY 10017-3288 800-344-4867
Fax: 212-986-7981

Traces the National Multiple Sclerosis Society's historic role in propelling MS research and explains current approaches for nonscientists.
10 minutes

Web Sites

6625 Healing Well
www.healingwell.com

An online health resource guide to medical news, chat, information and articles, newsgroups and message boards, books, disease-related web sites, medical directories, and more for patients, friends, and family coping with disabling diseases, disorders, or chronic illnesses.

6626 Health Finder
www.healthfinder.gov

Searchable, carefully developed web site offering information on over 1000 topics. Developed by the US Department of Health and Human Services, the site can be used in both English and Spanish.

6627 Healthlink USA
www.healthlinkusa.com

Health information concerning treatment, cures, prevention, diagnosis, risk factors, research, support groups, email lists, personal stories and much more. Updated regularly.

6628 Helios Health
www.helioshealth.com

Online resource for your health information. Detailed information about specific health topics, access to expert advice from our Medical Advisory Board, and up-to-date health news.

6629 MedicineNet
www.medicinenet.com

An online resource for consumers providing easy-to-read, authoritative medical and health information.

6630 Medscape
www.mywebmd.com

Medscape offers specialists, primary care physicians, and other health professionals the Web's most robust and integrated medical information and educational tools.

6631 Multiple Sclerosis Foundation
www.msfocus.org

Dedicated to helping create a brighter tomorrow for those with MS, the foundation offers a wide array of free services including: national toll-free support, educational programs, homecare, support groups, assitive technology, publications, a comprehensive website and more to improve the quality of life for those affected by MS.

6632 National Multiple Sclerosis Society
www.nmss.org

Provides research, public and professional education, advocacy and the design of rehabilitative and psychosocial programs.

6633 Neurology Channel
www.neurologychannel.com

Find clearly explained, medically accurate information regarding conditions, including an overview, symptoms, causes, diagnostic procedures and treatment options. On this site it is possible to ask questions and get information from a neurologist and connect to people who have similar health interests.

6634 WebMD
www.webmd.com

Information on Multiple Sclerosis, including articles and resources.

Description

6635 **Muscular Dystrophy**

Muscular dystrophy is a group of genetic disorders marked by progressive weakness and degeneration of the skeletal, or voluntary, muscles that control movement. The muscles of the heart and other involuntary muscles may also affected in some forms of muscular dystrophy, and a few forms of the disease involve other organs as well.

Muscular dystrophy can affect people of all ages. The most common form, Duchenne, appears in childhood, but others may not appear until middle age or later.

Duchenne muscular dystrophy affects males almost exclusively. By age five, those with Duchenne experience progressive weakness and difficulty in climbing, jumping and hopping. By ages eight to ten, leg braces are often required, and eventually walking is impossible. Duchenne is also associated with heart problems, although without symptoms, and intellectual impairment that affects verbal ability more than performance. Death usually occurs in the third decade of life, often as a result of pneumonia.

No specific treatment exists. Daily prednisone provides significant benefit but owing to the medication's numerous side effects, it should be reserved for patients with major functional decline. Other treatment includes physical therapy, which can help minimize the shortening of the muscles that occurs around joints; assistive devices; and avoidance of prolonged immobility. There are now techniques available to detect female carriers of the defective gene, enabling genetic counseling for families and couples considering conception.

Other forms of muscular dystrophy are myotonic, Becker, limb-girdle and facioscapulohumeral. Information about when and where muscle weakness first occurred, and its severity, is very helpful in classifying the type of muscular dystrophy. Studying a small piece of muscle tissue can indicate whether the disorder is muscular dystrophy and which form of the disease it is.

National Agencies & Associations

6636 **Muscular Dystrophy Association**
3300 E Sunrise Drive 520-529-2000
Tucson, AZ 85718-3299 800-572-1717
e-mail: mda@mdausa.org
www.mda.org
Primary objective of MDA is the support of scientific investigators seeking the causes of and effective treatments for muscular dystrophy and related neuromuscular disorders. The worldwide research program supports over 400 scientific investigations annually.
Robert Ross, President/CEO

6637 **Muscular Dystrophy Canada**
2345 Yonge Street 866-687-2538
Toronto, Ontario, M4P-2E5 Fax: 416-488-7523
e-mail: info@muscle.ca
www.muscle.ca
Since 1954, Muscular Dystrophy Canada has been committed to improving the quality of life for the tens of thousands of Canadians with neuromuscular disorders and funding leading research for the discovery of therapies and cures for neuromuscular disorders.

6638 **Parent Project: Muscular Dystrophy**
1012 N University Boulevard 513-424-0696
Middletown, OH 45042 800-714-5437
Fax: 513-425-9907
e-mail: pat@parentprojectmd.org
www.parentprojectmd.org
Organization of families around the world who have children diagnosed with DMD/BMD. Our goal is to invest significant amounts of money raised into medical research with clinical application.
Patricia Furlong, President
Kimberly Galberaith, Executive Vice President

6639 **Society for Muscular Dystrophy Information International**
PO Box 7490 902-685-3961
Bridgewater, Nova Scotia, B4V-2X6 Fax: 902-685-3962
e-mail: smdi@auracom.com
users.auracom.com
A registered Canadian charity founded in 1983 by us, to provide a non-technical worldwide information links via publications and now this web site, for neuromuscular disorders.

Research Centers

6640 **Baylor College of Medicine: Jerry Lewis Neuromuscular Disease Research**
Methodist Neurological Institute
Department of Neurology 713-798-5971
Houston, TX 77030 Fax: 713-798-3854
e-mail: neurons@bcm.edu
www.bcm.edu/neurology
Offers research into biochemistry molecular genetics and neuromuscular disorders.
Stanley Appe MD, Director

6641 **Columbia Presbyterian Medical Center Neurological Institute**
Columbia University
710 W 168th Street 212-305-2700
New York, NY 10032 Fax: 212-058-98
www.cumc.columbia.edu
Neuromuscular clinical research center.
Hiroshi Mits MD, Division Head Neuromuscular Division

6642 **Columbia University Clinical Research Center for Muscular Dystrophy**
College of Physicians & Surgeons
630 W 168th Street 212-305-3806
New York, NY 10032 Fax: 212-305-1343
www.columbia.edu
Salvatore DiMauro, Co Director

6643 **Hospital of the University of Pennsylvania University of Pennsylvania**
University of Pennsylvania
3400 Spruce Street 215-662-4000
Philadelphia, PA 19104 800-789-PENN
Fax: 215-903-09
e-mail: pleasure@email.chop.edu
www.pennhealth.com
Research program centering its efforts on finding better ways to prevent and treat neuromuscular disorders.
David E Pleasure MD, Director

6644 **Mayo Clinic and Foundation Mayo Foundation**
Mayo Foundation
201 W Center Street 507-284-2511
Rochester, MN 55905 Fax: 507-284-0161
TTY: 507-284-9786
www.mayo.edu
Neuromuscular clinical research center with a primary research interest in neuropathies.
Peter J Dyck MD, Director Nerve Studies
Andrew G Engel MD, Director Muscle Studies

6645 **Muscular Dystrophy Association**
3300 E Sunrise Drive 520-529-2000
Tucson, AZ 85718-3299 800-572-1717
Fax: 520-529-5300
e-mail: mda@mdausa.org
www.MDausa.org
Fights neuromuscular disease including all muscular dystrophies. Conducts extensive programs of research services and public education including 230 clinics.
Robert Ross, President/CEO

6646 **University of Utah Utah Genome Depot University of Utah**
University of Utah
20 S 2030 E 801-585-7606
Salt Lake City, UT 84112 Fax: 801-857-7177
e-mail: bob.weiss@genetics.utah.edu
www.genome.utah.edu
Focuses research on human muscular dystrophies.
Robert Weiss, Principal Investigator
Jackie Tyce, Program Coordinator

Support Groups & Hotlines

6647 **Facioscapulohumeral Muscular Dystrophy Soc iety (FSH Society)**
3 Westwood Road 781-860-0501
Lexington, MA 02420 Fax: 781-860-0599
e-mail: solvefshd@fshsociety.org
www.fshsociety.org
The Facioscapulohumeral Muscular Dystrophy Society (FSH Society) serves as a resource for individuals and families with FSHD, representing them and advocating on their behalf. Purposes of the organization are to accumulate, disseminate and encourage the exchange of information about FSHD, including educating the general public, relevant governmental bodies, and the medical and scientific professions about the existence, diagnosis and treatment of FSHD.
Daniel Paul Perez, President/CEO
Carol A Perez, Executive Director

6648 **National Health Information Center**
PO Box 1133 310-565-4167
Washington, DC 20013 800-336-4797
Fax: 301-984-4256
e-mail: info@nhic.org
www.health.gov/nhic
Offers a nationwide information referral service, produces directories and resource guides.

Books

6649 **Clinical Evaluation and Diagnostic Tests for Neuromuscular Disorders**
Butterworth-Heinemann Medical
200 Wheeler Road 781-221-2212
Burlington, MA 01803 Fax: 781-221-1615
e-mail: custserv.bh@elsevier.com
www.bh.com
Expert advice from leading authorities on how and when to use the numerous evaluation tests now available for diagnosis and management of neuromuscular disorders.
2002

6650 **Everyday Life with ALS: A Practical Guide**
Muscular Dystrophy Association
3300 E Sunrise Drive 520-529-2000
Tucson, AZ 85718-3299 800-572-1717
Fax: 520-529-5383
e-mail: publications@mdausa.org
www.mda.org
Advice and information addressing degrees of affliction of those with ALS. Ways to conserve energy, to modifying your home space, to medical devices and equipment. Consider using the Guide with your care team.
2005
Christina Medvescek, Director of Editorial Services

6651 **Journey of Love: Parent's Guide to Duchenne Muscular Dystrophy**
Muscular Dystrophy Association
3300 E Sunrise Drive 520-529-2000
Tucson, AZ 85718-3299 800-572-1717
Fax: 520-529-5383
e-mail: publications@mdausa.org
www.mda.org
Complete guide for parents with children diagnosed with DMD. Information includes explanation of the disease, treatments, research, services provided by MDA, guides to finding assistance and more.
170 pages Paperback
Bob Mackle, Director Public Information
Christina Medvescek, Director of Editorial Services

6652 **MDA ALS Caregiver's Guide**
Muscular Dystrophy Association
3300 E Sunrise Drive 520-529-2000
Tucson, AZ 85718-3299 800-572-1717
e-mail: publication@mdusa.org
www.mda.org
A comprehensive guide to caring for a person with ALS at home. Covers everything from physical care to psychological and emotional concerns to getting financial assistance. Companion to "Everyday Life with ALS: A Practical Guide"
2008 58 pages Paperback
Bob Mackle, Director Public Information
Christina Medvescek, Director of Editorial Services

6653 **Moonrise: One Family, Genetic Identity, & Muscular Dystrophy**
St. Martin's Press
175 5th Avenue 212-674-5151
New York, NY 10010 Fax: 212-420-9314
www.stmartins.com
A mother writes about her teen-age son who has Duchenne muscular dystrophy, the life he leads, and the one he can look forward to.
2003

6654 **Muscular Dystrophy & Other Neuromuscular Diseases: Psychological Issues**
Leon Charash, Robert Lovelace, author
Haworth Press
10 Alice Street 607-722-5857
Binghamton, NY 13904 800-429-6784
Fax: 607-722-0012
www.haworthpress.com
Thoughtful book from professionals who assist people with neuromuscular disorders to help them adapt to lifestyle changes accompanying these disorders.
250 pages Hardcover
ISBN: 1-560240-77-0

6655 **Muscular Dystrophy in Children: Guide for Families**
Demos Medical Publishing
386 Park Avenue S
New York, NY 10015 800-532-8663
Fax: 212-683-0118
e-mail: orderdept@demospub.com
www.demosmedpub.com
Addresses emotional as well as physical challenges that families and caregivers will have to face and gives readers information on muscular dystrophy, how to adapt to a child's needs, and present research being conducted. In addition, it gives parents and caregivers sources for additional support and suggestions for further reading.
1999

6656 **Neuromuscular Dis. of Infancy, Childhood & Adolesesce: A Clinician's Approach**
Butterworth-Heinemann Medical
200 Wheeler Road 781-221-2212
Burlington, MA 01803 Fax: 781-221-1615
e-mail: custserv.bh@elsevier.com
www.bh.com
Explains how childhood neuromuscular diseases differ from those in adult patients, and provides clinicians with all the knowledge they need to successfully diagnose and treat pediatric patients.
2003

6657 **Noninvasive Mechanical Ventilation**
John Bach, MD, author
Elsevier
Book Customer Service Department
St. Louis, MO 63146
800-545-2522
Fax: 800-535-9935
e-mail: usbkinfo@elsevier.com
www.elsevier.com
Describes the use of inspiratory and expiratory muscle aids to prevent the pulmonary complications of lung disease and conditions with muscle weakness. It also describes treatment and rehabilitation interventions specific for patients with these conditions. This book is unique in presenting the use of entirely noninvasive management alternatives to eliminate respiratory morbidity and avoid the need to resort to tracheostomy for the majority of patients with lung or neuromuscular disease.
2002 348 pages Paperback
ISBN: 1-560535-49-0

6658 **Physical Medicine & Rehabilitation**
WB Saunders/Elsevier Science/Harcourt
200 Wheeler Road
Burlington, MA 01803
781-221-2212
Fax: 781-221-1615
e-mail: custserv.bh@elsevier.com
www.us.elsevierhealth.com
Current aspects of physical medicine and rehabilitation in a single, readable volume. Completely updated and revised edition includes all the latest advances and techniques.
2001

Children's Books

6659 **Abby & the South Seas Adventure Series**
Tyndale House Publishers
PO Box 80
Wheaton, IL 60189
630-668-8300
Fax: 630-668-3245
www.tyndalecatalog.com
Delightful new series, focusing on the travels of Abby Kendall, who has muscular dystrophy, is a sure-fire hit for 8 to 12 year old girls. Lots of surprises will keep them coming back for each new Abby title.
2000

6660 **Heartsongs, Journey Through Heartsongs, Hope Through Heartsongs, Celebrate**
Hyperion Books
1344 Crossman Avenue
Sunnyvale, CA 94089
408-744-9500
Fax: 408-744-0400
www.hyperion.com
By the 2002-2003 National Goodwill Ambassador for the Muscular Dystrophy Association. The first two books of inspiring poems were both on the New York Times bestseller list. Mattie's struggle with muscular dystrophy has never kept him from feeling deep love for his family, friends, country and faith — heartfelt emotions that are reflected throughout these pages by a precociously brilliant boy.
2001-2003
Carol Sowell, Director Publications

6661 **Muscular Dystrophy**
Enslow Publishers
40 Industrial Road
Berkeley Heights, NJ 07922-0398
800-398-2504
Fax: 908-771-0925
e-mail: info@enslow.com
www.enslow.com
Written for children, this book follows two families with muscular dystrophy and describes various forms of the disease, who gets it, and how to learn to live with it.
2000

Magazines

6662 **Quest Magazine**
Muscular Dystrophy Association
3300 E Sunrise Drive
Tucson, AZ 85718-3299
520-529-2000
800-572-1717
Fax: 520-529-5300
e-mail: publications@mdusa.org
www.mda.org
Quarterly magazine. Contains stories about vital concerns of people with meuromuscular diseases and their community. Find tips, hobbies, resources, treatments, findings, and products. Available online.
30 pages Paperback
Bob Mackle, Director Public Information
Christina Medvescek, Director of Editorial Services

Pamphlets

6663 **Breathe Easy: Respiratory Care with Muscular Dystrophy**
Muscular Dystrophy Association
3300 E Sunrise Drive
Tucson, AZ 85718-3299
520-529-2000
800-572-1717
Fax: 520-529-5383
e-mail: publications@mdausa.org
www.mda.org
Members of a respiratory care team describe how muscular dystrophy can affect breathing, maintaining respiratory health and types of therapies. Also available in Spanish.
2006
Christina Medvescek, Director of Editorial Services

6664 **Everybody's Different Nobody's Perfect**
Muscular Dystrophy Association
3300 E Sunrise Drive
Tucson, AZ 85718-3299
520-529-2000
800-572-1717
Fax: 520-529-5300
e-mail: publications@mdusa.org
www.mda.org
Children's Book. Explains how muscular dystrophy affects children and describes how people are different from each other in many ways. Emphasizing fun, friendship and caring, this booklet is ideal for heightening awareness and encouraging understanding of persons with disabilities. Also available in Spanish.
1999 11 pages Paperback
Bob Mackle, Director Public Information
Christina Medvescek, Director of Editorial Services

6665 **Facts About Charcot-Marie-Tooth Disease**
Muscular Dystrophy Association
3300 E Sunrise Drive
Tucson, AZ 85718-3299
520-529-2000
800-572-1717
Fax: 520-529-5383
e-mail: publications@mdausa.org
www.mda.org
Covers the forms of the disease and outlines the characteristics and genetic patterns of the CMTs. Research efforts aimed at finding the causes, treatments and cures are also described. Also available in Spanish.
15 pages
Christina Medvescek, Director of Editorial Services

6666 **Facts About Duchenne & Becker Muscular Dystrophies**
Muscular Dystrophy Association
3300 E Sunrise Drive
Tucson, AZ 85718-3299
520-529-2000
800-572-1717
Fax: 520-529-5383
e-mail: publications@mdausa.org
www.mda.org
Introductory booklet describes the two disorders, testing, inheritance and treatments. Also available in Spanish.
Christina Medvescek, Director of Editorial Services

6667 **Facts About Facioscapulohumeral Muscular Dystrophy**
Muscular Dystrophy Association
3300 E Sunrise Drive
Tucson, AZ 85718-3299
520-529-2000
800-572-1717
Fax: 520-529-5383
e-mail: publications@mdausa.org
www.mda.org

Introductory booklet describes FSHD in easy-to-understand terms and answers commonly asked questions about the disease. Also available in Spanish.
Christina Medvescek, Director of Editorial Services

6668 Facts About Friedreich's Ataxia
Muscular Dystrophy Association
3300 E Sunrise Drive 520-529-2000
Tucson, AZ 85718-3299 800-572-1717
Fax: 520-529-5300
e-mail: publications@mdusa.org
www.mda.org
Explains Friedreich's ataxia in layman's terms and answers commonly asked questions about the disease. Also available in Spanish.
15 pages Paperback
Bob Mackle, Director Public Information
Christina Medvescek, Director of Editorial Services

6669 Facts About Limb-Girdle Muscular Dystrophy
Muscular Dystrophy Association
3300 E Sunrise Drive 520-529-2000
Tucson, AZ 85718-3299 800-572-1717
Fax: 520-529-5383
e-mail: publications@mdausa.org
www.mda.org
Introductory booklet provides basic facts about LGMD and contains information regarding the many forms, diagnostic tests and current treatments. Also available in Spanish.
Christina Medvescek, Director of Editorial Services

6670 Facts About Metabolic Diseases of Muscle
Muscular Dystrophy Association
3300 E Sunrise Drive 520-529-2000
Tucson, AZ 85718-3299 800-572-1717
Fax: 520-529-5300
e-mail: publications@mdusa.org
www.mda.org
Provides an overview of the 11 inheritable metabolic diseases of muscle encompassed by MDA's program. Addresses commonly asked questions and highlights MDA's research efforts aimed at finding the causes of and effective treatments for these disorders. Also available in Spanish.
20 pages Paperback
Bob Mackle, Director Public Information
Christina Medvescek, Director of Editorial Services

6671 Facts About Mitochondrial Myopathies
Muscular Dystrophy Association
3300 E Sunrise Drive 520-529-2000
Tucson, AZ 85718-3299 800-572-1717
Fax: 520-529-5300
e-mail: publications@mdusa.org
www.mda.org
Explains mitochondrial myopathies in layman's terms and answers the most frequently asked questions about this disease. Also available in Spanish.
24 pages Paperback
Bob Mackle, Director Public Information
Christina Medvescek, Director of Editorial Services

6672 Facts About Myasthenia Gravis
Muscular Dystrophy Association
3300 E Sunrise Drive 520-529-2000
Tucson, AZ 85718-3299 800-572-1717
Fax: 520-529-5300
e-mail: publications@mdusa.org
www.mda.org
Explains myasthenia gravis and Lambert-Eaton syndrome in layman's terms and answers the most frequently asked questions about these diseases. Also available in Spanish.
19 pages Paperback
Bob Mackle, Director Public Information
Carol Sowall, Director Publications

6673 Facts About Myopathies
Muscular Dystrophy Association
3300 E Sunrise Drive 520-529-2000
Tucson, AZ 85718-3299 800-572-1717
Fax: 520-529-5300
e-mail: publications@mdusa.org
www.mda.org
Overview of the myopathies encompassed by MDA's program. Addresses commonly asked questions and highlights MDA's research efforts aimed at finding the causes of and effective treatments for these disorders. Also available in Spanish.
18 pages Paperback
Bob Mackle, Director Public Information
Christina Medvescek, Director of Editorial Services

6674 Facts About Myotonic Muscular Dystrophy
Muscular Dystrophy Association
3300 E Sunrise Drive 520-529-2000
Tucson, AZ 85718-3299 800-572-1717
Fax: 520-529-5383
e-mail: publications@mdausa.org
www.mda.org
Introductory booklet provides basic facts about the disorder and explains the causes and effects, as well as tests used to diagnose and MDA's search for treatments and cures. Also available in Spanish.
Christina Medvescek, Director of Editorial Services

6675 Facts About Plasmapheresis
Muscular Dystrophy Association
3300 E Sunrise Drive 520-529-2000
Tucson, AZ 85718-3299 800-572-1717
Fax: 520-529-5300
e-mail: publications@mdusa.org
www.mda.org
Describes plasmapheresis, a plasma exchange procedure often utilized as a treatment for autoimmune disease such as myasthenia gravis and Lambert-Eaton syndrome.
Paperback
Bob Mackle, Director Public Information
Christina Medvescek, Director of Editorial Services

6676 Facts About Polymyostis/Dermatomyositis
Muscular Dystrophy Association
3300 E Sunrise Drive 520-529-2000
Tucson, AZ 85718-3299 800-572-1717
Fax: 520-529-5300
e-mail: publications@mdusa.org
www.mda.org
Outlines these two front forms of inflammatory myopathy. Current approaches to treatment and MDA's efforts in continued research are described. Also available in Spanish.
13 pages Paperback
Bob Mackle, Director Public Information
Christina Medvescek, Director of Editorial Services

6677 Facts About Rare Muscular Dsytrophies
Muscular Dystrophy Association
3300 E Sunrise Drive 520-529-2000
Tucson, AZ 85718-3299 800-572-1717
Fax: 520-529-5300
e-mail: publications@mdusa.org
www.mda.org
This brochure gives basic facts about four forms of muscular dystrophy (Congenital, Distal, Emery-Dreifuss and Oculopharyngeal) and addresses commonly asked questions. Also available in Spanish.
28 pages Paperback
Bob Mackle, Director Public Information
Christina Medvescek, Director of Editorial Services

6678 Facts About Spinal Muscular Atrophy
Muscular Dystrophy Association
3300 E Sunrise Drive 520-529-2000
Tucson, AZ 85718-3299 800-572-1717
Fax: 520-529-5300
e-mail: publications@mdusa.org
www.mda.org
Covers the four forms of the disease and outlines the characteristics and genetic patterns of the SMAs. Research efforts aimed at

finding the causes, treatments and cures are also described. Also available in Spanish.
15 pages Paperback
Bob Mackle, Director Public Information
Christina Medvescek, Director of Editorial Services

6679 Genetics and Neuromuscular Diseases
Muscular Dystrophy Association
3300 E Sunrise Drive 520-529-2000
Tucson, AZ 85718-3299 800-572-1717
Fax: 520-529-5383
e-mail: publications@mdausa.org
www.mda.org
Booklet describes what a genetic disorder is and explains how genetic testing and counseling can help people understand how disorders that may affect them or their children are inherited. Also available in Spanish.
Christina Medvescek, Director of Editorial Services

6680 Hey, I'm Here Too
Muscular Dystrophy Association
3300 E Sunrise Drive 520-529-2000
Tucson, AZ 85718-3299 800-572-1717
Fax: 520-529-5383
e-mail: publications@mdausa.org
www.mda.org
Help for siblings of boys with Duchenne muscular dystrophy. Explores how they feel about themselves, their brothers and their families. Also provides specific answers to some questions that siblings may wonder about. Also available in Spanish.
28 pages
Bob Mackle, Director Public Information
Christina Medvescek, Director of Editorial Services

6681 Learning to Live with Neuromuscular Desease: A Message to Parents
Muscular Dystrophy Association
3300 E Sunrise Drive 520-529-2000
Tucson, AZ 85718-3299 800-572-1717
Fax: 520-529-5383
e-mail: publications@mdausa.org
www.mda.org
Helps parents and families cope with the fact that their child has a neuromuscular disease and with the impact the disease will have on everyday life. Also available in Spanish.
Christina Medvescek, Director of Editorial Services

6682 MDA Camp: A Special Place
Muscular Dystrophy Association
3300 E Sunrise Drive 520-529-2000
Tucson, AZ 85718-3299 800-572-1717
Fax: 520-529-5300
e-mail: publications@mdusa.org
www.mdusa.org
Highlights the activities of MDA dummer camps for youngsters diagnosed with one of the more than 40 diseases in MDA's program. Shares camper and volunteer reactions. Also available in Spanish.
Paperback
Bob Mackle, Director Public Information
Carol Sowall, Director Publications

6683 MDA Fact Sheet
Muscular Dystrophy Association
3300 E Sunrise Drive 520-529-2000
Tucson, AZ 85718-3299 800-572-1717
Fax: 520-529-5383
e-mail: publications@mdausa.org
www.mda.org
Basic information on MDA's origins and purposes; the more than 40 neuromuscular diseases in MDA's program, and brief symptom descriptions by category. Also available in Spanish.
Christina Medvescek, Director of Editorial Services

6684 MDA Services for the Individual, Family and Community
Muscular Dystrophy Association
3300 E Sunrise Drive 520-529-2000
Tucson, AZ 85718-3299 800-572-1717
Fax: 520-529-5383
e-mail: publications@mdausa.org
www.mda.org
Lists the diseases covered by MDA as well as eligibility criteria for MDA's services program, a list of MDA-sponsored clinics nationwide, and the services available through local MDA offices. Also available in Spanish.
Christina Medvescek, Director of Editorial Services

6685 Teacher's Guide to Neuromuscular Disease
Muscular Dystrophy Association
3300 E Sunrise Drive 520-529-2000
Tucson, AZ 85718-3299 Fax: 520-529-5383
e-mail: publications@mdausa.org
www.mda.org
This publication provides a source of guidance and information to teachers, giving details about neuromuscular diseases, how they affect school participation, and ways that teachers can help meet the needs of students affected by these disorders.
2005
Christina Medvescek, Director of Editorial Services

6686 Travis, I Got Lots of Neat Stuff Children Living with Muscular Dystrophy
Muscular Dystrophy Association
3300 E Sunrise Drive 520-529-2000
Tucson, AZ 85718-3299 800-572-1717
Fax: 520-529-5383
e-mail: publications@mdausa.org
www.mda.org
Booklet illustrates that a child with muscular dystrophy can do many things. Adapted for MDA's Hop-a-Thon program, the booklet heightens awareness and understanding of people with disabilities. It's suitable for youngsters in elementary school. Also available in Spanish.
24 pages
Christina Medvescek, Director of Editorial Services

Audio & Video

6687 Muscular Dystrophy
Films for the Humanities & Sciences
Box 2053 609-419-8000
Princeton, NJ 08543-2053 800-257-5126
Fax: 609-275-3767
Video deals with how Muscular Dystrophy sufferers deal with the disease that has no cure. Three life stories dealing with surgery, medicine, therapy and bracing as a means to survive. Dr. Betty Banke discusses the need to find a cure while Richard Nordgren from the Dartmouth-Hitchcock Medical Center discusses treatment.
20 Minutes

Web Sites

6688 Healing Well
www.healingwell.com
An online health resource guide to medical news, chat, information and articles, newsgroups and message boards, books, disease-related web sites, medical directories, and more for patients, friends, and family coping with disabling diseases, disorders, or chronic illnesses.

6689 Health Finder
www.healthfinder.gov
Searchable, carefully developed web site offering information on over 1000 topics. Developed by the US Department of Health and Human Services, the site can be used in both English and Spanish.

6690 Healthlink USA
www.healthlinkusa.com
Health information concerning treatment, cures, prevention, diagnosis, risk factors, research, support groups, email lists, personal stories and much more. Updated regularly.

6691 Helios Health
www.helioshealth.com
Online resource for your health information. Detailed information about specific health topics, access to expert advice from our Medical Advisory Board, and up-to-date health news.

6692 **MedicineNet**

www.medicinenet.com

An online resource for consumers providing easy-to-read, authoritative medical and health information.

6693 **Medscape**

www.mywebmd.com

Medscape offers specialists, primary care physicians, and other health professionals the Web's most robust and integrated medical information and educational tools.

6694 **Muscular Dystrophy Association**

www.mdausa.org

Information on effective treatments for muscular dystrophy, related neuromuscular disorders and research programs. In addition, MDA offers a comprehensive program of patient and community services, with access to over 230 MDA-supported clinics nationwide.

6695 **Parent Project: Muscular Dystrophy**

www.parentdmd.org

Organization of families around the world who have children diagnosed with DMD/BMD. Our goal is to invest significant amounts of money raised into medical research with clinical application.

6696 **WebMD**

www.webmd.com

Information on Muscular Dystrophy, including articles and resources.

Description

6697 **Myasthenia Gravis**

Myasthenia gravis is a disease of the neuromuscular junction - the structure which carries the nerve's chemical signal that tells the muscle to contract. Circulating antibodies attack this junction, leading to weakness of voluntary muscles and muscle fatigue after exercise. Any muscle may be involved, but muscles in the face and throat are especially susceptible. The disease therefore especially affects chewing, swallowing, coughing and facial expressions. These manifestations fluctuate in intensity over hours to days.

Because this disease is caused by an overactive immune system, most treatments target this system. These include corticosteroids, immunosuppressive drugs such as azathioprine, plasmapheresis (filtration of the blood with retention of the cells and removal of the plasma), intravenous immunoglobulins and surgical removal of the thymus gland. In addition, anticholinesterase drugs like pyridostigmine increase the level of the messenger chemical at the neuromuscular junction, thereby increasing muscle strength.

Because of the progressive weakness associated with this disease, physical therapy and assistive devices are generally required.

National Agencies & Associations

6698 **Myasthenia Gravis Association of BC**
2805 Kingsway
Vancouver, BC, V5R-5H9
640-451-5511
e-mail: mgabc@centreforability.bc.ca
www.myastheniagravis.ca
Informs members about new treatment thods and research concerning myasthenia gravis.

6699 **Myasthenia Gravis Foundation**
1821 University Avenue W
St Paul, MN 55104
651-917-6256
800-541-5454
Fax: 651-917-1835
e-mail: mgfa@myasthenia.org
www.myasthenia.org
The mission of the Foundation is to facilitate the timely diagnosis end optimal care of individuals affected by myasthenia gravis and closely related disorders and to improve their lives through programs of patient services, public information and medical reports.
Marcia Lorimer, Executive Committee
Sam Schulhof, Chair

6700 **Myasthenia Gravis Foundation of America**
5841 Cedar Lake Road
Minneapolis, MN 55416
43- 29- 986
800-541-5454
Fax: 952-646-2028
e-mail: mgfa@myasthenia.org
www.myasthenia.org
Dedicated to the conquest of the disease through research education information and patient services. Offers over 34 chapters and over 100 support groups across the country as well as 8 international chapters.
Tor Holtan, CEO
Jennifer Heidelberge, Chapter Relations Manager

State Agencies & Associations

Alabama

6701 **Alabama Chapter of the Myasthenia Gravis Foundation of America**
PO Box 530623
Birmingham, AL 35253
205-868-1210
866-749-0844
Fax: 205-868-1211
e-mail: alabama@myasthenia.org
www.myasthenia.org
Michael Greene, President
Joyce Wood, Vice President

Arizona

6702 **Jim L Walker: Arizona Chapter of the Myasthenia Gravis Foundation of America**
PO Box 34173
Phoenix, AZ 85067-1136
480-451-3060
877-347-7905
Fax: 480-767-7029
e-mail: azmgfa@myastheniagravisfoundation.phxcox
www.azmgfa.org
Wayne Magee, CEO/ President
Edward C Kaps, Chairman

Arkansas

6703 **Arkansas Chapter of the Myasthenia Gravis Foundation of America**
5204 Crystal Hill Road
N Little Rock, AR 72118
501-753-5974
877-455-4442
Fax: 501-753-5978
e-mail: mgfoundationar@sbcglobal.net
www.myasthenia.org

Connecticut

6704 **Connecticut Chapter of the Myasthenia Gravis Foundation of America**
33 Patmar Drive
Monroe, CT 06468-4511
203-926-9910
866-329-8784
e-mail: conn@myasthenia.org
www.myasthenia.org
Irving Beck ED

Delaware

6705 **MD/DC/Delaware Chapter of Myasthenia Gravis Foundation of America**
PO Box 186
Pasedena, MD 21123-0186
866-437-2881
e-mail: lhwaltz@aol.com

District of Columbia

6706 **MD/DC/Delaware Chapter of Myasthenia Gravis Foundation of America**
PO Box 186
Pasedena, MD 21113-0186
866-437-2881
e-mail: lhwaltz@aol.com

Florida

6707 **East Central Florida Chapter of the Myasthenia Gravis Foundation of America**
14502 87 Avenue N
Seminole, FL 33776-0623
727-596-1491
877-596-1491
Fax: 727-596-1491
e-mail: wcflorida@myasthenia.org
www.myasthenia.org

6708 **South Florida Gold Coast Chapter of the Myasthenia Gravis Foundation of America**
6185 Winding Brook Way
Delray Beach, FL 33484
561-638-2636
e-mail: oldjack@gateway.net
www.4-mga.org/orgsNEW.html
Jack Moore, Chairman
Loise Cororan, Vice Chairman

6709 **West Central Florida Chapter of the Myasthenia Gravis Foundation of America**
13540 Andova Drive
Largo, FL 33774-4633
727-596-1491
e-mail: mpeters@aol.com
www.4-mga.org/orgsNEW.html
Marie Peters, Chairman

Georgia

6710 **Georgia Chapter of the Myasthenia Gravis Foundation of America**
PO Box 93604
Atlanta, GA 30318
770-973-3269
800-743-4339
Fax: 770-973-3269
e-mail: gachapter_mgfa@hotmail.com
www.ga-mgfa.or

Indiana

6711 **Greater Indianapolis Chapter of the Myasthenia Gravis Foundation of America**
8922 Haverstick Road
Indianapolis, IN 46240
317-846-1462
e-mail: Spknke@aol.com
www.4-mga.org/orgsNEW.html
Earl Zimmerman, Chair

Kentucky

6712 **Kentucky Chapter of the Myasthenia Gravis Foundation of America**
2628 Rush Trail
Owensboro, KY 42303
270-684-4555
Fax: 270-926-2234
e-mail: shlane@bellsouth.net
www.myasthenia.org

Maryland

6713 **MD/DC/Delaware Chapter of Myasthenia Gravis Foundation of America**
PO Box 186
Pasadena, MD 21123-0186
410-432-6193
866-437-2881
e-mail: maryland@myasthenia.org
www.myasthenia.org

Massachusetts

6714 **Mass./New Hampshire Chapter of the Myasthenia Gravis Foundation of America**
5 Alcott Drive
Northboro, MA 01532
978-562-4570
e-mail: djemery@juno.com

6715 **Massachusetts Chapter of the MG Foundation**
5 Alcott Drive
Northboro, MA 01532
508-393-1403
Fax: 508-393-1403
e-mail: djemery@juno.com
www.4-mga.org/orgsNEW.html

6716 **Myasthenia Gravis: Massachusetts Chapter**
28 Bayview Road
Wellesley, MA 02181
508-851-3218
www.4-mga.org/orgsNEW.html
Michelle Ronchetti

Michigan

6717 **Great Lakes Chapter of the Myasthenia Gravis Foundation of America**
2680 Horizon Drive SE
Grand Rapids, MI 49546-4800
616-956-0622
800-224-9180
Fax: 616-956-9234
e-mail: nfo@myasthenia-mi.org
www.myasthenia-mi.org
Autoimmune, neuromuscular disease manifest in weakness of voluntary muscles; arms, legs, eyes, facial expressions, severe cases of breathing.
Jaime Sheppard, Executive Director
Paulus Heule, President

6718 **Myasthenia Gravis Association**
17117 W Nine Mile Road
Southfield, MI 48075
248-423-9700
Fax: 248-423-9705
e-mail: mgadetroit1@hotmail.com
www.mgadetroit-easternmi.org
Agnes Wisner, Executive Director
Taylor Bleibtrey, Board Member

Minnesota

6719 **Minnesota State Chapter of the Myasthenia Gravis Foundation of America**
29234 Piney Way
Breezy Point, MN 56472-1715
218-562-4594
e-mail: minnesota@myasthenia.org
www.myasthenia.org

Missouri

6720 **Myasthenia Gravis Foundation: Greater St. Louis Chapter**
PO Box 58785
Renton, WA 98058
425-235-1435
877-252-0677
Fax: 425-204-2070
e-mail: washington@myasthenia.org
www.myasthenia.org
Babette Figler, President

New Hampshire

6721 **Mass./New Hampshire Chapter of the Myasthenia Gravis Foundation of America**
460 S River Street
Marshfield, MA 02050
508-435-3808
e-mail: massachusetts@myasthenia.org
www.ma-nhmgfa.org
Marilyn Buckner, Chair
Marc Weinberg, Treasurer

New Jersey

6722 **Garden State Chapter of the Myasthenia Gravis Foundation of America**
PO Box 4258
Wayne, NJ 07474-1362
973-633-6900
800-437-4949
Fax: 973-633-6908
e-mail: gsmg@webspan.net
www.mgnj.org

New Mexico

6723 **New Mexico Chapter of the Myasthenia Gravis Foundation of America**
PO Box 34173
Phoenix, AZ 85067-6873
480-451-3060
877-347-7905
Fax: 623-321-9032
e-mail: azmgfa@myastheniagravisfoundation.phxcox
www.azmgfa.org
Wayne Magee, CEO/President
Edward C Kaps, Chairman

New York

6724 **Metro New York Chapter of Myasthenia Gravis Foundation of America**
PO Box 40
Stony Brook, NY 11790
516-538-0738
800-667-9807
e-mail: MetroNY@myasthenia.org
www.metronymgfa.org
Cindie Killeen, Chairperson
Debbie Thompsen, Vice Chairperson

6725 **Myasthenia Gravis Support Group: Long Island**
N Shore University Hospital
Manhasset, NY
516-785-7538
e-mail: KARKENN@SPEC.NET
www.members.tripod.com/LIMGer/limgsuppor
Carol

6726 Upstate NY Chapter of the Myasthenia Gravis Foundation of America
14 Summit Road 518-439-5377
Delmar, NY 12054 800-581-5377
Fax: 518-439-8783
e-mail: upstatenewyork@myasthenia.org
www.myasthenia-gravis.com
Barry Levine, President/Chair

North Carolina

6727 Carolinas Chapter of the Myasthenia Gravis Foundation of America
506 E Forest Hills Boulevard 919-490-2937
Durham, NC 27707-1801 800-842-8711
Fax: 919-489-7564
e-mail: tvassar56@aol.com
www.med.unc.edu/mgfa/mgnc-hom.htm

Ohio

6728 Mahoning-Shenango Chapter of the Myasthenia Gravis Foundation of America
PO Box 282 330-539-5582
Girard, OH 44420-0282

6729 Ohio Chapter of the Myasthenia Gravis Foundation of America
2907 B Lincoln Way E 330-834-9066
Massillon, OH 44646 Fax: 330-834-9067
e-mail: ohiochaptermgf@att.net
www.ohiochaptermgf.org
Jackie Held, Executive Director

Oklahoma

6730 Oklahoma Chapter of the Myasthenia Gravis Foundation of America
6465 S Yale Avenue 918-494-4951
Tulsa, OK 74136 Fax: 918-494-4951
e-mail: oklahoma@myasthenia.org
www.myasthenia.org
Peggy Foust, Executive Director
Margret Feller, Vice-President/Treasurer

Pennsylvania

6731 Myasthenia Gravis Association of Western Pennsylvania
490 EN Avenue 412-566-1545
Pittsburgh, PA 15212 Fax: 412-566-1550
e-mail: mgaoffice@mgawpa.org
www.mgawpa.org
A neuromuscular disorder with no known cause or cure. The mission is to provide access to superior medical treatment and medications at reasonable cost providing those patients and their families adequate social and psychological support and education.
Barbara Lefler, Executive Director

6732 Pennsylvania Chapter of the Myasthenia Gravis Foundation of America
2665 Pinewood Road 717-581-1271
Lancaster, PA 17601 e-mail: PennaMGFA@aol.com
www.pamgfa.org

Rhode Island

6733 Rhode Island 'Hope' Chapter
33 Patmar Drive 203-926-9910
Monroe, CT 06468 866-329-8784
e-mail: conn@myasthenia.org
www.myasthenia.org

South Carolina

6734 Carolinas Chapter of the Myasthenia Gravis Foundation of America
506 E Forest Hills Boulevard 919-490-2937
Durham, NC 27707-1801 800-842-8711
Fax: 919-489-7564
e-mail: tvassar56@aol.com
www.med.unc.edu/mgfa/mgnc-hom.htm

Texas

6735 Greater South Texas Chapter of the Myasthenia Gravis Foundation of America
10592 Fuqua Street #A 281-987-9393
Houston, TX 77089-1402 Fax: 281-328-2430
e-mail: gowens@accesscomm.net

6736 Northwest Texas Chapter of the Myasthenia Gravis Foundation of America
3406 Manioca Road 806-749-3126
Lubbock, TX 79403 Fax: 915-554-7044
e-mail: nwtexas@myasthenia.org
www.nwtcmg.org
Lowell McBroom, Vice-Chairperson

Utah

6737 Utah State Intermountain Chapter of the Myasthenia Gravis Foundation of America
8717 S 910 E 801-816-2204
Sandy, UT 84094-1831 Fax: 801-572-1787
e-mail: dawnascheib@waterfordschool.org
www.myasthenia.org

Virginia

6738 Virginia Chapter of the Myasthenia Gravis Foundation of America
PO Box 71193 804-308-1674
Richmond, VA 23255 800-728-4405
Fax: 804-308-1674
e-mail: va-wvchapmgfa@comcast.net
www.myasthenia-va.org
Georgiann C Davis, President
Anita Steele, VP

Washington

6739 Pacific Northwest Chapter of the Myasthenia Gravis Foundation of America
PO Box 58785 425-235-1435
Renton, WA 98058-6562 877-252-0677
Fax: 425-204-2070
e-mail: washington@myasthenia.org
www.myasthenia.org

Wisconsin

6740 Wisconsin Chapter of the Myasthenia Gravis Foundation of America
2474 S 96 Street 262-938-9800
W Allis, WI 53227 800-541-5454
Fax: 262-789-3363
e-mail: wisconsin@myasthenia.org
www.myasthenia.org
The Myasthenia Gravis Foundation of America is the only national volunteer health agency dedicated solely to fight against myasthenoia gravis.
Patricia Lamp, Chairperson
Ellie Burbach, Vice-Chairperson

Support Groups & Hotlines

6741 Myasthenia Gravis Association of Colorado
PO Box 18567 303-360-7080
Denver, CO 80218 Fax: 303-360-7080
e-mail: 4mga@4-mga.org
Sharon Leahy, Chairperson

6742 Myasthenia Gravis Support Group
6465 S Yale Ave 918-494-4951
Tulsa, OK 74136-7808 Fax: 918-494-4951
e-mail: oklahoma@myasthenia.org
www.myasthenia.rg
Provides education and patient services to improve the lives of all people affected by MG and to promote awareness of the disease myasthenia gravis.
Peggy Foust, Executive Director/President

6743 **Myasthenia Gravis Support Group East Central Illinois**
Myasthenia Gravis Foundation of Illinois
310 W Lake Street 630-835-0153
Elmhurst, IL 60126 800-888-6208
e-mail: myastheniaill@aol.org
www.myastheniagravis.org
To facilitate the timely diagnosis and optimal care of individuals affected by myasthenia gravis and to improve their lives through programs of patient services, public awareness, medical research, professional education, advocacy and patient care

6744 **Myasthenia Gravis Support Group of Wiscons in**
2474 S 96 Street 262-938-9800
West Allis, WI 53227-2204 Fax: 262-789-3363
e-mail: wisconsin@myasthenia.org
www.myasthenia.org
Serves patients and their families throughout the state of Wisconsin. The goal is to help achieve the conquest of Myasthenia Gravis through research, education, public awareness, anf fundraising.

6745 **Myasthenia Gravis Support Group: Virginia/ West Virginia**
PO Box 71193 804-308-1674
Richmond, VA 23255 Fax: 804-308-1647
e-mail: va-wvchapmgfa@comcast.net
www.myasthenia-va.org
To facilitate the timely diagnosis and optimal care of individuals affected by MG and closely related disorders and to improve their lives with programs of patient services, public information, medical research, professional education, advocacy and patient care.
Georgiann Davis, President

6746 **National Health Information Center**
US Department of Health and Human Services
PO Box 1133 301-565-4167
Washington, DC 20013-1133 800-336-4797
Fax: 301-984-4256
e-mail: info@nhic.org
www.health.gov/nhic
Offers a nationwide referral service, produces directories and resource guides.

Books

6747 **Myasthenia Gravis**
CRC Press
2000 NW Corporate Boulevard 561-994-0555
Boca Raton, FL 33431-7385 Fax: 561-994-3625
1993
ISBN: 0-849363-43-8

Newsletters

6748 **Alabama Chapter of the Myasthenia Gravis Foundation of America**
Alabama Chapter of the Myasthenia Gravis Found
300 Office Park Drive 205-868-1210
Birmingham, AL 35223 Fax: 205-868-1211
e-mail: alchaptermgfa@aol.com
Three to four newsletters per year. Support Group Information, articles about MG and it's treatment, information about chapters operations.

6749 **Connecticut Nutmeg**
Myasthenia Gravis Foundation
113 Folly Brook Boulevard 860-529-8784
Wetherfield, CT 06109 Fax: 860-529-8784

6750 **Conquer**
Myasthenia Gravis Foundation of Illinois
2411 New Street 708-385-3888
Blue Island, IL 60406-2328 800-888-6208
Fax: 708-385-0447
e-mail: myastheniaill@aol.com
myastheniagravis.org
A quarterly newsletter containing articles and stories relating to myasthenia gravis.
16 pages Quarterly
Gerald Tarka, Executive Director

6751 **East Central Florida Chapter of the Myasthenia Gravis Foundation of America**
PO Box 623 904-672-2635
Ormond Beach, FL 32175-0623
Published bi-monthly, and contains information about latest research. area meetings, and topics of concern for our readers.

6752 **Facts About Myasthenia Gravis for Patients and Families**
Myasthenia Gravis Foundation of America
5841 Cedar Lake Road 952-545-9438
Minneapolis, MN 55416 800-541-5454
Fax: 952-646-2028
e-mail: myastheniagravis@msn.com
www.myasthenia.org
Offers information on the history, clinical symptoms and features, causes, diagnosis, treatment and prognosis of Myasthenia Gravis.
16 pages 4 per year
Debora K Boelz, CEO
Jennifer Heidelberger, Chapter Relations Manager

6753 **Myasthenia Gravis Association**
2300 E Meyer Boulevard 816-276-4585
Kansas City, MO 64132-1199 Fax: 816-276-4569
e-mail: mga@planetkc.org
A nonprofit, United Way agency offering a variety of programs. The programs include; individualized education and advocacy, specialized outpatient clinics, patient support group meetings and newsletters.
Carole Bowe Thompson, Executive Director
Danna Garabedian, Administrative Assistant

6754 **Myasthenia Gravis Association: Detroit Chapter**
17117 W Nine Mile Road 248-423-9700
Southfield, MI 48075
A quarterly newslatter containing medical articles, personal stories relating to myasthenia gravis.

6755 **Myasthenia Gravis Foundation: Geater South Texas**
10592-A Fuqua 281-987-9393
Houston, TX 77089-1402 Fax: 281-328-2430
e-mail: gowens@accesscomm.net
Six issues per year. Support Group Information, articles about MG and it's treatment, information about Chapter operations.
Gary Owens, Chair

6756 **Myasthenia Gravis Foundation: Northwest Texas Chapter**
281 County Road 135
Ovalo, TX 79541 e-mail: nwtxmg@hotmail.com
A quarterly newsletter containing articles and stories relating myasthenia gravis.
Jenne McVicker, Editor

6757 **Myasthenia Gravis Foundation: Ohio Chapter**
PO Box 6392 330-477-7727
Canton, OH 44706 e-mail: ohiochaptermgf@nci2000,net

6758 **Puget Sound Chapter Newsletter**
PO Box 587853 206-235-1435
Renton, WA 98058-1785 Fax: 206-204-2070
A quarterly newsletter containing the latest articles and stories relating to myasthenia gravis.

Web Sites

6759 **Healing Well**
www.healingwell.com
An online health resource guide to medical news, chat, information and articles, newsgroups and message boards, books, disease-related web sites, medical directories, and more for patients, friends, and family coping with disabling diseases, disorders, or chronic illnesses.

6760 **Health Finder**
www.healthfinder.gov
Searchable, carefully developed web site offering information on over 1000 topics. Developed by the US Department of Health and Human Services, the site can be used in both English and Spanish.

6761 **Healthlink USA**
www.healthlinkusa.com

Health information concerning treatment, cures, prevention, diagnosis, risk factors, research, support groups, email lists, personal stories and much more. Updated regularly.

6762 **Helios Health**

www.helioshealth.com

Online resource for your health information. Detailed information about specific health topics, access to expert advice from our Medical Advisory Board, and up-to-date health news.

6763 **MedicineNet**

www.medicinenet.com

An online resource for consumers providing easy-to-read, authoritative medical and health information.

6764 **Medscape**

www.mywebmd.com

Medscape offers specialists, primary care physicians, and other health professionals the Web's most robust and integrated medical information and educational tools.

6765 **Myasthenia Gravis Foundation of America**

www.myasthenia.org

Dedicated to the conquest of the disease through research, education, information and patient services. Offers over 54 chapters and over 100 support groups across the country as well as 8 international chapters.

6766 **Neurology Channel**

www.neurologychannel.com

Find clearly explained, medically accurate information regarding conditions, including an overview, symptoms, causes, diagnostic procedures and treatment options. On this site it is possible to ask questions and get information from a neurologist and connect to people who have similar health interests.

6767 **WebMD**

www.webmd.com

Information on Myasthenia Gravis, including articles and resources.

Description

6768 **Neurofibromatosis**

Neurofibromatosis, or von Recklinghausen disease, named after a German pathologist, is an inherited genetic disorder. The more common form occurs once in 4,000 births. The skin and the nervous system are the primary target organs. Characteristic skin lesions are large, flat brown freckles, called cafe au lait spots, owing to their light coffee color. They are apparent at birth or in infancy in more than 90 percent of patients. Flesh-colored tumors appear in late childhood. Abnormal growths may be detectable in the brain, perhaps accounting for the seizures and learning difficulties commonly seen in this syndrome. Tumors may appear on the nerves from the eyes or the ears, sometimes causing hearing loss or visual disturbance.

There is no specific therapy for this condition, but tumors that produce severe symptoms can be surgically removed or irradiated. Genetic counseling is important for the entire family.

National Agencies & Associations

6769 **Association for the Neurologically Disable d of Canada**
59 Clement Road 416-244-1992
Etobicoke, Ontario, M9R-1Y5 Fax: 416-244-4099
e-mail: info@and.ca
www.and.ca
Provides functional rehabilitation programs to individuals with neurological disabilities.
Basil Ziv, Executive Director
Dr John Unruh, Director of Rehabilitation

6770 **BC Centre for Ability**
2805 Kingsway 604-451-5511
Vancouver, BC, V5R-5H9 Fax: 604-451-5651
e-mail: home@centreforability.bc.ca
www.centreforability.bc.ca
Founded in 1969 by families who desired alternatives to hospital or institutional-based services. The centre provides education and promotes the rights of individuals with disabilities to participate as valued members of their communities.
Angie Kwok, Executive Director
Moses Gabriel, Director of Resource Development

6771 **Children's Tumor Foundation**
95 Pine Street 212-344-6633
New York, NY 10005 800-323-7938
Fax: 212-747-0004
e-mail: info@ctf.org
www.ctf.org
Dedicated to health and well being of individuals and families affected by the neurofibromatoses (NF).
Allison Walsh, Communications Officer
John Risner, President

6772 **NF Canada**
800-1010 Sherbrooke Street W 888-986-3876
Montreal, Quebec, H3A-2R7 e-mail: infocanada@nfcanada.ca
www.nfcanada.ca
To ensure that all Canadians living with neurofibromatosis benefit from support, understanding, appropriate medical treatment and the hope that a cure is on the horizon.

6773 **Neurofibromatosis**
Po Box 18246 651-225-1720
Minneapolis, MN 55418 800-942-6825
Fax: 301-918-0009
e-mail: info@nfinc.org
www.nfinc.org
A national nonprofit organization with independent and regional chapters that provides support and services to NF families. Simulates funds and encourages participation in NF research. Works closely with clinical and research professionals.
Miguel Lessing, President
Rosemary Anderson, Vice President

6774 **Neurofibromatosis Society of Ontario**
180 Circle Lake Road 705-685-1409
North Bay, Ontario, P1A-3T2 Fax: 705-685-1409
e-mail: info@nfon.ca
www.nfon.ca
Support individuals and families affected by NF, to educate its members, professionals, and the general public about NF, and support NF research.
Lynne Leyland, Director
Gladys Hamilton, Director

6775 **Neurological Science Federation**
7015 Macleod Trail SW 403-229-9544
Calgary, AB, T2H-2K6 Fax: 403-229-1661
e-mail: info@cnsfederation.org
www.ccns.org
To promote and encourage all aspects of neurology, including research, education, assessment and accreditation.

State Agencies & Associations

Alabama

6776 **NNFF Alabama Affiliate**
1205 Branchwater Lane 205-529-8006
Birmingham, AL 35216 e-mail: jeffalb@charter.net
www.ctf.org
Jeff Albright, Chairperson

Arizona

6777 **Neurofibromatosis Association of Arizona**
Po Box 2718 480-945-9650
Chandler, AZ 85244 Fax: 480-945-9650
e-mail: info@nfaz.org
www.nfaz.org
Nicole Hicks, Executive Director
Michael Sheedy, President

Arkansas

6778 **NNFF Arkansas Affilaite**
139 Rainbow Lne 501-759-2710
Bigelow, AR 72016 e-mail: lesleyo@arbbs.net
www.ctf.org
Lesley Oslica, Information and Support

Colorado

6779 **NNFF Colorado Chapter**
70 N Ranch Road 303-734-9942
Littleton, CO 80127 e-mail: mark.ebel@eyeris.com
www.ctf.org
Mark Ebel, Chapter President

Connecticut

6780 **NNFF Connecticut Chapter**
8 S Barn Hill Road 860-286-2705
Bloomfield, CT 06002-1622 Fax: 860-286-2705
TTY: 860-286-2705
TDD: 860-286-2705
e-mail: StevenSand@aol.com
Steve Sandler, Chapter President

Florida

6781 **NF Center: North Broward Medical Center Neurofibromatosis**
Neurofibromatosis
201 E Sample Road
Pompano Beach, FL 33064-3502 954-786-7346
www.nfinc.org

6782 **NNFF Florida Chapter**
PO Box 410684
Melbourne, FL 32941
321-253-1622
800-540-5721
e-mail: NNFFflorida@aol.com
www.ctf.org
Suzanne Earle, Chapter President

Georgia

6783 **NNFF Georgia Affiliate**
5 Ardmore Circle
Cartersville, GA 30120
678-428-9711
e-mail: ctfgeorgia@bellsouth.net
www.ctf.org
Randy Watkins, Chairman

Idaho

6784 **NNFF Idaho Chapter**
4419 E Linden Street
Caldwell, ID 83605-8037
208-459-6022
Suzy Crici, Chapter President

Illinois

6785 **Illinois Midwest Neurofibromatosis**
Neurofibromatosis
Po Box 1923
Lombard, IL 60148
630-932-8111
800-322-6363
Fax: 630-932-8119
e-mail: info@nfmidwest.org
nfmidwest.org

6786 **NNFF Illinois Chapter: Chicago Area**
5604 W Henderson 3 W
Chicago, IL 60634
e-mail: ilnfchapter@hotmail.com
www.ctf.org
Debbi Callahan, Vice President

6787 **NNFF Illinois Chapter: Silvis Area**
513 16th Street
Silvis, IL 61282
309-792-4195
e-mail: nfquadcities@juno.com
Sue Rockwell, Patient Information and Support

6788 **NNFF Illinois Chapter: Springfield Area**
5 Twilight Lane
Springfield, IL 62712
217-529-0834
e-mail: ma.miller@InsightBB.com
www.ctf.org
Marcia Miller, Treasurer

6789 **NNFF Illinois Chapter:Peoria Region**
PO Box 213
Emden, IL 62635
217-732-8568
e-mail: beachph@cs.com
www.ctf.org
Paul Beach, President

Indiana

6790 **NNFF Indiana Chapter**
1173 Hague Court
Franklinolis, IN 46131
317-736-7577
e-mail: pdavis@athensmed.org
www.ctf.org
Dottie Whitehurst, Chapter President

Iowa

6791 **NNFF Iowa Chapter**
321 Glenview Drive
De Moines, IA 50312
515-277-8494
e-mail: drev@aol.com
www.ctf.org
Sheila Drevyanko, Chapter President

Kansas

6792 **NNFF Kansas Affiliate**
12606 E 49th Terrace
Independence, MO 64055
816-737-8378
e-mail: annette_novak@yahoo.com
www.ctf.org
Annette Novak, Chairperson

6793 **Neurofibromatosis Kansas and Central Plains**
Neurofibromatosis
PO Box 1792
Hutchinson, KS 67504-1792
620-669-8453
800-942-6825
e-mail: nprieb@sbcglobal.net
www.nfinc.org

Louisiana

6794 **NNFF Louisiana Chapter**
PO Box 499
Baton Rouge, LA 70821
225-665-3547
e-mail: nflouisiana1@cox.net
www.ctf.org
Debbie Bouy, Chairperson

Maryland

6795 **Neurofibromatosis: Mid-Atlantic**
Neurofibromatosis
8855 Annapolis Road
Lanham, MD 20706-2924
301-577-8984
800-942-6825
Fax: 301-577-0016
e-mail: info@nfmidatlantic.org
www.nfmidatlantic.org
Mid-Atlantic Chapter serves the following states: Maryland Virginia District of Columbia Delaware New Jersey Pennsylvania West Virginia and North Carolina.
Barbra Levin, Executive Director
Beverly B Dobson, President

Massachusetts

6796 **Neurofibromatosis: New England**
Neurofibromatosis
9 Bedford Street
Burlington, MA 01803-3702
781-272-9936
Fax: 781-272-9937
e-mail: info@nfincne.org
www.nfincne.org
Karen Peluso, Executive Director
Dr Paul Epstein, President

Minnesota

6797 **Neurofibromatosis: Minnesota**
Neurofibromatosis
PO Box 18246
Minneapolis, MN 55418
651-225-1720
e-mail: JohnE@cipmn.org
www.nfincmn.org
John Everett, President
Steven Schutts, Vice-President

Nevada

6798 **NNFF Nevada Affiliate: Reno Area**
8065 White Falls Drive
Reno, NV 89506
775-972-1882
e-mail: daverenorice@yahoo.com
www.ctf.org
David Rice, Chairperson

New Hampshire

6799 **NNFF Northern New England Chapter**
75 McNeil Way
Dedham, MA 02026
508-879-5638
888-585-5316
Fax: 781-326-4940
e-mail: nfe.ed@verizon.net
www.ctf.org
The Northern New England Chapter serves these states: Maine, New Hampshire, Vermont, Connecticut, Massachusetts, and Rhode Island.
Michelle M Braden, Vice President

New York

6800 **Tri-State Region: New York, New Jersey, An d Connecticut.**
Tri-State Development
212-344-6633
800-323-7938
e-mail: jradziejewski@ctf,org
www.ctf.org
John Radziejewski, Vice President

North Dakota

6801 **NNFF Northern Plains Chapter: North Dakota South Dakota, And Nebraska**
The Childrens Tumor Foundation
310-216-9570
888-314-6633
e-mail: csilberstein@ctf.org
www.ctf.org
Cathy Silberstein, Director Training and Development
Kelly McGowan, Chapter and Affiliate Coordinator

Oregon

6802 **NNFF Oregon Affiliate Kaiser Permanente Northwest**
Kaiser Permanente Northwest
2806 SW Troy 503-331-6325
Portland, OR 97227 Fax: 503-331-6320
e-mail: crowkas@pop.mts.kpnw.org
www.ctf.org
Katie Crow, Genetic Counselor

South Carolina

6803 **NNFF South Carolina Chapter**
111 Oakview Drive 843-393-9672
Darlington, SC 29532 e-mail: pmschrisley@aol.com
www.ctf.org
Pat Chrisely, Chairperson

Virginia

6804 **NNFF Mid-Atlantic Region Affiliate: Virgin a, District Of Columbia, And Maryland**
The Childrens Tumor Foundation
800-323-7938
e-mail: csilberstein@ctf.org
www.ctf.org
Cathy Silberstein, Director Training and Development

Wisconsin

6805 **NNFF Wisconsin Chapter**
6562 W Glenbrook Road 414-362-0211
Brown Deer, WI 53223 e-mail: epankownf@aol.com
www.ctf.org
Elaine Pankow, President

Support Groups & Hotlines

6806 **Children's Tumor Foundation**
95 Pine Street 212-344-6633
New York, NY 10005 800-323-7938
Fax: 212-747-0004
e-mail: info@ctf.org
www.ctf.org
Sponsors critical research, public awareness and patient support services.
Allison Walsh, Communications Officer

6807 **NF Support Group of West Michigan**
Spectrum Health
230 Michigan Street NE 616-451-3699
Grand Rapids, MI 49503 e-mail: nfwestmich@aol.com
www.nfsupport.org
Rose Mary Anderson, Patient Advocate

6808 **National Health Information Center**
PO Box 1133 310-565-4167
Washington, DC 20013 800-336-4797
Fax: 301-984-4256
e-mail: info@nhic.org
www.health.gov/nhic
Offers a nationwide information referral service, produces directories and resource guides.

6809 **Neurofibromatosis**
9320 Annapolis Road 301-918-4600
Lanham, MD 20706-3123 800-942-6825
Fax: 301-918-0009
e-mail: nfinfo@nfinc.com
www.nfinc.org
Dedicated to individuals and families affected by the neurofibromatosis through educational, support, clinical and research programs.
Miguell Lessing, President
Rosemary Anderson, Vice President

6810 **Neurofibromatosis Foundation: Colorado**
2280 S Columbine Street 303-460-8313
Denver, CO 80210 800-323-7938
e-mail: UsRKids@aol.com
www.unitedwaydenver.org
Offers a support group to persons affected by neurofibromatosis. Offers panel discussion, sharing, fundraising, and fun activities. Also provides new patient information.
Charles Taylor
Jane Cahn

6811 **Neurofibromatosis Support Network**
Parents Helping Parents
3041 Olcott Street 408-727-5775
Santa Clara, CA 95054 Fax: 408-727-0182
www.php.com
Helping children with special needs receive the resources, love, hope, respect, health care, education and other services they need to achieve their full potential by providing them with strong families and dedicated professionals to serve them.
Sheri Sobrato, MA/MFC

6812 **Neuroscience Institute at Mercy Hospital**
4120N W Memorial Road
Oklahoma City, OK 73120 800-996-3729
Fax: 405-752-3977
www.okmercy.net
Mike Patt, Chief Executive Officer

6813 **Texas Neurofibromatosis Foundation**
415 Travis Street
Dallas, TX 75205 214-528-5557
www.texasnf.org

Newsletters

6814 **Neurofibromatosis**
9320 Annapolis Road 301-918-4600
Lanham, MD 20706-3123 800-942-6825
Fax: 301-918-0009
e-mail: nfinfo@nfinc.org
www.nfinc.org
Provides a variety of resources for NF families, professionals and researchers.
SemiAnnual
Gwen Charest, Executive Director

Pamphlets

6815 **Child with Neurofibromatosis 1**
Children's Tumor Foundation
95 Pine Street 212-344-NNFF
New York, NY 10005-1703 800-323-7938
e-mail: info@ctf.org
www.ctf.org

Offers information on the prognosis, management, complications, genetic implications, and sources of support for children with neurofibromatosis 1.
Allison Walsh, Communications Officer

6816 Guide for Teens
Children's Tumor Foundation
95 Pine Street 212-344-NNFF
New York, NY 10005-1703 800-323-7938
e-mail: info@ctf.org
www.ctf.org
Offers information for teenagers on how to face neurofibromatosis on a daily basis.
Allison Walsh, Communications Officer

6817 How NF-1 Affects the Body
Neurofibromatosis
9320 Annapolis Road 301-918-4600
Lanham, MD 20706-3123 800-942-6825
Fax: 301-918-0009
e-mail: nfinfo@nfinc.org
www.nfinc.org
A graphic showing the parts of the body where symptoms of NF-1 can occur.
Gwen Charest, Executive Director

6818 How NF-2 Affects the Body
Neurofibromatosis
9320 Annapolis Road 301-918-4600
Lanham, MD 20706-3123 800-942-6825
Fax: 301-918-0009
e-mail: nfinfo@nfinc.org
www.nfinc.org
A graphic showing the parts of the body where symptoms of NF-2 can occur.
Gwen Charest, Executive Director

6819 National NF Medical Resource Listing
Neurofibromatosis
9320 Annapolis Road 301-918-4600
Lanham, MD 20706-3123 800-942-6825
Fax: 301-918-0009
e-mail: nfinfo@nfinc.org
www.nfinc.org
A listing of medical centers in the US where geneticists and NF experts are located.
Gwen Charest, Executive Director

6820 Neurofibromatosis
March of Dimes
233 Park Avenue South 212-353-8353
New York, NY 10003 Fax: 212-254-3518
e-mail: NY639@marchofdimes.com
www.marchofdimes.com
Located on the website.

6821 Neurofibromatosis Type 2: Information for Patients and Families
Children's Tumor Foundation
95 Pine Street 212-344-6633
New York, NY 10005-1703 800-323-7938
e-mail: info@ctf.org
www.ctf.org
Offers extensive information on what NF2 is and answers the most asked about questions regarding the illness.
Allison Walsh, Communications Officer

6822 Understanding Neurofibromatosis
9320 Annapolis Road 301-918-4600
Lanham, MD 20706-3123 800-942-6825
Fax: 301-918-0009
e-mail: nfinfo@nfinc.org
www.nfinc.org
A handbook specifically designed for the newly diagnosed NF families.
Gwen Charest, Executive Director

Web Sites

6823 Healing Well
www.healingwell.com
An online health resource guide to medical news, chat, information and articles, newsgroups and message boards, books, disease-related web sites, medical directories, and more for patients, friends, and family coping with disabling diseases, disorders, or chronic illnesses.

6824 Health Finder
www.healthfinder.gov
Searchable, carefully developed web site offering information on over 1000 topics. Developed by the US Department of Health and Human Services, the site can be used in both English and Spanish.

6825 Healthlink USA
www.healthlinkusa.com
Health information concerning treatment, cures, prevention, diagnosis, risk factors, research, support groups, email lists, personal stories and much more. Updated regularly.

6826 Helios Health
www.helioshealth.com
Online resource for your health information. Detailed information about specific health topics, access to expert advice from our Medical Advisory Board, and up-to-date health news.

6827 MGH Neurology
www.mgh.harvard.edu
Provides both unmonderated message boards and chat rooms for specific neurological disorders including: amyloidosis, arachnoiditis, cerebellar ataxia, congenital fiber type disproportion, CFS leak, DeMorsiers syndrome, erythromealgia, Lewy body disease, meningitis, meralgia paresthetic, Norrie disease, periodic paralysis, phantom limb pain, Romberg disorder, Syndenhams chorea, tethered cord syndrome, and thoracic outlet syndrome.

6828 MedicineNet
www.medicinenet.com
An online resource for consumers providing easy-to-read, authoritative medical and health information.

6829 Medscape
www.mywebmd.com
Medscape offers specialists, primary care physicians, and other health professionals the Web's most robust and integrated medical information and educational tools.

6830 Neurology Channel
www.neurologychannel.com
Find clearly explained, medically accurate information regarding conditions, including an overview, symptoms, causes, diagnostic procedures and treatment options. On this site it is possible to ask questions and get information from a neurologist and connect to people who have similar health interests.

6831 WebMD
www.webmd.com
Information on Neurofibromatosis, including articles and resources.

Description

6832 **Obesity**

Obesity refers to a condition in which there is an excessive accumulation of fat in subcutaneous and other tissues of the body. Being obese and being overweight are not necessarily synonymous, as people who are overweight may have increased body size as a result of increased muscle or skeletal tissue mass. Obesity may develop at any age, but peak development periods occur during the first 12 months of life, between the ages of five and six years, and during the adolescent years in children. In adults, obesity may develop at any time, but many people may find that weight gain progresses through the 3rd-6th decade. It is clear from numerous medial, public health and sociologic studies that obesity in the United States occurs in a staggering proportion of the population and many consider it to be an epidemic.

Obesity may result from an increase in the actual number of fat cells or from an increase in the size of the individual fat cells. Researchers believe that fat cells increase in number in proportion to caloric intake increase and that this increase is particularly evident in the first 12 months of life. As children grow, increases in fat cell populations continue at a slower rate. Because the number of fat cells cannot be decreased, except surgically, later weight loss must result from the reduction of fat in individual cells.

Obesity usually results when caloric intake exceeds the energy demands of the body, thus increasing the storage of body fat. Fat accumulation is usually a progressive process, resulting from repeated episodes of food intake exceeding the body's demand for energy (calories). Many factors may influence appetite or obesity. Such factors may include environmental influences; psychosocial disturbances that may be induced by stress or emotional upset or trauma; brain lesions that may involve certain area of the brain such as the hypothalamus or the pituitary gland (both essential to hormone production); an overabundance of insulin in the body (hyperinsulinism); and genetic influences. In addition, in rare instances, obesity may be a feature of certain genetic disorders (see *Prader-Willi syndrome*). the most common cause in North America however, is the excessive intake of calories, particularly those from fats and sugars, and the concomitant lack of physical exercise and activity that uses calories.

Complications of obesity in the child and the adult may include respiratory difficulties such as shortness of breath and increased cardiovascular risk factors such as high blood pressure, elevated total cholesterol levels as well as increased bad or LDL cholesterol and decreased good or HDL cholesterol, and increased levels of fatty acid and glycerol compunds (triglycerides). These are risk factors for the development of coronary artery disease, one of the leading causes of morbidity and the mortality in North America. In addition, obesity may be associated with a resistance to the hormone insulin that aids in the metabolism of glucose, fats, carbohydrates, and proteins. This resistance may lead to excessive levels of circulating insulin in the body (hyperinsulinism); however, the body is not able to appropriately use insulin and high blood sugar (hyperglycemia) may occur. This condition is known as Type II Diabetes Mellitus and its incidence in the population is also increasing dramatically in both children and adults. The diagnosis of obesity in children, adolescents and adults is usually determined through the use of certain screening methods such as measurement of the body mass index (BMI) as well as the triceps skinfold thickness.

Patterns of behavior that may lead to obesity may be established as early as infancy. For example, if parents or caregivers persistently use a bottle to pacify a crying baby, the baby may learn that food is equivalent to relief of stress. Treatment for obesity should include the cooperation and suport of the entire family and may be directed toward psychologic considerations, as well as proper exercise and nutrition to psychological and emotional needs may include behavior modification, as well as individual and family counseling. See also *Eating Disorders*.

National Agencies & Associations

6833 **Active Healthy Kids Canada**
1185 Eglinton Avenue E 416-426-7120
Toronto, Ontario, M3C-3C6 888-446-7432
Fax: 416-426-7373
e-mail: info@activehealthykids.ca
www.activehealthykids.ca
Established in 1994 to advocate the importance of quality, accessible, and enjoyable physical activity participation experiences for children and youth.
Elio Antunes, Executive Director
Jennifer Crowie-Bonne, Director of Development/Programs

6834 **American Obesity Association**
1250 24th Street NW 202-776-7711
Washington, DC 20037 Fax: 202-776-7712
e-mail: executive@obesity.org
obesity1.tempdomainname.com
AOA provides obesity awareness and prevention information.
Morgan Downey, Executive Director
Richard L Atkinson, President

6835 **Canadian Obesity Network**
237 Barton Street E 905-527-4322
Hamilton, Ontario, L8L-2X2 Fax: 905-528-7114
e-mail: info@obesitynetwork.ca
www.obesitynetwork.ca
Focuses the expertise and deciation of more than 1,000 member researchers, clinicans, allied health care providers and other professionals with an interest in obesity in a unified effort to reduce the mental, physical and economic burden of obesity in Canadians.
Alice Bradbury, Manager

6836 **National Association to Advance Fat Acceptance**
PO Box 22510 916-558-6880
Oakland, CA 94609 Fax: 916-558-6881
e-mail: naafa@naafa.org
www.naafa.org
NAAFA provides educational information a newsletter and hosts a national conference.
Carole Cullum, Co-Chair
Kara Brewer Allen, Co-Chair

6837 **Overeaters Anonymous World Service Office**
World Service Office

PO Box 44020
Rio Rancho, NM 87174-4020
505-891-2664
Fax: 505-891-4320
e-mail: info@oa.org
www.oa.org

A fellowship of men and women from all walks of life who meet in order to help solve a common problem - compulsive overeating.
Naomi, Managing Director, Board Administrator

6838 **Research Chair on Obesity**
2725 Chemin Sainte-Foy
Quebec, Canada, G1V
418-656-8711
Fax: 418-656-4929
e-mail: obesite.chair@crhl.ulaval.ca
http://obesity.chair.ulaval.ca

Provides understanding of the pathophysiology of obesity. Promotes communication and interaction among basic scientists and clinicians, involved in nutrition, energy metabolism, obesity, lipid metabolism and cardiovascular research., Provides continuing education about the best possible knowledge on obesity to health professionals, physicians and to the public at large regarding the causes, the complications and the treatment of obesity.
Paul Boisvert, Coordinator

Libraries & Resource Centers

6839 **Weight-control Information Network**
1 WIN Way
Bethesda, MD 20892-3665
202-828-1025
877-946-4627
Fax: 202-828-1028
e-mail: win@info.niddk.nih.gov
http://win.niddk.nih.gov/

WIN addresses the health information needs of individuals through the production and dissemination of educational materials. In addition, WIN is developing communication strategies for a pilot program to encourage at-risk individuals to achieve and maintain a healthy weight by making changes in their lifestyle.

Research Centers

6840 **Harvard Clinical Nutrition Research Center**
Harvard Medical School
Boston, MA 02215
617-998-8803
Fax: 617-998-8804
e-mail: allan_walker@hms.harvard.edu
nutrition.med.harvard.edu

Mission is to derive the benefit of continuity in assessing the effectiveness of the Center from year to year while still allowing flexibility for new insights as the Center's activities evolve.
W Allan Walker, Director
George Blackburn, Associate Director

6841 **Minnesota Obesity Center**
1334 Eckles Avenue
St Paul, MN 55108
763-807-0559
e-mail: mnoc@tc.umn.edu
www1.umn.edu/mnoc

Mission is to find ways to prevent weight gain obesity and its complications. The Center incorporates 46 Participating Investigators who are studying the causes and treatments of obesity. Provides the general public with a source of information on the happenings of the Center and on the current developments in the field of obesity.
Catherine C Welch, Program Coordinator

6842 **New York Obesity/Nutrition Research Center**
31 Center Drive MSC 2560
Bethesda, MD 20892-2560
301-496-3583
www.niddk.nih.gov/fund/other/centers.htm
Griffin P Rodgers, Director

6843 **Obesity Research Center St. Luke's-Roosevelt Hospital**
St. Luke's-Roosevelt Hospital
1090 Amsterdam Avenue
New York, NY 10025
212-523-4196
Fax: 212-523-3416
e-mail: dg108@columbia.edu
www.nyorc.org

The mission of the New York Obesity Research Center is to help reduce the incidence of obesity and related diseases through leadership in basic research clinical research epidemiology and public health patient care and public education.
Dr Xavier Pi-Sunyer, Director
Janet Crane, Dietitians

Support Groups & Hotlines

6844 **Greater New York Metro Intergroup of Overe aters Anonymous**
Madison Square Station
New York, NY 10159-1235
212-946-4599
e-mail: office@oanyc.org
www.oanyc.org

6845 **Office of Chronic Disease Prevention and Nutrition Services**
Obesity Prevention Program
150 N. 18th Avenue
Phoenix, AZ 85007
602-542-1886
Fax: 602-542-1890
www.azdhs.gov/phs/oncdps/opp

Mission is to improve the health and quality of life of Arizona residents by reducing the incidence and severity of chronic disease and obesity through physical activity and nutrition interventions.
Renae Cunnien, Program Manager

Books

6846 **An Atlas of Obesity and Weight Control**
George A. Bray, author
212-216-7800
Fax: 212-564-7854
www.taylorandfrancisgroup.com

This informative guide is a clearly written, beautifully illustrated color atlas on obesity, including its etiology, development and treatment. Contains nearly 150 clinical pictures of obesity and its related conditions, as well as many pertinent clinical guidelines and up-to-the-minute data on assessment and treatment.
135 pages

6847 **Dietary Guidelines for Americans 2005**
U.S. Government Printing Office
200 Independence Avenue, S.W.
Washington, DC 20201
202-619-0257
877-696-6775
www.health.gov/dietaryguidelines

80 pages
Tommy G. Thompson, HHS-Secretary
Ann M. Veneman, USDA-Secretary

6848 **Encyclopedia of Obesity and Eating Disorders**
Facts on File
11 Penn Plaza
New York, NY 10001
212-967-8800
800-322-8755
Fax: 800-678-3633

From abdominoplasty to Zung Rating Scale, this volume defines and explains these disorders, along with medical and other problems associated with them.
272 pages Hardcover

6849 **Handbook of Obesity Treatment**
Guilford Press
72 Spring Street
New York, NY 10012
800-365-7006
Fax: 212-966-6708
e-mail: info@guilford.com
www.guilford.com

This comprehensive handbook guides mental, medical, and allied health professionals through the process of planning and delivering individualized treatment services for those seeking help for Obesity.
2001 624 pages Hardcover
ISBN: 1-572307-22-6

6850 **Obesity**
National Academies Press
500 Fifth Street, NW
Washington, DC 20055
202-334-3313
888-624-8373
Fax: 202-334-2451
www.nap.edu

A ground breaking report on childhood obesity providing indepth background and instructive case studies that illustrate just how serious and widespread the problem is; gives honest, authorative, based advice that consitute our best weapons in this critical battle.
280 pages

6851 **Overeaters Anonymous**
World Service Office

117 W 26th Street 505-891-2664
New York, NY 10001-6807 Fax: 505-891-4320
www.overeatersanonymous.org
World Service Office offers literature, provides information or meetings world wide.
204 pages Hardcover

6852 **Preventing Childhood Obesity: Health in the Balance**
National Academies Press
500 Fifth Street NW 202-334-3313
Washington, DC 20055 888-624-8373
Fax: 202-334-2451
www.nap.edu
Provides a broad-based examination of the nature, extent, and consequences of obesity. Also explores the underlying causes of this serious health problem and the actions needed to initiate support, and sustain the societal and lifestyle changes that can reverse the trend among our children and youth.
436 pages
ISBN: 0-309091-96-9

6853 **Shape Up America!**
6707 Democracy Boulevard
Bethesda, MD 20817 www.shapeup.org
A high profile national initiative to promote healthy weight and increased physical activity in America. Involves a broad based coalition of industry, medical/health, nutrition, physical fitness, and related organizations and experts.
C. Everett Koop, Founder
Barbara J. Moore, President And CEO

6854 **Understanding Childhood Obesity**
J Clinton Smith, MD, author
University Press of Mississippi
3825 Ridgewood Road 601-432-6205
Jackson, MS 39211-6492 Fax: 601-432-6217
e-mail: press@ihl.state.ms.us
www.upress.state.ms.us
A clear explanation of causes, diagnosis, and treatment of childhood obesity.
1999 120 pages Paperback
ISBN: 1-578061-34-2
Kathy Burgess, Advertising/Marketing Services Manager

6855 **Understanding Obesity: The Five Medical Causes**
Lance Levy, author
Firefly Books Ltd
66 Leek Crescent 416-499-8412
Richmond Hill, Ontario, L4B-1H1 Fax: 416-499-1142
www.fireflybooks.com
An authoritative book that focuses on the causes of, and the treatment for, obesity. Obesity is usually related to other health problems and treatment for them is the first step.
200 pages

Children's Books

6856 **I Was a Fifteen-Year-Old Blimp**
Harper & Row
10 E 53rd Street 212-207-7000
New York, NY 10022-5299
This story focuses on Gabby, a teenage girl who overhears others discuss her weight and takes radical steps to become popular.
Grades 6-9

Magazines

6857 **CheckUp**
Medical University of South Carolina
135 Cannon Street 843-792-1414
Charleston, SC 29425 800-424-6872
www.muschealth.com/weight
Provides health information about screenings, treatments, medical advances and services available through MUSC, as well as advice about nutrition and prevention.
Susan Kammeraad-Campbell, Managing Editor
Damon Simmons, Art Director

6858 **Official Journal of NAASO**
NAASO
Boston Med. Center, 650 Albany St. 617-638-7107
Boston, MA 02118 Fax: 617-638-6630
e-mail: teffk!niddk.nih.gov
www.naaso.org
Promotes research, education and advocacy to better understand, prevent and treat obesity and improve the lives of those affected.
Barbara E. Corkey, Editor-In-Chief
Deborah Moskowitz, Managing Editor

6859 **Progress Notes**
Medical University of South Carolina
135 Cannon Street 843-792-2200
Charleston, SC 29425 800-922-5250
www.muschealth.com/weight
Designed to inform the medical community developments at the Medical University of South Carolina and as a continuing medical education resource for practicing physicians and faculty.
Susan Kammeraad-Campbell, Managing Editor
Lynne Barber Associate Editor, Alex Sargent, Associate Editor

Newsletters

6860 **Trim & Fit**
Obesity Foundation
5600 S Quebec Street 303-850-0328
Englewood, CO 80111-2202
Offers nutrition facts and articles, low-fat recipes, medical information on heart disease and cancer relating to nutrition and more.
James F Merker CAE, Editor

Pamphlets

6861 **About Overeaters Anonymous**
Metro Intergroup of Overeaters Anonymous
117 W 26th Street 212-206-8621
New York, NY 10001-6807

6862 **An Inside View**
Metro Intergroup of Overeaters Anonymous
117 W 26th Street 212-206-8621
New York, NY 10001-6807

6863 **Anonymity**
Metro Intergroup of Overeaters Anonymous
117 W 26th Street 212-206-8621
New York, NY 10001-6807

6864 **Before You Take That First...**
Metro Intergroup of Overeaters Anonymous
117 W 26th Street 212-206-8621
New York, NY 10001-6807

6865 **Compulsive Overeaters in the Military**
Metro Intergroup of Overeaters Anonymous
117 W 26th Street 212-206-8621
New York, NY 10001-6807

6866 **Compulsive Overeating & Overaters Anonymous**
Metro Intergroup of Overeaters Anonymous
117 W 26th Street 212-206-8621
New York, NY 10001-6807

6867 **For the Obese Employee**
Metro Intergroup of Overeaters Anonymous
117 W 26th Street 212-206-8621
New York, NY 10001-6807

6868 **Guide to the 12 Steps for You**
Metro Intergroup of Overeaters Anonymous
117 W 26th Street 212-206-8621
New York, NY 10001-6807

6869 Hazelden Step Pamphlets for Overeaters
Hazelden
15251 Pleasant Valley Road 651-257-4010
Center City, MN 55012-9640 800-328-9000
Fax: 651-213-4426
www.hazelden.org
A 12 pamphlet collection that offers one person's interpretation of the Twelve Steps for overeaters.

6870 If God Spoke to Overeaters Anonymous
Metro Intergroup of Overeaters Anonymous
117 W 26th Street 212-206-8621
New York, NY 10001-6807

6871 Many Symptoms, One Disease
Metro Intergroup of Overeaters Anonymous
117 W 26th Street 212-206-8621
New York, NY 10001-6807

6872 Members in Relapse
Metro Intergroup of Overeaters Anonymous
117 W 26th Street 212-206-8621
New York, NY 10001-6807

6873 One Day at a Time
Metro Intergroup of Overeaters Anonymous
117 W 26th Street 212-206-8621
New York, NY 10001-6807

6874 Overeaters Anonymous Cares
Metro Intergroup of Overeaters Anonymous
117 W 26th Street 212-206-8621
New York, NY 10001-6807

6875 Overeaters Anonymous is Not a Diet Club
Metro Intergroup of Overeaters Anonymous
117 W 26th Street 212-206-8621
New York, NY 10001-6807

6876 Person to Person
Metro Intergroup of Overeaters Anonymous
117 W 26th Street 212-206-8621
New York, NY 10001-6807

6877 Program of Recovery
Metro Intergroup of Overeaters Anonymous
117 W 26th Street 212-206-8621
New York, NY 10001-6807

6878 Questions and Answers
Metro Intergroup of Overeaters Anonymous
117 W 26th Street 212-206-8621
New York, NY 10001-6807

6879 So You've Reached Goal Weight
Metro Intergroup of Overeaters Anonymous
117 W 26th Street 212-206-8621
New York, NY 10001-6807

6880 Think First...
Metro Intergroup of Overeaters Anonymous
117 W 26th Street 212-206-8621
New York, NY 10001-6807

6881 To the Family
Metro Intergroup of Overeaters Anonymous
117 W 26th Street 212-206-8621
New York, NY 10001-6807

6882 To the Man
Metro Intergroup of Overeaters Anonymous
117 W 26th Street 212-206-8621
New York, NY 10001-6807

6883 To the Newcomer
Metro Intergroup of Overeaters Anonymous
117 W 26th Street 212-206-8621
New York, NY 10001-6807

6884 To the Teen
Metro Intergroup of Overeaters Anonymous
117 W 26th Street 212-206-8621
New York, NY 10001-6807

6885 Tools of Recovery
Metro Intergroup of Overeaters Anonymous
117 W 26th Street 212-206-8621
New York, NY 10001-6807

6886 Twelve Traditions of Overeaters Anonymous
Metro Intergroup of Overeaters Anonymous
117 W 26th Street 212-206-8621
New York, NY 10001-6807

6887 Welcome Back
Metro Intergroup of Overeaters Anonymous
117 W 26th Street 212-206-8621
New York, NY 10001-6807

Audio & Video

6888 Obesity Online
NAASO
301-563-6526
Educational resource for clinicians, researchers and educators with an interest in obesity and its related disorders.
Samuel Klein, Editor
Christie M. Ballantyne, Editor

Web Sites

6889 Boston Obesity Nutrition Research Center (BONRC)
www.bmc.org
Provides resources and support for studies in the area of obesity and nutrition. Comprised of four research cores located within the Boston area. In the areas of adipocytes, epidemiology and statistics, body composition, energy expenditure and genetic analyses, and transgenic animal models.

6890 Center for Human Nutrition
www.uchsc.edu/nutrition
A interdisciplinary team encompassing basic and clinical research, post-graduate training and career development of nutrition professionals, and commuity outreach. The research conducted at the CHN focuses on obesity prevention and treatment, nutrient metabolism, and micronutrient status in children. Activities conducted aim to improve the quallity of life by promoting physical activity and nutritional awareness.

6891 Clinical Nutrition Research Unit (CNRU)
http://depts.washington.edu/uwcnru
Promotes and enhances the interdisciplinary nutrition research and education at the Univeristy of Washington. By providing a number of Core Facilities, the CNRU attempts to integrate and coordinate the abundant ongoing activities with the goals of fostering new interdiscilinary research collaborations, stimulating new research activities, improving nutrition education at multiple levels, and facilitating the nutritional management of patients.

6892 MedicineNet
www.medicinenet.com
An online resource for consumers providing easy-to-read, authoritative medical and health information.

6893 New York Obesity/Nutrition Research Center (ONRC)
www.niddk.nih.gov/fund/other/centers.htm
Funded by the National Institute of Diabetes and Digestive and Kidney Diseases (NIDDK). A combined effort of Columbia anc Cornell Universities. Provides participating investigators of funded projects relevant to obesity research with valuable laboratory, technical, and educational services that otherwise would not be available to them, thereby improving the productivity an efficiency of their operations.

6894 North American Association for the Study of Obesity
www.naaso.org
The leading scientific society dedicated to the study of obesity. Committed to encouraging research on the causes and treatment of obesity, and to keeping the medical community and public informed of new advances.

6895 **Research Chair on Obesity**
2725 Chemin Sainte Foy 418-656-8711
Quebec,Canada, e-mail: obesite.chair@crhl.ulaval.ca
http://obesity.chair.ulaval.ca
Expand our understanding of the pathophysiology of obesity, through scientific research program, to promote communication and interaction among basic scientists and clinicians, involved in nutrition, energy metabolism, obesity, lipid metabolism and cardiovascular research, and to provide continuing education about the best possible knowledge on obesity to health professionals, physicians and to the public at large regarding the causes, the complications and the treatment of obesity.

6896 **University of Pittsburgh Obesity/Nutrition Research Center**
www.pitt.edu/~onrc
Goal is to develop more effective interventions for the prevention and treatment of obesity. Exists to support research functions for investigators studying the broad areas of obesity and nutrition. Focuses on behavioral aspects of obesity and behavioral treatment of this disease.

6897 **Vanderbilt Clinical Nutrition Research Unit (CNRU)**
www.vanderbilt.edu/nutrition/index.html
A core center grant funded by the National Institute of Diabetes and Digestive and Kidney Diseases (NIDDK). Nutrition research is carried out by faculty members i most academic departments and extends from basic laboratory research to clinical and applied research. Maintains service facilities to support both basic and clinical research. Supports research cores that bring nutrition investigators together to discuss their work.

6898 **Weight-control Information Network**
www.niddk.nih.gov/health/nutrit/win.htm
WIN addresses the health information needs of individuals through the production and dissemination of educational materials. In addition, WIN is developing communication strategies for a pilot program to encourage at-risk individuals to achieve and maintain a healthy weight by making changes in their lifestyle.

Description

6899 **Osteogenesis Imperfecta**

Osteogenesis imperfecta, OI, often called "brittle bone" disease, is actually is a group of serious genetic disorders that are characterized by abnormally fragile bones that break or fracture easily. There are at least four distinct forms of the disorder, with neonatal (congenital) being the most severe. A person with OI has either less collagen, the major protein of the connective tissue, including bone, or a poorer quality collagen. Infants born with OI may have multiple bone fractures and hearing loss, and routine vaginal delivery may lead to significant bone fracture, hemorrhage into the brain and other major problems. Survivors develop shortened extremities and other bony abnormalities. If no injury to the brain occurs then mental and intellectual function should be unaffected. Hearing loss may occur.

At present, there is no effective treatment for this disorder. Careful handling of these infants is essential. Gentle exercise and physical therapy are directed at preventing fractures and increasing function. Surgical implants can provide stability to the skeletal structure. Genetic counseling is also important.

National Agencies & Associations

6900 **NIH Osteoporosis and Related Bone Diseases - National Resource Center**
2 AMS Circle 202-223-0344
Bethesda, MD 20892-3676 800-624-2663
Fax: 202-293-2356
TTY: 202-466-4315
e-mail: niamsboneinfo@mail.nih.gov
www.osteo.org
Provides patients, health professionals and the public with an important link to resources and information on osteoporosis, Paget's disease of bone, osteogenesis imperfecta, and other metabolic bone diseases. The National Resource Center's mission is to expand awareness and enhance knowledge and understanding of the prevention, early detection, and treatment of these diseases.

6901 **NIH Osteoporosis and Related Bone Disease**
2 AMS Circle 202-223-0344
Bethesda, MD 20892 800-624-2663
Fax: 202-293-2356
TTY: 202-466-4315
e-mail: niamsboneinfo@mail.nih.gov
www.niams.nih.gov
Provides patients health professionals and the public with an important link to resources and information on osteoporosis Paget's disease of bone osteogenesis imperfecta and other metabolic bone diseases.
Stephen I Katz, Director
John O'Shea, Scientific Director

6902 **National Institute of Child Health and Human Development**
National Institutes of Health
31 Center Drive 301-496-5133
Bethesda, MD 20892-0001 Fax: 301-496-7107
Supports several basic and clinical research projects on osteogenesis imperfecta.
Duane Alexander, Director

6903 **Osteogenesis Imperfecta Foundation**
804 W Diamond Avenue 301-947-0083
Gaithersburg, MD 20878-1414 800-981-2663
Fax: 301-947-0456
TTY: 202-466-4315
TDD: 202-466-4315
e-mail: BoneLink@oif.org
www.oif.org
Support and resources for families and medical professionals dealing with osteogeneis imperfecta.
Mary Beth Huber, Information/Resource Director
Tracy Smith Hart, CEO

Libraries & Resource Centers

6904 **NIH Osteoporosis and Related Bone Diseases - National Resource Center**
2 AMS Circle 202-223-0344
Bethesda, MD 20892-3676 800-624-2663
Fax: 202-293-2356
TTY: 202-466-4315
e-mail: niamsboneinfo@mail.nih.gov
www.osteo.org
Provides patients, health professionals and the public with an important link to resources and information on osteoporosis, Paget's disease of bone, osteogenesis imperfecta, and other metabolic bone diseases. The National Resource Center's mission is to expand awareness and enhance knowledge and understanding of the prevention, early detection, and treatment of these diseases.

Research Centers

6905 **American Society for Bone and Mineral Research**
2025 M Street NW 202-367-1161
Washington, DC 20036-3309 Fax: 202-672-2161
e-mail: asbmr@asbmr.org
www.asbmr.org
The mission of the ASBMR is to be the premier society in the field of bone and mineral metabolism through promoting excellence in bone and mineral research fostering integration of clinical and basic science and facilitating the translation of that science to health care and clinical practice.
Ann Elderkin, Executive Director
Douglas Fesler, Associate Executive Director

6906 **Children's Brittle Bone Foundation**
7701 95th Street 847-433-4981
Pleasant Pride, WI 53158 866-694-2223
Fax: 262-947-0724
e-mail: info@cbbf.org
www.cbbf.org
The mission of the Children's Brittle Bone Foundation is to provide for research into the causes diagnosis treatment prevention a eventual cure for Osteogenesis Imperfecta (OI) while supporting programs which improve the quality of life for people afflicted.

Support Groups & Hotlines

6907 **National Health Information Center**
PO Box 1133 310-565-4167
Washington, DC 20013 800-336-4797
Fax: 301-984-4256
e-mail: info@nhic.org
www.health.gov/nhic
Offers a nationwide information referral service, produces directories and resource guides.

6908 **Osteogenesis Imperfecta Foundation**
804 W Diamond Avenue 301-947-0083
Gaithersburg, MD 20878 800-981-2663
Fax: 301-947-0456
TDD: 202-466-4315
e-mail: BoneLink@oif.org
www.oif.org

Support and resources for families and medical professional dealing with osteogeneis imperfecta.
Marybeth Huber, Information Resource Director
Bill Bradner, Director Communication/Events

Books

6909 Children with Ostegogenesis Imperfecta: St raties to Enhance Performance
Holly Lea Cintas, Lynn Gerber, author
Osteogenesis Imperfecta Foundation
804 W Diamond Avenue 301-947-0083
Gaithersburg, MD 20878 800-981-2663
Fax: 301-947-0456
e-mail: BoneLink@oif.org
www.oif.org
This guide covers the same issues, but has been written especially for elementary school readers.
252 pages Paperback
ISBN: 0-964218-95-X
Mary Beth Huber, Information/Resource Director

6910 Growing Up with OI: A Guide for Children
Ellen Painter Dollar, author
Osteogenesis Imperfecta Foundation
804 W Diamond Avenue 301-947-0083
Gaithersburg, MD 20878 800-981-2663
Fax: 301-947-0456
e-mail: bonelink@oif.org
www.oif.org
This guide covers the same issues as the adult book, Growing Up with OI: A Guide for Families and Caregivers, but has been written especially for elementary school readers.
122 pages Paperback
ISBN: 0-964218-92-5
Mary Beth Huber, Information/Resource Director

6911 Growing Up with OI: A Guide for Families a nd Caregivers
Ellen Painter Dollar, author
Osteogenesis Imperfecta Foundation
804 W Diamond Avenue 301-947-0083
Gaithersburg, MD 20878-1414 800-981-2663
Fax: 301-947-0456
e-mail: BoneLink@oif.org
www.oif.org
This guide covers common questions parents, family members and caregivers have about raising a child with OI. The focus is onmaximizing abilities and proactive problem solving. Chapters cover medical, financial, emotional and school related issues.
295 pages Paperback
ISBN: 0-964218-91-7
Mary Beth Huber, Information/Resource Director

6912 Managing Osteogenesis Imperfecta: A Medical Manual
Priscilla Wacaster, MD, author
Osteogenesis Imperfecta Foundation
804 W Diamond Avenue 301-947-0083
Gaithersburg, MD 20878-1414 800-981-2663
Fax: 301-947-0456
e-mail: BoneLink@oif.org
www.oif.org
The manual is designed for physicians, physical and occupational therapists, orthopedic technologists, early intervention providers and others who come in contact with persons with OI. It covers a broad range of topics including genetics, diagnosis, pregnancy, arthritis, osteoperosis and rodding.
Mary Beth Huber, Information/Resource Director

6913 Therapeutic Strategies: A Guide for Occupational & Physical Therapists
Ellen Painter Dollar, author
Osteogenesis Imperfecta Foundation
804 W Diamond Avenue 301-947-0083
Gaithersburg, MD 20878-1414 800-981-2663
Fax: 301-947-0456
e-mail: BoneLink@oif.org
www.oif.org
This booklet is intended for medical professionals, or for families to use as a resource while working with a medical professional.
14 pages
Mary Beth Huber, Information/Resource Director

Newsletters

6914 Breakthrough
Osteogenesis Imperfecta Foundation
804 W Diamond Avenue 301-947-0083
Gaithersburg, MD 20878-1414 800-981-2663
Fax: 301-947-0456
e-mail: BoneLink@oif.org
www.oif.org
Newsletter of the Osteogenesis Imperfecta Foundation that provides information on current research and OIF fundraising activities as well as support features.
15 pages Quarterly
Mary Beth Huber, Information/Resource Director

Pamphlets

6915 Caring for Infants and Children with Osteogenesis Imperfecta
Osteogenesis Imperfecta Foundation
804 W Diamond Avenue 301-947-0083
Gaithersburg, MD 20878-1414 800-981-2663
Fax: 301-947-0456
e-mail: BoneLink@oif.org
www.oif.org
A companion to the videotape You Are Not Alone. Presents some basic information and unique tips on caring for a baby with OI. Available in Spanish.
24 pages
Mary Beth Huber, Information/Resource Director

6916 Osteogenesis Imperfecta: A Guide for Medic al Professionals, Individuals & Families
Osteogenesis Imperfecta Foundation
804 W Diamond Avenue 301-947-0083
Gaithersburg, MD 20878-1414 800-981-2663
Fax: 301-947-0456
e-mail: BoneLink@oif.org
www.oif.org
This pamphlet contains basic information about the types of OI, inheritance factors, diagnosis and treatment.
10 pages Paperback
Mary Beth Huber, Information/Resource Director

Audio & Video

6917 Going Places and Plan for Success: An Educ ator's Guide to Students with OI
Osteogenesis Imperfecta Foundation
804 W Diamond Avenue 301-947-0083
Gaithersburg, MD 20878-1414 800-981-2663
Fax: 301-947-0456
e-mail: BoneLink@oif.org
www.oif.org
A 15-minute video with booklet that guides educators and parents through planning steps that will help children with OI fully participate in school activities.
Mary Beth Huber, Information/Resource Director

6918 Within Reach
Osteogenesis Imperfecta Foundation
804 W Diamond Avenue 301-947-0083
Gaithersburg, MD 20878-1414 800-981-2663
Fax: 301-947-0456
TDD: 202-466-4315
e-mail: BoneLink@oif.org
www.oif.org

This 50-minute video features in-depth interviews with adults living with OI. They talk candidly about how they have achieved independent and satisfying lives, addressing such issues as travel, career, marriage and family.
VHS/DVD
Mary Beth Huber, Information/Resource Director

6919 You Are Not Alone
Osteogenesis Imperfecta Foundation
804 W Diamond Avenue 301-947-0083
Gaithersburg, MD 20878-1414 800-981-2663
Fax: 301-947-0456
TDD: 202-466-4315
e-mail: BoneLink@oif.org
www.oif.org
Explores the emotional turmoil of dealing with the diagnosis of OI and offers practical and uplifting solutions for caring for infants with Type II to severe Type III OI. Also valuable for new families with the more mild forms of OI. Available open captioned or with Spanish subtitles (specify if needed). Add $5.00 per video for Canadian orders and $11.00 per video for overseas orders.
Mary Beth Huber, Information/Resource Director

Web Sites

6920 Healing Well
www.healingwell.com
An online health resource guide to medical news, chat, information and articles, newsgroups and message boards, books, disease-related web sites, medical directories, and more for patients, friends, and family coping with disabling diseases, disorders, or chronic illnesses.

6921 Health Finder
www.healthfinder.gov
Searchable, carefully developed web site offering information on over 1000 topics. Developed by the US Department of Health and Human Services, the site can be used in both English and Spanish.

6922 Healthlink USA
www.healthlinkusa.com
Health information concerning treatment, cures, prevention, diagnosis, risk factors, research, support groups, email lists, personal stories and much more. Updated regularly.

6923 Helios Health
www.helioshealth.com
Online resource for your health information. Detailed information about specific health topics, access to expert advice from our Medical Advisory Board, and up-to-date health news.

6924 MedicineNet
www.medicinenet.com
An online resource for consumers providing easy-to-read, authoritative medical and health information.

6925 Medscape
www.mywebmd.com
Medscape offers specialists, primary care physicians, and other health professionals the Web's most robust and integrated medical information and educational tools.

6926 Osteogenesis Imperfecta Foundation
www.oif.org
A website for those who want to learn more about Osteogenesis Imperfecta, the OI Foundation, and what they do.

6927 Osteoporosis and Related Bone Diseases: National Resource Center (NIGH)
www.osteo.org
Provides patients, health professionals and the public with an important link to resources and information on osteoporosis and other metabolic bone diseases.

6928 WebMD
www.webmd.com
Information on Osteogenesis Imperfecta, including articles and resources.

Description

6929 **Osteoporosis**

Osteoporosis is a general term for many conditions which result in a reduction in bone mass. Most cases occur in post-menopausal women because estrogen loss is associated with decreased bone mass. These women are at risk for fractures of the wrist, spine and hip. Post-menopausal osteoporosis may also cause marked reduction in a woman's height, as multiple vertebral bodies in the spine compress downwards over the years. Risk factors for osteoporosis include white race, cigarette smoking, thin body build and early menopause. Men can develop a similar condition, but it is generally much less severe. Excessive activity of the adrenal glands (Cushing's syndrome), the thyroid gland (thyrotoxicosis), the parathyroid glands (hyperparathyroidism), and the pituitary gland (hyperprolactinemia) cause bones to thin, as does underactivity of the testes or ovaries. Anorexia nervosa and prolonged administration of cortisone or heparin will also thin the bones.

Treatment is in part nonspecific, and can include surgery or other immobilization to treat fractures of the hip or wrist, control of pain with medications and physical therapy to encourage return to pre-fracture function. Specific therapy includes calcium and Vitamin D supplementation and weight-bearing exercises. Biphosphonates, such as alendronate, have been approved for osteoporosis and other new therapies are being developed.

National Agencies & Associations

6930 **National Osteoporosis Foundation**
1232 22nd Street NW 202-223-2226
Washington, DC 20037-1292 800-223-9994
Fax: 202-223-2237
e-mail: communications@nof.org
www.nof.org
The nation's leading resource for people seeking up-to-date medically sound information on the causes prevention detection and treatment of osteoporosis.
Leo Schargorodski, Executive Director
Ethel Siris, President

6931 **Osteoporosis Canada**
1090 Don Mills Road 416-696-2663
Toronto, Ontario, M3C-3R6 800-463-6842
Fax: 416-696-2673
www.osteoporosis.ca
A registered charity, is the only national organization serving people who have, or are at risk for, osteoporosis.
Karen L Ormerod MM, President/CEO
Dr Famida Jiwa MHSc DC BSc, VP

Libraries & Resource Centers

6932 **NIH Osteoporosis and Related Bone Diseases - National Resource Center**
2 AMS Circle 202-223-0344
Bethesda, MD 20892-3676 800-624-2663
Fax: 202-293-2356
TTY: 202-466-4315
e-mail: niamsboneinfo@mail.nih.gov
www.osteo.org
Provides patients, health professionals and the public with an important link to resources and information on osteoporosis, Paget's disease of bone, osteogenesis imperfecta, and other metabolic bone diseases. The National Resource Center's mission is to expand awareness and enhance knowledge and understanding of the prevention, early detection, and treatment of these diseases.

Research Centers

6933 **Medical College of Pennsylvania Center for the Mature Woman**
3300 Henry Avenue 215-842-6000
Philadelphia, PA 19129
our purpose is to provide consumers information to help them get high quality services and products at the best possible prices.
Jon Schneider,MD, Director

6934 **Osteoporosis Center Memorial Hospital/Advanced Medical Diagn**
Memorial Hospital/Advanced Medical Diagnostic
1700 Coffee Road
Modesto, CA 95355 209-526-4500
www.memorialmedicalcenter.org
Memorial Medical Center is part of Memorial Hospitals Association a not-for-profit organization that exists to maintain and improve the health status of citizens in the greater Stanislaus County.
David Benn, Director
Bev Finley, Director

6935 **Regional Bone Center Helen Hayes Hospital**
Helen Hayes Hospital
51-55 Route 9W 845-786-4839
W Haverstraw, NY 10993 Fax: 845-947-3000
e-mail: info@helenhayeshospital.org
www.helenhayeshospital.org
The mission of the Regional Bone conduct a broad-based research program focused on the elucidation of cellular mechanisms underlying metabolic bone disease and the development of new treatments for bone disease.
David W Dempster PhD, Director
Adrienne Tewksbury, Grants Administrator

6936 **University of Connecticut Osteoporosis Center**
263 Farmington Avenue 860-679-7692
Farmington, CT 06030 800-535-6232
Fax: 860-679-1258
www.uchc.edu
Jay R Lieberman, Director

6937 **University of Connecticut: Exercise Research Laboratory**
Health Center
263 Farmington Avenue 860-679-1000
Farmington, CT 06032
Studies the effects of hormone treatment and exercise on osteoporosis in women.
Gail Dalsky PhD, Director

Support Groups & Hotlines

6938 **National Health Information Center**
PO Box 1133 310-565-4167
Washington, DC 20013 800-336-4797
Fax: 301-984-4256
e-mail: info@nhic.org
www.health.gov/nhic
Offers a nationwide information referral service, produces directories and resource guides.

6939 **National Osteoporosis Foundation (NOF)**
1232 22nd Street NW 202-223-2226
Washington, DC 20037-1292 Fax: 202-223-2237
e-mail: webmaster@nof.org
www.nof.org
Dedicated to reducing the widespread prevalence of osteoporosis through programs of research, education and advocacy. Provides referrals to existing support groups, as well as free resources, training and materials to assist people to start groups.
Leo Schargorodski, Executive Director
Daniel A Mica, Chairman of the Board

Books

6940 **One-Hundred-Fifty Most Asked Questions About Osteoporosis**
Hearst Books
1350 Avenue of the Americas 212-261-6500
New York, NY 10016 Fax: 212-261-6595
1993
ISBN: 0-688123-34-1

6941 **Preventing & Reversing Osteoporosis: Every Woman's Guide**
Prima Publishing
PO Box 1260
Rocklin, CA 95677-1260 916-624-5718
www.primapub.com
1993 275 pages
ISBN: 1-559582-98-7

6942 **Preventing and Managing Osteoporosis**
Springer Publishing Company
536 Broadway 212-431-4370
New York, NY 10012-3955 877-687-7476
Fax: 212-941-7842
e-mail: springer@springerpub.com
www.springerpub.com
This book will raise awareness and inform health professionals about this often preventable and treatable disease. Written by a team of authors from medicine, nursing, nutrition, exercise physiology, and physical therapy, the book provides an overview of the disease process.
216 pages Hardcover
ISBN: 0-826113-18-4
M Susan Burke MD, Editor
Helen Wright PhD, Editor

Newsletters

6943 **Osteoporosis Report**
National Osteoporosis Foundation
1232 22nd Street NW 202-223-2226
Washington, DC 20037-1292 800-223-9994
Fax: 202-223-2237
e-mail: communications@nof.org
www.nof.org
A benefit to members of the National Osteoporosis Foundation (NOF), the Osteoporosis Report includes updates on recent research, strategies for bone health and other information. NOF is the only nonprofit, voluntary health organization dedicated to reducing the widespread prevalence of osteoporosis through programs of research, education and advocacy. Contact the foundation for membership information.
Quarterly

Pamphlets

6944 **Boning Up on Osteoporosis**
National Osteoporosis Foundation
1232 22nd Street NW 202-223-2226
Washington, DC 20037-1292 800-223-9994
Fax: 202-223-2237
e-mail: communications@nof.org
www.nof.org
Risk factor card.

6945 **How Strong Are Your Bones?**
1232 22nd Street NW 202-223-2226
Washington, DC 20037-1292 800-223-9994
Fax: 202-223-2237
e-mail: communications@nof.org
www.nof.org
Describes the various methods for determining bone mass, including types of equipment and how bone density testing is used in the diagnosis and treatment of osteoporosis.
12 pages

6946 **Living with Osteoporosis**
1232 22nd Street NW 202-223-2226
Washington, DC 20037-1292 800-223-9994
Fax: 202-223-2237
e-mail: communications@nof.org
www.nof.org
A guide to preventing falls in the home and to protecting yourself from injury during your daily routine.

6947 **Medications and Bone Loss**
1232 22nd Street NW 202-223-2226
Washington, DC 20037-1292 800-223-9994
Fax: 202-223-2237
e-mail: communications@nof.org
www.nof.org
Designed for women dealing with menopause, this brochure provides information of estrogen replacement therapy and its relationship to bone health and osteoporosis prevention and treatment.

6948 **Men with Osteoporosis: In Their Own Words**
1232 22nd Street NW 202-223-2226
Washington, DC 20037-1292 800-223-9994
Fax: 202-223-2237
e-mail: communications@nof.org
www.nof.org

6949 **Official Prevention Month Poster**
1232 22nd Street NW 202-223-2226
Washington, DC 20037-1292 800-223-9994
Fax: 202-223-2237
e-mail: communications@nof.org
www.nof.org
Poster promotes public awareness about osteoporosis. It can be used as a compliment to the education kit, or by itself for exhibits, health fairs or community programs.

6950 **Official Prevention Week Poster**
1232 22nd Street NW 202-223-2226
Washington, DC 20037-1292 800-223-9994
Fax: 202-223-2237
e-mail: communications@nof.org
www.nof.org
Poster promotes public awareness about osteoporosis. It can be used as a compliment to the education kit, or by itself for exhibits, health fairs or community programs.

6951 **Osteoporosis Education Kit**
1232 22nd Street NW 202-223-2226
Washington, DC 20037-1292 800-223-9994
Fax: 202-223-2237
e-mail: communications@nof.org
www.nof.org
This kit is designed for preparing public and patient education programs. Updated annually and includes age-targeted materials, nutrition information and osteoporosis fact sheets that are easily duplicated.

6952 **Osteoporosis Education Poster**
1232 22nd Street NW 202-223-2226
Washington, DC 20037-1292 800-223-9994
Fax: 202-223-2237
e-mail: communications@nof.org
www.nof.org
Ideal for health care settings, the poster clearly illustrates the effect of osteoporosis on bone tissue and common fracture sites.

6953 **Osteoporosis Information Package**
NAMSIC/National Institutes of Health
1 AMS Circle 301-495-4484
Bethesda, MD 20892-0001 877-226-4267
Fax: 301-718-6366
TTY: 301-565-2966
e-mail: niamsinfo@mail.nih.gov
www.nih.gov/niams
19 pages

6954 **Osteoporosis International**
1232 22nd Street NW
Washington, DC 20037-1292
202-223-2226
800-223-9994
Fax: 202-223-2237
e-mail: communications@nof.org
www.nof.org
An international multidisciplinary, clinically oriented journal for the exchange of ideas concerning osteoporosis.

6955 **Osteoporosis in Men Information Package**
NAMSIC/National Institutes of Health
1 AMS Circle
Bethesda, MD 20892-0001
301-495-4484
877-226-4267
Fax: 301-715-6366
TTY: 301-565-2966
e-mail: niamsinfo@mail.nih.gov
www.nih.gov/niams
19 pages

6956 **Osteoporosis: Clinical Updates**
1232 22nd Street NW
Washington, DC 20037-1292
202-223-2226
800-223-9994
Fax: 202-223-2237
e-mail: communications@nof.org
www.nof.org
NOF's health profession newsletter provides an in depth focus on varying clinical topics.

6957 **Osteoporosis: The Silent Disease-Slide Lecture Presentation**
1232 22nd Street NW
Washington, DC 20037-1292
202-223-2226
800-223-9994
Fax: 202-223-2237
e-mail: communications@nof.org
www.nof.org
This 42-slide presentation is ideal for community, patient and worksite education progams. It covers basic bone biology, osteoporosis risk factors, diagnosis, prevention and treatment and concludes with a patient case history. A question and answer document is also provided to assist the presenter with audience questions.
Slide set

6958 **Patient Education Sample Pack**
1232 22nd Street NW
Washington, DC 20037-1292
202-223-2226
800-223-9994
Fax: 202-223-2237
e-mail: communications@nof.org
www.nof.org
This pack contains one of each of NOF's patient education brochures and a catalog; health professionals can select the brochures appropriate for their audience.
Ten brochures

6959 **Risk Factor Card: Can It Happen to You?**
National Osteoporosis Foundation
1232 22nd Street NW
Washington, DC 20037-1292
202-223-2226
800-223-9994
Fax: 202-223-2237
e-mail: communications@nof.org
www.nof.org
Explains osteoporosis, the causes, symptoms and preventions and high risk persons.

6960 **Stand Up to Osteoporosis**
National Osteoporosis Foundation
1232 22nd Street NW
Washington, DC 20037-1292
202-223-2226
800-223-9994
Fax: 202-223-2237
e-mail: communications@nof.org
www.nof.org
One of 25 educational brochures on all aspects of this chronic and debilitating disease. The National Osteoporosis Foundation (NOF) is the nation's only private, nonprofit organization dedicated to education, advocacy and public services. Memberships are available to health professionals and public. Quarterly newsletter and physician's guide.

6961 **Strategies for People with Osteoporosis**
1232 22nd Street NW
Washington, DC 20037-1292
202-223-2226
800-223-9994
Fax: 202-223-2237
e-mail: communications@nof.org
www.nof.org
This series of articles from NOF's newsletter helps patients learn how to cope with osteoporosis. Articles cover hip, vertebrae and wrist fracture recovery, fall-proofing your home, finding the right doctor, what to do after you've been diagnosed and more.

Audio & Video

6962 **Be BoneWise: Exercise**
National Osteoperosis Foundation
1232 22nd Street NW
Washington, DC 20037-1292
202-223-2226
800-223-9994
Fax: 202-223-2237
e-mail: communications@nof.org
www.nof.org
Take steps toward better bones, health, flexibility and balance with the offical weight bearing and strength training exercise video.

6963 **Osteoperosis: The Silent Disease**
National Osteoperosis Foundation
1232 22nd Street NW
Washington, DC 20037-1292
202-223-2226
800-223-9994
Fax: 202-223-2237
e-mail: communications@nof.org
www.nof.org
A scripted, visual presentation covers basic bone biology, osteoperosis risk factors, diagnosis, prevention and treatment. Available as a slide presentation or power point CD Rom.

6964 **Patient Education Video**
National Osteoperosis Foundation
1232 22nd Street NW
Washington, DC 20037-1292
202-223-2226
800-223-9994
Fax: 202-223-2237
e-mail: communications@nof.org
www.nof.org
Discusses treatment, exercise, nutrition and coping strategies for those already diagnoses with osteoporosis.
15 minutes

Web Sites

6965 **Healing Well**
www.healingwell.com
An online health resource guide to medical news, chat, information and articles, newsgroups and message boards, books, disease-related web sites, medical directories, and more for patients, friends, and family coping with disabling diseases, disorders, or chronic illnesses.

6966 **Health Finder**
www.healthfinder.gov
Searchable, carefully developed web site offering information on over 1000 topics. Developed by the US Department of Health and Human Services, the site can be used in both English and Spanish.

6967 **Healthlink USA**
www.healthlinkusa.com
Health information concerning treatment, cures, prevention, diagnosis, risk factors, research, support groups, email lists, personal stories and much more. Updated regularly.

6968 **Helios Health**
www.helioshealth.com
Online resource for your health information. Detailed information about specific health topics, access to expert advice from our Medical Advisory Board, and up-to-date health news.

6969 **MedicineNet**
www.medicinenet.com
An online resource for consumers providing easy-to-read, authoritative medical and health information.

6970 Medscape

www.mywebmd.com

Medscape offers specialists, primary care physicians, and other health professionals the Web's most robust and integrated medical information and educational tools.

6971 NIH Osteoporosis and Related Bone Disease

www.osteo.org

Information on prevention, early detection, and treatment of these diseases is also available. The Resource Center is operated by the National Osteoporosis Foundation, in collaboration with The Paget Foundation and the Osteogenesis Imperfecta Foundation.

6972 National Osteoporosis Foundation

www.nof.org

The nation's leading resource for people seeking up-to-date, medically sound information on the causes, prevention, detection and treatment of osteoporosis.

6973 WebMD

www.webmd.com

Information on osteoporosis, including articles and resources.

Description

6974 **Paget's Disease**

Paget's disease is a disorder of the bone, which typically results in enlarged and deformed bones in one or more regions of the skeleton. Excessive bone breakdown and formation cause new bone to be dense but fragile. Paget's disease occurs most frequently in the spine, skull, pelvis, and legs.

Early symptoms of Paget's disease include bone and joint pain and fatigability, as well as headaches and hearing loss, when the skull is affected. Deformities of bone such as enlargement of the forehead, bowing of a limb, and curvature of the spine may occur as the disease progresses.

The cause of Paget's disease is unknown. It is sometimes familial, but a specific genetic pattern is unclear.

The course of the disease varies greatly and may range from complete stability to rapid progression. Generally, symptoms progress slowly in affected bones with usually no spread to normal ones.

Although there is no cure for Paget's disease at the present, treatments include drugs that suppress disease activity. Orthopedic surgery for joint replacement or stabilization may also be beneficial.

National Agencies & Associations

6975 **Arthritis Foundation**
1330 W Peachtree Street 404-872-7100
Atlanta, GA 30309 800-283-7800
Fax: 404-872-0457
e-mail: help@arthritis.org
www.arthritis.org
A nonprofit organization that depends on volunteers to provide services to help people with arthritis. Supports research to find ways to cure and prevent arthritis and provides services to improve the quality of life for those affected by arthritis.
Cecile Perich, Chair
John H Klippel MD, President and CEO

6976 **Paget Foundation for Paget's Disease of Bone & Related Disorders**
120 Wall Street 212-509-5335
New York, NY 10005-4001 800-237-2438
Fax: 212-509-8492
e-mail: PagetFdn@aol.com
www.paget.org
Private voluntary health agency that provides information to patients and health professionals on several bone disorders including: Paget's disease of bone, primary hyperparathyroidism, fibrous dysplasia, osteoporosis (not osteoporosis) and complications of these conditions.
Charlene Waldman, Executive Director
Christal Sumpter, Administrator & Web Manager

Support Groups & Hotlines

6977 **National Health Information Center**
PO Box 1133 310-565-4167
Washington, DC 20013 800-336-4797
Fax: 301-984-4256
e-mail: info@nhic.org
www.health.gov/nhic
Offers a nationwide information referral service, produces directories and resource guides.

Newsletters

6978 **Update**
Paget Foundation
120 Wall Street 212-509-5335
New York, NY 10005-4001 800-237-2438
Fax: 212-509-8492
e-mail: PagetFdn@aol.com
www.paget.org
Provides information for consumers and health professionals on the following disorders: paget's disease of bone, primary hyperparathyroidism, fibrous dysplasia, osteopetrosis (not osteoporosis) and the complications of breast and prostate cancer metastic to the bone.
3 per year
Charlene Waldman, Executive Director

Pamphlets

6979 **Questions & Answers About Paget's Disease of Bone**
Paget Foundation
120 Wall Street 212-509-5335
New York, NY 10005-4001 800-237-2438
Fax: 212-509-8492
e-mail: pagetfdn@aol.com
www.paget.org
The Paget Foundation provides this and other question and answer booklets and fact sheets on Paget's disease of bone, primary hyperparathyroidism,, fibrous dysplasia, osteopetrosis (not osteoporosis) and breast and prostate cancer metastic to bone. These publications are available on the foundation websit and in print.
Charlene Waldman, Executive Director

Web Sites

6980 **Healing Well**
www.healingwell.com
An online health resource guide to medical news, chat, information and articles, newsgroups and message boards, books, disease-related web sites, medical directories, and more for patients, friends, and family coping with disabling diseases, disorders, or chronic illnesses.

6981 **Health Finder**
www.healthfinder.gov
Searchable, carefully developed web site offering information on over 1000 topics. Developed by the US Department of Health and Human Services, the site can be used in both English and Spanish.

6982 **Healthlink USA**
www.healthlinkusa.com
Health information concerning treatment, cures, prevention, diagnosis, risk factors, research, support groups, email lists, personal stories and much more. Updated regularly.

6983 **Helios Health**
www.helioshealth.com
Online resource for your health information. Detailed information about specific health topics, access to expert advice from our Medical Advisory Board, and up-to-date health news.

6984 **MedicineNet**
www.medicinenet.com
An online resource for consumers providing easy-to-read, authoritative medical and health information.

6985 **Medscape**
www.mywebmd.com
Medscape offers specialists, primary care physicians, and other health professionals the Web's most robust and integrated medical information and educational tools.

6986 **Paget Foundation for Paget's Disease of Bone & Related Disorders**

www.paget.org

Includes information for patients and health professionals on Paget's disease of bone, primary hyperparathyroidism, fibrous dysplasia, osteopetrosis (not osteoporosis) and the complications of certain cancers on the skeleton.

6987 **WebMD**

www.webmd.com

Information on Paget's disease, including articles and resources.

Description

6988 **Parkinson Disease**

Parkinson disease is a neurological condition characterized by slow and decreased movement. It affects about 1 percent of those over age 65. The cause of Parkinson disease is unknown, but both genetic and environmental factors may play a role. In a minority of cases, Parkinson disease develops after repeated head trauma, carbon monoxide poisoning, drug use, or viral infections that affect the brain.

In about 50 percent to 80 percent of patients, Parkinson disease begins with a slight tremor in the hands, resembling "pill-rolling." With fatigue and stress, the tremor becomes more pronounced. As the disease progresses, voluntary movements, such as walking and eating, become more and more difficult. Rigidity and postural instability (difficulty standing up) develop. Dementia affects approximately one third of patients with advanced Parkinson disease.

Because Parkinson disease is characterized by reduced levels of neurotransmitter chemicals, notably dopamine, in certain parts of the brain, therapy has focused on restoring these levels to normal. Monoamine oxidase type B inhibitors given early in the disease, may protect the cells that secrete these chemicals, and thus delay the need for other therapy. When it is necessary to directly manipulate the chemical levels because of progression of the disease, levodopa, related to dopamine, is the mainstay of treatment and is associated with improvement of all Parkinson symptoms. Anticholinergic medications are especially helpful in treating tremor.

Parkinson disease is the subject of intense research, and experimental surgical or drug treatments are frequently available to patients whose response to standard therapy has been unsatisfactory. General supportive care should not be neglected, and includes physical therapy and an exercise program to help optimize mobility.

National Agencies & Associations

6989 **American Parkinson Disease Association**
135 Parkinson Avenue 718-981-8001
Staten Island, NY 10305-1943 800-223-2732
Fax: 718-981-4399
e-mail: apda@apdaparkinson.org
www.apdaparkinson.org
Provides help advice and information about the brain disorder that causes muscle tremors, stiffness and weakness.
Mario J Esposito, Board of Director
Joel Gerste, Executive Director

6990 **Michael J. Fox Foundation for Parkinson's Research**
Grand Central Station
New York, NY 10163 800-708-7644
www.michaeljfox.org
The Michael J. Fox Foundation is dedicated to ensuring the development of a cure for Parkinson's disease within this lifetime through an aggressively funded research center.
Deborah W Brooks, Co-Founder
Katie Hood, CEO

6991 **National Institute of Neurological Disorders and Stroke**
PO Box 5801 301-496-5751
Bethesda, MD 20824-5801 800-352-9424
Fax: 301-402-2186
TTY: 301-468-5981
www.ninds.nih.gov
Offers a brochure on Parkinsons disease and America's focal point for support of research on brain and nervous system disorders.

6992 **National Parkinson Foundation**
1501 NW 9th Avenue 305-243-6666
Miami, FL 33136-1407 800-327-4545
Fax: 305-243-6824
e-mail: contact@parkinson.org
www.parkinson.org
A nonprofit organization dedicated to research, diagnosis, treatment and care for men and women suffering from Parkinson's and other related neurological diseases. The Foundation also supports the Bob Hope research and rehabilitation center.
Nathan Slewett, Chairman
Joyce A Oberdorf, President and Chief Executive Officer

6993 **Parkinson Society Canada**
4211 Yonge Street 416-227-9700
Toronto, Ontario, M2P-2A9 800-565-3000
Fax: 416-227-9600
e-mail: info@parkinson.ca
www.parkinson.ca
A not-for-profit, national charitable organization. The Society raises money through corporate sponsorships, public donations, and planned gifts. Finding the cause and cure for Parkinson's disease remains our mission.
Joyce Gordon, President/CEO
Beverly Crandell, National Director, Resource Development

6994 **Parkinson's Action Network (PAN)**
1025 Vermont Avenue NW 202-638-4101
Washington, DC 20005 800-850-4726
Fax: 202-638-7257
e-mail: info@parkinsonaction.org
www.parkinsonsaction.org
The Parkinson's Action Network is the unified voice of the Parkinson's disease community-advocating for more than one million Americans and their families.
Amy Comstock Rick, Chief Executive Officer
Michelle Duelley, Executive Assistant to the CEO

6995 **Parkinson's Institute**
675 Almanor Avenue 408-734-2800
Sunnyvale, CA 94085-1605 800-655-2273
Fax: 408-734-8522
e-mail: info@thepi.org
www.thepi.org
The mission of the Parkinson's Institute is to find the cause(s) and a cure for Parkinson's Disease and provide the best possible treatment to those afflicted with the disease.
J William Langston, Founder/CEO/Chief Scientific Officer
Melanie M Brandabur, Clinic Director

6996 **WE MOVE**
204 W 84th Street 212-875-8312
New York, NY 10024 e-mail: wemove@wemove.org
www.wemove.org
WE MOVE's mission is to raise awareness of neurologic movement disorder among healthcare professionals, patients and families and the public.
Susan B Bressman, President
Mo Moadeli, Vice President

State Agencies & Associations

Arizona

6997 **Arizona Chapter of the National Parkinson Foundation**
20280 N 59th Avenue 480-607-1960
Glendale, AZ 85308-6182 866-637-8772
Fax: 480-607-1957
e-mail: info@aznpf.org
www.aznpf.org

Affiliate chapter of The National Parkinson Foundation Inc.
Alan Marks, President
Kenneth Larkin, Vice President

California

6998 Los Angeles Alliance Against Parkinson's Disease
3251 Oakley Drive 323-851-3230
Los Angeles, CA 90068-1315 e-mail: Millard@millardtipp.com
www.parkinson.org/chapters.htm#
Affiliate of the National Parkinson Foundation.

6999 National Parkinson Foundation: California Office
4929 Wilshire Boulevard 323-442-8434
Los Angeles, CA 90010-3899

7000 National Parkinson Foundation: Orange County Chapter
PO Box 2207 949-764-6998
Newport Beach, CA 92659 Fax: 949-548-4624
e-mail: nfo@npfocc.org
www.npfocc.org
Affiliate of The National Parkinson Foundation.
Mignone M Trenary, President

7001 Northstate Parkinson's Chapter
1003 Yuba Street
Redding, CA 96001 530-229-0878
www.parkinson.org
Affiliate of The National Parkinson Foundation, Inc.
Craig Boyer

7002 Parkinson Association of the Sacramento Valley
900 Fulton Avenue 916-489-0226
Sacramento, CA 96825-4502 Fax: 916-489-0241
e-mail: parkanc@sbcglobal.net
www.parkinsonsacramento.org
Bernardine Ford, President
George Johnston, 2nd Vice President

7003 Parkinson Network of Mount Diablo
Po Box 3127 925-284-2189
Walnut Creek, CA 94598-0127 e-mail: mmhansell@hotmail.com
www.parkinson.org
Affiliate of the National Parkinson Foundation.
Mary Hansell

7004 Parkinson's Action Network (PAN) Parkinson's Action Network
Parkinson's Action Network
1025 Vermont Avenue NW 202-638-4101
Washington, DC 20005 800-850-4726
Fax: 202-638-7257
e-mail: info@parkinsonsaction.org
www.parkinsonsaction.org
Amy Comstock Rick, Chief Executive Officer
Anne Udall, Chair/Founding Chair

Colorado

7005 Colorado Parkinson Foundation
1155 Kelly Johnson Boulevard 719-884-0103
Colorado Springs, FL 90920-1494 800-327-4545
Fax: 719-495-909
e-mail: rpfarrer@msn.com
colorado.parkinson.org
The mission of the National Parkinson Foundation if to find the cause of the cure for Parkinson disease through research. To improve the quality if life for persons with Parkinson and their caregivers. To also educate persons with Parkinson their carecar
Ric Pfarrer, Chairperson

Florida

7006 Alzheimer/Parkinson Association of Indian River County
2501 27th Avenue 772-563-0505
Vero Beach, FL 32960 e-mail: alzsupport@fastmail.fm
www.parkinson.org
Toni Teresi, Chairperson

7007 Goodwill Industries-Suncoast
Goodwill Industries-Suncoast
10596 Gandy Boulevard 727-523-1512
St. Petersburg, FL 37023 888-279-1988
Fax: 727-563-9300
e-mail: gw.marketing@goodwill-suncoast.org
www.goodwill-suncoast.org
A nonprofit community based organization whose purpose is to improve the quality of life for people who are disabled, disadvantaged and/or aged. This mission is accomplished through a staff of over 1,200 employees providing independent living skills, affordable housing, career assessment and planning, job skills, training, placement, and job retention assistance with useful employment. Annually, Goodwill Industries-Suncoast serves over 30,000 people in Citrus, Hernando, Levy, Marion and more.
R Lee Waits, President/CEO
Martin W Gladysz, Chair

7008 Parkinson Association of Greater Daytona Beach
111 North Frederick Avenue 386-252-8959
Daytona Beach, FL 32114 e-mail: goatie@cfl.rr.com
www.parkinson.org
Nancy Dawson, Chairperson

7009 Parkinson Association of Greater Kansas
111 N Frederick Avenue
Daytona Beach, FL 32114 386-252-8959
www.parkinson.org
Nancy Dawson, Chairperson

7010 Parkinson Association of Southwest Florida
6226 Trail Boulevard 239-254-7791
Naples, FL 34108 Fax: 239-254-9421
e-mail: pasfi@aol.com
www.pasfi.org
Affiliate of the National Parkinson Foundation.
Jacqueline Urso, Executive Director
Ellen Chaney, Secretary

7011 South Palm Beach County Chapter of NFP
PO Box 880145
Boca Raton, FL 33433-0145 561-482-2867
www.parkinson.org
Irving Layton, Chairperson

7012 Southeast Parkinson Disease Association
6530 Metrowest Boulevard 407-489-4124
Orlando, FL 32835-6520 e-mail: srh_pres@sepda.org
www.sepda.org
Steve Hochberger, Chairperson

Georgia

7013 Northwest Georgia Parkinson Disease Association
708 Glen Milner Boulevard 706-235-3164
Rome, GA 30161 e-mail: webmaster@gaparkinsons.org
www.gaparkinsons.org
James Trussel, Chairperson

Hawaii

7014 Hawaii Parkinson Association Gwendolyn A Montibon President
Gwendolyn A Montibon, President
347 N Kuakini Street 808-528-0935
Honolulu, HI 96817 Fax: 808-528-1897
e-mail: kekim@hawaii.edu
www.parkinson.org
Affiliate of The National Parkinson Foundation.

Kansas

7015 Northeast Kansas Parkinson Association
PO Box 251
Topeka, KS 66601 785-228-1337
www.parkinson.org
Mary Hatke, Chairperson

7016 Parkinson Association of Greater Kansas City
8900 State Line Road 913-341-8828
Leawood, KS 66206 Fax: 913-341-8885
e-mail: meg@parkinsonheartland.org
www.parkinsonheartland.org

Affiliate of The National Parkinson Foundation.
Meg Duggan, Executive Director
Katie Fuchs, Program Coordinator

Louisiana

7017 **Eljay Foundation for Parkinson Syndrome Awareness**
715 Ryan Street 337-310-0083
Lake Charles, LA 70601 e-mail: info@eljayfd.org
www.eljayfd.org
Eligha Guillory, Chairperson

Massachusetts

7018 **Cape Cod Chapter National Parkinson Foundation**
33 Ships Way 508-385-2333
Buzzards Bay, MA 02532-0584 e-mail: meacapecod@yahoo.com
www.parkinson.org
Affiliate of The National Parkinson Foundation.
Joseph Wimbrow, President

7019 **National Parkinson Foundation:Cape Cod Chapter**
33 Ships Way 508-385-2333
Buzzards Bay, MA 02532-0584 e-mail: meacapecod@yahoo.com
www.parkinson.org
Garland Smith, Chairperson

7020 **Northeast Parkinson's and Caregivers**
27 Sutcliffe Road 508-756-7721
Brimfield, MA 01010 e-mail: rstake@northeastparkinsons.com
www.northeastparkinsons.com
Richard Stake, Chairperson

Minnesota

7021 **Parkinson Association of Minnesota**
2205 Zealand Avenue N 763-545-1272
Golden Valley, MN 55427-4602 800-327-4545
e-mail: info@parkinsonmn.org
www.parkinsonmn.org
Affiliate of The National Parkinson Foundation.
Paul Blom, President

New Jersey

7022 **Parkinson Alliance**
PO Box 308 609-688-0870
Kingston, NJ 08540 800-579-8440
Fax: 609-688-0875
e-mail: admin@parkinsonalliance.net
www.parkinsonalliance.net
The Princeton-New Jersey based Parkinson Alliance is a National nonprofit organization dedicated to raising funds to help finance the most promising research to find the cause and curefor Parkinson's disease.
Carol Walton, Executive Director

New York

7023 **National Parkinson Foundation: New York Office**
122 E 42nd Street
New York, NY 10017-5622 800-457-6676

7024 **Parkinsons Wellness Group of Western New York**
222 Seabert Avenue 716-684-0650
Depew, NY 14043 e-mail: coach71395@aol.com
www.parkinsonswny.com
Richard Lipka, Chairperson

Oklahoma

7025 **Parkinson Foundation of the Heartland Oklahoma Branch**
1000 W Wilshire 405-810-0695
Oklahoma City, OK 73116 e-mail: jimk@parkinsonheartland.org
www.parkinson.org
Satellite office of the Kansas Chapter
Jim Keating, Chairperson

Oregon

7026 **Parkinsons Resources of Oregon**
3975 Mercantile Drive 503-594-0901
Lake Oswego, OR 97035 800-426-6806
Fax: 503-594-0547
e-mail: info@parkinsonsresources.org
www.parkinsonsresources.org
Holly Chaimov, Executive Director

Pennsylvania

7027 **Parkinson Chapter of Greater Pittsburgh**
6507 Wilkins Avenue 412-365-2086
Pittsburgh, PA 15217 e-mail: info@pfwpa.org.
www.parkinsonpittsburgh.org
Doreen Grasso, Chairperson
Maggie Schmidt, Executive Director

7028 **Parkinson Council**
111 Presidential Boulevard 610-668-4292
Bala Cynwyd, PA 19004 Fax: 610-668-4275
e-mail: info@theparkinsoncouncil.org
www.theparkinsoncouncil.org
The Parkinson Council is dedicated to promoting research initiating to find the causes and cure for Parkinson Disease educating patients their caregivers healthcare professionals and the general public about Parkinson's and improving the quality of lif
Mark Vernon, Chairperson
Sally J Bellet, Executive Director

South Dakota

7029 **Parkinson Association of South Dakota**
PO Box 87952 605-328-4227
Sioux Falls, SD 57109-9938 Fax: 605-328-7150
e-mail: info@parkinsonsd.org
www.parkinsonsd.org
Affiliate of The National Parkinson Foundation.
Elaine Spader, President
Lori Jones, Vice President

Virginia

7030 **Parkinson Foundation of the National Capitol Area**
8300 Greensboro Drive 703-287-8729
McLean, VA 22102-4201 Fax: 703-918-4847
e-mail: pfnca@parkinsonfoundation.org
www.parkinsonfoundation.org
Susan D Hamburger, Chairperson

Washington

7031 **Parkinson Educational Society of Puget Sound**
Evergreen Nursing And Rehabilitation
1501 NW 9th Avenue 305-243-6666
Miami, FL 33136-1494 800-327-4545
Fax: 305-243-6824
e-mail: contact@parkinson.org
www.parkinson.org
The National Parkinson Foundation is the largest organization in the world serving persons affected by Parkinson disease. The Foundation supports research for a cure and programs dedicated to improving care and quality of life.
Bernard J Fogel, Chairman

Wisconsin

7032 **Wisconsin Parkinson Association**
945 N 12th Street 414-219-7061
Milwaukee, WI 53233 800-972-5455
Fax: 414-219-6564
www.parkcntr.org/
Affiliate of The National Parkinson Foundation.
Keith Brewer, President

Foundations

7033 **Parkinsons Disease Foundation**
1359 Broadway
New York, NY 10018
212-923-4700
800-457-6676
Fax: 212-923-4778
e-mail: info@pdf.org
www.pdf.org

The foundation has been one of teh leaders in subsidizing research into Parkinson's Disease. Offers many services including The Summer Fellowship Program, The Postdoctoral Fellowship Program, support groups nationwide, grants for clinical and laboratory studies, public awareness and government promotion of the disease.

Lewis P Rowland, MD, President
Robin A Elliott, Executive Director

Libraries & Resource Centers

7034 **Parkinson's Resource Organization**
74090 El Paseo
Palm Desert, CA 92260-4135
760-773-5628
877-775-4111
Fax: 760-773-9803
e-mail: info@parkinsonsresource.org
www.parkinsonsresource.org

Our mission is to help families affected by Parkinson's forge through the journey of the disease's progression with as much quality as life can provide. Working so no one is isolated because of Parkinson's

Jo Rosen, Visionary, President, Founder
Bonnie Shoemaker, Programs Director

Research Centers

7035 **California Institute for Medical Research**
2260 Clove Drive
San Jose, CA 95128
408-998-4554
Fax: 408-998-2723
e-mail: admin@clmr.org
www.cimr.org

Medical research including infectious diseases stroke and cancer specializing in Parkinson's Disease related studies.

David A Stevens, Researcher Infectious Diseases
J William Langston, Researcher Parkinson's Disease

7036 **Texas Tech University Tarbox Parkinson's Disease Institute**
3601 4th Street
Lubbock, TX 79430
806-743-1000
www.ttuhsc.edu

The current objectives of the Tarbox Institute are to provide services for Parkinson's disease patients and their families in the underserved West Texas area; to maintain a Parkinson's Disease Information and Referral Center to enable both healthcare professionals and affected families to obtain the latest information on services available new developments in research support groups and educational literature.

Joseph Green, Chairman

7037 **University of Alabama at Birmingham Parkinsons Disease Center**
1720 7th Avenue S
Birmingham, AL 35294
205-934-9100
Fax: 205-346-78
e-mail: apda@uab.edu
www.uab.edu

Offers educational emotional and political support to Parkinson disease patients and their families.

Ray Watts, Interim CEO
David G Standaert, Director

7038 **William T Gossett Parkinson's Disease Center**
Henry Ford Hospital
Department of Neurology
Detroit, MI 48202
313-972-1693

Jay M Gorell MD, Director

Support Groups & Hotlines

7039 **National Health Information Center**
PO Box 1133
Washington, DC 20013
310-565-4167
800-336-4797
Fax: 301-984-4256
e-mail: info@nhic.org
www.health.gov/nhic

Offers a nationwide information referral service, produces directories and resource guides.

California

7040 **Parkinson's Disease Association of San Die go (PDASD)**
8555 Arco Drive
San Diego, CA 92123-1746
858-273-6763
877-737-7576
Fax: 858-273-6764
e-mail: info@pdasd.org
www.pdasd.org

Information and referral research center for Parkinson's disease patients and their families.

Ronald C Hendrix, Executive Director
Kathleen Wescott, Program Director

Florida

7041 **Greater Daytona Area Parkinson Support Group**
Bishop's Glen Retirement Center
Daytona, FL
904-322-4748
e-mail: boba@n-jcenter.com
www.parkinson.org/shell/areacode.pl

Affiliate of the National Parkinson Foundation.

7042 **National Parkinson Foundation Hotline**
National Parkinson Foundation
1501 NW 9th Avenue Bob Hope Road
Miami, FL 33136
305-243-6666
800-327-4545
Fax: 305-243-5595
www.parkinson.org

Offers support and emergency information for persons with Parkinson's and their families.

Jose Garcia Pebrosa, Director

7043 **Pembroke Pines Parkinson Support Group**
Century Village, Club House
Pembroke Pines, FL 33027
954-433-0947
www.parkinson.org/shell/areacode.pl

Affiliate of the National Parkinson Foundation.

Hawaii

7044 **Kuakini Parkinson Disease (PD) Information & Referral**
Kuakini Medical Center
347 North Kuakini Street
Honolulu, HI 96817
808-528-0935
800-570-1101
Fax: 808-528-1897
e-mail: pr@kuakini.org
www.kuakini.org/SiteMap.asp

The Kuakini Parkinson Disease (PD) Information & Referral Office provides referrals to neurologists and other special services for Parkinson disease patients; provides information about community services to assist PD patients and their caregivers in finding optimal care; distributes educational materials; conducts educational conferences and other activities; and assists with support groups for PD patients and caregivers.

Gary K Kajiwara, President/Chief Executive Officer
Gregg Oishi, SVP/Chief Operating Officer

Illinois

7045 **Rockford Parkinson's Support Group**
5415 Watson Road
Rockford, IL 61108
815-654-0614
800-972-5455

Affiliate of The National Parkinson Foundation, Inc.

Maryland

7046 **Parkinson Support Groups of America**
11376 Cherry Hill Road
Beltsville, MD 20705
301-937-1545

Offers support networks and groups for persons with Parkinson's disease, families, friends and professionals.

Mississippi

7047 APDA Center for Advanced Parkinson Disease Research
Washington University School of Medicine
660 South Euclid 314-362-6909
St Louis, MO 63110 Fax: 314-362-0168
e-mail: joel@npg.wustl.edu
www.neuro.wustl.edu/parkinson/
Information and referral research center for Parkinson's disease patients and their families.
Joel Perlmutter, Director

Missouri

7048 Ozarks Parkinson Support Group
Po Box 50595
Springfield, MO 65805 417-885-9595
www.parkinson.org/shell/areacode.pl
Affiliate of the National Parkinson Foundation.
Monty Montgomery, Contact

New Jersey

7049 New Jersey Parkinson's Disease Information Center
Robert Wood Johnson University Hospital
One Robert Wood Johnson Place 732-745-7520
New Brunswick, NJ 08901 Fax: 732-745-3114
e-mail: elizabeth.schaaf@rwjuh.edu
www.rwjuh.edu/medical_services/
The New Jersey Parkinson's Disease Information and Referral Center reaches out to persons affected by Parkinson's disease, including patients, families and healthcare professionals. This Information and Referral Center is committed to providing community education and information as well as support groups for caregivers and persons with Parkinson's disease.
Elizabeth Schaaf, Parkinson's Disease Center Coordinator

New York

7050 American Parkinson Disease Association Hotline
1250 Hylan Boulevard
Staten Island, NY 10305 800-908-2732
Fax: 718-981-4399
www.attaparkinson.org
Offers information and physician referrals to patients and their families.
Joel Gerstel, Director

7051 New York College of Osteopathic Medicine
PO Box 8000 516-686-7516
Old Westbury, NY 11568-8000 800-345-6948
Fax: 516-686-7613
e-mail: Barbara
www.iris.nyit.edu/nycom/
Information and referral research center for Parkinson's disease patients and their families.
Rosslee Vice President

7052 Parkinson's Support Group of Upstate New York
PO Box 23204
Rochester, NY 14692-3204 716-377-6718
www.parkinson.org/upstate.htm
Affiliate of The National Parkinson Foundation, Inc.
David Look, President

7053 St. John's Episcopal Hospital
Rt 25A 631-361-4100
Smithtown, NY 11787
Information and referral research center for Parkinson's disease patients and their families.

7054 University of Rochester
500 Wilson Boulevard
Rochester, NY 14627 585-275-2121
www.rochester.edu/
Information and referral research center for Parkinson's disease patients and their families.

Oregon

7055 Oregon Health Sciences University
3181 SW Sam Jackson Park Road 503-494-5285
Portland, OR 97201 888-222-6478
Information and referral research center for Parkinson's disease patients and their families.

Pennsylvania

7056 University of Pittsburgh
Forbes Avenue 412-624-4141
Pittsburgh, PA 15260 e-mail: helpdesk+@pitt.edu
www.pitt.edu
Information and referral research center for Parkinson's disease patients and their families.
Mark Nordenderg, Counselor

Texas

7057 Presbyterian Hospital of Dallas
8200 Walnut Hill Lane
Dallas, TX 75231 214-345-6789
www.texashealth.org
Information and referral research center for Parkinson's disease patients and their families.
Mark H Merril

7058 University of Texas HSC at San Antonio
7703 Floyd Curl Drive
San Antonio, TX 78229-3900 512-567-6688
www.uthscsa.edu/
Information and referral research center for Parkinson's disease patients and their families.

Washington

7059 University of Washington
Box 355840 206-543-5369
Seattle, WA 98195-5840 e-mail: uwvic@u.washington.edu
www.washington.edu/
Information and referral research center for Parkinson's disease patients and their families.

Books

7060 Coping with Parkinson's Disease
American Parkinson's Disease Association
1250 Hylan Boulevard
Staten Island, NY 10305-1944 800-223-2732
88 pages

7061 Living with Parkinson's Disease
Demos Medical Publishing
386 Park Avenue S 212-683-0072
New York, NY 10016-8804 800-532-8663
Fax: 212-683-0118
e-mail: orderdept@demospub.com
www.demospub.com
Written specifically for anyone who has been diagnosed with Parkinson's disease, as well as family members and friends.
1996 150 pages
ISBN: 1-888799-10-2
Dr. Diana M Schneider, President

7062 Parkinson's - A Personal Story of Acceptance
Branden Publishing Company
17 Station Street Box 843 617-734-2045
Brookline Village, MA 02147 Fax: 617-734-2046
www.branden.com
1993 162 pages Paperback
ISBN: 0-828319-49-9

7063 Parkinson's Disease & Movement Disorders
Williams & Wilkins
351 W Camden Street 301-528-4000
Baltimore, MD 21201-7912 800-638-0672
1993 640 pages
ISBN: 0-683043-80-3

7064 **Parkinson's Disease Handbook**
National Parkinson Foundation
1501 NW 9th Avenue 305-547-6666
Miami, FL 33136-1407 800-327-4545
Fax: 305-548-4403
www.parkinson.org
A guide for patients and their families regarding the illness of Parkinson's.
Paperback

7065 **Parkinson's Disease: A Guide for Patient and Family**
Raven Press
1185 Avenue of the Americas 212-930-9500
New York, NY 10036-2601 800-777-2295
Recommended by patients, the medical community and the leading medical journals, this guide offers information on the most recent medical advances in the field of Parkinson's disease and answers the patients most frequently asked questions about the illness.
224 pages Hardcover
ISBN: 0-781703-12-3

7066 **Parkinsonian Syndromes**
John H Dekker & Sons
2941 Clydon Avenue SW 616-538-5160
Grand Rapids, MI 49509-2403 Fax: 616-538-0720
1993 584 pages
ISBN: 0-824788-38-9

7067 **The Comfort of Home for Parkinson Disease: A Guide for Caregivers**
Marie Meyer & Paula Derr, RN with Susa Imke, RN/MS, author
CareTrust Publications
PO Box 10283
Portland, OR 97296-0283 800-565-1533
Fax: 415-673-2005
e-mail: sales@comfortofhome.com
www.comfortofhome.com
Comfort will help caregivers be equipped with information about everything from the importance of and noticing "wearing off" signs to making difficult decisions to travel, equipment options, therapies and dietary guidelines. It offers caregivers mental and emotional support in coping with their challenging role, as well.
2007 298 pages
ISBN: 0-966476-77-8

Children's Books

7068 **Journey to Almost There**
Clarion Books
215 Park Avenue S 212-420-5800
New York, NY 10003-1603
An interesting tale that surrounds the relationship of Alison and her Granfather O'Brien when Alison's mother feels that he should enter an elderly home.
Grades 6-9

Newsletters

7069 **American Parkinson Disease Association Newsletter**
60 Bay Street 718-981-8001
Staten Island, NY 10301-2514 800-223-2732
Offers information on the association activities and events, convention and legislative information, medical updates and research reports for the Parkinson's patient and their families.
Quarterly

7070 **News & Review**
Parkinsons Disease Foundation
1359 Broadway 212-923-4700
New York, NY 10018 800-457-6676
Fax: 212-923-4778
e-mail: info@pdf.org
www.pdf.org
In each issue we include reports on scientific research and discoveries, treatments and therapies, commentary from physicians and insight from Parkinson's specialists. We also provide practical suggestions, tips and articles from people who live with the disease and wish to share their experiences.
Quarterly
Lewis P Rowland, MD, President
Robin A Elliott, Executive Director

7071 **Parkinson Report**
National Parkinson Foundation
1501 NW 9th Avenue 305-547-6666
Miami, FL 33136-1407 800-327-4545
Fax: 305-548-4403
www.parkinson.org
Offers association news and events, conference and symposia news, legislative and medical updates, research reports and more for the Parkinson's patient, their families and the general public.
Quarterly

7072 **Parkinson's Disease Foundation Newsletter**
Parkinson's Disease Foundation
650 W 168th Street 212-923-4700
New York, NY 10032-3702 800-457-6676
Provides information on Parkinson's Disease Foundation events, news stories of research findings, and technical advances in the field of patient care.

Pamphlets

7073 **A One-Stop Shop for Parkinson's Informatio n**
Parkinsons Disease Foundation
1359 Broadway 212-923-4700
New York, NY 10018 800-457-6676
Fax: 212-923-4778
e-mail: info@pdf.org
www.pdf.org
An explanation of PDF's services and resources that are available to answer your most important questions about Parkinson's disease. These services include a toll-free helpline, our Ask the Expert web service and print/video materials.
Lewis P Rowland, MD, President
Robin A Elliott, Executive Director

7074 **Adjustment, Adaptation and Accomodation: Psychological Approaches**
National Parkinson Foundation
1501 NW 9th Avenue 305-547-6666
Miami, FL 33136-1407 800-327-4545
Fax: 305-548-4403
www.parkinson.org
Coping strategies for Parkinson's disease.

7075 **Akathisia in Parkinson's Disease**
Parkinson United Foundation
833 W Washington Boulevard 312-733-1893
Chicago, IL 60607
1990

7076 **Answering Your Questions About PROPATH**
525 Middlefield Road
Menlo Park, CA 94025-3447 800-776-7284
This brochure explains and offers an introduction to PROPATH, a program for Parkinson's disease patients.

7077 **Autonomic Failure and Parkinson's Disease**
United Parkinson Foundation
833 W Washington Boulevard 312-733-1893
Chicago, IL 60607-2316
1990

7078 **Balance Disturbances and Parkinson's Disease**
United Parkinson Foundation
833 W Washington Boulevard 312-733-1893
Chicago, IL 60607-2316
1990

7079 **Basic Information About Parkinson's Disease**
American Parkinson's Disease Association
1250 Hylan Boulevard
Staten Island, NY 10305-1944 800-223-2732
Offers information on the illness, incidence, treatments, education and support for both patients and professionals.

7080 **Deep Brain Stimulation for Parkinson's Disease**
Parkinsons Disease Foundation
1359 Broadway 212-923-4700
New York, NY 10018 800-457-6676
Fax: 212-923-4778
e-mail: info@pdf.org
www.pdf.org
This booklet addresses the newest area of surgical options in the treatment of PD symptoms _ deep brain stimulation (or DBS) surgery _ while also describing older surgical approaches used to treat PD.
Lewis P Rowland, MD, President
Robin A Elliott, Executive Director

7081 **Dental Care for the Patient with Parkinson's Disease**
United Parkinson Foundation
833 W Washington Boulevard 312-733-1893
Chicago, IL 60607-2316
1987

7082 **Depression and Dementia in Parkinson's Disease**
United Parkinson Foundation
833 W Washington Boulevard 312-733-1893
Chicago, IL 60607-2316
1993

7083 **Diagnosis Parkinson's Disease: You Are Not Alone**
Parkinsons Disease Foundation
1359 Broadway 212-923-4700
New York, NY 10018 800-457-6676
Fax: 212-923-4778
e-mail: info@pdf.org
www.pdf.org
Designed for the person newly diagnosed with Parkinson's, this informational booklet serves as a reference for the many questions that may arise. It shares resources, medical expert testimony and the experiences of people who have dealt with the diagnosis of Parkinson's disease.
Booklet
Lewis P Rowland, MD, President
Robin A Elliott, Executive Director

7084 **Dietary Considerations for Parkinson's Disease Patients**
United Parkinson Foundation
833 W Washington Boulevard 312-733-1893
Chicago, IL 60607-2316

7085 **Differential Diagnosis of Parkinsonism**
United Parkinson Foundation
833 W Washington Boulevard 312-733-1893
Chicago, IL 60607-2316
1984

7086 **Driving and the Parkinson's Disease Patient: Some Considerations**
United Parkinson Foundation
833 W Washington Boulevard 312-733-1893
Chicago, IL 60607-2316
1994

7087 **Efficacy of Antiparkinson Medications**
United Parkinson Foundation
833 W Washington Boulevard 312-733-1893
Chicago, IL 60607-2316
1983

7088 **Equipment and Suggestions for Persons with Parkinson's Disease**
American Parkinson's Disease Association
1250 Hylan Boulevard
Staten Island, NY 10305-1944 800-223-2732
19 pages

7089 **Eyes and Parkinson's Disease**
United Parkinson Foundation
833 W Washington Boulevard 312-733-1893
Chicago, IL 60607-2316
1986

7090 **Fighting Back Against PD: One Women's Story**
National Parkinson Foundation
1501 NW 9th Avenue 305-547-6666
Miami, FL 33136-1407 800-327-4545
Fax: 305-548-4403
www.parkinson.org
One woman's battle against Parkinson's disease.

7091 **Fulfilling the Hope: Our Commitment to the Parkinson's Community**
Parkinsons Disease Foundation
1359 Broadway 212-923-4700
New York, NY 10018 800-457-6676
Fax: 212-923-4778
e-mail: info@pdf.org
www.pdf.org
This brochure provides an overview of Parkinsons Disease Foundations services and programs.
Lewis P Rowland, MD, President
Robin A Elliott, Executive Director

7092 **Good Nutrition in Parkinson's Disease**
American Parkinson Disease Association
60 Bay Street
Staten Island, NY 10301-2514 800-223-2732
Offers information on diet, nutrients, proteins and recipes for people with Parkinson's disease.

7093 **How to Start a Parkinson's Disease Support Group**
American Parkinson's Disease Association
1250 Hylan Boulevard
Staten Island, NY 10305-1944 800-223-2732
42 pages

7094 **MR Imaging in Parkinson's Disease**
United Parkinson Foundation
833 W Washington Boulevard 312-733-1893
Chicago, IL 60607-2316
1990

7095 **Micrographia**
United Parkinson Foundation
833 W Washington Boulevard 312-733-1893
Chicago, IL 60607-2316
1991

7096 **Neuropsychology and Parkinson's Disease**
United Parkinson Foundation
833 W Washington Boulevard 312-733-1893
Chicago, IL 60607-2316
1992

7097 **Neurotrophic Factors in Parkinson's Disease**
United Parkinson Foundation
833 W Washington Boulevard 312-733-1893
Chicago, IL 60607-2316
1992

7098 **One Step at a Time Brochure**
United Parkinson Foundationon
833 W Washington Boulevard 312-733-1893
Chicago, IL 60607-2316
An exercise manual for the Parkinsonian patient.
1985

7099 **Pain Syndromes and Parkinson's Disease**
United Parkinson Foundation
833 W Washington Boulevard 312-733-1893
Chicago, IL 60607-2316
1990

7100 **Parkinson Handbook: A Guide for Patients and Their Families**
National Parkinson Foundation
1501 NW 9th Avenue 305-547-6666
Miami, FL 33136-1407 800-327-4545
Fax: 305-548-4403
www.parkinson.org
Offers informative, up-to-date information on exercises, hobbies, treatments, speech impairments and psychological aspects.

7101 **Parkinson's Advocacy: The Keys to Empowerment**
Parkinsons Disease Foundation

1359 Broadway
New York, NY 10018
212-923-4700
800-457-6676
Fax: 212-923-4778
e-mail: info@pdf.org
www.pdf.org

Use this informational brochure to learn how to harness your power as a person living with Parkinson's and join the fight for a cure.

Lewis P Rowland, MD, President
Robin A Elliott, Executive Director

7102 **Parkinson's Disease Handbook**
American Parkinson's Disease Association
1250 Hylan Boulevard
Staten Island, NY 10305-1944
800-223-2732
40 pages

7103 **Parkinson's Disease Q&A: A Guide for Patients**
Parkinsons Disease Foundation
1359 Broadway
New York, NY 10018
212-923-4700
800-457-6676
Fax: 212-923-4778
e-mail: info@pdf.org
www.pdf.org

This booklet answers the most frequently asked questions about Parkinson's disease. Movement disorder specialists from the Columbia University Medical Center address topics ranging from signs of Parkinson's to treatment options to daily living issues.

Booklet
Lewis P Rowland, MD, President
Robin A Elliott, Executive Director

7104 **Parkinson's Disease and the Menstrual Cycle**
United Parkinson Foundation
833 W Washington Boulevard
Chicago, IL 60607-2316
312-733-1893
1990

7105 **Parkinson's Disease: The Patient Experience**
United Parkinson Foundation
833 W Washington Boulevard
Chicago, IL 60607-2316
312-733-1893

Booklet designed for patients with Parkinson's disease and their families to explain medical terminology and offer suggestions on how to deal with the disease more easily.

1986

7106 **Parkinson's Patient: What You and Your Family Should Know**
National Parkinson Foundation
1501 NW 9th Avenue
Miami, FL 33136-1407
305-547-6666
800-327-4545
Fax: 305-548-4403
www.parkinson.org

Offers a brief overview of Parkinson's Disease causes, symptoms and treatments as well as offering an insight into statistical information on the illness.

7107 **Patient Perspectives on Parkinson's**
National Parkinson Foundation
1501 NW 9th Avenue
Miami, FL 33136-1407
305-547-6666
800-327-4545
Fax: 305-548-4403
www.parkinson.org

Offers a brief overview of Parkinson's disease, the onset of the illness, depression, sexuality, exercise, sleep and nutrition information for daily living.

45 pages

7108 **Perioperative Management of Parkinson's Disease**
United Parkinson Foundation
833 W Washington Boulevard
Chicago, IL 60607-2316
312-733-1893
1989

7109 **Pet Scans: A New Look at Parkinson's Disease**
United Parkinson Foundation
833 W Washington Boulevard
Chicago, IL 60607-2316
312-733-1893
1989

7110 **Podiatry and Parkinson's Disease**
United Parkinson Foundation
833 W Washington Boulevard
Chicago, IL 60607-2316
312-733-1893
1983

7111 **Postural Hypotension**
United Parkinson Foundation
833 W Washington Boulevard
Chicago, IL 60607-2316
312-733-1893
1988

7112 **Practical Pointers for Parkinson Patients**
National Parkinson Foundation
1501 NW 9th Avenue
Miami, FL 33136-1407
305-547-6666
800-327-4545
Fax: 305-548-4403
www.parkinson.org

7113 **Role of Physical Therapy in Parkinson's Disease**
United Parkinson Foundation
833 W Washington Boulevard
Chicago, IL 60607-2316
312-733-1893
1985

7114 **Sexual and Bladder Difficulties in Parkinson's Disease**
United Parkinson Foundation
833 W Washington Boulevard
Chicago, IL 60607-2316
312-733-1893
1988

7115 **Sleep Problems with Parkinson's Disease**
United Parkinson Foundation
833 W Washington Boulevard
Chicago, IL 60607-2316
312-733-1893
1992

7116 **Speech & Swallowing Problems for Parkinsonians**
National Parkinson Foundation
1501 NW 9th Avenue
Miami, FL 33136-1407
305-547-6666
800-327-4545
Fax: 305-548-4403
www.parkinson.org

7117 **Speech Problems & Swallowing Problems in Parkinson's Disease**
American Parkinson Disease Association
60 Bay Street
Staten Island, NY 10301-2514
800-223-2732

Offers information on speech problems, swallowing problems, hearing impairments and facial mobility for the person with Parkinson's.

7118 **Speech and Voice Impairment**
United Parkinson Foundation
833 W Washington Boulevard
Chicago, IL 60607-2316
312-733-1893
1983

7119 **Stages of Parkinson's Disease**
United Parkinson Foundation
833 W Washington Boulevard
Chicago, IL 60607-2316
312-733-1893
1983

7120 **Suggested Exercise Program for People with Parkinson's Disease**
American Parkinson Disease Association
60 Bay Street
Staten Island, NY 10301-2514
800-223-2732

Exercise program pamphlet with full illustrations explaining each exercise.

23 pages

7121 **Treatment of Parkinson's Disease with Carbidopa-Levodopa**
National Parkinson Foundation
1501 NW 9th Avenue
Miami, FL 33136-1407
305-547-6666
800-327-4545
Fax: 305-548-4403
www.parkinson.org

Offers information on treating Parkinson's Disease.

Audio & Video

7122 **Diagnosis Parkinson's Disease: You Are Not Alone**
Parkinsons Disease Foundation
1359 Broadway 212-923-4700
New York, NY 10018 800-457-6676
Fax: 212-923-4778
e-mail: info@pdf.org
www.pdf.org

Designed for the person newly diagnosed with Parkinson's, this informational booklet and video serve as a reference for the many questions that may arise. It shares resources, medical expert testimony and the experiences of people who have dealt with the diagnosis of Parkinson's disease.
Video & Booklet
Lewis P Rowland, MD, President
Robin A Elliott, Executive Director

7123 **Motivating Moves for People with Parkinson's**
Parkinsons Disease Foundation
1359 Broadway 212-923-4700
New York, NY 10018 800-457-6676
Fax: 212-923-4778
e-mail: info@pdf.org
www.pdf.org

Motivating Moves is a unique program of 24 seated exercises designed especially for people with Parkinson's. Exercises address typical Parkinson's symptoms such as stability, flexibility, posture, vocal range and facial expressivity. The video is divided into three sections, "How to Do Motivating Moves" (45 minutes), "The Exercise Class" (36 minutes) and "Practical Tips for Daily Living" (4 minutes).
Video
Lewis P Rowland, MD, President
Robin A Elliott, Executive Director

7124 **PDF Exercise Program**
Parkinsons Disease Foundation
1359 Broadway 212-923-4700
New York, NY 10018 800-457-6676
Fax: 212-923-4778
e-mail: info@pdf.org
www.pdf.org

This program consists of three sets of exercises specifically designed for PD patients. Each exercise is clearly illustrated in a 3-ring binder with flip-chart pages and includes two cassette tapes, which provide verbal cues and music for timing.
Cassettes
Lewis P Rowland, MD, President
Robin A Elliott, Executive Director

7125 **Parkingson's: Lynda's Story**
David Tucker, author
Fanlight Productions
4196 Washington Street 617-469-4999
Boston, MA 02131 800-937-4113
Fax: 617-469-3379
e-mail: fanlight@fanlight.com
www.fanlight.com

Parkingson's disease is robbing Lynda McKenzie of normal coordination and movement. She's prepared to participate in a clinical study of surgery to transplant fetal cells directly into her brain, but she will have to live for a year not knowing whether she has received the actual cells or a placebo.
1999 46 Minutes
ISBN: 1-572954-22-1
Nicole Johnson, Publicity Coordinator

Web Sites

7126 **Healing Well**
www.healingwell.com

An online health resource guide to medical news, chat, information and articles, newsgroups and message boards, books, disease-related web sites, medical directories, and more for patients, friends, and family coping with disabling diseases, disorders, or chronic illnesses.

7127 **Health Finder**
www.healthfinder.gov

Searchable, carefully developed web site offering information on over 1000 topics. Developed by the US Department of Health and Human Services, the site can be used in both English and Spanish.

7128 **Healthlink USA**
www.healthlinkusa.com

Health information concerning treatment, cures, prevention, diagnosis, risk factors, research, support groups, email lists, personal stories and much more. Updated regularly.

7129 **Helios Health**
www.helioshealth.com

Online resource for your health information. Detailed information about specific health topics, access to expert advice from our Medical Advisory Board, and up-to-date health news.

7130 **MedicineNet**
www.medicinenet.com

An online resource for consumers providing easy-to-read, authoritative medical and health information.

7131 **Medscape**
www.mywebmd.com

Medscape offers specialists, primary care physicians, and other health professionals the Web's most robust and integrated medical information and educational tools.

7132 **National Parkinson Foundation**
www.parkinson.org

Information on research, diagnosis, treatment and care for men and women suffering from parkinson's and other related neurological diseases.

7133 **Neurology Channel**
www.neurologychannel.com

Find clearly explained, medically accurate information regarding conditions, including an overview, symptoms, causes, diagnostic procedures and treatment options. On this site it is possible to ask questions and get information from a neurologist and connect to people who have similar health interests.

7134 **WebMD**
www.webmd.com

Information on Parkinson's disease, including articles and resources.

Description

7135 **Post-Polio Syndrome**

Post-Polio syndrome, PPS, also known as the late effects of polio or post polio sequelae, is characterized by new symptoms that occur in people with a history of polio after a long period of stability during which whatever strength they had recovered remained unchanged. PPS affects approximately 60 percent of polio survivors, 20 to 40 years after the initial episode. The hallmark of PPS is new weakness. Other symptoms include fatigue, pain, difficulty breathing and swallowing, intolerance to cold, and new muscle atrophy.

While the cause of PPS is not clearly understood, two theories exist. One suggests that it is caused by normal muscle loss that accompanies aging. The other is that PPS is causd by the repeated over use of muscle groups. In both cases, muscle groups not previously known to have been affected by polio are weakened, and it is this weakness that is the major indicator of PPS. A polio survior with an affected leg may find that his or her arms are newly affected. Whether the arm problems are a result of undetected muscle damage that occurred at the time of the original polio or newer damage resulting from the over use of the remaining good muscles, or a combinatin of the two, is not clearly understood.

PPS is frequently emotionally difficult for polio survivors. Many feel they have triumphed over their initial polio, or have come to terms with their resulting disabilities. To think that the polio is coming back is often terrifying. These emotional issues are frequently made more difficult by the fact that PPS is often mis-diagnosed as other conditions or normal aging. Also, patients are often given misinformation about PPS.

Post-polio syndrome, like most diseases classified as syndromes, does not have a specific diagnostic test, but a diagnosis of exclusion. This means that other medical conditions that may present wtih symptoms similar to those found in PPS should be considered and excluded, if possible. Once diagnosis of PPS is determined, treatment is individualized by primary symptoms and may include medications, supervised therapy, injections and, in some cases, surgery.

National Agencies & Associations

7136 **Post Polio Awareness and Support Society o f British Columbia**
#2-2630 Ross Lane 250-477-8244
Victoria, BC, V8T-5L5 Fax: 250-477-8287
e-mail: ppass@ppass.bc.ca
www.ppass.bc.ca
A non-profit society that links area groups, through our board and our provincial office in Victoria.
Joan Toone, President

Support Groups & Hotlines

7137 **PostPolio Health International**
4207 Lindell Boulevard 314-534-0475
Saint Louis, MO 63108-2915 Fax: 314-534-5070
e-mail: info@postpolio.org
www.post-polio.org/
Post-Polio Health International's mission is to enhance the lives and independence of polio survivors and home ventilator users through education, advocacy, research and networking.
Joan L Headley, Executive Director
Sheryl Rudy, Webmaster

Books

7138 **Managing Post-Polio: A Guide for Polio Survivors and Their Families**
Yale University Press
PO Box 209040 203-732-0960
New Haven, CT 06520-9040 Fax: 203-432-0948
Diagnosis and management of polio-related health problems . Essential resources for polio survivors, their families and health care providers.

7139 **Managing Post-Polio: A Guide to Living Well with Post-Polio Syndrome**
ABI Professional Publications
PO Box 5243 703-525-5488
Arlington, VA 22205 Fax: 703-524-4105
Practical information resulting from a combination of professional knowledge and personal experience. A comprehensive array of topics are addressed: the diagnostic process, finding expert medical care, energy conservation, psychosocial aspects of disability, support groups, vocational strategies, managed care concerns, Social Security benefits, and internet resources.
256 pages

Newsletters

7140 **Polio Network News**
Post-Polio Health International
4207 Lindell Boulevard 314-534-0475
St. Louis, MO 63108-2915 Fax: 314-534-5070
e-mail: ventinfo@post-polio.org
www.post-polio.org/IVUN
Joan Headley, Executive Director

7141 **Post-Polio Health**
Post-Polio Health International
4207 Lindell Boulevard 314-534-0475
Saint Louis, MO 63108-2915 Fax: 314-534-5070
e-mail: ventinfo@post-polio.org
www.post-polio.org/IVUN
12 pages Quarterly
Joan Headley, Executive Director

7142 **Post-Polio Health International**
Joan L Headley, author
4207 Lindell Boulevard 314-534-0475
St. Louis, MO 63108-2915 Fax: 314-534-5070
e-mail: info@post-polio.org
www.post-polio.org
Provides educational materials, advocacy, networking and support research to enhance the lives and independence of polio survivors and users of home mechanical ventilators. Minimum $25.00 with membership.
12 pages
Joan Headley, Executive Director

7143 **Ventilator-Assisted Living**
Joan L Headley, author
4207 Lindell Boulevard 314-534-0475
St. Louis, MO 63108-2915 Fax: 314-534-5070
e-mail: info@post-polio.org
www.post-polio.org

Provides educational materials, advocacy, networking and support research to enhance the lives and independence of polio survivors and users of home mechanical ventilators. Minimum $25.00 with membership.
12 pages
Joan Headley, Executive Director

7144 Ventilator: Assisted Living
Post-Polio Health International
4207 Lindell Boulevard 314-534-0475
St. Louis, MO 63108-2915 Fax: 314-534-5070
e-mail: ventinfo@post-polio.org
www.post-polio.org/IVUN
The newsletter of the International Ventilator Users Network, an affiliate of Post-Polio Health International.
12 pages Newsletter
Joan Headley, Executive Director

Pamphlets

7145 Guidelines for People Who Have Had Polio
March of Dimes
PO Box 1657 717-820-8104
Wilkes-Barre, PA 18703 800-367-6630
Fax: 570-825-1987
Located on website as a PDF file. Information based on March of Dimes International Conference on Post-Polio Syndrome.

7146 Post-Polio Syndrome: Identifying Best Practices in Diagnosis and Care
March of Dimes
233 Park Avenue South 212-353-8353
New York, NY 10003 Fax: 212-254-3518
e-mail: NY639@marchofdimes.com
www.marchofdimes.com
Located on website as PDF file.

Web Sites

7147 EMedicine
www.emedicine.com/pmr/topic110.htm
EMedicine was launched in 1996 and is the largest and most current clinical knowledge base available to physicians and health professionals.

7148 International Rehabilitation Center for Polio
www.polioclinic.org
International Rehabilitation Center for Polio (IRCP) at Spaulding Rehabilitation HOspital website offers information about PPS and resources for polio survivors and others with an interest in post-polio syndrome.

7149 MedicineNet
www.medicinenet.com
An online resource for consumers providing easy-to-read, authoritative medical and health information.

7150 Polio Experience Network
www.polionet.org
The Polio Experience Network offers information, inspiration, ideas and resources for polio survivors and those seeking information on post-polio syndrome.

7151 Social Security Administration
www.ssa.gov/disability
The Social Security Administration website on disability benefits includes information about how to apply for benefits.

Description

7152 **Prader-Willi Syndrome**

Prader-Willi syndrome, PWS, is a group of abnormalities first described by Drs. Prader, Labart, and Willi in 1956. This uncommon condition occurs in about one in every 20,000 births. In about 50 percent of PWS patients, there is a missing piece (deletion) of part of chromosome 15.

PWS is characterized by obesity, short stature, small penis and testicles (hypogonadism), small hands and feet, mental retardation and decreased muscle tone. During the toddler years, many patients begin to overeat. Some persons with PWS may show signs of obsessive-compulsive disorder, apart from their obsessions with food. In addition to insatiable hunger, other behavioral features include emotional highs and lows, poor motor skills and cognitive impairment. Sexual development is halted, and facial and skeletal abnormalities develop.

Therapies for PWS are aimed at symptoms with an emphasis on specialized diets and customized exercise programs and support.

National Agencies & Associations

7153 **National Institute of Child Health and Human Development**
31 Center Drive
Bethesda, MD 20892
301-496-5133
Fax: 301-496-7101
www.nih.gov
Offers reprints, articles and various information on Prader-Willi Syndrome in children and adults.
Duane Alexander, Director

7154 **Prader-Willi Syndrome Association (USA) Prader-Willi Syndrome Association**
Prader-Willi Syndrome Association (USA)
8588 Potter Park Drive
Sarasota, FL 34238
941-312-0400
800-926-4797
Fax: 941-312-0142
e-mail: webmaster1@pwsausa.org
www.pwsausa.org
Provides to parents and professionals a national and international network of information, support services and research endeavors to expressly meet the needs of affected children and adults and their families. Offers 31 state chapters and published materials.
Janalee Heinemann, Executive Director

State Agencies & Associations

Arizona

7155 **Prader-Willi Syndrome Arizona Association: Phoenix Area**
Prader-Willi Syndrome Association
3920 East Bronco Trail
Phoenix, AZ 85044
480-598-0966
e-mail: shemc@netzero.net
www.pwsausa.org
Sheila McMahon, President

7156 **Prader-Willi Syndrome Arizona Association Prader-Willi Syndrome Association**
Prader-Willi Syndrome Association
13839 N Bentwater Drive
Tucson, AZ 85737
520-297-7025
e-mail: p.penta@comcast.net
www.pwsausa.org
Tammie Penta, President

Arkansas

7157 **Prader-Willi Arkansas Association Prader-Willi Syndrome Association**
Prader-Willi Syndrome Association
2504 S Drive
N Little Rock, AR 72118-4245
501-753-8715
e-mail: jpattpnlr@msn.com
www.pwsausa.org
Jim Patton, President

California

7158 **Prader-Willi California Foundation**
514 N Prospect Avenue
Redondo Beach, CA 90277
310-372-5053
800-400-9994
Fax: 310-372-4329
e-mail: PWCF1@aol.com
www.pwsausa.org
Lisa Graziano, Executive Director

7159 **Prader-Willi California Foundation: Newport Area**
419 Fullerton Avenue
Newport Beach, CA 92663
949-642-9772
e-mail: olsonbb@adelphia.net
www.pwsausa.org
Robert J Olsen, President

Colorado

7160 **Prader-Willi Colorado Association Prader-Willi Syndrome Association**
Prader-Willi Syndrome Association
8290 S Yukon Way
Littleton, CO 80128
303-973-4780
e-mail: hosler@dynamicsolutions.com
www.pwsausa.org
Lynette Hosler, President

Connecticut

7161 **Prader-Willi Connecticut Association Prader-Willi Syndrome Association**
Prader-Willi Syndrome Association
35 Ansonia Drive
N Haven, CT 06473-3306
203-239-9902
e-mail: pwsactchapter@yahoo.com
www.pwsausa.org
Vicki Knoph, President

Delaware

7162 **Prader-Willi Delaware Association Prader-Willi Syndrome Association**
Prader-Willi Syndrome Association
300 Bethel Circle Millwood
Middletown, DE 19709
302-378-7385
e-mail: swede455@aol.com
www.pwsausa.org
Karen Swanson, President

Florida

7163 **Prader-Willi Florida Assocition Prader-Willi Syndrome Association**
Prader-Willi Syndrome Association
17777 S W 285 Street
Homestead, FL 33030
305-245-6484
e-mail: pwfa2000@aol.com
www.pwsausa.org
Debbie Stallings, Co-President
John Stallings, Co-President

Georgia

7164 **PWSA of Georgia Prader-Willi Syndrome Association**
Prader-Willi Syndrome Association
562 Lakeland Plaza
Cumming, GA 30040
770-886-2334
877-866-2334
Fax: 770-886-2335
e-mail: pwsaga@earthlink.net
www.pwsausa.org
Debbie Lang, Executive Director

Hawaii

7165 **Prader-Willi Northwest Association**
Prader-Willi Syndrome Association
269 Kaha Street
Hailua, HI 96734
808-263-8177
e-mail: susanlundh@yahoo.com
www.pwsausa.org

Susan Lundh, President

Idaho

7166 **Prader-Willi Northwest Association**
Prader-Willi Syndrome Association
550 Lodgepole Road
Athol, ID 83801
208-683-2993
e-mail: idaho4ts@aol.com
www.pwsausa.org

Susan Lundh, President
Gene Todhunter, Local Contact

Illinois

7167 **PWSA Illinois Prader-Willi Syndrome Association**
Prader-Willi Syndrome Association
2128 N Sedgwick Street
Chicago, IL 60614
773-281-9170
e-mail: illinois@pwsausa.org
www.pwsausa.org

Jeffrey Fender, President

Indiana

7168 **PWSA of Indiana Prader-Willi Syndrome Association**
Prader-Willi Syndrome Association
7536 Moonbeam Drive
Indianapolis, IN 46259
317-527-9173
e-mail: pwsain@yahoo.com
www.pwsausa.org

Jacque McGuire, President

Iowa

7169 **PWSA of Iowa Prader-Willi Syndrome Association**
Prader-Willi Syndrome Association
15130 Holcomb Avenue
Clive, IA 50325-9695
515-987-0288
e-mail: ktcaedav@netins.net
www.pwsausa.org

Tammi Davis, President
Edie Bogaczyk, President

Kansas

7170 **PWSA of Kansas Prader-Willi Syndrome Association**
Prader-Willi Syndrome Association
14 NE Bayview Drive
Lees Summit, MO 64064-1624
816-350-1375
e-mail: national@pwsausa.org
www.pwsausa.org

Terri Douglas, Prader-Willi Syndrome Advocate
Barry Douglas, Prader-Willi Syndrome Advocate

Kentucky

7171 **Prader-Willi Kentucky Association Prader-Willi Syndrome Association**
Prader-Willi Syndrome Association
9213 Reigate Court
Louisville, KY 40222
502-339-7872
e-mail: national@pwsausa.org
www.pwsausa.org

Frank Beckles, President
Rick Settles

Maine

7172 **Prader-Willi New England Association**
Andover, MA 01757
978-475-5570
e-mail: pwsane@aol.com
www.pwsausa.org

Eileen Rullo, President

Massachusetts

7173 **Prader-Willi New England Association Prader-Willi Syndrome Association**
Prader-Willi Syndrome Association
Andover, MA 01757
978-475-5570
e-mail: pwsane@aol.com
www.pwsausa.org

Eileen Rullo, President

7174 **Prader-Willi Syndrome of Western Massachusetts**
Prader-Willi Syndrome Association
10 Cottage Avenue
Holyoke, MA 01040
413-533-8335
e-mail: national@pwsausa.org
www.pwsausa.org

Violet Gingras, President

Michigan

7175 **Prader-Willi Syndrome Association of Michigan**
10756 Woodbushe
Lowell, MI 49331
616-642-0017
e-mail: chrishendrick@cablespeed.com
www.pwsausa.org

Jon Hendrick, Co-Chairperson
Chris Hendrick, Co-Chairperson

Minnesota

7176 **PWSA of Minnesota Prader-Willi Syndrome Association**
Prader-Willi Syndrome Association
7209 Oaklawn Avenue
Woodbury, MN 55105
952-893-9318
e-mail: national@pwsausa.org
www.pwsausa.org

Jey Behnken, President

Missouri

7177 **PWSA Missouri Chapter Prader-Willi Syndrome Association**
Prader-Willi Syndrome Association
1465 S Grand Boulevard Missouri Str
Louis, MO 63104
314-268-4027
Fax: 314-935-7461
e-mail: national@pwsausa.org
www.pwsausa.org

Barbara Whitman, President

Montana

7178 **Prader-Willi Northwest Association**
3706 29th Avenue W
Seattle, WA 98199
206-285-7679
e-mail: susanlundh@yahoo.com
www.pwsausa.org

This association covers Washington, Oregon, Idaho, Montana, Alaska,and Hawaii.
Susan Lundh, President

Nebraska

7179 **PWSA Nebraska Chapter Prader-Willi Syndrome Association**
Prader-Willi Syndrome Association
302 S 49th Avenue
Omaha, NE 68132
402-551-9168
e-mail: national@pwsausa.org
www.pwsausa.org

Jennifer Varner, Local Contact

New Jersey

7180 **Prader-Willi New Jersey Association Prader-Willi Syndrome Association**
Prader-Willi Syndrome Association
514 Gatewod Road
Cherry Hill, NJ 08003
856-795-4229
e-mail: national@pwsausa.org
www.pwsausa.org

Sybil Cohen, President
Judy Livny, Vice-President

New York

7181 **Prader-Willi Alliance of New York Prader-Willi Syndrome Association**
Prader-Willi Syndrome Association
PO Box 1114 716-276-2211
Niagara Falls, NY 14304 800-442-1655
e-mail: alliance@prader-willi.org
www.prader-willi.org
Barbara McManus, President

North Carolina

7182 **Prader-Willi Syndrome Association of North Carolina**
Prader-Willi Syndrome Association
1404 Sutton Drive 252-527-1813
Kinston, NC 28501 e-mail: national@pwsausa.org
www.pwsausa.org
Sally St John, President

North Dakota

7183 **PWSA Fargo Chapter Prader-Willi Syndrome Association**
Prader-Willi Syndrome Association
2902 S University Drive 701-232-3301
Fargo, ND 58103-6032 Fax: 701-237-5775
e-mail: fraser@fraserltd.org
www.fraserltd.org

Ohio

7184 **PWSA Ohio Chapter Prader-Willi Syndrome Association**
Prader-Willi Syndrome Association
4075 W 226 Street 440-716-0552
Fairview Park, OH 44126 e-mail: pwsaohio@aol.com
www.pwsausa.org
Jennifer Bolander, President

Oklahoma

7185 **PWSA Oklahoma Chapter Prader-Willi Syndrome Association**
Prader-Willi Syndrome Association
3816 SE 89th Street 405-677-8089
Oklahoma City, OK 74135-6222 e-mail: national@pwsausa.org
www.pwsausa.org
Daphne Mosley, President

7186 **Prader-Willi Association: Tulsa Area**
4444 S Columbia Avenue 918-747-7848
Tulsa, OK 74105-5221 e-mail: marishack@aol.om
www.pwsausa.org
Curt Shacklett, Chairman

Oregon

7187 **PWSA Oregon Chapter Prader-Willi Syndrome Association**
Prader-Willi Syndrome Association
303 E Historic Columbia 503-669-7191
Troutdale, OR 97060 e-mail: national@pwsausa.org
www.pwsausa.org
Cory Eliason, President

Pennsylvania

7188 **PWSA Pennsylvania Chapter Prader-Willi Syndrome Association**
Prader-Willi Syndrome Association
104 Persimmon Place 724-779-4415
Cranberry Township, PA 16066 e-mail: national@pwsausa.org
www.pwsausa.org
Debbie Fabio, President

South Carolina

7189 **PWSA South Carolina Chapter Prader-Willi Syndrome Association**
Prader-Willi Syndrome Association
912 Lake Spur Lane 803-345-1379
Chapin, SC 29036 e-mail: national@pwsausa.org
www.pwsausa.org
Rhett Eleazer, Local Contact

Tennessee

7190 **PWSA Tennessee Chapter Prader-Willi Syndrome Association**
Prader-Willi Syndrome Association
105 Foxwood Lane 615-790-6659
Franklin, TN 37065 e-mail: national@pwsausa.org
www.pwsausa.org
Terry Bolander, Local Contact

Texas

7191 **PWSA Texas Chapter Prader-Willi Syndrome Association**
Prader-Willi Syndrome Association
14427 Perchin Drive 210-946-6789
San Antonio, TX 78247 e-mail: national@pwsausa.org
www.pwsausa.org
Susan Carvajal, Local Contact

Utah

7192 **Prader-Willi Utah Association Prader-Willi Syndrome Association**
Prader-Willi Syndrome Association
2652 Nottingham Way 801-582-0998
Salt Lake City, UT 84108 Fax: 801-768-3924
e-mail: national@pwsausa.org
www.pwsausa.org
Lisa Thornton, President

Virginia

7193 **PWSA of Maryland, Virginia & DC**
Prader-Willi Syndrome Association
2601 Chriswell Place 410-822-3752
Hernson, VA 20171-2940 e-mail: pwsausa@pwsausa.org
www.pwsausa.org
Linda Keder, President
Susie Wood, Maryland Contact

Washington

7194 **Prader-Willi Northwest Association Prader-Willi Syndrome Association**
Prader-Willi Syndrome Association
16208 SE 46th Place 206-285-7679
Bellevue, WA 98006 e-mail: jlubderwood@juno.com
www.pwsausa.org
Joanne Underwood, Co-President
Susan Lundh, Co-President

Wisconsin

7195 **PWSA of Wisconsin Prader-Willi Syndrome Association**
Prader-Willi Syndrome Association
2701 N Alexander Street 920-882-6371
Appleton, WI 54911-2512 866-797-2947
e-mail: wisconsion@pwsausa.org
www.pwsausa.org
Mary Lynn Larson, Program Director
Mike Larson, President

Support Groups & Hotlines

7196 **National Health Information Center**
PO Box 1133 310-565-4167
Washington, DC 20013 800-336-4797
Fax: 301-984-4256
e-mail: info@nhic.org
www.health.gov/nhic
Offers a nationwide information referral service, produces directories and resource guides.

7197 **PraderWilli Syndrome Association**
PraderWilli Syndrome Association
5700 Midnight Pass Road
Sarasota, FL 34242
941-312-0400
800-926-4797
Fax: 941-312-0142
e-mail: pwsuasa@aol.com
www.pwsausa.org

Jenalee Heinemann, Executive Director
Steve Dudrow, Business Manager

Books

7198 **Child with Prader-Willi Syndrome: Birth to Three**
Prader-Willi Syndrome Association (USA)
8588 Potter Park Drive
Sarasota, FL 34238
941-312-0400
800-926-4797
Fax: 941-312-0142
e-mail: info@pwsausa.com
www.pwsausa.org

Discusses the common concerns of the first three years and offers specific recommendations for early intervention strategies. A helpful and positive resource for families, physicians, early intervention workers and other care providers. Booklet
2004 34 pages
Craig Pulhemus, Executive Director

7199 **Early Years**
Prader-Willi Syndrome Association (USA)
8588 Potter Park Drive
Sarasota, FL 34238
941-312-0400
800-926-4797
Fax: 941-312-0142
e-mail: info@pwsausa.com
www.pwsausa.org

Collection of articles regarding young children with PWS — many from a parent's perspective.
1998 37 pages
Craig Polhemus, Executive Director

7200 **Growing Up with Prader-Willi Syndrome: Personal Reflections of a Mother**
Prader-Willi Syndrome Association (USA)
8588 Potter Park Drive
Sarasota, FL 34238
941-312-0400
800-926-4797
Fax: 941-312-0142
e-mail: info@pwsausa.com
www.pwsausa.org

Collection of 15 articles. Tips for managing family life on a practical level. Booklet
2003 37 pages
Craig Polhemus, Executive Director

7201 **Growth Hormone & Prader-Willi Syndrome: A Reference for Familes & Care Providers**
Linda S. Keder, author
Prader-Willi Syndrome Association (USA)
8588 Potter Park Drive
Sarasota, FL 34238
941-312-0400
800-926-4797
Fax: 941-312-0142
e-mail: info@pwsausa.com
www.pwsausa.org

Reference for families and care providers.
2001 52 pages
Craig Polhemus, Executive Director

7202 **Handbook for Parents**
Shirley Neason, author
Prader-Willi Syndrome Association (USA)
8588 Potter Park Drive
Sarasota, FL 34238
941-312-0400
800-926-4797
Fax: 941-312-0142
e-mail: info@pwsausa.com
www.pwsausa.org

Parent-to-Parent handbook for understanding and managing issues related to PWS, from birth to adulthood.
1999 75 pages
Craig Polhemus, Executive Director

7203 **Nutrition Care for Children with PWS: Infants and Toddlers**
J. Hovasi & D. Doorlag, with J. Loker & C. Loker, author
Prader-Willi Syndrome Association (USA)
8588 Potter Park Drive
Sarasota, FL 34238
941-312-0400
800-926-4797
Fax: 941-312-0142
e-mail: info@pwsausa.com
www.pwsausa.org

Provides answers to frequently asked questions about nutrition and feeding infants and toddlers with PWS.
2004 62 pages
Craig Polhemus, Executive Director

7204 **Sometimes I'm Mad, Sometimes I'm Glad - A Sibling Booklet**
Sarah Heinemann, author
Prader-Willi Syndrome Association (USA)
8588 Potter Park Drive
Sarasota, FL 34238
941-312-0400
800-926-4797
Fax: 941-312-0142
e-mail: info@pwsausa.com
www.pwsausa.org

Explains sibling relationships and how they are affected by Prader-Willi syndrome. Written in the voice of a sibling of someone with PWS. Ages 5-13
32 pages
Craig Polhemus, Executive Director

7205 **Supporting Adults with Prader-Willi Syndro me in a Residential Setting**
B.J. Goff, Ed.D, author
Prader-Willi Syndrome Association (USA)
8588 Potter Pass Drive
Sarasota, FL 34238
941-312-0400
800-926-4797
Fax: 941-312-0142
e-mail: info@pwsausa.com
www.pwsausa.org

Filling a large gap for care givers of those with Prader-Willi Sydrome, this is an extensive manual covering residential care issues; including management strategies, specifics for phase of life, and a number of additional ideas.
2002 121 pages
Craig Polhemus, Executive Director

Newsletters

7206 **Gathered View**
Prader-Willi Syndrome Association (USA)
8588 Potter Park Drive
Sarasota, FL 34238
941-312-0400
800-926-4797
Fax: 941-312-0142
e-mail: info@pwsausa.com
www.pwsausa.org

The official newsletter of PWSA, mailed 6 time/year to members. Offers current research findings, behavior and weight management techniques, educational news, articles and more.
BiMonthly
Craig Polhemus, Executive Director

Pamphlets

7207 **An Early Prader-Willi Syndrome Diagnosis & How to Make it Easier on Parents**
Prader-Willi Foundation
40 Holly Lane
Roslyn Hts, NY 11577-1533
516-944-8136
800-253-7993
Fax: 516-944-3173
e-mail: foundation@prader-willi.inter.net
www.prader-willi.org

A parent of a child with PWS and an advocate for others with the afflication speaks.

7208 **Behavior Management: Collection of Articless**
Prader-Willi Syndrome Association (USA)

8588 Potter Park Drive
Sarasota, FL 34238
941-312-0400
800-926-4797
Fax: 941-312-0142
e-mail: info@pwsausa.com
www.pwsausa.org

Includes general articles of behavior concerns, use of psychotropic medications, skin picking and teaching social skills.
2003 49 pages
Craig Polhemus, Executive Director

7209 **Educational Choices for Children with PWS**
Prader-Willi Foundation
40 Holly Lane
Roslyn Hts, NY 11577-1533
516-944-8136
800-253-7993
Fax: 516-944-3173
e-mail: foundation@prader-willi.inter.net
www.prader-willi.org

Parents of young children with Prader-Willi syndrome discuss their individual philosophies of educational choice - inclusion vs. specialized setting.

7210 **Nutrition Care for Adolescents and Adults with PWS**
Karenn H. Borgie, MA, RD, author
Prader-Willi Syndrome Association (USA)
8588 Potter Park Drive
Sarasota, FL 34238
941-312-0400
800-926-4797
Fax: 941-312-0142
e-mail: info@pwsausa.com
www.pwsausa.org

covers essential diet information for families, caregivers, and residential service providers.
Craig Polhemus, Executive Director

7211 **Nutrition Care for Children with PWS, Ages 3-9**
Karen H. Borgie, MA, RD, author
Prader-Willi Syndrome Association (USA)
8588 Potter Park Drive
Sarasota, FL 34238
941-312-0400
800-926-4797
Fax: 941-312-0142
e-mail: info@pwsausa.com
www.pwsausa.org

Discusses calorie needs, supplements, diet planning, food management, and exchange lists. Softvcover.
Craig Polhemus, Executive Director

7212 **What Educators Should Know About Prader-Willi Syndrome**
Prader-Willi Syndrome Association (USA)
8588 Potter Park Drive
Sarasota, FL 34238
941-312-0400
800-926-4797
Fax: 941-312-0142
e-mail: info@pwsausa.com
www.pwsausa.org

Offers guidelines and strategies for helping the student with PWS stay focused, develop skills and knowledge, and minimize problems associated with the syndrome in the school setting.
Craig Polhemus, Executive Director

Audio & Video

7213 **Prader-Willi Syndrome: An Overview for Health Professionals**
Prader-Willi Syndrome Association
5700 Midnight Pass Road
Sarasota, FL 34242-3000
941-312-0400
800-926-4797
Fax: 941-312-0142
e-mail: national@pwsausa.org
www.pwsausa.org

Essential viewing for all health care professionals who are not experts on prader-willi syndrome. It deals with all major genetics and health care issues of the child with PWS.
2002

7214 **Prader-Willi Syndrome: the Early Years**
Prader-Willi Syndrome Association
5700 Midnight Pass Road
Sarasota, FL 34242-3000
941-312-0400
800-926-4797
Fax: 941-312-0142
e-mail: national@pwsausa.org
www.pwsausa.org

Offers help and practical suggestions for those families with a young child newly diagnosed with PWS. Genetics, medical, early intervention and family issues are presented, personalized with family interviews. Although focusing on young children, this video is a wonderful resource for schools and families with children of all ages.
2002

Web Sites

7215 **Healthlink USA**
www.healthlinkusa.com

Health information concerning treatment, cures, prevention, diagnosis, risk factors, research, support groups, email lists, personal stories and much more. Updated regularly.

7216 **MedicineNet**
www.medicinenet.com

An online resource for consumers providing easy-to-read, authoritative medical and health information.

7217 **Medscape**
www.mywebmd.com

Medscape offers specialists, primary care physicians, and other health professionals the Web's most robust and integrated medical information and educational tools.

Description

7218 **Raynaud's Disease**

Raynaud's disease is the spasm of blood vessels to fingers and toes, resulting in restricted blood supply in response to cold or emotional upset. Symptoms include tingling and numbness. During an episode, which can last from minutes to hours, the arteries contract briefly and the skin, deprived of oxygen, turns pale and then blue. As arteries relax and blood begins to flow, reddening, tingling, or swelling may occur. While hands and feet are most commonly affected, the nose and ears can also be subject to Raynaud's.

Raynaud's most commonly affects women under 40, accounting for perhaps 90 percent of all cases. When the classic symptoms are present, without other complaints, the condition is referred to as Raynaud's disease (primary Raynaud's), and generally results in no serious consequences. The second form, Raynaud's phenomenon (secondary Raynaud's), is the result of other underlying medical conditions, including scleroderma, vascular disease, rheumatoid arthritis and lupus.

Certain drugs can also trigger Raynaud's, including ergotamine and a number of beta-blocking drugs that are used in the treatment of heart disease. About 10 percent of Raynaud's cases are related to specific repetitive stress activities such as the operation of pneumatic drills and other hand-held vibrating machinery. In most Raynaud's cases, symptoms are discomforting but not serious. In extreme cases, Raynaud's can result in tissue atrophy and gangrene. Preventative measures include protection from cold, even when taking food out of the refrigerator or freezer, and avoiding behavior that disrupts bloodflow, for instance, smoking cigarettes.

Medical treatment of Raynaud's is directed toward improving blood flow to the extremities. In many cases, simple exercises are prescribed, and relaxation techniques, such as biofeedback, teach the body to ignore trivial or transient signals of cold. In other cases, vasodilator drugs which are designed to relax and open blood vessels to improve blood flow are prescribed. In the most extreme cases, surgery may be performed to cut nerves that may be inappropriately triggering the contraction of arteries, although relief may last only 1 to 2 years. Herbal remedies have been used in the treatment of Raynaud's and other circulatory conditions, especially the Chinese herb Dong quai. There is also evidence that foods rich in vitamin E, and fish oils, may help to reduce or moderate the vascular spasms that produce Raynaud's symptoms.

National Agencies & Associations

7219 **Arthritis Foundation**
1330 W Peachtree Street 404-872-7100
Atlanta, GA 30309 800-283-7800
Fax: 404-872-0457
e-mail: help@arthritis.org
www.arthritis.org

A nonprofit organization that depends on volunteers to provide services to help people with arthritis. Supports research to find ways to cure and prevent arthritis and provides services to improve the quality of life for those affected by arthritis.
Cecile Perich, Chair
John H Klippel MD, President and CEO

7220 **Raynaud's Foundation**
PO Box 346176 773-622-9220
Chicago, IL 60634-6176 Fax: 773-622-9221
members.aol.com/raynauds/index.ht

The Raynaud's Foundation is a non-profit dedicated to the promotion of education and research Raynaud's Phenomenon and related diseases, both autoimmune and non-autoimmune.
Ida Therese Jablanovec, Executive Director

7221 **United Scleroderma Foundation**
300 Rosewood Drive 978-463-5843
Danvers, MA 01923-0350 800-722-4673
Fax: 978-463-5809
www.scleroderma.org

Offers materials and referrals conducts workshops and support groups for those with Raynaud's and their families.
Mary Ann Berman, Office Assistant
Liz Dorsett, Communications Manager

Libraries & Resource Centers

7222 **Arizona Telemedicine Program**
University of Arizona, Health Science Center
PO Box 245105 520-626-4785
Tucson, AZ 85724-5105 Fax: 520-626-1027
e-mail: kerps@email.arizona.edu
www.telemedicine.arizona.edu/index.html

The Arizona Telemedicine Program is a large, multidisciplinary, university-based program that provides telemedicine services, distance learning, informatics training, and telemedicine technology assessment capabilities to communities throughout Arizona, the sixth largest state in the United States, in square miles.
Ronald S Weinstein, MD, Director
Richard A McNeeley, Co-Director

Support Groups & Hotlines

7223 **National Health Information Center**
PO Box 1133 310-565-4167
Washington, DC 20013 800-336-4797
Fax: 301-984-4256
e-mail: info@nhic.org
www.health.gov/nhic

Offers a nationwide information referral service, produces directories and resource guides.

Books

7224 **Raynaud's Phenomenon**
Oxford University Press
This is a detailed and technical work on the physiology finger circulation, and on diagnosis and treatment of Raynaud's Phenomenon and Raynaud's Disease. Includes a chapter on Acrocyanosis and Livedo reticularis.
186 pages
ISBN: 0-195057-56-2

Pamphlets

7225 **Raynaud's Phenomenon**
Arthritis Foundation
PO Box 7669 404-872-7100
Atlanta, GA 30357-0669 800-283-7800
Fax: 404-872-0457

Web Sites

7226 **Health Finder**

www.healthfinder.gov

Searchable, carefully developed web site offering information on over 1000 topics. Developed by the US Department of Health and Human Services, the site can be used in both English and Spanish.

7227 **MedicineNet**

www.medicinenet.com

An online resource for consumers providing easy-to-read, authoritative medical and health information.

7228 **United Scleroderma Foundation**

www.scleroderma.org

Offers materials and referrals, conducts workshops and support groups for those with Raynaud's and their families.

Description

7229 **Sarcoidosis**

Sarcoidosis is a chronic disease that can affect almost any part of the body. It is characterized by the deposit of small masses of tissue (granulomas) in multiple organs. The cause is unknown, although it is speculated to be related to an immunologic defect or infection. Incidence varies widely between countries. In the United States, sarcoidosis is 10- to 18-fold higher in African Americans than in whites. Most cases start between the ages of 30 and 50 years.

Clinical features vary considerably, depending on the site and extent of involvement. Systemic symptoms may include fatigue, weight loss, loss of appetite and fever. Local symptoms may involve any organ, but the most commonly affected are the lungs, skin, eyes and lymph nodes. If the disease becomes severe and life-threatening, it is usually because of lung involvement. Patients develop cough, wheeze, chest pain and difficulty breathing.

Both the severity and the long-term outlook are extremely variable. In most patients, the disease regresses within 2 years and does not recur. In approximately 25 percent of patients, the disease progresses and causes serious disability. If progressive symptoms require treatment, corticosteroids are usually given. If these are not effective or tolerated, immuno suppressive drugs such as methotrexate or azathioprine may be tried. Approximately 5 percent of patients die of respiratory failure.

National Agencies & Associations

7230 **National Sarcoidosis Family Aid and Research Foundation**
268 Martin Luther King Boulevard 973-624-4703
Newark, NJ 07102 800-223-6429
Fax: 973-877-2850
www.php.com
Provides information on a rare disease involving inflammation in lymph nodes and other body tissues, usually in young adults.
Mary Ellen Peterson, Executive Director
Melissa King, Program Coordinator

7231 **National Sarcoidosis Resource Center**
PO Box 1593 732-699-0733
Piscataway, NJ 08855-1593 Fax: 732-699-0882
www.nsrc-global.net
The center provides a national computer database with statistical information and studies, telephone support for patients, subscriptions to national magazines and newsletters and public information provided by mail.
Sandra Conroy, President

7232 **Sarcoidosis Networking Program National Sarcoidosis Resource Center**
National Sarcoidosis Resource Center
437 Rivercrest Drive 732-699-0733
Piscataway, NJ 08855-1593 800-223-6429
Fax: 732-699-0882
A program meant to educate give encouragement and build public awareness of the illness. Also provides information to encourage the formation of self-help groups and to eliminate the isolation that is often felt by the Sarcoidosis sufferer.

Research Centers

7233 **Sarcoidosis Center**
6005 Park Avenue 901-761-5877
Memphis, TN 38119 866-727-2643
Fax: 901-761-2280
e-mail: sarcoid@sarcoidcenter.com
www.sarcoidcenter.com
A nonprofit tax exempt organization dedicated to increasing knowledge of the disease sarcoidosis. This broad goal encompasses three main areas: Disseminating information to professionals who assist with treatment of the disease obtaining and dispersing funds to assist with investigation into the cause and treatment of the disease and providing support for individuals afflicted with the disease.

7234 **Sarcoidosis Treatment and Research Center Thomas Jefferson University Hospital**
Thomas Jefferson University Hospital
111 S 11th Street 215-955-6590
Philadelphia, PA 19107-5092

Support Groups & Hotlines

7235 **Better Breather's Clubs**
American Lung Association of Virginia
9221 Forest Hill Avenue 804-267-1900
Richmond, VA 23235 800-586-4872
Fax: 804-267-5634
e-mail: chamm@lungva.org
www.lungusa.org
Support Groups for those suffering from chronic obstructive pulmonary disease (COPD) such as emphysema, chronic bronchitis and asthma. In these meetings members give and receive support, and learn more about chronic lung disease from health care professionals who share trends in therapy, medication and other topics, or simply answer members' questions.
Catherine G Hamm, President/Chief Excutive Officer
Michelle LaRose, Development Director

7236 **Let's Breathe Sarcoidosis Support Group**
2225 Foster Street 708-328-9410
Evanston, IL 60201-3353 e-mail: bharris354@aol.com
Brenda Harris, Facilitator

7237 **Middle Tennessee Sarcoidosis Support Group**
PO Box 1342
Cookesville, TN 38503 931-528-7826
www.tennesseesarcoidosisawareness.org
Becky Robertson, Group Leader

7238 **Mount Sinai Sarcoidosis Support Group**
One Gustave L. Levy Place
New York, NY 10029 212-241-8733
www.mountsinai.org

7239 **National Health Information Center**
PO Box 1133 310-565-4167
Washington, DC 20013 800-336-4797
Fax: 301-984-4256
e-mail: info@nhic.org
www.health.gov/nhic
Offers a nationwide information referral service, produces directories and resource guides.

7240 **Pacific NW Support Group**
Providence Hospital
Casey Room 500 17th Avenue 206-784-9365
Seattle, WA 98107
Ed Girvan, Facilitator

7241 **Sarcoidosis HelpNet**
PO Box 022642 718-802-1970
Brooklyn, NY 11202 Fax: 212-241-8733
Soneni B Smith, Contact

7242 **Sarcoidosis Research Institute (SRI)**
3475 Central Avenue
Memphis, TN 38111
901-766-6951
Fax: 901-774-7294
e-mail: sarcoid@sarcoidcenter.com
www.sarcoidcenter.com/saradd.htm
The Sarcoidosis Research Institute is a non-profit, tax-exempt organization dedicated to increasing knowledge of the disease sarcoidosis. This broad goal encompasses three main areas: Disseminating information to professionals who assist with treatment of the disease; Obtaining and dispersing funds to assist with investigation into the cause and treatment of the disease; and, providing support for individuals afflicted with the disease.
Paula Yette Polite, Board of Directors President
Wayne Crook, Vice President Board of Directors

7243 **Sarcoidosis Self-Help Group: New York**
Nassau County Medical Center
2201 Hempstead Turnpike
East Meadow, NY 11554
516-483-2666
Robert Schoenfeld, Facilitator

7244 **Sarcoidosis Self-Help Group: Virginia**
American Lung Association of Northern Virginia
9735 Main Street
Fairfax, VA 22031
703-591-4131
Carolyn Thomas, Facilitator

7245 **Sarcoidosis Support Group Delaware**
American Lung Association of Delaware
1021 Gilpin Avenue
Wilmington, DE 19806
302-655-7258
800-586-4872
Fax: 302-655-8546
e-mail: dbrown@alade.org
www.alade.org
Peter Shanley, Chairman
Martha Bogdan, President/CEO

7246 **Sarcoidosis Support Group: New Jersey**
268 Dr. ML King Boulevard
Newark, NJ 07106
201-374-7570
Jean Curlin-Miller, Facilitator

7247 **Sarcoidosis Support Group: Washington DC**
110 Irving Street
Washington, DC 20010
202-877-6286
Fax: 202-877-5779
Carol Bartlett

7248 **Triangle Area Sarcoidosis Support Group**
Soapstone UM Church
12837 Norwood Road
Raleigh, NC 27613
919-676-6498
e-mail: fairleyl@bellsouth.net
Priscilla Fairley, Facilitator

7249 **Understanding Sarcoidosis Self-Help Group**
2112 Highland Avenue
New Castle, PA 16105
412-652-6089
Della Emmanuel

7250 **University of North Carolina Sarcoidosis Support Group**
UNC Chapel Hill Healthcare
130 Mason Farm Road
Chapel Hill, NC 27599
919-966-2531
e-mail: sharikia_burt@med.unc.edu
Sharikia Burt, Clinical Coordinator

7251 **West Tennessee Sarcoidosis Support Group**
1670 McLemoresville Road
Huntington, TN 38344
731-986-9832
www.tennesseesarcoidosisawareness.org
Patricia Coleman, Group Leader

Books

7252 **Sarcoidosis Resource Guide and Directory**
PC Publications
PO Box 1593
Piscataway, NJ 08855-1593
732-699-0733
Fax: 732-699-0882
1993 304 pages Paperback
ISBN: 0-963122-25-8

Newsletters

7253 **Online Sarcoidosis Newsletter**
National Sarcoidosis Resource Center
PO Box 1593
Piscataway, NJ 08855-1593
732-699-0733
Fax: 732-699-0882
Offers information on the center's activities and events, medical and legislative updates for the patients and their families.
Quarterly

Pamphlets

7254 **Anemia of Sarcoidosis**
PC Publications
PO Box 1593
Piscataway, NJ 08855-1593
732-699-0733
800-223-6429
Fax: 732-699-0882

7255 **Bronchoalveolar Lymphocytes in Sarcoidosis**
PC Publications
PO Box 1593
Piscataway, NJ 08855-1593
732-699-0733
800-223-6429
Fax: 732-699-0882

7256 **Case Report: MR Imaging of Myocardial Sarcoidosis**
PC Publications
PO Box 1593
Piscataway, NJ 08855-1593
732-699-0733
800-223-6429
Fax: 732-699-0882

7257 **Case Report: Osseous Sarcoidosis and Chronic Polyarthritis**
PC Publications
PO Box 1593
Piscataway, NJ 08855-1593
732-699-0733
800-223-6429
Fax: 732-699-0882

7258 **Case Report: Overlap of Granulomatous Vasculitis and Sarcoidosis**
PC Publications
PO Box 1593
Piscataway, NJ 08855-1593
732-699-0733
800-223-6429
Fax: 732-699-0882

7259 **Case Report: Rapidly Dev. Confusion, Impaired Memory and Unsteady Gait**
PC Publications
PO Box 1593
Piscataway, NJ 08855-1593
732-699-0733
800-223-6429
Fax: 732-699-0882

7260 **Coping with Sarcoidosis**
National Sarcoidosis Resource Center
PO Box 1593
Piscataway, NJ 08855-1593
732-699-0733
800-223-6429
Fax: 732-699-0882
A pamphlet offering information on how to manage and live with sarcoidosis.

7261 **Disability Law: A Legal Primer**
PC Publications
PO Box 1593
Piscataway, NJ 08855-1593
732-699-0733
800-223-6429
Fax: 732-699-0882

7262 **Drugs That Have Been Used for the Treatment of Sarcoidosis**
PC Publications
PO Box 1593
Piscataway, NJ 08855-1593
732-699-0733
800-223-6429
Fax: 732-699-0882

7263 **Effect of Corticosteroid or Methotrexate Therapy on Lung Lymphocytes**
PC Publications
PO Box 1593
Piscataway, NJ 08855-1593
732-699-0733
800-223-6429
Fax: 732-699-0882

7264 **Effects of Sarcoid and Steroids on Angiotensin-Converting Enzyme**
PC Publications

PO Box 1593
Piscataway, NJ 08855-1593
732-699-0733
800-223-6429
Fax: 732-699-0882

7265 Evaluation of the Efficacy and Toxicity of the Cyclosporine
PC Publications
PO Box 1593
Piscataway, NJ 08855-1593
732-699-0733
800-223-6429
Fax: 732-699-0882

7266 Gastrointestinal Presentation of Churg Strauss Syndrome
PC Publications
PO Box 1593
Piscataway, NJ 08855-1593
732-699-0733
800-223-6429
Fax: 732-699-0882

7267 Governor New Jersey Proclamation: Sarcoidosis Awareness Day
PC Publications
PO Box 1593
Piscataway, NJ 08855-1593
732-699-0733
800-223-6429
Fax: 732-699-0882

7268 How to Get the Most Out of Your Doctor: A Neurologist's Perspective
PC Publications
PO Box 1593
Piscataway, NJ 08855-1593
732-699-0733
800-223-6429
Fax: 732-699-0882

7269 Ideas and Considerations for Starting a Self-Help Mutual Aid Group
PC Publications
PO Box 1593
Piscataway, NJ 08855-1593
732-699-0733
800-223-6429
Fax: 732-699-0882

7270 Masqueraders of Sarcoidosis
PC Publications
PO Box 1593
Piscataway, NJ 08855-1593
732-699-0733
800-223-6429
Fax: 732-699-0882

7271 Mayor Piscataway, NJ Proclamation: Sarcoidosis Awareness Day
PC Publications
PO Box 1593
Piscataway, NJ 08855-1593
732-699-0733
800-223-6429
Fax: 732-699-0882

7272 Multidisciplinary Clinico-Pathologic Conference
PC Publications
PO Box 1593
Piscataway, NJ 08855-1593
732-699-0733
800-223-6429
Fax: 732-699-0882

7273 National Sarcoidosis Resource Center
PC Publications
PO Box 1593
Piscataway, NJ 08855-1593
732-699-0733
Fax: 732-699-0882
www.nsrc-global.net

A booklet offering a brief introduction to the illness and offers information on the role of the Center in finding a cure and educating the public on Sarcoidosis.

7274 Neurosarcoidosis
PC Publications
PO Box 1593
Piscataway, NJ 08855-1593
732-699-0733
800-223-6429
Fax: 732-699-0882

7275 Neurosarcoidosis or Multiple Sclerosis?
National Sarcoidosis Resource Center
PO Box 1593
Piscataway, NJ 08855-1593
732-699-0733
800-223-6429
Fax: 732-699-0882

7276 Paranoid Psychosis Due to Neurosarcoidosis
PC Publications
PO Box 1593
Piscataway, NJ 08855-1593
732-699-0733
800-223-6429
Fax: 732-699-0882

7277 Patient Information Package
National Sarcoidosis Resource Center
PO Box 1593
Piscataway, NJ 08855-1593
732-699-0733
800-223-6429
Fax: 732-699-0882

Contains various brochures and pamphlets offering information about Sarcoidosis.

7278 Physician Listings
PC Publications
PO Box 1593
Piscataway, NJ 08855-1593
732-699-0733
800-223-6429
Fax: 732-699-0882

7279 Possible Association of Rheumatoid Arthritis & Sarcoidosis
PC Publications
PO Box 1593
Piscataway, NJ 08855-1593
732-699-0733
800-223-6429
Fax: 732-699-0882

7280 Presidential Proclamation - National Sarcoidosis Awareness Day
PC Publications
PO Box 1593
Piscataway, NJ 08855-1593
732-699-0733
800-223-6429
Fax: 732-699-0882

7281 Psychological Factors in Sarcoidosis
PC Publications
PO Box 1593
Piscataway, NJ 08855-1593
732-699-0733
800-223-6429
Fax: 732-699-0882

7282 Public Law 102-94
PC Publications
PO Box 1593
Piscataway, NJ 08855-1593
732-699-0733
800-223-6429
Fax: 732-699-0882

7283 Pulmonary Sarcoidosis: Evaluation with High Resolution
PC Publications
PO Box 1593
Piscataway, NJ 08855-1593
732-699-0733
800-223-6429
Fax: 732-699-0882

7284 Pulmonary Sarcoidosis: What We Are Learning
PC Publications
PO Box 1593
Piscataway, NJ 08855-1593
732-699-0733
800-223-6429
Fax: 732-699-0882

7285 Questionnaire Responses for Demographics and Symptoms from 1000 Patients
PC Publications
PO Box 1593
Piscataway, NJ 08855-1593
732-699-0733
800-223-6429
Fax: 732-699-0882

7286 Right & Left Ventricular Function at Rest in Patients with Sarcoidosis
PC Publications
PO Box 1593
Piscataway, NJ 08855-1593
732-699-0733
800-223-6429
Fax: 732-699-0882

7287 Role of Magnetic Resonance Imaging in Neurosarcoidosis
PC Publications
PO Box 1593
Piscataway, NJ 08855-1593
732-699-0733
800-223-6429
Fax: 732-699-0882

7288 Sarcoidosis
PC Publications
PO Box 1593
Piscataway, NJ 08855-1593
732-699-0733
800-223-6429
Fax: 732-699-0882

Offers information on the illness, causes, symptoms and treatments.

7289 Sarcoidosis Diagnosed in a Patient with Known HIV Infection
PC Publications
PO Box 1593
Piscataway, NJ 08855-1593
732-699-0733
800-223-6429
Fax: 732-699-0882

7290 **Sarcoidosis Patient Questionnaire**
PC Publications
PO Box 1593 732-699-0733
Piscataway, NJ 08855-1593 800-223-6429
Fax: 732-699-0882

7291 **Sarcoidosis Questionnaire: Demographics and Symptomatology-The Patients Respond**
PC Publications
PO Box 1593 732-699-0733
Piscataway, NJ 08855-1593 800-223-6429
Fax: 732-699-0882

7292 **Sarcoidosis and Pregnancy: Clinical Observation**
PC Publications
PO Box 1593 732-699-0733
Piscataway, NJ 08855-1593 800-223-6429
Fax: 732-699-0882

7293 **Sarcoidosis and You: A Listing of Possible Symptoms**
PC Publications
PO Box 1593 732-699-0733
Piscataway, NJ 08855-1593 800-223-6429
Fax: 732-699-0882

7294 **Sarcoidosis in India: A Review of 125 Biopsy-Proven Cases from India**
PC Publications
PO Box 1593 732-699-0733
Piscataway, NJ 08855-1593 800-223-6429
Fax: 732-699-0882

7295 **Sarcoidosis of the Liver**
PC Publications
PO Box 1593 732-699-0733
Piscataway, NJ 08855-1593 800-223-6429
Fax: 732-699-0882

7296 **Sarcoidosis: A Multisystem Disease**
PC Publications
PO Box 1593 732-699-0733
Piscataway, NJ 08855-1593 800-223-6429
Fax: 732-699-0882

Explains the effects of the illness on the lungs and joints.

7297 **Sarcoidosis: International Review**
PC Publications
PO Box 1593 732-699-0733
Piscataway, NJ 08855-1593 800-223-6429
Fax: 732-699-0882

7298 **Sarcoidosis: Pleural Involvement Mimicking a Coin Lesson**
PC Publications
PO Box 1593 732-699-0733
Piscataway, NJ 08855-1593 800-223-6429
Fax: 732-699-0882

7299 **Sarcoidosis: Usual and Unusual Manifestations**
PC Publications
PO Box 1593 732-699-0733
Piscataway, NJ 08855-1593 800-223-6429
Fax: 732-699-0882

7300 **Seasonal Clustering of Sarcoidosis**
National Sarcoidosis Resource Center
PO Box 1593 732-699-0733
Piscataway, NJ 08855-1593 800-223-6429
Fax: 732-699-0882

7301 **Successful Treatment of Myocardial Sarcoidosis with Steriods**
PC Publications
PO Box 1593 732-699-0733
Piscataway, NJ 08855-1593 800-223-6429
Fax: 732-699-0882

7302 **Support Group Listing**
PC Publications
PO Box 1593 732-699-0733
Piscataway, NJ 08855-1593 800-223-6429
Fax: 732-699-0882

7303 **Use of Low Dose Methotrexate in Refractory Sarcoidosis**
PC Publications
PO Box 1593 732-699-0733
Piscataway, NJ 08855-1593 800-223-6429
Fax: 732-699-0882

7304 **World Association Sarcoidosi Other Granulatomous**
PC Publications
PO Box 1593 732-699-0733
Piscataway, NJ 08855-1593 800-223-6429
Fax: 732-699-0882

Audio & Video

7305 **Dialogue with Doris**
PC Publications
PO Box 1593 732-699-0733
Piscataway, NJ 08855-1593 800-223-6429
Fax: 732-699-0882

7306 **Help with a Hidden Disease Update**
PC Publications
PO Box 1593 732-699-0733
Piscataway, NJ 08855-1593 800-223-6429
Fax: 732-699-0882

7307 **Of Their Own: Person to Person Show**
PC Publications
PO Box 1593 732-699-0733
Piscataway, NJ 08855-1593 800-223-6429
Fax: 732-699-0882

7308 **Sarcoidosis Conference 2**
PC Publications
PO Box 1593 732-699-0733
Piscataway, NJ 08855-1593 800-223-6429
Fax: 732-699-0882

7309 **Sarcoidosis Conference 3**
PC Publications
PO Box 1593 732-699-0733
Piscataway, NJ 08855-1593 800-223-6429
Fax: 732-699-0882

7310 **Sarcoidosis and Lyme Disease**
PC Publications
PO Box 1593 732-699-0733
Piscataway, NJ 08855-1593 800-223-6429
Fax: 732-699-0882

7311 **Sarcoidosis: What's That?**
PC Publications
PO Box 1593 732-699-0733
Piscataway, NJ 08855-1593 800-223-6429
Fax: 732-699-0882

7312 **XIV International World Conference on Sarcoidosis: Patient Symposium**
PC Publications
PO Box 1593 732-699-0733
Piscataway, NJ 08855-1593 800-223-6429
Fax: 732-699-0882

Cassette.

Web Sites

7313 **Healing Well**
www.healingwell.com

An online health resource guide to medical news, chat, information and articles, newsgroups and message boards, books, disease-related web sites, medical directories, and more for patients, friends, and family coping with disabling diseases, disorders, or chronic illnesses.

7314 **Health Finder**
www.healthfinder.gov

Searchable, carefully developed web site offering information on over 1000 topics. Developed by the US Department of Health and Human Services, the site can be used in both English and Spanish.

7315 **Healthlink USA**

www.healthlinkusa.com

Health information concerning treatment, cures, prevention, diagnosis, risk factors, research, support groups, email lists, personal stories and much more. Updated regularly.

7316 **Helios Health**

www.helioshealth.com

Online resource for your health information. Detailed information about specific health topics, access to expert advice from our Medical Advisory Board, and up-to-date health news.

7317 **MedicineNet**

www.medicinenet.com

An online resource for consumers providing easy-to-read, authoritative medical and health information.

7318 **Medscape**

www.mywebmd.com

Medscape offers specialists, primary care physicians, and other health professionals the Web's most robust and integrated medical information and educational tools.

7319 **National Sarcoidosis Resource Center**

www.nsrc-global.net

Provides the general public with sarcoidosis information, for patients to obtain medical and emotional help and to provide government officials with the information they need.

7320 **WebMD**

www.webmd.com

Information on sarcoidosis, including articles and resources.

Description

7321 **Scleroderma**

Scleroderma, literally "hard skin", is a form of systemic sclerosis, a generalized disturbance of connective and vascular tissue which leads to scarring (sclerosis). Scleroderma is a rare disease, with about 5,000 new cases in the United States each year. Women are 3 or 4 times as likely as men to get the disease, which typically begins between the ages of 30 and 50 years. It is comparatively rare in children. The cause of the disease is unknown.

Since almost any organ may be involved, the list of possible symptoms is extensive. Important ones include weakness, fatigue, stiffness, weight loss, shortness of breath, abdominal bloating and pain, diarrhea and irritation of the eyes. Kidney involvement usually causes abrupt acceleration of high blood pressure. A very characteristic symptom, although not unique to this disease, is Raynaud's phenomenon. On exposure to cold, the arteries of the patient's hands and feet contract, causing the skin color to change from red, to white (blanch), to blue (cyanosis), accompanied by pain and numbness.

If the disease is limited to the skin the outlook is good, but involvement of lung and kidney in the systemic form may be fatal. Use of the ACE inhibitor class of anti-hypertensive drugs has helped preserve kidney function. Many immunosuppressive drugs have been tried without clear success. Clinical trials of new agents are often available to patients. When end-stage kidney disease cannot be prevented, dialysis and transplant can be used, although the death rate remains high.

National Agencies & Associations

7322 **Canadian Dermatology Association**
1385 Bank Street
Ottawa, Ontario, K1H-8N4
613-738-1748
800-267-3376
Fax: 613-738-4695
e-mail: contact.cda@dermatology.ca
www.dermatology.ca
Ensure the Canadian public has equal access to timely and exemplary dermatologic care, by advocating on dermatologic issues, providing leadership in continuing medical and public education, and promoting and disseminating dermatologic knowledge and research.
Dr Louis Weatherhead, President of the Board
Dr Laurence Warshawski, President of the Board

7323 **Scleroderma Foundation**
300 Rosewood Drive
Danvers, MA 01923
978-463-5843
800-722-4673
Fax: 978-463-5809
e-mail: sfinfo@scleroderma.org
www.scleroderma.org
A national nonprofit organization serving the interests of persons with Scleroderma. The Foundation's 26 chapters and 135 support groups nationwide help to carry out its three-fold mission of support, education and research.
Joseph Camerino, Chair
Carol Feghali-Bostwi, Vice Chair

7324 **Scleroderma Society of Ontario**
393 University Avenue
Toronto, Ontario, M5G-1E6
800-321-1433
Fax: 416-979-8366
www.sclerodermaontario.ca
Committed to promoting increased public awareness, advancing patient wellness and supporting research in scleroderma.
Carroll Vapsva, Scleroderma Society Canada Liaison
Peter Woolcott, President of the Board

State Agencies & Associations

Arizona

7325 **Scleroderma Foundation: Arizona Chapter**
18402 N 19th Avenue
Phoenix, AZ 85023
623-847-3757
e-mail: carolnader@cox.net
Local chapter of the national Scleroderma Foundation in Byfield, Massachusetts. Please contact this group for information on area support groups.
Carol Nader, President

California

7326 **Scleroderma Foundation: Greater San Diego Chapter**
8748 Cherry Hills Road
Santee, CA 92071
619-448-6301
e-mail: GSDchapter@scleroderma.org
www.scleroderma.org
Local chapter of the national Scleroderma Foundation in Byfield, Massachusetts. Please contact this group for information on area support groups.
Fletcher Diehl, President
Carol Ireland, Vice President

7327 **Scleroderma Foundation: Northern California Chapter**
PO Box 601313
Sacramento, CA 95860-1313
916-832-1102
e-mail: NoCAchapter@scleroderma.org
www.scleroderma.org
Local chapter of the national Scleroderma Foundation in Byfield, Massachusetts. Please contact this group for information on area support groups.
Cathy Eddy, President
Cheryl George, Vice President

7328 **Scleroderma Foundation: Southern California Chapter (& LA Area)**
11704 Wilshire Boulevard
Los Angeles, CA 90025
310-477-8225
877-443-5755
Fax: 310-477-8774
e-mail: SoCAchapter@scleroderma.org
www.scleroderma.org
Local chapter of the national Scleroderma Foundation in Byfield, Massachusetts. Please contact this group for information on area support groups.
Brian Ross Adams, Executive Director
Dan Furst, President

Colorado

7329 **Scleroderma Foundation: Colorado Chapter**
PO Box 460940
Aurora, CO 80046-0940
303-806-6686
e-mail: COchapter@scleroderma.org
www.scleroderma.org
Local chapter of the national Scleroderma Foundation in Byfield, Massachusetts. Please contact this group for information on area support groups.
Rita Miller, President
Fran Penk, Vice President

Connecticut

7330 **Scleroderma Foundation: Tri-State Chapter**
Binghamton, NY
201-837-9826
800-867-0885
e-mail: sdtristate@aol.com
Local chapter of the national Scleroderma Foundation in Byfield, Massachusetts. Please contact this group for information on area support groups.
Rosemary Markoff, President

Delaware

7331 **Scleroderma Foundation: Delaware Valley Chapter**
385 Kings Highway N 732-449-7001
Cherry Hill, NJ 08034 866-675-5545
e-mail: DVchapter@scleroderma.org
www.scleroderma.org
Local chapter of the national Scleroderma Foundation in Byfield, Massachusetts. Please contact this group for information on area support groups.
Melissa Kuscher, Executive Director
Colleen Ferara, Administrative Assistant

District of Columbia

7332 **Scleroderma Foundation: Greater Washington DC Chapter**
2010 Corporate Ridge
McLean, VA 22102 888-233-4779
e-mail: carolsod@att.net
Local chapter of the national Scleroderma Foundation in Byfield, Massachusetts. Please contact this group for information on area support groups.
Carol Sodetz, President

Florida

7333 **Scleroderma Foundation: Southeast Florida Chapter**
6145 NW 123rd Lane 954-255-8335
Coral Springs, FL 33076-3913 Fax: 954-255-8081
e-mail: SEFLchapter@scleroderma.org
www.scleroderma.org
Local chapter of the national Scleroderma Foundation in Byfield, Massachusetts. Please contact this group for information on area support groups.
Berna Falkoff, President
Ruth Greenspan, Vice - Chair

Georgia

7334 **Scleroderma Foundation: Georgia Chapter Scleroderma Foundation**
Scleroderma Foundation
800-722-4673
e-mail: swright@cleroderma.org
www.scleroderma.org
Local chapter of the national Scleroderma Foundation in Byfield, Massachusetts. Call the national office for contact information on the Georgia Chapter. Please contact this group for information on area support groups.
Stacy Wright, Contact
Mary Haulk, Contact

Illinois

7335 **Scleroderma Foundation: Greater Chicago Chapter**
203 N Wabash Street 312-660-1131
Chicago, IL 60601 Fax: 312-660-1133
e-mail: GCchapter@scleroderma.org
www.scleroderma.org
Local chapter of the national Scleroderma Foundation in Byfield, Massachusetts. Please contact this group for information on area support groups.
Mike Robbins, President
Greg Marion, Vice President

Maine

7336 **Scleroderma Foundation: New England Chapter**
462 Boston Street
Topsfield, MA 01983 888-525-0658
e-mail: sclfndne@aol.com
Local chapter of the national Scleroderma Foundation in Byfield, Massachusetts. Please contact this group for information on area support groups. Includes MA, ME, NH, VT, & RI.
Marie Coyle, President

Maryland

7337 **Scleroderma Foundation: Greater Washington DC Chapter**
2010 Corporate Ridge
McLean, VA 22102 888-233-4779
e-mail: carolsod@att.net
Local chapter of the national Scleroderma Foundation in Byfield, Massachusetts. Please contact this group for information on area support groups.
Carol Sodetz, President

Massachusetts

7338 **Scleroderma Foundation: New England Chapter**
462 Boston Street
Topsfield, MA 01983 888-525-0658
e-mail: sclfndne@aol.com
Local chapter of the national Scleroderma Foundation in Byfield, Massachusetts. Please contact this group for information on area support groups.
Marie Coyle, President

Michigan

7339 **Scleroderma Foundation: Michigan Chapter**
30301 Northwestern Highway 248-865-7259
Farmington Hills, MI 48334 800-716-6554
Fax: 248-865-7523
e-mail: MIchapter@scleroderma.org
www.scleroderma.org
Local chapter of the national Scleroderma Foundation in Byfield, Massachusetts. Please contact this group for information on area support groups.
Laura Dyas, Executive Director
Janus Landrum, Executive Assistant

Minnesota

7340 **Scleroderma Foundation: Minnesota Chapter**
5775 Wayzata Boulevard 952-525-2273
Saint Louis Park, MN 55416 877-794-0347
e-mail: MNChapter@scleroderma.org
www.scleroderma.org
Local chapter of the national Scleroderma Foundation in Byfield, Massachusetts. Please contact this group for information on area support groups.
Lee Roy Jones, President
Chris Woo, Executive Director

Missouri

7341 **Scleroderma Foundation: Missouri Chapter**
Springfield, MO 65808 417-887-3269
e-mail: MOchapter@scleroderma.org
www.scleroderma.org
Local chapter of the national Scleroderma Foundation in Byfield, Massachusetts. Please contact this group for information on area support groups.
Mary Blades, President
Ben Blades, Vice President

Nevada

7342 **Scleroderma Foundation: Nevada Chapter**
6760 Surrey Street 702-368-1572
Las Vegas, NV 89119 e-mail: NVchapter@scleroderma.org
www.scleroderma.org
Local chapter of the national Scleroderma Foundation in Byfield, Massachusetts. Please contact this group for information on area support groups.
Barbara Dempsey, President
Sheila Gray, VP Support Group

New Hampshire

7343 **Scleroderma Foundation: New England Chapter**
462 Boston Street
Topsfield, MA 01983 888-525-0658
e-mail: sclfndne@aol.com

Local chapter of the national Scleroderma Foundation in Byfield, Massachusetts. Please contact this group for information on area support groups.
Marie Coyle, President

New Jersey

7344 Scleroderma Foundation: Tri-State Chapter
59 Front Street 607-723-2239
Binghamton, NY 13905 800-867-0885
Fax: 607-723-2039
e-mail: chribar@scleroderma.org
www.scleroderma.org
Local chapter of the national Scleroderma Foundation in Byfield, Massachusetts. Please contact this group for information on area support groups.
Jeff Mace, President
Corey Hribar, Executive Director

New York

7345 Scleroderma Foundation: Central New York Chapter
59 Front Street 607-723-2239
Binghamton, NY 13905 e-mail: chribar@scleroderma.org
www.scleroderma.org
Local chapter of the national Scleroderma Foundation in Byfield, Massachusetts. Please contact this group for information on area support groups.
Corey Hribar, Executive Director
Tom Knapp, Office Manage

7346 Scleroderma Foundation: Tri-State Chapter
59 Front Street 607-723-2239
Binghamton, NY 13905 800-867-0885
Fax: 607-723-2039
e-mail: chribar@scleroderma.org
www.scleroderma.org
Local chapter of the national Scleroderma Foundation in Byfield, Massachusetts. Please contact this group for information on area support groups.
Jeff Mace, President
Corey Hribar, Executive Director

7347 Scleroderma Foundation: Western New York Chapter
PO Box 708 716-627-2283
Hamburg, NY 14075 877-969-2478
e-mail: wnychpt@aol.com
www.scleroderma.org
Local chapter of the national Scleroderma Foundation in Byfield, Massachusetts. Please contact this group for information on area support groups.
Laura Henry, Co-President

Ohio

7348 Scleroderma Foundation: Ohio Chapter
PO Box 846 614-334-0846
Hilliard, OH 43026-0846 866-849-9030
e-mail: OHchapter@scleroderma.org
www.scleroderma.org
Local chapter of the national Scleroderma Foundation in Byfield, Massachusetts. Please contact this group for information on area support groups.
Mariann Boyanowski, President
Amelia Yaussy, Past President

Oregon

7349 Scleroderma Foundation: Oregon Chapter
PO Box 19296 503-246-0235
Portland, OR 97280-0296 e-mail: ORchapter@scleroderma.org
www.scleroderma.org
Local chapter of the national Scleroderma Foundation in Byfield, Massachusetts. Please contact this group for information on area support groups.
Liz Orem-Bedel, Vice President
Richard Bates, President

Pennsylvania

7350 Scleroderma Foundation: Delaware Valley Chapter
385 Kings Highway N 732-449-7001
Cherry Hill, NJ 08034 866-675-5545
e-mail: DVchapter@scleroderma.org
www.scleroderma.org
Local chapter of the national Scleroderma Foundation in Byfield, Massachusetts. Please contact this group for information on area support groups.
Melissa Kuscher, Executive Director
Colleen Ferara, Administrative Assistant

7351 Scleroderma Foundation: Western Pennsylvania Chapter
3500 Terrace Street 724-869-2515
Pittsburgh, PA 15261 800-722-4673
e-mail: WPAchapter@scleroderma.org
www.scleroderma.org
Local chapter of the national Scleroderma Foundation in Byfield, Massachusetts. Please contact this group for information on area support groups.
Betty Aquino, President
Thomas A Medsger Jr, Treasurer

Rhode Island

7352 Scleroderma Foundation: New England Chapter
462 Boston Street
Topsfield, MA 01983 888-525-0658
e-mail: sclfndne@aol.com
Local chapter of the national Scleroderma Foundation in Byfield, Massachusetts. Please contact this group for information on area support groups.
Marie Coyle, President

South Carolina

7353 Scleroderma Foundation: South Carolina Chapter
1027 S Pendleton Street 843-832-9486
Easley, SC 29642 866-557-3729
e-mail: SCchapter@scleroderma.org
www.scleroderma.org
Local chapter of the national Scleroderma Foundation in Byfield. Massachusetts. Please contact this group for information on area support groups.
Amy Parrish, President
Dolores Collins, Vice President

Tennessee

7354 Scleroderma Foundation: Tennessee Chapter
PO Box 2844 615-792-4610
Hendersonville, TN 37077 800-497-5193
Fax: 615-792-4610
e-mail: TNchapter@scleroderma.org
www.scleroderma.org
Local chapter of the national Scleroderma Foundation in Byfield, Massachusetts. Please contact this group for information on area support groups.
April Simpkins, President
Charles Cowell, Vice President

Texas

7355 Scleroderma Foundation: Bluebonnet Chapter
PO Box 1836 972-396-9400
Allen, TX 75013-1894 866-532-7673
Fax: 972-649-7910
e-mail: TXchapter@scleroderma.org
www.scleroderma.org
Local chapter of the national Scleroderma Foundation in Byfield, Massachusetts. Please contact this group for information on area support groups.
Cindi Brannum, President
Peggy Brown, Vice President

Vermont

7356 Scleroderma Foundation: New England Chapter
462 Boston Street 978-887-0658
Topsfield, MA 01983 888-525-0658
Fax: 978-887-0659
e-mail: sclfndne@aol.com
www.scleroderma.org

Local chapter of the national Scleroderma Foundation in Byfield, Massachusetts. Please contact this group for information on area support groups.
Marie Coyle, President
Tom Curran, Executive Director

Virginia

7357 Scleroderma Foundation: Greater Washington DC Chapter
2010 Corporate Ridge 703-938-2191
McLean, VA 22102 888-233-4779
e-mail: GWDCchapter@scleroderma.org
www.scleroderma.org

Local chapter of the national Scleroderma Foundation in Byfield, Massachusetts. Please contact this group for information on area support groups.
Carol Sodetz, President
Fi Fi J Lin, Vice President

Washington

7358 Scleroderma Foundation: Evergreen Chapter
PO Box 84506 206-285-9822
Seattle, WA 98124-5806 e-mail: WAchapter@scleroderma.org
www.scleroderma.org

Local chapter of the national Scleroderma Foundation in Byfield, Massachusetts. Please contact this group for information on area support groups.
Bunny Garthe, President
Nic Evans, Vice President

Foundations

7359 Juvenile Scleroderma Network
1204 W 13th Street 310-519-9511
San Pedro, CA 90731 866-338-5892
e-mail: OutreachJSDN@jsdn.org
www.jsdn.org

Organization that is working to provide educational programs about JSD, and to help children and their families to gain a better understanding.
Jerry Gaither, Chairman
Kathy Gaither, President

Research Centers

7360 Boston University University Medical Center
University Medical Center
One Boston Medical Center Place 617-638-8000
Boston, MA 02118 Fax: 617-385-26
www.bmc.org

Ongoing clinical trials and studies in scleroderma. Office hours by appointment.
Melynn Nuite RN, Clinical Trails Contact
Elaine Ullian, President/CEO

7361 Center for Rheumatology
1367 Washington Avenue 518-489-4471
Albany, NY 12206 e-mail: cbarr@joint-docs.com
www.joint-docs.com

This is a committed research facility as well as a medical practice. Our research practice is made up of seven physicians a certified physician's assistant and four research coordinators. We may have as many as 20 ongoing trails at a time in various indications within the study of rheumatology. Investigational treatment of interstitial lung disease associated with systemic sclerosis.
Norman R Romanoff, Practitioner
Joel M Kremer, Practitioner

7362 Georgetown University Hospital: Department of Rheumatology
3800 Reservoir Road NW 202-444-8233
Washington, DC 20007 Fax: 202-444-8579
www.medicine.georgetown.edu

Research is based on clinical trials and special interest in scleroderma and kidney pulmonary hypertension pregnancy epidemiology and natural history of scleroderma subsets.
Thomas R Cupps, Division Chief
James N Baraniuk, Associate Professor

7363 Johns Hopkins University: Scleroderma Center
Johns Hopkins Bayview Medical Center
5501 Hopkins Bayview Circle 410-550-7715
Baltimore, MD 21224 Fax: 410-550-1363
www.scleroderma.jhmi.edu

Specializes in the management of systemic sclerosis (scleroderma) Raynaud's phenomenon and related disorders. In addition to patient care the center is involved in both basic and clinical research projects.
Frederick M Wigley MD, Director
Barbara Whit MD, Director

7364 Mayo Clinic Scottsdale Center for Scleroderma Care & Research
Mayo Clinic
13400 E Shea Boulevard 480-301-8000
Scottsdale, AZ 85259 Fax: 480-301-7006
www.mayoclinic.org/rheumatology

Integrates multiple medical as well as surgical specialties under the direction of the Division of Rheumatology to provide coordinated and comprehensive evaluations and treatment. New clinical trails are in development.
Lester Mertz MD, Assistant Professor of Medicine
April Chang-Miller, Assistant Professor of Medicine

7365 Medical University of South Carolina Medical University of South Carolina
Medical University of South Carolina
96 Johnathan Lucas Street 843-792-2300
Charleston, SC 29403 800-424-MUSC
Fax: 843-792-2601
e-mail: wickman@musc.edu
www.musc.edu

Actively engaged in basic and clinical research of scleroderma.
Richard M Silver, Director of Rheumatology and Immunology
W Stuart Smith, Vice President for Clinical Operations a

7366 Scleroderma Clinical & Research Center State University of New York at Stonybro
State University of New York at Stonybrook
26 Research Way 631-444-6345
E Setauket, NY 01173-9260 Fax: 631-444-0562
Ongoing research of scleroderma.

7367 Scleroderma Research Foundation
220 Montgomery Street 415-834-9444
San Francisco, CA 94104 800-637-4005
Fax: 415-834-9177
e-mail: info@sclerodermaresearch.org
www.srfcure.org

Mission is to find a cure for scleroderma a life threatening and degenerative illness by funding and facilitating the most promising highest quality research and placing the disease and its need for a cure in the public eye.
Luke Evnin PhD, Chairman
Nancy Bechtle, Member of Board of Directors

7368 Thomas Jefferson University Hospital
111 S 11th Street 215-955-6000
Philadelphia, PA 19107 Fax: 215-923-5828
www.jeffersonhospital.org

Provides diagnostic evaluations treatment and access to the latest research studies for more than one thousand patients with scleroderma and related diseases.
Oscar Irigoyen, Director Division of Rheumatology
Sergio Jimen MD, Professor

7369 University of Alabama Birmingham
6th Avenue S 205-934-4011
Birmingham, AL 35294 Fax: 205-755-54
www.uab.edu

Located in the Clinical Immunology and Rheumatology department Oral Type 1 Collagen in Scleroderma is studied.
Carol Garrison, President
William Ferniany, CEO

7370 **University of Chicago Center for Advanced Medicine Duchossis Center**
University of Chicago hospital
5841 S Maryland Avenue
Chicago, IL 60637
773-702-1000
888-UCH-0200
Fax: 773-028-02
e-mail: orogers@medicine.bsd.uchicago.edu
www.uchospitals.com
Scleroderma clinic.
Michael Ellm MD, Clinic Contact
Ornery Rogers, Clinic Contact

7371 **University of Illinois at Chicago Medical Center Outpatient Clinical Center**
University of Illinois
600 S Hoyne Avenue
Chicago, IL 60612
312-996-7000
800-UIC-1002
Fax: 312-633-3434
TTY: 312-413-0123
e-mail: info@iMDc.org
www.uic.edu
Scleroderma clinic held on the first and third Thursdays of every month.
Sylvia Manning, Chancellor
Michael R Tanner, Provost and Vice Chancellor for Academic

7372 **University of Pittsburgh**
3500 Terrance Street
Pittsburgh, PA 15261
412-624-4141
Fax: 412-383-2264
www.pitt.edu
Clinic and research of scleroderma.
Carol Blair RN, Clinic Contact

7373 **University of Tennessee Medical Group**
956 Court Avenue
Memphis, TN 38103
901-448-5775
Fax: 901-448-7265
www.utmedicalgroup.com
Ongoing research protocols.
Arnold E Postlewaite MD, Research Contact

7374 **University of Texas Health Science Center**
7000 Fannin
Houston, TX 77030
713-500-4472
Fax: 713-500-3026
e-mail: sclerodermaregister@uth.tmc.edu
www.uthouston.edu
Clinic research and clinical trials concerning scleroderma.
Maureen Mayes, Research Contact

Support Groups & Hotlines

7375 **National Health Information Center**
PO Box 1133
Washington, DC 20013
310-565-4167
800-336-4797
Fax: 301-984-4256
e-mail: info@nhic.org
www.health.gov/nhic
Offers a nationwide information referral service, produces directories and resource guides.

7376 **Rhode Island Scleroderma Support Group**
18 Talbot Manor
Cranston, RI 02905
401-781-5013
e-mail: scleroderma@hotmail.com
www.angelfire.com/ri/scleroderma
Meets on the fourth Wednsday of every month at Roger Williams Hospital.
Carole Cowell, President

7377 **Scleroderma Support Groups**
Scleroderma Foundation
12 Kent Way
Byfield, MA 01922
978-463-5843
800-722-4633
Fax: 978-463-5809
e-mail: sfinfo@scleroderma.org
www.scleroderma.org
Please contact the Scleroderma Foundation or visit our web site for a listing of support groups in your area.

Books

7378 **Best of the Beacon**
Scleroderma Foundation
12 Kent Way
Byfield, MA 01922
978-463-5843
800-722-4673
Fax: 978-463-5809
e-mail: sfinfo@scleroderma.org
www.scleroderma.org/store.html#books
Interesting, readable and highly practical collection of articles of particular interest to those living with scleroderma. This mini encyclopedia includes 11 medical articles, 358 most frequently asked questions, 34 sharing stories, 62 articles of special interest on a variety of useful topics and a glossary that defines 240 words you may encounter when reading about scleroderma.
Marie Coyle, Editor

7379 **Handout on Health: Scleroderma**
NAMSIC/National Institutes of Health
1 AMS Circle
Bethesda, MD 20892-0001
301-495-4484
877-226-4267
Fax: 301-718-6366
TTY: 301-565-2966
e-mail: niamsinfo@mail.nih.gov
www.nih.gov/niams
143 pages

7380 **Helpful Hints for Living with Scleroderma**
Scleroderma Foundation
12 Kent Way
Byfield, MA 01922
978-463-5843
800-722-4673
Fax: 978-463-5809
e-mail: sfinfo@scleroderma.org
www.scleroderma.org/store.html#books
Booklet of helpful suggestions from our chapters and members, for the comfort and convienience of others who share the same challenges.
57 pages

7381 **Perspectives on Living with Scleroderma**
Scleroderma Foundation
12 Kent Way
Byfield, MA 01922
978-463-5843
800-722-4673
Fax: 978-463-5809
e-mail: sfinfo@scleroderma.org
www.scleroderma.org/store.html#books
Insightful articles on coping with scleroderma come from not only from Dr. Flapan's counseling and volunteer work, but also from his personal experience as a scleroderma patient.
233 pages

7382 **Scleroderma Book**
Scleroderma Foundation
12 Kent Way
Byfield, MA 01922
978-463-5843
800-722-4673
Fax: 978-463-5809
e-mail: sfinfo@scleroderma.org
www.scleroderma.org/store.html#books
Definitive guide to scleroderma for patients and their families, with easy to understand explanations.
182 pages

7383 **Scleroderma: Surviving a Seventeen-Year Itch**
Scleroderma Foundation
978-463-5809
800-722-4673
Fax: 978-463-5809
e-mail: sfinfo@scleroderma.org
www.scleroderma.org
Self-help manual including history, diagnosis, daily routines and exercise programs for persons with scleroderma.

7384 **Scleroderma: a New Role for Patients and Families**
Scleroderma Foundation

12 Kent Way
Byfield, MA 01922
978-463-5843
800-722-4673
Fax: 978-463-5809
e-mail: sfinfo@scleroderma.org
www.scleroderma.org/store.html#books

Provides an overview of key issues and offers resources that enable patients and their families to find more resources on thier own.

168 pages

7385 **Understanding & Managing Scleroderma**
Scleroderma Foundation
12 Kent Way
Byfield, MA 01923
978-463-5843
800-722-4633
Fax: 978-463-5809
e-mail: sfinfo@scleroderma.org
www.scleroderma.org

Booklet intended to help persons with scleroderma, their families and others interested in scleroderma to better understand what scleroderma is, what effects it may have, and what those with scleroderma can do to help themselves and their physicians manage the disease. It answers some of the most frequently asked questions about scleroderma.

Magazines

7386 **Scleroderma Voice**
Scleroderma Foundation
12 Kent Way
Byfield, MA 01922
978-463-5843
800-722-4673
Fax: 978-463-5809
e-mail: sfinfo@scleroderma.org
www.scleroderma.org

Feautures the latest information available on scleroderma treatments and research. Subscription to the Voice includes a one-year membership in the Scleroderma Foundation.

Quarterly

Pamphlets

7387 **If You Have Scleroderma You Need Not Feel Alone**
Scleroderma Foundation
12 Kent Way
Byfield, MA 01922
978-463-5843
800-722-4673
Fax: 978-463-5809
e-mail: sfinfo@scleroderma.org
www.scleroderma.org/store.html#brochures

Scleroderma Foundation's membership brochure. Free of charge, also available in Spanish.

7388 **Scleroderma: an Overview**
Scleroderma Foundation
12 Kent Way
Byfield, MA 01922
978-463-5843
Fax: 978-463-5809
e-mail: sfinfo@scleroderma.org
www.scleroderma.org/store.html#brochures

Concise genral overview of sytemic scleroderma. Also available in Spanish, and downloadable in Portugese.

7389 **What Causes Scleroderma?**
Scleroderma Foundation
12 Kent Way
Byfield, MA 01922
978-463-5843
800-722-4673
Fax: 978-463-5809
e-mail: sfinfo@scleroderma.org
www.scleroderma.org/store.html#brochures

Discusses the puzzling nature of scleroderma. Also available in Spanish, and downloadable in Portugese.

Web Sites

7390 **Healing Well**
www.healingwell.com

An online health resource guide to medical news, chat, information and articles, newsgroups and message boards, books, disease-related web sites, medical directories, and more for patients, friends, and family coping with disabling diseases, disorders, or chronic illnesses.

7391 **Health Finder**
www.healthfinder.gov

Searchable, carefully developed web site offering information on over 1000 topics. Developed by the US Department of Health and Human Services, the site can be used in both English and Spanish.

7392 **Healthlink USA**
www.healthlinkusa.com

Health information concerning treatment, cures, prevention, diagnosis, risk factors, research, support groups, email lists, personal stories and much more. Updated regularly.

7393 **Helios Health**
www.helioshealth.com

Online resource for your health information. Detailed information about specific health topics, access to expert advice from our Medical Advisory Board, and up-to-date health news.

7394 **MedicineNet**
www.medicinenet.com

An online resource for consumers providing easy-to-read, authoritative medical and health information.

7395 **Medscape**
www.mywebmd.com

Medscape offers specialists, primary care physicians, and other health professionals the Web's most robust and integrated medical information and educational tools.

7396 **Scleroderma Foundation**
www.scleroderma.org

501 (c)3 national nonprofit organization serving the interests of persons with scleroderma. The Foundation's 26 chapters and 135 support groups nationwide help to carry out its three-fold mission of support, education and research. The Scleroderma Foundation is a leading nonprofit supporter of scleroderma research — funding over $1 million of new grants each year to find the cause and cure of scleroderma.

7397 **WebMD**
www.webmd.com

Information on scleroderma, including articles and resources.

Description

7398 **Scoliosis**

Scoliosis is a lateral curvature of the spine, with 60 to 80 percent of the cases occurring in girls. It may first be suspected when one of the teenager's shoulders appears higher than the other or clothes don't hang straight. The spinal curve is more pronounced when the adolescent bends forward. More than 80 percent of scoliosis is idiopathic, that is, there is no known cause.

Symptoms include prominent shoulder blades, uneven hip levels, and fatigue in the lower back after sitting or standing for prolonged periods of time. In many cases there are no symptoms unless the scoliosis is severe.

The prognosis depends on the site and severity of the curve, and the age of onset of symptoms. Early detection through school screening provides more treatment options, and prompt referral to an orthopedist is indicated. The majority of cases require only observation for progression. Approximately 20 percent of those with scoliosis will require an orthopedic brace or spinal fusion surgery.

National Agencies & Associations

7399 **American Academy of Orthopaedic Surgeons**
6300 N River Road
Rosemont, IL 60018-4238
847-823-7186
800-346-2267
Fax: 847-823-8125
e-mail: custserv@aaos.org
www.aaos.org
The American Academy of Orthopaedic Surgeons provides education and practice management services for orthopaedic surgeons and allied health professionals. The Academy also serves as an advocate for improved patient care and informs the public.
Karen L Hackett FACHE CAE, CEO
Richard J Stewart, Chief Financial Officer

7400 **International Federation of Spine Associations**
Howard M Shulman
9908 Cape Scott Court
Raleigh, NC 27614-9025
919-846-2204
www.scoliosisrx.com
IFOSA is a federation of various national Spine Associations from countries in North America Europe and Australia. These organizations principally represent the spine patients and their families.

7401 **National Scoliosis Foundation**
5 Cabot Place
Stoughton, MA 02072
781-341-6333
800-673-6922
Fax: 781-341-8333
e-mail: NSF@scoliosis.org
www.scoliosis.org
Promotes school screening offers public awareness materials to promote public education maintains a resource center for professional information conducts scoliosis conferences and offers support groups to people affected by the disease.
Joseph P O'Brien, President/CEO
Dennis J Fusco, Treasurer

7402 **Scoliosis Association**
PO Box 811705
Boca Raton, FL 33481-1705
561-994-4435
800-800-0669
Fax: 561-994-2455
e-mail: normlipin@aol.com
www.scoliosis-assoc.org
Sponsors and encourages spinal screening programs. Disseminates information throughout the country and raises funds for scoliosis research. Membership fee includes subscription to newsletter. Videos and printed information available.

7403 **Spinal Connection National Scoliosis Foundation**
National Scoliosis Foundation
5 Cabot Place
Stoughton, MA 02072
781-341-6333
800-673-6922
Fax: 781-341-8333
e-mail: NSF@scoliosis.org
www.scoliosis.org
Offers updated information and the latest medical advances in the area of spinal cord injury and spina bifida. Includes resources reviews support group and meeting information.
Joseph P O'Brien, President/CEO
Dennis J Fusco, Treasurer

Research Centers

7404 **Scoliosis Research Society**
555 E Wells Street
Milwaukee, WI 53202
414-289-9107
Fax: 414-276-3349
e-mail: info@srs.org
www.srs.org
This society provides an international forum for those interested in the management of spinal deformities. It holds a yearly meeting at which health professionals meet to share observations and results and to explore new avenues of research.
Tressa Goulding, Executive Director
Kathryn Agard, Administrative Assistant

7405 **Shriners Hospital for Crippled Children Chicago Unit**
Chicago Unit
2211 N Oak Park Avenue
Chicago, IL 60707
773-622-5400
Fax: 773-855-88
www.shrinersplural2hopitals.org
A 60-bed orthopedic hospital providing comprehensive spinal cord injury care to children. Provides care for spinal deformities Cerebral Palsy Osteoeneisis Imperfecta and Scoliosis as well as others.
Chara Jones, Administrator
Diether Sturm, Chief of Staff

Support Groups & Hotlines

7406 **National Health Information Center**
PO Box 1133
Washington, DC 20013
310-565-4167
800-336-4797
Fax: 301-984-4256
e-mail: info@nhic.org
www.health.gov/nhic
Offers a nationwide information referral service, produces directories and resource guides.

Books

7407 **Adult Scoliosis Surgery...It Can Be Done**
St. Luke's Spine Center
11311 Shaker Boulevard
Cleveland, OH 44104-3805
216-368-7000
Describes various types of surgery and procedures used in adult scoliosis patients.
21 pages

7408 **Coalition Index**
American School Health Association
PO Box 708
Kent, OH 44240
330-678-1601
800-445-2742
Fax: 330-678-4526
e-mail: asha@ashaweb.org
www.ashaweb.org
A professional membership organization dedicated to promoting the health and well being of children and youth through coordinated school health programs.
Susan Wooley, Executive Director

7409 **Getting Ready, Getting Well**
National Scoliosis Foundation
5 Cabot Place 781-341-6333
Stoughton, MA 02072 800-673-6922
Fax: 781-341-8333
e-mail: NSF@scoliosis.org
www.scoliosis.org
Guide for those anticipating surgery. Divided into three sections: Making up Your Mind, Taking Charge, and Home Again.
73 pages
Joseph P O'Brien, President/CEO

7410 **Handbook of Scoliosis**
Scoliosis Research Society
555 East Wells Street 414-289-9107
Milwaukee, WI 53202 Fax: 414-276-3349
www.srs.org
Tressa Goulding, Executive Director

7411 **Stopping Scoliosis**
National Scoliosis Foundation
5 Cabot Place 781-341-6333
Stoughton, MA 02072 800-673-6922
Fax: 781-341-8333
e-mail: NSF@scoliosis.org
www.scoliosis.org
Filled with accurate, currently researched information for adults concerned with their condition or that of a young person.
Joseph P O'Brien, President/CEO

7412 **Twenty Years at Hull House**
New American Library
375 Hudson Street 212-366-2000
New York, NY 10014
Book dealing with Scoliosis.
Grades 7-12

Children's Books

7413 **Deenie**
Bradbury Press
866 3rd Avenue 212-702-2000
New York, NY 10022-6221 800-257-5755
Deenie, a beautiful thirteen-year-old girl, had a mother who was pushing her to become a model. The agency representatives told Deenie she had the looks but walked differently. Deenie's main wish was to become a cheerleader. Her close friend, Janet, made the cheerleading squad but Deenie didn't make the finalist list. After this her gym teacher noticed her posture and called her family. After seeing therapists, the diagnosis of adolescent idiopathic scoliosis was made.
159 pages Hardcover
ISBN: 0-027110-20-6

7414 **Tina's Story...Scoliosis and Me**
Alfred I DuPont Institute
PO Box 269 302-651-4000
Wilmington, DE 19801
Suggested for parents of children anticipating surgery. This outstanding book, written as an eighth grade project by a gifted thirteen year old writer and scoliosis patient, relates her experiences and emotions while wearing a brace for three years prior to surgery.

7415 **What Young People and Parents Need to Know about Scoliosis**
American Physical Therapy Association
1111 N Fairfax Street 703-684-2782
Alexandria, VA 22314
A physical therapist's perspective.

Newsletters

7416 **Backtalk**
Scoliosis Association
PO Box 811705 561-994-4435
Boca Raton, FL 33481-1705 800-800-0669
Fax: 561-994-2455
e-mail: scolioassn@aol.com
www.scoliosis.org
Information for families, patients and health care professionals.

Pamphlets

7417 **1 in Every 10 Persons Has Scoliosis**
National Scoliosis Foundation
5 Cabot Place 781-341-6333
Stoughton, MA 02072 800-673-6922
Fax: 781-341-8333
e-mail: NSF@scoliosis.org
www.scoliosis.org
Explains what scoliosis is and illustrates how to screen for it. It also contains facts about the Foundation.
Joseph P O'Brien, President/CEO

7418 **Adolescent Idiopathic Scoliosis: Prevelance, Natural History, Treatments**
National Scoliosis Foundation
5 Cabot Place 781-341-6333
Stoughton, MA 02072 800-673-6922
Fax: 781-341-8333
e-mail: NSF@scoliosis.org
www.scoliosis.org
Expert overview of a condition that affects many young people.
Joseph P O'Brien, President/CEO

7419 **Boston Bracing System for Idiopathic Scoliosis**
National Scoliosis Foundation
5 Cabot Place 781-341-6333
Stoughton, MA 02072 800-673-6922
Fax: 781-341-8333
e-mail: NSF@scoliosis.org
www.scoliosis.org
Explaination of an available option.
Joseph P O'Brien, President/CEO

7420 **Brace & Her Brace is No Handicap**
National Scoliosis Foundation
5 Cabot Place 781-341-6333
Stoughton, MA 02072 800-673-6922
Fax: 781-341-8333
e-mail: NSF@scoliosis.org
www.scoliosis.org
Contains two illustrated short stories, each about a teenage girl coping successfully with scoliosis.
Joseph P O'Brien, President/CEO

7421 **Getting a Second Opinion**
National Scoliosis Foundation
5 Cabot Place 781-341-6333
Stoughton, MA 02072 800-673-6922
Fax: 781-341-8333
e-mail: NSF@scoliosis.org
www.scoliosis.org
Reprinted from Health Tips.
Joseph P O'Brien, President/CEO

7422 **Going Home**
University Hospital Spine Center
2074 Abington Road 216-844-1616
Cleveland, OH 44106
Instructions for pediatric and adult patients who have had a spinal fusion.

7423 **Medical Update Column**
National Scoliosis Foundation
5 Cabot Place 781-341-6333
Stoughton, MA 02072 800-673-6922
Fax: 781-341-8333
e-mail: NSF@scoliosis.org
www.scoliosis.org
Reprints from past issues of the Spinal Connections Medical Update Column available on various topics.
Joseph P O'Brien, President/CEO

7424 **NSF Packets**
National Scoliosis Foundation

5 Cabot Place
Stoughton, MA 02072
781-341-6333
800-673-6922
Fax: 781-341-8333
e-mail: NSF@scoliosis.org
www.scoliosis.org

Packet contains information for parents and young people, adults, and healthcare professionals.
Joseph P O'Brien, President/CEO

7425 **Patient with Scoliosis**
Educational Services, Division of AJV Company
555 W 57th Street
New York, NY 10019-2925
212-996-6473
A reprint from the American Journal of nursin.

7426 **Postural Screening Program**
National Scoliosis Foundation
5 Cabot Place
Stoughton, MA 02072
781-341-6333
800-673-6922
Fax: 781-341-8333
e-mail: NSF@scoliosis.org
www.scoliosis.org

Guidelines for physicians and school nurses.
Joseph P O'Brien, President/CEO

7427 **Questions Most Often Asked the NSF**
National Scoliosis Foundation
5 Cabot Place
Stoughton, MA 02072
781-341-6333
800-673-6922
Fax: 781-341-8333
e-mail: NSF@scoliosis.org
www.scoliosis.org

Answers the most frequently asked questions about scoliosis and the foundation in general.
Joseph P O'Brien, President/CEO

7428 **Scoliosis**
Scoliosis Research Society
611 E Wells Street
Milwaukee, WI 53202
414-289-9107
Fax: 414-276-3349
www.srs.org

Brochure describing scoliosis, kyphosis, lordosis; causes, prevention, treatment and adult scoliosis.
Tressa Goulding, Executive Director

7429 **Scoliosis Patient Becomes a Model**
National Scoliosis Foundation
5 Cabot Place
Stoughton, MA 02072
781-341-6333
800-673-6922
Fax: 781-341-8333
e-mail: NSF@scoliosis.org
www.scoliosis.org

Reprinted from Children's Today.
Joesph P O'Brien, President/CEO

7430 **Scoliosis Road Map**
University Hospital Spine Center
2074 Abington Road
Cleveland, OH 44106
216-844-1616
Written for teenagers affected by this illness.

7431 **Scoliosis Screening: The Carlsbad Program**
National Scoliosis Foundation
5 Cabot Place
Stoughton, MA 02072
781-341-6333
800-673-6922
Fax: 781-341-8333
e-mail: NSF@scoliosis.org
www.scoliosis.org

Exceptional scoliosis screening program.
Joseph P O'Brien, President/CEO

7432 **Scoliosis Surgery, What's It All About?**
University Hospital Spine Center
2074 Abington Road
Cleveland, OH 44106
216-844-1616
This pamphlet answers many of the questions patients ask before having surgery.

7433 **Scoliosis and Kyphosis**
Scoliosis Research Society
555 East Wells Street
Milwaukee, WI 53202
414-289-9107
Fax: 414-276-3349
www.srs.org

Information and advice from parents.
Tressa Goulding, Executive Director

7434 **Scoliosis, Me?**
North Dallas Scoliosis Center
1910 N Collins Boulevard
Richardson, TX 75080-3525
972-644-1930
Detailed answers to questions most asked by parents and teens.

7435 **Scoliosis... Now it Can Be Treated in Adults as Well as Children**
National Scoliosis Foundation
5 Cabot Place
Stoughton, MA 02072
781-341-6333
800-673-6922
Fax: 781-341-8333
e-mail: NSF@scoliosis.org
www.scoliosis.org

Reprinted from Cleveland Magazine.
Joseph P O'Brien, President/CEO

7436 **Scoliosis: Handbook for Patients**
National Scoliosis Foundation
5 Cabot Place
Stoughton, MA 02072
781-341-6333
800-673-6922
Fax: 781-341-8333
e-mail: NSF@scoliosis.org
www.scoliosis.org

Information on detection and treatment of adolescent scoliosis, kyphosis and lordosis and adult scoliosis.
Joseph P O'Brien, President/CEO

7437 **Screening Procedure Guidelines for Spinal Deformity**
Scoliosis Research Society
555 East Wells Street
Milwaukee, WI 53202
414-289-9107
Fax: 414-276-3349
www.srs.org

Seven page brochure covers reasons, organizations and procedures for spinal screening. Signs of spinal deformity, as seen in both standing and forward bending positions are illustrated and discussed. Includes sample screening form.
7 pages
Tressa Goulding, Executive Director

7438 **Spinal Deformity: Congenital Scoliosis and Kyphosis**
Scoliosis Research Society
555 East Wells Street
Milwaukee, WI 53202
414-289-9107
Fax: 414-276-3349
www.srs.org

Discusses signs and causes of congenital spinal deformities, associated conditions, treatment options and a glossary of terms.
12 pages
Tressa Goulding, Executive Director

7439 **Spinal Deformity: Scoliosis and Kyphosis**
Scoliosis Research Society
555 East Wells Street
Milwaukee, WI 53202
414-289-9107
Fax: 414-276-3349
www.srs.org

Twelve page brochure discusses signs and causes of scoliosis and kyphosis, indications for treatment, treatment options, commonly asked questions and a glossary of terms.
12 pages
Tressa Goulding, Executive Director

7440 **What Young People & Their Parents Need to Know About Scoliosis**
American Physical Therapy Association
1111 N Fairfax Street
Alexandria, VA 22314-1488
703-684-2782
A physical therapists' perspective.

7441 **What if You Need an Operation for Scoliosis?**
St. Luke's Spine Center
11311 Shaker Boulevard
Cleveland, OH 44104-3805
216-368-7000

7442 **When the Spine Curves**
National Scoliosis Foundation

5 Cabot Place 781-341-6333
Stoughton, MA 02072 800-673-6922
Fax: 781-341-8333
e-mail: NSF@scoliosis.org
www.scoliosis.org

Joseph P O'Brien, President/CEO

7443 **You and Your Brace**
University Hospital Spine Center
2074 Abington Road 216-844-1616
Cleveland, OH 44106

Audio & Video

7444 **Cutting Edge Medical Report**
National Scoliosis Foundation
5 Cabot Place 781-341-6333
Stoughton, MA 02072 800-673-6922
Fax: 781-341-8333
e-mail: NSF@scoliosis.org
www.scoliosis.org
As seen on the Discovery Channel, this video is an indepth examination of the latest developments in the diagnosis and treatment of scoliosis.
Joseph P O'Brien, President/CEO

7445 **Growing Straighter and Stronger**
National Scoliosis Foundation
5 Cabot Place 781-341-6333
Stoughton, MA 02072 800-673-6922
Fax: 781-341-8333
e-mail: NSF@scoliosis.org
www.scoliosis.org
Fifteen-minute presentation available in VHS video format, for the pre-screening education of students in grades 5 through 7.
Videotape
Joseph P O'Brien, President/CEO

7446 **Preparing Yourself for Spinal Surgery for Teenagers with Severe Scoliosis**
National Scoliosis Foundation
5 Cabot Place 781-341-6333
Stoughton, MA 02072 800-673-6922
Fax: 781-341-8333
e-mail: NSF@scoliosis.org
www.scoliosis.org
Patient education video helping to reduce anxiety for teenagers facing surgery by giving a sense of what to expect before, during, and after surgery.
Joseph P O'Brien, President/CEO

7447 **School Screening with Dr. Robert Keller**
National Scoliosis Foundation
5 Cabot Place 781-341-6333
Stoughton, MA 02072 800-673-6922
Fax: 781-341-8333
e-mail: NSF@scoliosis.org
www.scoliosis.org
Training video that teaches the proper technique for doing spinal screening. Defines scoliosis and kyphosis. Four teenagers, three with curves and one without, are examined and the findings explained.
Videotape
Joseph P O'Brien, President/CEO

7448 **Scoliosis: An Adult Perspective**
National Scoliosis Foundation
5 Cabot Place 781-341-6333
Stoughton, MA 02072 800-673-6922
Fax: 781-341-8333
e-mail: NSF@scoliosis.org
www.scoliosis.org
Dr. Blackman and five women patients provide an overall perspective of what scoliosis is, who gets it, the types of devices, myths about the disorder, and options for treatment.
Joseph P O'Brien, President/CEO

7449 **Sharing Scoliosis: You're Not Alone**
National Scoliosis Foundation
5 Cabot Place 781-341-6333
Stoughton, MA 02072 800-673-6922
Fax: 781-341-8333
e-mail: NSF@scoliosis.org
www.scoliosis.org
The Missouri chapter of the NSF, shares their experience with scoliosis including diagnosis, wearing a brace, surgery, and recovery. It is a good source of support for patients of all ages and their families.
Joseph P O'Brien, President/CEO

7450 **Spinal Screening Program**
Scoliosis Research Society
555 East Wells Street 414-289-9107
Milwaukee, WI 53202 Fax: 414-276-3349
www.srs.com
Twenty minute videotape designed to instruct screeners in the spinal screening program. It demonstrates methods of screening, showing adolescents with normal and abnormal spines. Includes sample screening form.
VHS Video Tape
Tressa Goulding, Executive Director

7451 **Taking the Mystery Out of Spinal Deformities**
Children's Hospital of LA, Div. of Orthopaedics
4650 Sunset Boulevard 213-660-2450
Los Angeles, CA 90027 800-841-7439
e-mail: RWETZEL@chla.usc.edu
Answers questions most often asked by screeners, patients and parents.
Videotape

7452 **Understanding Scoliosis**
National Scoliosis Foundation
5 Cabot Place 781-341-6333
Stoughton, MA 02072 800-673-6922
Fax: 781-341-8333
e-mail: NSF@scoliosis.org
www.scoliosis.org
Kaiser Permanente's educational video clearly and positively addresses the patient community. In this video four teenagers at various stages of treatment talk about their life with scoliosis.
Joseph P O'Brien, President/CEO

7453 **What's This Thing Called Scoliosis**
National Scoliosis Foundation
5 Cabot Place 781-341-6333
Stoughton, MA 02072 800-673-6922
Fax: 781-341-8333
e-mail: NSF@scoliosis.org
www.scoliosis.org
Comprehensive overview of scoliosis using the latest computer technology. The anatomical spine and animated model work together to truly show the 3D aspects of scoliosis and the corresponding impact on the patient.
Joseph P O'Brien, President/CEO

7454 **You Are Not Alone**
Minnesota Spine Center
606 24th Avenue S 612-332-3843
Minneapolis, MN 55454-1438
A video presenting two women's experiences with surgery. Personal life, concerns, hospital experience, recovery and improved lifestyle are openly discussed.
Videotape

Web Sites

7455 **American Association of Neurological Surgeons**
www.neurosurgery.org/
Official web site of the American Association of Neurological Surgeons and Congress of Neurological Surgeons. Whether you are a patient, physician, health care professional, or member of the media, this site is your online resource for neurosurgical information.

7456 **British Scoliosis Research Society**
www.ndos.ox.ac.uk/pzs/
This site contains: background to the meeting, Scoliosis Research Society review papers on the aetiology of idiopathic scoliosis, a

list of participants, abstracts classified by discussion group and the chairman's conclusions for each group.

7457 Healing Well

www.healingwell.com

An online health resource guide to medical news, chat, information and articles, newsgroups and message boards, books, disease-related web sites, medical directories, and more for patients, friends, and family coping with disabling diseases, disorders, or chronic illnesses.

7458 Health Finder

www.healthfinder.gov

Searchable, carefully developed web site offering information on over 1000 topics. Developed by the US Department of Health and Human Services, the site can be used in both English and Spanish.

7459 Healthlink USA

www.healthlinkusa.com

Health information concerning treatment, cures, prevention, diagnosis, risk factors, research, support groups, email lists, personal stories and much more. Updated regularly.

7460 Helios Health

www.helioshealth.com

Online resource for your health information. Detailed information about specific health topics, access to expert advice from our Medical Advisory Board, and up-to-date health news.

7461 MedicineNet

www.medicinenet.com

An online resource for consumers providing easy-to-read, authoritative medical and health information.

7462 Medscape

www.mywebmd.com

Medscape offers specialists, primary care physicians, and other health professionals the Web's most robust and integrated medical information and educational tools.

7463 Patients Rate Their Scoliosis Doctors

This web site is a free internet service for communicating subjective impressions of medical doctor (MD) reputations among scoliosis patients. Please use this system to learn some of the subjective impressions of the treatment other patients have received from their doctors.

7464 Scoliosis Association

www.sauk.org.uk/

The Scoliosis Association (UK) was founded in 1981. It is the only independent support group for scoliosis in the UK. SAUK aims to provide information about scoliosis, eliminate fear and stigma, and offer contacts for shared experiences.

7465 WebMD

www.webmd.com

Information on scoliosis, including articles and resources.

Description

7466 **Seizure Disorders**

There are two types of seizure disorders: an isolated, nonrecurring attack, such as may occur with high fevers in children, head trauma, or from other diseases (metabolic abnormalities or brain tumor) and epilepsy, which is characterized by recurrent, sudden, rapid changes in brain function caused by abnormalities in the electrical activity of the brain. Roughly 2 million Americans suffer from epilepsy, with half of the cases found in children and adolescents.

Seizures can be classified as generalized, affecting the whole brain at once, or partial, affecting a part of the brain. Absence (petit mal) attacks are generalized seizures in which there is only a brief (10-30 second) loss of consciousness, with eye and muscle fluttering but no loss of muscle tone. A generalized tonic-clonic seizure (grand mal) usually lasts 1-2 minutes, and includes loss of consciousness, falling, and involuntary contractions of the arms and legs. Some patients report that they see flashing lights and experience a heightened sense of taste and smell (known as an aura) that indicates they are about to have a seizure.

In many cases there is no apparent cause of the disorder, and it is therefore called idiopathic epilepsy.

Treatment aims primarily to control seizures. Causative or precipitating factors should be eliminated. Drug treatment is the mainstay of therapy for most types of seizures. In order to limit toxic effects, an attempt is made to use only a single drug. Some patients may need to take more than one drug. In most cases, acceptable control can be achieved with medications alone. Rarely, seizures will not respond to drugs, and surgery on the brain will be recommended. In this procedure, the surgeon tries to identify and destroy the part of the brain that is triggering the seizures.

National Agencies & Associations

7467 **American Epilepsy Society**
342 N Main Street — 860-586-7505
W Hartford, CT 06117-2500 — Fax: 860-568-7550
e-mail: ctubby@aesnet.org
www.aesnet.org
Fosters treatment of epilepsy in its biological clinical and social phases.
M Suzanne C Berry, Executive Director
Cheryl-Ann Tubby, Assistant Executive Director

7468 **Epilepsy Foundation**
8301 Professional Place — 301-459-3700
Landover, MD 20785 — 800-332-1000
Fax: 301-577-2684
e-mail: postmaster@efa.org
www.epilepsyfoundation.org
A national charitable nonprofit volunteer agency in the US dedicated to the welfare of people with epilepsy. Its goals are the prevention and cure of seizure disorders, the alleviation of their effects and the promotion of independence.
Steven T Sabatini, Chair of the Board of Directors
Eric R Hargis, President & CEO

7469 **National Association of Epilepsy Centers**
5775 Wayzata Boulevard — 612-525-4526
Minneapolis, MN 55416-1222 — 888-525-6232
Fax: 612-525-1560
e-mail: info@naec-epilepsy.org
www.naec-epilepsy.org
A nonprofit organization that encourages and supports professional and technical education in the treatment of epilepsy. Over 50 centers nationwide are members of the trade association which will make referrals to its member centers.
Robert J Gumnit MD, President
Gregory L Barkley, VP

7470 **National Institute of Neurological Disorders and Stroke**
31 Center Drive, Building 31 — 301-496-5751
Bethesda, MD 20892-0001 — 800-352-9424
Fax: 301-402-2186
www.ninds.nih.gov
America's focal point for support of research on brain and nervous system disorders.
Zach Hall, Director

State Agencies & Associations

California

7471 **Epilepsy Foundation of Northern California**
5700 Stoneridge Mall Road — 925-224-7760
Pleasanton, CA 94588-2824 — 800-632-3532
Fax: 925-224-7770
e-mail: efnca@epilepsynorcal.org
www.epilepsynorcal.org
Nonprofit organization serving families affected by epilepsy.
Neva Hirschkorn, Executive Director
Bill Stack, Associate Director

Florida

7472 **Epilepsy Association of Big Bend**
1215 Lee Avenue — 850-222-1777
Tallahassee, FL 32303-2651 — Fax: 850-222-7440
e-mail: epilepsyassoc@embarqmail.com
www.epilepsyassoc.org
Services include: Case management, prevention education, counseling and advocacy, information and referral.

7473 **Epilepsy Foundation of South Florida**
7300 N Kendall Drive — 305-670-4949
Miami, FL 33156-7840 — Fax: 305-670-0904
e-mail: information@epilepsysofla.org
www.epilepsyfound.org
A twenty five year old nonprofit community based organization dedicated to enhancing the personal and social adjustments of individuals with seizure disorders and their families.
Karen Basha Egozi, Executive Director
Ana Alfonso, Executive Administrator

7474 **Epilepsy Services Foundation**
4618 N Armenia Avenue — 813-870-3414
Tampa, FL 33603-2706 — Fax: 813-870-1321
e-mail: info@epilepsysf.org
www.epilepsysf.org
Information on medical and supportive services for persons affected by epilepsy living in West Central Florida. Raise funds to provide medical and supportive services and to build an endowment to make a difference in the lives of generations to come.
Thomas Orth, Executive Director

7475 **Epilepsy Services of North Central Florida**
11200 NW 8th Avenue — 352-392-6449
Gainesville, FL 32601-4946 — 800-330-9746
Fax: 352-392-5792
e-mail: jlyons@college.med.ufl.edu
www.floridaepilepsy.org/northcentral.htm
Jim Lyons, Program Director
Mike Dorsey, PE Coordinator

7476 **Epilepsy Services of Northeast Florida**
5209 San Jose Boulevard 904-731-3751
Jacksonville, FL 32207-2267 e-mail: epilepsy@bellsouth.net
Services include: Program case management, program prevention and education, employment services, children's summer camp, counseling and advocacy, and information and referrals.

7477 **Epilepsy Services of Southwest Florida**
1900 Main Street 941-953-5988
Sarasota, FL 34236 Fax: 941-366-5890
www.epilepsyservicesofswfl.org
Dedicated to providing case management and medical services for individuals with seizure disorders who meet eligibility criteria. Provides employment education for individuals and families affected by seizure disorders and prevention education to the com
Thomas Garrity, Executive Director

7478 **Manattee County Office Epilepsy Services of Southwest Florida**
1701 14th Street W 941-746-6488
Bradenton, FL 34205-7132 Fax: 941-746-8382
e-mail: bardentonep@aol.com
Brian Larocque, Social Worker

New Jersey

7479 **Epilepsy Foundation of New Jersey**
429 River View Plaza 609-392-4900
Trenton, NJ 08611-3420 800-336-5843
Fax: 609-392-5621
TTY: 800-852-7899
TDD: 800-852-7899
e-mail: efnj@efnj.com
www.efnj.com
Eric M Joice, Executive Director
Liza Gundell, Deputy Director

New York

7480 **Epilepsy Foundation of Long Island**
506 Stewart Avenue 516-739-7733
Garden City, NY 11530-4700 888-672-7154
Fax: 516-794-2180
e-mail: info@epil.org
www.efli.org
Robert A Karson, President
John Savarese, Vice President

Pennsylvania

7481 **Epilepsy Foundation of Western Pennsylvania**
1323 Forbes Avenue 412-261-5880
Pittsburgh, PA 15219-4725 Fax: 412-261-5361
e-mail: staff@efwp.org
www.efwp.org

Washington

7482 **Epilepsy Foundation of North West Washington**
2311 N 45th Street 206-547-4551
Seattle, WA 98103 800-752-3509
Fax: 206-547-4557
e-mail: mail@epilepsynw.org
www.epilepsyfoundation.org
Brent Herrmann, President/CEO
Alta C Hancock, Associate Director

Research Centers

7483 **Baylor College of Medicine: Epilepsy Research Center**
Texas Medical Center
6550 Fannin 713-798-8259
Houston, TX 77030 Fax: 713-798-7533
e-mail: neurochair@bcm.edu
www.bcm.edu/neurology
The clinical program at Baylor College of Medicine for the comprehensive evaluation of those with epilepsy or those suspected of having seizures or epilepsy.
Eli Mizrahi MD, Director

7484 **Duke University Center for the Advanced Study of Epilepsy**
Duke Neuroscience Clinic
200 Trent Drive 919-668-7600
Durham, NC 27710 888-ASK-DUKE
www.dukehealth.org
Clinical and research unit that experiments in limbic epilepsy.
James McNama MD, Director
William B Gallentine

7485 **Duke University Epilepsy Research Center**
Trent Drive 919-684-8111
Durham, NC 27710 888-275-3853
www.mc.duke.edu
Dr James McNamara, Director

7486 **Neurology Research Center Helen Hayes Hospital**
Helen Hayes Hospital
53-55 Route 9W 845-786-4535
W Haverstraw, NY 10993 888-70R-EHAB
Fax: 845-947-3097
e-mail: info@helenhayeshospital.org
www.helenhayeshospital.org
Robert Linds MD, Chief Internal medicine
Jason P Greenberg, Assistant Clinical Professor of Neurolog

7487 **University of Illinois at Chicago Consultation Clinic for Epilepsy**
912 S Wood Street 312-996-6906
Chicago, IL 60612-7330 Fax: 312-996-4169
e-mail: neu50@uic.edu
www.uic.edu
Dr. John R Hughes, Director

7488 **University of Tennessee: Center for Neuroscience**
875 Monroe Avenue 901-448-5960
Memphis, TN 38163-0001 Fax: 901-448-4685
www.utmem.edu/neuroscience
Epilepsy research and studies.
William E Armstrong, Director
Anton J Reiner, Co-Director

7489 **University of Wisconsin Madison Neurophysiology Laboratory**
UW Hospital and Clinics
600 Highland Avenue 608-263-6400
Madison, WI 53792 800-323-8942
Fax: 608-265-5512
www.uwhealth.org
Epilepsy research.
Thomas P Sutula, Chairman of Neurology
Paul A Rutecki, Vice Chairman of Neurology

Support Groups & Hotlines

7490 **Epilepsy Foundation of America Helpline**
Epilepsy Foundation of America
4351 Garden City Drive 301-459-3700
Landover, MD 20785-7223 800-332-1000
Fax: 301-577-4941
e-mail: postmaster@esa.org
www.epilepsyfoundation.org
A toll free information and referral service staffed by specially trained people who will answer questions and discuss concerns about seizure disorders and their treatment. Staff will direct callers to local affiliates of the EFA and tell about a broad range of medical services that respond to the needs of people with seizure disorders.
Eric Hargis, Chief Executive Officer

7491 **National Health Information Center**
PO Box 1133 310-565-4167
Washington, DC 20013 800-336-4797
Fax: 301-984-4256
e-mail: info@nhic.org
www.health.gov/nhic
Offers a nationwide information referral service, produces directories and resource guides.

Books

7492 **Americans with Disabilities Act**
Epilepsy Foundation of America
4351 Garden City Drive 301-459-3700
Landover, MD 20785-2267 800-332-1000
Fax: 301-577-9056
Learn how the Americans With Disabilities Act of 1990 can benifit you. Excellent comprehensive resource for individuals with seizure disorders.
46 pages Softcover
ISBN: 0-802774-65-2

7493 **Bomb in the Brain: A Heroic Tale of Science, Surgery and Survival**
MacMillan Publishing Company
866 3rd Avenue 212-702-2000
New York, NY 10022
The autobiographical account of this author's struggle with epilepsy and the debilitating effects it has on health, emotions, and mental stability.
Grades 10-12

7494 **Brainstorms: Epilepsy in Our Words**
4351 Garden City Drive 301-459-3700
Landover, MD 20785-2267 800-332-1000
Fax: 301-577-9056
Patients describe their experiences with seizures. Sixty-eight in-depth personal accounts of actual seizures are followed by a short section on how epilepsy affects the lives of the patients.
197 pages Paperback
ISBN: 0-802774-65-2

7495 **Children with Epilepsy**
Epilepsy Foundation of America
4351 Garden City Drive 301-459-3700
Landover, MD 20785-2267 800-332-1000
Fax: 301-577-9056
Offers direction and support to parents of a child with epilepsy, by first educating them about epilepsy and then helping them cope with the effects this disorder will have on their child and family.
314 pages Paperback
ISBN: 0-933149-19-0

7496 **Does Your Child Have Epilepsy?**
4351 Garden City Drive 301-459-3700
Landover, MD 20785-2267 800-332-1000
Fax: 301-577-9056
This book establishes Ten Basic Rules for parents of children with epilepsy.
201 pages Softcover

7497 **Embrace the Dawn**
Epilepsy Foundation of America
4351 Garden City Drive 301-459-3700
Landover, MD 20785-2267 800-332-1000
Fax: 301-577-9056
A moving biographical account of one person's lifelong experience with epilepsy.
127 pages Softcover

7498 **Epilepsy A to Z**
4351 Garden City Drive 301-459-3700
Landover, MD 20785-2267 800-332-1000
Fax: 301-577-9056
This book is designed to give health-care personnel a convenient way to find brief answers to questions about epilepsy. It includes definitions of terms, ranging all the way from abdominal epilepsy to Zonisimide.
322 pages Softcover

7499 **Epilepsy Diet Treatment: An Introduction to the Ketogenic Diet**
Epilepsy Foundation of America
4351 Garden City Drive 301-459-3700
Landover, MD 20785-2267 800-332-1000
Fax: 301-577-9056
The only book devoted exclusively to the ketogenic diet - a rigid, mathematically calculated, doctor-supervised diet that is high in fat and low in carbohydrate and protein with strictly limited calories and liquid intake. Gives all the facts about the diet, plus quotes from parents showing what the experience is really like and 30 sample recipes.
1996 200 pages
ISBN: 0-939957-86-8

7500 **Epilepsy Surgery**
Raven Press
1185 Avenue of the Americas 212-930-9500
New York, NY 10036-2601
The most complete and current references on surgical treatments of the epilepsies.
880 pages
ISBN: 0-881678-21-0

7501 **Epilepsy and the Family: A New Guide**
Harvard University Press
79 Garden Street
Cambridge, MA 02138 800-448-2242
www.hup.harvard.edu/catalog/LECEPF.html

ISBN: 0-674258-97-5

7502 **Epilepsy: 199 Answers**
Demos Medical Publishing
386 Park Avenue S 212-683-0072
New York, NY 10016-8804 800-532-8663
Fax: 212-683-0118
e-mail: orderdept@demosmed.com
www.demosmedpub.com
Addresses the needs of everyone with epilepsy. A helpful guide to the most common questions asked by people with epilepsy and will help the reader to work with his physician and take charge of the epilepsy.
1996 152 pages
ISBN: 1-888799-09-9
Dr. Diana M Schneider, President

7503 **Epilepsy: A Behavior Medicine Approach to Assessment & Treatment in Children**
Hogrefe & Huber Publications
PO Box 51 716-282-1610
Lewiston, NY 14092-0051 Fax: 716-484-4200
1993 200 pages
ISBN: 0-889371-06-7

7504 **Epilepsy: Current Approaches to Diagnosis and Treatment**
Raven Press
1185 Avenue of the Americas 212-930-9500
New York, NY 10036-2601
288 pages
ISBN: 0-881676-15-2

7505 **Epilepsy: I Can Live with That**
4351 Garden City Drive 301-459-3700
Landover, MD 20785-2267 800-332-1000
Fax: 301-577-9056
The experience of epilepsy as recorded by a group of ordinary men and women living in Australia. Each story focuses on personal growth, triumph over disability and emphasizes individual courage and hope.
Softcover
ISBN: 0-802774-65-2

7506 **Epilepsy: Models, Mechanisms & Concepts**
Cambridge University Press
40 W 20th Street 212-924-3900
New York, NY 10011-4211 800-221-4512
Fax: 212-691-3239
e-mail: customerservice@cup.org
www.cup.org
1993 400 pages
ISBN: 0-521392-98-5
Alice Ra, Assistant Marketing Manager

7507 **Epilepsy: Patient and Family Guide**
O Devinsky, MD, author
FA Davis Company

1915 Arch Street
Philadelphia, PA 19103
215-568-2172
800-523-4049
Fax: 215-568-5065
e-mail: mrt@fadavis.com
www.fadavis.com

Epilepsy expert Dr. Orrin Devinsky provides an easy-to-read guide to understanding the disease so that patients can achieve — and maintain — a higher quality of life. This book will educate recently-diagnosed patients, as well as those who have been living with epilepsy for years.

434 pages Paperback
ISBN: 0-803604-98-X
Michael Torso, Marketing Manager

7508 Equal Partners
Epilepsy Foundation of America
4351 Garden City Drive
Landover, MD 20785-2267
301-459-3700
800-332-1000
Fax: 301-577-9056

This book tells the story of a young Harvard-trained doctor whose experiences with seizures, brain surgery and subsequent epilepsy turns her from physician to patient.

257 pages Hardcover
ISBN: 0-802774-65-2

7509 Guide to Understanding and Living with Epilepsy
4351 Garden City Drive
Landover, MD 20785-2267
301-459-3700
800-332-1000
Fax: 301-577-9056

Easy-to-understand resource for people with epilepsy and their families. Covers a wide range of medical, social and legal issues. Topics include expanation of seizures and epilepsy; information about medication, side effects and risks; and getting the best medical care.

7510 Ketogenic Diet: A Treatment for Epilepsy
Demos Medical Publishing
386 Park Avenue S
New York, NY 10016
212-683-0072
Fax: 212-683-0118
e-mail: orderdept@demopub.com
www.demosmedpub.com

256 pages
ISBN: 1-888799-39-0
Dr. Diana M Schneider

7511 Living Well with Epilepsy
Epilepsy Foundation of America
4351 Garden City Drive
Landover, MD 20785-2267
301-459-3700
800-332-1000
Fax: 301-577-9056

Designed to help both health-care professionals and patients to understand all aspects of diagnosis and of pharmacologic and surgical management; to enable patients to participate more knowledgeably in interactions with their health care team and to help steer them toward a more normal, fulfilling life.

166 pages Softcover
ISBN: 1-888799-11-0

7512 Managing Seizure Disorder
Epilepsy Foundation of America
4351 Garden City Drive
Landover, MD 20785-2267
301-459-3700
800-332-1000
Fax: 301-577-9056

Provides health professionals with detailed information, on a variety of subjects, designed to help them help people with epilepsy live the kind of life they desire.

276 pages Softcover
ISBN: 0-802774-65-2

7513 Miles to Go Before I Sleep
Epilepsy Foundation of America
4351 Garden City Drive
Landover, MD 20785-2267
301-459-3700
800-332-1000
Fax: 301-577-9056

This book tells the story of a hijacking in which the author sustained a severe brain injury that, among other things, affected her vision, her memory, and left her with epilepsy.

230 pages Hardcover
ISBN: 0-802774-65-2

7514 Students with Seizures: A Manual for School Nurses
Epilepsy Foundation of America
4351 Garden City Drive
Landover, MD 20785-2267
301-459-3700
800-332-1000
Fax: 301-577-9056

A professional text with the sole purpose of creating a more accepting and understanding school environment for children with seizure disorders.

131 pages Paperback

Children's Books

7515 Dotty the Dalmatian has Epilepsy
Epilepsy Foundation of America
4351 Garden City Drive
Landover, MD 20785-2267
301-459-3700
800-332-1000
Fax: 301-577-9056

This is the story of Dotty the Dalmatian who discovers she has epilepsy.

16 pages Softcover
ISBN: 0-802774-65-2

7516 Epilepsy
Franklin Watts Grolier
90 Old Sherman Tpke
Danbury, CT 06816-0001
203-797-3500
800-621-1115
Fax: 203-797-3197
www.grolier.com

This book explains what epilepsy is, causes of epileptic seizures, diagnosis and treatments.

96 pages Grades 7-12
ISBN: 0-531108-07-4

7517 Lee the Rabbit with Epilepsy
4351 Garden City Drive
Landover, MD 20785-2267
301-459-3700
800-332-1000
Fax: 301-577-9056

Written for children ages 3-6, this illustrated picture book follows the adventures of a small rabbit who has seizures during a fishing trip with her Grandpa.

23 pages Hardcover

7518 Season of Secrets
Little, Brown & Company
3 Center Plz
Boston, MA 02108
617-227-0730
800-759-0190
Fax: 800-286-9471

Grades 4-6

Newsletters

7519 Epilepsia: Journal of the International League Against Epilepsy
Blackwell Publishing, Inc.
Commerce Place
Malden, MA 02148
781-388-8200
800-862-6657
Fax: 781-388-8210
www.blackwellpublishing.com

The leading international journal on the epilepsies for more than 30 years, Epilepsia provides comprehensive coverage of current clinical and research results.

7520 Epilepsy Services Foundation Newsletter
4618 N Armenia Avenue
Tampa, FL 33603-2706
813-870-3414
Fax: 813-870-1321
e-mail: eswcf@epilepsyservices.com
www.epilepsyservices.com

Information on medical and supportive services for persons affected by epilepsy living in West Central Florida. Raise funds to provide medical and supportive services to build and endowment to make a difference in the lives of generations to come.

2 pages 2-3 x/year
Thomas Orth, Executive Director

Pamphlets

7521 Child with Epilepsy at Camp
Epilepsy Foundation of America
4351 Garden City Drive 301-459-3700
Landover, MD 20785-2267 800-332-1000
Fax: 301-577-9056
Helps to explain why the child with epilepsy should be included in the camping experience.
14 pages Pamphlet

7522 Children and Seizures: Information for Babysitters
Epilepsy Foundation of America
4351 Garden City Drive 301-459-3700
Landover, MD 20785-2267 800-332-1000
Fax: 301-577-9056
Explains seizures, routine and special care, emergency aid and first aid to babysitters. Also offers a graph to write down important information about the child with seizure disorders for a quick reference.

7523 Epilepsy Medicines and Dental Care
Epilepsy Foundation of America
4351 Garden City Drive 301-459-3700
Landover, MD 20785-2267 800-332-1000
Fax: 301-577-9056
Explains dental care and includes instructions for brushing and flossing.

7524 Epilepsy: Legal Rights, Legal Issues
Epilepsy Foundation of America
4351 Garden City Drive 301-459-3700
Landover, MD 20785-2267 800-332-1000
Fax: 301-577-9056
Offers persons diagnosed with epilepsy information on their legal rights in employment, education, insurance and general disability benefits.
9 pages

7525 Epilepsy: Part of Your Life Series
Epilepsy Foundation of America
4351 Garden City Drive 301-459-3700
Landover, MD 20785-2267 800-332-1000
Fax: 301-577-9056
Provides information for staying healthy, describes various tests and diagnostic procedures, includes information for parents of children with epilepsy and provides general answers to questions about epilepsy.
Series of 4

7526 Epilepsy: You and Your Child, a Guide for Parents
Epilepsy Foundation of America
4351 Garden City Drive 301-459-3700
Landover, MD 20785-2267 800-332-1000
Fax: 301-577-9056
This instructional booklet offers information on emotional aspects of epilepsy, how to handle seizures, medication, diet and nutrition, and offers referral organizations for parents.

7527 Epilepsy: You and Your Treatment
Epilepsy Foundation of America
4351 Garden City Drive 301-459-3700
Landover, MD 20785-2267 800-332-1000
Fax: 301-577-9056
Reviews medical tests and diagnostic procedures used by physicians in diagnosing epilepsy.

7528 Facts About Epilepsy
Epilepsy Foundation of America
4351 Garden City Drive 301-459-3700
Landover, MD 20785-2267 800-332-1000
Fax: 301-577-9056
Designed for use by physicians and other health professionals with an interest in or who deal with the problems of people with epilepsy.
16 pages Softcover

7529 Finding Out About Seizures: A Guide to Medical Tests
Epilepsy Foundation of America
4351 Garden City Drive 301-459-3700
Landover, MD 20785-2267 800-332-1000
Fax: 301-577-9056
Introduces adults and children with epilepsy to the types of tests they may have to undergo.

7530 Kits for Adults with Epilepsy
Epilepsy Foundation of America
4351 Garden City Drive 301-459-3700
Landover, MD 20785-2267 800-332-1000
Fax: 301-577-9056
A variety of informative pamphlets for persons with epilepsy or seizure disorders.

7531 Management by Common Sense
Epilepsy Foundation of America
4351 Garden City Drive 301-459-3700
Landover, MD 20785-2267 800-332-1000
Fax: 301-577-9056
Promotes the employability of people with seizure disorders. Provides employers with information about epilepsy, customer/client reactions, workers' compensation issues, side effects of medication and other information relevant to employing a person with epilepsy.
46 pages Paperback
ISBN: 0-802774-65-2

7532 Me and My World Packet for Children
Epilepsy Foundation of America
4351 Garden City Drive 301-459-3700
Landover, MD 20785-2267 800-332-1000
Fax: 301-577-9056
Collection of pamphlets designed for children with epilepsy.

7533 Medicines for Epilepsy
Epilepsy Foundation of America
4351 Garden City Drive 301-459-3700
Landover, MD 20785-2267 800-332-1000
Fax: 301-577-9056
Offers information on medication and treatments, generic drugs, side effects, drug abuse and more. Contains a color chart with picyures of the most common medications for epilepsy.

7534 Mom I Have a Staring Problem
Epilepsy Foundation of America
4351 Garden City Drive 301-459-3700
Landover, MD 20785-2267 800-332-1000
Fax: 301-577-9056
Tiffany, a seven-year-old, describes her experience with petit mal seizures; her feelings, wishes and fears. Written to help adults recognize a hidden problem that could be occuring with a child who has learning problems.
24 pages Softcover
ISBN: 0-802774-65-2

7535 My Brother Matthew
Woodbine House
4351 Garden City Drive 301-459-3700
Landover, MD 20785-2267 800-332-1000
Fax: 301-577-9056
A picture and text book for children who have a brother or sister with developmental delay.
25 pages Harcoverr
ISBN: 0-802774-65-2

7536 My Friend Emily
Epilepsy Foundation of America
4351 Garden City Drive 301-459-3700
Landover, MD 20785-2267 800-332-1000
Fax: 301-577-9056
A story about Emily and her best friend Katy. Emily, a self confident child who enjoys life, shows that kids with epilepsy are just like other kids.
35 pages Softcover
ISBN: 0-802774-65-2

7537 Patient's Guide to Everyday Life
Epilepsy Foundation of America
4351 Garden City Drive 301-459-3700
Landover, MD 20785-2267 800-332-1000
Fax: 301-577-9056

Provides information for the newly diagnosed individual with epilepsy.

7538 Preventing Epilepsy
Epilepsy Foundation of America
4351 Garden City Drive 301-459-3700
Landover, MD 20785-2267 800-332-1000
Fax: 301-577-9056

Examines some known causes of seizures and suggests precautionary measures which may prevent the occurrence of epilepsy.
16 pages

7539 Recognizing the Signs of Childhood Seizures
Epilepsy Foundation of America
4351 Garden City Drive 301-459-3700
Landover, MD 20785-2267 800-332-1000
Fax: 301-577-9056

Explains what seizures are and what to look for in your child.

7540 Seizure Recognition and First Aid
Epilepsy Foundation of America
4351 Garden City Drive 301-459-3700
Landover, MD 20785-2267 800-332-1000
Fax: 301-577-9056

Helps you recognize a seizure when it happens and give basic first aid.

7541 Surgery for Epilepsy
Epilepsy Foundation of America
4351 Garden City Drive 301-459-3700
Landover, MD 20785-2267 800-332-1000
Fax: 301-577-9056

Describes current surgical treatment and the testing that precedes it.
12 pages

7542 Talking to Your Doctor About Seizure Disorders
Epilepsy Foundation of America
4351 Garden City Drive 301-459-3700
Landover, MD 20785-2267 800-332-1000
Fax: 301-577-9056

Designed to help the patient talk with medical personnel about treatment of epilepsy.
Pamphlet

7543 Teacher's Role, A Guide for School Personnel
Epilepsy Foundation of America
4351 Garden City Drive 301-459-3700
Landover, MD 20785-2267 800-332-1000
Fax: 301-577-9056

Provides tips on recognizing seizures and handling a seizure in the classroom.
14 pages

Audio & Video

7544 Comprehensive Clinical Management of the Epilepsies
Epilepsy Foundation of America
4351 Garden City Drive 301-459-3700
Landover, MD 20785-2267 800-332-1000
Fax: 301-577-9056

Excellent reference on the treatment of epilepsy.
17 minutes

7545 How to Recognize and Classify Seizures
Epilepsy Foundation of America
4351 Garden City Drive 301-459-3700
Landover, MD 20785-2267 800-332-1000
Fax: 301-577-9056

Discusses the classification of seizures and epileptic syndromes.
25 minutes

7546 Just Like You and Me
TASH
1025 Vermont Avenue 202-263-5600
Washington, DC 20005 Fax: 202-637-0138
e-mail: btrader@tash.org
www.tash.org/index.html

A video/print package on successful living with epilepsy.
Lu Zeph, Executive of Board Operating Committee
Barbara A Trader, Human Resources Director

7547 Meeting the Challenge: Employment Issues and Epilepsy
Epilepsy Foundation of America
4351 Garden City Drive 301-459-3700
Landover, MD 20785-2267 800-332-1000
Fax: 301-577-2684

This video answers the fquestions most often asked by emloyers. It covers issues such as driving, absenteeism, productivity, accidents and first aid, and emphasized that most people with epilepsy can be gainfully employed.
9 minutes

7548 Rest of the Family
Epilepsy Foundation of America
4351 Garden City Drive 301-459-3700
Landover, MD 20785-2267 800-332-1000
Fax: 301-577-9056

Presents the feelings and concerns of other family members including siblings, of children with epilepsy.
Video cassette

7549 Seizure First Aid
Epilepsy Foundation of America
4351 Garden City Drive 301-459-3700
Landover, MD 20785-2267 800-332-1000
Fax: 301-577-9056

This video combines footage of real seizures with reenactments to demonstrate proper first aid procedures. In addition, people with epilepsy talk about how they feel when they have a seizure, discuss how they would like friends, family and the general public to react when a seizure occurs.
10 minutes

7550 Understanding Seizure Disorders
Epilepsy Foundation of America
4351 Garden City Drive 301-459-3700
Landover, MD 20785-2267 800-332-1000
Fax: 301-577-9056

Provides an explanation of seizure disorders in everyday language and dispels many misconceptions about epilepsy with medically accurate information.
Video cassette

7551 Voices from the Workplace
Epilepsy Foundation of America
Epilepsy Foundation of America 301-459-3700
4351 Garden City Drive, MD 20785 800-332-1000
Fax: 301-577-2684

Inspirational tape to help people with epilepsy cope with employment challenges. Individuals with epilepsy describe personal and social challenges in the workplace. They explain how they cope with their seizures and the reactions of co-workers and the public.

Web Sites

7552 American Epilepsy Society
www.aesnet.org

Fosters treatment of epilepsy in its biological, clinical and social phases.

7553 Epilepsy Foundation of America
www.efa.org

Information on the prevention and cure of seizure disorders, the alleviation of their effects, and the promotion of independence and optimal quality of life for people who have these disorders.

7554 Healing Well
www.healingwell.com

An online health resource guide to medical news, chat, information and articles, newsgroups and message boards, books, disease-related web sites, medical directories, and more for patients, friends, and family coping with disabling diseases, disorders, or chronic illnesses.

7555 Health Finder
www.healthfinder.gov

Searchable, carefully developed web site offering information on over 1000 topics. Developed by the US Department of Health and Human Services, the site can be used in both English and Spanish.

7556 **Healthlink USA**

www.healthlinkusa.com

Health information concerning treatment, cures, prevention, diagnosis, risk factors, research, support groups, email lists, personal stories and much more. Updated regularly.

7557 **Helios Health**

www.helioshealth.com

Online resource for your health information. Detailed information about specific health topics, access to expert advice from our Medical Advisory Board, and up-to-date health news.

7558 **MedicineNet**

www.medicinenet.com

An online resource for consumers providing easy-to-read, authoritative medical and health information.

7559 **Medscape**

www.mywebmd.com

Medscape offers specialists, primary care physicians, and other health professionals the Web's most robust and integrated medical information and educational tools.

7560 **National Institute of Neurological Disorders and Stroke**

www.aamc.org

America's focal point for support of research on brain and nervous system disorders.

7561 **Neurology Channel**

www.neurologychannel.com

Find clearly explained, medically accurate information regarding conditions, including an overview, symptoms, causes, diagnostic procedures and treatment options. On this site it is possible to ask questions and get information from a neurologist and connect to people who have similar health interests.

7562 **WebMD**

www.webmd.com

Information on seizure disorders, including articles and resources.

Description

7563 **Sexually Transmitted Diseases**

Sexually transmitted diseases, STDs, are among the most common infectious diseases in the U.S. More than 20 STDs have been identified, and roughly 13 million persons are affected. Fortunately, most STDs are curable with prompt treatment, and do not become chronic. These include bacterial vaginosis, gonorrhea, syphilis, trichomoniasis and chlamydia. People who suffer from these diseases over long periods almost always do so because of re-infection rather than treatment failure. HIV and hepatitis B are commonly transmitted through sexual intercourse; see also *AIDS* and *Hepatitis*.

Fortunately, behavioral changes in sexual practices can drastically reduce the risk of STDs. Abstinence from intercourse or having a long-term mutually faithful monogamous relationship with an uninfected partner give essentially complete protection. Risk rises with multiple partners, unprotected intercourse between males, anonymous sex and contact with high-risk individuals, such as prostitutes. Barrier methods, notably condoms, give significant but not complete protection.

Until recently, no vaccines were available for any common STD except hepatitis B. However, researchers developed a vaccine for human papilloma virus (HPV) that is, amazingly, 100 percent effective. The vaccine is such a critical discovery because one specific type of HPV causes cervical cancer. Common STDs which may become chronic despite treatment are described below.

Genital herpes is a virus of the herpes family characterized by blisters (vesicles) in the genital area. The appearance of the blisters is often preceded by low-grade fever and by burning pain in the affected area. The first episode is often the most painful. Specific anti-viral therapy will shorten the duration and intensity of an attack. Herpes infections are self-limited but recurrent because the virus chronically infects nerves that radiate from the spinal column. Under certain conditions, such as febrile illness and physical or emotional stress, the virus reactivates and causes another outbreak. People with frequent recurrences can lower the risk of repeat attacks by taking a low dose of the anti-viral medication every day.

Genital warts are caused by the human papilloma virus (HPV.) There are roughly 750,000 new cases each year in the United States. The warts may appear anywhere in the genital and rectal area, making transmission difficult to prevent with a condom. Genital warts in the male, unless quite large, are often just a cosmetic nuisance, although a wart inside the urinary passage may cause discomfort. Women with genital warts not only need to have the warts removed, but to be observed for pre-cancerous changes in the cervix. Warts are generally destroyed by application of chemicals, but doctors have also used laser beams, freezing and electrical currents to destroy them. Recurrence after treatment is common, even in the absence of re-infection.

Pelvic inflammatory disease (PID) is not always sexually transmitted, but it is included here because chlamydia and gonorrhea, which are sexually transmitted, are commonly the cause of PID. In this condition, the sensitive pelvic reproductive organs are attacked, leading to fever and lower abdominal pain and occasionally collection of pus in a pelvic abscess. Even after the attack is treated with high doses of antibiotics, residual scarring may lead to chronic pelvic pain, pain with intercourse, infertility and ectopic pregnancy, in which the fertilized egg implants in other pelvic structures outside the uterus. Prompt recognition and vigorous treatment of the acute attack of PID are important.

National Agencies & Associations

7564 **American Foundation for the Prevention of Venereal Disease**
799 Broadway
New York, NY 10003
212-759-2069
www.chclibrary.org
Encourages every individual to assume responsible sexual relations and proper personal hygiene.
Mary O'Connell, Secretary

7565 **American Social Health Association**
PO Box 13827
Research Triangle Park, NC 27709-3827
919-361-8400
800-227-8922
Fax: 919-361-8425
www.ashastd.org
Provides resources to local communities to improve STD control programs through citizen action.
Lynn Barclay, President CEO
Deborah Arrindell, Vice President Health Policy

7566 **American Venereal Disease Association**
PO Box 1753
Baltimore, MD 21203-1753
301-955-3150
www.alternativemedicine.com
Primary interest of this organization is in the reduction of the prevalence of the diseases.
Edward Hook III MD, Secretary

7567 **Centers for Disease Control and Prevention**
1600 Clifton Road
Atlanta, GA 30333
404-639-3111
800-232-4636
TTY: 888-232-6348
e-mail: cdcinfo@cdc.gov
www.cdc.gov
Offers reprints reports public awareness and educational materials and research on sexually transmitted diseases.
Richard E Besser, Director

7568 **Citizens Alliance for VD Awareness**
5002 W Madison
Chicago, IL 60644
773-379-1000
Fax: 773-379-1342
e-mail: info@cfhcn.org
www.circlefamilycare.org
Seeks to increase commitment of health professionals to venereal disease and AIDS control.
Bruce Peoples, President/CEO
Patrick C Nwaezeigwe, CFO

7569 **Herpes Resource Center**
PO Box 13827
Research Triangle Park, NC 27709-3827
919-361-8400
800-227-8922
Fax: 919-361-8425
www.ashastd.org
Gives emotional support to individuals and provides information to the public about herpes.
Carolyn Mabry, Coordinator
Lynn Barclay, President CEO

7570 **National Institute of Allergy and Infectious Diseases**
6610 Rockledge Drive
Bethesda, MD 20892-6612 301-496-5717
www.niaid.nih.gov

Research Centers

7571 **Herpes Resource Center**
PO Box 13827 919-361-8400
Research Triangle Park, NC 27709 800-227-8922
Fax: 919-361-8425
www.ashastd.org
Offers information and referrals for persons affected by herpes and other sexually transmitted disease prevention.
Lynn Barclay, President and Chief Executive Officer
Deborah Arrindell, Vice President Health Policy

7572 **International Union Against Venereal Diseases**
New York Hospital - Cornell Medical Center
1153 York Avenue 212-746-1200
New York, NY 10021 Fax: 212-746-1202
e-mail: ajacobso@myp.org
Encourages campaigns medical and social against venereal disease.
Lewis Drusin MD, Director

7573 **University of Chicago Committee on Virology**
Marjorie B Kovler Viral Oncology Laboratories
910 E 58th Street 773-702-1898
Chicago, IL 60637 Fax: 773-702-1631
mgcb.bsd.uchicago.edu
Focuses research into the area of sexually transmitted disease.
Bernard Roizman, Chairman
Olaf Schneewind, Professor and Chairman

Support Groups & Hotlines

7574 **National Health Information Center**
PO Box 1133 310-565-4167
Washington, DC 20013 800-336-4797
Fax: 301-984-4256
e-mail: info@nhic.org
www.health.gov/nhic
Offers a nationwide information referral service, produces directories and resource guides.

7575 **STI Resource Center Hotline**
919-361-8488
800-227-8922
www.ashastd.org
Provides information, materials and referrals to anyone concerned about sexually transmitted infections.
Lynn Barclay, President/CEO
Deborah Arrindell, VP Health Policy

Books

7576 **Herpes and Papilloma Viruses Volume I & II**
Raven Press
1185 Avenue of the Americas 212-930-9500
New York, NY 10036-2601
382 pages
ISBN: 0-881671-95-9

7577 **Sexually Transmitted Diseases**
Raven Press
1185 Avenue of the Americas 212-930-9500
New York, NY 10036-2601
Focuses on the clinically important subject of the immune response to sexually transmitted diseases.
350 pages
ISBN: 0-881678-82-1

7578 **Understanding Helps**
University Press of Mississippi
3825 Ridgewood Road 601-432-6205
Jackson, MS 39211-6492 800-737-7788
Fax: 601-432-6217
e-mail: press@ihl.state.ms.us
www.upress.state.ms.us
This book is for people who wish to learn about herpes simplex viruses, two remarkably complex microbes capable of causing a wide variety of infections. These include genital herpes, a very common chronic sexually transmitted disease.
120 pages Hardcover
ISBN: 1-578060-40-0
Kathy Burgess, Advertising Manager/Marketing Assistant

7579 **Understanding Herpes: Revised Second Edition**
Lawrence R Stanberry, MD; PhD, author
University Press of Mississippi
3825 Ridgewood Road 601-432-6205
Jackson, MS 39211-6492 Fax: 601-432-6217
e-mail: kburgess@ihl.state.ms.us
www.upress.state.ms.us
A concise overview of advances and resources.
2006 144 pages Paperback
ISBN: 1-578068-68-1
Kathy Burgess, Advertising/Marketing Services Manager

7580 **Women at Risk**
Bristol Publishing
PO Box 1737 415-895-4461
San Leandro, CA 94577-0811 Fax: 415-895-4459
1993 159 pages
ISBN: 0-917851-62-5

Children's Books

7581 **Teen Guide to Safe Sex**
Franklin Watts Grolier
90 Old Sherman Tpke 203-797-3500
Danbury, CT 06816-0001 800-621-1115
Fax: 203-797-3197
www.grolier.com
A basic book about sexually transmitted diseases. Describes what they are, what causes them, how to recognize them and how teenagers can protect against them.
64 pages Grades 9-12
ISBN: 0-531105-92-0

Newsletters

7582 **Sexually Transmitted Diseases: Journal**
Julius Scachter, PhD, author
Lippincott Wiliiams & Wilkins
PO Box 1600
Hagerstown, MD 21741-1600 800-638-3030
Fax: 301-223-2400
e-mail: orders@lww.com
www.lww.com
This timely, scholarly journal publishes original, peer-reviewed articles on clinical, laboratory, immunologic, epidemiologic, sociologic, and historical topics pertaining to sexually transmitted diseases and related fields.
Monthly

7583 **Step Perspective**
Seattle Treatment Education Project
127 Broadway E 206-329-4857
Seattle, WA 98102-5711 800-869-7837
A publication of the Seattle Treatment Education Project. Published three times a year.
Michael Auch, Executive Director

Pamphlets

7584 **AIDS...What We Need To Know Pamphlet**
March of Dimes

233 Park Avenue South
New York, NY 10003
212-353-8353
Fax: 212-254-3518
e-mail: NY639@marchofdimes.com
www.marchofdimes.com
Discusses the facts about HIV/Æinfection and AIDS and how you can reduce your risk.
Pkg of 50
ISBN: 0-923500- -

7585 Chlamydial Infection
National Institute of Allergy/Infectious Diseases
National Institutes of Health
Bethesda, MD 20892-0001
301-496-5717
Offers information on diagnosis, treatment, effects, prevention and research.

7586 Genital Herpes
National Institute of Allergy/Infectious Diseases
National Institutes of Health
Bethesda, MD 20892-0001
301-496-5717
Offers information on symptoms, causes, diagnosis and reccurences.

7587 Genital Herpes Fact Sheet
March of Dimes
233 Park Avenue South
New York, NY 10003
212-353-8353
Fax: 212-254-3518
e-mail: NY639@marchofdimes.com
www.marchofdimes.com
Fact Sheets: one to two page review written for the general public. Also available electronically from our website www.marchofdimes.com

7588 Gonorrhea
National Institute of Allergy/Infectious Diseases
National Institutes of Health
Bethesda, MD 20892-0001
301-496-5717
Offers information on the symptoms, diagnosis, treatment, complications, prevention and research.

7589 Human Papillomavirus and Genital Warts
National Institute of Allergy/Infectious Diseases
National Institutes of Health
Bethesda, MD 20892-0001
301-496-5717
Offers information on diagnosis, treatment, complications and prevention of the diseases.

7590 Introduction to Sexually Transmitted Diseases
National Institute of Allergy/Infectious Diseases
National Institutes of Health
Bethesda, MD 20892-0001
301-496-5717
Offers information on STDs, various types and symptoms, research, and referral services.

7591 Other Important STD's
National Institute of Allergy/Infectious Diseases
National Institutes of Health
Bethesda, MD 20892-0001
301-496-5717
Lists over ten of the most common sexually transmitted diseases. Offers information on what they are, the causes and treatments, research being done in these areas and referral numbers of where to call for more information on the diseases.

7592 Pelvic Inflammatory Disease
National Institute of Allergy/Infectious Diseases
National Institutes of Health
Bethesda, MD 20892-0001
301-496-5717
Offers information on the causes, symptoms, risk factors, diagnosis, treatment, and prevention.

7593 Syphilis
National Institute of Allergy/Infectious Diseases
National Institutes of Health
Bethesda, MD 20892-0001
301-496-5717
Offers information on what syphilis is, the symptoms, complications, diagnosis, prevention and treatment methods available.

7594 Vaginal Infections
National Institute of Allergy/Infectious Diseases
National Institutes of Health
Bethesda, MD 20892-0001
301-496-5717
Lists three specific types of vaginitis, with information on their symptoms, prevention, complications and treatments.

Web Sites

7595 American Social Health Association
sunsite.unc.edu/asha
Provides resources to local communities to improve STD control programs through citizen action.

7596 Centers for Disease Control
www.cdc.gov
Offers reprints, reports, public awareness and educational materials and research on sexually transmitted diseases.

7597 Healing Well
www.healingwell.com
An online health resource guide to medical news, chat, information and articles, newsgroups and message boards, books, disease-related web sites, medical directories, and more for patients, friends, and family coping with disabling diseases, disorders, or chronic illnesses.

7598 Health Finder
www.healthfinder.gov
Searchable, carefully developed web site offering information on over 1000 topics. Developed by the US Department of Health and Human Services, the site can be used in both English and Spanish.

7599 Healthlink USA
www.healthlinkusa.com
Health information concerning treatment, cures, prevention, diagnosis, risk factors, research, support groups, email lists, personal stories and much more. Updated regularly.

7600 Helios Health
www.helioshealth.com
Online resource for your health information. Detailed information about specific health topics, access to expert advice from our Medical Advisory Board, and up-to-date health news.

7601 MedicineNet
www.medicinenet.com
An online resource for consumers providing easy-to-read, authoritative medical and health information.

7602 Medscape
www.mywebmd.com
Medscape offers specialists, primary care physicians, and other health professionals the Web's most robust and integrated medical information and educational tools.

7603 WebMD
www.webmd.com
Information on sexually transmitted diseases, including articles and resources.

Description

7604 **Sickle Cell Disease**

Sickle cell disease (also called sickle cell anemia) is an inherited defect of hemoglobin, the oxygen-carrying element in the blood. Under some circumstances, the normally disc-shaped red blood cell takes on a crescent or sickle shape. It then becomes lodged in small capillaries and prevents normal oxygen flow to the tissues. This oxygen deprivation can cause sickle cell crises, with symptoms of severe pain in the back, joints, hands, and feet, and may even include neurologic changes. Severe abdominal pain and vomiting may also occur.

Sickle cell anemia occurs almost exclusively in African Americans. There are approximately 55,000 people in the United States with this condition. These children have sickle cell trait, occurring when one receives a copy of the sickle cell gene from only one parent. Only if a child receives a copy of the defective gene from both parents will the full-blown disease develop.

Therapy for sickle cell disease is aimed at preventing and treating infections, maintaining an adequate diet and fluid intake, and managing acute attacks with painkillers, oxygen, antibiotics and blood transfusion. Hydroxyurea has been shown to reduce the number of attacks by 50 percent as well as the need for transfusion. In the past, death typically occurred because of overwhelming infection or from organ destruction brought about by multiple sickling crises. Modern therapy has imporved life expectancy dramatically, but some level of disability is common. Geneticcounseling is important for the patient and all family members.

National Agencies & Associations

7605 **American Sickle Cell Anemia**
10300 Carnegie Avenue 216-229-8600
Cleveland, OH 44106-0171 Fax: 216-229-4500
e-mail: irabragg@ascaa.org
www.ascaa.org
Provides education testing counseling and supportive services for sickle cell anemia and its hemoglobinopathy variants.
Ira Bragg-Grant, Executive Director
Leslie Carter, Newborn Screening Coordinator

7606 **Comprehensive Sickle Cell Center**
80 Jesse Hill Jr Drive SE 404-616-3572
Atlanta, GA 30303 Fax: 404-616-5998
e-mail: aplatt@emory.edu
www.scinfo.org
The mission of Sickle Cell Information Center is to provide sickle cell patient and professional education, news, research updates and world wide sickle cell resources, as well as world class compassionate care.
James R Eckman, Medical Director
Lewis Hsu, Interim Director

7607 **Sickle Cell Anemia Foundation**
503 S Center Street 704-878-0732
Statesville, NC 28687
This program is designed to provide information about sickle cell disease symptoms available treatments and service facilities by distributing literature and dispatching foundation members to address organizations church or school groups.
Priscilla Dudley

7608 **Sickle Cell Association of Ontario**
3199 Bathurst Street 416-789-2855
Toronto, Ontario, M6A-2B2 Fax: 416-789-1903
e-mail: sicklecell@look.ca
www.sicklecellontario.com
A voluntary, non-profit, charitable organization which is funded by donations from individuals, organizations and employee charitable funds.
Dotty Nicholas RN, President

7609 **Sickle Cell Disease Association of America**
231 E Baltimore Street 410-528-1555
Baltimore, MD 21202 800-421-8453
Fax: 410-528-1495
e-mail: scdaa@sicklecelldisease.org
www.sicklecelldisease.org
Purpose is to promote leadership on a national level in order to create awareness in all circles of the impact of sickle cell disease on emotional and economic well-being of families and the individual.
Willarda V Edwards, President/COO
Jeannine Knight, Executive Assistant to the President/COO

7610 **Sickle Cell Information Center Grady Memorial Hospital**
Grady Memorial Hospital
80 Jesse Hill Jr Drive SE 404-616-3572
Atlanta, GA 30303 Fax: 404-616-5998
e-mail: aplatt@emory.edu
www.SCInfo.org
Our mission is to provide sickle cell patient and professional education news research updates and world wide sickle cell resources. It is the mission of our organizations to provide world class compassionate care.
James R Eckman, Medical Director
Lewis Hsu, Interim Director

Foundations

7611 **James R Clark Memorial Sickle Cell Foundation**
1420 Gregg Street 803-765-9916
Columbia, SC 29201 800-506-1273
Fax: 803-799-6471
e-mail: sicklecell@sc.rr.com
Genetic Blood Disorder Disease.
Melodie A Hunnicutt, Executive Director
Saundra Kidwell, Director Finance

7612 **Northeast Louisiana Sickle Cell Anemia Foundation**
1604 Winnsboro Road 318-322-0896
Monroe, LA 71202 Fax: 318-387-4740
e-mail: sickle@bayou.com
The Foundation is a community-based non-profit, tax-exempt organization whose purpose is to provide services to sickle cell patients and their families, as well as be a resource in the communities we serve (12 northeast parishes) We provide education, trait counseling, patient assistance and social services. Our services are free.
Lasandre R Starks, Executive Director
Cheryl Minor, Registered Social Worker

7613 **Sickle Cell Foundation of Georgia**
2391 Benjamin E Mays Drive 404-755-1641
Atlanta, GA 30311 800-326-5287
Fax: 404-755-7955
e-mail: n_nichols@sicklecellatlaga.org
www.sicklecellatlaga.org
Our mission is dedicated to providing education, screening and counseling programs for Sickle Cell and other abnormal hemoglobin.
D Jean Brannan, President
Nesby Gibson, Project Director

7614 **Sickle Cell Foundation of Greater Montgomery**
3180 US Highway 8 West 334-286-9122
Montgomery, AL 36108 800-742-5534
e-mail: sicklec2@aol.com
www.scfgm.org
The main objectives of the Foundation are to give accurate information about sickle cell disease and related hemoglobinopathies, to provide testing and diagnostic services to interested persons, to

counsel individuals with positive test results so they can make informed decisions about their lives and to provide supportive services for clients and their family members.
Willie Owens, Executive Director

Research Centers

7615 **Boston Sickle Cell Center Boston Medical Center**
Boston Medical Center
88 E Newton Street 617-414-1020
Boston, MA 02118-2999 Fax: 617-414-1021
e-mail: mhsteinb@bu.edu
www.bu.edu/sicklecel
The treatment facility of choice for Boston-area patients with sickle cell disease. The Center also promotes interactive basic and clinical research and patient and professional educational activities.
Martin Steinberg, Director
Shawn H Eung, Program Manager

7616 **Columbia University: Comprehensive Sickle Cell Center**
Harlem Hospital
506 Lenox Avenue
New York, NY 10037-1000 212-939-1426
www.nyc.gov/html/hhc/html/facilities/har
Research into sickle cell disease.
Dr Jeanne Smith, Director

7617 **Comprehensive Sickle Cell Center Children's Hospital Research Foundation**
Children's Hospital Research Foundation
3333 Burnet Avenue 513-636-4541
Cincinnati, OH 5229—3039 800-344-2462
Fax: 513-636-5562
e-mail: blood@cchmc.org
www.cincinnatichildrens.org
Offers research and statistical information in the area of sickle cell disease.
Clinton Joiner, Director
Karen Kalinyak, Clinical Director

7618 **Howard University Center for Sickle Cell Disease**
1840 7th Street NW 202-865-8292
Washington, DC 20001 Fax: 202-232-6719
e-mail: sicklecell@howard.edu
www.sicklecell.howard.edu
Victor R Gordeuk, Director
Catherine Nwokolo, Clinical Staff Member

7619 **Medical College of Georgia: Sickle Cell Center**
1521 Pope Avenue 706-721-2171
Augusta, GA 30912-0002 Fax: 706-721-4575
www.mcg.edu/centers/sicklecel
Offers research into sickle cell disease.
Abdullah Kutlar, Director
Kavita Natarajan

7620 **Philadelphia Biomedical Research Institute**
100 Ross and Royal Road 610-962-0615
King of Prussia, PA 19406 Fax: 610-254-9332
e-mail: stohmishi@aol.com
members.aol.com/stohinishi/phila_biomed
Study on the management of sickle cell anemia through nutrition.
S Tsuyoshi Ohinishi PhD, Director

7621 **SUNY Health Science Center at Brooklyn Sickle Cell Center**
450 Clarkson Avenue 718-270-1000
Brooklyn, NY 11203 Fax: 718-270-7592
www.hscbklyn.edu
John C LaRosa, President
Paul J Davis, Interim Chief Financial Officer

7622 **Sickle Cell Anemia Research Foundation**
2625 3rd Street 318-487-8019
Alexandria, LA 71309 877-722-7370
Fax: 318-487-9990
e-mail: scarf@sicklecelldisease.org
www.kumc.edu
The Sickle Cell Anemia Research Foundation provides a comprehensive program on Sickle Cell Disease. We offer education training counseling and help with prescriptions.

7623 **Sickle Cell Association of the Texas Gulf Coast**
2626 S Loop W 713-666-0300
Houston, TX 77054-2649 Fax: 713-660-17
Rebecca Jasso, Executive Director

7624 **University of California Northern Comprehensive Sickle Cell Center**
Childrens Hospital Research Center
747 50 2nd Street 510-428-3651
Oakland, OK 94609-3594
Sickle cell disease research.
Elliot Vichinsky, Director

7625 **University of Southern California: Comprehensive Sickle Cell Center**
2025 Zonal Avenue 213-342-1259
Los Angeles, CA 90033-1034
Dr Cage S Johnson, Director

7626 **University of Texas Southwestern Medical Center/Sickle Cell Management**
Southwestern Medical Center
1935 Medical District Drive 214-456-7000
Dallas, TX 75235-7701 Fax: 214-648-3122
e-mail: jsquires@childmed.dallas.tx.us
www.childrens.com
Focuses on the prevention of disease complications and management using the newest treatment strategies including hydroxyurea chronic transfusions stem cell (bone marrow) transplantation and state-of-the-art approaches to infection prevention pain management and treatment of specific organ-related complications (chest syndrome priapism avascular necrosis of the femoral head etc.).
George Bucha MD, Director
James F Amatruda

7627 **Wayne State University: Comprehensive Sickle Cell Center**
Curricular Affairs Office
Scott Hall 313-577-1546
Detroit, MI 48201 Fax: 313-577-8777
wayne.edu
Charles F Whitten MD, President

Support Groups & Hotlines

7628 **Keon Paschal Perry Sickle Cell Anemia Disease Awareness**
7510 Granby Street, Perry Building
Norfolk, VA 23505 888-406-5111
e-mail: keon4u@aol.com
International Sickle Cell Anemia Disease Awareness Campaign.
Roy L Perry-Bey, CEO/Executive Director

7629 **Lehigh Valley Sickle Cell Support Group**
PO Box 1711 610-706-0636
Allentown, PA 18105-1711 e-mail: SororW@aol.com
www.members.aol.com/SororW/index.html
Anyone affected/effected by Sickle Cell and all interested persons. Our mission is to educate the local community about Sickle Cell.

7630 **National Health Information Center**
PO Box 1133 310-565-4167
Washington, DC 20013 800-336-4797
Fax: 301-984-4256
e-mail: info@nhic.org
www.health.gov/nhic
Offers a nationwide information referral service, produces directories and resource guides.

7631 **Sickle Cell Anemia Association of Austin: Marc Thomas Chapter**
PO Box 201092 512-335-2306
Austin, TX 78720-1092 e-mail: llthomas@austin.cc.tx.us
www.tdh.state.tx.us
To raise awareness, resources and support for clients with sickle cell disease.
Linda L Thomas

7632 **Sickle Cell Disease Association of America Philadelphia/Delaware Valley Chapter**
4601 Market Street 215-471-8686
Philadelphia, PA 19139 Fax: 215-471-7441
e-mail: scdaa.pdvc@verizon.net
www.sicklecelldisorder.com
The Philadelphia/Delaware Valley Chapter of the Sickle Cell Disease Association of America (SCDAA/PDVC) assists the sickle cell community by serving as a vehicle and resource center for the psycho-social and social service needs of those individuals affected by the disease through the following services: case management; counseling; hospital/clinic visits; advocacy; career/vocational assistance; newborn screening follow-up; transportation; and outreach/community education.
Stanley A Simpkins, Executive Director
Karin Darius, Program Director

Pamphlets

7633 **Sickle Cell Disease**
March of Dimes
233 Park Avenue South 212-353-8353
New York, NY 10003 Fax: 212-254-3518
e-mail: NY639@marchofdimes.com
www.marchofdimes.com
Fact Sheets: one to two page review written for the general public. Also available electronically from the website www.marchofdimes.com

Web Sites

7634 **American Sickle Cell Anemia**
www.ascaa.org
Provides education, testing, counseling and supportive services for sickle cell anemia and its hemoglobinopathies variants.

7635 **Healing Well**
www.healingwell.com
An online health resource guide to medical news, chat, information and articles, newsgroups and message boards, books, disease-related web sites, medical directories, and more for patients, friends, and family coping with disabling diseases, disorders, or chronic illnesses.

7636 **Health Finder**
www.healthfinder.gov
Searchable, carefully developed web site offering information on over 1000 topics. Developed by the US Department of Health and Human Services, the site can be used in both English and Spanish.

7637 **Healthlink USA**
www.healthlinkusa.com
Health information concerning treatment, cures, prevention, diagnosis, risk factors, research, support groups, email lists, personal stories and much more. Updated regularly.

7638 **Helios Health**
www.helioshealth.com
Online resource for your health information. Detailed information about specific health topics, access to expert advice from our Medical Advisory Board, and up-to-date health news.

7639 **MedicineNet**
www.medicinenet.com
An online resource for consumers providing easy-to-read, authoritative medical and health information.

7640 **Medscape**
www.mywebmd.com
Medscape offers specialists, primary care physicians, and other health professionals the Web's most robust and integrated medical information and educational tools.

7641 **Sickle Cell Disease Association of America**
sicklecelldisease.org
Purpose is to promote leadership on a national level in order to create awareness in all circles of the impact of sickle cell disease on emotional and economic well-being of families and the individual.

7642 **WebMD**
www.webmd.com
Information on Sickle Cell disease, including articles and resources.

Description

7643 **Sjogren's Syndrome**

Sjogren's syndrome (also called sicca syndrome) is an autoimmune disorder characterized by dryness of the mouth, eyes and mucous membranes. Variable enlargement of the lacrimal (tear) or salivary gland can occur. The disorder has no known cause, but many researchers believe that it has a genetic basis. Sjogren's syndrome is divided into primary (affecting only the eyes and mouth) and secondary (generalized) forms which may be associated with connective tissue diseases such as rheumatoid arthritis, systemic lupus erythematosus, polymyositis or scleroderma.

Patients who suffer from Sjogren's syndrome often complain initially of a gritty sensation in the eyes or severe dryness of the mouth. Patients may develop kidney, skin, neurologic, pulmonary or joint problems.

Treatment for Sjogren's is mainly symptomatic in the form of artificial tears, sipping fluids throughout the day, chewing gum and using special mouthwash. Pilocarpine may be used to stimulate saliva production. Severe cases, especially if they affect parts of the body outside of the glands, may require corticosteroid therapy. Dental caries (cavities) are a complication of dry mouth, so close dental follow-up is important.

National Agencies & Associations

7644 **National Sjogren's Syndrome Foundation NSSA**
NSSA
5815 N Blk Canyon Highway
Phoenix, AZ 85015-2200
602-433-9844
800-395-6772
Fax: 602-433-9838
e-mail: NSSA@aol.com
www.sjogrens.org
Provides educational materials to members about medical developments and research concerning SS nationally and internationally. Membership also includes assorted discounts on additional materials and events.
Steven Taylor, National Executive Director
Sheriese DeFruscio, Vice President of Development

7645 **Sjogren's Syndrome Foundation**
6707 Democracy Boulevard
Bethesda, MD 20817-2025
301-530-4420
800-475-6473
Fax: 301-530-4415
e-mail: tms@sjogrens.org
www.sjogrens.org
A non-profit voluntary health organization whose purposes are to educate patients and their families about Sjogren's syndrome and help them cope with the problems and frustrations of living with Sjogren's syndrome and to increase public and medical awareness.
Philip C Fox, President
Steven Taylor, CEO

Support Groups & Hotlines

7646 **National Health Information Center**
PO Box 1133
Washington, DC 20013
310-565-4167
800-336-4797
Fax: 301-984-4256
e-mail: info@nhic.org
www.health.gov/nhic
Offers a nationwide information referral service, produces directories and resource guides.

Books

7647 **New Sjogren's Syndrome Handbook**
Sjogren's Syndrome Foundation
366 N Broadway
Jericho, NY 11753-2025
516-933-6365
800-475-4736
Fax: 516-933-6368
www.sjogrens.org
An authoritative guide for patients and health care providers on the many aspects of Sjogren's syndrome written by renowned experts, plus practical suggestions for living more comfortably with this chronic illness.
Hardcover
ISBN: 0-195117-24-7
Steven Carsons MD, Editor
Elaine K Harris, Editor

Newsletters

7648 **Moisture Seekers Newsletter**
Sjogren's Syndrome Foundation
366 N Broadway
Jericho, NY 11753-2025
516-933-6365
800-475-4736
Fax: 516-933-6368
www.sjogrens.org
Contains up-to-date information on Sjogren's syndrome including new treatments, new products, and clinical trails; also features articles on the ways members cope with this chronic disease.
9x Year
Linda Saslow, Editor

Pamphlets

7649 **Dry Eyes? Dry Mouth? Dry Nose? Arthritis? If Two or More: Sjogren's Syndrome**
Sjogren's Syndrome Foundation
382 Main Street
Port Washington, NY 11050-3136
516-767-2866
Fax: 516-767-7156
Offers a brief overview of what the illness is, a history, statistical information, causes, symptoms and treatments.

7650 **Sjogren's Syndrome**
NAMSIC/National Institutes of Health
1 AMS Circle
Bethesda, MD 20892-0001
301-495-4484
Fax: 301-587-4352
TTY: 301-565-2966
www.nih.gov/niams/
14 pages

Audio & Video

7651 **SjoGren's Syndrome Survival Guide**
6707 Democracy Boulevard
Bethesda, MD 20817
301-530-4420
800-475-6473
Fax: 301-530-4415
e-mail: staylor@sjogrens.org
www.sjogrens.org
A complete resource for Sjogren's sufferers providing the newest medical information, research results, and treatment methods available, as well as the most effective and practical self-help strategies. Sjogren's syndrome is an autoimmune disease in which the body's immune system mistakenly attacks its own moisture producing glands.
Steven Taylor, Chief Executive Officer
Sheriese DeFruscio, Vice President of Development

Web Sites

7652 **Healing Well**
www.healingwell.com
An online health resource guide to medical news, chat, information and articles, newsgroups and message boards, books, disease-related web sites, medical directories, and more for patients, friends,

and family coping with disabling diseases, disorders, or chronic illnesses.

7653 Health Finder

www.healthfinder.gov

Searchable, carefully developed web site offering information on over 1000 topics. Developed by the US Department of Health and Human Services, the site can be used in both English and Spanish.

7654 Healthlink USA

www.healthlinkusa.com

Health information concerning treatment, cures, prevention, diagnosis, risk factors, research, support groups, email lists, personal stories and much more. Updated regularly.

7655 Helios Health

www.helioshealth.com

Online resource for your health information. Detailed information about specific health topics, access to expert advice from our Medical Advisory Board, and up-to-date health news.

7656 MedicineNet

www.medicinenet.com

An online resource for consumers providing easy-to-read, authoritative medical and health information.

7657 Medscape

www.mywebmd.com

Medscape offers specialists, primary care physicians, and other health professionals the Web's most robust and integrated medical information and educational tools.

7658 National Sjogren's Syndrome Association

www.sjogrens.org

Provides educational materials to members about medical developments and research concerning SS nationally and internationally. Membership also includes assorted discounts on additional materials and events.

7659 Sjogren's Syndrome Foundation

www.sjogrens.org

Information on Sjogren's Syndrome, the SS Foundation, and links to other related sites.

7660 WebMD

www.webmd.com

Information on Sjogren's Syndrome, including articles and resources.

Description

7661 **Skin Disorders**

The three most common chronic skin disorders are acne, psoriasis and eczema. Although these conditions do not shorten one's life, or cause significant disability, they can have a profound effect on one's quality of life and self-esteem.

Acne is probably the most common skin disorder, and can affect all age groups. It typically occurs in adolescents and young adults. Acne involves the sebaceous glands - glands that produce sebum, a substance that preserves the skin's natural oiliness. In acne, the glands' pores become plugged, trapping the sebum and bacteria. Inflammation follows, resulting in small red tender bumps with a corresponding blackhead or whitehead. These lesions can become pus-filled or even cystic ranging from 1 mm to 5 mm. Acne is seen most commonly on the face, neck, back and shoulders. Treatment starts with keeping affected areas clean. Locally-applied creams include retinoic acid, benzoyl peroxide and various antibiotics. Oral antibiotics (tetracycline) are especially effective for large, deep pimples. Oral tretinoin (Accutane) is very affective, but causes birth defects and other side effects and should be used only as a last resort and in consultation with a dermatologist. Oral contraceptives are often helpful in young women.

Psoriasis usually begins in early adult life, and affects 2 to 4 percent of the white population. A family history is common. The disease is characterized by scaly patches, some as small rain drop, others a few inches in diameer. Typical locations are the scalp, knees and elbows, but any part of the body may be affected. The patches are extremely itchy, and compulsive scratching may further damage the skin. In roughly 10 percent there is an associated arthritis. Milder cases are treated with steroid creams applied to skin and tar preparations or oral psoralen drugs, is effective in more severe cases. The most severe cases may require immunomodulating drugs like methotrexate or cyclosporine.

Eczema is a catchall term for many diseases which involve skin inflammation in response to some irritant. The irritant may be a direct one, such as contact dermatitis from the metal in a belt buckle, or an indirect one, as in atopic dermatitis triggered by various environmental agents (inhalants) and factors (certain foods). Atopic dermatitis is frequently associated with a personal or family history of allergic disorders (hay fever, asthma). For either situation, treatment consists of identifying and eliminating the offending agent(if possible) and local application of corticosteroid creams or nonspecific soothin and hydrating substances. Topical tacrolimus, approved by the FDA in 2000, is an immunosuppressive ointment effective for severe eczema without damaging the skin in the way that long-term topical steriods sometimes do.

National Agencies & Associations

7662 **American Academy of Dermatology**
PO Box 4014 847-330-0230
Schaumburg, IL 60168-4014 866-503-7546
Fax: 847-240-1859
e-mail: volunteer@aad.org
www.aad.org
The largest, most influential dermatologic association in the world. The Academy is committed to the highest quality standards in continuing medical education and plays a major role in formulating socioeconomic solutions.
Cyndi Del Boccio, Board of Director
Barbara Greenan, Advisory Board

7663 **American Board of Dermatology American Society for Dermatologic Surger**
American Society for Dermatologic Surgery
5550 Meadowbrook Drive 847-956-0900
Rolling Meadows, IL 60008 Fax: 847-956-0999
e-mail: info@asds.net
www.asds-net.org
Sole mission is to ensure competence for patients with cutaneous diseases through board representation.
Katherine J Svedman, Executive Director
Debra Kennedy, Associate Executive Director

7664 **American Dermatological Association University of Iowa Hospital and Clinics**
University of Iowa Hospital and Clinics
Department of Dermatology 319-356-2274
Iowa City, IA 52242 Fax: 319-356-8317
Professional society of physicians specializing in dermatology. Promotes teaching, practice, public education and research into dermatology.
John S Strauss MD, Secretary

7665 **American Society for Dermatologic Surgery**
5550 Meadowbrook Drive 847-956-0900
Rolling Meadows, IL 60008-2005 Fax: 847-956-0999
e-mail: info@asds.net
www.asds.net
Seeks to improve the quality of abnormal skin conditions especially the structural changes produced by skin cancer and other disease.
Katherine J Svedman, Executive Director
Robert A Weiss, President

7666 **American Society of Plastic and Reconstructive Surgeons**
444 E Algonquin Road 847-228-9900
Arlington Heights, IL 60005-4654 800-475-2784
e-mail: media@plasticsurgery.org
www.plasticsurgery.org
This Society sends free information about various surgical procedures and also provides the names of board certified plastic surgeons in a patient's area.

7667 **Dermatology Foundation**
1560 Sherman Avenue 847-328-2256
Evanston, IL 60201-4808 Fax: 847-328-0509
e-mail: dfgen@dermatologyfoundation.org
www.dermfnd.org
Raises funds for the control of skin diseases through research improved education and better patient care. Supports basic clinical investigations.

7668 **Eczema Association for Science and Education**
4460 Redwood Highway 415-499-3474
San Rafael, CA 94903 800-818-7546
Fax: 415-472-5345
e-mail: info@nationaleczema.org
www.nationaleczema.org
Offers research and information to persons with eczema and other skin disorders.
Donald S Young, Chair
John [Jack] R Crossen, CFO

7669 **International Society of Dermatology**
2323 N State Street 386-437-4405
Bunnell, FL 32110-0001 Fax: 386-437-4427
e-mail: info@intsocderm.org
www.intsocderm.org
Promotes interest education and research in dermatology.
Sigfrid A Muller MD, President
Luitgard Wie MD, Executive Vice President

7670 **National Arthritis and Musculoskeletal & Skin Diseases Information Clearinghouse**
National Institutes of Health
31 Center Drive - MSC 2350 301-496-8190
Bethesda, MD 20892-2350 Fax: 301-480-2814
e-mail: niamsinfo@mail.nih.gov
www.niams.nih.gov
Our mission is to support research into the causes, treatment and prevention of arthritis and musculoskeletal and skin diseases, the training of basic and clinical scientists to carry out this research and the dissemination of information on research.
Stephen I Katz MD PhD, Director

7671 **National Institute of Arthritis and Musculoskeletal and Skin Disease (NIAMS)**
1 AMS Circle 301-495-4484
Bethesda, MD 20892 888-226-4267
Fax: 301-718-6366
TTY: 301-565-2966
e-mail: niamsinfo@mail.nih.gov
www.niams.nih.gov
The NIAMS Information Clearinghouse provides information about various forms of arthritis and rheumatic disease and bone, muscle and skin diseases. It distributes patient and professional education materials and refers people to other sources of information.
Stephen I Katz MD PhD, Director

Foundations

7672 **National Psoriasis Foundation**
6600 SW 92nd Avenue 503-244-7404
Portland, OR 97223-7195 800-723-9166
Fax: 503-245-0626
e-mail: getinfo@psoriasis.org
www.psoriasis.org
Misson: To find a cure for psoriasis arthritis and to eliminate their devastating effects through research, advocacy, and education. Provides: patient services; public and professional education; community services; government affairs; research.
Randy Beranek, President/CEO
Catie Coman, Director Communications

Research Centers

7673 **Agromedicine Program Medical University of South Carolina**
Medical University of South Carolina
295 Calhoun Street 843-792-2281
Charleston, SC 29425-0100 Fax: 843-792-1798
www.musc.edu
Does research into the effects of pesticides on humans including epidemiology and skin diseases.
Dr Stanley Schuman, Director
W Stuart Smith, Vice President for Clinical Operations a

7674 **Duke University Plastic Surgery Research Laboratories**
Medical Center
Box 3974 919-681-8555
Durham, NC 27710-1 e-mail: elizabeth.yundt@duke.edu
plastic.surgery.duke.edu
Conducts studies on skin cancer and aging skin.
L Scott Levin, Chief Division of Plastic and Reconstru
Detlev Erdmann, Associate Professor of Surgery

7675 **Laboratory of Dermatology Research Memorial Sloane-Kettering Cancer Center**
Memorial Sloane-Kettering Cancer Center
1275 York Avenue 212-639-2000
New York, NY 10065-6007 Fax: 212-717-3363
www.mskcc.org/mskcc
Specific studies on the identification of skin disorders and dermatology.
Allan C Halpern, Chief Dermatology Service

7676 **Massachusetts General Hospital: Harvard Cutaneous Biology Research Center**
Massachusetts General Hospital
55 Fruit Street 617-726-5254
Boston, MA 02114 Fax: 617-726-1875
TTY: 617-724-8800
www.massgeneral.org
Dermatology research.
Dr John Parrish, Director

7677 **Orentreich Foundation for the Advancement of Science**
855 Route 301 212-606-0836
Cold Spring, NY 10516-4155 Fax: 845-265-4210
e-mail: ofas@orentreich.org
Conducts biomedical research on dermatology.
Norman Orentreich, Founder and Co-Director
David S Orentreich, Co-Director

7678 **Psoriasis Research Institute**
600 Town & Country Center 650-326-1848
Palo Alto, CA 94301 Fax: 650-326-1262
Studies the causes symptoms and treatments of psoriasis.

7679 **Rockefeller University Laboratory for Investigative Dermatology**
Rockefeller University
1230 York Avenue 212-327-7458
New York, NY 10021-6399 Fax: 212-708-32
www.rockefeller.edu
Research into skin disorders and the whole specialty of dermatology in general.

7680 **Rockefeller University, Laboratory for Investigative Dermatology**
1230 York Avenue 212-327-7458
New York, NY 10021-6399 Fax: 212-570-8232
D Martin Carter MD, PhD, Head

7681 **Scripps Clinic and Research Foundation: Autoimmune Disease Center**
10550 N Torrey Pines Road 858-784-1000
La Jolla, CA 92037-1092 Fax: 619-554-6805
www.scripps.edu
Research into dermatomyostis and polymyositis.
Eng Tan, Professor Emeritus

7682 **Sulzberger Institute for Dermatologic Education**
PO Box 94020 847-330-0230
Palatine, IL 60094-4020 Fax: 847-330-0050
A nonprofit research center whose sole goal is to enhance patient care through the development and promotion of quality educational programs on the care and disorders of the skin, hair, nails and mucous membranes.

7683 **Sulzberger Institute for Dermatologic Educ**
PO Box 94020 847-330-0230
Palatine, IL 60094 Fax: 847-330-0050
A nonprofit research center whose sole goal is to enhance patient care through the development and promotion of quality educational programs on the care and disorders of the skin hair nails and mucous membranes.

7684 **University of California: San Francisco Dermatology Drug Research**
515 Spruce 415-476-2001
San Francisco, CA 94143-0001 Fax: 415-221-4751
www.ucsf.edu
Conducts clinical testing of new or existing pharmalogic agents used in the treatment of skin disorders.
John Koo MD, Director

7685 **University of Texas: Southwestern Medical Center at Dallas, Immunodermatology**
5323 Harry Hines Boulevard 214-648-3111
Dallas, TX 75390-7208 Fax: 214-688-8275
www.utsouthwestern.edu

Provides a focus for research into the causes prevention and management of diseases such as immune deficiencies and infections. Studies are aimed at increasing basic-level understanding of immunologic skin diseases.
Paul Bergtresser, Chair in Dermatology
Kiyoshi Ariizumi, Associate Professor

Support Groups & Hotlines

7686 **National Health Information Center**
PO Box 1133 310-565-4167
Washington, DC 20013 800-336-4797
Fax: 301-984-4256
e-mail: info@nhic.org
www.health.gov/nhic
Offers a nationwide information referral service, produces directories and resource guides.

Books

7687 **Managing Your Psoriasis**
MasterMedia
33 Beecker Street 212-260-5600
New York, NY 10012 800-334-8232
1993 Paperback
ISBN: 0-942361-83-0

7688 **Psoriasis and Psoriatic Arthritis Pocket G uide**
National Psoriasis Foundation
6600 SW 92nd Avenue 503-244-7404
Portland, OR 97223-7195 800-723-9166
Fax: 503-245-0626
e-mail: getinfo@psoriasis.org
www.psoriasis.org
The Pocket Guide includes algorithms for therapy_including combination and biologic treatments_based on patient types. This second edition was revised to provide guidance for managing patients with severe psoriasis and to put the roll of new biologics into perspective.
2005 79 pages

7689 **Q&A's About Psoriasis**
NAMSIC/National Institutes of Health
1 AMS Circle 301-495-4484
Bethesda, MD 20892-0001 877-226-4267
Fax: 301-718-6366
TTY: 301-565-2966
e-mail: niamsinfo@mail.nih.gov
www.nih.gov/niams
Offers various information for the psoriasis patient and their family regarding treatments, risks, nutrition and more.
24 pages

7690 **Therapy of Moderate-to-Severe Psoriasis**
National Psoriasis Foundation
6600 SW 92nd Avenue 503-244-7404
Portland, OR 97223-7195 800-723-9166
Fax: 503-245-0626
e-mail: getinfo@psoriasis.org
www.psoriasis.org
Edited by Gerald D. Weinstein, MD, and Alice Gottlieb, MD, PhD, this book includes information on state-of-the-art clinical management through contributions from national experts on psoriasis.
2002
Gail M Zimmerman, President/CEO
Paula Fasano, Director Marketing/Communications

7691 **Treatment Guide for the Health Insurance Industry**
National Psoriasis Foundation
6600 SW 92nd Avenue 503-244-7404
Portland, OR 97223-7195 800-723-9166
Fax: 503-245-0626
e-mail: getinfo@psoriasis.org
www.psoriasis.org
This easy-to-read general overview is a valuable tool for the insurer or any health professional interested in detailed information about psoriasis and psoriatic arthritis, patient quality of life issues, and many available treatments.
Gail M Zimmerman, President/CEO
Paula Fasano, Director Marketing/Communications

Magazines

7692 **International Journal of Dermatology**
International Society of Dermatology
200 1st Street SW 507-284-3736
Rochester, MN 55905-0001
Focuses on information for dermatologists and the whole specialty of dermatology research and education.
10x Year

7693 **Journal of Dermatologic Surgery and Oncology**
International Society for Dermatologic Surgery
930 N Meachan Road 847-330-9830
Schaumburg, IL 60173 Fax: 847-330-1135
Focuses on medical updates and information on dermatology.
Monthly

7694 **Journal of the Academy of Dermatology**
American Academy of Dermatology
PO Box 94020 847-330-0230
Palatine, IL 60094-4020 Fax: 847-330-0050
A scientific publication serving the clinical needs of the specialty and provides a wide selection of articles on various topics important to continuing medical education of Academy members and the international dermatologic community.
Monthly

7695 **Psoriasis Advance**
National Psoriasis Foundation
6600 SW 92nd Avenue 503-244-7404
Portland, OR 97223-7195 800-723-9166
Fax: 503-245-0626
e-mail: getinfo@npfusa.org
www.psoriasis.org
Written especially for the psoriatis community four times a year. Provides current articles to keep you up to date with treatmetnt and research information, pave the way to empowerment, and connect you with others.
40 pages BiMonthly
Sheri Decker, Director Communication

7696 **Psoriasis Forum**
National Psoriasis Foundation
6600 SW 92nd Avenue 503-244-7404
Portland, OR 97223-7195 800-723-9166
Fax: 503-245-0626
e-mail: getinfo@psoriasis.org
www.psoriasis.org
Dedicated to providing up-to-date and practical information to health care providers on the frontline of psoriasis treatment. Professional Members only.
Quarterly
Gail M Zimmerman, President/CEO
Paula Fasano, Director Marketing/Communications

Newsletters

7697 **Dermatology Focus**
Dermatology Foundation
1560 Sherman Avenue 847-328-2256
Evanston, IL 60201-4808 Fax: 847-328-0509
e-mail: dfgen@dermatologyfoundation.org
www.dermfnd.org
Designed to communicate to practitioners the latest advances in medical and surgical dermatology. The publication also serves as the Foundation's newsletter, recognizing the accomplishments and activities of the many dermatologists who give not only their monetary support, but countless hours to develop the research and teaching careers of future leaders throughout the specialty.
Quarterly
Sandra Rahn Benz, Executive Director

7698 **Dermatology Focus**
Dermatology Foundation
1560 Sherman Avenue 847-328-2256
Evanston, IL 60201-4808 Fax: 847-328-0509
e-mail: dfgen@dermatologyfoundation.org
www.dermfnd.org
Designed to communicate to practitioners the latest advances in medical and surgical dermatology. The publication also serves as the Foundation's newsletter recognizing the accomplishments and activities of the many dermatologists who give not only their monetary support, but countless hours to develop the research and teaching careers of future leaders throughout the specialty.
Quarterly
Sandra Rahn Benz, Executive Director

7699 **Dermatology World**
American Academy of Dermatology
PO Box 94020 847-330-0230
Palatine, IL 60094-4020 Fax: 847-330-0050
Offers Academy members information outside the clinical realm. It carries news of government actions, reports of socioeconomic issues, societal trends and other events which impinge on the practice of dermatology.
Monthly

7700 **Progress in Dermatology**
Dermatology Foundation
1560 Sherman Avenue 847-328-2256
Evanston, IL 60201-4808 Fax: 847-328-0509
e-mail: dfgen@dermatologyfoundation.org
www.dermfnd.org
The journal provides in-depth coverage of clinically relevant topics as well as basic scientific advances affecting all of dermatology. Distributed exclusively to members of the Foundation.
Quarterly
Sandra Rahn Benz, Executive Director

7701 **Psoriasis Newsletter**
Psoriasis Research Institute
600 Town & Country Center 650-326-1848
Palo Alto, CA 94301 Fax: 650-326-1262
e-mail: emfpri@aol.com
Offers information and medical updates on the disease of psoriasis, events, fundraising and more.
4 pages Quarterly

Pamphlets

7702 **Acne**
American Academy of Dermatology
PO Box 4014 847-330-0230
Schaumburg, IL 60168-4014 Fax: 847-330-0050
Explains the causes of acne. Treatments are explored, including diet, medications, antibiotics, and sun exposure. Available in Spanish.
1996

7703 **Allergic Contact Rashes**
American Academy of Dermatology
PO Box 4014 847-330-0230
Schaumburg, IL 60168-4014 Fax: 847-330-0050
Lists the common causes of skin rashes, including jewelry and hidden ingredients in fabrics and household products.
1997

7704 **Athlete's Foot**
American Academy of Dermatology
PO Box 4014 847-330-0230
Schaumburg, IL 60168-4014 Fax: 847-330-0050
This common fungal infection is not only a problem for athletics. Discusses what causes it and how to treat it.
1994

7705 **Black Skin**
American Academy of Dermatology
PO Box 4014 847-330-0230
Schaumburg, IL 60168-4014 Fax: 847-330-0050
Explains the skin diseases common with black skin and how they are diagnosed and treated.
1996

7706 **Conception, Pregnancy & Psoriasis**
National Psoriasis Foundation
6600 SW 92nd Avenue 503-244-7404
Portland, OR 97223-7195 800-723-9166
Fax: 503-245-0626
e-mail: getinfo@npfusa.org
www.psoriasis.org
Explains pregnancy factors for persons with psoriasis.

7707 **Cosmetics & Skin Care**
American Academy of Dermatology
PO Box 4014 847-330-0230
Schaumburg, IL 60168-4014 Fax: 847-330-0050
Discusses skin reactions to fragrances, makeup, and bath and body care products.
1994

7708 **Darker Side of Tanning**
American Academy of Dermatology
PO Box 4014 847-330-0230
Schaumburg, IL 60168-4014 Fax: 847-330-0050
Discusses the dangers of ultraviolet radiation from the sun, tanning beds, and sun lamps. Includes descriptions of the different skin types and tips to help minimize the sun's damage to the skin and eyes.
1996

7709 **Eczema/Atopic Dermatitis**
American Academy of Dermatology
PO Box 4014 847-330-0230
Schaumburg, IL 60168-4014 Fax: 847-330-0050
Explains how to recognize and treat dermatitis.
1995

7710 **For Parents**
National Psoriasis Foundation
6600 SW 92nd Avenue 503-244-7404
Portland, OR 97223-7195 800-723-9166
Fax: 503-245-0626
e-mail: getinfo@npfusa.org
www.psoriasis.org
Offers advice and resources on how to educate yourself about psoriasis and your child, as well as treatment information and summer camps.

7711 **Genital Psoriasis**
National Psoriasis Foundation
6600 SW 92nd Avenue 503-244-7404
Portland, OR 97223-7195 800-723-9166
Fax: 503-245-0626
e-mail: getinfo@npfusa.org
www.psoriasis.org
Introduces the reader to the basics of genital psoriasis, and treatment options.

7712 **Hand Eczema**
American Academy of Dermatology
PO Box 4014 847-330-0230
Schaumburg, IL 60168-4014 Fax: 847-330-0050
Shows examples of hand rashes, explains causes, lists protective measures and treatments.
1993

7713 **Hives**
American Academy of Allergy, Asthma and Immunology
611 E Wells Street 414-272-6071
Milwaukee, WI 53202-3889 800-822-2762
Fax: 414-272-6070
www.aaaai.org
This brochure offers information on what causes hives, what is Angioedema, and how hives can be treated.

7714 **Home Phototherapy**
National Psoriasis Foundation

6600 SW 92nd Avenue
Portland, OR 97223-7195
503-244-7404
800-723-9166
Fax: 503-245-0626
e-mail: getinfo@npfusa.org
www.psoriasis.org

Talks about the use of a home UVB unit to treat psoriasis.

7715 **Methotrexate (MTX)**
National Psoriasis Foundation
6600 SW 92nd Avenue
Portland, OR 97223-7195
503-244-7404
800-723-9166
Fax: 503-245-0626
e-mail: getinfo@npfusa.org
www.psoriasis.org

An introductions to MTX treatment.

7716 **Oral Retinoid Therapy (Soriatane)**
National Psoriasis Foundation
6600 SW 92nd Avenue
Portland, OR 97223-7195
503-244-7404
800-723-9166
Fax: 503-245-0626
e-mail: getinfo@npfusa.org
www.psoriasis.org

Explains Soriatane treatment options.

7717 **PUVA (Psoralen Plus Ultraviolet Light A)**
National Psoriasis Foundation
6600 SW 92nd Avenue
Portland, OR 97223-7195
503-244-7404
800-723-9166
Fax: 503-245-0626
e-mail: getinfo@npfusa.org
www.psoriasis.org

Explains PUVA treatment options, pros, cons, and potential side-effects.

7718 **Pityriasis Rosea**
American Academy of Dermatology
PO Box 4014
Schaumburg, IL 60168-4014
847-330-0230
Fax: 847-330-0050

Discusses the appearance, symptoms, and causes of this common rash. Diagnosis and treatment are also explained.
1996

7719 **Psoriasis on Specific Skin Sites**
National Psoriasis Foundation
6600 SW 92nd Avenue
Portland, OR 97223-7195
503-244-7404
800-723-9166
Fax: 503-245-0626
e-mail: getinfo@npfusa.org
www.psoriasis.org

Including nails, ears, eyelids, face, mouth and lips, hands and feet.

7720 **Psoriasis: How It Makes You Feel**
National Psoriasis Foundation
6600 SW 92nd Avenue
Portland, OR 97223-7195
503-244-7404
800-723-9166
Fax: 503-245-0626
e-mail: getinfo@npfusa.org
www.psoriasis.org

7721 **Psoriatic Arthritis**
National Psoriasis Foundation
6600 SW 92nd Avenue
Portland, OR 97223-7195
503-244-7404
800-723-9166
Fax: 503-245-0626
e-mail: getinfo@npfusa.org
www.psoriasis.org

7722 **Rosacea**
American Academy of Dermatology
PO Box 4014
Schaumburg, IL 60168-4014
847-330-0230
Fax: 847-330-0050

The condition, do's and don'ts for rosacea patients, and treatment are explained.
1995

7723 **Scabies**
American Academy of Dermatology
PO Box 4014
Schaumburg, IL 60168-4014
847-330-0230
Fax: 847-330-0050

Explains the nature of the scabies parasite, symptoms, at-risk groups, individual and large group treatments. Available in Spanish.
1997

7724 **Scalp Psoriasis**
National Psoriasis Foundation
6600 SW 92nd Avenue
Portland, OR 97223-7195
503-244-7404
800-723-9166
Fax: 503-245-0626
e-mail: getinfo@npfusa.org
www.psoriasis.org

7725 **Seborrheic Dermatitis**
American Academy of Dermatology
PO Box 4014
Schaumburg, IL 60168-4014
847-330-0230
Fax: 847-330-0050

Answers the most frequently asked questions about this common, easily treatable skin condition.
1995

7726 **Seborrheic Keratoses**
American Academy of Dermatology
PO Box 4014
Schaumburg, IL 60168-4014
847-330-0230
Fax: 847-330-0050

Describes seborrheic keratosis growths, causes, and treatments.
1997

7727 **Skin Cancer**
American Academy of Dermatology
PO Box 4014
Schaumburg, IL 60168-4014
847-330-0230
Fax: 847-330-0050

Warning signs and how to perform self-examinations are discussed.
1994

7728 **Skin Conditions Related to AIDS**
American Academy of Dermatology
PO Box 4014
Schaumburg, IL 60168-4014
847-330-0230
Fax: 847-330-0050

What AIDS is, who's at risk, and other important information about this major health problem are discussed.
1997

7729 **Specific Forms of Psoriasis**
National Psoriasis Foundation
6600 SW 92nd Avenue
Portland, OR 97223-7195
503-244-7404
800-723-9166
Fax: 503-245-0626
e-mail: getinfo@npfusa.org
www.psoriasis.org

Pustular, Guttate, Inverse, and Erythrodermic.

7730 **Spider Veins, Varicose Vein Therapy**
American Academy of Dermatology
PO Box 4014
Schaumburg, IL 60168-4014
847-330-0230
Fax: 847-330-0050

Discusses the latest methods for removing unsightly and unwanted blood vessels that appear mostly on the legs.
1995

7731 **Sun & Water Therapy**
National Psoriasis Foundation
6600 SW 92nd Avenue
Portland, OR 97223-7195
503-244-7404
800-723-9166
Fax: 503-245-0626
e-mail: getinfo@npfusa.org
www.psoriasis.org

7732 **Sun Protection for Children**
American Academy of Dermatology
PO Box 4014
Schaumburg, IL 60168-4014
847-330-0230
Fax: 847-330-0050

Teaches parents how to protect their children from the sun's harmful rays.
1996

7733 **Sun and Your Skin**
American Academy of Dermatology
PO Box 4014
Schaumburg, IL 60168-4014
847-330-0230
Fax: 847-330-0050

Information on acute sunburn, premature aging of the skin, allergies, and skin cancer. Tips on how to be sun smart.
1994

7734 **Sunlight, Ultraviolet Radiation and the Skin**
National Cancer Institute
Building 31
Bethesda, MD 20892-0001 800-422-6237

7735 **Tinea Versicolor**
American Academy of Dermatology
PO Box 4014 847-330-0230
Schaumburg, IL 60168-4014 Fax: 847-330-0050
Discusses the symptoms, diagnosis, and treatment of this often misunderstood fungal infection.
1995

7736 **Treatment Overview**
National Psoriasis Foundation
6600 SW 92nd Avenue 503-244-7404
Portland, OR 97223-7195 800-723-9166
Fax: 503-245-0626
e-mail: getinfo@npfusa.org
www.psoriasis.org
Discusses a number of available psoriasis treatments, what is considered by the doctor when developing a treatment plan, and treatment resources.

7737 **Vascular Birthmarks**
American Academy of Dermatology
PO Box 4014 847-330-0230
Schaumburg, IL 60168-4014 Fax: 847-330-0050
Includes descriptions and treatments for most common types of vascular birthmarks - macular stains, hemangiomas, and port-wine stains.
1997

7738 **Vitiligo**
American Academy of Dermatology
PO Box 4014 847-330-0230
Schaumburg, IL 60168-4014 Fax: 847-330-0050
Discusses lost skin pigmentation and what can be done about it, including repigmentation therapy.
1994

7739 **Young People and Psoriasis**
National Psoriasis Foundation
6600 SW 92nd Avenue 503-244-7404
Portland, OR 97223-7195 800-723-9166
Fax: 503-245-0626
e-mail: getinfo@npfusa.org
www.psoriasis.org
Infancy through adolescence.

7740 **Your Diet & Psoriasis**
National Psoriasis Foundation
6600 SW 92nd Avenue 503-244-7404
Portland, OR 97223-7195 800-723-9166
Fax: 503-245-0626
e-mail: getinfo@npfusa.org
www.psoriasis.org
A discussion of particular diets, foods and supplements and the effect they have on psoriasis.

7741 **Your Skin and Your Dermatologist**
American Academy of Dermatology
PO Box 4014 847-330-0230
Schaumburg, IL 60168-4014 Fax: 847-330-0050
Explains why a dermatologist is the appropriate specialist for the care of diseases of the skin, hair, nails, and mucous membranes.
1997

Audio & Video

7742 **Allergic Skin Reactions**
American Academy of Allergy, Asthma and Immunology
611 E Wells Street 414-272-6071
Milwaukee, WI 53202-3889 800-822-2762
Fax: 414-272-6070
www.aaaai.org
In some people, allergy symptoms include itching redness, rashes, or hives. This video describes the symptoms, triggers, and treatment for common skin reactions such as dermatitis, hives and angioedema.
10-13 minutes

7743 **Basic Science Series**
American Academy of Dermatology
PO Box 4014 847-330-0230
Schaumburg, IL 60168-4014 Fax: 847-330-0050
Combines high-quality 35mm slides and accompanying narration on audiocassette and features topics that underline and support clinical dermatology. The series is useful for residents in training as well as practicing dermatologists.
Slides

7744 **CME Video Library**
American Academy of Dermatology
PO Box 4014 847-330-0230
Schaumburg, IL 60168-4014 Fax: 847-330-0050
A series of video programs developed by AAD experts recognized for their continued efforts in dermatologic advancement.
Videotapes

7745 **Facts About Acne**
American Academy of Dermatology
PO Box 4014 847-330-0230
Schaumburg, IL 60168-4014 Fax: 847-330-0050
The etiology of acne and treatment choices are explained by consultants, with patient encounters.
13 minutes

7746 **Mystery of Contact Dermatitis**
American Academy of Dermatology
PO Box 4014 847-330-0230
Schaumburg, IL 60168-4014 Fax: 847-330-0050
The causes and treatment of some common forms of contact dermatitis are shown with consultation and commentary.
10 minutes

7747 **National Library of Dermatologic Teaching Slides**
American Academy Of Dermatology
PO Box 94020 847-330-0230
Palatine, IL 60094-4020 Fax: 847-330-0050
A collection of dermatologic teaching slides offering the most comprehensive series ever assembled. Each set offers a realistic presentation of classic clinical skin conditions encountered by the dermatologist.

7748 **Skin Cancer: The Undeclared Epidemic**
American Academy of Dermatology
PO Box 4014 847-330-0230
Schaumburg, IL 60168-4014 Fax: 847-330-0050
Examples of skin cancer lesions, interviews with patients at screenings, and comments from Academy members.
9 minutes

7749 **Skin Care Under the Sun**
American Academy of Dermatology
PO Box 4014 847-330-0230
Schaumburg, IL 60168-4014 Fax: 847-330-0050
Dramatization of the dangers of overexposure to the sun, providing explanations of the effects of ultraviolet radiation on the skin.
7 minutes

Web Sites

7750 **American Academy of Dermatology**
www.aad.org
Promotes and advances the science and art of medicine and surgery related to the skin, promotes the highest possible standards in clinical practice, education and research.

7751 **American Society of Plastic and Reconstructive Surgeons**
www.plasticsurgery.org
This Society sends free information about various surgical procedures and also provides the names of board certified plastic surgeons in a patient's area.

7752 Derma Doctor

www.dermadoctor.com

The most informative skin care site on the Web. An extensive library of newsletters to help answer your questions.

7753 Dermatology Foundation

www.dermfnd.org

Raises funds for the control of skin diseases through research, improved education and better patient care. Supports basic clinical investigations.

7754 Healing Well

www.healingwell.com

An online health resource guide to medical news, chat, information and articles, newsgroups and message boards, books, disease-related web sites, medical directories, and more for patients, friends, and family coping with disabling diseases, disorders, or chronic illnesses.

7755 Health Finder

www.healthfinder.gov

Searchable, carefully developed web site offering information on over 1000 topics. Developed by the US Department of Health and Human Services, the site can be used in both English and Spanish.

7756 Healthlink USA

www.healthlinkusa.com

Health information concerning treatment, cures, prevention, diagnosis, risk factors, research, support groups, email lists, personal stories and much more. Updated regularly.

7757 Helios Health

www.helioshealth.com

Online resource for your health information. Detailed information about specific health topics, access to expert advice from our Medical Advisory Board, and up-to-date health news.

7758 MedicineNet

www.medicinenet.com

An online resource for consumers providing easy-to-read, authoritative medical and health information.

7759 Medscape

www.mywebmd.com

Medscape offers specialists, primary care physicians, and other health professionals the Web's most robust and integrated medical information and educational tools.

7760 Nat'l Arthritis and Musculoskeletal Skin

www.niams.nih.gov

Supports and provides clinical and public information and research to increase understanding of the many skin diseases and related disorders. Also provides lists and order forms for their resources and materials.

7761 Nat'l Institute of Arthritis

www.nih.gov

Handles inquiries on the following - arthritis, bone diseases and skin diseases. Consumer and professional education materials are available.

7762 National Psoriasis Foundation

www.psoriasis.org

Offers information, support and referrals for victims of psoriasis and their families.

7763 Skin Store

www.skinstore.com

Carries over 500 of the finest skincare products, available at the lowest prices, delivered immediately to your home.

7764 WebMD

www.webmd.com

Information on skin disorders, including articles and resources.

Description

7765 **Sleep Disorders**

Sleep disorders are defined as disturbances that affect the ability to fall or stay asleep, that involve sleeping too much, or that result in abnormal sleep-related behavior. They can be categorized into primary sleep disorders; sleep disorders related to another mental disorder or a general medical condition; and substance induced sleep disorder. The two conditions discussed here, narcolepsy and obstructive sleep apnea, are both primary sleep disorders.

Narcolepsy is a rare disorder of abnormal and irresistible daytime drowsiness. Excessive daytime sleepiness with involuntary daytime sleep episodes, disturbed nighttime sleep, and cataplexy (sudden weakness or loss of muscle tone, often triggered by emotion), are the most common symptoms of narcolepsy. Generally, symptoms appear between the onset of puberty and age 25, and worsen as the patient ages. There are 100,000 people in the US with this condition.

Although the exact cause of narcolepsy is unknown, there appears to be a genetic link.

Oral medication, including stimulant agents, as well as specific sleep schedules and other forms of behavioral therapy are also prescribed.

Obstructive sleep apnea is a serious and common sleep disorder that features heavy snoring and breathing irregularities. It is chronic and relapsing, and varies in severity from mild to lethal. Almost 90 percent of the estimated 12 million sleep apnea sufferers are male. Obstructive sleep apnea is biomechanical and usually occurs when tissues in the back of the throat collapse and close the breathing passage. Sufferers experience heavy snoring, periods during sleep when breathing halts for 10 seconds or more, and many short awakenings which they do not remember. In the worst cases, sufferers may cease breathing for more than half of total sleeping time, which can result in daytime fatigue, oxygen deprivation and hypertension.

Signs of sleep apnea or a related sleeping disorder include loud, habitual snoring, fatigue on waking, daytime sleepiness, and choking, gasping or holding one's breath while asleep. Overweight persons and smokers are more prone to develop this disorder. Heavy eating, late-night snacking, sedative use, and alcohol consumption are often contributing factors.

The diagnosis of sleep apnea often requires a polysomnography, or sleep study, which monitors brain waves, muscle tension, eye movement, respiration and blood-oxygen levels. Obviously, a partner can easily help to confirm these symptoms; single people can arrange for sleep observation in a hospital or clinic setting. Behavior modification is frequently sufficient to reduce or eliminate many snoring problems, as is sleeping on one's side and/or without a pillow. In addition to behavioral changes, mild cases are often responsive to oral devices that help to keep airways open by bringing the jaw forward, elevating the soft palate, or repositioning the tongue. More severe cases can be treated with a C-PAP (continuous positive airway pressure) machine, or a Bi-Level (Bi-PAP) machine, both of which blow air into the patient's airways in a regulated manner. Surgery is sometimes indicated, when facial or oral irregularities, such as jaw irregularities, small throat openings, enlarged tonsils, a large tongue or other tissue in front of the airway, or a deviated septum, impede proper airflow.

National Agencies & Associations

7766 **American Narcolepsy Association**
PO Box 26230
San Francisco, CA 94126-6230 800-222-6085
Offers help and information to persons with narcolepsy and their families.

7767 **American Sleep Apnea Association**
6856 E Avenue 202-293-3650
Washington, DC 20012 Fax: 202-293-3656
e-mail: asaa@sleepapnea.org
www.sleepapnea.org
Offers help and information to persons with sleep apnea and their families.
Rochelle Goldberg, President and Chief Medical Officer
Kathe Henke, Secretary

7768 **Association of Professional Sleep Societies**
One Westbrook Corporate Center 708-492-0930
Westchester, IL 60154 Fax: 708-273-9354
www.apss.org
Works to facilitate the research and development of sleep disorders medically by encouraging exchange of information among members.
Jerome A Barrett, Executive Director
Jennifer Markkanen, Assistant Executive Director

7769 **Lung Association**
Station S 780-488-6819
Edmonton, AB, T6E-6K2 Fax: 780-488-7195
e-mail: lasa@sleep-apnea.ab.ca
www.sleep-apnea-ab.ca
The Lung Association - Sleep Apnea (LASA) is a patient and professional coalition providing support through improved care for patients with respiratory disorders of sleep.

7770 **NIH/National Institute of Neurological Disorders and Stroke**
PO Box 5801 301-496-5751
Bethesda, MD 20824 800-352-9424
TTY: 301-468-5981
www.ninds.nih.gov
Mission is to reduce the burden of neurological disease, a burden borne by every age group, by every segment of society, by people all over the world.
Story C Landis, Director
Walter J Koroshetz, Deputy Director

7771 **Narcolepsy Institute/Montefiore Medical Center**
111 E 210th Street 718-920-6799
Bronx, NY 10467-2490 Fax: 718-654-9580
e-mail: MGoswami@aol.com
www.montefiore.org
Offers services such as screening, information on narcolepsy, counseling and referrals for individuals and their families with problems arising as a consequence of narcolepsy, and adult and teenage support groups to help individuals develop positive self-images.
Dr Meeta Goswami, Director

7772 **Narcolepsy Network**
PO Box 294
Pleasantville, NY 10570
410-667-2523
888-292-6522
Fax: 401-633-6567
e-mail: narnet@aol.com
www.narcolepsynetwork.org
Nonprofit organization consisting of memberships by people who have narcolepsy (or related sleep disorders), their families and friends and professionals involved in treatment, research and public education.
Eveline Honig, Executive Director
Collen A Rettig, Office Manager

7773 **National Sleep Foundation**
1522 K Street NW
Washington, DC 20005-1253
202-347-3471
Fax: 202-347-3472
e-mail: nsf@sleepfoundation.org
www.sleepfoundation.org
The National Sleep Foundation (NSF) is an independent nonprofit organization dedicated to improving public health and safety by achieving understanding of sleep and sleep disorders and by supporting education sleep-related research and advocacy.
Meir H Kryger, Chairman
Thomas J Balkin, Vice Chairman

7774 **Sleep Research Society American Academy of Sleep Medicine**
American Academy of Sleep Medicine
One Westbrook Corporate Center
Westchester, IL 60154
708-492-1093
Fax: 708-492-0943
e-mail: ncekosh@srsnet.org
www.sleepresearchsociety.org
Facilitates communication among research workers in this field but does not sponsor research investigations on its own.
Michael V Vitiello, President
Ronald Szymusiak, Secretary/Treasurer

Research Centers

7775 **Baylor College of Medicine: Sleep Disorder and Research Center**
10019 S Main Street
Houston, TX 77025-3498
713-798-3300
Fax: 713-796-9718
www.baylorclinic.com
Internal unit of the College that focuses on research into sleep and sexual dysfunction in males.
Shyam Subramanian, Medical Director
Charlie Lan, Assistant Professor of Medicine

7776 **Capital Regional Sleep-Wake Disorders Center**
St. Peter's Hospital and Albany Medical Center
25 Hackett Boulevard
Albany, NY 12208-3420
518-436-9253
Cheryl Carlu MD

7777 **Center for Narcolepsy Research at the University of Illinois at Chicago**
University of Illinois
845 S Damen Avenue
Chicago, IL 60612-7350
312-996-5176
Fax: 312- 99- 700
e-mail: julielaw@uic.edu
www.uic.edu/depts/cnr
Provides information to health professionals and people with sleep disorders regarding diagnosis and treatment. Maintain national network with sleep professionals throughout the US.
6-8 pages 2 per year
David W Carley, Director
Julie Law, Center Administrator

7778 **Center for Research in Sleep Disorders Affiliated with Mercy Hospital**
Mercy Hospital of Hamilton/Fairfield
1275 E Kemper Road
Cincinnati, OH 45246
513-671-3101
Martin Schar PhD

7779 **Center for Sleep & Wake Disorders: Miami Valley Hospital**
One Wyoming Street
Dayton, OH 45409-2722
513-220-2515
www.miamivalleyhospital.org
Offering the largest variety of sleep disorder testing available in the area it also offers comprehensive sleep care and care of related issues with a sleep lab clinical treatment pulmonary treatment and behavioral treatment in the same facility.
Kevin Huban, Director
Amy Cline, Administrative Director of Respiratory C

7780 **Center for Sleep Medicine of the Mount Sinai Medical Center**
1176 Fifth Avenue
New York, NY 10029-6500
212-241-5098
Fax: 212-875-84
www.mountsinai.org
The Center for Sleep Medicine at The Mount Sinai Medical Center is a comprehensive program dedicated to the diagnosis and treatment of all aspects of sleep pathology including breathing related sleep disorders periodic limb movements in sleep insomnia and narcolepsy. Mechanical (CPAP BiPAP ventilator) surgical dental and pharmacologic therapies are available.
E Neil Schachter, Professor
Gwen S Skloot, Associates Professor

7781 **Geisinger Wyoming Valley Medical Center: Sleep Disorders Center**
1000 E Mountain Drive
Wilkes-Barre, PA 18711
570-819-5770
www.geisinger.org
Our dedicated sleep team operates service sleep centers and laboratories to diagnose and treat a broad range of sleep disorders.ÿ Geisinger sleep centers are conveniently located in Danville Bloomsburg Shamokin Wilkes-Barre and Mt. Pocono.
Andrew Paul Matragrano, Director
Stephanie Schaefer, Nurse Practitioner

7782 **Johns Hopkins University: Sleep Disorders Francis Scott Key Medical Center**
Francis Scott Key Medical Center
601 N Caroline Street
Baltimore, MD 21287
410-550-0545
www.hopkinshospital.org
The Johns Hopkins University Sleep Disorders Center is a tertiary care center for patients with sleep/wake disorders and medical disorders associated with sleep.
Phillip L Smith, Director

7783 **Knollwoodpark Hospital Sleep Disorders Center**
5600 Girby Road
Mobile, AL 36693-3398
334-660-5757
Fax: 334-660-5254
e-mail: 71054.2530@compuserve.com

7784 **Knollwoodpark Hospital Sleep Disorders Cen**
5600 Girby Road
Mobile, AL 36693
334-660-5757
Fax: 334-660-5254
e-mail: 71054.2530@compuserve.com
www.southalabama.edu/usakph

7785 **Loma Linda University Sleep Disorders Clinic**
VA Hospital Medical Services Center
11201 Benton Street
Loma Linda, CA 92357-1
909-825-7084
800-741-8387
Fax: 909-963-64
www.lom.med.va.gov
Ralph Downey III MD, Director

7786 **Methodist Hospital Sleep Center Winona Memorial Hospital**
Rehab Centers
3232 N Meridian Street
Indianapolis, IN 46208-8126
317-927-2100
Fax: 317-927-2914
Kenneth Wies MD

7787 **MidWest Medical Center: Sleep Disorders Center**
Winona Memorial Hospital
3232 N Meridian Street
Indianapolis, IN 46208-4688
317-927-2100
Fax: 317-927-2914
Kenneth Wiesert MD

7788 **Northwest Ohio Sleep Disorders Center Toledo Hospital**
Toledo Hospital
2142 N Cove Boulevard
Toledo, OH 43606-3896
419-471-5629
Frank O Horton III MD, Director

7789 Ohio Sleep Medicine Institute
4975 Bradenton Avenue 614-766-0773
Dublin, OH 43017-3521 Fax: 614-766-2599
e-mail: info@sleepmedicine.com
www.sleepohio.com
Betty Palmer, Director

7790 Penn Center for Sleep Disorders: Hospital of the University of Pennsylvania
3400 Spruce Street 215-662-7772
Philadelphia, PA 19104-4204 Fax: 215-349-8038
Joanne Getsy MD, Director

7791 Presbyterian-University Hospital: Pulmonary Sleep Evaluation Center
DeSoto At O'Hara Street 412-647-3475
Pittsburgh, PA 15213
Mark Sanders MD, Director

7792 Scripps Clinic Sleep Disorders Center Scripps Clinic
Scripps Clinic
10666 N Torrey Pines Road 858-455-9100
La Jolla, CA 92037-1027 Fax: 858-828-64
e-mail: malcoRN@scrippsclinic.com
www.scripps.org
The Scripps Clinic Sleep Center provides evaluation diagnosis and treatment of a full range of sleep disorders such as Circadian rhythm disorders Insomnia Narcolepsy Night terror Nightmares Restless legs syndrome Sleep apnea Sleepwalking and Snoring.
Dan Dworsky MD, Medical Director
Merrill M Mitler MD, Scientific Director

7793 Sleep Alertness Center: Lafayette Home Hospital
2400 S Street 765-447-6811
Lafayette, IN 47904-3027 e-mail: glenda.eberhard@glhsi.org
Frederick Ro MD

7794 Sleep Center: Community General Hospital
4900 Broad Road
Syracuse, NY 13215-5100 315-492-5877
www.cgh.org
The Sleep Center at Community General Hospital is a specialized facility providing accurate diagnosis and recommending treatment of sleep-related problems.
Robert Westl MD, Medical Director
Antonio Cule MD, Neurology Consultant

7795 Sleep Disorders Center Bethesda Oak Hospital
619 Oak Street
Cincinnati, OH 45206-1613 513-569-6320
www.trihealth.com
Milton Krame MD

7796 Sleep Disorders Center Columbia Presbyterian Medical Center
The University Hospital of Columbia & Cornell
161 Fort Washington Avenue 212-305-1860
New York, NY 10032 Fax: 212-305-5496
e-mail: inquire@sleepNYP.com
www.sleepnyp.com
A Highly specialized outpatient facility for the evaluation and treatment of patients with problems related to sleep and wakefulness.
Neil B Kavey, Medical Director
Andrew Tucker, Director

7797 Sleep Disorders Center Dartmouth Hitchcock Medical Center
Darthmouth Hitchcock medical Center
One Medical Center Drive 603-650-7534
Lebanon, NH 03756-1 866-346-2362
Fax: 603-650-7820
e-mail: Joanne.MacQuarrie@dartmouth.edu
dms.dartmouth.edu
Provides consultation and testing for all varieties of sleep-related disturbances including snoring sleep apnea narcolepsy restless legs syndrome periodic limb movement disorder insomnia parasomnias and circadian rhythm disorders.
Glen Greenough, Fellowship Director
Michael Sate MD, Director

7798 Sleep Disorders Center Lankenau Hospital
100 E Lancaster Avenue 610-645-3400
Wynnewood, PA 19096-3498 Fax: 610-645-2291

7799 Sleep Disorders Center Ohio State University Medical Center
1492 E Broad Street 614-257-2500
Columbus, OH 43205-1228 800-293-5123
Fax: 614-257-2551
medicalcenter.osu.edu
Ulysses J Magalang MD, Medical Director

7800 Sleep Disorders Center at California: Pacific Medical Center
2340 Clay Street 415-923-3336
San Francisco, CA 94115-1932 Fax: 415-923-3584
e-mail: 76307.2221@compuserve.com

7801 Sleep Disorders Center at California: Paci
2340 Clay Street 415-923-3336
San Francisco, CA 94115 Fax: 415-923-3584
e-mail: 76307.2221@compuserve.com

7802 Sleep Disorders Center of Metropolitan Toronto
2888 Bathurst Street 416-785-1128
Toronto Ontario, M6B-4H6 Fax: 416-782-2740
e-mail: sleep@compuserve.com
www.sdc.ca
Jeffrey Lips MD, Director

7803 Sleep Disorders Center of Rochester: St. Mary's Hospital
2110 Clinton Avenue S 716-442-4141
Rochester, NY 14618-2616
Donald Green MD

7804 Sleep Disorders Center of Western New York Millard Fillmore Hospital
3 Gates Circle 716-887-5337
Buffalo, NY 14209-1120 Fax: 716-887-5332
gates.kaleidahealth.org
Daniel Rifkin, Director

7805 Sleep Disorders Center: Cleveland Clinic Foundation
9500 Euclid Avenue 216-636-5860
Cleveland, OH 44195-0001 800-588-2264
Fax: 216-445-1022
my.clevelandclinic.org
Accredited by the American Academy of Sleep Medicine the Cleveland Clinic Sleep Disorders Center is staffed by physicians specializing in sleep disorders from a variety of disciplines including adult and child neurology pulmonary and critical care medicine psychology psychiatry otolaryngology and dentistry.
Nancy Foldva Schaefer DO, Director
Petra Podmor RPSGT, Laboratory Manager

7806 Sleep Disorders Center: Community Medical Center
1822 Mulberry Street 717-969-8931
Scranton, PA 18510-2375
John Goodnow, Director

7807 Sleep Disorders Center: Crozer-Chester Medical Center
Sleep Disorders Center
175 E Chester Pike
Ridley Park, PA 19078-3975 610-447-2689
www.crozer.org
A multidisciplinary facility for the investigation and treatment of sleep problems
Calvin Staff MD, Medical Director

7808 Sleep Disorders Center: Good Samaritan Medical Center
1020 Franklin Street 814-533-1661
Johnstown, PA 15905-4109
Richard Parc DO, Director

7809 Sleep Disorders Center: Kettering Medical Center
3935 Southern Boulevard 937-395-8805
Kettering, OH 45439-1295 Fax: 937-395-8821
www.kmcnetwork.org
Donna Arand PhD, Clinical Director
George G Burton MD, Medical Director

7810 Sleep Disorders Center: Medical College of Pennsylvania
3200 Henry Avenue 215-842-4250
Philadelphia, PA 19129-1137
June M Fry MD PhD, Director

7811 Sleep Disorders Center: Newark Beth Israel Medical Center
201 Lyons Avenue at Osborne Terrace
Newark, NJ 07112-2027 973-926-2973
www.sbhcs.com
Evaluates a wide range of disorders including sleep apnea snoring insomnia narcolepsy sleep-wake schedule disorders and male impotency. The center also provides board-certified consultants in sleep medicine neurology urology endocrinology psychiatry cardiology and ear nose and throat surgery in addition to certified sleep technologists.
Monroe S Karetzky MD

7812 Sleep Disorders Center: Rhode Island Hospital
70 Catamore Boulevard 401-431-5420
E Providence, RI 02914 Fax: 401-431-5429
www.lifespan.org
Richard Mill MD, Director

7813 Sleep Disorders Center: St. Vincent Medical Center
2213 Cherry Street 419-321-4980
Toledo, OH 43608-2691
Joseph Schaf PhD, Director

7814 Sleep Disorders Center: University Hospital, SUNY at Stony Brook
240 Middle Country Road 631-444-2500
Smithtown, NY 11787-0001 Fax: 631-444-2580
uhmc-xweb1.uhmc.sunysb.edu/sleepdisorder
Wallace Mend MD

7815 Sleep Disorders Center: Winthrop, University Hospital
222 Station Plaza N
Mineola, NY 11501-3808 516-663-3907
www.winthrop.org
Steven H Feinsilver MD

7816 Sleep Disorders Unit Beth Israel Deaconess Medical Center
330 Brookline Avenue
Boston, MA 02215-5400 617-667-3237
www.bidmc.org
Jean K Matheson MD

7817 Sleep Laboratory St Joseph's Hospital
St Joseph's Hospital
945 E Genesee Street 315-475-3379
Syracuse, NY 13210 Fax: 315-755-77
www.sjhsyr.org
The Sleep Lab focuses on diagnosing and treating Obstructive Sleep Apnea and sleep-related breathing disorders and has the largest number of sleep-credentialed physicians and registered sleep technologists of any sleep lab in the area.
Edward T Downing, Director

7818 Sleep Laboratory, Maine Medical Center
22 Bramhall Street 207-871-2279
Portland, ME 04102-3134
George E Bokinsky Jr

7819 Sleep Medicine Associates of Texas
5477 Glen Lakes Drive 214-750-7776
Dallas, TX 13210-4353 Fax: 214-750-4621
e-mail: smat@sleepmed.com
www.sleepmed.com
First largest and longest standing accredited sleep center in North Texas.
Philipp Becker, President and Founding Partner
Andrew O Jamieson MD, Chairman of the Board and Founding Partn

7820 Sleep Research Foundation
170 Morton Street 617-522-9270
Boston, MA 02130-3735
Ernest Hartm MD, Director

7821 Sleep Wake Disorders Center Montefiore Sleep Disorders Center
111 E 210th Street 718-920-4841
Bronx, NY 10467-2401 Fax: 718-798-4352
www.montefiore.org
Provide outstanding clinical care for patients with disorders that affect the sleep-wake cycle and are committed to performing high quality research and to making outstanding contributions to the areas of clinical research that includes the entire spectrum of sleep medicine.
Michael J Thorpy MD, Director
Karen Ballab MD, Associate Director

7822 Sleep and Chronobiology Center: Western Psychiatric Institute and Clinic
3811 Ohara Street 412-624-2246
Pittsburgh, PA 15213-2593
Charles F Reynolds III MD, Director

7823 Sleep-Wake Disorders Center: New York Hospital-Cornell Medical Center
520 E 70th Street 212-746-2623
New York, NY 10021-1504 Fax: 212-746-5509
www.weillcornell.org
Charles Poll MD, Director

7824 Sleep/Wake Disorders Center: Community Hospitals of Indianapolis
1500 N Ritter Avenue 317-355-4275
Indianapolis, IN 46219-3027 Fax: 317-351-2785
e-mail: mevollmer@pol.net
Marvin E Vollmer MD

7825 Sleep/Wake Disorders Center: Hampstead Hospital
E Road 603-329-5311
Hampstead, NH 03841
Deborah Sewi PhD

7826 Stanford University Center for Narcolepsy Dept of Psychiatry & Behavioral Sciences
450 Broadway Street 650-725-6517
Redwood City, CA 94063-5102 Fax: 650-498-7761
e-mail: jck@stanford.edu
med.stanford.edu
Dr Emanuel Mignot, Director
Marlene Iry, Admin Associate

7827 Thomas Jefferson University: Sleep Disorders Center
Jefferson Medical College
211 S Ninth Street 215-955-6175
Philadelphia, PA 19107-5083 800-JEF-FNOW
Fax: 215-955-9783
www.jefferson.edu
A comprehensive clinical research and educational program in sleep and sleep disorders medicine.
Karl Doghram MD, Medical Director

7828 University of Texas Sleep/Wake Disorders Center
Southwestern Medical Center
5323 Harry Hines Boulevard 214-648-7350
Dallas, TX 75390-9070 Fax: 214-487-59
Studies sleep/wake disorders including insomnia apnea and narcolepsy.
Howard Roffw MD, Director

Support Groups & Hotlines

7829 Narcolepsy Institute/Montefiore Medical Center
111 E 210th Street 718-920-6799
Bronx, NY 10467-2490 Fax: 718-654-9580
e-mail: MGoswami@aol.com
www.narcolepsyinstitute.org
The Narcolepsy Institute provides psychosocial support services for narcolepsy.
Dr. Meeta Goswami, Director

7830 Narcolepsy Network
110 Ripple Lane 401-667-2523
North Kingstown, RI 02852 888-292-6522
Fax: 401-633-6567
e-mail: narnet@narcolepsynetwork.org
www.narcolepsynetwork.org
Provides advocacy and education, supports research. Newsletter, conferences, phone support and group development guidelines.
Patricia Higgins, President
Eveline V. Honig, Md, MPh, Executive Director

7831 National Health Information Center
PO Box 1133 310-565-4167
Washington, DC 20013 800-336-4797
Fax: 301-984-4256
e-mail: info@nhic.org
www.health.gov/nhic
Offers a nationwide information referral service, produces directories and resource guides.

Books

7832 ABC of ZZZs
National Sleep Foundation
1522 K Street NW 202-347-3471
Washington, DC 20005-1235 Fax: 202-347-3472
www.sleepfoundation.org
A primer on sleep basics, including getting enough sleep, why sleep is important, and ' sleep stealers.'
Emerson Darbonne, Communications Coordinator

7833 Doctor, I Can't Sleep: Insomnia Training Manual
Narcolepsy Network
PO Box 42460 513-891-3522
Cincinnati, OH 45242-0460 Fax: 513-891-9936
e-mail: narnet@aol.com
Comprehensive course manual for primary care physicians and the public. Outlines basic facts about epidemiology, sleep hygiene, relaxation techniques, diagnosis, and treatment.
100+ pages

7834 International Classification of Sleep Disorders
American Academy of Sleep Medicine
One Westbrook Corporate Center 708-492-0930
Westchester, IL 60154 Fax: 708-492-0943
www.aasmnet.org
A comprehensive manual for physicians and other healthcare professionals containing information on 84 sleep disorders. The extensive text describes the diagnostic features of each disorder and includes specific diagnostic and severity criteria for each disorder.
396 pages Paperback

7835 Living with Narcolepsy
National Sleep Foundation
1522 K Street 202-347-3471
Washington, DC 20005-1235 Fax: 202-347-3472
www.sleepfoundation.org
Defines and describes narcolepsy and what can be expected after diagnosis, including effects on education, career, social and family life.
Emerson Darbonne, Communications Coordinator

7836 Melatonin: The Basic Facts
National Sleep Foundation
1522 K Street 202-347-3471
Washington, DC 20005-1235 Fax: 202-347-3472
www.sleepfoundation.org
If you're curious about melatonin, it's not suprising. There has been a lot of attention paid to the hormone in popular magazines and books, scholarly journals, and advertisements. You may habe heard claims that malatonin cures everything from jet lag to insomnia to aging.
Emerson Darbonne, Communications Coordinator

7837 Narcolepsy Primer
Meeta Goswami, Michael Thorpy, author
Narcolepsy Institute/Montefiore Medical Center
111 E 210th Street 718-920-6799
Bronx, NY 10467-2401 Fax: 718-654-9580
e-mail: MGsowami@aol.com
narcolepsyinstitute.org
A guide for physicians, patients and their families on the affects, causes and prevention of narcolepsy.
Dr. Meeta Goswami, Director

7838 Narcolepsy Primer Package
Meeta Goswami, Michael Thorpy, author
Narcolepsy Institute/Montefiore Medical Center
111 E 210th Street 718-920-6799
Bronx, NY 10467-2401 Fax: 718-654-9580
e-mail: MGsowami@aol.com
narcolepsyinstitute.org
The package includes: Narcolepsy Primer; Manuel on Narcolepsy and A Counseling Service for Narcolepsy: A Sociomedical Model.
Dr. Meeta Goswami, Director

7839 Pain and Sleep
National Sleep Foundation
1522 K Street NW 202-347-3471
Washington, DC 20005-1235 Fax: 202-347-3472
www.sleepfoundation.org
Whether pain results from headache, backache, arthritis, or other conditions, it frequently occurs with sleep difficulty. This overview of the pain and sleep connection describes behavioral and pharmacological approaches to pain management.
Emerson Darbonne, Communications Coordinator

7840 Sleep Aids: Everything You Wanted To Know But Were Too Tired To Ask
National Sleep Foundation
1522 K Street NW 202-347-3471
Washington, DC 20005-1235 Fax: 202-347-3472
www.sleepfoundation.org
If you have trouble falling or staying asleep, or you wake up feeling unrefreshed, you may be suffering from insomnia. Insomnia is a symptom. It may be caused by stress, anxiety, depression, disease, pain, medications, sleep disorders or poor sleep habits.
Emerson Darbonne, Communications Coordinator

7841 Sleep Apnea
National Sleep Foundation
1522 K Street, NW 202-347-3471
Washington, DC 20005-1235 Fax: 202-347-3472
www.sleepfoundation.org
A brochure about sleep apnea, a breathing disorder characterized by brief interruptions of breathing during sleep. Brochure explains what it is, who gets it, and how it is diagnosed and treated.
Emerson Darbonne, Communications Coordinator

7842 Snoring and Sleep Apnea
Demos Medical Publishing
386 Park Avenue S 212-683-0072
New York, NY 10016 Fax: 212-683-0118
e-mail: orderdept@demopub.com
www.demosmedpub.com
A straightforward, jargon-free approach to dealing with snoring and sleep problems.
222 pages
ISBN: 1-888799-29-3
Dr. Diana M Schneider, President

7843 You Don't LOOK Sick!: Living Well with Invisible Chronic Illness
Joy Selak, Steven Overman, author
Haworth Press
10 Alice Street 607-722-5857
Binghamton, NY 13904-1580 800-429-6784
Fax: 607-722-0012
www.haworthpress.com
Chronicles a patient's true-life stories and her physician's compassionate commentary as they take a journey through the three stages of chronic illness - Getting Sick, Being Sick, and Living Well. Hardcover $29.95 (ISBN): 978-0-7890-2488-0, Paperback $14.95 (ISBN): 978-0-7890-2499-7.
145 pages Hrdcover/Ppbck

Magazines

7844 **SleepMatters**
National Sleep Foundation
1522 K Street NW 202-347-3471
Washington, DC 20005-1235 Fax: 202-347-3472
www.sleepfoundation.org
Covering hot sleep news, profiles, advice from experts and much more!
Quarterly
Cameron Darbonne, Communications Coordinator

Newsletters

7845 **Eye Opener**
American Narcolepsy Association
425 California Street, Suite 201 415-788-4793
San Francisco, CA 94126-6230
Offers information on sleep disorders including a question and answer column for persons suffering from disorders.

7846 **Narcolepsy Institute/Montefiore Medical Center**
Meeta Goswami, author
Narcolepsy Institute
111 E 210th Street 718-920-6799
Bronx, NY 10467-2490 Fax: 718-654-9580
e-mail: MGsowami@aol.com
narcolepsyinstitute.org
The Narcolepsy Institute provides psychosocial support services for narcolepsy and has a newsletter, a video, and a primer on narcolepsy.
8 pages Bi-Annual
Dr. Meeta Goswami, Director

7847 **Sleep Medicine Alert**
Nationa Sleep Foundation
1522 K Street NW 202-347-3471
Washington, DC 20005-1235 Fax: 202-347-3472
www.sleepfoundation.org
This quearterly newsletter is for healthcare professionals. It offers updates on sleep research and its clinical implications, information on diagnosing and treating a variety of sleep disorders.

Pamphlets

7848 **Get the Facts About Sleep Apnea**
American Sleep Apnea Association
1424 K Street NW 202-293-3650
Washington, DC 20005 Fax: 202-293-3656
e-mail: asaa@sleepapnea.org
www.sleepapnea.org

7849 **Helping Yourself to a Good Night's Sleep**
Nantional Sleep Foundation
1522 K Street NW 202-347-3471
Washington, DC 20005-1253 Fax: 202-347-3472
www.sleepfoundation.org
About half of Americans report sleep difficulty at least occasionally, according to National Sleep Foundation surveys. These woescalled insomnia by doctors-have far reaching effects. This brochure details the many things you can do to improve your sleep.

7850 **Narcolepsy**
American Academy of Sleep Medicine
One Westbrook Corporate Center 708-492-0930
Westchester, IL 60154 Fax: 708-492-0943
www.aasmnet.org
Describes the causes, symptoms and treatments of a disorder characterized by excessive sleepiness.
Lot of 50

7851 **Sleep Diary**
National Sleep Foundation
1522 K Street, NW 202-347-3471
Washington, DC 20005-1235 Fax: 202-347-3472
www.sleepfoundation.org
It includes sections on sleep schedules, quality and quantity of sleep, sleep disturbances, sleep hygiene and daytime sleepiness. It enables people to identify their sleep and health habits and note any sleep problems they may have.
Emerson Darbonne, Communications Coordinator

7852 **Sleep Strategies for Shift Workers**
National Sleep Foundation
1522 K Street NN 202-347-3471
Washington, DC 20005-1235 Fax: 202-347-3472
www.sleepfoundation.org
This brochure outlines the common effects of shift work on health, workplace alertness and productivity and offers tips about diet, sleep environment, medications, light therapy and sleep hygiene.
Cameron Darbonne, Communications Coordinator

7853 **Wake Up! Brochure**
National Sleep Foundation
1522 K Street NW 202-347-3471
Washington, DC 20005-1235 Fax: 202-347-3472
www.sleepfoundation.org
A blooklet dedicated to the drowsy driving problem, including the risks, the myths, the danger signals and recommendations.
Cameron Darbonne, Communications Coordinator

7854 **When You Can't Sleep**
Narcolepsy Network
Po Box 294 401-667-2523
Pleasantville, NY 10570-0460 888-292-6522
Fax: 401-633-6567
e-mail: narnet@aol.com
A primer on sleep basics, including getting enough sleep, why sleep is important, and sleep stealers. Plus a sleep quotient quiz.

7855 **Women and Sleep**
National Sleep Foundation
1522 K Street NW 202-347-3471
Washington, DC 20005-1235 Fax: 202-347-3472
www.sleepfoundation.org
A brochure dealing with the effects of sleep on women which explores reasons for tiredness, increased accidents, problems concentrating, and poor performance on the job and in school, and possible increased sickness.
Cameron Darbonne, Communications Coordinator

Audio & Video

7856 **Narcolepsy**
American Academy of Sleep Medicine
One Westbrook Corporate Center 708-492-0930
Westchester, IL 60154 Fax: 708-492-0943
www.aasmnet.org
Addresses the etiology, pathophysiology, diagnosis and management of narcolepsy.
58 slides

7857 **Narcolepsy: Fanlight Productions**
Jason Margolis, author
Fanlight Productions
4196 Washington Street 617-469-4999
Boston, MA 02131-1731 800-937-4113
Fax: 617-469-3379
e-mail: fanlight@fanlight.com
www.fanlight.com
This remarkable film presents the experiences of three individuals whose lives and relationships have been disrupted by narcolepsy.
2000 25 Minutes
ISBN: 1-572953-23-2

7858 **Video on Narcolepsy**
Narcolepsy Institute/Montefiore Medical Center
111 E 210th Street 718-920-6799
Bronx, NY 10467 Fax: 718-654-9580
e-mail: MGsowami@aol.com
www.narcolepsyinstitute.org
Clinical symptoms, genetics, diagnosis, effects of Narcolepsy, support groups.
Dr. Meeta Goswami, Director

Web Sites

7859 **American Sleep Apnea Association**

www.sleeppapnea.org

The ASAA is a 501(c)(3) organization dedicated to reducing injury, disability, and depth from sleep apnea and to enhancing the well-being of those affected by this common disorder. The ASAA promotes education and awareness, the ASAA A.W.A.K.E. network of voluntary mutual support groups, research, and continuous improvement of care.

7860 **American Sleep Disorders Association**

Provides full diagnostic and treatment services to improve the quality of care for patients with all types of sleep disorders.

7861 **Healing Well**

www.healingwell.com

An online health resource guide to medical news, chat, information and articles, newsgroups and message boards, books, disease-related web sites, medical directories, and more for patients, friends, and family coping with disabling diseases, disorders, or chronic illnesses.

7862 **Health Finder**

www.healthfinder.gov

Searchable, carefully developed web site offering information on over 1000 topics. Developed by the US Department of Health and Human Services, the site can be used in both English and Spanish.

7863 **Healthlink USA**

www.healthlinkusa.com

Health information concerning treatment, cures, prevention, diagnosis, risk factors, research, support groups, email lists, personal stories and much more. Updated regularly.

7864 **Helios Health**

www.helioshealth.com

Online resource for your health information. Detailed information about specific health topics, access to expert advice from our Medical Advisory Board, and up-to-date health news.

7865 **MGH Neurology WebForums**

Online. Provides both unmoderated message boards and chat rooms for specific neurological disorders.

7866 **MedicineNet**

www.medicinenet.com

An online resource for consumers providing easy-to-read, authoritative medical and health information.

7867 **Medscape**

www.mywebmd.com

Medscape offers specialists, primary care physicians, and other health professionals the Web's most robust and integrated medical information and educational tools.

7868 **National Sleep Foundation**

www.sleepfoundation.org

Information for millions of Americans who suffer from sleep disorders, and to prevent the catastrophic accidents that are related to poor or disordered sleep through research, education and the dissemination of information.

7869 **Neurology Channel**

www.neurologychannel.com

Find clearly explained, medically accurate information regarding conditions, including an overview, symptoms, causes, diagnostic procedures and treatment options. On this site it is possible to ask questions and get information from a neurologist and connect to people who have similar health interests.

7870 **Sleep Research Society**

www.sleepresearchsociety.org

Facilitates communication among research workers in this field, but does not sponsor research investigations on its own.

7871 **WebMD**

www.webmd.com

Information on Narcolepsy, including articles and resources.

Description

7872 **Spina Bifida**

Spina bifida refers to conditions which result in an incomplete closure of the spinal column during fetal development. It is the most serious of a group of disorders called neural tube defects. The severity of spina bifida ranges from mild to severe.

Spina bifida occulta is an opening in one or more vertebrae without damage to the spinal cord. Meningocele is when the protective covering around the spinal cord (meninges) has protruded into the vertebrae, with little, if any, damage. Myelomeningocele, the most severe form of spina bifida, is when part of the actual spinal cord pushes through the back and exposes nerves and tissues.

The effects of spina bifida, in its most extreme state, are serious. They can include paralysis, loss of bowel and bladder control and hydrocephalus. Other inherited abnormalities may be present. Open spina bifida can be diagnosed in utero by finding elevations of a specific protein in maternal amniotic fluid. Prevention involves supplementation with folic acid. Treatments for spina bifida require a united effort by a team of specialists, and depend on the severity of the defects. With proper care, many children with spina bifida live fairly normal lives. See also *Birth Defects*.

National Agencies & Associations

7873 **Canadian & American Spinal Research Organi zation**
120 Newkirk Road
Richmond Hill, ON, L4C-9S7
905-508-4000
Fax: 905-508-4002
e-mail: info@csro.com
www.csro.com

Dedicated to the improvement of the physical quality of life for persons with a spinal cord injury and those with related neurological deficits, through targeted medical and scientific research.
Barry Munro, Chair
Dave Lostchuk, Treasurer

7874 **Easter Seals**
230 W Monroe Street
Chicago, IL 60606-4703
312-726-6200
800-221-6827
Fax: 312-726-1494
TTY: 312-726-4258
e-mail: info@easter-seals.org
www.easter-seals.org

Provides serves to children and adults with disabilities as well as support to their families.
Reenie Kavalar, VP Medical/Rehabilitation Services

7875 **March of Dimes Birth Defects Foundation**
1275 Mamaroneck Avenue
White Plains, NY 10605
914-949-7166
www.marchofdimes.com

Our mission is to improve the health of babies by preventing birth defects premature birth and infant mortality. The March of Dimes carries out this mission through programs of research community services education and advocacy to save babies' lives.

7876 **Spina Bifida Association of America**
4590 Macarthur Boulevard NW
Washington, DC 20007-4226
202-944-3285
800-621-3141
Fax: 202-944-3295
e-mail: sbaa@sbaa.org
www.sbaa.org

The association works for people with spina bifida and their families through education advocacy research and service. There is also an annual conference and publications available.
Cindy Brownstein, CEO
Maya House, Resource Center Manager

7877 **Spina Bifida and Hydrocephalus Association of Canada**
#977-167 Lombard Avenue
Winnipeg, Manitoba, R3B-0V3
204-925-3650
Fax: 204-925-3654
e-mail: spinab@mts.net
www.sbhac.ca

To improve the quality of life of all individuals with spina bifida and/or hydrocephalus and their families, through awareness, education, research, and advocacy, and to reduce the incidence of neural tube defects.
Lorelei Fletcher, President
Gene Layton, VP

State Agencies & Associations

Alabama

7878 **Spina Bifida Association of Alabama**
PO Box 13254
Birmingham, AL 35202-0538
256-617-1414
e-mail: info@sbaofal.org
www.sbaofal.org

Lori Turner, President
David Little, Executive Director

Arizona

7879 **Spina Bifida Association of Arizona**
1001 E Fairmount Avenue
Phoenix, AZ 85014-4806
602-274-3323
Fax: 602-274-7632
e-mail: office@sbglobal.net
www.sbaaz.org

Benjaman D Scanlan, President
Ron Whiteside, Treasurer

Arkansas

7880 **Spina Bifida Association of Arkansas**
PO Box 24663
Little Rock, AR 72221-4663
501-978-7222
Fax: 501-320-6805
e-mail: sigmondr@sbglobal.net
www.sbaa.org

James Rucker, President

California

7881 **Spina Bifida Association of Greater San Diego**
PO Box 232272
San Diego, CA 92193-2272
619-491-9018
Fax: 619-275-3361
e-mail: sbaofgsd@hotmail.com
www.sbaa.org

Erika Jorquera, President

Colorado

7882 **Spina Bifida Association of Colorado**
PO Box 22994
Denver, CO 80222-0994
303-797-7870
Fax: 303-730-8032
e-mail: sbacolorado@gmail.com
www.coloradospinabifida.org

Marge Hayes, Equipment Swap
Marie Arroyo, President

Connecticut

7883 **Spina Bifida Association of Connecticut**
PO Box 2545
Hartford, CT 06146-2545
860-832-8905
800-574-6274
Fax: 860-832-6260
e-mail: sbac@sbac.org
www.sbac.org

Mary Attardo, President
Kiley J Carlson, Executive Director

Delaware

7884 Spina Bifida Association of Delaware
PO Box 807 302-478-4805
Wilmington, DE 19899-0807 e-mail: kbasar@aol.com
www.angelfire.com/de/sbaofde/

Blake Heath, Vice President
Andy Anderso Jr, Treasurer

Florida

7885 Spina Bifida Association of Florida Space Coast
3685 Starlight Avenue 321-454-9737
Merrit Island, FL 32953-2549 Fax: 321-454-9737
e-mail: sbafscearthlink.com
www.sbaa.org

Robin Reinarts, President

7886 Spina Bifida Association of Jacksonville
807 Childrens Way 904-390-3686
Jacksonville, FL 32207-8426 800-722-6355
Fax: 904-390-3466
e-mail: sbaj@sbaj.org
www.sbaj.org

Michael Erhard, Chairperson

7887 Spina Bifida Association of Tampa
PO Box 151038 813-933-4827
Tampa, FL 33684-1038 Fax: 813-872-9845
e-mail: sbatampabay@aol.com
www.sbaj.org

Dianne Gore, President

Georgia

7888 Spina Bifida Association of Georgia
1448 Mclendon Drive 770-939-1044
Decatur, GA 30033 Fax: 770-939-1049
e-mail: info@spinabifidaga.org
www.spinabifidaofgeorgia.org

Provides referrals, evaluation, treatment and therapeutic activities for children and teens afflicted with spina bifida. The goal of this center is to help children or teenagers prepare for life.
William Turnispeed, President
Judy Thibadeau, Vice President

Illinois

7889 Illinois Spina Bifida Association
8765 W Higgins Road 773-444-0305
Chicago, IL 60631-1693 800-969-4722
Fax: 630-637-1066
e-mail: sbail@sbail.org
www.sbail.org

Dedicated to improving the quality of life of people with spina bifida through direct services, information and referral and public awareness. Direct services include a residential summer camp for children with spina bifida over the age of seven.
Scott J Munkvold, President
Amy Maggio, CEO

Indiana

7890 Spina Bifida Association of Central Indiana
PO Box 19814 317-592-1630
Indianapolis, IN 46279-0814 Fax: 317-351-2010
e-mail: pres@sbaci.org
www.sbaci.org

James Zetzl, President

Iowa

7891 Spina Bifida Association of Iowa
PO Box 1456 515-964-8810
Des Moines, IA 50305-1456 e-mail: spinabifidaiowa@yahoo.com
www.spinabifidaia.com

Rod Tressel, President

Kentucky

7892 Spina Bifida Association of Kentucky Kosair Charities Center
Kosair Charities Center
982 Eastern Parkway 502-637-7363
Louisville, KY 40217-1568 866-340-7225
Fax: 502-637-1010
e-mail: sbak@sbak.org
www.sbak.org

Angela Cosby, President
Patty Dissell, Executive Director

Louisiana

7893 Spina Bifida Association of Greater New Orleans
PO Box 1346 504-737-5181
Kenner, LA 70063-1346 Fax: 504-538-9046
e-mail: sbagno@sbagno.com
www.sbagno.org

Al Hitt, President
Judy Otto, Vice-President

Maryland

7894 Spina Bifida Association of Maryland
2416 Lampost Lane 410-665-1543
Baltimore, MD 21234-1460 Fax: 410-833-1700
e-mail: sbamaryland@comcast.net ÿÿ
www.home.comcast.net/~sbamaryland

7895 Spina Bifida Association of the Eastern Shore
316 Prospect Avenue 410-822-8609
Easton, MD 21601-4046 Fax: 410-822-5455
www.spinabifidaassociation.org

Massachusetts

7896 Spina Bifida Association of Massachusetts
321 Fortune Boulevard 617-742-2574
Milford, MA 01757-2741 888-479-1900
Fax: 978-649-8725
e-mail: bsullivan@sbaMass.org
www.msbaweb.org

Brendan Sullivan, President
Cara Packard, Vice President

Michigan

7897 Spina Bifida Association of Grand Rapids
235 Wealthy Street SE 616-240-9672
Grand Rapids, MI 49503-5299 Fax: 616-222-1541
e-mail: WMiSBA@hotmail.comÿ
www.spinabifidaassociation.org

Carol Carpenter, President

7898 Spina Bifida Association of Upper Peninsula Michigan
1220 N 3rd Street 906-485-5127
Ishpeming, MI 44849-1108 Fax: 906-225-7230
e-mail: cbengson@chartermi.net
www.sba-up.8m.com

Lois Bengson, President

7899 Spina Bifida and Hydrocephalus Association of Southwestern Michigan
PO Box 212 269-385-3959
Mattawan, MI 49071-0212 Fax: 269-392-9765
e-mail: marenhorkness@yahoo.com

Richard Benthnin, President

7900 Spina Bifida and Hydrocephalus Association
PO Box 212 269-385-3959
Mattawan, MI 49071 Fax: 269-392-9765
e-mail: marenharkness@yahoo.com
www.spinabifidasupport.com

Richard Benthnin, President

Minnesota

7901 **Spina Bifida Association of Minnesota**
PO Box 29323 651-222-6395
Minneapolis, MN 55429-0212 Fax: 952-591-0246
e-mail: sbamn@hotmail.com
www.sbamn.com

Wendy Swanson, President
Jim Thayer, Executive Director

Missouri

7902 **Spina Bifida Association of Greater St. Louis**
8050 Watson Road 314-843-2244
Saint Louis, MO 63119-2000 800-784-0983
Fax: 314-353-1446
e-mail: sbastl@charter.net
www.sbstl.com

Mark Abbott, President

Nebraska

7903 **Spina Bifida Association of Nebraska**
7612 Maple Street 402-932-5826
Omaha, NE 68134-2153 Fax: 402-572-3002
www.spinabifidanebraska.org

LeAnn Karman, President

New Jersey

7904 **Spina Bifida Association of the Tri-State Region**
84 Park Avenue 908-782-7475
Flemington, NJ 08822-1174 877-722-8774
Fax: 908-782-6102
e-mail: info@thesbrn.org
www.sbatsr.org

Serves New Jersey, New York Metro Area and Southern Connecticut.
Jane Horowitz, Executive Director and President
K David Holmes, Chairman of the Board

New Mexico

7905 **Spina Bifida Association of New Mexico**
1127 University Boulevard NE
Albuquerque, NM 87102-1740 505-242-1184
www.sbanm.com

Rey Garduno, Executive Director
Ann Beddingfield, Interim Treasurer

New York

7906 **Spina Bifida Association of Albany/Capital District**
100 Spring 518-399-9151
Scotia, NY 12302-3312 e-mail: sbaalbany102@aol.com
www.abaalbany.org

Kevin Chamberlain, Co-President
Vanessa Chamberlain, Co-President

7907 **Spina Bifida Association of Greater Rochester**
PO Box 3 585-381-5471
Fairport, NY 14450-0003 Fax: 585-264-9547
e-mail: jarmst4459@aol.com

JoAnn Armstrong, President

7908 **Spina Bifida Association of Nassau County**
12 Hampton Road 631-821-9028
Sound Beach, NY 11789 e-mail: kid3418@optonline.net
www.spinabifidaassociation.org

Leslieann Sussman, President

North Carolina

7909 **Spina Bifida Association of North Carolina**
3915 Grace Court 704-882-0988
Indian Trail, NC 28079 800-847-2262
Fax: 704-882-0988
e-mail: sbanc@mindspring.com
www.spinabifidaassociation.org

Julie Yindra, President
Kin Gates, Executive Director

Ohio

7910 **Spina Bifida Association of Canton**
S Cherokee Trail 330-863-2531
Malvern, OH 44644 Fax: 330-863-1172
e-mail: cmgriffin@nero.rr.com
www.spinabifidasupport.com

Connie Griffin, President

7911 **Spina Bifida Association of Central Ohio**
7239 Upper Cambridge Way 614-818-3840
Westerville, OH 43082 e-mail: sbaco@sbaco.net
www.sbaco.net

Laurie Schulze, Treasurer
Chrissy Zepfel, President

7912 **Spina Bifida Association of Cincinnati**
3245 Deborah Lane 513-923-1378
Cincinnati, OH 45239-0152 e-mail: sbacincy@sbacincy.org
www.sbacincy.org

Brady Sellet, President
Diane Burns, Executive Director

7913 **Spina Bifida Association of Greater Dayton**
4801 Springfield Street 937-236-1122
Dayton, OH 45431 Fax: 937-434-4899
e-mail: mvspinabifida@yahoo.com
www.sbadayton.org

David Skinner, President
Lisa Maas, Vice President

7914 **Spina Bifida Association of Northwest Ohio**
2211 River Road 419-794-0561
Maumee, OH 43537 Fax: 419-533-3952
e-mail: sba@sbaofnorthwestohio.org
www.sbaofnorthwestohio.org

Ginnette Clark, President
Julie Harley, Vice President

Pennsylvania

7915 **Spina Bifida Association of Central Pennsylvania**
209 E State Street 717-786-9280
Quarryville, PA 17566-1242 888-770-SBPA
Fax: 717-786-8821
e-mail: SBAofPA@aol.com
www.geocities.com/sbaofgpa

Patricia Fulvio, President
Amy Graver, Chairman

7916 **Spina Bifida Association of Delaware Valley**
PO Box 859 610-584-5530
Worcester, PA 19490-0289 Fax: 215-412-9396
e-mail: info@sbadv.org
www.sbadv.org

Marilyn Lieb, President
Keri Mascaro, Executive Director

7917 **Spina Bifida Association of Greater Pennsylvania**
209 E State Street 717-786-9280
Quarryville, PA 17566-9614 Fax: 717-786-8821
e-mail: sbaofpa@aol.com
www.spinabifidasupport.com

Amy Graver, President
Patricia Fulvio, Executive Director

Rhode Island

7918 Spina Bifida Association of Rhode Island
PO Box 6948
Warwick, RI 02887-6948
401-732-7862
Fax: 401-732-7862
www.spinabifidaassociation.org

Tennessee

7919 Spina Bifida Association of Tennessee
PO Box 23056
Nashville, TN 37202-5529
615-791-8117
Fax: 615-791-1518
e-mail: lynnhess56@comcast.net
www.spinabifidasupport.com

Lynn Cook, President

Texas

7920 Spina Bifida Association of Austin
9301 Bradner Drive
Austin, TX 78748
512-292-6317
Fax: 512-479-3845
e-mail: austinspinabifida@yahoo.com
www.spinabifidasupport.com

Kelley Hively, President

7921 Spina Bifida Association of Dallas
705 W Avenue B
Garland, TX 75040
972-238-8755
Fax: 972-414-3772
e-mail: sbdal@aol.com
www.sbdallas.org

Robin Leeÿ, President
Ryan McCoy, Vice President

7922 Spina Bifida Association of Texas, Gulf Coast
440 Benmar
Houston, TX 77060-2460
281-493-4349
Fax: 281-997-2278
e-mail: Yvonne.Horner@sbahgc.org
www.sbahgc.org

Yvonne Horner, President
Donnis Collier, Vice President

Washington

7923 Spina Bifida Association of Evergreen
2128 N Pines Road
Spokane, WA 99208
253-589-3700
888-289-3700
Fax: 775-766-1654
e-mail: patti_logan04@yahoo.com
www.evergreenspinabifida.org

Patti Logan, Secretary
Ed Kennedy, President

Wisconsin

7924 Spina Bifida Association of Northern Wisconsin
PO Box 421
Schofield, WI 54476-0421
715-798-3944
e-mail: dtackley@chegnet.net
David Blanchard, President

7925 Spina Bifida Association of Northwest Ohio
PO Box 421
Schofield, WI 54476
715-359-9674
e-mail: thutton@cheqnet.net
www.spinabifidasupport.com

Teresa Vullings, President

7926 Spina Bifida Association of Southeastern Wisconsin
830 N 109th Street
Wauwatosa, WI 53226
414-607-9061
Fax: 414-607-9602
e-mail: sbawi@sbawi.org
www.sbawi.org

Karen Drzewiecki, President
Heather Lynn Flohr, Executive Director

7927 Spina Bifida Association of the Greater Fox Valley
325 N John Street
Kimberly, WI 54136
920-687-0801
e-mail: fus1234@athenet.net
www.spinabifidasupport.com

Kelly Richard, President

Support Groups & Hotlines

7928 National Health Information Center
PO Box 1133
Washington, DC 20013
310-565-4167
800-336-4797
Fax: 301-984-4256
e-mail: info@nhic.org
www.health.gov/nhic

Offers a nationwide information referral service, produces directories and resource guides.

Books

7929 Answering Your Questions About Spina Bifida
Spina Bifida Association of America
4590 Macarthur Boulevard NW
Washington, DC 20007-4226
202-944-3285
800-621-3141
Fax: 202-944-3295
e-mail: sbaa@sbaa.org
www.sbaa.org

Provides information to help people understand the basic medical, educational and social issues which commonly affect people with Spina Bifida.

7930 Bowel Continence and Spina Bifida
Spina Bifida Association of America
4590 Macarthur Boulevard NW
Washington, DC 20007-4226
202-944-3285
800-621-3141
Fax: 202-944-3295
e-mail: sbaa@sbaa.org
www.sbaa.org

An excellent book aimed at anyone (infant or adult) trying to attain bowel continence. Focuses on continence programs, bowel management development and techniques.

7931 Clinic Directory
Spina Bifida Association of America
4590 Macarthur Boulevard NW
Washington, DC 20007-4226
202-944-3285
800-621-3141
Fax: 202-944-3295
e-mail: sbaa@sbaa.org
www.sbaa.org

A directory of health care clinics throughout the United States for children and adults with spina bifida.
200 pages 3-Ring Binder

7932 Complete IEP Guide: How to Advocate for Your Special Ed Child
Spina Bifida Association
4590 Macarthur Boulevard NW
Washington, DC 20007-4226
202-944-3285
800-621-3141
e-mail: sbaa@sbaa.org
www.sbaa.org

This all-in-one guide will help you understand special education law, identify your child's needs, prepare for meetings, develop the IEP and resolve disputes.

7933 Confronting the Challenges of Spina Bifida
Spina Bifida Association of America
4590 Macarthur Boulevard NW
Washington, DC 20007-4226
202-944-3285
800-621-3141
Fax: 202-944-3295
e-mail: sbaa@sbaa.org
www.sbaa.org

A group curriculum addressing self-care, self-esteem, and social skills in 8 to 13 year olds.

7934 Healthcare Guidelines
Spina Bifida Association of America
4590 Macarthur Boulevard NW
Washington, DC 20007-4226
202-944-3285
800-621-3141
Fax: 202-944-3295
e-mail: sbaa@sbaa.org
www.sbaa.org

7935 Learning Disabilities and the Person with Spina Bifida
Spina Bifida Association of America

4590 Macarthur Boulevard NW
Washington, DC 20007-4226
202-944-3285
800-621-3141
Fax: 202-944-3295
e-mail: sbaa@sbaa.org
www.sbaa.org

7936 **Negotiating the Special Education Maze: A Guide for Parents and Teachers**
Spina Bifida Association
4590 Macarthur Boulevard NW
Washington, DC 20007-4226
202-944-3285
800-621-3141
e-mail: sbaa@sbaa.org
www.sbaa.org
An excellent aid for the development of an effective special education program.

7937 **New Language of Toys: Teaching Communication Skills to Children...**
Spina Bifida Association
4590 Macarthur Boulevard NW
Washington, DC 20007-4226
202-944-3285
800-621-3141
e-mail: sbaa@sbaa.org
www.sbaa.org
A guide for parents and teachers, this reader-friendly resource guide provides a wealth of information on how play activities affect a child's language development (with a focus on special needs) and where to get the toys and materials to use in these activities.

7938 **Nick Joins In**
Spina Bifida Association
4590 Macarthur Boulevard NW
Washington, DC 20007-4226
202-944-3285
800-621-3141
e-mail: sbaa@sbaa.org
www.sbaa.org
When Nick, who is in a wheelchair, enters a regular classroom, for the first time he realizes that he has much to contribute.

7939 **Princess Pooh**
Spina Bifida Association
4590 Macarthur Boulevard NW
Washington, DC 20007-4226
202-944-3285
800-621-3141
e-mail: sbaa@sbaa.org
www.sbaa.org
Jealous of her disabled sister's royal treatment as she sits on her throne with wheels, Patty Jean borrows it and discovers that life in a wheelchair isn't so easy.

7940 **SBAA General Information Packet**
Spina Bifida Association of America
4590 Macarthur Boulevard NW
Washington, DC 20007-4226
202-944-3285
800-621-3141
Fax: 202-944-3295
e-mail: sbaa@sbaa.org
www.sbaa.org

7941 **Sexuality and the Person with Spina Bifida**
Spina Bifida Association of America
4590 Macarthur Boulevard NW
Washington, DC 20007-4226
202-944-3285
800-621-3141
Fax: 202-944-3295
e-mail: sbaa@sbaa.org
www.sbaa.org
Focuses on sexuality, sexual development, sexual activity, and other important issues.

7942 **Social Development and the Person with Spina Bifida**
Spina Bifida Association of America
4590 Macarthur Boulevard NW
Washington, DC 20007-4226
202-944-3285
800-621-3141
Fax: 202-944-3295
e-mail: sbaa@sbaa.org
www.sbaa.org

7943 **Steps to Independence: Teaching Everyday Skills to Children with Special Needs**
Spina Bifida Association
4590 Macarthur Boulevard NW
Washington, DC 20007-4226
202-944-3285
800-621-3141
e-mail: sbaa@sbaa.org
www.sbaa.org
A guide to help parents teach life skills to their disabled child.

7944 **Taking Charge**
Spina Bifida Association of America
4590 Macarthur Boulevard NW
Washington, DC 20007-4226
202-944-3285
800-621-3141
Fax: 202-944-3295
e-mail: sbaa@sbaa.org
www.sbaa.org
Teenagers talk about life and physical disabilities.

7945 **Unlocking Potential: College and Other Choices for People with LD and AD/HD**
Spina Bifida Association
4590 Macarthur Boulevard NW
Washington, DC 20007-4226
202-944-3285
800-621-3141
e-mail: sbaa@sbaa.org
www.sbaa.org
An indispensible tool for high school students with learning disabilities and AD/HD. Includes a comprehensive listing of resources.

Children's Books

7946 **Margaret's Moves**
Dutton Children's Books
375 Hudson Street
212-366-2000
New York, NY 10014-3658
This story deals with all the nuances and impairments that children afflicted with spina bifida must encounter and succeed in overcoming.
Grades 4-6

7947 **Rolling Along with Goldilocks and the Three Bears**
Spina Bifida Association
4590 Macarthur Boulevard NW
Washington, DC 20007-4226
202-944-3285
800-621-3141
e-mail: sbaa@sbaa.org
www.sbaa.org
The familiar folktale with a special-needs twist.

7948 **Views from Our Shoes: Growing Up with a Brother or Sister with Special Needs**
Spina Bifida Association
4590 Macarthur Boulevard NW
Washington, DC 20007-4226
202-944-3285
800-621-3141
e-mail: sbaa@sbaa.org
www.sbaa.org
A balanced view of the positives and negatives of living with a disabled sibling. Written for siblings ages nine and up.

Newsletters

7949 **Insights Into Spina Bifida**
Spina Bifida Association of America
4590 Macarthur Boulevard NW
Washington, DC 20007-4226
202-944-3285
800-621-3141
Fax: 202-944-3295
e-mail: sbaa@sbaa.org
www.sbaa.org
Includes articles on the latest research, the latest up-dates on legislation, features and emotional aspects specific to Spina Bifida, educational information and information on the Association's national conference.
BiMonthly

7950 **NASS News**
222 S Prospect Avenue
847-698-1628
Park Ridge, IL 60068-4037
Association activities newsletter.

Pamphlets

7951 **Educational Issues Among Children with Spina Bifida**
Spina Bifida Association of America

4590 Macarthur Boulevard NW 202-944-3285
Washington, DC 20007-4226 800-621-3141
Fax: 202-944-3295
e-mail: sbaa@sbaa.org
www.sbaa.org

1995

7952 **Learning Among Children with Spina Bifida**
Spina Bifida Association of America
4590 Macarthur Boulevard NW 202-944-3285
Washington, DC 20007-4226 800-621-3141
Fax: 202-944-3295
e-mail: sbaa@sbaa.org
www.sbaa.org

1995

7953 **Monetary Allowance, Health Care and Vocational Training**
National Veterans Services Fund
PO Box 2465 203-656-0003
Darien, CT 06820-0465 Fax: 203-656-1957
e-mail: NatVetSvc@aol.com

Monetary allowance, health care and vocational training and rehabilitation for Vietnam Veterans' children with spine bifida.
Pamphlet

7954 **Sexual Issues in Spina Bifida**
Spina Bifida Association of America
4590 Macarthur Boulevard NW 202-944-3285
Washington, DC 20007-4226 800-621-3141
Fax: 202-944-3295
e-mail: sbaa@sbaa.org
www.sbaa.org

1993

7955 **Urologic Care of the Child with Spina Bifida**
Spina Bifida Association of America
4590 Macarthur Boulevard NW 202-944-3285
Washington, DC 20007-4226 800-621-3141
Fax: 202-944-3295
e-mail: sbaa@sbaa.org
www.sbaa.org

1994

Audio & Video

7956 **Protecting Against Latex Allergy**
Spina Bifida Association of America
4590 Macarthur Boulevard NW 202-944-3285
Washington, DC 20007-4226 800-621-3141
Fax: 202-944-3295
e-mail: sbaa@sbaa.org
www.sbaa.org

Audio-visual resource focusing on the awareness of latex allergies.
Audio-Visual
Cindy Brownstein, Chief Executive Officer
Caroline Alston, Program Director

7957 **Raising a Child with Spina Bifida: An Introduction**
Ajn Company
New York, NY 10019 212-582-8820
800-226-6256
Fax: 212-586-5462

Offers information parents need when their child is born with spina bifida. Uses clear explanations to define spina bifida and discuss its implications for the child. Covers procedures the child may face, such as a ventricular shunt. Emphasizes the importance of early intervention and contains footage of happy and healthy children and interviews with parents.
29 minutes

7958 **The Challenge**
Spina Bifida Association of America
4590 Macarthur Boulevard NW 202-944-3285
Washington, DC 20007-4226 800-621-3141
Fax: 202-944-3295
e-mail: sbaa@sbaa.org
www.sbaa.org

A human look of how people come to grips with and overcome the challenges related to living with Spina Bifida.
14 minutes
Cindy Brownstein, Chief Executive Officer
Caroline Alston, Program Director

Web Sites

7959 **Healing Well**
www.healingwell.com

An online health resource guide to medical news, chat, information and articles, newsgroups and message boards, books, disease-related web sites, medical directories, and more for patients, friends, and family coping with disabling diseases, disorders, or chronic illnesses.

7960 **Health Finder**
www.healthfinder.gov

Searchable, carefully developed web site offering information on over 1000 topics. Developed by the US Department of Health and Human Services, the site can be used in both English and Spanish.

7961 **Healthlink USA**
www.healthlinkusa.com

Health information concerning treatment, cures, prevention, diagnosis, risk factors, research, support groups, email lists, personal stories and much more. Updated regularly.

7962 **Helios Health**
www.helioshealth.com

Online resource for your health information. Detailed information about specific health topics, access to expert advice from our Medical Advisory Board, and up-to-date health news.

7963 **March of Dimes Birth Defects Foundation**
www.modimes.org

Information on the treatment and prevention of birth defects, including spina bifida.

7964 **MedicineNet**
www.medicinenet.com

An online resource for consumers providing easy-to-read, authoritative medical and health information.

7965 **Medscape**
www.mywebmd.com

Medscape offers specialists, primary care physicians, and other health professionals the Web's most robust and integrated medical information and educational tools.

7966 **Spina Bifida Association of America**
www.sbaa.org

Represents approximately 60 chapters of parents and other members of families having children born with spina bifida, individuals with spina bifida, and health professionals who work with them.

7967 **WebMD**
www.webmd.com

Information on Spina Bifida, including articles and resources.

Description

7968 **Spinal Cord Injuries**

Spinal cord injury results from trauma to or disease of the spinal cord. Depending on where the spinal cord was injured, paraplegia (paralysis affecting the legs and lower part of the body) or quadriplegia (paralysis affecting all muscles below the neck and therefore all four limbs), may occur. Bladder and/or sexual function may be damaged. Each year, 12,000 people, mostly teenage males, sustain a spinal cord injury as a result of motor vehicle or sports-related accidents, or violent crimes.

Modern medical and surgical care has dramatically increased both long-term survival and quality of life in victims of spinal cord injury. This improvement reflects intensive medical care and appropriate surgical stabilization at the time of the injury, and in later years, attention to preventing the complications, such as skin breakdown, bladder infection and lung dysfunction. One of the greatest challenges is helping persons with spinal cord injuries to live as productive and independent a life as possible. Rehabilitation should begin as soon as possible after the injury. It usually starts with several weeks at a specialized inpatient facility, then transitions to family-assisted or independent living, depending on the extent of the disability. The multidisciplinary team provides education, emotional support, physical and occupational therapy, assistive devices, braces, and beds, and helps arrange special vans or modifications to the patient's home. Many voluntary societies and government agencies can help with the transition to life in the community.

National Agencies & Associations

7969 **American Association of Spinal Cord Injury Nurses**
801 18th Street NW — 202-416-7704
Washington, DC 20006 — Fax: 202-416-7641
e-mail: aascin@pva.org
www.aascin.org
Comprised of nurses who specialize in spinal cord research nursing and education.
Sara Lerman MPH, Program Manager
Maurice L Jordan, Acting Executive Director

7970 **American Paraplegic Society**
801 18th Street NW — 202-416-7704
Washington, DC 20006-1131 — Fax: 202-416-7641
e-mail: aps@pva.org
www.apssci.org
A professional membership organization for physicians scientists and allied health care professionals.
Maurice L Jordan, Acting Executive Director
Brenda Finkel, Administrative Assistant

7971 **American Spinal Cord Injury Association**
2020 Peachtree Road NW — 404-355-9772
Atlanta, GA 30309 — Fax: 404-355-1826
e-mail: ASIA_Office@shepherd.org
www.asia-spinalinjury.org
Provides a forum for doctors, nurses, rehabilitation professionals and others to exchange information through seminars and workshops. Scientific conferences include workshops on chronic SCI problems, neurophysiology, bioengineering and outpatient care.
Lesley M Hudson, Executive Director
Patricia Duncan, Administrative Coordinator

7972 **American Spinal Injury Association (ASIA)**
2020 Peachtree Road NW — 404-355-9772
Atlanta, GA 30309 — Fax: 404-355-1826
e-mail: ASIA_Office@shepherd.org
www.asia-spinalinjury.org
Professional association for physicians and other clinicians working in the field of spinal cord injury research prevention and care delivery.
Lesley Hudson, Director Meetings/Publications
Patricia Duncan, Administrative Coordinator

7973 **Association of Spinal Cord Injury Psychologists and Social Workers**
801 18th Street NW — 202-416-7704
Washington, DC 20006-1131 — Fax: 202-416-7641
e-mail: aascipsw@epua.org
www.aascipsw.org
Formed in 1986 to provide a forum for the exchange of ideas and information with assistance of the Eastern Paralyzed Veterans Association.
Maurice L Jordan, Acting Executive Director
Brenda Finkel, Administrative Assistant

7974 **Christopher & Dana Reeve Foundation Paralysis Resource Center**
636 Morris Turnpike — 973-467-8270
Short Hills, NJ 07078 — 800-225-0292
e-mail: info@paralysis.org
www.paralysis.org
The Paralysis Resource Center is a national clearinghouse of information referral and educational materials on paralysis. Services include a free lending library of books and videos and quality of life grants to qualifying non-profit organizations.
Paul Daversa, CEO
John McConnell, Senior Vice President of Programming

7975 **Eastern Paralyzed Veterans Association of America**
7520 Astoria Boulevard — 718-803-3782
E Elmhurst, NY 11370-1177 — 800-444-0120
Fax: 718-803-0414
Dedicated to serving veterans with a spinal cord injury or disease in New York New Jersey Connecticut or Pennsylvania. Based in New York City EPVA is the leader in funding SCI research and care.
Angela Wu, Director of Library Information

7976 **FES Information Center WO Walker Industrial Rehabilitation Cent**
WO Walker Industrial Rehabilitation Center
11000 Cedar Avenue
Cleveland, OH 44106-3052 — 800-666-2353
FES offers technology to persons with neuromuscular disorders resulting from spinal cord injury, head injury or stroke. The most widely known use of FES in the spinal community is for exercise.

7977 **International Medical Society of Paralegia: US Office**
T Giles
1333 Moursend Avenue — 713-797-5910
Houston, TX 77030 — Fax: 713-799-7017
National non-profit organization offers information resources and research for people with spinal cord injury or dysfunction. Professional organization for physicians.

7978 **International Spinal Cord Regeneration Center**
Po Box 451 — 619-463-5350
Bonita, CA 91908 — Fax: 619-460-2699
e-mail: spinal@mailutopia.net
spinal.siteutopia.net
Specializes in spinal cord regeneration as well as Embryonic Cell Transplant Therapy.
Fernando C Ramirez del Rio, Medical Director
Wolfram W Kuhnau, Associate

7979 **Kent Waldrep National Paralysis Foundation Main Office**
Main Office
16415 Addison Road — 972-248-7100
Addison, TX 75001 — 800-925-2873
Fax: 972-248-7313

National non-profit organization offers information referral resources and research for people with spinal cord injury their family members or service providers.

7980 **National Spinal Cord Injury Association: Metropolitan Washington Chapter**
6701 Democracy Boulevard 301-214-4006
Bethesdae, MD 20817 800-962-9629
Fax: 301-881-9817
e-mail: stevetowle@cs.com
The mission of the National Spinal Cord Injury A ssociation is to enable people with spinal cord injury and disease to achieve their highest level of indepedence, health, and personal fulfillment by providing resources, services, and peer support.
Harley Thomas, President

7981 **National Spinal Cord Injury Statistical Center**
University of Alabama, Dept. of Physical Medicine
619 19th Street S 205-934-3283
Birmingham, AL 35249 Fax: 205-975-4691
e-mail: sciweb@uab.edu
www.spinalcord.uab.edu
Supervises and directs the collection management and analysis of an extensive spinal cord injury database.
Amie Jackson, Project Director & Medical Director
Pam Mott, Director Research Services

7982 **Paralysis Society of America**
801 Eighteenth Street NW 202-973-8420
Washington, DC 20006-3517 888-772-1711
Fax: 202-973-8421
TTY: 2029738422
e-mail: info@psa.org
www.psa.org
Membership organization for people who have sustained a spinal cord injury or who have contracted a spinal cord disease; provides information services and advocacy.
Randy L Pleva, National President
Gene A Crayton, National Senior Vice President

7983 **Paralyzed Veterans of America**
801 18th Street NW 202-872-1300
Washington, DC 20006-3517 800-424-8200
Fax: 202-785-4452
e-mail: info@pva.org
www.pva.org
A congressionally chartered veterans service organization founded in 1946 has developed a unique expertise in a wide variety of issues involving the special needs of members - veterans of the armed forces who have experienced spinal cord injury or dysfunction.
Randy L Pleva, National President
Gene A Crayton, National Senior Vice President

7984 **Rick Hansen Foundation**
520 W 6th Avenue 604-876-6800
Vancouver, BC, V5Z-1A1 800-213-2131
Fax: 604-876-6666
e-mail: info@rickhanse.com
www.rickhansen.com
To inspire others to share in the achievement of big dreams that accelerate improvements in the quality of life of people with spinal cord injury.

7985 **Spinal Cord Injury Network International**
3911 Princeton Drive 707-577-8796
Santa Rosa, CA 95405-7013 800-548-2673
Fax: 707-577-0605
e-mail: spinal@sonic.net
www.spinalcordinjury.org
Provides information and referral for spinal cord injured individuals and their families. Video lending library with information about spinal cord injuries. Provides answers to many questions about disability and spinal cord injury and disease.
Lennice Ambrose, Executive Director
Sharon E Hunt, Medical Librarian

7986 **Spinal Cord Society**
19051 County Highway 1 218-739-5252
Fergus Falls, MN 56537 Fax: 218-739-5262
www.scsus.org
Funds research for spinal cord injuries and provides physician referrals.

State Agencies & Associations

Arizona

7987 **Arizona United Spinal Cord Association Samaritan Rehab Institute R-2**
Samaritan Rehab Institute R-2
901E Willetta Street 602-239-5929
Phoenix, AZ 85006 877-778-6588
Fax: 602-239-6268
e-mail: info@azspinal.org
www.azspinal.org
Organization dedicated to improving the quality of life for persons with spinal cord injuries and related disorders and their families. Seeks to fulfill this mission by raising awareness about spinal cord injury through education and injury prevention.
Paul Mortensen, Executive Director
Vangie Mortenson, Office Manager

California

7988 **National Spinal Cord Injury Association: San Diego County Chapter**
6645 Alvarado Road 619-229-7001
San Diego, CA 92120 e-mail: rehabdsg@gte.net
Organization dedicated to improving the quality of life for persons with spinal cord injury and related disorders and their families. Seeks to fufill this mission by raising awareness about spinal cord injury through education, injury prevention, improvement of medical, rehabilitative and supportive services, research and public policy formulation.
Royce Hamrick

7989 **National Spinal Cord Injury Association: Los Angeles Chapter**
311 Robertson Boulevard 310-553-4833
Beverly Hills, CA 90211 Fax: 310-230-0999
spinalcord.org
Organization dedicated to improving the quality of life for persons with spinal cord injury and related disorders and their families. Seeks to fulfill this mission by raising awareness about spinal cord injury through education, injury prevention, improvement of medical, rehabilitative and supportive services, research and public policy formulation.
Paul Berns MD, President

Connecticut

7990 **National Spinal Cord Injury Association: Connecticut Chapter**
PO Box 400 203-284-1045
Wallingford, CT 06492 e-mail: nscia@sciact.org
www.sciat.org
Organization dedicated to improving the quality of life for persons with spinal cord injury and related disorders and their families. Seeks to fufill this mission by raising awareness about spinal cord injury through education, injury prevention, improvement of medical, rehabilitative and supportive services, research and public policy formulation.
Bill Mancini, President

Florida

7991 **Goodwill Industries-Suncoast**
Goodwill Industries-Suncoast
10596 Gandy Boulevard 727-523-1512
Saint Petersburg, FL 33702 888-279-1988
Fax: 727-579-0850
TTY: 727-579-1068
e-mail: gw.marketing@goodwill-suncoast.com
www.goodwill-suncoast.org
A nonprofit community based organization whose purpose is to improve the quality of life for people who are disabled, disadvantaged and/or aged. This mission is accomplished through a staff of over 1,200 employees providing independent living skills.
R Lee Waits, President/Chief Executive Officer
Chris Ward, Marketing and Media Relations Manager

Georgia

7992 Shepherd Spinal Center
2020 Peachtree Road NW 404-352-2020
Atlanta, GA 30309 e-mail: webmaster@shepherd.org
www.shepherd.org
A nationally recognized facility in the United States dedicated exclusively to the care of patients with paralyzing spinal cord injuries and neuromuscular diseases.
David F Apple Jr, Medical Director Emeritus
Brock K Bowman, Assistant Medical Director

Illinois

7993 Spinal Cord Injury Association of Illinois
1032 S LaGrange Road 708-352-6223
LaGrange, IL 60525 877-373-0301
Fax: 708-352-9065
e-mail: sciinjury@aol.com
www.sci-illinois.org
Organization dedicated to improving the quality of life for persons with spinal cord injury and related disorders and their families. Seeks to fulfill this mission by raising awareness about spinal cord injury through education and injury prevention.
Mercedes Rauen, Executive Director

Indiana

7994 National Spinal Cord Injury Association: Central Indiana Chapter
2109 Cleveland Street 219-944-8037
Garyanapolis, IN 46404 Fax: 317-329-2530
e-mail: rjackson@ci.gary.in.us
Organization dedicated to improving the quality of life for persons with spinal cord injury and related disorders and their families. Seeks to fulfill this mission by raising awareness about spinal cord injury through education, injury prevention, improvement of medical, rehabilitative and supportive services, research and public policy formulation.
Lucille Hightower

Kentucky

7995 National Spinal Cord Injury Association: Derby City Area Chapter
Center for Accessible Living
1518 Herr Lane 502-589-6620
Louisville, KY 40222 e-mail: dallgood@calky.org
Organization dedicated to improving the quality of life for persons with spinal cord injury and related disorders and their families. Seeks to fulfill this mission by raising awareness about spinal cord injury through education, injury prevention, improvement of medical, rehabilitative and supportive services, research and public policy formulation.
David Allgood, President

Louisiana

7996 National Spinal Cord Injury Association: Louisiana Chapter
3650 18th Street 504-455-1178
Metairie, LA 70002 Fax: 504-455-7315
Organization dedicated to improving the quality of life for persons with spinal cord injury and related disorders and their families. Seeks to fulfill this mission by raising awareness about spinal cord injury through education, injury prevention, improvement of medical, rehabilitative and supportive services, research and public policy formulation.
Yadi Mark

Maryland

7997 National Spinal Cord Injury Association
6701 Democracy Blvd. 301-214-4006
Bethesda, MD 20817 800-962-9629
Fax: 301-990-0445
e-mail: nscia2@aol.com
www.spinalcord.org
The missionof The National Spimal Cord Injury Association is to enable people with spinal cord injury and diesease to achieve their highest level of independence, health, and peronal fulfillment by providing resourcces, services, and peer support.
Steven A Towle, Contact

Massachusetts

7998 National Spinal Cord Injury Association
545 Concord Avenue 301-588-6959
Cambridge, MA 02138-1173 800-962-9629
Fax: 301-588-9414
e-mail: nscia2@aol.com
www.spinalcord.org
Organization dedicated to improving the quality of life for persons with spinal cord injury and related disorders and their families. Seeks to fulfill this mission by raising awareness about spinal cord injury through education, injury prevention, improvement of medical, rehabilitative and supportive services, research and public policy formulation.

7999 National Spinal Cord Injury Association: Greater Boston Chapter
New England Rehabilitation Hospital
Two Rehabilitation Way 781-933-8666
Woburn, MA 01801 Fax: 781-933-0043
e-mail: sciboston@aol.com
www.sciboston.com
Organization dedicated to improving the quality of life for persons with spinal cord injury and related disorders and their families. Seeks to fulfill this mission by raising awareness about spinal cord injury through education and injury prevention.
Kevin Gibson, Coordinator
Dave Estrada, Director

New Hampshire

8000 New Hampshire Chapter NSCIA
Northeast Rehabilitation Hospital
PO Box 197 North Salem 603-479-0560
Salem, NH 03079-3974 Fax: 928-438-9607
www.nhspinal.org
Lisa Thompson, President

New York

8001 Greater Rochester Area Chapter NSCIA
PO Box 20516 716-275-6345
Rochester, NY 14602-0076 e-mail: ascaram4@frontier.net
Karen Genet, Contact

Pennsylvania

8002 Philadelphia Unit of Shriners Hospital
3551 N Broad Street 215-430-4000
Philadelphia, PA 19140 800-281-4050
Fax: 215-430-4079
www.shrinershq.org
Studies and research done on children with spinal cord injuries.
Richard B Gallier, Chairman
Randal R Betz, Chief of Staff and Medical Director

8003 Spinal Cord Injury Program at Harmarville Rehabilitation Center
PO Box 11460 412-828-1300
Pittsburgh, PA 15238 800-624-4673
Most comprehensive center for the treatment of spinal cord injury and disease.

Texas

8004 Rio Grande Chapter: NSCIA Rio Vista Rehabilitation Hospital
Rio Vista Rehabilitation Hospital
1395 George Dieter
El Paso, TX 79936-2901 915-532-3004
www.spinalcord.org
Sukie Armendariz, Contact
Ron Prieto, Contact

Virginia

8005 **Old Dominion Area Chapter: NSCIA**
5206 Markel Road 804-726-4990
Richmond, VA 23226 Fax: 888-752-7857
e-mail: info@odcnscia.org
www.odcnscia.org

Steve Fetrow, President
Craig Fabian, Vice President

West Virginia

8006 **West Virginia Mountaineer Chapter: NSCIA**
PO Box 1004 304-766-4751
Institute, WV 25112-1004 Fax: 304-766-4849
www.spinalcord.org

Steve Hill, President

Wisconsin

8007 **Greater Milwaukee Area Chapter: NSCIA Sacred Heart Rehabilitation Hospital**
Sacred Heart Rehabilitation Hospital
1545 S Layton Boulevard 414-384-4022
Milwaukee, WI 53215-1993 Fax: 414-384-7820
e-mail: someone@example.com
www.nsciagmac.org

John Dziewa, President

Research Centers

8008 **Miami Project to Cure Paralysis**
1095 NW 14th Terrace 305-243-6001
Miami, FL 33136 800-STA-NDUP
Fax: 205-243-6017
e-mail: miamiproject@med.miami.edu
www.miamiproject.miami.edu
The Project which began in 1985 is on the leading edge of basic science and clinical research to restore function after spinal cord injury. The Project is divided into three areas. The primary emphasis is on basic science research under the direction of Dr. Richard Bunge an eminent researcher. The second area is under the direction of Barth Green M.D. a neurosurgeon. The third area is rehabilitation research.
Suzie M Fayfie, Executive Director
Marc A Buoniconti, President

8009 **Paralysis Project**
PO Box 56141
Sherman Oaks, CA 91413-1141 818-785-5555
www.venturablvd.com
Funds scientific research and clinical studies that focus on spinal nerve repair and regeneration. The Project distributes current research data regarding paralysis and scientific projects public awareness and community information referral and support services for paralyzed individuals.

8010 **Pushin On: RRTC on Secondary Conditions of Spinal**
UAB Office of Research Services
619 19th Street S 205-934-3283
Birmingham, AL 35249-7330 Fax: 205-975-4691
e-mail: rtc@sun.rehabm.uab.edu
www.spinalcord.uab.edu
A federally funded rehabilitation research and training center.
8 pages 2 per year
Phil Klebine, Project Coordinator/Editor
Pamela Mott, Director Research Services

8011 **RRTC on Aging with a Disability Los Amigos Research and Education Instit**
Los Amigos Research and Education Institute
800 W Annex 562-401-7402
Downey, CA 90242-3456 Fax: 562-401-7011
e-mail: lcarrothers@agingwithdisability.org
www.agingwithdisability.org
A federally funded rehabilitation research and training center.
Leanne Carro Pt PhD, Training Director
Bryan Kemp PhD, Director

Support Groups & Hotlines

8012 **Georgia National Spinal Cord Injury Association Support Group Network**
PO Box 2645
Columbus, GA 31920 800-422-3352
Support group dedicated to improving the quality of life for persons with spinal cord injury and related disorders and their families. Seeks to fufill this mission by raising awareness about spinal cord injury through rehabilitative and supportive services, research and public policy formulation.
Andy Harp

8013 **HEALTHSOUTH Capital Rehabilitation Hospital**
1675 Riggins Road 850-656-4800
Tallahassee, FL 32308 Fax: 850-656-4809
www.healthsouth.com
Support group dedicated to improving the quality of life for persons with spinal cord injury and related disorders and their families. Seeks to fufill this mission by raising awareness about spinal cord injury through rehabilitative and supportive services, research and public policy formulation.
Lynn Streetman, Chief Executive Officer

8014 **Maryland National Spinal Cord Injury Association Support Group Network**
Kerman Hospital
2200 Kerman Drive 410-448-6307
Baltimore, MD 21207 800-962-9629
Support group dedicated to improving the quality of life for persons with spinal cord injury and related disorders and their families. Seeks to fufill this mission by raising awareness about spinal cord injury through rehabilitative and supportive services, research and public policy formulation.
Jessica Richard

8015 **National Health Information Center**
PO Box 1133 310-565-4167
Washington, DC 20013 800-336-4797
Fax: 301-984-4256
e-mail: info@nhic.org
www.health.gov/nhic
Offers a nationwide information referral service, produces directories and resource guides.

8016 **National Spinal Cord Injury Hotline**
2200 Kerman Drive 410-448-6824
Baltimore, MD 21207 800-492-5538
Fax: 410-448-6825
www.kernanhospital.com/pain
Provides information and referral services and peer support for people affected by a traumatic paralyzing injury.

8017 **National Spinal Cord Injury Support Goups**
Florida Rehabilitation and Sports Medicine
5165 Adanson Street 407-895-7991
Orlando, FL 32804
Support group dedicated to improving the quality of life for persons with spinal cord injury and related disorders and their families. Seeks to fufill this mission by raising awareness about spinal cord injury through rehabilitative and supportive services, research and public policy formulation.
Robin Kohn

8018 **VIVA!**
Health Enhancement Learning Programs
PO Box 543065 972-986-2977
Dallas, TX 75354-3065 800-334-4403
A computer-based patient education system on spinal cord injury.

8019 **National Spinal Cord Injury Support Groups**
Healthsouth Central Georgia Rehab Hospital
3351 Northside Drive 478-201-6500
Macon, GA 31210 800-491-3550
Fax: 478-633-5134
e-mail: tamboli.sara@mccg.org
www.centralgarehab.com/
Support group dedicated to improving the quality of life for persons with spinal cord injury and related disorders and their families. Seeks to fufill this mission by raising awareness about spinal

cord injury through rehabilitative and supportive services, research and public policy formulation.
Kathy Parks Combs RN, SCI Support Group Coordinator

8020 **National Spinal Cord Injury Support Groups**
HEALTHSOUTH, Sea Pines Rehabilitation Hospital
101 E Florida Avenue 407-984-4600
Melbourne, FL 32901
Support group dedicated to improving the quality of life for persons with spinal cord injury and related disorders and their families. Seeks to fufill this mission by raising awareness about spinal cord injury through rehabilitative and supportive services, research and public policy formulation.
Dorn Williamson

8021 **National Spinal Cord Injury Support Groups**
115 Alpine Street 334-456-1768
Chickasaw, AL 36611
Support group dedicated to improving the quality of life for persons with spinal cord injury and related disorders and their families. Seeks to fufill this mission by raising awareness about spinal cord injury through rehabilitative and supportive services, research and public policy formulation.
Marilyn McPherson

Books

8022 **Body Silent: An Anthropologist Embarks into the World of the Disabled**
WW Norton Publishing
500 Fifth Avenue 212-354-5500
New York, NY 10110 Fax: 212-869-0856
www.wwnorton.com
Diagnosed at midlife in the early 1980s with an inoperable (and, at the time, untreatable) ependymona of the spine, an anthropologist frankly discusses his progressive disability.

ISBN: 0-393307-02-6
RF Murphy

8023 **Climbing Back**
Miramar Communications
PO Box 8987
Malibu, CA 90265-8987 800-543-4116
The author broke his back after a climbing fall. With his sights at the top of the mountain he climbs back in this inspiring story.
256 pages Hardcover

8024 **Occupational Therapy Practice Guidelines for Adults with Spinal Cord Injury**
American Occupational Therapy Association
4720 Montgomery Lane 301-652-2682
Bethesda, MD 20824-1220 Fax: 301-652-7711
TDD: 800-377-8555
www.aota.org

31 pages
ISBN: 1-569001-54-5

8025 **Options: Spinal Cord Injury and the Future**
National Spinal Cord Injury Association
8300 Colesville Road 301-588-6959
Silver Spring, MD 20910-3243 800-962-9629
Fax: 301-588-9414
e-mail: nscia2@aol.com
www.spinalcord.org
A collection of conversations with people who have had spinal cord injuries who share some of their experiences and emotions.
150 pages

8026 **Spinal Cord Injury Home Care Manual**
Santa Clara Valley Medical Center
751 S Bascom Avenue
San Jose, CA 95128-2699 408-885-5000
www.scvmed.org
Provides people with spinal cord injury, their families and professionals with information about physical care, independent living, psychosocial issues, attendant care and supplies.

8027 **Spinal Network**
Miramar Communications
PO Box 8987
Malibu, CA 90265 800-543-4116
Total wheelchair resource book.

Children's Books

8028 **Follow Your Dreams**
National Spinal Cord Injury Association
8300 Colesville Road 301-588-6959
Silver Spring, MD 20910-3243 800-962-9629
Fax: 301-588-9414
e-mail: nscia2@aol.com
www.spinalcord.org
JT, born with spina bifida, goes on an adventure. Written for and by children with SCI, for children ages 9-12.
30 pages

8029 **Tell it Like it is**
National Spinal Cord Injury Association
8300 Colesville Road 301-588-6959
Silver Spring, MD 20910-3243 800-962-9629
Fax: 301-588-9414
e-mail: nscia2@aol.com
www.spinalcord.org
Written by teenagers with SCI for teenagers with SCI.

Magazines

8030 **SCI Life**
National Spinal Cord Injury Association
8300 Colesville Road 301-588-6959
Silver Spring, MD 20910-3243 800-962-9629
Fax: 301-588-9414
e-mail: nscia2@aol.com
www.spinalcord.org
Official magazine of NSCIA. Updates on topics such as research, medical issues, prevention, new products, books, and Association activities.
Quarterly

8031 **Spinal Column**
Shepherd Spinal Center
2020 Peachtree Road NW 404-352-2020
Atlanta, GA 30309-1465
This quarterly magazine from the spinal center offers information on the newest treatments, therapies, referral centers, assistive devices and much more for persons living with spina bifida, multiple sclerosis and other chronic physical ailments.
Quarterly

Newsletters

8032 **Progress in Research**
American Paralysis Association
500 Morris Avenue 973-379-2690
Springfield, NJ 07081-1020 800-225-0292
Fax: 973-912-9433
Offers information on the association, news, reviews, books, and information on the latest medical and technological advances in spinal cord injury research.
Quarterly
Susan P Howley, Research Director
Mitchell R Stoller, President/CEO

8033 **Pushing on: University of Alabama**
Christopher Reeve Association
500 Morris Avenue 973-379-2690
Springfield, NJ 07081 800-225-0292
Fax: 973-912-9433
A research newsletter regarding spinal cord injuries.
Quarterly
Mitchell R Stoller, President/CEO

8034 **Spinal Cord Society Newsletter**
Spinal Cord Society
19051 County Highway 1 — 218-739-5252
Fergus Falls, MN 56537 — Fax: 218-739-5262
www.members.aol.com/scsweb

Offers medical reports, articles, convention news, chapter news and more for persons with spinal cord injury.
Monthly

8035 **Walking Tomorrow: University of Alabama**
Christopher Reeve Association
500 Morris Avenue — 973-379-2690
Springfield, NJ 07081-1020 — 800-225-0292
Fax: 973-912-9433

A research newsletter regarding spinal cord injuries.
Quarterly
Mitchell R Stoller, President/CEO

Pamphlets

8036 **Autonomic Dysreflexia**
National Spinal Cord Injury Association
8300 Colesville Road — 301-588-6959
Silver Spring, MD 20910-3243 — 800-962-9629
Fax: 301-588-9414
e-mail: nscia2@aol.com
www.spinalcord.org

8037 **Choosing A Spinal Cord Injury Rehabilitation Program**
National Spinal Cord Injury Association
8300 Colesville Road — 301-588-6959
Silver Spring, MD 20910-3243 — 800-962-9629
Fax: 301-588-9414
e-mail: nscia2@aol.com
www.spinalcord.org

Includes a listing of programs accredited by CARF & Model Centers designated by NIDRR.

8038 **Fun and Games**
National Spinal Cord Injury Association
8300 Colesville Road — 301-588-6959
Silver Spring, MD 20910-3243 — 800-962-9629
Fax: 301-588-9414
e-mail: nscia2@aol.com
www.spinalcord.org

8039 **Functional Electrical Stimulation: Clinical Applications**
National Spinal Cord Injury Association
8300 Colesville Road — 301-588-6959
Silver Spring, MD 20910-3243 — 800-962-9629
Fax: 301-588-9414
e-mail: nscia2@aol.com
www.spinalcord.org

8040 **Importance of Basic Science in Research**
National Spinal Cord Injury Association
8300 Colesville Road — 301-588-6959
Silver Spring, MD 20910-3243 — 800-962-9629
Fax: 301-588-9414
e-mail: nscia2@aol.com
www.spinalcord.org

8041 **Male Reproductive Function After Spinal Cord Injury**
National Spinal Cord Injury Association
8300 Colesville Road — 301-588-6959
Silver Spring, MD 20910-3243 — 800-962-9629
Fax: 301-588-9414
e-mail: nscia2@aol.com
www.spinalcord.org

8042 **Medical Facilities and Resources for Ventilator Users**
National Spinal Cord Injury Association
8300 Colesville Road — 301-588-6959
Silver Spring, MD 20910-3243 — 800-962-9629
Fax: 301-588-9414
e-mail: nscia2@aol.com
www.spinalcord.org

8043 **Reading Resources on Spinal Cord Injury**
National Spinal Cord Injury Association
8300 Colesville Road — 301-588-6959
Silver Spring, MD 20910-3243 — 800-962-9629
Fax: 301-588-9414
e-mail: nscia2@aol.com
www.spinalcord.org

8044 **Sexuality After Spinal Cord Injury**
National Spinal Cord Injury Association
8300 Colesville Road — 301-588-6959
Silver Spring, MD 20910-3243 — 800-962-9629
Fax: 301-588-9414
e-mail: nscia2@aol.com
www.spinalcord.org

8045 **Spinal Cord Injury Awareness**
National Spinal Cord Injury Association
8300 Colesville Road — 301-588-6959
Silver Spring, MD 20910-3243 — 800-962-9629
Fax: 301-588-9414
e-mail: nscia2@aol.com
www.spinalcord.org

Understanding the importance of language and images.

8046 **Spinal Cord Injury: Statistical Information**
National Spinal Cord Injury Association
8300 Colesville Road — 301-588-6959
Silver Spring, MD 20910-3243 — 800-962-9629
Fax: 301-588-9414
e-mail: nscia2@aol.com
www.spinalcord.org

8047 **Starting a Support Group**
National Spinal Cord Injury Association
8300 Colesville Road — 301-588-6959
Silver Spring, MD 20910-3243 — 800-962-9629
Fax: 301-588-9414
e-mail: nscia2@aol.com
www.spinalcord.org

8048 **Tendon Transfer Surgery**
National Spinal Cord Injury Association
8300 Colesville Road — 301-588-6959
Silver Spring, MD 20910-3243 — 800-962-9629
Fax: 301-588-9414
e-mail: nscia2@aol.com
www.spinalcord.org

8049 **Travel After Spinal Cord Injury**
National Spinal Cord Injury Association
8300 Colesville Road — 301-588-6959
Silver Spring, MD 20910-3243 — 800-962-9629
Fax: 301-588-9414
e-mail: nscia2@aol.com
www.spinalcord.org

8050 **Understanding Spinal Muscular Atrophy**
Families of Spinal Muscular Atrophy
PO Box 196 — 847-367-7620
Libertyville, IL 60048-0196 — 800-886-1762
Fax: 847-367-7623
e-mail: info@fsma.org
www.curesma.com

Offers a brief overview of Spinal Muscular Atrophy, causes, treatments, symptoms and unknowns.
Kenneth Hobby, Executive Director

8051 **What is Spinal Cord Injury?**
National Spinal Cord Injury Association
8300 Colesville Road — 301-588-6959
Silver Spring, MD 20910-3243 — 800-962-9629
Fax: 301-588-9414
e-mail: nscia2@aol.com
www.spinalcord.org

8052 **What is a Physiatrist?**
National Spinal Cord Injury Association
8300 Colesville Road — 301-588-6959
Silver Spring, MD 20910-3243 — 800-962-9629
Fax: 301-588-9414
e-mail: nscia2@aol.com
www.spinalcord.org

8053 **What's New in Spinal Cord Injury Research?**
National Spinal Cord Injury Association
8300 Colesville Road
Silver Spring, MD 20910-3243
301-588-6959
800-962-9629
Fax: 301-588-9414
e-mail: nscia2@aol.com
www.spinalcord.org

Audio & Video

8054 **Living with Spinal Cord Injury**
Barry Corbet, author
Fanlight Productions
4196 Washington Street
Boston, MA 02131-1731
617-469-4999
800-937-4113
Fax: 617-469-3379
e-mail: fanlight@fanlight.com
www.fanlight.com
A series of three videos produced by an individual who has experienced spinal cord injury himself. Changes is about coming to terms with spinal cord injury and beginning rehabilitation. Outside looks at the life-long process by which some injured people have created active and rewarding lives. Survivors explores the problems of growing old with a disability.
1973 84 Minutes

8055 **SCI and Lower Extremity Orthoses**
Health Enhancement Learning Programs
PO Box 543065
Dallas, TX 75354-3065
214-902-8277
800-334-4403
A video presenting an overview of indications and use of HKAFO, KAFO and AFO. Perfect resource for medical presentations and professional workshops.

8056 **Spinal Cord Injury Video Access**
Spinal Cord Injury Access International
39111 Princeton Drive
Santa Rosa, CA 95405
800-548-2673
Offers informational videotapes on spinal cord injury.

8057 **Spinal Injury Slide Series**
Health Enhancement Learning Programs
PO Box 543065
Dallas, TX 75354-3065
214-902-8277
800-334-4403
A slide series based on the VIVA program, a patient education system on spinal cord injury.

Web Sites

8058 **American Association of Spinal Cord Injury Nurses**
www.aascin.org
Comprised of nurses who specialize in spinal cord research, nursing and education.

8059 **American Paraplegic Society**
www.apssci.org
A professional membership organization for physicians, scientists and allied health care professionals.

8060 **Christopher Reeve Paralysis Foundation**
www.apacure.com
Dedicated to finding a cure for paralysis caused by spinal cord injury, head injury and stroke. A network of chapters across the country formed to provide comfort to the paralyzed but primarily to help raise funds to find a paralysis cure.

8061 **Healing Well**
www.healingwell.com
An online health resource guide to medical news, chat, information and articles, newsgroups and message boards, books, disease-related web sites, medical directories, and more for patients, friends, and family coping with disabling diseases, disorders, or chronic illnesses.

8062 **Health Finder**
www.healthfinder.gov
Searchable, carefully developed web site offering information on over 1000 topics. Developed by the US Department of Health and Human Services, the site can be used in both English and Spanish.

8063 **Healthlink USA**
www.healthlinkusa.com
Health information concerning treatment, cures, prevention, diagnosis, risk factors, research, support groups, email lists, personal stories and much more. Updated regularly.

8064 **Helios Health**
www.helioshealth.com
Online resource for your health information. Detailed information about specific health topics, access to expert advice from our Medical Advisory Board, and up-to-date health news.

8065 **MedicineNet**
www.medicinenet.com
An online resource for consumers providing easy-to-read, authoritative medical and health information.

8066 **Medscape**
www.mywebmd.com
Medscape offers specialists, primary care physicians, and other health professionals the Web's most robust and integrated medical information and educational tools.

8067 **Miami Project to Cure Paralysis**
www.miamiproject.miami.edu
Science and clinical research to restore function after spinal cord injury. The primary emphasis is on basic science research, under the direction of Dr. Richard Bunge, an eminent researcher.

8068 **Sexual Health Network**
www.sexualhealth.com
Informative site dealing with disability, sexuality and fertility.

8069 **Spinal Cord Injury Information Network Center**
www.spinalcord.uab.edu
Supervises and directs the collection, management and analysis of an extensive spinal cord injury database.

8070 **Spinal Cord Injury Network International**
www.sonic.net/~spinal
A non-profit organization that provides information and referral services and lends videos.

8071 **University of Alabama, (UAB)**
www.spinalcord.uab.edu
Up-to-date statistical information as well as extensive fact sheets on many aspects of Spinal Cord Injury.

8072 **WebMD**
www.webmd.com
Information on spinal cord injuries, including articles and resources.

Description

8073 **Stroke**

Strokes are caused by an interruption of blood flow in the brain, and usually — 80 percent of cases — are the result of a blocked blood vessel. The incidence increases with age, is higher in men than in women, and is higher in blacks than in whites. Depending on the severity and location of the damage, symptoms of stroke may include sudden weakness or paralysis (especially on one side of the body), blurred vision, difficulty speaking, slurred speech, dizziness and falling, extreme headache, stiff neck, altered level of alertness, and loss of bladder control. High blood pressure, atherosclerosis (fatty deposits), heart disease, diabetes, cigarette smoking, and heavy alcohol use are the major risk factors predisposing someone to stroke.

Preventive therapy is aimed at treatment of high blood pressure, heart disease, and diabetes. If someone has had a stroke they may be treated with blood thinning agents and/or other medication to prevent brain swelling. Research has shown that patients who are given one of these agents within three hours of stroke symptoms may have some or total restoration of neurologic function. To that end, the Golden Hour program was developed in which emergency medical personnel can initite therapy in certain patients on the way to the hospital. Rehabilitation after the stroke involves physical and occupational therapy. Many stroke survivors experience depression and difficulty regaining independence, so it is important to provide emotional support for both survivors and their families.

National Agencies & Associations

8074 **American Heart Association**
7272 Greenville Avenue 214-373-6300
Dallas, TX 75231 800-242-8721
www.americanheart.org
A national organization whose primary concern is the reduction of death and disability due to cardiovascular diseases and stroke.
M Cass Wheeler, CEO

8075 **American Stroke Association**
7272 Greenville Avenue
Dallas, TX 75231 888-478-7653
www.strokeassociation.org
The American Stroke Association is a division of the American Heart Association that focuses on reducing risk, disability and death from stroke through research, education, fund raising and advocacy.

8076 **Heart and Stroke Foundation of Canada**
222 Queen Street 613-569-4361
Ottawa, Ontario, K1P-5V9 Fax: 613-569-3278
ww2.heartlandstroke.ca
Volunteer-based health charity, leads in eliminating heart disease and stroke and reducing their impact through the advancement of research and its application, the promotion of healthy living and advocacy.

8077 **National Heart, Lung & Blood Institute**
PO Box 301051 301-592-8573
Bethesda, MD 20824 Fax: 240-629-3296
TTY: 240-629-3255
e-mail: nhlbiinfo@nhlbi.nih.gov
www.nhlbi.nih.gov
Primary responsibility of this organization is the scientific investigation of heart, blood vessel, lung and blood disorders. Oversee research, demonstration, prevention, education and training activities in these fields and emphasizes the control of stroke.
Elizabeth G Nabel, Director

8078 **National Institute of Neurological Disorders and Stroke**
PO Box 5801 301-496-5751
Bethesda, MD 20824 800-352-9424
TTY: 301-468-5981
www.ninds.nih.gov
Offers a brochure on stroke. A leading supporter of research on brain and nervous system disorders, including stroke.

8079 **National Stroke Association**
9707 E Easter Lane 303-649-9299
Centennial, CO 80112-3747 800-787-6537
Fax: 303-649-1328
e-mail: Info@stroke.org
www.stroke.org
A national organization whose sole purpose is to reduce the incidence and impact of stroke through prevention treatment rehabilitation and research and support for stroke survivors and their families.
James Baranski, Chief Executive Officer
Mike Stefanski, Controller

8080 **Neurology Institute**
P O Box 5801 301-496-5751
Bethesda, MD 20824 Fax: 301-402-2186
TTY: 301-468-5981
www.ninds.nih.gov
Offers information support and resources for persons with neurological disorders heart disease and stroke victims.
Story Landis, Director
Walter J Koroshetz, Deputy Director

8081 **Stroke Recovery Canada**
10 Overlea Boulevard 888-540-6666
Toronto, Ontario, M4H-1A4 Fax: 416-425-1920
e-mail: info@strokerecoverycanada.com
www.strokerecoverycanada.com
National service offering post-recovery support, education and programs for stroke survivors, their families and health care providers.

Foundations

8082 **American Stroke Foundation**
5960 Dearborn 913-649-1776
Mission, KS 66202 866-549-1776
Fax: 913-649-6661
www.americanstroke.org
The American Stroke Foundation helps those who can't help themseles. They offer compassionate-but practical-knowledge and service in a comfortable,"home-like" environment. Stroke survivors get the continued assistance and suppoort they need to reach their full potential.
Rita Griffith, Executive Director
Mark Bertrand, Director Development

Research Centers

8083 **Bowman Gray School of Medicine**
Medical Center Boulevard 919-716-7461
Winston Salem, NC 27157-0001 Fax: 919-716-5639
www.web.bgsm.edu
James Toole MD, Professor

8084 **Cerebral Blood Flow Laboratories Veterans Administration Medical Center**
Veterans Administration Medical Center
2002 Holcombe Boulevard 713-795-5807
Houston, TX 77030-4211 Fax: 713-957-01
Offers research in cerebrovascular disorders and risk factors for stroke.
John S Meyer MD, Director

8085 Comprehensive Stroke Center of Oregon University of Oregon Health Sciences Cen
University of Oregon Health Sciences Center
3181 SW Sam Jackson Park Road
Portland, OR 97239-3098
503-949-8311
www.ohsu.edu
Provide comprehensive treatment and prevention services to adults who have had a stroke or at risk of stroke.
Bruce Coull MD, Professor

8086 Departments of Neurology & Neurosurgery: University of California, San Francisco
UCSF Medical Center
505 Parnassus Avenue
San Francisco, CA 94143
415-353-1668
Fax: 415-353-8593
e-mail: bill.dillon@radiology.ucsf.edu
www.neurorad.ucsf.edu
Suzie M Fayfie, Professor

8087 Hospital of the University of Pennsylvania
3400 Spruce Street
Philadelphia, PA 19104
215-662-4000
800-789-PENN
Fax: 215-903-09
e-mail: pleasure@email.chop.edu
www.pennhealth.com
Research program centering its efforts on finding better ways to prevent and treat neuromuscular disorders.
David E Pleasure MD, Director

8088 Massachusetts General Departments of Neurology and Neurosurgery
Massachusetts General Hospital
55 Fruit Street
Boston, MA 02114
617-726-2000
www.massgeneral.org
Peter Slavin, Director

8089 Stroke Research and Treatment Center UAB Medical Center
Medical Center
1813 6th Avenue S
Birmingham, AL 35294-7
205-975-8569
800-822-6478
Fax: 205-975-6785
main.uab.edu/neurology
An interdisciplinary program specializing in the prevention diagnosis and treatment of stroke and stroke-related disorders. The CSRC integrates the latest in medical technology with a multi-faceted approach.
Andrei V Alexandrov MD, Director and Professor
James D Halsey Jr MD, Director Stroke Residency Program

8090 University of Iowa College of Medicine
200 CMAB
Iowa City, IA 52242
319-335-6707
e-mail: webmaster@mail.medicine.uiowa.edu
www.medicine.uiowa.edu
Donald D Heistad MD, Professor

8091 University of Maryland Center for Studies of Cerebrovascular Disease & Stroke
16 S Utah Street
Baltimore, MD 21201
410-328-4323
Fax: 410-328-1149
Thomas R Price MD, Principal Investor

8092 University of Miami School of Medicine Department of Neurology
1120 NW 14th Street
Miami, FL 33136
305-243-6732
877-243-4340
Fax: 305-243-1632
e-mail: RSacco@med.miami.edu
www.med.miami.edu
Myron D Ginsberg MD, Professor
Ralph L Sacco MD, Chairman Department of Neurology

8093 Wake Forest University: Cerebrovascular Research Center
Department of Neurology
300 S Hawthorne Road
Winston-Salem, NC 27103-2732
336-748-2338
Fax: 336-748-5477
Cerebrovascular research.
Dr James Toole, Director

8094 Washington University School of Medicine
660 S Euclid Avenue
Saint Louis, MO 63110-1016
314-362-5000
e-mail: web@medicine.wustl.edu
www.medicine.wustl.edu
Marcus Raich MD

Support Groups & Hotlines

8095 National Health Information Center
PO Box 1133
Washington, DC 20013
310-565-4167
800-336-4797
Fax: 301-984-4256
e-mail: info@nhic.org
www.health.gov/nhic
Offers a nationwide information referral service, produces directories and resource guides.

8096 Stroke Clubs International
805 12th Street
Galveston, TX 77550
409-762-1022
e-mail: strokeclubs@earthlink.net
www.ninds.nih.gov
Organization of persons who have experienced strokes, their families and friends for the purpose of mutual support, education, social and recreational activities. Provides information and assistance to Stroke Clubs (which are usually sponsored by local organizations).
Ellis Williamson

Books

8097 Alzheimer's, Stroke and 29 Other Neurological Disorders Sourcebook
Omnigraphics
615 Griswold Street
Detroit, MI 48226-3993
313-961-1340
800-234-1340
Fax: 800-875-1340
www.omnigraphics.com
Provides vital information for the nontechnical reader focusing on Alzheimer's disease, stroke and various neurological disorders. Answers thousands of questions related to afflications of the central nervous system with each chapter reviwing a particular disorder and offers in-depth discussions.

8098 Courage: Poems & Positive Thoughts for Stroke Survivors
National Stroke Association
9707 E Easter Lane
Englewood, CO 80112-3747
303-649-9299
800-787-6537
Fax: 303-649-1328
www.stroke.org
Words of inspiration from survivors and caregivers.
83 pages
Colette Lafosse, Director Rehabilitation/Recovery Program

8099 Discovery Circles
National Stroke Association
9707 E Easter Lane
Englewood, CO 80112-3747
303-649-9299
800-787-6537
Fax: 303-649-1328
www.stroke.org
NSA's guide to organizing and facilitating stroke support groups. This detailed manual describes the support group structure and the facilitator's role.
213 pages
Colette Lafosse, Director Rehabilitation/Recovery Program

8100 Magic of Humor in Caregiving
National Stroke Association
9707 E Easter Lane
Englewood, CO 80112-3747
303-649-9299
800-787-6537
Fax: 303-649-1328
www.stroke.org
A dynamic researching tool focusing on the necessity of humor in daily caregiving interaction.
Colette Lafosse, Director Rehabilitation/Recovery Program

8101 November Days
National Stroke Association

9707 E Easter Lane 303-649-9299
Englewood, CO 80112-3747 800-787-6537
Fax: 303-649-1328
www.stroke.org

A caregiver's story of her struggle with a loved one's stroke.
225 pages

8102 Occupational Therapy Practice Guidelines for Adults with Stroke
American Occupational Therapy Association
4720 Montgomery Lane 301-652-2682
Bethesda, MD 20824-1220 Fax: 301-652-7711
TDD: 800-377-8555
www.aota.org

15 pages
ISBN: 1-569001-55-3

8103 Stroke Book
William Morrow & Company
1350 Avenue of the Americas 212-261-6500
New York, NY 10019-4702
1993
ISBN: 0-688090-55-9

8104 Stroke: A Clinical Approach
Butterworth-Heinemann
225 Wildwood Avenue 617-928-2500
Woburn, MA 01801-2079 800-366-2665
1993 584 pages
ISBN: 0-750691-81-6

8105 Stroke: A Guide for Patient and Family
Raven Press
1185 Avenue of the Americas 212-930-9500
New York, NY 10036-2601
224 pages
ISBN: 0-881672-79-3

8106 Stroke: Your Complete Exercise Guide
Human Kinetics Publishers
PO Box 5076 217-351-1549
Champaign, IL 61825-5076 800-747-4457
Fax: 217-351-5076

Part of the Cooper Clinic and Research Institute Fitness Series providing exercise rehabilitation for persons suffering from strokes.
126 pages Paperback
ISBN: 0-873224-28-0

8107 Ted's Stroke: The Caregiver's Story
National Stroke Association
9707 E Easter Lane 303-649-9299
Englewood, CO 80112-3747 800-787-6537
Fax: 303-649-1328
www.stroke.org

Personal experiences, guidance and tips for caregivers.
175 pages
ISBN: 0-962487-61-9

8108 The Comfort of Home for Stroke: A Guide fo r Caregivers
Marie Meyer & Paula Derr, RN with Jon Caswell, author
CareTrust Publications
PO Box 10283
Portland, OR 97296-0283 800-565-1533
Fax: 415-673-2005
e-mail: sales@comfortofhome.com
www.comfortofhome.com

Comfort guides readers through every caregiving stage, from understanding personality changes, preparing the home, equipment, the healthcare team, and the activities of daily living. It helps take the fear out of home care and assists caregivers in maintaining peace of mind.
2007 344 pages
ISBN: 0-966476-78-6

8109 Women in Your Life: Protect Yourself, Protect Your Family
National Stroke Association
9707 E Easter Lane 303-649-9299
Englewood, CO 80112-3747 800-787-6537
Fax: 303-649-1328
www.stroke.org

Valuable information about the unique toll stroke takes on women.
Colette Lafosse, Director Rehabilitation/Recovery Program

Magazines

8110 Stroke Connection
American Stroke Foundation
8700 Lamar 913-649-1776
Overland Park, KS 66207 Fax: 913-649-6661
www.americanstroke.org

Official magazine of the American Stroke Foundation. Supports stroke survivors, their families, caregivers and friends by providing resources, services, education and information that improves the quality of life.

Pamphlets

8111 African-Americans and Stroke
National Stroke Association
9707 E Easter Lane 303-649-9299
Englewood, CO 80112-3747 800-787-6537
Fax: 303-649-1328
www.stroke.org

Colette Lafosse, Director Rehabilitation/Recovery Program

8112 Aneurysm Answers
National Stroke Association
9707 E Easter Lane 303-649-9299
Englewood, CO 80112-3747 800-787-6537
Fax: 303-649-1328
www.stroke.org

Colette Lafosse, Director Rehabilitation/Recovery Program

8113 Check Your Pulse, America: Atrial Fibrillation
National Stroke Association
9707 E Easter Lane 303-649-9299
Englewood, CO 80112-3747 800-787-6537
Fax: 303-649-1328
www.stroke.org

Colette Lafosse, Director Rehabilitation/Recovery Program

8114 Cholesterol and Stroke
National Stroke Association
9707 E Easter Lane 303-649-9299
Englewood, CO 80112-3747 800-787-6537
Fax: 303-649-1328
www.stroke.org

Colette Lafosse, Director Rehabilitation/Recovery Program

8115 Facts on Heart Disease, Heart Attack, Stroke and Risk Factors
American Heart Association
7272 Greenville Avenue 214-373-6300
Dallas, TX 75231-5129 Fax: 214-706-1341

Offers information on how to recognize a heart attack or stroke, recovery and rehabilitation techniques and risk factors.

8116 High Blood Pressure and Stroke
National Stroke Association
9707 E Easter Lane 303-649-9299
Englewood, CO 80112-3747 800-787-6537
Fax: 303-649-1328
www.stroke.org

Colette Lafosse, Director Rehabilitation/Recovery Program

8117 Mobility: Issues Facing Stroke Survivors and Their Families
National Stroke Association
9707 E Easter Lane 303-649-9299
Englewood, CO 80112-3747 800-787-6537
Fax: 303-649-1328
www.stroke.org

Colette Lafosse, Director Rehabilitation/Recovery Program

8118 Recurrent Stroke
National Stroke Association

9707 E Easter Lane
Englewood, CO 80112-3747
303-649-9299
800-787-6537
Fax: 303-649-1328
www.stroke.org
Colette Lafosse, Director Rehabilitation/Recovery Program

8119 **Smoking Cessation: Be Smoke Free in 3 Minutes**
National Stroke Association
9707 E Easter Lane
Englewood, CO 80112-3747
303-649-9299
800-787-6537
Fax: 303-649-1328
www.stroke.org
Colette Lafosse, Director Rehabilitation/Recovery Program

8120 **Stroke: Hope Through Research**
Office of Scientific & Health Reports
Building 31
Bethesda, MD 20892-0001
301-496-5751
800-352-9424
Offers information on stroke, research and advances in treatments and rehabilitation programs to help patients.

8121 **Transient Ischemic Attack**
National Stroke Association
9707 E Easter Lane
Englewood, CO 80112-3747
303-649-9299
800-787-6537
Fax: 303-649-1328
www.stroke.org
Colette Lafosse, Director Rehabilitation/Recovery Program

Audio & Video

8122 **Secret Life of the Brain**
PBS Home Video
PO Box 751089
Charlotte, NC 28275
877-727-7467
Fax: 703-739-8131
www.pbs.org/wnet/brain/about.html
Reveals the facinating processes involved in brain development across a lifetime. The five-part series informs viewers of exciting new information in the brain sciences, introduces the foremost researchers in the field, and utilizes dynamic visual imagry and compelling human stories to help a general audience understand otherwise difficult scientific concepts.
5 Tapes
Paula Kerger, President/CEO
Wayne Godwin, Chief Operating Officer

8123 **Stroke: Touching the Soul of Your Family**
National Stroke Association
9707 E Easter Lane
Englewood, CO 80112-3747
303-649-9299
800-787-6537
Fax: 303-649-1328
www.stroke.org
Fifteen minute video chronicling three stroke survivors and their courageous struggle to overcome daily challenges and educate others about stroke.
Colette Lafosse, Director Rehabilitation/Recovery Program

Web Sites

8124 **American Heart Association**
www.americanheart.org
A national organization whose primary concern is the reduction of death and disability due to cardiovascular diseases and stroke.

8125 **Healing Well**
www.healingwell.com
An online health resource guide to medical news, chat, information and articles, newsgroups and message boards, books, disease-related web sites, medical directories, and more for patients, friends, and family coping with disabling diseases, disorders, or chronic illnesses.

8126 **Health Finder**
www.healthfinder.gov
Searchable, carefully developed web site offering information on over 1000 topics. Developed by the US Department of Health and Human Services, the site can be used in both English and Spanish.

8127 **Healthlink USA**
www.healthlinkusa.com
Health information concerning treatment, cures, prevention, diagnosis, risk factors, research, support groups, email lists, personal stories and much more. Updated regularly.

8128 **Helios Health**
www.helioshealth.com
Online resource for your health information. Detailed information about specific health topics, access to expert advice from our Medical Advisory Board, and up-to-date health news.

8129 **MedicineNet**
www.medicinenet.com
An online resource for consumers providing easy-to-read, authoritative medical and health information.

8130 **Medscape**
www.mywebmd.com
Medscape offers specialists, primary care physicians, and other health professionals the Web's most robust and integrated medical information and educational tools.

8131 **National Heart, Lung & Blood Institute**
www.nhlbi.nih.gov/nhlbi/nhlbi.htm
Primary responsibility of this organization is the scientific investigation of heart, blood vessel, lung and blood disorders. Oversee research, demonstration, prevention, education and training activities in these fields and emphasizes the control of stroke.

8132 **National Institute of Neurological Disorders and Stroke**
www.ninds.nih.gov
Offers a brochure on stroke. A leading supporter of research on brain and nervous system disorders, including stroke.

8133 **National Stroke Association**
www.stroke.org
A national organization whose sole purpose is to reduce the incidence and impact of stroke through prevention, treatment, rehabilitation and research, and support for stroke survivors and their families. Educational resources on all aspects of stroke available on website.

8134 **Neurology Channel**
www.neurologychannel.com
Find clearly explained, medically accurate information regarding conditions, including an overview, symptoms, causes, diagnostic procedures and treatment options. On this site it is possible to ask questions and get information from a neurologist and connect to people who have similar health interests.

8135 **WebMD**
www.webmd.com
Information on stroke, including articles and resources.

Description

8136 **Substance Abuse**

Substance abuse is a broad term that refers to any illegal, dangerous or destructive use of some substance. This use may be legal (binge drinking by an adult) or illegal (smoking marijuana). Abused substances include alcohol, nicotine, marijuana, heroin, prescription painkillers and tranquilizers, stimulants such as amphetamines and cocaine, and hallucinogens such as LSD. The abuse may be a danger to the user, family members, business associates, close friends or even total strangers. Substance dependence refers to a state of strong compulsion to use the substance, in many cases accompanied by physical withdrawal symptoms if the substance is not regularly available.

The cause of substance abuse is very complex, and involves an interplay between the individual's behavioral choices, their genetic background and past and present social environment. Some substance abusers also have a definable psychiatric disorder such as depression or schizophrenia; treatment of these dual-disorder patients is especially challenging.

The consequences of substance abuse are well-known, and include job loss, arrest, family breakup, automobile and other accidents, birth defects (fetal alcohol syndrome), direct toxic effects (cirrhosis of the liver from alcohol or lung cancer from smoking), and infections (HIV or hepatitis B from sharing needles). Substance abuse, unless it occurs in extremely isolated persons, greatly affects family members and loved ones. Family members often deny the reality of the abuse, and may help, or enable, the abuser to cover up the problem and avoid its consequences.

There is no quick and universally effective treatment for substance abuse. Options range from inexpensive peer-based organizations such as Alcoholics Anonymous to very expensive long-term inpatient programs. Some peer-based programs appeal to a niche defined by sex, race, age or religious affiliation. Treatment is much more likely to succeed if it is freely chosen by the individual rather than mandated by a court. Dropout during treatment and relapse after initial success are common, but many people do achieve life-long cures with abstinence from further substance abuse. Family members should look for education and support through groups like Al-Anon, which bring them together with people facing similar situations.

National Agencies & Associations

8137 **AAA Foundation for Traffic Safety**
607 14th Street NW 202-638-5944
Washington, DC 20005-6001 Fax: 202-638-5943
e-mail: info@aaafoundation.org
www.aaafoundation.org

This national organization publishes drinking and traffic safety programs for K-6 and junior high students. Courses offered are taught by school district teachers who have participated in two-hour in-service training seminars.
J Peter Kissinger, President
Kristin Backstrom, Senior Manager Development

8138 **African American Family Services**
2616 Nicollet Avenue 612-871-7878
Minneapolis, MN 55408 Fax: 612-871-2567
e-mail: contact@aafs.net
www.aafs.net

This institute provides training and technical assistance to programs that want to serve African-American/black clients and others of color more effectively.
Terry J Ticey, Chairman of the Board
Robert S Bradley, Treasurer

8139 **Al-Anon Family Group Headquarters**
1600 Corporate Landing Parkway 757-563-1600
Virginia Beach, VA 23454-5617 888-425-2666
Fax: 757-563-1655
e-mail: wso@al-anon.org
www.al-anon.alateen.org

A fellowship of relatives and friends of alcoholics who believe their lives have been affected by someone else's drinking and a mutual support group recovery program based on the 12 steps of Alcoholics Anonymous.
Caryn Johnson, Director Communications

8140 **Alateen Al-Anon Family Group Headquarters**
Al-Anon Family Group Headquarters
1600 Corporate Landing Parkway 757-563-1600
Virginia Beach, VA 23454-5617 800-425-2666
Fax: 757-563-1655
e-mail: wso@al-anon.org
www.al-anon.alateen.org

A part of the Al-Anon program Alateen is for teenagers who have been affected by someone else's drinking whether it be a family member or a friend.
Caryn Johnson, Director Communications

8141 **Alcoholics Anonymous General Service Office/Grand Central Sta**
General Service Office/Grand Central Station
PO Box 459 212-870-3400
New York, NY 10163-0459 Fax: 212-870-3003
e-mail: www.aa.org
www.aa.org

Founded in 1935 Alcoholics Anonymous is a world-wide fellowship of men and women who have found solutions to their drinking problems. The only requirement for A.A. membership is a desire to stop drinking. There are no dues.

8142 **American Council for Drug Education**
50 Jay Street 718-222-6641
Brooklyn, NY 11201-2301 800-488-3784
Fax: 212-595-2553
e-mail: acde@phoenixhouse.org
www.acde.org

This organization provides information on drug use publishes books and offers films and curriculum materials for prevention.
J David Hawkins, Director
George E Woody, Chief of Staff

8143 **American Council on Alcohol Problems**
1000 E Indian School Road 602-264-7897
Phoenix, AZ 85014 800-527-5344
Fax: 602-264-7403
e-mail: info@aca-usa.org
www.aca-usa.org

Provides the forum and the mechanism through which concerned people can find common ground on alcohol and other drug problems and address these issues with a united voice.
Lloyd Vocovsky, Executive Director
Percy Menzies, Acting Chairman

8144 **American Dental Association Department of Library Services**
Department of Library Services
211 E Chicago Avenue 312-440-2500
Chicago, IL 60611-2637 Fax: 312-440-2822
e-mail: kittelson@ada.org
www.ada.org

Referrals to Chemical Dependency Support Groups that offer intervention services, referrals to dentists for treatment centers and doctors' support groups and assists with state licensing boards questions.
Linda Kittel MS RN, Manager
Brandon R Maddox, Representative

8145 **Associate Administrator for Alcohol Prevention and Treatment Policy**
Substance Abuse & Mental Health Services Offices
200 Independance Avenue 301-443-8956
Washington, DC 20201-0001 e-mail: info@samhsa.gov
www.samhsa.gov
Promotes monitors evaluates and coordinates programs for the prevention and treatment of alcoholism and alcohol abuse.

8146 **Association of Halfway House Alcoholism Programs of North America**
401 E Sangamon Avenue 217-523-0527
Springfield, IL 62702 Fax: 217-698-8234
e-mail: president@ahhap.org
www.ahhap.org
Acts as a clearinghouse of the latest literature on alcoholism assists chemical dependency counselors in placing post treatment individuals in halfway houses and helps in setting up halfway houses.
Olivia Howard, President
David Logan, Vice President

8147 **BACCHUS of the US**
PO Box 100430 303-871-0901
Denver, CO 80250 Fax: 303-871-0907
e-mail: admin@bacchusnetwork.org
www.bacchusgamma.org
Boosts alcohol consciousness concerning the health of university students.
Drew Hunter, President
Janet Cox, Vice President/COO

8148 **CSAP State Liason Program CSAP Division of Communications Programs**
CSAP Division of Communications Programs
7200 Wisconsin Avenue
Bethesda, MD 20857-0001 301-941-8500
www.covesoft.com/csap.html
This program is designed to support alcohol and other drug abuse prevention efforts in the States.

8149 **Center for Substance Abuse Prevention**
Substance Abuse and Mental Health Services Admin.
PO Box 2345
Rockville, MD 20847-2345 800-279-6686
TTY: 800-487-4886
TDD: 800-487-4886
e-mail: info@health.org.
ncadi.samhsa.gov
This organization's goal is to connect people and resources with innovative ideas strategies and programs designed to encourage creative and effective efforts aimed at reducing and eliminating alcohol tobacco and other drug problems in our society.

8150 **Chemical People Project Public Television Outreach Alliance**
Public Television Outreach Alliance
4802 5th Avenue 412-391-0900
Pittsburgh, PA 15213-2957
The project supplies information in the form of tapes literature and seminars.

8151 **Cocaine Anonymous: World Service Office**
3740 Overland Avenue 310-559-5833
Los Angeles, CA 90034-6337 800-999-9951
Fax: 310-559-2554
e-mail: cawso@ca.org
www.ca.org
A support group based on the twelve steps of Alcoholics Anonymous that focuses specifically on problems of cocaine addiction.

8152 **Drug Abuse Resistance Education of America**
PO Box 512090 310-215-0575
Los Angeles, CA 90051-0090 800-223-3273
www.dare.com
Provides information, resources, tips, warning signs and other information for parents and kids to help keep children off drugs.
Herb Kleber, Chairman
Carol J Boyd, Director

8153 **Drugs Anonymous**
PO Box 473 212-874-0700
New York, NY 10023
A twelve-step program that holds more than 30 meetings for drug addicts in the Greater New York Area including several in hospitals and institutions.

8154 **Families Anonymous**
PO Box 3475 310-313-5800
Culver City, CA 90231-3475 800-736-9805
Fax: 310-815-9682
e-mail: famanon@familiesanonymous.org
www.familiesanonymous.org
Addresses the needs of families who are concerned about a relative with a drug problem and with related behavioral problems. Offers informational packets meetings and support networks for these families.

8155 **Families in Action National Drug Information Center**
2957 Clairmont Road NE 404-248-9676
Atlanta, GA 30329 Fax: 404-248-1312
e-mail: nfia@nationalfamilies.org
www.nationalfamilies.org
Offers news and information for persons interested in drug abuse prevention.
Sue Rusche, President
Paula Kemp, Executive Vice President

8156 **Hazelden**
PO Box 11 651-213-4200
Center City, MN 55012-0011 800-257-7810
Fax: 651-213-4411
e-mail: info@hazeldon.org
www.hazelden.com
A nonprofit organization dedicated to providing quality rehabilitation education and professional services for chemical dependency and related addictive behaviors. Services offered include assessment and rehabilitation and family services.
Ellen Breyer, President

8157 **Indian Health Service**
801 Thompson Avenue
Rockville, MD 20852-1627 605-226-7456
www.ihs.gov
Charged with providing a comprehensive program of alcoholism and substance abuse prevention and treatment for Native Americans and Alaskan natives.

8158 **Lawyers Concerned for Lawyers**
2550 University Avenue W 651-646-5590
Saint Paul, MN 55114-4127 866-525-6466
Fax: 651-646-2364
e-mail: lcl.org@aol.com
www.mnlcl.org
A nonprofit organization of recovering lawyers and judges and concerned others. Educates lawyers and judges about the disease of chemical dependency assists in assessments and arranging interventions and offers lawyer-only AA meetings.
Joan Bibelhausen, Executive Director
Ellen Murphy-Fritsch, Case Manager

8159 **Marijuana Anonymous: World Services**
Marijuana Anonymous World Services
PO Box 2912
Van Nuys, CA 91404-2318 800-766-6779
e-mail: office@marijuana-anonymous.org
www.marijuana-anonymous.org
A fellowship of men and women who share our experience strength and hope with each other that we may solve our common problem and help others to recover from marijuana addiction.

8160 **Mothers Against Drunk Driving (MADD)**
511 E John Carpenter Freeway 214-744-6233
Irving, TX 75062 800-438-6233
Fax: 972-869-2206
www.madd.org

Founded by a small group of mothers and has turned into one of the largest crime victims organizations in the world.
Paul D Folkemer, Chairman of the Board
Charles A (Chuck) Hurley, Chief Executive Officer

8161 Narcotics Anonymous World Service Office
World Service Office
PO Box 9999 — 818-773-9999
Van Nuys, CA 91409-9099 — Fax: 818-700-0700
e-mail: fsmail@na.org
www.na.org
Similar to Alcoholics Anonymous this program is a fellowship of men and women who meet to help one another with their drug dependency problems.

8162 National Association for Children of Alcoholics
11426 Rockville Pike — 301-468-0985
Rockville, MD 20852-3007 — 888-554-2627
Fax: 301-468-0987
e-mail: nacoa@nacoa.org
www.nacoa.org
Advocates for all children and families affected by alcohol and other drug dependencies.
Sis Wenger, President/CEO
Judy Galloway, Coordinator-Affiliate Services

8163 National Association for Native American Children of Alcoholics
Seattle Indian Health Board
1402 Third Avenue — 206-467-7686
Seattle, WA 98114-3364 — 800-322-5601
Fax: 206-467-7689
e-mail: nanacoa@aol.com
Formed to facilitate positive change in individuals and communities in order to break the intergenerational cycle of addiction among Native Americans.

8164 National Association of Alcoholism and Drug Abuse Counselors
1001 N Fairfax Street — 703-741-7686
Alexandria, VA 22314 — Fax: 800-377-1136
e-mail: naadac@naadac.org
www.naadac.org
Largest membership organization serving addiction counselors educators and other addiction-focused health care professionals who specialize in addiction prevention treatment and education.
Patricia M Greer, President
Sharon DeEsch, Secretary

8165 National Association on Drug Abuse Problems
Director of Corporate and Community Services
355 Lexington Avenue — 212-986-1170
New York, NY 10017 — Fax: 212-697-2939
e-mail: info@nadap.org
www.nadap.org
Provides skills evaluation job training and job placement to recovering drug addicts in the metropolitan New York area.
John A Darin, President & CEO
Gary Stankowski, Senior Vice President

8166 National Clearinghouse for Alcohol and Drug Information
11420 Rockville Pike Suite 200 — 301-468-2600
Rockville, MD 20847-2345 — 800-729-6686
Fax: 240-221-4292
TTY: 800-487-4889
TDD: 800-487-4889
e-mail: webmaster@health.org
www.health.org
Nation's one-stop resource for information about substance abuse prevention and addiction treatment.

8167 National Council on Alcoholism and Drug Dependence
244 E 58th Street — 212-269-7797
New York, NY 10022-3128 — 800-622-2255
Fax: 212-269-7510
e-mail: national@ncadd.org
www.ncadd.org
Provides education information help and hope in the fight against addictions. Founded in 1944 NCADD with its nationwide network of affiliates advocates prevention intervention and treatment and is committed to ridding the disease of its stigma.
Robert Lindsey, President
Leah Brock, Director of Affiliate Relations

8168 National Crime Prevention Council
2345 Crystal Drive — 202-466-6272
Arlington, VA 22202 — Fax: 212-269-7510
www.ncpc.org
This organization works to prevent crime and drug use in many ways including developing materials for parents and children.
Alfonso E Lenhardt, President/CEO
David A Dean, Executive Committee Chair

8169 National Families in Action
2957 Clairmont Road NE — 404-248-9676
Atlanta, GA 30329 — Fax: 404-248-1312
e-mail: nfia@nationalfmailies.org
www.nationalfamilies.org
Mission is to help families and communities prevent drug use among children by promoting policies based on science.
Joseph A Califano Jr, Chairman and President
Susan P Brown, Vice President/Director of Finance

8170 National Organization on Fetal Alcohol Syndrome
900 17th Street NW — 202-785-4585
Washington, DC 20006 — 800-666-6327
Fax: 202-466-6456
e-mail: information@nofas.org
www.nofas.org
Dedicated to eliminating birth defects caused by alcohol consumption during pregnancy and to improving the quality of life for those affected individuals and families.
Terry Lierman, Chairperson
Tom Donaldson, President

8171 National Parents Resources Institute for Drug Education
4 W Oak Street — 231-924-1662
Fermont, MI 49412 — 800-668-9277
Fax: 231-924-5663
e-mail: info@prideyouthprograms.org
www.prideyouthprograms.org
A provider of prevention services in the area of alcohol and other drugs. Mission is to build a drug-free America.
Jay Dewispelaere, President/CEO
Lou Anne Wheater, Membership Coordinator

8172 Office of Applied Studies Substance Abuse & Mental Health Services
Substance Abuse & Mental Health Services Offices
5600 Fishers Lane
Rockville, MD 20857-0001 — 301-443-8956
www.oas.samhsa.gov
Provides the leadership needed for collecting data on mental illness and substance abuse including incidence and prevalence studies.

8173 Office of Substance Abuse Prevention
5600 Fishers Lane
Rockville, MD 20857-0001 — 301-443-0373
www.samhsa.gov
Reviews the government's alcohol and drug abuse policy operates a grant program supports development of model programs and conducts prevention workshops.

8174 Office of Women's Services Substance Abuse & Mental Health Services
Substance Abuse & Mental Health Services Offices
5600 Fishers Lane — 301-443-8956
Rockville, MD 20857-0001
Provides leadership and guidance in creating and maintaining an agency-wide focus for addressing the substance abuse and mental health needs of women.

8175 Office on Smoking and Health: CDCP
Centers for Disease Control And Prevention
1600 Clifton Road — 404-639-3311
Atlanta, GA 30333 — TTY: 888-232-6348
e-mail: tobaccoinfo@cdc.gov
www.cdc.gov/tobacco

Offers reference services to researchers through the Technical Information Center. Publishes and distributes a number of titles in the field of smoking and health.

8176 Partnership for a Drug-Free America
405 Lexington Avenue 212-922-1560
New York, NY 10174-0002 Fax: 212-922-1570
www.drugfreeamerica.org
Non-profit coalition of communication health medical and educational professionals working to reduce illicit drug use and help people live health drug-free lives.
Stephen J Pasierb, President & CEO
Roy J Bostock, Chairman

8177 Remove Intoxicated Drivers (RID-USA)
PO Box 520 518-372-0034
Schenectady, NY 12301 Fax: 518-310-4917
e-mail: dwi@rid-usa.org
rid-usa.org
Volunteers working to deter impaired driving, to help its victims obtain justice, restitution and peace of mind when faced with the maze of criminal justice systems, and to curb the alcohol abuse which leads to drunken driving.
Doris Aiken, Founder/President
Bill Aiken, VP/Manager

8178 Safe Homes
4 Mann Street 508-366-4305
Worcester, MA 01602-0702 Fax: 508-836-5560
e-mail: safehomes@thebridgecm.org
www.safehomesma.org
This national organization encourages parents to sign a contract stipulating that when parties are held in one another's homes they will adhere to a strict no-alcohol/no-drug-use rule.

8179 Students Against Destructive Decisions
255 Main Street 508-481-3568
Marlborough, MA 01752 877-723-3462
Fax: 508-481-5759
e-mail: info@sadd.org
www.sadd.org
Offers materials to improve students' knowledge of and attitudes toward alcohol and other drugs and to help them plan their behavior so they can reduce the chances of becoming involved in drunk driving situations.
Penelope Wells, President and Executive Director
Stephen Wallace, Chairman and Chief Executive Officer

8180 Substance Abuse and Mental Health Services Administration
P O Box 2345 877-726-4727
Rockville, MD 20847-0001 877-696-6775
TTY: 800-487-4889
www.samhsa.gov
The goal of this organization is to reduce incidence and prevalence of mental disorders and substance abuse and improve treatment outcomes for persons suffering from addictive and mental health problems and disorders.

8181 Workplace Program CSAP Division of Communication Programs
CSAP Division of Communication Programs
5600 Fishers Lane 301-443-9936
Rockville, MD 20857-0001
This program sets standards for drug testing in workplace settings.

State Agencies & Associations

Alabama

8182 Division of Mental Illness and Substance Abuse Community Programs
Department of Mental Health
100 N Union Street 334-242-3456
Montgomery, AL 36130-1410 800-832-0952
Fax: 334-242-0759
e-mail: DMHMR@MH.Alabama.GOV
www.mh.alabama.gov
Kent Hunt, Associate Commissioner Substance Abuse
Susan P Chambers, Associate Commissioner Mental Illness

Alaska

8183 Office of Alcohol and Substance Abuse Department of Health and Social Services
Department of Health and Social Services
PO Box 110620 907-465-3370
Juneau, AK 99811 800-465-4828
Fax: 907-465-2668
e-mail: Stacy.Toner@Alaska.gov
www.hss.state.ak.us
Stacy Toner, Deputy Director
Cheryl Lowenstein, Administrative Operations Manager II

Arizona

8184 Alcoholism and Drug Abuse: Office of Community Behavioral Health
Department of Health Services
150 N 18th Avenue 602-364-4558
Phoenix, AZ 85007-3228 Fax: 602-364-4570
e-mail: cancerlr@azdhs.gov
www.azdhs.gov
January Contreras, Acting Director

Arkansas

8185 Office of Alcohol and Drug Abuse Prevention
4313 West Markham 501-686-9866
Little Rock, AR 72205 Fax: 501-686-9035
e-mail: linda.baker@arkansas.gov
www.state.ar.us

California

8186 California Women's Commission on Alcohol and Drug Dependencies
14622 Victory Boulevard 818-376-0470
Van Nuys, CA 91411
Dedicated to improving the quality and increasing the quantity of services to women with alcohol-related problems.

8187 Department of Alcohol and Drug Programs
1700 K Street 916-445-0834
Sacramento, CA 95811-4037 800-879-2772
Fax: 916-323-1270
e-mail: resourcecenter@adp.state.ca.us
www.adp.state.ca.us
Kathryn P Jett, Director

Colorado

8188 Alcohol and Drug Abuse Division Department of Human Services
Department of Human Services
4055 S Lowell Boulevard 303-866-7480
Denver, CO 80236-3120 Fax: 303-866-7481
e-mail: jaqueline.enriques@state.co.us
www.cdhs.state.co.us
Janet Wood, Director
Mary McCann, Acting Manager

Connecticut

8189 Connecticut Alcohol and Drug Abuse Commission
410 Capitol Avenue 860-418-7000
Hartford, CT 06134 800-446-7348
Fax: 860-418-6780
TTY: 860-418-6707
e-mail: ronna.keil@pa.state.ct.us
www.dmhas.state.ct.us
Thomas A Kirk Jr, Commissioner
Pat Rehmer, Deputy Commissioner

Delaware

8190 Delaware Division of Alcoholism, Drug Abuse and Mental Health
Alcohol And Drug Services

1901 North DuPont Highway
New Castle, DE 19720
303-255-9399
Fax: 302-255-4428
e-mail: DHSSInfor@state.de.us
www.dhss.delware.gov

Renata J. Henry, Director

District of Columbia

8191 Health Planning and Development
825 N Capitol Street NE
Washington, DC 20002
202-422-5875
Fax: 202-442-4827
www.dchealth.dc.gov

Florida

8192 Alcohol and Drug Abuse Program Department Of Children And Families
Department Of Children And Families
1317 Winewood Boulevard
Tallahassee, FL 32399-6570
850-487-2920
Fax: 850-414-7474
www.dcf.state.fl.us/mentalhealth/sa

Cynthea Panzarino, Director

Georgia

8193 Alcohol and Drug Services Addictive Diseases Program
Addictive Diseases Program
Two Peachtree Street NW
Atlanta, GA 30303-3171
404-657-2331
Fax: 404-657-2160
www.mhddad.dhr.georgia.gov

Hawaii

8194 Alcohol and Drug Abuse Division Department of Health
Department of Health
601 Kamokila Boulevard
Kapoleiu, HI 96707
808-692-7506
Fax: 808-692-7521
e-mail: ATRINFO@doh.hawaii.gov
www.hawaii.gov/health

Chiyome Fukino, Director
Bernie Strand, Program Director

Idaho

8195 Department of Health and Welfare Department Of Health And Welfare
Department Of Health And Welfare
1720 Westgate Drive
Boise, ID 83704-0036
208-334-6747
800-926-2588
Fax: 208-334-6738
e-mail: rossil@dhw.idaho.gov
www.healthandwelfare.idaho.gov

Landis Rossi, Regional Director
Richard Armstrong, Director

Illinois

8196 Department of Alcoholism and Substance Abuse
Department Of Human Services
100 W Randolph Street
Chicago, IL 60601
312-814-3840
800-843-6154
Fax: 312-814-2419
TTY: 800-447-6404
e-mail: dhsas16@dhs.state.il.us
www.dhs.state.il.us

Theodora Binion-Tayl, Director

8197 Illinois Church Action on Alcohol Problems
1132 W Jefferson Street
Springfields, IL 62702
217-546-6871
Fax: 217-546-2814
e-mail: mail@ilcaaap.org
www.ilcaaap.org

An interdenominational Christian agency representing church groups in Illinois. Works to prevent alcohol and other drug-related problems through education legislative action and public awareness.

8198 Parkside Medical Services Corporation
205 W Touhy Avenue
Park Ridge, IL 60068-4256
847-698-9866
800-727-5723

This establishment offers treatment and hope for the alcoholic/substance abuser. A resource center that provides information books and resources pertaining to substance abuse and offers treatment facilities in various states across the country.

Indiana

8199 Division of Addiction Services Department of Mental Health
Department of Mental Health
402 W Washington Street
Indianapolis, IN 46204-3614
317-232-7800
800-662-4357
Fax: 317-233-3472
www.in.gov/fssa

Gina Eckart, Director
Alma Burrus, Operations Manager

Iowa

8200 Department of Public Health: Division of Substance Abuse and Health
Lucas State Office Building
321 E 12th Street
Des Moines, IA 50319-0075
515-281-7689
866-227-9878
Fax: 515-281-4535
e-mail: jzwick@idphstate.ia.us
www.idph.state.ia.us

Kathy Stone, Director

Kansas

8201 Alcohol and Drug Abuse Services
915 Harrison Street
Topeka, KS 66612
785-296-3959
800-586-3690
Fax: 785-296-7275
TTY: 785-296-1491
e-mail: dxmd@srskansas.org
www.srskansas.org

Don Jordan, Secretary
Laura Howard, Deputy Secretary and CFO

Kentucky

8202 Division of Substance Abuse: Department of Mental Health
Department For MH/MR Services
100 Fair Oaks Lane
Frankfort, KY 40621
502-564-2880
Fax: 502-564-7152
TTY: 502-564-5777
www.mhmr.ky.gov

Louisiana

8203 Office of Human Services: Division of Alcohol and Drug Abuse
628 N 4th Street
Baton Rouge, LA 70821-2790
225-342-6717
877-664-2248
Fax: 225-342-3875
e-mail: jbordeln@dhh.la.gov
www.dhh.louisiana.gov

Maine

8204 Office of Alcohol and Drug Abuse Prevention
Office Of Substance Abuse
AMHI Complex, Marquardt Building
Augusta, ME 04333-0159
207-289-2595
Fax: 207-287-4334
e-mail: osa.ircosa@state.me.us
www.maine.gove

Kimberly A. Johnson, Director

Maryland

8205 Maryland State Alcohol and Drug Abuse Administration
55 Wade Avenue
Catonsville, MD 21228
410-402-8600
Fax: 410-402-8601
e-mail: adaainfo@dhmh.state.md.us
www.maryland-adaa.org

Kathleen Rebbert-Fra, Acting Director
Steve Bocian, Acting Deputy Director

Massachusetts

8206 **Division of Substance Abuse**
250 Washington Street
Boston, MA 02108-4619
617-624-5111
800-327-5050
Fax: 617-624-5185
TTY: 617-536-5872
e-mail: bsas.questions@state.ma.us
www.mass.gov

Michael Botticelli, Director

Michigan

8207 **Office of Substance Abuse Services Department of Public Health**
Department of Public Health
320 S Walnut Street
Lansing, MI 48913
517-373-4700
888-736-0253
Fax: 517-335-2121
TTY: 517-373-3573
www.michigan.gov

Yvonne Blackmond, Director

Minnesota

8208 **Chemical Dependency Program Division Department of Human Services**
Department of Human Services
444 Lafayette Road
Saint Paul, MN 55155-3899
651-431-2460
800-627-3529
Fax: 651-582-1865
e-mail: DHS.ADAD@state.mn.us
www.dhs.state.mn.us

8209 **Dentists Concerned for Dentists**
450 N Syndicate
Saint Paul, MN 55104
651-641-0730
www.medhelp.org/amshc/amshc53.htm
A nonprofit organization for chemically dependent Minnesota dentists and concerned others.

Mississippi

8210 **Division of Alcohol & Drug Abuse: Mississippi**
Department of Mental Health
Robert E Lee State Office Building
Jackson, MS 39201
601-359-1288
Fax: 601-359-6295
www.dmh.state.ms.us

8211 **Division of Alcohol & Drug Abuse: South Department of Mental Health**
1101 Robert E Lee Building
Jackson, MS 39201
601-359-1288
Fax: 601-359-6295
TTY: 601-359-6230
www.dmh.state.ms.us

Edwin C LeGrand III, Executive Director

Missouri

8212 **Missouri Division of Alcohol and Drug Abuse**
Department of Mental Health
1706 E Elm Street
Jefferson City, MO 65102
573-751-4122
800-364-9687
Fax: 573-751-8224
TTY: 573-526-1201
e-mail: dmhmail@dmh.mo.gov
www.dmh.missouri.gov

Mark G Stringer, Director
Heidi DiBiaso, Administrative Assistant

Montana

8213 **Department of Institutions, Alcohol and Drug Abuse Division**
PO Box 202905nue
Helena, MT 59620-2905
406-444-3964
Fax: 406-444-9389
e-mail: jcassidy@mt. gov
www.dphhs.st.mt.us

Nebraska

8214 **Department of Public Instruction: Division of Alcoholism and Drug Abuse**
Division Of Behavioral Health
PO Box 98925
Lincoln, NE 68509-8925
402-471-7818
800-648-4444
Fax: 402-479-5162
e-mail: richard.deliberty@hhss.ne.gov
www.hhs.state.ne.us

Scot Adams, Director
GibsonBlaine Shaffer, CEO

Nevada

8215 **Alcohol and Drug Abuse Bureau: Department of Human Resources**
4126 Technology Way
Carson City, NV 89706
775-684-4190
Fax: 775-684-4185
e-mail: mcanfiel@nvhd.state.nv.us
www.mhds.nv.gov

Maria Canfield, Chief

New Hampshire

8216 **Office of Alcohol and Drug Abuse Prevention**
State Office Park South
105 Pleasant Street
Concord, NH 03301-3852
800-804-0909
Fax: 603-271-6105
e-mail: rosemary.shannon@dhhs.sate.nh.us
www.dhhs.state.nh.us

8217 **Office of Alcohol and Drug Abuse Programs State Office Park South**
105 Pleasant Street
Concord, NH 03301
603-271-6100
Fax: 603-271-6105
TTY: 800-735-2964
e-mail: rosemary.shannon@dhhs.sate.nh.us
www.dhhs.state.nh.us

New Jersey

8218 **Department of Health**
120 S Stockton Street
Trenton, NJ 08625-0362
609-292-7837
800-367-6543
Fax: 609-292-3816
e-mail: georgene.rhodunda@dhs.state.nj.us
www.state.nj.us

Heather Howard, Commissioner
Mary E O'Dowd, Chief of Staff

8219 **Division of Narcotic and Drug Abuse Control**
120 S Stockton Street
Trenton, NJ 08625-0362
609-292-5760
800-238-2333
Fax: 609-292-3816
www.state.nj.us/humanservices

Jeffers, Director

New Mexico

8220 **Substance Abuse Bureau**
1190 Saint Francis Drive
Santa Fe, NM 87502
505-827-2601
800-362-2013
Fax: 505-827-0097
www.nmcares.org

New York

8221 **Division of Substance Abuse Services Substance Abuse Services**
Substance Abuse Services
1450 Western Avenue
Albany, NY 12203-3526
518-473-3460
Fax: 518-457-5474
e-mail: communications@oasas.state.ny.us
www.oasas.state.ny.us

Karen M Carpenter-Palumbo, Commissioner
Kathleen Caggiano-Si, Executive Deputy Commissioner

North Carolina

8222 **Alcohol and Drug Abuse Section Division of Mental Health & Mental Retar**
Division of Mental Health & Mental Retardation
3001 Mail Service Center 919-733-7011
Raleigh, NC 27699-3007 800-662-7030
Fax: 919-508-0951
www.dhhs.state.nc.us

Leza Wainwright, Director
Michael S Lancaster, Director

North Dakota

8223 **Division of Alcoholism & Drug Abuse: Department of Human Services**
Department Of Human Services
1237 W Divide Avenue 701-328-8920
Bismarck, ND 58501 800-755-2719
Fax: 701-328-8969
e-mail: dhsmhsas@state.nd.us
www.state.nd.us

Ohio

8224 **Bureau on Alcohol Abuse and Recovery Ohio Department of Health**
Ohio Department of Health
280 N Hight Street 614-466-3445
Columbus, OH 43215-2550 Fax: 614-752-8645
e-mail: INFO@ada.ohio.gov
www.odadas.state.oh.us

Angela Corne Dawson, Director
Jewel Neely, Deputy Director

8225 **Bureau on Drug Abuse: Ohio Department of Health**
Ohio Department of Health
280 N High Street 614-466-3445
Columbus, OH 43215 Fax: 614-752-8645
e-mail: INFO@ada.ohio.gov
www.odadas.state.oh.us

Angela Corne Dawson, Director
Jewel Neely, Deputy Director

Oklahoma

8226 **Oklahoma Department of Mental Health and Substance Abuse Services**
Substance Abuse Program
1200 NE 13th Street 405-522-3908
Oklahoma City, OK 73152-3277 800-522-9054
Fax: 405-522-3650
TTY: 405-522-3851
e-mail: jglover@odmhsas.org
www.odmhsas.org

Terri White, Commissioner

Oregon

8227 **Office of Alcohol and Drug Abuse Programs**
500 Summer Street NE 503-945-5763
Salem, OR 97301-1118 Fax: 503-378-8467
TTY: 800-375-2863
e-mail: omhas.web@state.or.us
www.oregon.gov

Pennsylvania

8228 **Drug and Alcohol Programs Department Of Health**
Department Of Health
02 Kline Plaza 717-783-8200
Harrisburg, PA 17104-0090 877-724-3258
Fax: 717-787-6285
e-mail: rkauffman@state.pa.us
www.dsf.health.state.pa.us

Rhode Island

8229 **Division of Substance Abuse: Department of Mental Health and Hospitals**
Department Of Mental Health And Retardation
14 Harrington Road 401-462-4680
Cranston, RI 02920-0944 800-622-7422
Fax: 401-462-6078
www.mhrh.state.ri.us

Craig S Stenning, Executive Director

South Carolina

8230 **South Carolina Commission on Alcohol and Drug Abuse**
Department Of Alcohol And Drug Abuse Services
101 Executive Center Drive 803-896-5555
Columbia, SC 29210-9498 Fax: 803-896-5557
www.daodas.org

W Lee Catoe, Director
Lillian Roberson, Manager of Operation Division

South Dakota

8231 **Division of Alcohol & Drug Abuse: South Dakota**
Department Of Human Services
3800 E Highway 34 605-773-5990
Pierre, SD 57501-5070 800-265-9684
Fax: 605-773-5483
TTY: 605-773-6412
e-mail: infodhs@state.sd.us
www.dhs.sd.gov

Gilbert Sudbeck, Director

Tennessee

8232 **Department of Mental Health and Mental Retardation, Alcohol & Drug Service**
Bureau Of Alcohol And Drug Abuse Services
425 Fifth Avenue N 615-532-6500
Nashville, TN 37243-4401 800-560-5767
Fax: 615-532-2419
e-mail: oca.mhdd@tn.gov
www.state.tn.us

Virginia Tro Betts, Commissioner

Texas

8233 **Texas Commission on Alcohol and Drug Abuse Department Of State Health**
Department Of State Health
PO Box 149347 512-206-5000
Austin, TX 78714 866-378-8440
Fax: 512-458-7477
TTY: 800-735-2989
e-mail: contact@dshs.state.tx.us
www.tcada.state.tx.us

Utah

8234 **Department of Social Services: Division of Substance Abuse**
Department Of Human Services
120 N 200 W Street 801-538-3939
Salt Lake City, UT 84103 Fax: 801-538-9892
e-mail: dsamhwebmaster@utah.gov
www.hsdsa.utah.gov

Paula Bell, Chairperson
Darryl Wagner, Vice Chairman

Vermont

8235 **Alcohol and Drug Abuse Programs of Vermont Department Of Health**
Department Of Health
108 Cherry Street 802-651-1550
Burlington, VT 05402-1531 Fax: 802-651-1573
e-mail: vtadap@vdh.state.vt.us
www.healthvermont.gov

Virginia

8236 Substance Abuse Services Office of Virginia
Department of Mental Health & Mental Retardation
PO Box 1797 804-786-3921
Richmond, VA 23218-1797 800-451-5544
Fax: 804-371-6638
TTY: 804-371-8977
e-mail: wglover@co.dmhmrsas.virginia.gov
www.dmhmrsas.virginia.gov
James Reinhard, Commissioner
Heidi Dix, Deputy Commissioner

Washington

8237 Washington Department of Social and Health Services, Alcohol and Drug Prog.
Department Of Social And Health Services
PO Box 45130 877-301-4557
Olympia, WA 98504-5330 800-562-1240
Fax: 360-438-8078
TTY: 877-301-4557
e-mail: starkkd@dshs.wa.gov
www1.dshs.wa.gov

West Virginia

8238 West Virginia Division of Alcohol & Drug Abuse
Department Of Health And Human Resources
350 Capitol Street 304-558-2276
Charleston, WV 25301-3702 Fax: 304-558-1008
e-mail: obhs@wvdhhr.org
www.wvdhhr.org
Eugenie Taylor, Acting Commissioner

Wisconsin

8239 Office of Alcohol and Other Drug Abuse
1 W Wilson Street 608-266-1865
Madison, WI 53703-7851 Fax: 608-266-1533
TTY: 608-267-7371
e-mail: DHSwebmaster@wisconsin.gov
www.dhfs.state.wi.us
John Easterday, Administrator
Susan Gadacz, Contact

Wyoming

8240 Alcohol & Drug Abuse Programs of Wyoming Department Of Health
Department Of Health
6101 Yellowestone Road 307-777-6494
Cheyenne, WY 82002-0480 800-535-4006
Fax: 307-777-5849
e-mail: aburde@state.wy.us
wdh.state.wy.us
Korin Schmidt, Administrator
Rodger McDaniel, Deputy Director

Libraries & Resource Centers

8241 National Clearinghouse for Alcohol and Drug Information
PO Box 2345 240-221-4019
Rockville, MD 20847-2345 800-729-6686
Fax: 240-221-4292
TDD: 800-487-4889
e-mail: info@health.org
www.ncadi.samhsa.gov
A resource for alcohol and other drug information. It carries a wide variety of publications dealing with alcohol and other drug abuse.
John Noble, Director

8242 Parents Resource Institute for Drug Education
160 Vanderbilt Court
Bowling Green, KY 42103 800-279-6361
Fax: 270-746-9598
e-mail: janie.pitcock@pridesurveys.com
www.pridesurveys.com
Offers national information and educational materials pertaining to alcohol and drug dependency.
Thomas J Gleaton, EdD, President
Janie Pitcock, Director Operations

Research Centers

8243 Alcohol Disease Foundation
33 Eglantine Avenue 609-737-0088
Pennington, NJ 08534-2308
Founded in 1988 to promote research on testing systems that could diagnose the metabolic aspects of alcoholism. Seeks to educate the public on the validity of the disease concept of alcoholism.

8244 Alcohol Research Group Public Health Institute
Public Health Institute
6475 Christie Avenue 510-597-3440
Emeryville, CA 94608-1324 Fax: 510-985-6459
e-mail: info@arg.org
www.arg.org
One of ten national research centers funded by the National Institute on Alcohol Abuse and Alcoholism. Its alcoholism library carries 5 500 books 130 journals 150 newsletters and 60 000 other materials.
Dominique La MPH, Executive Director
Debbie Gill, Manager Administrative Services

8245 Boston University Laboratory of Neuropsychology
Dept of Behavioral Neuroscience
80 E Concord Street M9 617-638-4803
Boston, MA 02118 Fax: 617-638-4806
www.bu.edu
Offers research and studies into the effects of Alcoholism pertaining to aphasia apraxia dementia memory disorders and various other neurological malfunctions.
Marlene Osca Berman PhD, Director

8246 Center for Alcohol & Addiction Studies Brown University
Brown University
Box G-S121-5 401-863-6600
Providence, RI 02912-0001 Fax: 401-863-6697
e-mail: CAAS@brown.edu
www.caas.brown.edu
The Center for Alcohol and Addiction Studies through its affiliation with the Brown Medical School occupies a unique position within the University. The Center brings together more that 90 faculty and professional staff members from 11 University departments and eight affiliated hospitals to promote the identification prevention and effective treatment of alcohol and other substance abuse.
Peter M Monti PhD, Center Director
Damaris Rohs PhD, Associate Director

8247 Cornerstone Medical Arts Center Hospital
Medical Arts Center Hospital
159-05 Union Turnpike 718-906-6700
Fresh Meadows, NY 11366-2802 800-233-9999
Fax: 718-906-6840
www.cornerstoneny.com
Offers a complete integrated program for alcohol assessment alcohol and drug rehabilitation continuing care community education and comprehensive family recovery.

8248 Do it Now Foundation
PO Box 27658 480-736-0599
Tempe, AZ 85285-7658 Fax: 480-736-0599
e-mail: info@dci-deitnaw.com
www.doitnow.org
An information clearinghouse for service providers that publishes well-written pamphlets booklets and materials on chemical dependency and recovery.

8249 Dorothea Dix Hospital Clinical Research Unit
809 Ruggles Drive 919-733-5227
Raleigh, NC 27603 866-349-5627
Fax: 919-733-5351
www.med.unc.edu

Researches the biological risk factors of alcoholism using young adults without the disease but with history of familial alcoholism.
Terry Spell, Director

8250 Ernest Gallo Clinic and Research Center
5858 Horton Street 510-985-3100
Emeryville, CA 94608 Fax: 510-985-3101
e-mail: ngreen@gallo.ucsf.edu
www.galloresearch.org
Alcoholism studies with a special emphasis on genetics.
Raymond L White PhD, Director
William R Sawyers JD, Chief Administrative Officer

8251 Families in Action National Drug Abuse Center
National Drug Abuse Center
PO Box 3553 252-237-1242
Wilson, NC 27895 Fax: 252-237-6544
e-mail: wfapmooring@simflex.com
www.familiesinaction.org
Publish prevention materials and serves as an information clearinghouse for families with a member suffering from a drug or alcohol addiction.
Phillip A Mooring, Executive Director
Elizabeth Bunn, Coordinator

8252 Friends Medical Science Research Center
11075 Santa Monica Boulevard 310-479-9330
Los Angeles, CA 90025 Fax: 310-477-9601
Studies narcotic addictions.
Meta P Barton, President

8253 Hahnemann University Laboratory of Human Pharmacology
Department of Pharmacology
Broad and Vine 215-854-8100
Philadelphia, PA 19102 Fax: 215-762-8109
www.hahnemannhospital.com
Benjamin Cal MD, Director

8254 Harvard Cocaine Recovery Project
1493 Cambridge Street 617-498-1000
Cambridge, MA 02139-1099 Fax: 617-642-58
Six-year study of relapse and recovery in cocaine addicts.
William McAu MD, Principal Investigator

8255 Interdisciplinary Program in Cell and Molecular Pharmacology
Medical University of South Carolina
173 Ashley Avenue BSB 358 843-792-2471
Charleston, SC 29425 Fax: 843-792-2475
www.musc.edu/pharm
Research into pharmacology and toxicology.
Kenneth D Tew, Professor and Chairman
Belinda Andersen, Administrative Coordinator

8256 Johns Hopkins University: Behavioral Pharmacology Research Unit
John Hopkins Bay View Campus
5510 Nathan Shock Drive 410-550-1686
Baltimore, MD 21224-2735 Fax: 410-550-0030
e-mail: bigelow@jhmi.edu
www.hopkinsmedicine.org
An internationally recognized center of excellence in research on psychoactive drugs. As the name implies BPRU's orientation is behavioral and pharmacological emphasizing a behavioral analysis of drug action.
George E Bigelow PhD, Scientific Director
Eric C Strain MD, Medical Director

8257 Kettering-Scott Magnetic Resonance Laboratory
Wright State University, School of Medicine
PO Box 927
Dayton, OH 45401-0927 937-296-7839
www.med.wright.edu
No information found on the website.
Joseph Manti MD, Director

8258 Marin Institute
24 Belvedere Street 415-456-5692
San Rafael, CA 94901-4817 Fax: 415-456-0491
www.marinInstitute.org
The mission of this Institute is to reduce the toll of alcohol and other drug problems on Marin County and society in general. The Institute fulfills this mission by developing implementing evaluating and disseminating innovative approaches to prevention locally nationally and internationally.
Bruce Lee Livingston MPP, Executive Director
Michele Simo JD MPH, Research & Policy Director

8259 Narcotic and Drug Research
11 Beach Street 212-966-8700
New York, NY 10013-2429 Fax: 212-334-8058
Nonprofit organization that is devoted to drug abuse education treatment and prevention.
Douglas S Lipton PhD, Director

8260 National Center on Addiction and Substance Abuse
Columbia University
633 3rd Avenue 212-841-5200
New York, NY 10017-6706 800-622-4357
Fax: 212-956-8020
www.casacolumbia.org
The only nation-wide organization that brings together under one roof all the professional disciplines needed to study and combat abuse of all substances - alcohol nicotine as well as illegal prescription and performance enhancing drugs - in all sectors of society.
Susan Brown, Vice President
Joseph A Califano Jr, Chairman and President

8261 National Prevention Resource Center CSAP Division of Communications Programs
CSAP Division of Communications Programs
5600 Fishers Lane 301-443-9936
Rockville, MD 20857-0001
Supports an array of prevention program evaluation approaches including individual grantee evaluations program evaluations and a National Evaluation Project. Also offers a National Data Base to provide information on programs for prevention of substance abuse.

8262 National Treatment Consortium for Alcohol and Other Drugs
PO Box 1294
Washington, DC 20013 202-434-4780
www.ntc-usa.org

8263 National Volunteer Training Center for Substance Abuse Prevention
CSAP Division of Communications Programs
5600 Fishers Lane 301-443-9936
Rockville, MD 20857
Volunteers are always on hand to provide answers, information, referrals and resources pertaining to alcohol, drugs and substance abuse.

8264 National Volunteer Training Center for Sub CSAP Division of Communications Programs
5600 Fishers Lane 301-443-9936
Rockville, MD 20857
Volunteers are always on hand to provide answers information referrals and resources pertaining to alcohol drugs and substance abuse.

8265 Ohio State University Clinical Pharmacology Division
College of Medicine
333 Western 9th Avenue 614-292-8600
Columbus, OH 43210-1239 800-252-3636
Fax: 614-292-4293
www.medicine.osu.edu
Substance abuse and alcohol related research.

Glen Apsloss, Director

8266 Ohio State University Clinical Pharmacolog College of Medicine
333 Western 9th Avenue 614-292-6908
Columbus, OH 43210 800-252-3636
Fax: 614-292-4293
www.medicine.osu.edu
Substance abuse and alcohol related research.

Glen Apsloss, Director

8267 RADAR Network National Clearinghouse for Alcohol & Dru
National Clearinghouse for Alcohol & Drug Info

PO Box 2345
Rockville, MD 20847-2345
301-468-2600
877-SAM-HSA7
Fax: 240-221-4292
TTY: 800-487-4889
ncadi.samhsa.gov

Consists of state clearinghouses specialized information centers of national organizations and the Department of Education Regional Training Centers. Each RADAR member can offer the public a variety of information services.
John Noble, Director

8268 Research Institute on Alcoholism State University of New York at Buffalo
State University of New York at Buffalo
1021 Main Street
Buffalo, NY 14203
716-887-2566
Fax: 716-872-52
e-mail: connors@ria.buffalo.edu
www.ria.buffalo.edu

Integral part of the New York State Division of Alcoholism and Alcohol Abuse.
Gerard Conno MD, Director
Kimberly S Walitzer, Deputy Director

8269 Rockefeller University Laboratory of Biology
1230 York Avenue
New York, NY 10021
212-327-7458
Fax: 212-277-54
www.rockefeller.edu

Vincent P Doyle, Head

8270 Rutgers University Center of Alcohol Studies
Busch Campus
607 Allison Road
Piscataway, NJ 08854
732-445-2190
Fax: 732-445-5300
e-mail: alclib@rci.rutgers.edu
alcoholstudies.rutgers.edu

Causes and treatment of alcoholism.
Robert Pandi PhD, Director
Marsha E Bates PhD, Research Professor I of Psychology

8271 Rutgers University: Controlled Drug- Delivery Research Center
College of Pharmacy
PO Box 789
Piscataway, NJ 08855-0789
732-932-3834
Fax: 732-932-5767
Yie W Chien, Director

8272 Ruth E Golding Clinical Pharmacokinetics Laboratory
College of Pharmacy
1703 E Mabel
Tucson, AZ 85721-1427
520-626-1938
e-mail: webmaster@pharmacy.arizona.edu
www.pharmacy.arizona.edu

Conducts studies of drugs in humans and animals.
Michael Maye MD, Head

8273 Southern California Research Institute
7065 Hayvenhurst Avenue
Van Nuys, CA 91406
310-390-8481
Fax: 310-390-8482
www.scri.org

Effects of alcohol and drugs on behavior studies.
Dary Fiorent PhD, Executive Director
Bergetta Die BA, Research Associate

8274 Stanford Center for Research in Disease Prevention
Stanford University School of Medicine
1070 Arastradero Road
Palo Alto, CA 94304
650-725-6906
Fax: 650-723-6254
prevention.stanford.edu

Prevention and control of alcohol and drug abuse related disorders.
John W Farquhar MD, Director

8275 State University of New York at Buffalo Toxicology Research Center
3435 Main Street
Buffalo, NY 14214
716-831-2125
Fax: 716-829-2806
www.smbs.buffalo.edu

Toxicology-related research and services including the development of tests to evaluate toxins chemicals and drugs.
Paul Kostyni PhD, Director
Dr James R Olson, Assistant Director

8276 University of California: Los Angeles Alcohol Research Center
760 Westwood Plaza
Los Angeles, CA 90095-8353
310-825-1891
Fax: 310-206-7309
www.ucla.edu

Causes of alcoholism including genetics.
Dr Ernest Noble, Director

8277 University of Michigan: Alcohol Research Center
400 E Eisenhower Parkway
Ann Arbor, MI 48108-3318
734-763-7952
Fax: 734-998-7994
www.umich.edu

Alcohol abuse studies among the elderly including the relationship between alcohol and aged disorders.
Robert A Zucker PhD, Contact

8278 University of Michigan: Psychiatric Center
1500 E Medical Center Drive
Ann Arbor, MI 48109-0001
734-936-4960
Fax: 734-936-9761
www.umich.edu

Psychiatric disease research pertaining to the effects of alcoholism and drug abuse.
John F Greden, Chairman

8279 University of Minnesota: Program on Alcohol/Drug Control
Stadium Gate 27
Minneapolis, MN 55455
612-624-6861
Alcohol tobacco and drug research.
Dr James Schaefer, Director

8280 University of Missouri: Kansas City Drug Information Service
2464 Charlotte
Kansas City, MO 64108-2640
816-235-5490
Fax: 816-235-5491
dic.umkc.edu

Literature research and evaluation of clinical drug problems and questions.
Pat Bryant PhD, Director
Heather A Pace PhD, Assistant Director

8281 University of Tennessee Drug Information Center
875 Monroe Avenue
Memphis, TN 38163-1
901-528-5555
Fax: 901-448-5419
e-mail: utdic@utmem.edu
dop.utmem.edu/dic

Katie Suda, Director
Camille Thornton, Assistant Professor

8282 University of Texas Health Science Center Neurophysiology Research Center
Speech & Hearing Institute
1343 Moursund Street
Houston, TX 77030-3405
713-792-4542
Fax: 713-792-4513
Conducts clinical and animal studies aimed at combating alcohol drug and tobacco dependence.
Malcolm Skol PhD, Director

8283 University of Texas at Austin: Drug Synamics Institute
1 University Station
Austin, TX 78712
512-475-9746
Fax: 512-471-2746
www.utexas.edu

Pharmaceutical and drug research.
Janet C Walkow PhD, Director
Carla Van Den Berg PhD, Associate Professor

8284 University of Utah: Center for Human Toxicology
417 Wakara Way
Salt Lake City, UT 84112-1210
801-581-5117
Fax: 801-581-5034
e-mail: dwilkins@alanine.pharm.utah.edu
www.pharmacy.utah.edu

Clinical forensic and toxicology research.
Douglas Roll MD, Associate Director
Dennis Crouch, Director

8285 University of Wisconsin Milwaukee Medicinal Chemistry Group
University of Wisconsin
PO Box 413
Milwaukee, WI 53201-413
414-229-1122
www4.uwm.edu

Research on drugs including studies of valium receptors.
Carlos Santiago, Chancellor

Support Groups & Hotlines

8286 **Al-Anon Alateen Family Group Hotline**
1600 Corporate Landing Parkway 757-563-1600
Virginia Beach, VA 10018-970 888-425-2666
Fax: 757-563-1655
e-mail: wso@alanon.org
www.alanon.org
A mutual support program with groups meeting worldwide to provide hope and help to the families of alcoholics. Although a seperate entity from Alcoholics Anonymous, our program is based upon the twelve steps.
Ric Buchanan, Executive Director

8287 **Alcohol Drug Treatment Referral**
1316 South Coast Highway
Laguna Beach, CA 92651-3118 800-454-8966
Fax: 949-281-1933
National Help and Referral Network, a nonprofit organization available 24 hours a day to assist people troubled by drug or alcohol abuse. Here to provide information on addiction treatment and support services and to help save lives and mend broken dreams.
Mike Cohan, Director

8288 **Alcoholics Anonymous World Services**
PO Box 459 212-870-3400
New York, NY 10163-4059 Fax: 212-870-3003
www.aa.org
Alcoholics Anonymous is a fellowship of men and women who share their experience, strength and hope with each other that they may solve their common problem and help others to recover from alcoholism. The only requirement for membership is a desire to stop drinking. There are no dues or fees for AA membership; they are self-supporting through their own contributions.
Greg M, General Manager

8289 **Drug Free Workplace Hotline**
Division of Workplace Programs
Samhsa Diagonal CSAP 1 Choke Cherry 240-276-2612
Rockville, MD 20857 800-967-5752
Fax: 240-276-1210
www.drugfreeworkplace.gov
A hotline for businesses to obtain information on a wide range of drug abuse related problems, issues and services.
Robert Stephenson II, Director

8290 **Friday Night Live**
California Dept of Drug & Alcohol Programs
1700 K Street 916-445-7456
Sacramento, CA 95814 Fax: 916-230-59
e-mail: laura@tcoe.org
www.communitycounseling.org/fnl
These groups, located in California, are all run by students with a faculty adviser. They arrange local alcohol and drug free events, from dances and movies to visiting hospitalized children. Students not only have fun but they learn to have fun sober.
Jim Kooler, Administrator
Laura Purcellabuzo, Project Coordinator

8291 **Images Within: A Child's View of Parental Alcoholism**
Children of Alcoholics Foundation
PO Box 4185 212-595-5810
New York, NY 10163-4185 800-359-2623
e-mail: coaf@phoenixhouse.org
www.coaf.org
An innovative program designed to teach all children about family alcoholism. Middle-school-aged children learn how to get help for themselves or give help to their friends.

8292 **International Lawyers in Alcoholics Anonymous**
39 Smith Neck Road 860-529-7474
Old Lyme, CT 6371 e-mail: bert@bertwitehead.com
www.ilaa.org
Provides 40 independent local groups.

8293 **National Health Information Center**
PO Box 1133 310-565-4167
Washington, DC 20013 800-336-4797
Fax: 301-984-4256
e-mail: info@nhic.org
www.health.gov/nhic
Offers a nationwide information referral service, produces directories and resource guides.

8294 **ToughLove International**
PO Box 1069 215-348-7090
Doylestown, PA 18901-0019 800-333-1069
www.toughlove.org
This national self-help group for parents, children and communities emphasizes cooperation, personal initiative and action. Publishes books, brochures and promotional information and holds workshops and seminars across the country.

8295 **WFS' New Life Program**
Women for Sobriety
PO Box 618 215-536-8026
Quakertown, PA 18951-0618 Fax: 215-538-9026
e-mail: newlife@nni.com
www.womenforsobriety.org
A self-help program for women that can be used independent from AA or with AA. Groups are in many states in the United States. Donations suggested.
Rebecca M Fenner, Director

Books

8296 **AA Comes of Age**
Alcoholics Anonymous
PO Box 459 212-870-3400
New York, NY 10163-0459 Fax: 212-870-3137
Tells how AA was started, how the Steps and Traditions evolved and how the AA Fellowship grew and spread overseas.

8297 **AA in Prison: Inmate to Inmate**
Alcoholics Anonymous
PO Box 459 212-870-3400
New York, NY 10163-0459 Fax: 212-870-3137
Thirty-two stories that share the experience of men and women who found AA while in prison.
128 pages

8298 **Accepting Ourselves & Others**
Hazelden
15251 Pleasant Valley Road 651-257-4010
Center City, MN 55012-9640 800-328-9000
Fax: 651-213-4426
www.hazelden.org
Fully revised and expanded second edition. Examines recovery as it affects the gay, lesbian, and bisexual community, as well as their friends, family, and therapists. Addresses the relationship between substance abuse and being a sexual minority, and discusses the impact of other issues such as anxiety, depression, sexual abuse, and learning disabilities.
379 pages Paperback
ISBN: 1-568381-20-4

8299 **Addiction and Responsibility**
The Crossroad Publishing Company
370 Lexington Avenue 212-532-3650
New York, NY 10017-6503 800-395-0690
Fax: 212-532-4922
Anyone who has wrestled with such basic questions about addiction such as: Is drug addiction a behavior disorder or a character flaw? Is it genetic or learned? What is it like to be addicted? will find welcome answers in this groundbreaking philosophical inquiry into the addictive mind. The author helps readers understand addiction.
192 pages
ISBN: 0-824513-65-7

8300 **Addictions Counseling**
The Crossroad Publishing Company

370 Lexington Avenue 212-532-3650
New York, NY 10017-6503 800-395-0690
Fax: 212-532-4922

A practical guide to counseling people with chemical and other addictions.
144 pages Paperback
ISBN: 0-824513-86-0

8301 **Addictive Personality**
Hazelden
15251 Pleasant Valley Road 651-257-4010
Center City, MN 55012-9640 800-328-9000
Fax: 651-213-4426
www.hazelden.org

Understanding how an individual becomes an addict through examination of addiction's causes, stages of development, and consequences. Second edition further refines these ideas and includes the most recent information on the addictive process, cultural influences on addictive behaviors, recovery, genetic factors in addiction, mental health issues, and new research findings.
130 pages Paperback
ISBN: 1-568381-29-8

8302 **Addictive Thinking Understanding Self-Deception**
Hazelden
15251 Pleasant Valley Road 651-257-4010
Center City, MN 55012-9640 800-328-9000
Fax: 651-213-4426
www.hazelden.org

Illustrates the irrational perspective and complicated, contradictory thinking patterns of addictive thinking, and demonstrates how they lead to low self-esteen, addiction, and relapse. Revised edition includes expanded information on depression and affective disorders, the relationship between addictive thinking and relapse, and the new research related to the origins of addictive thinking.
140 pages Paperback
ISBN: 1-568381-38-7

8303 **Adult Children of Alcoholics**
Hazelden
15251 Pleasant Valley Road 651-257-4010
Center City, MN 55012-9640 800-328-9000
Fax: 651-213-4426
www.hazelden.org

Written to and for adult children of dysfunctional families.
138 pages Paperback

8304 **Al-Anon Family Groups**
Al-Anon Family Group Headquarters
1600 Corporate Landing Parkway 757-563-1600
Virginia Beach, VA 23454-5617 800-425-2666
Fax: 757-563-1655
e-mail: wso@al-anon.org
www.al-anon.alateen.org

Basic book that explains the purpose of fellowship, how it works and how it is held in unity. Includes real life stories by husbands, wives, parents and children of those who suffer from alcoholism.
177 pages
ISBN: 0-910034-54-0
Caryn Johnson, Director Communications

8305 **Al-Anon's Twelve Steps and Twelve Traditions**
Al-Anon Family Group Headquarters
1600 Corporate Landing Parkway 757-563-1600
Virginia Beach, VA 23454-5617 800-425-2666
Fax: 757-563-1655
e-mail: wso@al-anon.org
www.al-anon.alateen.org

Written for people whose lives have been affected by alcoholism.
142 pages Hardcover
ISBN: 0-910034-24-9
Caryn Johnson, Director Communications

8306 **Alateen: A Day at a Time**
Al-Anon Family Group Headquarters
1600 Corporate Landing Parkway 757-563-1600
Virginia Beach, VA 23454-5617 800-425-2666
Fax: 757-563-1655
e-mail: wso@al-anon.org
www.al-anon.alateen.org

A collection of positive, daily sharings written by teenagers around the world.
384 pages
ISBN: 0-910034-53-2
Caryn Johnson, Director Communications

8307 **Alateen: Hope for Children of Alcoholics**
Al-Anon Family Group Headquarters
1600 Corporate Landing Parkway 757-563-1600
Virginia Beach, VA 23454-5617 800-425-2666
Fax: 757-563-1655
e-mail: wso@al-anon.org
www.al-anon.alateen.org

A gold mine of information written by Alateens themselves. It covers the history of Alateen, understanding alcoholism and personal stories.
115 pages
ISBN: 0-910034-20-6
Caryn Johnson, Director Communications

8308 **Alcohol and Other Drug Services: Dir. of California's Community Services**
Department of Alcohol and Drug Programs
1700 K Street 916-445-0834
Sacramento, CA 95814-4022

A directory listing agencies, alcohol and drug providers, county 504 coordinators and county program administrators for the state of California.
136 pages

8309 **Alcohol, Drug and Other Addictions: A Directory of Treatment Centers**
Oryx Press
4041 N Central Avenue 602-265-2651
Phoenix, AZ 85012-3397 800-279-4663

Lists 18,000 federal, state and local addiction treatment regimens that include public and private centers.

8310 **Alcohol, Tobacco and Other Drugs May Harm the Unborn**
National Clearinghouse for Alcohol and Drug Info.
PO Box 2345
Rockville, MD 20847-2345 800-729-6686

Presents the most recent findings of basic research and clinical studies conducted on the effects of alcohol, drugs and tobacco on the unborn.

8311 **Alcoholics Anonymous**
Alcoholics Anonymous
PO Box 459 212-870-3400
New York, NY 10163-0459 Fax: 212-870-3137

Third edition of the Big Book, basic text of AA. Chapters describe the AA recovery program and personal histories have been added.

8312 **Alcoholics Anonymous: The Big Book**
Hazelden
15251 Pleasant Valley Road 651-257-4010
Center City, MN 55012-9640 800-328-9000
Fax: 651-213-4426
www.hazelden.org

Classic text that guides Alcoholics Anonymous programs and describes how millions of men and women have recovered from alcoholism.
575 pages Paperback

8313 **American Academy of Psychiatrists in Alcoholism and Addiction Directory**
Box 376 301-220-0951
Greenbelt, MD 20768 Fax: 301-220-0941

Lists 900 member professionals who are concerned with drug and alcohol abuse.

8314 **An Annotated Bibliography of Recent Empirical Research In Methadone**
National Clearinghouse for Alcohol and Drug Info.
PO Box 2345
Rockville, MD 20847-2345 800-729-6686

Provides guidelines and suggestions to investigators engaged in the demanding and essential task of followup research on intravenous drug users who have contracted AIDS.
97 pages

8315 As Bill Sees It
Alcoholics Anonymous
PO Box 459 212-870-3400
New York, NY 10163-0459 Fax: 212-870-3137
This collection of Bill W's writings offers a daily source of comfort and inspiration.

8316 As We Understood...
Al-Anon Family Group Headquarters
1600 Corporate Landing Parkway 757-563-1600
Virginia Beach, VA 23454-5617 800-425-2666
Fax: 757-563-1655
e-mail: wso@al-anon.org
www.al-anon.alateen.org
Al-Anon members share their understanding of a higher power, fellowship, spiritual awakening, prayer, meditation and letting go.
269 pages
ISBN: 0-910034-56-7
Caryn Johnson, Director Communications

8317 Black, Beautiful and Recovering
African American Family Services
2616 Nicollet Avenue S 612-871-7878
Minneapolis, MN 55408
A helpful guide for Black people who are in the process of recovering from alcohol or other substance abuse problems.
10 pages

8318 Body, Mind, and Spirit
Hazelden
15251 Pleasant Valley Road 651-257-4010
Center City, MN 55012-9640 800-328-9000
Fax: 651-213-4426
www.hazelden.org
Addressing such issues as self-esteem, fear, anger, and spirituality, these 366 daily meditations and affirmations integrate the physical, mental, and spiritual aspects of healing from addiction.
410 pages Paperback
ISBN: 1-568380-77-1

8319 Came to Believe
Alcoholics Anonymous
PO Box 459 212-870-3400
New York, NY 10163-0459 Fax: 212-870-3137
A collection of stories by AA members who write about what the phrase spiritual awakening means to them.
120 pages

8320 Chemically Dependent Older Adults
Hazelden
15251 Pleasant Valley Road 651-257-4010
Center City, MN 55012-9640 800-328-9000
Fax: 651-213-4426
www.hazelden.org
Reviews the importance of considering the older adult's health, living conditions and social and economic resources when developing treatment and aftercare plans.
136 pages Paperback

8321 Childhood and Adolescent Drug Abuse: A Physician's Guide
American Council on Drug Education
204 Monroe Street
Rockville, MD 20850-4425 800-488-3784
A scientific monograph which educates and sensitizes doctors to the dimensions of drug problems.
68 pages

8322 Circle of Hope
Hazelden
15251 Pleasant Valley Road 651-257-4010
Center City, MN 55012-9640 800-328-9000
Fax: 651-213-4426
www.hazelden.org
Spirituality, acceptance, and living one day at a time are show through personal stories of individuals living with HIV and AIDS and dealing with adiction and recovery.
364 pages Paperback
ISBN: 0-894866-10-9

8323 Citizen's Alcohol and Other Drug Prevention Directory
National Clearinghouse for Alcohol and Drug Info.
PO Box 2345
Rockville, MD 20847-2345 800-729-6686
National directory of over 3,000 state, local and government agencies dealing with alcohol and other drug-related topics.
276 pages

8324 Cocaine Today
American Council on Drug Education
204 Monroe Street
Rockville, MD 20850-4425 800-488-3784
A recent revision of this popular book. Cocaine Today takes a new look at cocaine and its derivative, crack.

8325 Codependent No More
Hazelden
15251 Pleasant Valley Road 651-257-4010
Center City, MN 55012-9640 800-328-9000
Fax: 651-213-4426
www.hazelden.org
Explains codependent behaviors in clear, simple terms.
208 pages Paperback

8326 Color of Light
Hazelden
15251 Pleasant Valley Road 651-257-4010
Center City, MN 55012-9640 800-328-9000
Fax: 651-213-4426
www.hazelden.org
These 366 meditations speak to both the practical and spiritual journey of living with HIV/AIDS, and demonstrate how to integrate personal values with those offered in chemical dependency recovery and the Twelve Steps.
400 pages Paperback
ISBN: 0-894865-11-0

8327 Confusion is a State of Grace
Hazelden
15251 Pleasant Valley Road 651-257-4010
Center City, MN 55012 800-328-9000
Fax: 651-213-4426
www.hazelden.org
Compilation of quotes that captures the wisdom, humor, and healing found in Al-Anon and other Twelve Step groups.
153 pages Paperback
ISBN: 1-568380-89-5

8328 Courage to Be Me: Living with Alcoholism
Al-Anon Family Group Headquarters
1600 Corporate Landing Parkway 757-563-1600
Virginia Beach, VA 23454-5617 800-425-2666
Fax: 757-563-1655
e-mail: wso@al-anon.org
www.al-anon.alateen.org
Written for and by Alateens of all ages who will treasure the honesty and strength of recovery shown.
326 pages
ISBN: 0-910034-30-3
Caryn Johnson, Director Communications

8329 Daily Reflections: A Book of Reflections by AA Members for AA Members
Alcoholics Anonymous
PO Box 459 212-870-3400
New York, NY 10163-0459 Fax: 212-870-3137
AAs reflect on favorite quotations from A.A. literature. A reading for each day of the year.

8330 Day at a Time: Daily Reflections for Recovering People
Hazelden
15251 Pleasant Valley Road 651-257-4010
Center City, MN 55012-9640 800-328-9000
Fax: 651-213-4426
www.hazelden.org
Offers inspiration and hope for people recovering from chemical dependency or other addictions. Each daily passage reinforces the message of Twelve Step recovery.
384 pages Paperback
ISBN: 1-568380-36-4

8331 **Day by Day**
Hazelden
15251 Pleasant Valley Road
Center City, MN 55012
651-257-4010
800-328-9000
Fax: 651-213-4426
www.hazelden.org
A book of daily meditations for recovering addicts that reinforce Narcotics Anonymous principles and objectives.
400 pages Paperback

8332 **Days of Healing, Days of Joy**
Hazelden
15251 Pleasant Valley Road
Center City, MN 55012-9640
651-257-4010
800-328-9000
Fax: 651-213-4426
www.hazelden.org
Three hundred and sixty-six daily quotes, meditations and affirmations to help adult children in their search for serenity.
400 pages Paperback

8333 **Developing Chemical Dependency Services for Black People**
African American Family Services
2616 Nicollet Avenue S
612-871-7878
Minneapolis, MN 55408
This manual has been developed to address many of the questions asked by new or expanding programs as they establish new culturally specific initiatives for African-American clients.
78 pages

8334 **Dilemma of the Alcoholic Marriage**
Al-Anon Family Group Headquarters
1600 Corporate Landing Parkway
Virginia Beach, VA 23454-5617
757-563-1600
800-425-2666
Fax: 757-563-1655
e-mail: wso@al-anon.org
www.al-anon.alateen.org
This book explores the problem of alcoholism in marriage and includes questions for applying the twelve steps to relationships.
100 pages
ISBN: 0-910034-18-4
Caryn Johnson, Director Communications

8335 **Dr. Bob and the Good Oldtimers**
Alcoholics Anonymous
PO Box 459
New York, NY 10163-0459
212-870-3400
Fax: 212-870-3137
The life story of the fellowship's co-founder, interwoven wth recollections of early AA in the Midwest.

8336 **Drug Abuse and Addiction Information/Treatment Programs**
American Business Directories
5711 S 86th Circle
Omaha, NE 68127-4146
402-593-4600
Fax: 402-331-1505
Number of entries is 9,425.

8337 **Drug Use Among American High School Seniors, College Students & Youth**
National Clearinghouse for Alcohol and Drug Info.
PO Box 2345
Rockville, MD 20847-2345
800-729-6686
Comprehensive reports presenting the results of the 16th national survey of the drug use and related attitudes of American high school seniors.
199 pages Volumes I & II

8338 **Drugs and Pregnancy: It's Not Worth the Risk**
American Council on Drug Education
204 Monroe Street
Rockville, MD 20850
800-488-3784
A scientific monograph for health care providers which teaches them to identify alcohol and drug problems in their patients.
48 pages

8339 **Dual Diagnosis**
Hazelden
15251 Pleasant Valley Road
Center City, MN 55012-9640
651-257-4010
800-328-9000
Fax: 651-213-4426
www.hazelden.org
Focuses on the issues surrounding the treatment of clients with co-existing chemical dependency and psychiatric conditions.
191 pages Paperback

8340 **Dual Disorders**
Hazelden
15251 Pleasant Valley Road
Center City, MN 55012-9640
651-257-4010
800-328-9000
Fax: 651-213-4426
www.hazelden.org
Presents case histories and analyses of psychiatric disorders.
140 pages Paperback

8341 **Dual Disorders Recovery Book**
Hazelden
15251 Pleasant Valley Road
Center City, MN 55012-9640
651-257-4010
800-328-9000
Fax: 651-213-4426
www.hazelden.org
Helps individuals with dual disorders develop a plan for daily living through a specially-designed Twelve-Step program.
242 pages Paperback
ISBN: 1-568380-34-8

8342 **Each Day a New Beginning**
Hazelden
15251 Pleasant Valley Road
Center City, MN 55012-9640
651-257-4010
800-328-9000
Fax: 651-213-4426
www.hazelden.org
Promotes the development of a significant spiritual core for recovery that can be enhanced throughout the rest of life.
400 pages Paperback

8343 **Elephant in the Living Room: A Leader's Guide**
Hazelden
15251 Pleasant Valley Road
Center City, MN 55012-9640
651-257-4010
800-328-9000
Fax: 651-213-4426
www.hazelden.org
The adult companion to the classic children's book. Caretakers learn how to explain addiction and its effect on the family to small children who's parents or siblings are chemically dependent.
129 pages Paperback
ISBN: 1-568380-34-8

8344 **Encyclopedia of Drug Abuse**
Facts on File
11 Penn Plaza
New York, NY 10001
212-967-8800
800-322-8755
Fax: 800-678-3633
More that 500 entries explore: specific drugs, countries, organizations, treatment programs, laws, medical terms, and psychosocial concepts.
496 pages Hardcover

8345 **Ethics for Addiction Professionals**
Hazelden
15251 Pleasant Valley Road
Center City, MN 55012-9640
651-257-4010
800-328-9000
Fax: 651-213-4426
www.hazelden.org
Probes crucial, complex ethical issues including counselor relapse, paid referrals and discrimination.
60 pages

8346 **Extent and Adequacy of Insurance Coverage for Substance Abuse I & II**
National Clearinghouse for Alcohol and Drug Info.
PO Box 2345
Rockville, MD 20847-2345
800-729-6686
These volumes examine the extent to which the cost of alcohol and other drug treatments is covered by private insurance, public financing and other sources.

8347 **Eye Opener**
Hazelden
15251 Pleasant Valley Road
Center City, MN 55012-9640
651-257-4010
800-328-9000
Fax: 651-213-4426
www.hazelden.org

Daily meditations about understanding the Alcoholics Anonymous program, writen by a favorite early AA member and author.
380 pages Cloth
ISBN: 0-894860-23-2

8348 Fact Is...Hispanic Parents Can Help Their Children Avoid Alcohol/Drugs
National Clearinghouse for Alcohol and Drug Info.
PO Box 2345
Rockville, MD 20847-2345 800-729-6686

8349 Feeding the Hungry Heart, the Experience of Compulsive Eating
Gurze Books
PO Box 2238
Carlsbad, CA 92018-2238 800-756-7533
Fax: 760-434-5476
e-mail: gzcatl@aol.com
www.bulimia.com
This is a widely respected, extremely readable book from Ms. Roth and the many participants of early breaking free workshops. It is an intimate, vulnerable sharing of experiences which continues to touch and change lives.
212 pages Paperback

8350 Food for Thought: Daily Meditations for Overeaters
Hazelden
15251 Pleasant Valley Road 651-257-4010
Center City, MN 55012-9640 800-328-9000
Fax: 651-213-4426
www.hazelden.org
Offers guidance in the early days of living a Twelve Step program.
400 pages Paperback
ISBN: 0-894860-90-9

8351 Forum Favorites: Volumes 1, 2, 3 & 4
Al-Anon Family Group Headquarters
1600 Corporate Landing Parkway 757-563-1600
Virginia Beach, VA 23454-5617 800-425-2666
Fax: 757-563-1655
e-mail: wso@al-anon.org
www.al-anon.alateen.org
Personal sharings show how the fundamentals of the Al-Anon programs are applied to everyday situations.
428 pages Set of 4
ISBN: 0-910034-51-6
Caryn Johnson, Director Communications

8352 Freedom from Smoking at Work Program
American Lung Association
1740 Broadway
New York, NY 10017 212-315-8700
www.lungusa.org
ALA program for organizations interested in creating a healthier workplace environment through a comprehensive, multicomponent smoking education, cessation and policy development program designed for the workplace.

8353 Future by Design/A Community Framework
National Clearinghouse for Alcohol and Drug Info.
PO Box 2345
Rockville, MD 20847-2345 800-729-6686
Provides communities with a manageable framework for getting involved in alcohol and other drug prevention.
234 pages

8354 Gentle Path Through the Twelve Steps
Hazelden
15251 Pleasant Valley Road 651-257-4010
Center City, MN 55012-9640 800-328-9000
Fax: 651-213-4426
www.hazelden.org
This workbook provides a unique set of structured forms and exercises to help recoving people integrate the Twelve Steps in all aspects of their lives.
224 pages Paperback
ISBN: 1-568380-58-5

8355 Getting Started in AA
Hazelden
15251 Pleasant Valley Road 651-257-4010
Center City, MN 55012-9640 800-328-9000
Fax: 651-213-4426
www.hazelden.org
Practical suggestions for staying sober, summaries of AA principles, concepts, and slogans, and a historical overview to help the reader understand the spirit of the program.
211 pages Paperback
ISBN: 1-568380-91-7

8356 Getting Tough on Gateway Drugs: A Guide for the Family
American Council On Drug Education
204 Monroe Street
Rockville, MD 20850-4425 800-488-3784
Gateway drugs including marijuana, alcohol and tobacco are those which open doors into all drug abuse. This family survival guide helps parents understand the consequences of drug dependence and suggests actions the family can take to prevent and solve drug problems.
332 pages

8357 Getting it Together: Promoting Drug Free Communities
National Clearinghouse for Alcohol and Drug Info.
PO Box 2345
Rockville, MD 20847 800-729-6686
Provides resources and step-by-step information on how local communities and organizations can work effectively with young people who are committed to preventing alcohol and other drug abuse.
71 pages

8358 God Grant Me the Laughter: A Treasury of Twelve Step Humor
Hazelden
15251 Pleasant Valley Road 651-257-4010
Center City, MN 55012-9640 800-328-9000
Fax: 651-213-4426
www.hazelden.org
Hearty cartoons and humorous anecdotes clearly demonstrate how readers' lives today contrast with their drinking and drug using in the past.
200 pages Paperback
ISBN: 1-568380-38-0

8359 Good First Step
Hazelden
15251 Pleasant Valley Road 651-257-4010
Center City, MN 55012-9640 800-328-9000
Fax: 651-213-4426
www.hazelden.org
Features a structured format and emphasis on the meaning of the First Step to help build a solid foundation for recovery.
60 pages Paperback
ISBN: 1-568381-13-1

8360 Goodbye Hangovers, Hello Life
Women for Sobriety
PO Box 618 215-536-8026
Quakertown, PA 18951-0618 Fax: 215-536-8026
e-mail: NewLife@nni.com
www.womenforsobriety.org
A book about recovery - how it happens, what problems arise and how to overcome these problems.
250 pages Paperback

8361 Grateful to Have Been There
Hazelden
15251 Pleasant Valley Road 651-257-4010
Center City, MN 55012 800-328-9000
Fax: 651-213-4426
www.hazelden.org
Aide and executive secretary to AA's co-founder Bill W. for 20 years, Wing shares her memories and impressions of 42 years of involvement with the Fellowship.
150 pages Paperback
ISBN: 0-942421-44-2

8362 Growing Up Drug Free: A Parent's Guide to Prevention
National Clearinghouse for Alcohol and Drug Info.
PO Box 2345
Rockville, MD 20852 800-729-6686

Offers information on what parents can do to prevent their child from becoming a substance abuser/alcoholic. Focuses on counseling, peer pressure issues, education, school-parent cooperation and offers an introduction to each drug, symptoms and how to spot the warning signs of drug addiction.
47 pages

8363 Handle with Care
Hazelden
15251 Pleasant Valley Road 651-257-4010
Center City, MN 55012-9640 800-328-9000
Fax: 651-213-4426
www.hazelden.org
A comprehensive look at how parents, teachers and other care givers of children ages 10 and younger can identify and meet their special needs.

8364 Help for Helpers: Daily Meditations for Counselors
Hazelden
15251 Pleasant Valley Road 651-257-4010
Center City, MN 55012-9640 800-328-9000
Fax: 651-213-4426
www.hazelden.org
Written by addiction treatment center staff members from across the country, these daily meditations encourage, comfort, and challenge helpers to understand others and themselves.
400 pages Paperback
ISBN: 1-568380-61-5

8365 Helping Homeless People with Alcohol and Other Drug Problems
National Clearinghouse for Alcohol and Drug Info.
PO Box 2345
Rockville, MD 20847 800-729-6686
Developed by professionals who work directly with homeless people, this manual provides basic information about homeless people with AOD problems.
50 pages

8366 Helping Your Students Say No Teacher's Guide
National Clearinghouse for Alcohol and Drug Info.
PO Box 2345
Rockville, MD 20847-2345 800-729-6686
Explains the effects of alcohol on the body, why children start to drink, how teachers can help their students refuse alcohol and deal with the first signs of drinking.
13 pages

8367 How to Manage Your Drug-Free Workplace Programs
American Council on Drug Education
204 Monroe Street
Rockville, MD 20850-4425 800-488-3784
Step-by-step process for introducing and managing a drug awareness program that includes a variety of additional tips to complement messages in the drug awareness pamphlet series.
48 pages

8368 I'm Black and I'm Sober
Hazelden
15251 Pleasant Valley Road 651-257-4010
Center City, MN 55012-9640 800-328-9000
Fax: 651-213-4426
www.hazelden.org
An autobiography written by a recovering African American woman who discusses the impact of discrimination and the obstacles faced through the journey back to sobriety.
279 pages Paperback
ISBN: 1-568380-71-2

8369 If Only I Could Quit
Hazelden
15251 Pleasant Valley Road 651-257-4010
Center City, MN 55012-9640 800-328-9000
Fax: 651-213-4426
www.hazelden.org
Promotes the Twelve Step process for recovery from nicotine addiction.
320 pages Paperback

8370 In God's Care
Hazelden
15251 Pleasant Valley Road 651-257-4010
Center City, MN 55012-9640 800-328-9000
Fax: 651-213-4426
www.hazelden.org
Excellent relaxation and education tool for clients working on their Second and Third Steps.
400 pages Paperback

8371 Keep Quit
Hazelden
15251 Pleasant Valley Road 651-257-4010
Center City, MN 55012-9640 800-328-9000
Fax: 651-213-4426
www.hazelden.org
Daily motivational guide to help the new nonsmoker understand the craving for nicotine and learn how to break the rituals and patterns associated with relapse.
300 pages Paperback
ISBN: 1-568381-04-2

8372 Keep it Simple
Hazelden
15251 Pleasant Valley Road 651-257-4010
Center City, MN 55012-9640 800-328-9000
Fax: 651-213-4426
www.hazelden.org
Daily prayers that help clients learn to ask for help and to turn their self-will over to a Higher Power.
400 pages Paperback

8373 Learning to Live Drug Free: A Curriculum Model for Prevention
National Clearinghouse for Alcohol and Drug Info.
PO Box 2345
Rockville, MD 20847-2345 800-729-6686
Provides a flexible framework for classroom-based prevention efforts for kindergarten through grade 12.
52 pages

8374 Let's Talk About Alcohol Abuse
Rosen Publishing Group's PowerKids Press
29 E 21st Street 212-777-3017
New York, NY 10010 800-237-9932
Fax: 888-436-4643
e-mail: customerservice@rosenpub.com
www.rosenpublishing.com
In gentle and sensitive terms this book talks about when a parent drinks and what alcohol can do to the body. Kids are told about the illegality of drinking as minors. Recommended for grade K-4.

ISBN: 0-823923-03-7
Marianne Johnston, Author

8375 Life of My Own: Daily Meditations on Hope and Acceptance
Hazelden
15251 Pleasant Valley Road 651-257-4010
Center City, MN 55012-9640 800-328-9000
Fax: 651-213-4426
www.hazelden.org
Offers daily access to strength, serenity, and insight in our relationships with chemically dependent people.
400 pages Paperback
ISBN: 0-894868-63-2

8376 Little Red Book
Hazelden
15251 Pleasant Valley Road 651-257-4010
Center City, MN 55012-9640 800-328-9000
Fax: 651-213-4426
www.hazelden.org
A primer for members of Alcoholics Anonymous. Each page acts as a study guide to the Big Book and its teachings.
164 pages Paperback
ISBN: 0-894869-85-X

8377 Living Sober
Hazelden
15251 Pleasant Valley Road 651-257-4010
Center City, MN 55012-9640 800-328-9000
Fax: 651-213-4426
www.hazelden.org

Offers clients sound advice about how to stay sober.
88 pages Paperback

8378 Lois Remembers
Al-Anon Family Group Headquarters
1600 Corporate Landing Parkway 757-563-1600
Virginia Beach, VA 23454-5617 800-425-2666
Fax: 757-563-1655
e-mail: wso@al-anon.org
www.al-anon.alateen.org
The memoirs of a co-founder of Al-Anon. Lois tells her personal story and recalls the eventful years before and after the founding of AA and Al-Anon.
204 pages
ISBN: 0-910034-23-0
Caryn Johnson, Director Communications

8379 Marijuana
Branden Publishing Company
17 Station Street 617-734-2045
Brookline Village, MA 02147 Fax: 617-734-2046
www.branden.com
Paperback
ISBN: 0-828319-49-9

8380 Marijuana Smoking Prevention Program for Schools
American Lung Association
1740 Broadway 212-315-8700
New York, NY 10017
Cast of the TV show FAME enlivens highly motivational program to inform parents about the dangers of pot and discourages 9-11 year olds from using it.

8381 Marijuana Today
American Council on Drug Education
204 Monroe Street
Rockville, MD 20850-4425 800-488-3784
A revision of the long time bestseller, this book examines the history of marijuana, its use, the risks associated with use and the short and long-term effects of use.

8382 Marijuana and Reproduction
American Council on Drug Education
204 Monroe Street
Rockville, MD 20850-4425 800-488-3784
A scientific monograph for physicians which describes marijuana, profiles the users and discusses the effects on the reproductive system.
30 pages

8383 Marketing Booze to Blacks
African American Family Services
2616 Nicollet Avenue S 612-871-7878
Minneapolis, MN 55408
This controversial book details how liquor industries target the black population with its advertising.
55 pages

8384 Mistaken Beliefs About Relapse
Hazelden
15251 Pleasant Valley Road 651-257-4010
Center City, MN 55012-9640 800-328-9000
Fax: 651-213-4426
www.hazelden.org
Examines mistaken beliefs people have about relapse.
30 pages Paperback

8385 My Mind is Out to Get Me: Humor and Wisdom in Recovery
Hazelden
15251 Pleasant Valley Road 651-257-4010
Center City, MN 55012 800-328-9000
Fax: 651-213-4426
www.hazelden.org
Five hundred inspirational sayings and slogans that reflect both the lighter side of living a sober life and the profound wisdom offered in recovery. Each quote has been drawn from the wisdom of Alcoholics Anonymous.
180 pages Paperback
ISBN: 1-568380-10-0

8386 Narcotics Anonymous
Hazelden
15251 Pleasant Valley Road 651-257-4010
Center City, MN 55012-9640 800-328-9000
Fax: 651-213-4426
www.hazelden.org
Men and women describe the N.A. program and how it works.
289 pages Paperback

8387 National Conference on Drug Abuse Researcg & Practice
National Clearinghouse for Alcohol and Drug Info.
PO Box 2345
Rockville, MD 20847 800-729-6686
Offers summaries of workshops, forums, dinner speeches and sessions presented at the National Conference on Drug Abuse Research and Practice.
275 pages

8388 National Directory of Drug Abuse and Alcoholism Treatment and Programs
US National Institute On Drug Abuse
5600 Fishers Lane
Rockville, MD 20857 202-625-8400
www.nida.nih.gov
Eleven thousand listings of agencies that administer treatment and services on the federal, state and local levels.

8389 Night Light: A Book of Nighttime Meditations
Hazelden
15251 Pleasant Valley Road 651-257-4010
Center City, MN 55012-9640 800-328-9000
Fax: 651-213-4426
www.hazelden.org
Three hundred and sixty-six meditations designed to help relax and encourage prayer. Reminds readers to look to their Higher Power for strength, reassurance, comfort, and guidance.
400 pages Paperback
ISBN: 0-894863-81-9

8390 Not God: A History of Alcoholics Anonymous
Hazelden
15251 Pleasant Valley Road 651-257-4010
Center City, MN 55012-9640 800-328-9000
Fax: 651-213-4426
www.hazelden.org
Documenting AA's philosophical and social development within the larger context of American culture, this book follows the remarkable story of the evolution of a small group of Depression-era alcoholics into a worldwide movement.
436 pages Paperback
ISBN: 0-894860-65-8

8391 Occupational Therapy Practice Guidelines for Adults with Substance Use Disorders
American Occupational Therapy Association
4720 Montgomery Lane 301-652-2682
Bethesda, MD 20824-1220 Fax: 301-652-7711
TDD: 800-377-8555
www.aota.org
22 pages
ISBN: 1-569001-60-X

8392 Of Course You're Angry
Hazelden
15251 Pleasant Valley Road 651-257-4010
Center City, MN 55012-9640 800-328-9000
Fax: 651-213-4426
www.hazelden.org
Revised edition dealing with the nature and resolution of anger. Demonstrates how to make anger work in a positive and effective way that can ease, rather than exacerbate, the challenges of early recovery.
120 pages Paperback
ISBN: 1-568381-41-7

8393 One Day at a Time in Al-Anon
Al-Anon Family Group Headquarters

1600 Corporate Landing Parkway 757-563-1600
Virginia Beach, VA 23454-5617 800-425-2666
Fax: 757-563-1655
e-mail: wso@al-anon.org
www.al-anon.alateen.org

Inspirational daily readings cover various aspects of the Al-Anon philosopha and relate it to everyday situations.

376 pages
ISBN: 0-910034-21-4
Caryn Johnson, Director Communications

8394 **Operation PAR**
National Clearinghouse for Alcohol and Drug Info.
PO Box 2345
Rockville, MD 20847-2345 800-729-6686

Describes successful community alcohol and other drug abuse prevention and treatment programs.

40 pages

8395 **Parent Training is Prevention**
National Clearinghouse for Alcohol and Drug Info.
PO Box 2345
Rockville, MD 20847-2345 800-729-6686

Contains information to help communities identify and carry out programs on parenting.

184 pages

8396 **Pass it On**
Alcoholics Anonymous
World Services 212-870-3400
New York, NY 10163 Fax: 212-870-3137

The story of Bill Wilson, the co-founder of AA and the development of the Fellowship.

8397 **Passages Through Recovery**
Hazelden
15251 Pleasant Valley Road 651-257-4010
Center City, MN 55012-9640 800-328-9000
Fax: 651-213-4426
www.hazelden.org

Guides clients through the six stages of recovery.

130 pages Paperback

8398 **Peer Pressure Reversal**
Human Resource Development Press
22 Amherst Road 413-253-3488
Amherst, MA 01002-9730

8399 **Pregnancy and Exposure to Alcohol and Other Drug Use**
National Clearinghouse for Alcohol and Drug Info.
PO Box 2345
Rockville, MD 20847-2345 800-729-6686
www.health.org

This report is for health care professionals presenting the state-of-the-art information about preventing ATOD use among women of childbearing age.

8400 **Preparing for the Drug-Free Years: A Family Activity Book**
Developmental Research and Programs
130 Nickerson Street 206-286-1805
Seattle, WA 98145-1746 800-736-2630
Fax: 206-286-1462
www.drp.org

8401 **Presence at the Center**
Hazelden
15251 Pleasant Valley Road 651-257-4010
Center City, MN 55012-9640 800-328-9000
Fax: 651-213-4426
www.hazelden.org

About a new way of life that addresses transformation, change, the presence of a Higher Power, letting go of reluctance and fear, and the freedom commitment can bring.

76 pages Paperback
ISBN: 1-568380-01-1

8402 **Prevention Plus II: Tools for Creating & Sustaining a Drug-Free Community**
National Clearinghouse for Alcohol and Drug Info.
PO Box 2345
Rockville, MD 20847-2345 800-729-6686
www.health.org

Provides a framework for organizing or expanding community alcohol and other drug problem prevention activities for youth into a coordinated, complimentary system.

541 pages

8403 **Prevention Plus III: Assessing Alcohol & Other Prevention Programs**
National Clearinghouse for Alcohol and Drug Info.
PO Box 2345
Rockville, MD 20847-2345 800-729-6686
www.health.org

Provides tools and techniques for alcohol and other drug prevention, planning and implementation.

470 pages

8404 **Prevention Resource Guide: Alcohol and Other Drug Related Periodicals**
National Clearinghouse for Alcohol and Drug Info.
PO Box 2345
Rockville, MD 20847-2345 800-729-6686
www.health.org

Provides a concise annotated bibliography of journals, newsletters and other publications related to the AOD prevention field.

12 pages

8405 **Prevention Resource Guide: American Indian/Native Alaskans**
National Clearinghouse for Alcohol and Drug Info.
PO Box 2345
Rockville, MD 20847-2345 800-729-6686
www.health.org

This resource guide is a survey of current data on alcohol abuse among American Indians and Native Alaskans.

24 pages

8406 **Prevention Resource Guide: Asian and Pacific Islander Americans**
National Clearinghouse for Alcohol and Drug Info.
PO Box 2345
Rockville, MD 20847-2345 800-729-6686
www.health.org

Contains facts and figures about Asian and Pacific Islander Americans and alcohol and other drug prevention.

13 pages

8407 **Prevention Resource Guide: Elementary Youth**
National Clearinghouse for Alcohol and Drug Info.
PO Box 2345
Rockville, MD 20847-2345 800-729-6686
www.health.org

This resource guide includes materials specifically developed for youth that may be used in an elementary school setting.

23 pages

8408 **Prevention Resource Guide: Pregnant Postpartum Women and Their Infants**
National Clearinghouse for Alcohol and Drug Info.
PO Box 2345
Rockville, MD 20847-2345 800-729-6686
www.health.org

This resource guide targets health care providers, prevention program planners and counselors of pregnant and postpartum women between the ages of 15 and 44.

30 pages

8409 **Prevention Resource Guide: Secondary School Students**
National Clearinghouse for Alcohol and Drug Info.
PO Box 2345
Rockville, MD 20847-2345 800-729-6686
www.health.org

This resource guide targets teachers, administrators and program leaders who come in contact with secondary school youth.

27 pages

8410 **Prevention Resource Guide: Women**
National Clearinghouse for Alcohol and Drug Info.

PO Box 2345
Rockville, MD 20847-2345 800-729-6686
www.health.org
This resource guide provides the latest information about the effects of drugs and alcohol on women.
32 pages

8411 Prevention in Action
National Clearinghouse for Alcohol and Drug Info.
PO Box 2345
Rockville, MD 20847-2345 800-729-6686
Provides descriptions selected by representatives of national organizations and State alcohol and drug agency representatives.
20 pages

8412 Program for You
Hazelden
15251 Pleasant Valley Road 651-257-4010
Center City, MN 55012-9640 800-328-9000
Fax: 651-213-4426
www.hazelden.org
Study guide interpreting the original AA program as described in Alcoholics Anonymous and helps apply the wisdom to everyday life.
183 pages Paperback
ISBN: 0-894867-41-5

8413 Promise of a New Day: A Book of Daily Meditations
Hazelden
15251 Pleasant Valley Road 651-257-4010
Center City, MN 55012-9640 800-328-9000
Fax: 651-213-4426
www.hazelden.org
Simple, inspiring wisdom about creating and maintaining inner peace. Each of the 366 daily meditations expresses the essence of Twelve Step spirituality without the program jargon.
400 pages Paperback
ISBN: 0-894862-03-0

8414 Quit & Stay Quit: A Personal Program to Stop Smoking
Hazelden
15251 Pleasant Valley Road 651-257-4010
Center City, MN 55012-9640 800-328-9000
Fax: 651-213-4426
www.hazelden.org
Guide to nicotine recovery offerring an effective long-term program to quit by showing readers how smoking has subtly shaped their values, attitudes, and lives.
196 pages Paperback
ISBN: 1-568381-09-3

8415 Quit Smoking Manual
American Lung Association
1740 Broadway 212-315-8700
New York, NY 10019-4315
Original self-help smoking cessation manual showing the public how to quit smoking in 20 days.
64 pages

8416 Recovery Journal for Exploring Who I Am
Hazelden
15251 Pleasant Valley Road 651-257-4010
Center City, MN 55012-9640 800-328-9000
Fax: 651-213-4426
www.hazelden.org
Introduces clients to journal writing as an effective therapeutic adjunct for addiction recovery.
48 pages

8417 School Answers Back: Responding to Student Drug Use
American Council on Drug Education
204 Monroe Street
Rockville, MD 20850 800-488-3784
Provides teachers, counselors, administrators and parents with a model for schools to use in confronting drug and alcohol abuse.
145 pages

8418 Search for Serenity
Hazelden
15251 Pleasant Valley Road 651-257-4010
Center City, MN 55012-9640 800-328-9000
Fax: 651-213-4426
www.hazelden.org
Provides clients with practical inspiration to change their feelings toward people and situations.
152 pages Paperback

8419 Shame Faced
Hazelden
15251 Pleasant Valley Road 651-257-4010
Center City, MN 55012-9640 800-328-9000
Fax: 651-213-4426
www.hazelden.org
Discusses the relationship between shame and chemical dependency.
28 pages

8420 Skeptic's Guide to the 12 Steps
Hazelden
15251 Pleasant Valley Road 651-257-4010
Center City, MN 55012-9640 800-328-9000
Fax: 651-213-4426
www.hazelden.org
Investigates each of the 12 steps to gain a deeper understanding of a Higher Power.
241 pages Paperback

8421 Smoking and Pregnancy Kit for Health Care Providers
American Lung Association
1740 Broadway 212-315-8700
New York, NY 10019-4315
A program kit for health care providers designed to educate pregnant women not to smoke and to help them kick the habit.

8422 Smoking, Drinking & Illicit Drug Use
National Clearinghouse for Alcohol and Drug Info.
PO Box 2345
Rockville, MD 20847-2345 800-729-6686
Comprehensive reports representing the results of the 12th national survey on drug use and analyzing data collected from young Americans from 1975-1991.

8423 Sober But Stuck
Hazelden
15251 Pleasant Valley Road 651-257-4010
Center City, MN 55012-9640 800-328-9000
Fax: 651-213-4426
www.hazelden.org
Collection of personal stories by men and women who are long-time members of Alcoholics Anonymous. Each story shares the anecdotes and resources which helped members break through the barriers that limited their enjoyment of a sober life.
215 pages Paperback
ISBN: 1-568380-78-X

8424 Social Policy Prevention Handbook
African American Family Services
2616 Nicollet Avenue S 612-871-7878
Minneapolis, MN 55408
A manual that details IBCA's community based approach to the development of alcohol and drug abuse prevention strategies.
24 pages

8425 Staying Clean
Hazelden
15251 Pleasant Valley Road 651-257-4010
Center City, MN 55012-9640 800-328-9000
Fax: 651-213-4426
www.hazelden.org
Each section focuses on one of 33 proven ideas for staying drug-free, such as professional help, prayer, support groups and meditation.
76 pages Paperback

8426 Staying Sober
Hazelden
15251 Pleasant Valley Road 651-257-4010
Center City, MN 55012-9640 800-328-9000
Fax: 651-213-4426
www.hazelden.org

Discusses addictive diseases and its physical, psychological and social effects.
228 pages Paperback

8427 Step Zero: Getting to Recovery
Hazelden
15251 Pleasant Valley Road 651-257-4010
Center City, MN 55012-9640 800-328-9000
Fax: 651-213-4426
www.hazelden.org
Explains the concepts of Step Zero, when clients drop their defenses, begin to face themselves and start to assess their behavior and the reasons for it.
170 pages Paperback

8428 Stools and Bottles
Hazelden
15251 Pleasant Valley Road 651-257-4010
Center City, MN 55012-9640 800-328-9000
Fax: 651-213-4426
www.hazelden.org
Depicts the first Three steps using a three-legged stool and eight whiskey bottles representing character defects revealed when working Step Four.
160 pages Hardcover

8429 Substance Abuse and Physical Disability
Allen Heinemann, PhD, author
Haworth Press
10 Alice Street 607-722-5857
Binghamton, NY 13904-1580 800-429-6784
Fax: 607-722-0012
www.haworthpress.com
This book offers information on alcohol and drug abuse being a contributing factor in traumatic and disabling injuries.
1993 289 pages Hardcover
ISBN: 1-560242-89-3

8430 Success Stories from Drug-Free Schools
National Clearinghouse for Alcohol and Drug Info.
PO Box 2345
Rockville, MD 20847-2345 800-729-6686
www.health.org
Salutes the 107 schools honored by the US Department of Education's Drug-Free Recognition Program.
59 pages

8431 Tackling Alcohol Problems on Campus: Tools for Media Advocacy
National Clearinghouse for Alcohol and Drug Info.
PO Box 2345
Rockville, MD 20847-2345 800-729-6686
Reviews the role of alcohol on campus and shows how to use the media to get attention and support.
38 pages

8432 Team Up for Drug Prevention with America's Young Athletes
Drug Enforcement Administration, Demand Reduction
1405 I Street NW
Washington, DC 20537-0001 202-307-5550
www.usdoj.gov/dea/programs/demand.htm

8433 Ten Steps to Help Your Child Say No: A Parent's Guide
National Clearinghouse for Alcohol and Drug Info.
PO Box 2345
Rockville, MD 20847-2345 800-729-6686

8434 Things My Sponsors Taught Me
Hazelden
15251 Pleasant Valley Road 651-257-4010
Center City, MN 55012-9640 800-328-9000
Fax: 651-213-4426
www.hazelden.org
Features AA philosophy, quotes, slogans and refreshing reminders.
76 pages Paperback

8435 Today I Will Do One Thing: Daily Readings for Awareness & Hope
Hazelden
15251 Pleasant Valley Road 651-257-4010
Center City, MN 55012-9640 800-328-9000
Fax: 651-213-4426
www.hazelden.org
Specially designed to integrate recovery from addiction with the treatment of emotional or psychiatric illness. Each meditation focuses on a task or goal to be completed each day.
400 pages Paperback
ISBN: 1-568380-83-6

8436 Today's Gift
Hazelden
15251 Pleasant Valley Road 651-257-4010
Center City, MN 55012-9640 800-328-9000
Fax: 651-213-4426
www.hazelden.org
Inspiring meditations bringing families together and strengthening family bonds.
400 pages Paperback

8437 Touchstones
Hazelden
15251 Pleasant Valley Road 651-257-4010
Center City, MN 55012-9640 800-328-9000
Fax: 651-213-4426
www.hazelden.org
A book of daily meditations for men in the Twelve-Step program.
400 pages Paperback

8438 Turnabout
Women for Sobriety
PO Box 618 215-536-8026
Quakertown, PA 18951-0618 Fax: 215-536-8026
e-mail: WFSobriey@aol.com
www.mediapulse.com/wfs/
This is the story of the founder of Women for Sobriety and her struggle to quit drinking.
183 pages

8439 Turning Awareness Into Action: What Your Community Can Do About Drug Use
National Clearinghouse for Alcohol and Drug Info.
PO Box 2345
Rockville, MD 20847-2345 800-729-6686
www.health.org
This bilingual booklet is designed to show leaders at the grassroots level how to make the most of their talents and their community's resources.
73 pages

8440 Twelve Step Sponsorship: How it Works
Hazelden
15251 Pleasant Valley Road 651-257-4010
Center City, MN 55012-9640 800-328-9000
Fax: 651-213-4426
www.hazelden.org
Complete handbook for working with a newcomer. Based on Twelve Step traditions and knowledge passed orally through the generations, this working manual defines the sponsorship role and guides sponsors through the rewards and pitfalls of reaching out to help new program members.
260 pages Paperback
ISBN: 1-568381-22-0

8441 Twelve Steps and Traditions
Hazelden
15251 Pleasant Valley Road 651-257-4010
Center City, MN 55012-9640 800-328-9000
Fax: 651-213-4426
www.hazelden.org
Outlines the core principles by which AA members recover and by which the fellowship functions.
192 pages Paperback

8442 Twelve Steps and Twelve Traditions
Alcoholics Anonymous
PO Box 459 212-870-3400
New York, NY 10163-0459 Fax: 212-870-3137
Twenty-four essays on the Steps and Traditions that discuss the principles of individual recovery and group unity.

8443 Twelve Steps and Twelve Traditions for Alateen
Al-Anon Family Group Headquarters
1600 Corporate Landing Parkway 757-563-1600
Virginia Beach, VA 23454-5617 800-425-2666
Fax: 757-563-1655
e-mail: wso@al-anon.org
www.al-anon.alateen.org
Questions, discussions and personal reflections of Alateen members.
60 pages
Caryn Johnson, Director Communications

8444 Twelve Steps for Everyone...Who Really Wants Them
Hazelden
15251 Pleasant Valley Road 651-257-4010
Center City, MN 55012-9640 800-328-9000
Fax: 651-213-4426
www.hazelden.org
A basic primer outlining how spiritual and emotional health can be found by working and living the Twelve Steps. Emphasizes that the Twelve Steps are for anyone who wants to change.
208 pages Paperback
ISBN: 1-568380-47-X

8445 Twelve Steps of Alcoholics Anonymous
Hazelden
15251 Pleasant Valley Road 651-257-4010
Center City, MN 55012-9640 800-328-9000
Fax: 651-213-4426
www.hazelden.org
A series of short discussions that interpret each of the Twelve Steps, from admission of individual powerlessness outlined in Step One to the moral inventory of Step Four and the spiritual awakening of Step Twelve.
130 pages Paperback
ISBN: 0-894869-04-3

8446 Twenty Four Hours a Day
Hazelden
15251 Pleasant Valley Road 651-257-4010
Center City, MN 55012-9640 800-328-9000
Fax: 651-213-4426
www.hazelden.org
Offers a resource that serves as a solid foundation in a spiritual program. Simple, yet effective resource that helps clients relate to the Twelve-Step program.
400 pages Paperback

8447 Walk in Dry Places
Hazelden
15251 Pleasant Valley Road 651-257-4010
Center City, MN 55012-9640 800-328-9000
Fax: 651-213-4426
www.hazelden.org
Core-recovery book filled with practical spiritual advice and time-honored Twelve Step philosophy. Insightful explorations of the deeper issues of living in recovery address the daily concerns of those new to life without alcoholism, as well as those with long-term sobriety.
400 pages Paperback
ISBN: 1-568381-27-1

8448 Wasted Tales of a Gen X Drunk
Hazelden
15251 Pleasant Valley Road 651-257-4010
Center City, MN 55012-9640 800-328-9000
Fax: 651-213-4426
www.hazelden.org
Cynicism and black humor underscore this hard-edged memoir of a young journalist's alcoholism and subsequent recovery. Captures the ethos of a generation often suspicious and alienated by the Twelve-Step approach.
250 pages Cloth
ISBN: 1-568381-42-5

8449 What Works: Schools Without Drugs
National Clearinghouse for Alcohol and Drug Info.
PO Box 2345
Rockville, MD 20847-2345 800-729-6686

8450 What You Can Do About Drug Use in America
National Clearinghouse for Alcohol and Drug Info.
PO Box 2345 301-468-2600
Rockville, MD 20847-2345 800-729-6686
www.health.org
Offers information on what parents and professionals can do to prevent drug use in America.

8451 Why Am I Afraid to Tell You Who I Am?
Hazelden
15251 Pleasant Valley Road 651-257-4010
Center City, MN 55012-9640 800-328-9000
Fax: 651-213-4426
www.hazelden.org
Outlines types of interpersonal relationships.

8452 Woman's Way Through the Twelve Steps
Hazelden
15251 Pleasant Valley Road 651-257-4010
Center City, MN 55012-9640 800-328-9000
Fax: 651-213-4426
www.hazelden.org
How women understnad and work the Twelve Steps of AA, including reflections of spirituality, powerlessness, and the emergence of a sense of the feminine soul.
228 pages Paperback
ISBN: 0-894869-93-0

8453 Young Teens: Who They Are and How to Talk to Them About Alcohol & Drugs
National Clearinghouse for Alcohol and Drug Info.
PO Box 2345
Rockville, MD 20847-2345 800-729-6686
Offers information on how parents, educators and concerned citizens can work together to help youngsters avoid alcohol and other drugs by understanding the risks and dangers.
57 pages

Children's Books

8454 Alcoholism
Franklin Watts Grolier
90 Old Sherman Tpke 203-797-3500
Danbury, CT 06816-0001 800-621-1115
Fax: 203-797-3197
www.grolier.com
This comprehensive overview describes the different types of alcoholism, the addictive personality and the warning signs.
112 pages Grades 7-12
ISBN: 0-531108-79-1

8455 Alcoholism and the Family
Franklin Watts Grolier
90 Old Sherman Tpke 203-797-3500
Danbury, CT 06816-0001 800-621-1115
Fax: 203-797-3197
www.grolier.com
This book, after discussing what alcoholism is, its effects on health and behavior modifications through alcohol, starts addressing one of the most important aspects of alcoholism, the effects on the family.
32 pages Grades 3-5
ISBN: 0-531125-48-3

8456 America's War on Drugs
Franklin Watts Grolier
90 Old Sherman Tpke 203-797-3500
Danbury, CT 06816 800-621-1115
Fax: 203-797-3197
www.grolier.com
An overview of the United States' attempts to combat illegal drugs on the supply side, from stopping the supply of drugs into the country.
160 pages Grades 7-12
ISBN: 0-531109-54-2

8457 Buzzy's Rebound
National Clearinghouse for Alcohol and Drug Info.

PO Box 2345
Rockville, MD 20847-2345 800-729-6686
A Fat Albert comic book that describes the pressure on a new kid in town to drink.
18 pages

8458 Caffeine and Nicotine
Hazelden
15251 Pleasant Valley Road 651-257-4010
Center City, MN 55012-9640 800-328-9000
Fax: 651-213-4426
www.hazelden.org
Simple, clear, and accurate presentation of nicotine and caffeine dependency. How to avoid these addictions, and why teens ought to do so.
64 pages Paperback
ISBN: 1-568381-68-9

8459 Christy's Chance
Crestridge Corporate Center
10155 York Road 410-628-0390
Hunt Valley, MD 21030 Fax: 410-628-0398
e-mail: cboyce@networkpub.com
www.networkpub.com
A story geared to younger teens that allows the reader to make a nonuse decision about marijuana.

8460 Cocaine
Hazelden
15251 Pleasant Valley Road 651-257-4010
Center City, MN 55012-9640 800-328-9000
Fax: 651-213-4426
www.hazelden.org
The information that teens need to stay drug-free, promoting understanding of the ramifications, both social and personal.
64 pages Paperback
ISBN: 1-568381-64-6

8461 Coping with Codependency
Hazelden
15251 Pleasant Valley Road 651-257-4010
Center City, MN 55012-9640 800-328-9000
Fax: 651-213-4426
www.hazelden.org
Explains the cycle of codependency, describes its destructive effects on all involved, and suggests ways to break free and live in more healthy relationships.
64 pages Paperback
ISBN: 1-568381-85-9

8462 Coping with Depression
Hazelden
15251 Pleasant Valley Road 651-257-4010
Center City, MN 55012-9640 800-328-9000
Fax: 651-213-4426
www.hazelden.org
Practical ways to cope with depression. Provides clear suggestions for handling life's downers, and encourages readers to seek professional help when they feel they can't deal with problems themselves.
64 pages Paperback
ISBN: 1-568381-79-4

8463 Coping with Drinking and Driving
Hazelden
15251 Pleasant Valley Road 651-257-4010
Center City, MN 55012-9640 800-328-9000
Fax: 651-213-4426
www.hazelden.org
Addressing teens' illusion of invulnerability, the author describes exactly how alcohol affects the body and one's driving skills, emphasizing that teens are not immune to alcohol's effects.
64 pages Paperback
ISBN: 1-568381-80-8

8464 Coping with Peer Pressure
Hazelden
15251 Pleasant Valley Road 651-257-4010
Center City, MN 55012-9640 800-328-9000
Fax: 651-213-4426
www.hazelden.org
Discussion of the positive and negative effects that members of a peer group can have on each other and explores ways teens can handle the pressure they face.
64 pages Paperback
ISBN: 1-568381-83-2

8465 Coping with Stress
Hazelden
15251 Pleasant Valley Road 651-257-4010
Center City, MN 55012-9640 800-328-9000
Fax: 651-213-4426
www.hazelden.org
Outlines positive strategies to help teens learn to cope more effectively with stress, rather than turning to destructive outlets such as drugs and even suicide.
64 pages Paperback
ISBN: 1-568381-76-X

8466 Coping with a Drug-Abusing Parent
Hazelden
15251 Pleasant Valley Road 651-257-4010
Center City, MN 55012-9640 800-328-9000
Fax: 651-213-4426
www.hazelden.org
Describes steps that teens, powerless to stop a drug-abusing parent from continuing on that destructive path, can take to to learn to take better care of themselves. Includes coping strategies and who to call for help.
64 pages Paperback
ISBN: 1-568381-78-6

8467 Crack Down on Drugs
National Clearinghouse for Alcohol and Drug Info.
PO Box 2345
Rockville, MD 20847 800-729-6686
Coloring book for children featuring McGruff, the crime dog, that teaches young children the importance of refusing alcohol and drug abuse.
Ages 5-8

8468 Different Like Me: A Book for Teens Who Worry About Their Parents' Using
Johnson Institute
Ohms Lane 612-831-1630
Edina, MN
Provides support and information for teens who are concerned, confused, scared and angry because their parents abuse alcohol and other drugs.
110 pages

8469 Drug Abuse: The Impact on Society
Franklin Watts Grolier
90 Old Sherman Tpke 203-797-3500
Danbury, CT 06816 800-621-1115
Fax: 203-797-3197
www.grolier.com
Discusses all major aspects of illegal drug usage and the health and personality effects they cause.
144 pages Grades 7-12
ISBN: 0-531105-79-2

8470 Drugs and AIDS
Hazelden
15251 Pleasant Valley Road 651-257-4010
Center City, MN 55012-9640 800-328-9000
Fax: 651-213-4426
www.hazelden.org
Covers many topics through case studies, including the effects of the disease on the body, transmission, homosexuality, condom use, drug treatment, and peer pressure.
64 pages Paperback
ISBN: 1-568381-72-7

8471 Drugs and Anger
Hazelden

15251 Pleasant Valley Road 651-257-4010
Center City, MN 55012-9640 800-328-9000
Fax: 651-213-4426
www.hazelden.org

True-to-life scenarios and practical techniques found here can help teens cope constructively with their anger.
64 pages Paperback
ISBN: 1-568381-73-5

8472 **Drugs and Depression**
Hazelden
15251 Pleasant Valley Road 651-257-4010
Center City, MN 55012-9640 800-328-9000
Fax: 651-213-4426
www.hazelden.org

Describes positive ways of handling depression, as well as suggesting resources for receiving assistance.
64 pages Paperback
ISBN: 1-568381-74-3

8473 **Drugs and Domestic Violence**
Hazelden
15251 Pleasant Valley Road 651-257-4010
Center City, MN 55012-9640 800-328-9000
Fax: 651-213-4426
www.hazelden.org

Describes valuable coping tactics that can help teens stay safe in situations involving domestic violence and drug use.
64 pages Paperback
ISBN: 1-568381-75-1

8474 **Drugs and Your Friends**
Hazelden
15251 Pleasant Valley Road 651-257-4010
Center City, MN 55012-9640 800-328-9000
Fax: 651-213-4426
www.hazelden.org

Helps teens make sound decisions on vital choices and provides many suggestions for resisting peer pressure.
64 pages Paperback
ISBN: 1-568381-70-0

8475 **Drugs and Your Parents**
Hazelden
15251 Pleasant Valley Road 651-257-4010
Center City, MN 55012-9640 800-328-9000
Fax: 651-213-4426
www.hazelden.org

Practical advice for teenage children of parents addicted to alcohol or other drugs. How to cope initially with the situation as well as long-term survival strategies.
64 pages Paperback
ISBN: 1-568381-71-9

8476 **Drugs in the Body: Effects of Abuse**
Franklin Watts Grolier
90 Old Sherman Tpke 203-797-3500
Danbury, CT 06816 800-621-1115
Fax: 203-797-3197
www.grolier.com

Traces the effects of cocaine and crack, opium, morphine, heroine, marijuana and hashish, LSD and PCP in a person's system. Special emphasis is placed on long-term adverse effects in the body.
144 pages Grades 7-12
ISBN: 0-531125-07-6

8477 **Elephant in the Living Room: The Children's Book**
Hazelden
15251 Pleasant Valley Road 651-257-4010
Center City, MN 55012-9640 800-328-9000
Fax: 651-213-4426
www.hazelden.org

An activity book to help children understand and cope with the problem of chemical dependency in the family.
88 pages Paperback
ISBN: 1-568380-35-6

8478 **Facts on Alcohol**
Franklin Watts Grolier
90 Old Sherman Tpke 203-797-3500
Danbury, CT 06816 800-621-1115
Fax: 203-797-3197
www.grolier.com

Offers various information on alcohol so young children can have an opportunity to form their own opinions and the ability to make their own decisions when it comes to alcoholism.
32 pages Grades 5-7
ISBN: 0-531108-21-0

8479 **Facts on the Crack and Cocaine Epidemic**
Franklin Watts Grolier
90 Old Sherman Tpke 203-797-3500
Danbury, CT 06816 800-621-1115
Fax: 203-797-3197
www.grolier.com

Offers young children information on these deadly drugs to help them become informed.
32 pages Grades 5-7
ISBN: 0-531108-22-8

8480 **Feed Your Head**
Hazelden
15251 Pleasant Valley Road 651-257-4010
Center City, MN 55012-9640 800-328-9000
Fax: 651-213-4426
www.hazelden.org

Offers practical guidance for young people.
137 pages Paperback

8481 **Gangs and Drugs**
Hazelden
15251 Pleasant Valley Road 651-257-4010
Center City, MN 55012-9640 800-328-9000
Fax: 651-213-4426
www.hazelden.org

Encouraging and helpful message that goes beyond Just say no.
240 pages Paperback
ISBN: 1-568381-35-2

8482 **How to Say No and Keep Your Friends**
Hazelden
15251 Pleasant Valley Road 651-257-4010
Center City, MN 55012-9640 800-328-9000
Fax: 651-213-4426
www.hazelden.org

Ideas to help teens deal with negative peer pressure.
112 pages

8483 **I Can Talk About What Hurts**
Hazelden
15251 Pleasant Valley Road 651-257-4010
Center City, MN 55012-9640 800-328-9000
Fax: 651-213-4426
www.hazelden.org

Written and illustrated for children whose lives have been affected by someone else's chemical dependency.
56 pages Paperback

8484 **I Wish Daddy Didn't Drink So Much**
Judith Vigna, author
Albert Whitman & Company
6340 Oakton Street 847-581-0033
Morton Grove, IL 60053-2723 800-255-7675
Fax: 847-581-0039
e-mail: mail@awhitmanco.com
www.albertwhitman.com

A young girl shres her feelings and frustrations about her alcoholic father's behavior.
1993 32 pages Grades P-3
ISBN: 0-807535-23-0
Pat McPartland, Sales
Joe Campbell, Customer Service

8485 **If Drugs Are So Bad, Why Do So Many People Use Them?**
Hazelden
15251 Pleasant Valley Road 651-257-4010
Center City, MN 55012-9640 800-328-9000
Fax: 651-213-4426
www.hazelden.org

Uses direct language to explain drugs and their effects.
29 pages Grades 5-9

8486 In a Perfect World
Hazelden
15251 Pleasant Valley Road
Center City, MN 55012-9640
651-257-4010
800-328-9000
Fax: 651-213-4426
www.hazelden.org
Kevin thinks his world will be perfect when his father stops drinking, but Kevin is in for a few surprises.
160 pages Softcover

8487 Inhalants
Hazelden
15251 Pleasant Valley Road
Center City, MN 55012-9640
651-257-4010
800-328-9000
Fax: 651-213-4426
www.hazelden.org
Clear, straightforward explanation of the dangers and consequences of using seemingly harmless chemicals, such as model airplane glue, hair spray, whipping cream, and cleaning and lighter fluids, as well as sources of help for those who need it.
64 pages Paperback
ISBN: 1-568381-69-7

8488 Inside Out
Hazelden
15251 Pleasant Valley Road
Center City, MN 55012-9640
651-257-4010
800-328-9000
Fax: 651-213-4426
www.hazelden.org
Offers open-ended sentences for readers to fill in their responses.
97 pages Paperback

8489 Kids and Alcohol: Get High on Life
Health Communications
1721 Blount Road
Pompano Beach, FL 33069
954-360-0909
A workbook designed to help children make important decisions in their lives and feel good about themselves.
Ages 11-14

8490 Let's Talk About Drug Abuse
Rosen Publishing Group's PowerKids Press
29 E 21st Street
New York, NY 10010
212-777-3017
800-237-9932
Fax: 888-436-4643
e-mail: customerservice@rosenpub.com
www.rosenpublishing.com
A first step in a child's education about the dangers of drugs. Recommended for grade K-4.

ISBN: 0-823923-02-9
Anna Kreiner, Author

8491 McGruff's Surprise Party
National Clearinghouse for Alcohol and Drug Info.
PO Box 2345
Rockville, MD 20847-2345
800-729-6686
A comic book that helps children understand the importance of refusing alcohol and other drugs.
14 pages Ages 8-10

8492 My Body is My House
Hazelden
15251 Pleasant Valley Road
Center City, MN 55012
651-257-4010
800-328-9000
Fax: 651-213-4426
www.hazelden.org
A coloring book about alcohol, drugs and health.
16 pages

8493 Sad Story of Mary Wanna or How Marijuana Harms You
Woodmere Press
PO Box 20190
New York, NY 10025-1518
Activity book for children that contains pictures of the damage that marijuana does to the body
40 pages Grades 1-4

8494 Should Drugs Be Legalized?
Franklin Watts Grolier
90 Old Sherman Tpke
Danbury, CT 06816-0001
203-797-3500
800-621-1115
Fax: 203-797-3197
www.grolier.com
Presents a discussion of this controversial subject.
160 pages Grades 7-12

8495 Smoking-At Issues Series
Greenhaven Press
Thomson Gale
Farmington Hills, MI 48333-9187
800-877-4253
Fax: 800-414-5043
e-mail: gale.customerservice@thomson.com
www.gale.com/greenhaven
Written in a straightforward manner, this book answers questions most young adults are asking regarding smoking and health.

ISBN: 0-737701-57-9

8496 Stand Strong
African American Family Services
2616 Nicollet Avenue S
Minneapolis, MN 55408
612-871-7878
Comic book prevention for young adults. Profiles two African-American teens as they go through the hazards and risks of drug use and sexual behavior.
16 pages

8497 Summer of Sassy Jo
Houghton Mifflin
Wayside Road
Burlington, MA 01803
800-225-3362
A story of a thirteen-year-old girl faced with reconciliation with her recovered alcoholic mother after eight years of abandonment.
192 pages Grades 7+
ISBN: 0-395669-56-1

8498 Teen Alcoholism-Teen Issues
Lucent Books
Thomson Gale
San Diego, CA 48333-9187
800-877-4253
Fax: 800-414-5043
e-mail: gale.customerservice@thomson.com
www.gale.com/lucent
Offers readable interviews for reports and answers the most frequently asked questions about alcohol.

ISBN: 1-590185-01-3

8499 Teen Guide to Pregnancy, Drugs and Smoking
Franklin Watts Grolier
90 Old Sherman Tpke
Danbury, CT 06816-0001
203-797-3500
800-621-1115
Fax: 203-797-3197
www.grolier.com
Outlines the risks of smoking and drug taking while pregnant and answers teenagers' questions about the use of legal, illegal and prescription drugs.
64 pages Grades 9-12
ISBN: 0-531108-35-0

8500 Understanding Drugs
Franklin Watts Grolier
90 Old Sherman Tpke
Danbury, CT 06816-0001
203-797-3500
800-621-1115
Fax: 203-797-3197
www.grolier.com
This series of books explains the current drug phenomenon at a high-interest, low-vocabulary level. Gives in-depth information about all aspects of commonly abused substances, including their negative mental, physical and social effects. Each book features photographs, diagrams, a glossary, an index and list of addresses for futher information and help. Set of seven volumes.
Grades 5-7

8501 Violence and Drugs
Franklin Watts Grolier

90 Old Sherman Tpke 203-797-3500
Danbury, CT 06816-0001 800-621-1115
Fax: 203-797-3197
www.grolier.com
This informative book studies the fascinating link between drug use and violent behavior.
112 pages Grades 9-12
ISBN: 0-531108-18-0

8502 What's Drunk Mama?
Al-Anon Family Group Headquarters
1600 Corporate Landing Parkway 757-563-1600
Virginia Beach, VA 23454-5617 800-425-2666
Fax: 757-563-1655
e-mail: wso@al-anon.org
www.al-anon.alateen.org
Large print illustrated booklet for use as a shared reading experience to help younger children understand alcoholism.
32 pages
Caryn Johnson, Director Communications

8503 Whiskers Says No to Drugs
Weekly Reader Skills Books
245 Long Hill Road
Middletown, CT 06457-4063 860-346-7157
www.weeklyreader.com
This book contains stories and follow-up activities for students to provide information and form attitudes before they face peer pressure to experiment.
Grades 2-3

8504 Why Do People Drink Alcohol?
Franklin Watts Grolier
90 Old Sherman Tpke 203-797-3500
Danbury, CT 06816-0001 800-621-1115
Fax: 203-797-3197
www.grolier.com
Answers young children's questions about alcoholism.
32 pages Grades 3-5
ISBN: 0-531171-34-5

8505 Why Do People Smoke?
Franklin Watts Grolier
90 Old Sherman Tpke 203-797-3500
Danbury, CT 06816-0001 800-621-1115
Fax: 203-797-3197
www.grolier.com
Raises and answers questions of specific interest to seven-to-ten year olds about smoking.
32 pages Grades 3-5
ISBN: 0-531171-92-2

8506 Why Do People Take Drugs?
Franklin Watts Grolier
90 Old Sherman Tpke 203-797-3500
Danbury, CT 06816-0001 800-621-1115
Fax: 203-797-3197
www.grolier.com
Raises important questions and offers some answers for young children on the aspects and everyday living with a drug addiction.
32 pages Grades 3-5
ISBN: 0-531171-13-2

8507 Winning the Battle Against Drugs: Rehabilitation Programs
Franklin Watts Grolier
90 Old Sherman Tpke 203-797-3500
Danbury, CT 06816-0001 800-621-1115
Fax: 203-797-3197
www.grolier.com
Programs contained in this book will help adolescents see that drug and alcohol addiction can be successfully treated.
160 pages Grades 7-12
ISBN: 0-531110-63-0

8508 Young Person's Guide to the Twelve Steps
Hazelden
15251 Pleasant Valley Road 651-257-4010
Center City, MN 55012-9640 800-328-9000
Fax: 651-213-4426
www.hazelden.org
Explains the Twelve Steps in the best way young people can understand: in their own language.
168 pages Paperback

8509 Young, Sober & Free
Hazelden
15251 Pleasant Valley Road 651-257-4010
Center City, MN 55012-9640 800-328-9000
Fax: 651-213-4426
www.hazelden.org
Features young peoples' personal experiences of living with addiction.
137 pages Paperback

Magazines

8510 ACAP Recap
American Council on Alcohol Problems
3426 Bridgeland Drive 314-739-5944
Bridgeton, MO 63044-2603 Fax: 314-739-0848
Offers information on organization activities and events, updates on resources and publications and legislative information for affiliate executives.
Monthly

8511 American Issue
American Council on Alcohol Problems
3426 Bridgeland Drive 314-739-5944
Bridgeton, MO 63044-2603 Fax: 314-739-0848
Offered to contributors of the organization.
Monthly

8512 Drug Abuse Update
2296 Henderson Mill Road 770-934-6364
Atlanta, GA 30345-2739
A journal of news and information for persons interested in drug prevention.
Quarterly

8513 Lead Line
Grapevine
PO Box 1980 212-870-3400
New York, NY 10163-1980 Fax: 212-870-3301
AA members all over the world communicate with each other through the pages of this magazine. It contains: insight into how AAs stay sober; readers' views; old-timers corner, beginners meeting, youth enjoying sobriety, and spotlight on service.
Monthly

Newsletters

8514 ADPA Professional
Alcohol/Drug Problems Association of North America
307 N Main Street 314-589-6702
St. Charles, MO 63301 Fax: 314-940-2358
Offers information to members on events, conferences and activities, reviews the newest resources and technology pertaining to alcoholism and drug addiction.

8515 Drug-Free Workplace Educator
American Council on Drug Education
204 Monroe Street
Rockville, MD 20850-4425 800-488-3784
Offers continuing education for employers and their supervisors responsible for substance abuse prevention. Practical articles feature information to help employers design, implement and maintain a drug-free workplace.
BiMonthly

8516 Just Say Notes
Just Say No International
2101 Webster Street 510-451-6666
Oakland, CA 94612-3065 800-258-2766
Offers information on the organizations, activities, programs, conferences and events.
BiMonthly

8517 **RID-USA Newsletter**
Remove Intoxicated Drivers (RID-USA)
PO Box 520 518-393-4357
Schenectady, NY 12301-0520 Fax: 518-370-4917
Membership news.
3x Year
Doris Aiken, President & CEO

8518 **Sobering Thoughts**
Women for Sobriety
PO Box 618 215-536-8026
Quakertown, PA 18951-0618 800-333-1606
Fax: 215-536-8026
e-mail: NewLife@nni.comcom
wwww.womenforsobriety.com
A monthly membership newsletter for women with an addiction problem who wish for recovery and start a new life.
16 pages Monthly
Rebecca Fenner, Director

8519 **Substance Abuse Funding News**
CD Publications
8204 Fenton Street 301-588-6380
Silver Spring, MD 20910-4571 800-666-6380
Fax: 301-588-6385
e-mail: chf@cdpublications.com
www.cdpublications.com
Detailed coverage of private and federal funding opportunities for alcohol, tobacco and drug abuse programs. Plus advice on successful grantseeking strategies and news affecting your programs.
18 pages BiWeekly
Mike Gerecht, Publisher
Amy Bernstein, Editor

Pamphlets

8520 **AA Member: Medications and Other Drugs**
Alcoholics Anonymous
PO Box 459 212-870-3400
New York, NY 10163-0459 Fax: 212-870-3137
Report from a group of doctors in Alcoholics Anonymous.

8521 **AA Service Manual: Twelve Concepts for World Service**
Alcoholics Anonymous
PO Box 459 212-870-3400
New York, NY 10163-0459 Fax: 212-870-3137
This manual opens with a history of AA services.

8522 **AA and the Armed Services**
Alcoholics Anonymous
PO Box 459 212-870-3400
New York, NY 10163-0459 Fax: 212-870-3137
Personal stories tell how men and women in the military can beat a drinking problem.

8523 **AA and the Gay/Lesbian Alcoholic**
Alcoholics Anonymous
PO Box 459 212-870-3400
New York, NY 10163-0459 Fax: 212-870-3137
Excerpts from experience, strength and hope of sober gay and lesbian alcoholics.

8524 **AA as a Resource for Health Care Professionals**
Alcoholics Anonymous
PO Box 459 212-870-3400
New York, NY 10163-0459 Fax: 212-870-3137
Information about the Fellowship and describes some approaches that health care professionals use in referring problem drinkers to AA.

8525 **AA for the Native North American**
Alcoholics Anonymous
PO Box 459 212-870-3400
New York, NY 10163-0459 Fax: 212-870-3137
Addressed to and contains stories by Native American AA members.

8526 **AA for the Woman**
Alcoholics Anonymous
PO Box 459 212-870-3400
New York, NY 10163-0459 Fax: 212-870-3137
Relates the experiences of alcoholic women, all ages and from all walks of life.

8527 **AA in Correctional Facilities**
Alcoholics Anonymous
PO Box 459 212-870-3400
New York, NY 10163-0459 Fax: 212-870-3137
Experience based on the functioning of AA groups in prisons, with institutional opinions recommending AA as a helpful ally.

8528 **AA in Treatment Facilities**
Alcoholics Anonymous
PO Box 459 212-870-3400
New York, NY 10163-0459 Fax: 212-870-3137
Shares experiences of treatment facility administrators and of AA's who have carried the message into these facilities.

8529 **Acceptance**
Hazelden
15251 Pleasant Valley Road 651-257-4010
Center City, MN 55012-9640 800-328-9000
Fax: 651-213-4426
www.hazelden.org
Addresses issues such as facing life, the kindness of God, suffering and contentment.

8530 **Adult Children of Alcoholics Newcomer Packet**
Al-Anon Family Group Headquarters
1600 Corporate Landing Parkway 757-563-1600
Virginia Beach, VA 23454-5617 800-425-2666
Fax: 757-563-1655
e-mail: wso@al-anon.org
www.al-anon.alateen.org
For those who have grown up with parental alcoholism, this is a loving introduction to Al-Anon and the twelve steps.
9 pieces
Caryn Johnson, Director Communications

8531 **African Americans in Treatment**
Hazelden
15251 Pleasant Valley Road 651-257-4010
Center City, MN 55012 800-328-9000
Fax: 651-213-4426
www.hazelden.org
Helps African American clients understand treatment from a cultural standpoint.
23 pages

8532 **Al-Anon Newcomers Packet**
Al-Anon Family Group Headquarters
1600 Corporate Landing Parkway 757-563-1600
Virginia Beach, VA 23454-5617 800-425-2666
Fax: 757-563-1655
e-mail: wso@al-anon.org
www.al-anon.alateen.org
Material specifically for the newcomer to Al-Anon packed in a handsome sleeve.
8 pieces
Caryn Johnson, Director Communications

8533 **Al-Anon Spoken Here**
Al-Anon Family Group Headquarters
1600 Corporate Landing Parkway 757-563-1600
Virginia Beach, VA 23454-5617 800-425-2666
Fax: 757-563-1655
e-mail: wso@al-anon.org
www.al-anon.alateen.org
Why are Al-Anon meetings the way they are? Questions and answers that lead to a better understanding of the importance of keeping Al-Anon principles.
8 pages
Caryn Johnson, Director Communications

8534 **Al-Anon is for Men**
Al-Anon Family Group Headquarters

1600 Corporate Landing Parkway 757-563-1600
Virginia Beach, VA 23454-5617 800-425-2666
Fax: 757-563-1655
e-mail: wso@al-anon.org
www.al-anon.alateen.org

Straight forward questions to help men identify their reactions to alcoholism in another person.
6 pages
Caryn Johnson, Director Communications

8535 Al-Anon, You and the Alcoholic
Al-Anon Family Group Headquarters
1600 Corporate Landing Parkway 757-563-1600
Virginia Beach, VA 23454-5617 800-425-2666
Fax: 757-563-1655
e-mail: wso@al-anon.org
www.al-anon.alateen.org

Answers the most frequently asked questions about Al-Anon and how it helps families deal with problems brought about by alcoholism.
12 pages
Caryn Johnson, Director Communications

8536 Alateen Newcomer Packet
Al-Anon Family Group Headquarters
1600 Corporate Landing Parkway 757-563-1600
Virginia Beach, VA 23454-5617 800-425-2666
Fax: 757-563-1655
e-mail: wso@al-anon.org
www.al-anon.alateen.org

Helpful leaflets assembled in a sleeve ready to give to the new young member.
13 pieces
Caryn Johnson, Director Communications

8537 Alcohol Alert #11: Estimating the Cost of Alcohol Abuse
National Clearinghouse for Alcohol and Drug Info.
PO Box 2345
Rockville, MD 20847-2345 800-729-6686
www.health.org

Discusses the various problems of estimating the cost of alcohol abuse.

8538 Alcohol Alert #15: Alcohol and AIDS
National Clearinghouse for Alcohol and Drug Info.
PO Box 2345
Rockville, MD 20847-2345 800-729-6686
www.health.org

Discusses the relationship between alcohol consumption and HIV infection and AIDS.

8539 Alcohol Alert #16: Moderate Drinking
National Clearinghouse for Alcohol and Drug Info.
PO Box 2345
Rockville, MD 20847-2345 800-729-6686
www.health.org

Defines moderate drinking and explores the benefits and risks associated with moderate drinking.

8540 Alcohol Alert #17: Treatment Outcome Research
National Clearinghouse for Alcohol and Drug Info.
PO Box 2345
Rockville, MD 20847-2345 800-729-6686
www.health.org

Discusses purpose, methodology, randomization, blinding, followup and what treatment outcome research reveals.

8541 Alcohol Alert #18: The Genetics of Alcoholism
National Clearinghouse for Alcohol and Drug Info.
PO Box 2345
Rockville, MD 20847-2345 800-729-6686
www.health.org

Presents the results of studies that investigate the role of genes and the environment in the development of alcoholism.

8542 Alcohol Alert #21: Alcohol and Cancer
National Clearinghouse for Alcohol and Drug Info.
PO Box 2345
Rockville, MD 20847-2345 800-729-6686
www.health.org

8543 Alcohol Alert #23: Alcohol and Minorities
National Clearinghouse for Alcohol and Drug Info.
PO Box 2345
Rockville, MD 20847-2345 800-729-6686
www.health.org

8544 Alcohol Alert #24: Animal Models in Alcohol Research
National Clearinghouse for Alcohol and Drug Info.
PO Box 2345
Rockville, MD 20847-2345 800-729-6686
www.health.org

8545 Alcohol Alert #25: Alcohol-Related Impairment
National Clearinghouse for Alcohol and Drug Info.
PO Box 2345
Rockville, MD 20847-2345 800-729-6686
www.health.org

8546 Alcohol Alert #26: Alcohol and Hormones
National Clearinghouse for Alcohol and Drug Info.
PO Box 2345
Rockville, MD 20847-2345 800-729-6686
www.health.org

8547 Alcohol Alert #27: Alcohol Medication Interactions
National Clearinghouse for Alcohol and Drug Info.
PO Box 2345
Rockville, MD 20847-2345 800-729-6686
www.health.org

8548 Alcohol and Drug Abuse in Black America: A Guide for Community Action
African American Family Services
2616 Nicollet Avenue S 612-871-7878
Minneapolis, MN 55408

A booklet giving a description of the history and the current manifestations of alcohol and drug problems in Black America with a discussion of strategies for fundamental change.
24 pages

8549 Alcohol and Pregnancy
March of Dimes
233 Park Avenue South 212-353-8353
New York, NY 10003 Fax: 212-254-3518
e-mail: NY639@marchofdimes.com
www.marchofdimes.com

8550 Alcoholics Anonymous and Employee Assistance Program
Alcoholics Anonymous
PO Box 459 212-870-3400
New York, NY 10163-0459 Fax: 212-870-3137

Of interest to management and union officials, this pamphlet gives concise descriptions of the help AA can offer to the alcoholic employee.

8551 Alcoholism Tends to Run in Families
National Clearinghouse for Alcohol and Drug Info.
PO Box 2345
Rockville, MD 20847-2345 800-729-6686
www.health.org

Provides answers and questions about how to help children of alcoholics and where to find resources for additional information.

8552 Alcoholism: A Merry-Go-Round Named Denial
Al-Anon Family Group Headquarters
1600 Corporate Landing Parkway 757-563-1600
Virginia Beach, VA 23454-5617 800-425-2666
Fax: 757-563-1655
e-mail: wso@al-anon.org
www.al-anon.alateen.org

Dramatic explanations that help family members and friends see the roles they play in the problems of alcoholism.
18 pages
Caryn Johnson, Director Communications

8553 Alcoholism: The Family Disease
Al-Anon Family Group Headquarters

1600 Corporate Landing Parkway
Virginia Beach, VA 23454-5617
757-563-1600
800-425-2666
Fax: 757-563-1655
e-mail: wso@al-anon.org
www.al-anon.alateen.org

A treasury of information and inspiration with the purpose of the Al-Anon program, actual stories of people who found serenity in Al-Anon, questions/answers, slogans, evaluations and thoughts to live by.

48 pages

Caryn Johnson, Director Communications

8554 **Anabolic Steroids: A Threat to Body and Mind**
National Clearinghouse for Alcohol and Drug Info.
PO Box 2345
Rockville, MD 20847
800-729-6686

Summarizes the findings of recent studies on the use of anabolic steroids in the United States.

11 pages

8555 **Anonymity**
Al-Anon Family Group Headquarters
1600 Corporate Landing Parkway
Virginia Beach, VA 23454-5617
757-563-1600
800-425-2666
Fax: 757-563-1655
e-mail: wso@al-anon.org
www.al-anon.alateen.org

Offers information on Al-Anon and Alateen traditions and what a big factor anonymity plays for members.

6 pages

Caryn Johnson, Director Communications

8556 **Are You Concerned About Someone's Drinking**
Al-Anon Family Group Headquarters
1600 Corporate Landing Parkway
Virginia Beach, VA 23454-5617
757-563-1600
800-425-2666
Fax: 757-563-1655
e-mail: wso@al-anon.org
www.al-anon.alateen.org

12 pages

Caryn Johnson, Director Communications

8557 **Be Kind to Nonsmokers**
American Lung Association
1740 Broadway
New York, NY 10019-4315
212-315-8700

Explains why smoke hurts nonsmokers.

8558 **Best of Public Outreach**
Al-Anon Family Group Headquarters
1600 Corporate Landing Parkway
Virginia Beach, VA 23454-5617
757-563-1600
800-425-2666
Fax: 757-563-1655
e-mail: wso@al-anon.org
www.al-anon.alateen.org

Helps groups, committees and individuals carry out their PI institutions and CPC activities; includes suggested activities and open letters to various professionals.

24 pages

Caryn Johnson, Director Communications

8559 **Black, Beautiful and Recovering**
Hazelden
15251 Pleasant Valley Road
Center City, MN 55012-9640
651-257-4010
800-328-9000
Fax: 651-213-4426
www.hazelden.org

20 pages

8560 **Chemical Dependency and the African American**
Hazelden
15251 Pleasant Valley Road
Center City, MN 55012-9640
651-257-4010
800-328-9000
Fax: 651-213-4426
www.hazelden.org

Reviews the impact alcohol and other drug abuse has on African American communities.

66 pages

8561 **Chemical Dependency: An Acceptable Disease**
Hazelden
15251 Pleasant Valley Road
Center City, MN 55012-9640
651-257-4010
800-328-9000
Fax: 651-213-4426
www.hazelden.org

Help persons identify and acknowledge their chemical dependency.

14 pages

8562 **Chew or Snuff is Real Bad Stuff**
National Cancer Institute
Building 31
Bethesda, MD 20892
301-496-4000

A pamphlet describing the hazards of using smokeless tobacco.

8 pages

8563 **Cigarette Smoking**
American Lung Association
1740 Broadway
New York, NY 10019-4315
212-315-8700

Leaflet presenting the facts about how cigarette smoke is related to lung disease.

8564 **Communication Skills**
Hazelden
15251 Pleasant Valley Road
Center City, MN 55012-9640
651-257-4010
800-328-9000
Fax: 651-213-4426
www.hazelden.org

Helps clients discover how to become better listeners.

8565 **Community Campaign Brochure**
National Clearinghouse for Alcohol and Drug Info.
PO Box 2345
Rockville, MD 20847-2345
800-729-6686

Information and promotional brochure discusses key prevention concepts and messages and details how to plan campaign events.

8566 **Crack**
Hazelden
15251 Pleasant Valley Road
Center City, MN 55012-9640
651-257-4010
800-328-9000
Fax: 651-213-4426
www.hazelden.org

Explains history, use and effects of crack cocaine.

8567 **Crack Cocaine: The Big Lie**
National Clearinghouse for Alcohol and Drug Info.
PO Box 2345
Rockville, MD 20847-2345
800-729-6686
www.health.org

Offers information on what crack and cocaine are, how strong the addictions are from these drugs, how they affect the body and other risks in taking cocaine and crack.

8568 **Crossing the Line Between Social Drinking and Alcoholism**
Hazelden
15251 Pleasant Valley Road
Center City, MN 55012-9640
651-257-4010
800-328-9000
Fax: 651-213-4426
www.hazelden.org

20 pages

8569 **Denial**
Hazelden
15251 Pleasant Valley Road
Center City, MN 55012-9640
651-257-4010
800-328-9000
Fax: 651-213-4426
www.hazelden.org

Describes denial and its role in the five-stage acceptance process.

8570 **Depression and Recovery from Chemical Dependency**
Hazelden
15251 Pleasant Valley Road
Center City, MN 55012-9640
651-257-4010
800-328-9000
Fax: 651-213-4426
www.hazelden.org

Outlines depression's warning signs.

8571 **Detaching with Love**
Hazelden
15251 Pleasant Valley Road 651-257-4010
Center City, MN 55012-9640 800-328-9000
Fax: 651-213-4426
www.hazelden.org
Addresses the essential recovery tools clients need to cope with addiction and detach from the problem.

8572 **Detachment**
Al-Anon Family Group Headquarters
1600 Corporate Landing Parkway 757-563-1600
Virginia Beach, VA 23454-5617 800-425-2666
Fax: 757-563-1655
e-mail: wso@al-anon.org
www.al-anon.alateen.org
Everything you always wanted to know about detachment in an easy-to-use leaflet.
Caryn Johnson, Director Communications

8573 **Did You Grow Up with a Problem Drinker?**
Al-Anon Family Group Headquarters
1600 Corporate Landing Parkway 757-563-1600
Virginia Beach, VA 23454-5617 800-425-2666
Fax: 757-563-1655
e-mail: wso@al-anon.org
www.al-anon.alateen.org
Twenty personal questions help individuals decide if they can benefit from Al-Anon.
Caryn Johnson, Director Communications

8574 **Do You Think You're Different?**
Alcoholics Anonymous
PO Box 459 212-870-3400
New York, NY 10163-0459 Fax: 212-870-3137
Speaks to newcomers who may wonder how AA can work for someone different.

8575 **Don't Let Your Dreams Go Up in Smoke**
American Lung Association
1740 Broadway 212-315-8700
New York, NY 10019-4315
Photos, testimonials and clear language to deliver the message that everyone can and should stop smoking.

8576 **Don't Lose a Friend to Drugs**
National Crime Prevention Council
1000 Connecticut Avenue NW 202-466-6272
Washington, DC 20036-3802 Fax: 202-296-1356
www.ncpc.org
Offers practical advice to teenagers on how to say no to drugs, how to help a friend who uses drugs and how to initiate community efforts to prevent drug use.

8577 **Drinking Alcohol During Pregnancy**
March of Dimes
233 Park Avenue South 212-353-8353
New York, NY 10003 Fax: 212-254-3518
e-mail: NY639@marchofdimes.com
www.marchofdimes.com
Fact Sheets: one to two page review written for the general public. Also available electronically from the website www.marchofdimes.com

8578 **Drug Free Zones: A Manual**
African American Family Services
2616 Nicollet Avenue S 612-871-7878
Minneapolis, MN 55408
This booklet describes a variety of strategies concerned citizens are using to reclaim their neighborhoods from rampant drug abuse and dealing.
24 pages

8579 **Drugs and Pregnancy**
March of Dimes
233 Park Avenue South 212-353-8353
New York, NY 10003 Fax: 212-254-3518
e-mail: NY639@marchofdimes.com
www.marchofdimes.com
Brochures: 3 panel color brochures written for the general public.
pkg 50

8580 **Employer's Guide to Dealing with Substance Abuse**
National Clearinghouse for Alcohol and Drug Info.
PO Box 2345
Rockville, MD 20847-2345 800-729-6686
www.health.org
Instructs employers in setting up comprehensive alcohol and other drug programs in the workplace.
18 pages

8581 **Enabling**
Hazelden
15251 Pleasant Valley Road 651-257-4010
Center City, MN 55012-9640 800-328-9000
Fax: 651-213-4426
www.hazelden.org
Describes problems families encounter when they focus their lives on their chemically dependent family member.

8582 **Facts About Alateen**
Al-Anon Family Group Headquarters
1600 Corporate Landing Parkway 757-563-1600
Virginia Beach, VA 23454-5617 800-425-2666
Fax: 757-563-1655
e-mail: wso@al-anon.org
www.al-anon.alateen.org
Offers information on Alateen member services.
4 pages
Caryn Johnson, Director Communications

8583 **Facts About Alcohol Abuse**
Medical Arts Center Hospital
57 W 57th Street 212-838-2169
New York, NY 10019-2802 Fax: 212-755-0200
A question and answer pamphlet that offers information on alcohol abuse and the effects the abuse has on the family unit.

8584 **Family Denial**
Hazelden
15251 Pleasant Valley Road 651-257-4010
Center City, MN 55012-9640 800-328-9000
Fax: 651-213-4426
www.hazelden.org
Describes ways for families to recognize denial, examine common fears that cause denial and develop methods for overcoming it.

8585 **Fetal Alcohol Syndrome**
Hazelden
15251 Pleasant Valley Road 651-257-4010
Center City, MN 55012-9640 800-328-9000
Fax: 651-213-4426
www.hazelden.org
A source of information about the effects of drinking while pregnant.

8586 **Fight Drug Abuse at Home, Work, School and in the Community**
American Council for Drug Education
204 Monroe Street
Rockville, MD 20850-4425 800-488-3784
A catalog of print and video materials pertaining to substance abuse, alcoholism and drugs.

8587 **For a Strong and Healthy Baby**
National Clearinghouse for Alcohol and Drug Info.
PO Box 2345
Rockville, MD 20847-2345 800-729-6686
www.health.org
Recommends that women not drink or use other drugs if pregnant or planning to become pregnant.

8588 **Free to Care**
Hazelden
15251 Pleasant Valley Road 651-257-4010
Center City, MN 55012-9640 800-328-9000
Fax: 651-213-4426
www.hazelden.org
Explores today's definition of family and new attitudes about gender, technology, single-parents, relatives and friends.

8589 **Freedom from Despair**
Al-Anon Family Group Headquarters

1600 Corporate Landing Parkway 757-563-1600
Virginia Beach, VA 23454-5617 800-425-2666
Fax: 757-563-1655
e-mail: wso@al-anon.org
www.al-anon.alateen.org

A message of hope for those faced with a problem they can't solve alone.
4 pages
Caryn Johnson, Director Communications

8590 Freedom from Smoking Flyer
American Lung Association
1740 Broadway 212-315-8700
New York, NY 10019-4315
4 color flyer describing all FFS programs.

8591 Getting in Touch with Al-Anon/Alateen
Al-Anon Family Group Headquarters
1600 Corporate Landing Parkway 757-563-1600
Virginia Beach, VA 23454-5617 800-425-2666
Fax: 757-563-1655
e-mail: wso@al-anon.org
www.al-anon.alateen.org

A listing of Al-Anon information services throughout the world. Helps members, the public and professionals located nearby Al-Anon or Alateen groups.
Caryn Johnson, Director Communications

8592 Grieving
Hazelden
15251 Pleasant Valley Road 651-257-4010
Center City, MN 55012-9640 800-328-9000
Fax: 651-213-4426
www.hazelden.org

Outlines the five-phase grieving process for clients and the significance of each.

8593 Guidance on Our Journeys
Hazelden
15251 Pleasant Valley Road 651-257-4010
Center City, MN 55012-9640 800-328-9000
Fax: 651-213-4426
www.hazelden.org

Examines the relationship between the recovering person and his or her sponsor.

8594 Guide for the Family of the Alcoholic
Al-Anon Family Group Headquarters
1600 Corporate Landing Parkway 757-563-1600
Virginia Beach, VA 23454-5617 800-425-2666
Fax: 757-563-1655
e-mail: wso@al-anon.org
www.al-anon.alateen.org

A clear and realistic look at alcoholism, problems encountered by those close to the alcoholic and choices available to the family.
16 pages
Caryn Johnson, Director Communications

8595 Have Fun! Figure Out the Smoking Puzzle
American Lung Association
1740 Broadway 212-315-8700
New York, NY 10019-4315
Crossword puzzles make stimulating points on the effects of smoking.

8596 Healthy Beginning, Promotional Flyers
American Lung Association
1740 Broadway 212-315-8700
New York, NY 10019-4315
Flyer offers tips to help protect newborn and young children from the harmful effects of passive smoking.

8597 Help a Friend to Stop Smoking
American Lung Association
1740 Broadway 212-315-8700
New York, NY 10019-4315
This original guide to helping family members and friends support a smoker who is trying to quit smoking.
12 pages

8598 Helping Smokers Get Ready to Quit
American Lung Association
1740 Broadway 212-315-8700
New York, NY 10019-4315
Offers suggestions on how to get smokers to think about quitting and how to open up a dialogue on the issue.

8599 Helping Your Child Say No: A Parent's Guide
National Clearinghouse for Alcohol and Drug Info.
PO Box 2345
Rockville, MD 20847-2345 800-729-6686
Explains to parents how alcohol affects the body, how to tell if your child has been drinking and why children start to drink.

8600 Homeward Bound
Al-Anon Family Group Headquarters
1600 Corporate Landing Parkway 757-563-1600
Virginia Beach, VA 23454-5617 800-425-2666
Fax: 757-563-1655
e-mail: wso@al-anon.org
www.al-anon.alateen.org

A booklet designed to help beginners make the transition from the family treatment setting to Al-Anon. Contains forty members' personal sharings, a basic glossary of Al-Anon terms, brief explanations of Al-Anon slogans and helpful suggestions for newcomers.
48 pages
Caryn Johnson, Director Communications

8601 How Can I Help My Children?
Al-Anon Family Group Headquarters
1600 Corporate Landing Parkway 757-563-1600
Virginia Beach, VA 23454-5617 800-425-2666
Fax: 757-563-1655
e-mail: wso@al-anon.org
www.al-anon.alateen.org

Parents can help their children achieve a healthier attitude. Improving our own attitudes and behavior will help the entire family.
20 pages
Caryn Johnson, Director Communications

8602 How Drug Abuse Takes Profit Out of Business
National Clearinghouse for Alcohol and Drug Info.
PO Box 2345
Rockville, MD 20847-2345 800-729-6686
Answers employers questions about substance abuse in the workplace.

8603 How to Get the Most Out of Group Therapy
Hazelden
15251 Pleasant Valley Road 651-257-4010
Center City, MN 55012-9640 800-328-9000
Fax: 651-213-4426
www.hazelden.org

Answers clients' questions about going to and getting help from group therapy.

8604 How to Help a Friend Quit Smoking
American Lung Association
1740 Broadway 212-315-8700
New York, NY 10019-4315
Discusses how friends, family and co-workers can assist smokers with their concerns about quitting smoking.

8605 How to Take Care of Your Baby Before Birth
National Clearinghouse for Alcohol and Drug Info.
PO Box 2345
Rockville, MD 20847-2345 800-729-6686
www.health.org

A low-literacy brochure aimed at pregnant women that describes what they should and should not do during pregnancy.

8606 I Can't Be Addicted Because...
Hazelden
15251 Pleasant Valley Road 651-257-4010
Center City, MN 55012-9640 800-328-9000
Fax: 651-213-4426
www.hazelden.org

Focuses on denial and elaborates on its most common forms.

8607 Ice Storm
Hazelden

15251 Pleasant Valley Road 651-257-4010
Center City, MN 55012-9640 800-328-9000
Fax: 651-213-4426
www.hazelden.org

Prepares treatment professionals for the complications of one of the most recently synthesized drugs - ice.

8608 If Someone Close to You Has a Problem with Alcohol or Other Drugs
National Clearinghouse for Alcohol and Drug Info.
PO Box 2345
Rockville, MD 20847-2345 800-729-6686
www.health.org

This booklet is aimed at the general public and gives support and suggestions on coping with someone close who has an alcohol or drug problem.

8609 If You Are a Professional, AA Wants to Work with You
Alcoholics Anonymous
PO Box 459 212-870-3400
New York, NY 10163-0459 Fax: 212-870-3137

Directed at professionals of all types who deal with alcoholics.

8610 If Your Parents Drink Too Much
Al-Anon Family Group Headquarters
1600 Corporate Landing Parkway 757-563-1600
Virginia Beach, VA 23454-5617 800-425-2666
Fax: 757-563-1655
e-mail: wso@al-anon.org
www.al-anon.alateen.org

Alateen's cartoon booklet.
24 pages
Caryn Johnson, Director Communications

8611 Illicit Drug Use During Pregnancy
March of Dimes
233 Park Avenue South 212-353-8353
New York, NY 10003 Fax: 212-254-3518
e-mail: NY639@marchofdimes.com
www.marchofdimes.com

Fact Sheets: one to two page review for the general public. Also available electronically from the website www.marchofdimes.com

8612 Index to Alcoholics Anonymous
Hazelden
15251 Pleasant Valley Road 651-257-4010
Center City, MN 55012-9640 800-328-9000
Fax: 651-213-4426

Features page and line references to the topics discussed in Alcoholics Anonymous, the Big Book.

8613 Is AA for Me?
Alcoholics Anonymous
PO Box 459 212-870-3400
New York, NY 10163-0459 Fax: 212-870-3137

An illustrated easy to read version of the 12 questions in Is AA for You? pamphlet.
32 pages

8614 Is AA for You?
Alcoholics Anonymous
PO Box 459 212-870-3400
New York, NY 10163-0459 Fax: 212-870-3137

Symptoms of alcoholism are summed up in 12 questions most AA's had answered to identify themselves as alcoholics.

8615 Is There a Safe Tobacco?
American Lung Association
1740 Broadway 212-315-8700
New York, NY 10019-4315

Offers information on the health risks of cigarette smoking, pipes and cigars.

8616 Is There an Alcoholic in Your Life?
Alcoholics Anonymous
PO Box 459 212-870-3400
New York, NY 10163-0459 Fax: 212-870-3137

Explains the AA program as it affects anyone close to an alcoholic.

8617 It Happened to Alice
Alcoholics Anonymous
PO Box 459 212-870-3400
New York, NY 10163-0459 Fax: 212-870-3137

Easy to read comic-book style format for women alcoholics.

8618 It Sure Beats Sitting in a Cell
Alcoholics Anonymous
PO Box 459 212-870-3400
New York, NY 10163-0459 Fax: 212-870-3137

An illustrated pamphlet which presents the experience of seven inmates who found AA while in prison. It also offers suggested dos and don'ts for staying sober after release.

8619 Kids and Drugs: A Handbook for Parents & Professionals
PANDAA Press
4111 Watkins Trl 703-750-9285
Annandale, VA 22003-2051

8620 Let's Solve the Smokeword Puzzle
American Lung Association
1740 Broadway 212-315-8700
New York, NY 10019-4315

Fifth graders will love getting an antismoking message through solving a crossword puzzle.

8621 Let's Talk
Hazelden
15251 Pleasant Valley Road 651-257-4010
Center City, MN 55012-9640 800-328-9000
Fax: 651-213-4426
www.hazelden.org

Offers 12 guidelines to promote effective communication between parent and child.

8622 Letter to a Woman Alcoholic
Alcoholics Anonymous
PO Box 459 212-870-3400
New York, NY 10163-0459 Fax: 212-870-3137

Describes with sensitive understanding the problem of the alcoholic woman.

8623 Letting Go of the Need to Control
Hazelden
15251 Pleasant Valley Road 651-257-4010
Center City, MN 55012-9640 800-328-9000
Fax: 651-213-4426
www.hazelden.org

Discusses how control issues are common among chemically dependent people.

8624 Lifetime of Freedom from Smoking: Maintenance Manual
American Lung Association
1740 Broadway 212-315-8700
New York, NY 10019-4315

Companion manual helps persons stay quit once they have stopped smoking.
28 pages

8625 Little More About Alcohol
Alcohol Research Information Service
1120 E Oakland Avenue 517-485-9900
Lansing, MI 48906-5513 Fax: 517-485-1928
e-mail: alcoholisadrugtoo@yoyoger.net

A cartoon character explains the facts about alcohol and its effects on the body.

8626 Living Sober
Alcoholics Anonymous
PO Box 459 212-870-3400
New York, NY 10163-0459 Fax: 212-870-3137

Practical book demonstrating through simple examples, how AA members throughout the world live and stay sober one day at a time.
88 pages

8627 Living in a Shelter?
Al-Anon Family Group Headquarters

1600 Corporate Landing Parkway
Virginia Beach, VA 23454-5617
757-563-1600
800-425-2666
Fax: 757-563-1655
e-mail: wso@al-anon.org
www.al-anon.alateen.org

100 pieces
Caryn Johnson, Director Communications

8628 Look at Cross-Addiction
Hazelden
15251 Pleasant Valley Road
Center City, MN 55012-9640
651-257-4010
800-328-9000
Fax: 651-213-4426
Discusses cross-addiction, denial, coping skills and avoidance.

8629 Look at Relapse
Hazelden
15251 Pleasant Valley Road
Center City, MN 55012-9640
651-257-4010
800-328-9000
Fax: 651-213-4426
Addresses emotional consequences of relapse, such as decreased feelings of self-esteem and self-confidence.

8630 Managing Cocaine Cravings
Hazelden
15251 Pleasant Valley Road
Center City, MN 55012-9640
651-257-4010
800-328-9000
Fax: 651-213-4426
www.hazelden.org
Offers clients hands-on plan to help them stay away from cocaine.

8631 Marijuana
Hazelden
15251 Pleasant Valley Road
Center City, MN 55012-9640
651-257-4010
800-328-9000
Fax: 651-213-4426
www.hazelden.org
Outlines the physical and psychological effects of marijuana unique to episodic and chronic use.
65 pages

8632 Media Kit
Al-Anon Family Group Headquarters
1600 Corporate Landing Parkway
Virginia Beach, VA 23454-5617
757-563-1600
800-425-2666
Fax: 757-563-1655
e-mail: wso@al-anon.org
www.al-anon.alateen.org
An attractive silver folder containing information necessary to work with radio and TV stations.
Caryn Johnson, Director Communications

8633 Member's Eye View of Alcoholics Anonymous
Alcoholics Anonymous
PO Box 459
New York, NY 10163-0459
212-870-3400
Fax: 212-870-3137
Designed to explain to people in the helping professionals how AA works.
30 pages

8634 Members of the Clergy Ask About Alcoholics Anonymous
Alcoholics Anonymous
PO Box 459
New York, NY 10163-0459
212-870-3400
Fax: 212-870-3137
Introduction to AA for members of the clergy unfamiliar with the Fellowship.

8635 Memo to an Inmate Who May Be an Alcoholic
Alcoholics Anonymous
PO Box 459
New York, NY 10163-0459
212-870-3400
Fax: 212-870-3137
A message from AA's who have themselves been inmates. Their personal stories offer a new outlook to inmate alcholics who want to know who AA can help.

8636 Men Newcomer Packet
Al-Anon Family Group Headquarters
1600 Corporate Landing Parkway
Virginia Beach, VA 23454-5617
757-563-1600
800-425-2666
Fax: 757-563-1655
e-mail: wso@al-anon.org
www.al-anon.alateen.org
For men who are not sure Al-Anon is for them, this collection offers a realistic look at alcoholism and straight forward answers to frequently asked questions.
8 pieces
Caryn Johnson, Director Communications

8637 Message to Correctional Facilities Administrators
Alcoholics Anonymous
PO Box 459
New York, NY 10163-0459
212-870-3400
Fax: 212-870-3137
Information about what AA is and can do, and how groups function in correctional facilities.

8638 Message to Teenagers
Alcoholics Anonymous
PO Box 459
New York, NY 10163-0459
212-870-3400
Fax: 212-870-3137
This brochure offers a simple, 12-question quiz designed to help teenagers decide when drinking is becoming a problem in their lives.

8639 Military Packet
Al-Anon Family Group Headquarters
1600 Corporate Landing Parkway
Virginia Beach, VA 23454-5617
757-563-1600
800-425-2666
Fax: 757-563-1655
e-mail: wso@al-anon.org
www.al-anon.alateen.org
For those in the armed services with loved ones or colleagues who are alcoholic, here's a collection that says, Al-Anon can help.
7 pieces
Caryn Johnson, Director Communications

8640 Moment to Reflect on Codependency
Hazelden
15251 Pleasant Valley Road
Center City, MN 55012-9640
651-257-4010
800-328-9000
Fax: 651-213-4426
A collection of four booklets offering meditations that emphasize and reinforce self-esteem for young people recovering from addiction.

8641 Moment to Reflect on Self-Esteem
Hazelden
15251 Pleasant Valley Road
Center City, MN 55012-9640
651-257-4010
800-328-9000
Fax: 651-213-4426
Focuses on the fundamental recovery issue of self-esteem.
4 Booklets

8642 Moving On! From Alateen to Al-Anon
Al-Anon Family Group Headquarters
1600 Corporate Landing Parkway
Virginia Beach, VA 23454-5617
757-563-1600
800-425-2666
Fax: 757-563-1655
e-mail: wso@al-anon.org
www.al-anon.alateen.org
Former Alateen members experience the joy of continued recovery in Al-Anon.
12 pages
Caryn Johnson, Director Communications

8643 NIDA Capsules
National Clearinghouse for Alcohol and Drug Info.
PO Box 2345
Rockville, MD 20847-2345
800-729-6686
www.health.org

8644 Newcomer Asks
Alcoholics Anonymous
PO Box 459
New York, NY 10163-0459
212-870-3400
Fax: 212-870-3137
Gives straightforward answers on 15 points that once puzzled many of us.

8645 **Nicotine Addiction and Cigarettes**
American Lung Association
1740 Broadway 212-315-8700
New York, NY 10019-4315
Offers information on nicotine and cigarette smoking.

8646 **No Smoking Coloring Book**
American Lung Association
1740 Broadway 212-315-8700
New York, NY 10019-4315
Preschool and primary grade children will enjoy drawing and coloring while getting an antismoking message.

8647 **No Smoking: Lungs At Work**
American Lung Association
1740 Broadway 212-315-8700
New York, NY 10019-4315
Describes how lungs work and how they are affected by smoking.

8648 **Now What Do I Do for Fun?**
Hazelden
15251 Pleasant Valley Road 651-257-4010
Center City, MN 55012-9640 800-328-9000
Fax: 651-213-4426
www.hazelden.org
Explores the dilemma of finding new interests in recovery after completing treatment.

8649 **Older Adults After Treatment**
Hazelden
15251 Pleasant Valley Road 651-257-4010
Center City, MN 55012-9640 800-328-9000
Fax: 651-213-4426
www.hazelden.org
Discusses aftercare issues, such as family relations, health, medication and relapse.

8650 **Older Adults in Treatment**
Hazelden
15251 Pleasant Valley Road 651-257-4010
Center City, MN 55012-9640 800-328-9000
Fax: 651-213-4426
www.hazelden.org
Examines past beliefs about addiction and defines chemical dependency as a disease.

8651 **On the Air: A Guide to Creating A Smoke-Free Workplace**
American Lung Association
1740 Broadway 212-315-8700
New York, NY 10019-4315
A step-by-step guide for organizations interested in developing and implementing a successful workplace smoking control policy.
24 pages

8652 **Parents Newcomer Packet**
Al-Anon Family Group Headquarters
1600 Corporate Landing Parkway 757-563-1600
Virginia Beach, VA 23454-5617 800-425-2666
Fax: 757-563-1655
e-mail: wso@al-anon.org
www.al-anon.alateen.org
For parents who realize their child is an alcoholic, this is a compassionate and reassuring welcome to Al-Anon.
9 pieces
Caryn Johnson, Director Communications

8653 **Points for Parents Perplexed About Drugs**
Hazelden
15251 Pleasant Valley Road 651-257-4010
Center City, MN 55012-9640 800-328-9000
Fax: 651-213-4426
www.hazelden.org
Clear guidelines to help adults recognize, evaluate and deal with adolescent drug abuse.
16 pages

8654 **Preventing Relapse**
Hazelden
15251 Pleasant Valley Road 651-257-4010
Center City, MN 55012-9640 800-328-9000
Fax: 651-213-4426
www.hazelden.org
Offers practical information and personal stories to help clients better understand the relapse process.
28 pages

8655 **Program Booklet**
Women for Sobriety
PO Box 618 215-536-8026
Quakertown, PA 18951-0618 Fax: 215-536-8026
e-mail: WFSobriety@aol.com
www.womenforsobriety.org
Purse size booklet that explains the Thirteen Statements of Dr. Kirkpatrick's New Life program, statement by statement.

8656 **Put on the Brakes Bulletin: Take a Look at College Drinking**
National Clearinghouse for Alcohol and Drug Info.
PO Box 2345
Rockville, MD 20847-2345 800-729-6686
www.health.org
This second edition continues CSAP's campaign to raise awareness about the problems of college drinking.

8657 **Q&A About Smoking and Health**
American Lung Association
1740 Broadway 212-315-8700
New York, NY 10019-4315
Gives fact-crammed answers to questions on smoking and health.

8658 **Quick List to Build Pride in Your Communities**
National Clearinghouse for Alcohol and Drug Info.
PO Box 2345
Rockville, MD 20847-2345 800-729-6686
This parent guide is an adaptation of CSAP's Be Smart! Quick List: 10 Steps to Help Your Child Say No.

8659 **Reducing the Health Risks of Secondhand Smoke**
American Lung Association
1740 Broadway 212-315-8700
New York, NY 10019-4315
What a person can do at home, work and in public places to reduce the health risks of secondhand smoke.

8660 **Relapse and the Addict**
Hazelden
15251 Pleasant Valley Road 651-257-4010
Center City, MN 55012-9640 800-328-9000
Fax: 651-213-4426
www.hazelden.org
Identifies specific stages and triggers of relapse.

8661 **Releasing Anger**
Hazelden
15251 Pleasant Valley Road 651-257-4010
Center City, MN 55012-9640 800-328-9000
Fax: 651-213-4426
www.hazelden.org
Discusses anger as a normal feeling and how anger can endanger recovery.

8662 **Research on Drugs and the Workplace**
National Clearinghouse for Alcohol and Drug Info.
PO Box 2345
Rockville, MD 20847-2345 800-729-6686
Discusses prevalence and costs to society of drug use in the workplace, along with information on employee assistance programs, drug testing, grants and additional resources.

8663 **Secondhand Smoke**
American Lung Association
1740 Broadway 212-315-8700
New York, NY 10019-4315
Documents the effects of tobacco smoke on nonsmokers.

8664 **Seven Reasons Not to Use Drugs and Alcohol**
American Council On Drug Education
204 Monroe Street
Rockville, MD 20850-4425 800-488-3784

A series of five pamphlets offering information on the hazards of alcohol, crack, cocaine, steroids and tobacco products.
Grades 4-6

8665 Sexual Intimacy and the Alcoholic Relationship
Al-Anon Family Group Headquarters
1600 Corporate Landing Parkway 757-563-1600
Virginia Beach, VA 23454-5617 800-425-2666
Fax: 757-563-1655
e-mail: wso@al-anon.org
www.al-anon.alateen.org
Sex and alcohol? Al-Anon members face this personal problem when they apply to the Al-Anon program indexed.
48 pages
Caryn Johnson, Director Communications

8666 Should Tobacco Advertising and Promotion Be Banned?
American Lung Association
1740 Broadway 212-315-8700
New York, NY 10019-4315
Answers many questions about tobacco advertising and promotion, and explains how ads are targeted to vulnerable populations.

8667 Smoke Free Family Promotional Leaflet
American Lung Association
1740 Broadway 212-315-8700
New York, NY 10019-4315
Leaflet and order form describe an entire range of ALA's smoking-related materials.

8668 Smokeless Tobacco: No Way
American Lung Association
1740 Broadway 212-315-8700
New York, NY 10019-4315
Written for junior and senior high school students, this booklet presents the facts about health risks of smokeless tobacco use.

8669 Smoking and Pregnancy
American Lung Association
1740 Broadway 212-315-8700
New York, NY 10019-4315
Written in a question/answer format, this pamphlet discusses many issues relating to smoking and pregnancy.

8670 Stop Smoking, Stay Trim
American Lung Association
1740 Broadway 212-315-8700
New York, NY 10019-4315
Outlines how to avoid gaining weight while quitting smoking.

8671 Stop Smoking: A Guide to Your Options
American Lung Association
1740 Broadway 212-315-8700
New York, NY 10019-4315
Describes a variety of approaches to smoking cessation. Offers guidance on how to choose a program.

8672 Straight Back Home
Hazelden
15251 Pleasant Valley Road 651-257-4010
Center City, MN 55012-9640 800-328-9000
Fax: 651-213-4426
www.hazelden.org
Written for adolescents completing inpatient treatment and returning home.

8673 Stress in Recovery
Hazelden
15251 Pleasant Valley Road 651-257-4010
Center City, MN 55012-9640 800-328-9000
Fax: 651-213-4426
www.hazelden.org
Outlines methods for clients to overcome stress in their daily lives.

8674 This Is AA
Alcoholics Anonymous
PO Box 459 212-870-3400
New York, NY 10163-0459 Fax: 212-870-3137
A pamphlet offering an introduction to the AA recovery program.

8675 Three Talks to Medical Societies
Alcoholics Anonymous
PO Box 459 212-870-3400
New York, NY 10163-0459 Fax: 212-870-3137
Contains Bill Wilson's, the co-founder of AA, principles borrowed from medicine and religion and a summary of AA's first 23 years.

8676 Time to Start Living
Alcoholics Anonymous
PO Box 459 212-870-3400
New York, NY 10163-0459 Fax: 212-870-3137
Addresses the older alcoholic, with nine stories of men and women who came to AA after the age of 60 (large print edition is also available).

8677 Too Many Young People Drink and Know Too Little About the Consequences
National Clearinghouse for Alcohol and Drug Info.
PO Box 2345
Rockville, MD 20847-2345 800-729-6686
Provides up-to-date resources and statistics on the widespread use of alcohol by youth under 21 years of age.

8678 Too Young?
Alcoholics Anonymous
PO Box 459 212-870-3400
New York, NY 10163-0459 Fax: 212-870-3137
This cartoon pamphlet speaks to teenagers in their own language, telling the varied drinking stories of six youn people (13 to 18).

8679 Treating Nicotine Addiction
Hazelden
15251 Pleasant Valley Road 651-257-4010
Center City, MN 55012-9640 800-328-9000
Fax: 651-213-4426
www.hazelden.org
Describes the success of one chemical dependency treatment center that began treating nicotine as an addiction.

8680 Twelve Steps Illustrated
Alcoholics Anonymous
PO Box 459 212-870-3400
New York, NY 10163-0459 Fax: 212-870-3137
An easy-to-read version of AA's twelve steps.

8681 Twelve Steps for Tobacco Users
Hazelden
15251 Pleasant Valley Road 651-257-4010
Center City, MN 55012-9640 800-328-9000
Fax: 651-213-4426
www.hazelden.org
Presents the Surgeon General's findings that classify nicotine as an addictive substance.
25 pages

8682 Understanding Depression and Addiction
Hazelden
15251 Pleasant Valley Road 651-257-4010
Center City, MN 55012-9640 800-328-9000
Fax: 651-213-4426
www.hazelden.org
29 pages

8683 Understanding Major Anxiety Disorders and Addiction
Hazelden
15251 Pleasant Valley Road 651-257-4010
Center City, MN 55012-9640 800-328-9000
Fax: 651-213-4426
www.hazelden.org
36 pages

8684 Understanding Ourselves and Alcoholism
Al-Anon Family Group Headquarters
1600 Corporate Landing Parkway 757-563-1600
Virginia Beach, VA 23454-5617 800-425-2666
Fax: 757-563-1655
e-mail: wso@al-anon.org
www.al-anon.alateen.org

Explains how compulsion, obsession and denial affect those close to an alcoholic as well as the alcoholic.
6 pages
Caryn Johnson, Director Communications

8685 Understanding Personality Problems and Addiction
Hazelden
15251 Pleasant Valley Road 651-257-4010
Center City, MN 55012-9640 800-328-9000
Fax: 651-213-4426
www.hazelden.org
Describes common features of personality problems, such as self-centeredness and setting boundaries.
28 pages

8686 Understanding Post-Traumatic Stress Disorder and Addiction
Hazelden
15251 Pleasant Valley Road 651-257-4010
Center City, MN 55012-9640 800-328-9000
Fax: 651-213-4426
www.hazelden.org
17 pages

8687 Unpuffables Promotional Brochure
American Lung Association
1740 Broadway 212-315-8700
New York, NY 10019-4315
Describes the ALA Unpuffables program.

8688 What Are the Signs of Alcoholism?
Hazelden
15251 Pleasant Valley Road 651-257-4010
Center City, MN 55012-9640 800-328-9000
Fax: 651-213-4426
www.hazelden.org
Self-test for clients to review the role of alcohol in their lives.

8689 What Happened to Joe?
Alcoholics Anonymous
PO Box 459 212-870-3400
New York, NY 10163-0459 Fax: 212-870-3137
Dramatic story of a young construction worker and his drinking problem, told in brightly colored comic book style.

8690 What Happens After Treatment?
Al-Anon Family Group Headquarters
1600 Corporate Landing Parkway 757-563-1600
Virginia Beach, VA 23454-5617 800-425-2666
Fax: 757-563-1655
e-mail: wso@al-anon.org
www.al-anon.alateen.org
100 pieces
Caryn Johnson, Director Communications

8691 What is AA?
Hazelden
15251 Pleasant Valley Road 651-257-4010
Center City, MN 55012-9640 800-328-9000
Fax: 651-213-4426
www.hazelden.org
Answers the basic questions about Alcoholics Anonymous.

8692 What is NA?
Hazelden
15251 Pleasant Valley Road 651-257-4010
Center City, MN 55012-9640 800-328-9000
Fax: 651-213-4426
www.hazelden.org
Helps clients evaluate their addiction to narcotics and answers their questions about N.A.

8693 What's Your Cigarette Smoking IQ?
American Lung Association
1740 Broadway 212-315-8700
New York, NY 10019-4315
Brief true-or-false quiz that tests a person's knowledge of the effects of smoking.

8694 When You Go Back to Work
Hazelden
15251 Pleasant Valley Road 651-257-4010
Center City, MN 55012-9640 800-328-9000
Fax: 651-213-4426
www.hazelden.org
Stories demonstrating co-workers' attitudes clients may face upon their return to work.

8695 When Your Teen is in Treatment
Hazelden
15251 Pleasant Valley Road 651-257-4010
Center City, MN 55012-9640 800-328-9000
Fax: 651-213-4426
www.hazelden.org
A guide for parents.

8696 Where Do I Go from Here?
Alcoholics Anonymous
PO Box 459 212-870-3400
New York, NY 10163-0459 Fax: 212-870-3137
For people leaving treatment facilities, single-sheet flyer tells of continuing help offered by outside AAs.

8697 Why Anonymity in Al-Anon?
Al-Anon Family Group Headquarters
1600 Corporate Landing Parkway 757-563-1600
Virginia Beach, VA 23454-5617 800-425-2666
Fax: 757-563-1655
e-mail: wso@al-anon.org
www.al-anon.alateen.org
12 pages
Caryn Johnson, Director Communications

8698 Workers at Risk: Drugs and Alcohol on the Job
National Clearinghouse for Alcohol and Drug Info.
PO Box 2345
Rockville, MD 20847-2345 800-729-6686
Gives facts about drugs in the workplace and suggests appropriate behavior for employees who are confronted with a coworker's use of alcohol or other drugs.

8699 You Can Help Your Community Get Rid of Drugs
National Clearinghouse for Alcohol and Drug Info.
PO Box 2345
Rockville, MD 20847-2345 800-729-6686
Supports drug abuse treatment and explains how drug use can create problems for your community.

8700 Young Children and Drugs: What Parents Can Do
Wisconsin Clearinghouse
106 E. Washington Avenue
Madison, WI 53704-5275

8701 Youth and the Alcoholic Parent
Al-Anon Family Group Headquarters
1600 Corporate Landing Parkway 757-563-1600
Virginia Beach, VA 23454-5617 800-425-2666
Fax: 757-563-1655
e-mail: wso@al-anon.org
www.al-anon.alateen.org
Questions and suggestions to help young people improve their own lives.
12 pages
Caryn Johnson, Director Communications

Audio & Video

8702 AA: Rap with Us
Alcoholics Anonymous
PO Box 459 212-870-3400
New York, NY 10163-0459 Fax: 212-870-3137
Features four anonymous young AA members. Rap music and lyrics bridge these four young people's stories of alcoholic despair and A.A. recovery.
16 minutes

8703 Al-Anon Video
Al-Anon Family Group Headquarters

1600 Corporate Landing Parkway
Virginia Beach, VA 23454-5617
757-563-1600
800-425-2666
Fax: 757-563-1655
e-mail: wso@al-anon.org
www.al-anon.alateen.org

12 pages
Caryn Johnson, Director Communications

8704 **Al-Anon is for African Americans...and All People of Color**
Al-Anon Family Group Headquarters
1600 Corporate Landing Parkway
Virginia Beach, VA 23454-5617
757-563-1600
800-425-2666
Fax: 757-563-1655
e-mail: wso@al-anon.org
www.al-anon.alateen.org

12 pages
Caryn Johnson, Director Communications

8705 **Al-Anon's Path to Recovery: Al-Anon is for Americans/Aboriginals**
Al-Anon Family Group Headquarters
1600 Corporate Landing Parkway
Virginia Beach, VA 23454-5617
757-563-1600
800-425-2666
Fax: 757-563-1655
e-mail: wso@al-anon.org
www.al-anon.alateen.org

12 pages
Caryn Johnson, Director Communications

8706 **Alcoholics Anonymous: An Inside View**
Alcoholics Anonymous
PO Box 459
New York, NY 10163-0459
212-870-3400
Fax: 212-870-3137

Depicts alcoholics, recovering in A.A., going about their daily lives, attending A.A. meetings, and other gatherings.
28 minutes

8707 **Art of Living with Change: Turning Your Good Intentions Into Progress...**
Hazelden
15251 Pleasant Valley Road
Center City, MN 55012-9640
651-213-4030
800-328-0094
Fax: 651-213-4426
www.hazelden.org

45 minutes
ISBN: 0-894868-40-3

8708 **Bill Discusses the Twelve Traditions**
Alcoholics Anonymous
PO Box 459
New York, NY 10163-0459
212-870-3400
Fax: 212-870-3137

Bill W. tells how the principles safe-guarding A.A. unity developed.
60 minutes

8709 **Bill's Own Story**
Alcoholics Anonymous
PO Box 459
New York, NY 10163-0459
212-870-3400
Fax: 212-870-3137

Co-founder Bill W. tells of his drinking and recovery.
60 minutes

8710 **Caring for Ourselves: Hope for Healthy Relationships**
Hazelden
15251 Pleasant Valley Road
Center City, MN 55012-9640
651-213-4030
800-328-0094
Fax: 651-213-4426
www.hazelden.org

50 minutes
ISBN: 0-894866-38-9

8711 **Hope: Alcoholics Anonymous**
Alcoholics Anonymous
PO Box 459
New York, NY 10163-0459
212-870-3400
Fax: 212-870-3137

Explains the principles of AA: what it is, steps, traditions, sponsorship, and basic recovery tools.
15 minutes

8712 **It Sure Beats Sitting in a Cell**
Alcoholics Anonymous
PO Box 459
New York, NY 10163-0459
212-870-3400
Fax: 212-870-3137

Filmed inside correctional facilities in the United States and Canada, this film tells the story of four young AA's who were in prison as a result of drinking, yet today are sober.
17 minutes

8713 **Markings on the Journey**
Alcoholics Anonymous
PO Box 459
New York, NY 10163-0459
212-870-3400
Fax: 212-870-3137

Videocassette depicts 45 years of AA history, using rare materials from our archives.
35 minutes

8714 **Men's Work: How to Stop the Violence that Tears Our Lives Apart**
Hazelden
15251 Pleasant Valley Road
Center City, MN 55012-9640
651-213-4030
800-328-0094
Fax: 651-213-4426
www.hazelden.org

50 minutes
ISBN: 0-894868-28-4

8715 **Secret to a Satisfied Life: The Way You Encounter Life Can Bring Happiness...**
Hazelden
15251 Pleasant Valley Road
Center City, MN 55012-9640
651-213-4030
800-328-0094
Fax: 651-213-4426
www.hazelden.org

45 minutes
ISBN: 0-894868-17-9

8716 **Women: Coming Out of the Shadows**
Elyse A Williams, author
Fanlight Productions
4196 Washington Street
Boston, MA 02131-1731
617-469-4999
800-937-4113
Fax: 617-469-3379
e-mail: fanlight@fanlight.com
www.fanlight.com

Ten women share their personal stories of addiction and recovery.
1991 27 Minutes
ISBN: 1-572950-84-6

8717 **Young People and AA**
Alcoholics Anonymous
PO Box 459
New York, NY 10163-0459
212-870-3400
Fax: 212-870-3137

Four young AA members describe what it is like drinking, what happened to bring them to AA, and what their lives are like sober today.
28 minutes

Web Sites

8718 **AAA Foundation for Traffic Safety**
www.aaafts.org

This national organization publishes drinking and traffic safety programs for K-6 and junior high students.

8719 **Al-Anon**
www.al-anon.alateen.org

The single purpose of this organization is to help families and friends of alcoholics, whether the alcoholic is still drinking or not.

8720 **Alateen**
A part of the Al-Anon program, Alateen is for teenagers who have been affected by someone else's drinking, whether it be a family member or a friend.

8721 **American Council for Drug Education**
www.acde.org/

This organization provides information on drug use, publishes books and offers films and curriculum materials for prevention.

8722 CSAP State Liason Program
www.samhsa.gov/centers/csap/csap.html
This program is designed to support alcohol and other drug abuse prevention efforts in the States.

8723 Center for Substance Abuse Prevention
www.samhsa.gov/centers/csap/csap.html
This organization's goal is to connect people and resources with innovative ideas, strategies and programs designed to encourage creative and effective efforts aimed at reducing and eliminating alcohol, tobacco and other drug problems in our society.

8724 Cocaine Anonymous
www.ca.org
A support group based on the twelve steps of Alcoholics Anonymous that focuses specifically on problems of cocaine addiction.

8725 Dentists Concerned for Dentists
www.medhelp.org/amshc/amshc53.htm
A nonprofit organization for chemically dependent Minnesota dentists and concerned others.

8726 Families Anonymous
www.familiesanonymous.org/
Addresses the needs of families who are concerned about a relative with a drug problem and with related behavioral problems.

8727 Hazelden
www.hazelden.com
Organization dedicated to providing quality rehabilitation, education and professional services for chemical dependency and related addictive behaviors.

8728 Healing Well
www.healingwell.com
An online health resource guide to medical news, chat, information and articles, newsgroups and message boards, books, disease-related web sites, medical directories, and more for patients, friends, and family coping with disabling diseases, disorders, or chronic illnesses.

8729 Health Finder
www.healthfinder.gov
Searchable, carefully developed web site offering information on over 1000 topics. Developed by the US Department of Health and Human Services, the site can be used in both English and Spanish.

8730 Healthlink USA
www.healthlinkusa.com
Health information concerning treatment, cures, prevention, diagnosis, risk factors, research, support groups, email lists, personal stories and much more. Updated regularly.

8731 Helios Health
www.helioshealth.com
Online resource for your health information. Detailed information about specific health topics, access to expert advice from our Medical Advisory Board, and up-to-date health news.

8732 Indian Health Service
www.ihs.gov
Charged with providing a comprehensive program of alcoholism and substance abuse prevention and treatment for Native Americans and Alaskan natives.

8733 Lawyers Concerned for Lawyers
www.mnlcl.org/
Organization of recovering lawyers and judges and concerned others. Educates lawyers and judges about the disease of chemical dependency, assists in assessments and arranging interventions and offers lawyer-only AA meetings.

8734 MedicineNet
www.medicinenet.com
An online resource for consumers providing easy-to-read, authoritative medical and health information.

8735 Medscape
www.mywebmd.com
Medscape offers specialists, primary care physicians, and other health professionals the Web's most robust and integrated medical information and educational tools.

8736 National Clearinghouse for Alcohol and Drug Information
www.health.org

8737 National Council on Alcoholism and Drug Dependence
www.ncadd.org
Provides education, information, help and hope in the fight against addictions. Nationwide network of affiliates, advocates prevention, intervention and treatment, and is committed to ridding the disease of its stigma and its sufferers of their denial and shame.

8738 National Crime Prevention Council
www.ncpc.org
This organization works to prevent crime and drug use in many ways, including developing materials for parents and children.

8739 Office on Smoking and Health
www.cdc.gov/tobacco/
Offers reference services to researchers through the Technical Information Center. Publishes and distributes a number of titles in the field of smoking and health.

8740 Safe Homes
www.yescap.org/safehomes/safehomes.htm
This national organization encourages parents to sign a contract stipulating that when parties are held in one another's homes they will adhere to a strict no-alcohol/no-drug-use rule.

8741 Substance Abuse and Mental Health Services Administration
www.samhsa.gov
The goal of this organization is to reduce incidence and prevalence of mental disorders and substance abuse and improve treatment outcomes for persons suffering from addictive and mental health problems and disorders.

8742 WebMD
www.webmd.com
Information on substance abuse, including articles and resources.

Description

8743 **Sudden Infant Death Syndrome**

Sudden Infant Death Syndrome, SIDS, is the sudden death of an infant or young child that is unexpected and for which there is no demonstrable cause. It is the most common cause of death in children between 1 and 12 months of age, with a peak incidence between the second and fourth month of life. Almost all SIDS deaths occur when the infant is thought to be sleeping.

Despite extensive research, no cause for SIDS has been found, although evidence suggests that it may be related to malfunction of the mechanisms that control the heart function and breathing process. The diagnosis cannot be made without an adequate investigation of the infant after its death. The incidence of SIDS is greater in babies born to mothers who are young, unwed, smoke, have had many births, did not complete high school and have had poor prenatal care. Other possible factors include exposure to cigarette smoke, cold months, soft bedding (lamb's wool), waterbed mattresses, an overheated environment, and being a sibling of a SIDS victim.

Recent studies have indicated that having babies sleep on their backs reduces the risks of SIDS. The American Academy of Pediatrics recommends that infants be placed on their back for sleep. It further advises to avoid overwrapping the infant, remove soft bedding, and avoid smoking during and after pregnancy. In 1994, the Back to Sleep Campaign was launched, a national campaign that encourages that infants be placed to sleep on their backs. Between 1992 and 1996,the rate of SIDS dropped 38 percent and has continued to decrease since then.

Parents who lose a child to SIDS are grief-stricken and, because no definitive cause can be found for their seemingly healthy baby's death, usually have excessive guilt feelings. Bereavement support is necessary not only during the days immediately following the infant's death, but also for at least several months.

National Agencies & Associations

8744 **American SIDS Institute**
509 Augusta Drive 770-426-8746
Marietta, GA 30067-8657 800-232-7437
Fax: 770-426-1369
e-mail: prevent@sids.org
www.sids.org
Dedicated to the prevention of sudden infant death and the promotion of infant health through research clinical services education and family support.
Betty McEnti PhD, Executive Director
Marc Peterzell, Chairman

8745 **Center for Research for Mothers & Children**
National Institute of Child Health & Development
PO Box 3006 800-370-2943
Rockville, MD 20847 800-370-2943
Fax: 301-984-1477
TTY: 888-320-6942
e-mail: NICHDinformationresourcecenter@mail.nih
www.nichd.nih.gov
Mission is to ensure that every person is born healthy and wanted, that women suffer no harmful effects from reproductive processes, and that all children have the chance to achieve their full potential for healthy and productive lives free from disease.
Duane F Alexander, Director
Christine Ma Banks, Secretary

8746 **Compassionate Friends**
PO Box 3696 630-990-0010
Oak Brook, IL 60522-3696 877-969-0010
Fax: 630-990-0246
e-mail: nationaloffice@compassionatefriends.org
www.compassionatefriends.org
A national organization that offers 600 local chapters that give support to parents and siblings who have experienced the death of a child. Offers monthly support meetings to get through the difficult times and learn how to cope.
Patricia Loder, Executive Director
Terry Novy, Chapter Services Coordinator

8747 **National Center for Education in Maternal and Child Health**
Georgetown University
Box 571272 202-784-9770
Washington, DC 20057-1272 Fax: 202-784-9777
e-mail: mchlibrary@ncemch.org
www.ncemch.org
Provides national leadership to the maternal and child health community in three key areas—program development education and state-of-the-art knowledge—to improve the health and well-being of the nation's children and families.
Rochelle Mayer, Director

8748 **National Organization for Rare Disorders (NORD)**
55 Kenosia Avenue 203-744-0100
Danbury, CT 06813 800-999-6673
Fax: 203-798-2291
TDD: 203-797-9590
e-mail: orphan@rarediseases.org
www.rarediseases.org
The NORD is a unique federation of voluntary health organizations dedicated to helping people with rare orphan diseases and assisting the organizations that serve them.
Carolyn Asbury, PhD, Chair
Frank Sasinowski, Vice Chair

8749 **Parent Care**
9041 Colgate Street
Indianapolis, IN 46268-1210 Fax: 317-872-5464
This organization was formed in 1982 to improve the neonatal intensive care experience for families and care providers. Provides leadership to promote the development of effective parent support services at the local level.
Sarah Killion, Administrative Director

8750 **Pregnancy and Infant Loss Center**
1421 E Wayzata Boulevard
Wayzata, MN 55391 612-473-9372
www.bloomington.in.us
Purpose is to offer support, resources and education on miscarriage, stillborn and newborn death.

8751 **Sudden Infant Death Syndrome (SIDS) Network**
PO Box 520 86- 89- 704
Ledyard, CT 06339 Fax: 860-887-7309
e-mail: sidsnet1@sids-network.org
www.sids-network.org
Dedicated to eliminate Sudden Infant Death Syndrome through the support of SIDS research projects. Provides support for those who have been touched by the tragedy of Sudden Infant Death Syndrome and to raise public awareness of this event.
Chuck Mihalko, Co-founder and President

8752 **Sudden Infant Death Syndrome Alliance**
1314 Bedford Avenue 410-653-8226
Baltimore, MD 21208-6605 800-221-7437
Fax: 410-653-8709
e-mail: info@firstcandle.org
www.sidsalliance.org
The purpose of the Alliance is to help parents educate the community about SIDS and to support SIDS research. The Alliance assists

parents to organize local chapters and provides services including a newsletter and other literature.
Marian Sokol, President
Deborah Boyd, Executive Director

State Agencies & Associations

Alabama

8753 **Bureau of Family Health Services: Alabama Department of Public Health**
19 South Jackson Street
201 Monroe Street 334-206-5300
Montgomery, AL 36104 800-ALA-1818
Fax: 334-269-5200
e-mail: llee@aap.net
www.adph.org
Linda P Lee, Executive Director

Alaska

8754 **SIDS Information and Counseling Program: Alaska Department of Health**
550 W 8th Street 907-296-3900
Anchorage, AK 99501-3553 Fax: 907-296-3901
e-mail: william.hogan@alaska.gov
www.hss.state.ak.us
Joel Bill Hogan, Commissioner
Jay Butler, Chief Medical Officer

Arizona

8755 **Arizona SIDS Founation**
PO Box 1111 520-297-6013
Phoenix, AZ 85001 800-597-7437
e-mail: info@azsidf.org
www.azsidf.org
Vanessa Seaney, President

8756 **Office of Womens And Childrens Health: Alabama Department of Health**
State Dapartment of Healths Services
150 N 18th Avenue 602-542-1000
Phoenix, AZ 85007-2602 Fax: 602-542-0883
e-mail: newbers@azdhs.gov
www.azdhs.gov
Susan Newber RN, Manager

Arkansas

8757 **Arkansas Department of Health: SIDS Information & Counseling Program**
4815 W Markham Street
Little Rock, AR 72205-3866 501-280-4560
www.healthyarkansas.com
Jackie Whitfield, Program Coordinator
Dawn Graziani

California

8758 **California SIDS Program**
11344 Coloma Road 916-851-7437
Gold River, CA 95670-6052 800-369-7437
Fax: 916-851-5937
e-mail: info@californiasids.com
www.californiasids.com
Gwen Edelstein, Program Director
Cheryl McBride, Program Manager

8759 **Region IX Office Program Consultants for Maternal and Child Health**
90 7th Street 415-437-7873
San Francisco, CA 94103 Fax: 415-437-8336
e-mail: reginald.louie@acf.hhs.gov
www.mchoralhealth.org
Reginald Lou DDS MPH, Oral Health Consultant

8760 **SIDS Alliance Of Northern California**
1547 Palos Verdes Mall 925-274-1109
Walnut Creek, CA 94597 877-938-7437
e-mail: info@sidsnc.org
www.sidsnc.org
Lorie Gehrke, President

8761 **SIDS Foundation of Southern California**
10811 Washington Boulevard 310-558-4511
Culver City, CA 90232 Fax: 310-558-7075
e-mail: sidsfsc@aol.com
sidsfoundationofsoutherncalifornia.org
Margot Stern Bennett, Executive Director

Colorado

8762 **Colorado SIDS Program**
425 S Cherry Street 303-320-7771
Denver, CO 80224 888-285-7437
Fax: 303-320-7827
e-mail: rlouie@hrsa.gov
www.coloradosids.org
Tena Saltzman, Executive Director

8763 **Colordao Department of Health and Environment**
4300 Cherry Creek Drive S 303-692-2000
Denver, CO 80246-1530 800-886-7689
Fax: 303-782-5576
TTY: 303-691-7700
e-mail: cdphe.information@state.co.us
www.cdphe.state.co.us
Bill Letson, Director

8764 **Region VIII Office Program Consultants for Maternal and Child Health**
1961 Stout Street 303-844-1482
Denver, CO 80294-1961 Fax: 303-844-3642
e-mail: valeri.orlando@acf.hhs.gov
www.mchoralhealth.org
Valerie Orla RDH BS, Oral Health Consultant

Connecticut

8765 **Connecticut SIDS Alliance**
PO Box 486 860-626-1542
Torrington, CT 06790 866-574-7437
Fax: 860-496-9919
e-mail: ctsids@aol.com
www.ctsids.org
Shannon Strandberg, Secretary

8766 **SIDS Program: Connecticut Department of Health**
410 Capitol Avenue 860-509-8074
Hartford, CT 06134 Fax: 860-509-7720
e-mail: marilyn.binns@po.state.ct.us
www.sidsalliance.org
Marilyn Binns, Program Coordinator

Delaware

8767 **Delaware SIDS Alliance**
PO Box 5449 302-996-9464
Wilmington, DE 19808 Fax: 302-255-2273
www.sidsalliance.org
Linda Hawthorne, President

8768 **SIDS Information & Counseling: Division of Public Health**
1901 N DuPont Highway 302-255-9040
New Castle, DE 19720 Fax: 302-255-4429
e-mail: dhssinfo@state/de/us
www.dhss.delaware.gov
Elaine Marke LCSW BCD, Program Coordinator

District of Columbia

8769 **DC Department of Health Maternal and Family Health Administration**
Maternal And Family Health Administration

825 N Capitol Street NE
Washington, DC 20002
202-442-5955
Fax: 202-645-6491
e-mail: drena.reaves@dc.gov
www.dchealth.dc.gov

Pierre Vigilance, Director
Rosie McLaren, Program Manager

Florida

8770 **Children's Medical Services Program: Florida SIDS Program**
4052 Bald Cypress Way
Tallahassee, FL 32399
850-245-4444
Fax: 904-488-2341
e-mail: Health@doh.state.fl.us
www.doh.state.fl.us

Susan Potts

8771 **Florida Department of Health**
4052 Bald Cypress Way
Tallahassee, FL 32399
850-245-4444
Fax: 850-245-4047
e-mail: Health@doh.state.fl.us
www.doh.state.fl.us

Susan Potts, Coordinator

8772 **Florida SIDS Alliance**
4185 W Lake Mary Boulevard
Lake Mary, FL 32746
305-232-1640
800-SID-SFLA
e-mail: flasidsalliance@yahoo.com
www.flasids.com

Steve Bonwit, Officer
Roy Bagley, President

Georgia

8773 **Georgia Department of Human Resources: Center for Family Resource Planning**
2 Peach Tree Street NW
Atlanta, GA 30319
404-651-7371
Fax: 404-463-6729
e-mail: kotto@dhr.state.ga.us

Provides grief support for parents.
Katherine Ottoel, Coordinator

8774 **Georgia Department of Human Resources: Inf ant and Child Health**
2 Peach Tree Street NW
Atlanta, GA 30303
404-651-7371
Fax: 404-463-6729
e-mail: kotto@dhr.state.ga.us

Katherine Otto, Coordinator

8775 **Georgia SIDS Project**
4112-2 E Ponce De Leon Avenue
Clarkston, GA 30021
678-342-3360
Fax: 404-296-7211
e-mail: gasids@mindspring.com
www.sidsga.org

Sudden Infant Death Syndrome is the sudden death of an infant under one year of age which remains unexplained after a thorough case investigation.
Diane Manheim, Director

8776 **Region IV Office Program Consultants for Maternal and Child Health**
61 Forsyth Street SW
Atlanta, GA 30303-8909
404-562-2935
Fax: 404-562-2984
e-mail: ejalderman@comcast.net
www.mchoralhealth.org

E Joseph Alderman DDS MPH, Oral Health Consultant

Hawaii

8777 **Hawaii Department of Health: Family Health Division**
Child Wellness Program r
1250 Punchbowl Street
Honolulu, HI 96813
808-586-4400
Fax: 808-733-9032
e-mail: gwen.palmer@fshd.health.state.hi.us
ww.hawaii.gov/health

Gwen Palmer, Coordinator

Idaho

8778 **Child Health Improvement Program: Idaho Department of Health**
450 W State Street
Boise, ID 83720
208-334-5507
www.healthandwelfare.idao.gov

Simonne deGl MS PNP, SIDS Coordinator

8779 **Idaho Department of Health and Welfare**
590 W Washington Street
Boise, ID 83720
208-334-4000
800-632-8000
Fax: 208-334-4015
e-mail: gainord@idhw.state.id.us
www.healthandwelfare.idaho.gov

Richard F Hudson PhD, Bureau Chief

Illinois

8780 **SIDS of Illinois**
710 E Ogden Avenue
Naperville, IL 60563
630-305-7300
Fax: 630-305-4773
e-mail: pam@sidsillinois.org
www.sidsillinois.org

Pam Borchardt, Facilitator

8781 **Statewide SIDS Program: Illinois Department of Public Health**
500 E Monroe Street
Springfield, IL 62761
217-557-2931
Fax: 217-524-2831
e-mail: bbreiden@idph.state.il.us

Babara Breidenbaugh, Program Specialist

Indiana

8782 **Indiana State Board of Health: SIDS Project**
2 N Meridian Street
Indianapolis, IN 46204-2829
317-233-1325
800-457-8283
e-mail: hpb6@hpb.in.gov.in.us
www.in.gov/hpb

Jayma Ellerbrook, Project Director

8783 **Indiana State Department of Health Maternal And Child Health Services**
Maternal And Child Health Services
2 N Meridian Street
Indianapolis, IN 46204
317-233-1325
800-457-8283
Fax: 317-233-1300
e-mail: bmjohnso@isdh.state.in.us
www.in.gov/hpb

Beth Johnson, Nurse Consultant

8784 **SIDS Center of Indiana**
1810 Broad Ripple Avenue
Indianapolis, IN 46220
317-484-1500
e-mail: sidscenter@insids.org

John Schutt, Chairperson

Iowa

8785 **Iowa Department of Public Health Center for Congenital and Inherited Disorders**
Center For Congenital And Inherited Disorders
321 E 12th Street
Des Moines, IA 50319
515-281-7689
Fax: 515-242-6384
e-mail: kipper@idph.state.ia.us
www.idph.state.ia.us

Patricia Young, Prevention Coordinator
Rob Walker, Surveillance Officer

8786 **Iowa SIDS Alliance**
406 SW School Street
Ankeny, IA 50023
515-965-7655
866-480-4741
Fax: 515-964-7506
e-mail: info@iowasids.org
www.iowasids.org

Patty Keeley, Executive Director
Jennifer Atzen, President

8787 **Iowa SIDS Program Iowa Department of Public Health**
Iowa Department of Public Health

321 E 12th Street
Des Moines, IA 50319-0075
515-281-7689
866-227-9878
www.idph.state.ia.us

Jane Borst, Bureau Chief
Sally Clausen

Kansas

8788 Kansas Department of Health & Environment Bureau of Family Health
Bureau Of Children, Youth And Families
1000 SW Jackson Street
Topeka, KS 66612-1274
785-291-3368
800-332-6262
Fax: 785-296-6553
e-mail: info@kdheks.gov
www.kdheks.gov

Linda kenney, Director
Kobi Gomel, Administrative Specialist

8789 SIDS Network of Kansas
1148 S Hillside
Wichita, KS 67211
316-682-1301
866-399-7437
Fax: 316-682-1274
e-mail: info@sidsks.org
www.sidsks.org

Ellen Patterson, Program Director

Kentucky

8790 Department of Public Health: Adult and Child Health Division
275 E Main Street
Frankfort, KY 40621
502-564-3236
800-372-2973
Fax: 502-564-8389
TTY: 800-627-4702
e-mail: marcia.burkow@ky.gov

Marcia Burkow, SIDS Coordinator

8791 SIDS Network of Kentucky
PO Box 186
Caneyville, KY 42721-3555
800-928-7437
Fax: 859-245-0717
e-mail: info@sidsky.org
www.sidsky.org

Adrienne Grizzell, Executive Director

Louisiana

8792 Office of Public Health
628 N 4th Street
Baton Rouge, LA 70802
225-342-9500
Fax: 225-342-5568
e-mail: hhwebadmin@la.gov
www.dhh.louisiana.gov/offices/?ID=79

Tracy Hubbard, Coordinator

8793 Public Health Services of Louisiana
628 N 4th Street
Baton Rouge, LA 70802-0629
225-342-9500
Fax: 225-342-5568
e-mail: dhhwebadmin@la.gov
www.dhh.state.la.us/

Jamie Roques RNC, SIDS Coordinator

Maine

8794 Department of Human Services
221 State Street
Augusta, ME 04333-0001
207-287-3707
Fax: 207-287-3005
TTY: 800-606-0215
www.state.me.us/dhs/

Brenda Harvey, Commissioner

8795 Maine SIDS Foundation
14 Charlonate Drive
Gray, ME 04039
207-657-2220
Fax: 207-657-3737
e-mail: roybagley@aol.com
www.sidsalliance.org

Roy Bagley, Chairperson

8796 Maine SIDS Program Department Of Human Services
Department Of Human Services
200 Main Street
Lewiston, ME 04240
207-795-4450
Fax: 207-795-4445
e-mail: luanne.crinion@maine.gov

Luanne Crinion, Program Coordinator

Maryland

8797 Maryland SIDS Information & Counseling Program
22 S Green Street
Baltimore, MD 21201
410-328-8667
800-492-5538
TTY: 410-328-9600
TDD: 410-328-9600
e-mail: webmaster@umm.edu
www.marylandsids.com

Jeffrey A Rivest, President and Chief Executive Officer
R Keith Allen, Senior Vice President

Massachusetts

8798 Massachusetts Chapter of SIDS Alliance Boston Medical Center
Boston Medical Center
PO Box 520
Ledyard, CT 06339-2908
617-414-SIDS
800-641-7437
Fax: 617-534-5555
e-mail: sidsnet1@sids-network.org
www.sids-network.org

State chapter offering educational resources and information on SIDS, parent groups, support networks, monthly meetings and workshops to the community.

Frederick Mandell, Co Director
Michael Corwin, Co Director

8799 Region I Office Program: Consultants for Maternal and Child Health
John F Kennedy Building
Boston, MA 02203
617-899-1355
Fax: 202-833-8288
e-mail: Mary.Foley@mcphs.edu
www.mchoralhealth.org

Mary Foley RDH MPH, Oral Health Consultant

Michigan

8800 Apnea Identification Program Children's Hospital of Michigan
Children's Hospital of Michigan
3901 Beaubien Street
Detroit, MI 48201-2196
313-745-9048
888-DMC-2500
Fax: 313-745-5848
www.childrensdmc.org

Karen Branif RN MSW, Nurse Specialist

8801 Genesee County Health Department
630 S Saignaw Street
Flint, MI 48502-3915
810-257-3612
Fax: 810-257-3147
e-mail: gchd-info@gchd.us
www.gchd.us

John Northrup, Chairperson
Michael Boucree, Vice-Chairperson

8802 Kent County Health Department
300 Monroe Avenue NE
Grand Rapids, MI 49503-1996
616-632-7590
www.accesskent.com

Colleen Jill RN, SIDs Coordinator
David Kraker

8803 Michigan Department of Community Health
3423 MLK Boulevard
Lansing, MI 48909
517-373-1820
Fax: 517-373-2129
e-mail: lauberc@michigan.gov
www.michigan.gov

Cheryl Lauber, Coordinator

8804 Oakland County Health Division: SIDS Project
1200 N Telegraph
Pontiac, MI 48341-0482
248-858-1280
800-774-4542
Fax: 248-858-0178
TTY: 248-452-2247
TDD: 248-452-2247
e-mail: oakllbph@oakland.lib.mi.us
www.oakgov.com
David Conklin, Librarian
George J Miller Jr MA, Director

8805 SIDS LEAD: Children's Special Health Care Services
Michigan Department of Public Health
201 Townsend Street
Lansing, MI 48913-2934
517-373-3740
TTY: 517-373-3573
TDD: 517-373-3573
e-mail: norris@michigan.gov
www.michigan.gov/mdch
Janet Olszewski, Director
Ed Dore, Chief Deputy Director

Minnesota

8806 Minnesota Sudden Infant Death Center Minneapolis Children's Medical Center
Minneapolis Children's Medical Center
2525 Chicago Avenue
Minneapolis, MN 55404-4518
612-813-6000
Fax: 612-813-7344
e-mail: kathleen.fernbach@childreansHC.org
www.childrensmn.org/Communities/SIDs.asp
Sara Schumacher, Project Coordinator

8807 STOP-SIDS Minnesota
2873 Upper 138th Street
Rosemont, MN 55068
Fax: 651-310-2106
www.sidsalliance.org
Trish LaVictoire, President

Mississippi

8808 Mississippi SIDS Alliance
PO Box 2170
Madison, MS 39130-2170
877-471-7437
e-mail: mssids@jam.rr.com
www.sidsalliance.org
Cathy Files, Chairperson

8809 Mississippi State Department of Health and Child Health Services
570 E Woodrow Wilson
Jackson, MS 39216
601-576-7400
866-458-4948
Fax: 601-576-7498
e-mail: Linda.Proctor@msdh.state.ms.us
www.msdh.state.ms.us
Linda Proctor, Coordinator

Missouri

8810 Region VII Office Program: Consultants for Maternal and Child Health
Federal Building
10031 Perry Drive
Overland Park, KS 66212-2826
913-888-1377
Fax: 816-426-3633
e-mail: lwalker17@kc.rr.com
www.mchoralhealth.org
Lawrence Wal DDS MPH, Oral Health Consultant

8811 SIDS Resources
1120 S Sixth Street
Saint Louis, MO 63104
314-822-2323
800-421-3511
Fax: 314-822-2098
e-mail: lahrens@sidsresources.org
www.sidsresources.org
Lori Behrens, Executive Director
Teresa Buehler, Program Coordinator

8812 Western Region SIDS Resources
5700 Broadmoor
Mission, MO 66202
913-671-1818
Fax: 816-753-6906
e-mail: slogan@sidsresources.org
www.sidsalliance.org
Shay Logan, Program Coordinator

Montana

8813 Department of Public Health and Human Services
1400 Broadway
Helena, MT 59620
406-444-3565
800-232-4636
Fax: 406-444-2606
e-mail: WMcGraw@state.mt.us
www.dphhs.mt.gov
Brad Pickhardt, Chairperson
Peggy Baker, Administrative Aide

8814 Montana Department of Health & Environmental Sciences
Health Plannin Program
PO Box 200901
Helena, MT 59620-0901
406-444-4473
Charles Aagenes

Nebraska

8815 Nebraska Department of Health Perinatal Child and Adolescent Health
301 Centennial Mall South
Lincoln, NE 68509
402-471-0165
Fax: 402-471-7049
e-mail: jan.heusinkvelt@hhss.ne.gov
Jan Heusinkvelt, RN, BSN, Community Health Nurse

8816 Nebraska SIDS Foundation University of Nebraska Medical Center
University of Nebraska Medical Center
PO Box 460905
Papillion, NE 68046
402-431-8076
e-mail: board@nesids.org
www.nesids.com
Tammy Dawdy

Nevada

8817 Nevada State Health Division Bureau of Family Health Services
Bureau Of Family Health Services
3427 Goni Road
Carson City, NV 89706
775-684-4285
Fax: 775-684-4245
e-mail: chuth@nvhd.state.nv.us
www.health2k.state.nv.us
Cynthia Huthht, Health Program Specialist

New Hampshire

8818 New Hampshire SIDS Alliance
13 Drew Road
Derry, NH 03038
617-828-4996
e-mail: declan4204@comcast.net
www.sidsalliance.org
Charlie Foote, Chairperson

8819 New Hampshire SIDS Program
New Hampshire Division of Public Health Services
29 Hazen Drive
Concord, NH 03301
603-271-4536
Fax: 603-271-4519
e-mail: sidsnet1@sids-network.org
www.sids-network.org
Audrey Knigh MSN CPNP, SIDS Coordinator

New Jersey

8820 New Jersey Department of Health: Child Health Program
PO Box 360
Trenton, NJ 08625
609-292-7837
800-367-6543
e-mail: lindajones@doh.state.nj.us
www.state.nj.us/health
Linda Jones Hicks, Director
Shirley White-Walker, Chair

8821 New Jersey SIDS Alliance
15 Meadowbrook Road
Boonton Township, NJ 07005
973-299-6523
e-mail: njsids@yahoo.com
www.sidsalliance.org
Genny Elias-Warren, Chairperson

8822 SIDS Center of New Jersey
1 Robert Wood Johnson Place
New Brunswick, NJ 08903-1766
732-249-2160
800-704-7437
Fax: 732-235-6609
e-mail: hegyith@umdnj.edu
www2.umdnj.edu/sids
Thomas Hegyi MD, Co-Medical Director
Barbara Ostf PhD, Program Director

8823 SIDS Center of New Jersey: Northern Site
Hackensack Medical Center
30 Prospect Avenue
Hackensack, NJ 07601
201-996-5328
800-704-7437
Fax: 201-996-0754
e-mail: rhinnen@humed.com
www2.umdnj.edu/sids
Barbara Ostf PhD, Program Director
Thomas Hegyi MD, Co-Medical Director

New Mexico

8824 New Mexico SIDS Information and Counseling Program
University of New Mexico School of Medicine
2500 Marble NE
Albuquerque, NM 87131
505-277-3053
Fax: 505-272-3601
e-mail: sidsnet1@sids-network.org
www.sids-network.org
Beverly Whit RN MS, Director

New York

8825 NYS Center for SIDS
990 7th N Street
Liverpool, NY 13088-6148
315-634-2191
Fax: 315-634-1118
e-mail: csquillace@hospice-pca.org
www.sidsprojectimpact.com
Cynthia Squillace, Chairperson

8826 NYS Center for Sudden Infant Death: Eastern Satellite Office
Albany Medical College
47 New Scotland Avenue
Albany, NY 12208
518-262-5918
Fax: 518-262-7237
e-mail: whittrm@mail.amc.edu
Mary Whittredge, Regional Coordinator

8827 New York City Center for SIDS
New York City Satellite Office
520 1st Avenue
New York, NY 10016
212-686-8854
800-522-5006
Fax: 212-532-6564
e-mail: evelyne.longchamp@sids1.ssw.sunysb.edu
Judith Gaine CSW PhD, SIDS Program Director

8828 New York State Center for SIDS: School of Social Welfare
Stony Brook University
Health Sciences Center Level 2
Stony Brook, NY 11794-0001
631-444-1441
800-336-7437
Fax: 631-444-6475
e-mail: marie.chandick@stonybrook.edu
www.hsc.stonybrook.edu
Marie Chandi CSW, Associate Project Director

8829 Region II Office Program: Consultants for Maternal and Child Health
345 E 24th Street
New York, NY 10010-0004
212-998-9654
Fax: 212-995-4364
e-mail: ngh1@nyu.edu
www.mchoralhealth.org
Neal Herman DDS, Oral Health Consultant

8830 WNYS Center for SIDS
3580 Harlem Road
Buffalo, NY 14215
716-837-5189
Fax: 716-836-1578
e-mail: jwalkden@palliativecare.org
www.sidsalliance.org
Jan Walkden, Family Service Coordinator

North Carolina

8831 Department of Health and Human Services
200 Independence Avenue SW
Washington, DC 20201
919-715-8430
Fax: 919-715-3410
e-mail: april.ellis@ncmail.net
www.hhs.gov
April Ellis, SIDS Program Manager

8832 SIDS Alliance of the Carolinas
306 Lucas Park Drive
Greensboro, NC 27455
336-545-3348
e-mail: sandylkennedy@hotmail.com
www.sidsalliance.org
Sandy Kennedy, Chairperson

North Dakota

8833 North Dakota SIDS Alliance
128 Apollo Avenue
Bismarck, ND 58503
701-530-2507
Fax: 701-223-0440
e-mail: ndsids@btinet.net
www.sidsalliance.org
Barb Delvo, Chairperson

8834 North Dakota SIDS Management Program
Division of Maternal and Child Health
600 E Boulevard Avenue
Bismarck, ND 58505-0200
701-328-2493
800-472-2286
Fax: 701-328-1412
e-mail: kchintz@nd.gov
www.ndhealth.gov
Provides support education and follow-up to parents/caregivers family and childcare providers suffering a sudden infant death
Kjersti Hintz, Program Director

Ohio

8835 District Board of Health: Mahoning County
50 Westchester Drive
Youngstown, OH 44515
330-270-2855
800-873-MCHD
Fax: 330-270-2860
e-mail: mchealth@cboss.com
www.mahoning-health.org
Lisa Weiss MD, Forum Health
Bev Fisher, Manager

8836 Ohio Department of Health
Child Fatality Review
246 N High Street
Columbus, OH 43215
614-728-0773
866-634-7654
Fax: 614-564-2433
e-mail: SmkInfo@odh.ohio.govÿ
www.odh.ohio.gov
Alvin D Jackson, Director

8837 SIDS Network of Ohio
421 Graham Road
Cuyahoga Falls, OH 44221
Fax: 330-929-0593
e-mail: SIDNetwork@sidsohio.org
www.sidsohio.org
Pat Marquis, Chairperson

Oklahoma

8838 Oklahoma State Department of Health: Maternal and Child Health Services
1000 NE 10th Street
Oklahoma City, OK 73117-1207
405-271-5600
800-522-0203
Fax: 405-271-9202
e-mail: paulaw@health.ok.gov
www.ok.gov
Paula Wood, Executive Assistant
Suzanna Dooley

Oregon

8839 Oregon Department of Human Services
500 Summer Street NE
Salem, OR 97301
503-945-5944
Fax: 503-378-2897
TTY: 503-945-6214
e-mail: dhs.info@state.or.us
www.oregon.gov
Joyce Edmonds, Public Nurse Consultant

Pennsylvania

8840 Pennsylvania Department of Health Bureau of Family Health
Bureau of Family Health
7th & Forster Streets
Harrisburg, PA 17120
717-772-2762
877-PAH-EALT
Fax: 717-772-0323
e-mail: bcaboot@state.pa.us
www.dsf.health.state.pa.us
Robert Torres, Deputy Secretary for Administration

8841 Region III Office Program: Consultants for Maternal and Child Health
Public Ledger Building
2115 Wisconsin Avenue NW
Washington, DC 20007-3309
202-784-9771
Fax: 202-784-9777
www.mchoralhealth.org
Jolene Bertness, Health Education Specialist
Katrina Holt, Director

8842 SIDS of Pennsylvania
810 River Avenue
Pittsburgh, PA 15212
412-322-5680
800-721-7437
Fax: 412-481-5968
e-mail: sidspa@aol.com
www.sids-pa.org
Judy Bannon, Executive Director
Joseph Dominick, Chairman

Rhode Island

8843 Rhode Island Department of Health
3 Capitol Hill
Providence, RI 02908
401-222-4606
800-942-7434
Fax: 401-222-6548
TTY: 711
e-mail: DOH@health.ri.gov
www.health.state.ri.us
David R Gifford MD MPH, Director
Donald L Carcieri, Governor

8844 Rhode Island Department of Health: National SIDS Foundation
29 Hannah Drive
Warwick, RI 02888
401-461-2162
e-mail: wilksme@aol.com
www.sidsalliance.org
Mary Wilks, Area Contact

South Carolina

8845 Division of Perinatal Systems Mills Jarret Complex
Mills Jarret Complex
Box 101106
Columbia, SC 29211
803-898-0734
Fax: 803-898-2065
e-mail: swansokm@dhec.sc.gov
Kathy Swanson, State FIMR Director

South Dakota

8846 South Dakota Department of Health
Health Building
600 E Capitol Avenue
Pierre, SD 57501
605-773-3361
800-738-2301
Fax: 605-773-5509
e-mail: DOH.info@state.sd.us
www.doh.sd.gov
Nancy Shoup, Program Coordinator

Tennessee

8847 Tenessee Department of Health
Division of Maternal & Child Health
425 5th Avenue N
Nashville, TN 37243-4701
615-741-3111
Fax: 615-741-1063
e-mail: tn.health@tn.gov
health.state.tn.us
Susan R Cooper MSN RN, Commissioner

8848 Tennessee SIDS Alliance
7603 Moon Crest Court
Powell, TN 37849
423-947-6669
e-mail: lisasids@cs.com
ww.sidsalliance.org
Lisa Hunt, Chairperson

Texas

8849 Department of State Health Offices
Title V And Health Resources
PO Box 149347
Austin, TX 78714
512-458-7111
888-963-7111
Fax: 512-458-7650
e-mail: chan.mcdermott@dshs.state.tx.us
www.dshs.state.tx.us
Mary Chan Mcdermott, Prenatal Coordinator

8850 Greater Houston Chapter SIDS Alliance
916 Satsuma Street
Pasadena, TX 77506
713-924-1419
Fax: 281-541-5340
e-mail: anita.carmona@us.rhodia.com
www.sidsalliance.org
Anita Carmona, Chairperson

8851 Harris County Public Health and Environmental Services
2223 W Lop S
Houston, TX 77027
713-439-6000
e-mail: publicinfo@hd.co.harris.tx.us
www.hcphes.org
Herminia Palacio, Executive Director

8852 Region VI Office Program Consultants for Maternal and Child Health
1301 Young Street
Dallas, TX 75202-4325
214-767-3003
Fax: 214-767-3038
e-mail: geurink@zeecon.com
www.mchoralhealth.org
Kathy Geurin RDH BS MA, Oral Health Consultant

8853 Southwest SIDS Research Institute
Brazosport Memorial Hospital
100 Medical Drive
Lake Jackson, TX 77566
409-297-4411
www.swsids.com
ISBN: 9-792992-81-4
CF Hogan, President
Loretta Washington, Vice-President

Utah

8854 Utah Department of Health
Child Adolescent & School Health Program
288 N 1460 W
Salt Lake City, UT 84114-3231
801-538-6870
Fax: 801-538-6200
www.health.utah.gov
David Sundwa MD, Executive Director
A Richard Melton, Deputy Director

8855 Utah SIDS Alliance
1760 American Park Circle
W Valley City, UT 84119
801-487-7800
Fax: 801-487-4477
e-mail: lisa.hughes@fnwmail.com
www.sidsalliance.org
Lisa Hughes, President
Troy Hughes, Co-President

Vermont

8856 Vermont Department of Health: SIDS Information and Counseling Program
108 Cherry Street 802-652-2000
Burlington, VT 05402 Fax: 802-652-2005
TTY: 800-253-0191
e-mail: kkelehe@vdh.state.vt.us
healthvermont.gov
Kathy Keleher, Assistant Director Public Health

Virginia

8857 SIDS Mid-Atlantic
PO Box 799 703-955-6899
Haymarket, VA 20168 Fax: 703-933-9101
e-mail: bconnal@aol.com
www.sidsma.org
Betty Connal, Executive Director

8858 Virginia SIDS Alliance
PO Box 752
Mechanicsville, VA 23111 Fax: 757-548-7074
e-mail: mail@vasids.org
www.vasids.org
Terri Newman, President
Mark Ferraro, Vice President

8859 Virginia SIDS Program: Virginia Department of Health
Virginia Department of Health
109 Governor Street 804-846-7772
Richmond, VA 23219 Fax: 804-973-9498
e-mail: WomensAndInfantsHealth@vdh.virginia.gov
www.vdh.virginia.gov
Robert Stroube, Commissioner
Rosanne Kolesar, Deputy Commissioner Public Health

Washington

8860 Region X Office Program Consultants for Maternal and Child Health
2201 Sixth Avenue 206-615-2518
Seattle, WA 98121-1857 Fax: 206-615-2500
e-mail: rslayton@acf.hhs.gov
www.mchoralhealth.org
Rebecca Slay DDS PhD, Oral Health Consultant

8861 SIDS Foundation of Washington
4649 Sunnyside Avenue N 206-548-9290
Seattle, WA 98103 800-533-0376
Fax: 206-548-9445
e-mail: execdirector@sidsofwa.org
www.nisa-sids.org
Inga Paige, Executive Director
Lindsey Hulet, Office Administrator

8862 SIDS Northwest Regional Center
Washington Department of Health
111 Israel Rd SE 360-236-3502
Olympia, WA 98501-7880 800-533-0376
Fax: 360-236-2323
e-mail: mch.support@doh.wa.gov
www.doh.wa.gov
Lorrie Grevstad

8863 Washington State Department of Health Maternal & Child Health Office
111 Israel Rd SE 360-236-3502
Olympia, WA 98501 Fax: 360-236-2323
e-mail: mch.support@doh.wa.gov
www.doh.wa.gov
Shumei Yun, Manager Maternal and Child Health
Riley Peters, Director

West Virginia

8864 Office of Maternal, Child & Family Health
Bureau For Public Health
350 Capitol Street 304-558-7997
Charelston, WV 25301 Fax: 304-558-3510
e-mail: annmunson@wvdhhr.org
Ann Munson, SIDS Coordinator

Wisconsin

8865 Counseling and Research Center for SIDS
9000 W Wisconsin Avenue 414-266-2746
Wauwatosa, WI 53226 Fax: 414-266-3338
e-mail: aharvieux@chw.org
www.idcw.org
Anne Harvieux, Program Administrator

8866 Infant Death Center of Wisconsin Childrens Hospital Of Wisconsin
Childrens Hospital Of Wisconsin
PO Box 1997 414-266-2746
Milwaukee, WI 53201 Fax: 414-266-3140
e-mail: aharvieux@chw.org
www.idcw.org
Anne Harvieux, Program Administrator

Wyoming

8867 Wyoming Department of Health
Community & Family Health Section
6101 Yellowstone Road 307-777-6326
Cheyenne, WY 82002 Fax: 307-777-7215
e-mail: mirandie.peterson@health.wyo.gov
wdh.state.wy.us
Molly M Bruner MSN RNC, Administrator

Research Centers

8868 Massachusetts Sudden Infant Death Syndrome Boston City Hospital
Boston City Hospital
1 Boston Medical Center Place 617-534-7434
Boston, MA 02118 Fax: 617-534-5555
www.bmc.org
A joint program of Boston City Hospital and Children's Hospital. Services provided include around-the-clock availability for consultation to health professionals and families counseling of families parent group meetings and supportive home visits.

8869 Pediatric Pulmonary Unit Massachusetts General Hospital
Massachusetts General Hospital
55 Fruit Street 617-726-0336
Boston, MA 02114 Fax: 617-242-03
www.massgeneral.org
Sudden infant death syndrome and childhood disorders research.
T Bernard Kinane MD, Head Physician

8870 Sudden Infant Death Syndrome Institute of the University of Maryland
22 S Green Street 410-538-3363
Baltimore, MD 21201 800-492-5538
www.umm.edu
Dr M John O'Brien MB, Director

8871 USC: Neonatology Research Units
1240 Mission Road 213-226-3408
Los Angeles, CA 90033 Fax: 213-226-3440
Focuses on clinical problems of the newborn and premature infant.
Paul YK Wu MD, Director

Support Groups & Hotlines

8872 National Center for the Prevention of SIDS
1314 Bedford Avenue
Baltimore, MD 21208-6605 800-638-7437
Offers medical updates and information on prevention of SIDS and other disorders to parents and professionals.

8873 **National Health Information Center**
PO Box 1133
Washington, DC 20013
310-565-4167
800-336-4797
Fax: 301-984-4256
e-mail: info@nhic.org
www.health.gov/nhic
Offers a nationwide information referral service, produces directories and resource guides.

8874 **Parents Helping Parents A Family Resource Center**
3041 Olcott Street
Santa Clara, CA 95054
408-727-5775
866-747-4040
Fax: 408-727-0182
www.php.com
A group of parents and professionals committed to alleviating some of the problems, hardships and concerns of families with children having special needs.
Mary Ellen Peterson, Director

8875 **SIDS Information and Referral Hotline**
SIDS Alliance
1314 Bedford Avenue
Baltimore, MD 21208
410-653-8226
800-221-7437
Fax: 410-653-8709
www.firstcandle.org
Twenty-four hour information and referral line for parents who wish to discuss their concerns with a SIDS counselor, request additional information about SIDS and to receive referrals to the local SIDS affiliate in their area.
Deborah Boyd, Director

8876 **SIDS Support Group**
Massachusetts Center for SIDS
Boston Medical Center
Boston, MA 02118
617-414-SIDS
800-641-7437
www.bmc.org
Aids in the resolution of the early trauma of grief experienced by parents following the sudden unexpected death of their infant. The purposes are to provide a safe environemnt for parents to express their feelings, to provide contact with others who share their grief and are at various stages of resolution, to provide a reliable source of information about SIDS and to provide the opportunity to go on to help others.

Books

8877 **Apparent Life-Threatening Event and Sudden Infant Death Syndrome**
National Maternal and Child Health Clearinghouse
2070 Chain Bridge Road
Vienna, VA 22182-2588
703-442-9051
888-275-4772
Fax: 703-821-2098
e-mail: ask@hrsa.gov
www.ask.hrsa.gov
Provides information about ALTE and its relationship to SIDS.

8878 **Hospice Care for Children**
Oxford University Press
2001 Evans Road
Cary, NC 27513-2010
212-726-6000
800-451-7556
Fax: 919-677-1303
www.oup-usa.org
A comprehensive book offering the most inclusive and up-to-date information about caring for terminally ill children and their families.
304 pages
ISBN: 0-195073-12-6
Ann Armstrong-Dailey, Editor

8879 **Professional's Role in Sudden Infant Death Syndrome**
National Maternal and Child Health Clearinghouse
2070 Chain Bridge Road
Vienna, VA 22182-2588
703-442-9051
888-275-4772
Fax: 703-821-2098
e-mail: ask@hrsa.gov
www.ask.hrsa.gov
Contains abstracts of articles on the role of professionals in SIDS.

8880 **Smoking and Sudden Infant Death Syndrome**
National Maternal and Child Health Clearinghouse
2070 Chain Bridge Road
Vienna, VA 22182-2588
703-442-9051
888-275-4772
Fax: 703-821-2098
e-mail: ask@hrsa.gov
www.ask.hrsa.gov
Contains abstracts of materials about tobacco use, its relationship to SIDS and the dangers to the unborn and the newly born from passive and secondary smoking.

Newsletters

8881 **Newsletter: SIDS**
Massachusetts Center For SIDS
1 Boston Medical Center Place
Boston, MA 02118-2905
617-414-8504
www.bmc.org/program/sids/
Offers information on SIDS, articles pertaining to the latest information available on the mystery condition, latest research and fund-raising news and professional resources available.
Monthly

8882 **Parent Care News Brief**
Parent Care
303 Watts Branch Parkway
Rockville, MD 20850-1210
301-294-9338
Fax: 301-294-8848
e-mail: drscott@parentcare.com
www.parentcare.com
Features articles and medical updates pertaining to the care of the critically ill child.
Quarterly

Pamphlets

8883 **Crib Death: The Sudden Infant Death Syndrome**
US Department Of Health & Human Services
202 Independence Avenue SW
Washington, DC 20201-0001
202-619-0257
877-696-6775
e-mail: hhsmail@os.dhhs.gov
www.os.dhhs.gov
Offers information on the most frequently asked questions pertaining to SIDS and crib death.
Kristen Brett
Kathy McKnight

8884 **Developmental Delays and Developmental Disorders**
National Maternal and Child Health Clearinghouse
2070 Chain Bridge Road
Vienna, VA 22182-2588
703-442-9051
888-275-4772
Fax: 703-821-2098
e-mail: ask@hrsa.gov
www.ask.hrsa.gov
Contains abstracts of selected articles on developmental delays and developmental disorders and the relationship to SIDS.
1997

8885 **Facts About SIDS**
Sudden Infant Death Syndrome Alliance
1314 Bedford Avenue
Baltimore, MD 21208-6605
410-653-8226
800-221-7437
Fax: 410-653-8709
Offers information on basic facts, answers to the most frequently asked questions about SIDS and information on numbers to call and referral centers for more help.

8886 **Grief of Children After the Loss of a Sibling or Friend**
National Maternal and Child Health Clearinghouse
2070 Chain Bridge Road
Vienna, VA 22182-2588
703-442-9051
888-275-4772
Fax: 703-821-2098
e-mail: ask@hrsa.gov
www.ask.hrsa.gov
Discusses some of the common expressions of childrens grief and offers ways adults can help during the grieving process.
1995

8887 **Infant Positioning and Sudden Infant Death Syndrome**
National Maternal and Child Health Clearinghouse
2070 Chain Bridge Road 703-442-9051
Vienna, VA 22182-2588 888-275-4772
Fax: 703-821-2098
e-mail: ask@hrsa.gov
www.ask.hrsa.gov
Contains abstracts of selected articles on the topic of sleep position and SIDS.
1994

8888 **Nationwide Survey of Sudden Infant Death Syndrome (SIDS) Service**
National Maternal and Child Health Clearinghouse
2070 Chain Bridge Road 703-442-9051
Vienna, VA 22182-2588 888-275-4772
Fax: 703-821-2098
e-mail: ask@hrsa.gov
www.ask.hrsa.gov
Analysis of availability of SIDS services.
1994

8889 **Parents and the Grieving Process**
National Maternal and Child Health Clearinghouse
2070 Chain Bridge Road 703-442-9051
Vienna, VA 22182-2588 888-275-4772
Fax: 703-821-2098
e-mail: ask@hrsa.gov
www.ask.hrsa.gov
Defines grief, presents common reactions and emotions expressed by the bereaved.
1992

8890 **SIDS Information for the EMT**
National Maternal and Child Health Clearinghouse
2070 Chain Bridge Road 703-442-9051
Vienna, VA 22182-2588 888-275-4772
Fax: 703-821-2098
e-mail: ask@hrsa.gov
www.ask.hrsa.gov
Provides suggestions for first response of emergency medical technicians and others at the time of sudden infant death.
1983

8891 **SIDS Research: An Analysis in Three Parts**
National Maternal and Child Health Clearinghouse
2070 Chain Bridge Road 703-442-9051
Vienna, VA 22182-2588 888-275-4772
Fax: 703-821-2098
e-mail: ask@hrsa.gov
www.ask.hrsa.gov
Contains articles from a three part series on SIDS research.
1993

8892 **SIDS: Toward Prevention and Improved Infant Health**
American SIDS Institute
2480 Windy Hill Road SE 770-612-1030
Marietta, GA 30067-8657 800-232-7437
Fax: 770-612-8277
e-mail: prevent@sids.org
www.sids.org
A practical guide for those planning a pregnancy, for parents to be and for new parents.
Betty McEntire PhD, Executive Director

8893 **Selected Book on Sudden Infant Death Syndrome**
National Maternal and Child Health Clearinghouse
2070 Chain Bridge Road 703-442-9051
Vienna, VA 22182-2588 888-275-4772
Fax: 703-821-2098
e-mail: ask@hrsa.gov
www.ask.hrsa.gov
Provides a list of selected titles on SIDS covering topics such as research, support information and the professionals role.
1993

8894 **Selected Resources for Children Grieving the Loss of Another Child**
National Maternal and Child Health Clearinghouse
2070 Chain Bridge Road 703-442-9051
Vienna, VA 22182-2588 888-275-4772
Fax: 703-821-2098
e-mail: ask@hrsa.gov
www.ask.hrsa.gov
Provides a list of materials suitable for grieving children and teenagers.
1995

8895 **Sudden Infant Death Syndrome and Risk Reduction**
National Maternal and Child Health Clearinghouse
2070 Chain Bridge Road 703-442-9051
Vienna, VA 22182-2588 888-275-4772
Fax: 703-821-2098
e-mail: ask@hrsa.gov
www.ask.hrsa.gov
Contains abstracts of selected articles on risk reduction.
1997

8896 **What Every Parent Should Know About SIDS**
SIDS Alliance
1314 Bedford Avenue 410-653-8226
Baltimore, MD 21208-6605 800-221-7437
Fax: 410-653-8709
Pamphlet offering information on what SIDS is, causes, prevention techniques and what parents can do.

8897 **What is SIDS?**
National Maternal and Child Health Clearinghouse
2070 Chain Bridge Road 703-442-9051
Vienna, VA 22182-2588 888-275-4772
Fax: 703-821-2098
e-mail: ask@hrsa.gov
www.ask.hrsa.gov
Provides basic facts about SIDS and answers some of the most commonly asked questions.
1993

8898 **When Sudden Infant Death Syndrome Occurs in Childcare Settings**
National Maternal and Child Health Clearinghouse
2070 Chain Bridge Road 703-442-9051
Vienna, VA 22182-2588 888-275-4772
Fax: 703-821-2098
e-mail: ask@hrsa.gov
www.ask.hrsa.gov
Presents information about SIDS for child care providers.
1993

Web Sites

8899 **American SIDS Institute**
sids.org/
Dedicated to the prevention of sudden infant death and the promotion of infant health through research, clinical services, education and family support.

8900 **Center for Research for Mothers & Children**
cdrwww.who.ch/
Mission is to make sure everyone is born healthy and wanted, that women suffer no harmful effects from reproductive processes, and that all children have the chance to achieve their full potential for healthy and productive lives, free from disease or disability, and to ensure the health, productivity, independence, and well-being of all people through optimal rehabilitation.

8901 **Compassionate Friends**
www.compassionatefriends.org/
A national organization that offers 600 local chapters that give support to parents and siblings who have experienced the death of a child.

8902 **Healing Well**
www.healingwell.com
An online health resource guide to medical news, chat, information and articles, newsgroups and message boards, books, disease-related web sites, medical directories, and more for patients, friends, and family coping with disabling diseases, disorders, or chronic illnesses.

8903 **Healthlink USA**

www.healthlinkusa.com

Health information concerning treatment, cures, prevention, diagnosis, risk factors, research, support groups, email lists, personal stories and much more. Updated regularly.

8904 **Helios Health**

www.helioshealth.com

Online resource for your health information. Detailed information about specific health topics, access to expert advice from our Medical Advisory Board, and up-to-date health news.

8905 **MedicineNet**

www.medicinenet.com

An online resource for consumers providing easy-to-read, authoritative medical and health information.

8906 **Medscape**

www.mywebmd.com

Medscape offers specialists, primary care physicians, and other health professionals the Web's most robust and integrated medical information and educational tools.

8907 **National Center for Education in Maternal and Child Health**

www.ncemch.org

The National Center for Education in Maternal and Child Health provides national leadership to the maternal and child health community in three key areas - program development, policy analysis and education, and state-of-the-art knowledge to improve the health and well-being of the nation's children and families.

8908 **WebMD**

www.webmd.com

Information on Sudden Infant Death Syndrome, including articles and resources.

Description

8909 **Tay-Sachs Disease**

Tay-Sachs disease results from an absence of an enzyme (hexosaminidase A) which leads to an accumulation of fat (lipid) in the specific brain tissues (cerebral neurons). The disease is genetic and is autosomal recessive; if two carriers have children, the disease would have a 1 in 4 chance of being passed on. The disease is most prevalent in those of Jewish families, particularly those of Eastern European (Ashkenazi) background.

Symptoms usually present between 3-6 months of age. Early symptoms include mild muscle weakness, muscle spasms, and feeding difficulties. As the disease progresses, the patient may experience vision loss, seizures and eventually paralysis. Death usually occurs by the age of 4 years.

Treatment for Tay-Sachs disease is supportive and there is no cure. Genetic and premarital counseling is important to those at high risk.

National Agencies & Associations

8910 **National Foundation for Jewish Genetic Diseases**
Fifth Avenue at 100th Street 212-659-6774
New York, NY 10029 Fax: 212-241-6947
www.mssm.edu/jewish_genetics
Offers information and support for persons suffering from Tay-Sachs Disease as well as their families and professionals working with them. The Foundation supports research into all areas of genetic disorders.
R J Desnick PhD MD, Center Director

8911 **National Institute of Child Health and Human Development**
31 Center Drive 301-496-5133
Bethesda, MD 20892 800-370-2943
Fax: 866-760-5947
TTY: 888-320-6942
e-mail: mcgrathj@mail.nih.gov
www.nichd.nih.gov
Offers reprints, articles and various information on Tay-Sachs Disease for patients and professionals.
Duane Alexan MD, Director
John McGrath, Coordinator

8912 **National Institute of Neurological Disorders and Stroke**
P O Box 5801 301-496-5751
Bethesda, MD 20824 800-352-9424
TTY: 301-468-5981
Offers advice and information on treatments and care of individual patients with neurological disorders.

8913 **National Organization for Rare Disorders**
55 Kenosia Avenue 203-744-0100
Danbury, CT 06813 800-999-6673
Fax: 203-746-2291
TTY: 203-797-9590
TDD: 203-797-9590
e-mail: orphan@rarediseases.org
www.rarediseases.org
Serves as a clearinghouse for information about rare disorders and brings together families with similar disorders for mutual support; fosters communication among rare disease voluntary agencies, Government agencies, industry scientific researchers and academia.
Carolyn Asbu PhD, Chair
Frank Sasinowski, Vice Chair

8914 **National Tay-Sachs and Allied Diseases Association (NTSAD)**
2001 Beacon Street
Brighton, MA 02135 800-906-8723
Fax: 617-277-0134
e-mail: info@ntsad.org
www.ntstad.org
Offers programs of public and professional education prevention services testing research and family services and promotion of TSD genetic screening programs nationally.
Fran Berkwits, Director
Bradley L Campbell, President

Foundations

8915 **National Tay-Sachs and Allied Diseases Association (NTSAD)**
2001 Beacon Street
Brighton, MA 02135 800-906-8723
Fax: 617-277-0134
e-mail: info@ntsad.org
www.ntsad.org
Dedicated to the treatment and preventin of Tay Sachs, Canavan, and related diseases, and to provide information and support services to individuals and families affected by these diseases, as well as the public at large.
John F Crowley MBA, JD, President

Support Groups & Hotlines

8916 **National Health Information Center**
PO Box 1133 310-565-4167
Washington, DC 20013 800-336-4797
Fax: 301-984-4256
e-mail: info@nhic.org
www.health.gov/nhic
Offers a nationwide information referral service, produces directories and resource guides.

8917 **National Tay-Sachs Association: Delaware Valley (NTSAD-DV)**
720 Greenwood Avenue 215-887-0877
Jenkintown, PA 19046 877-599-9293
Fax: 215-887-1931
e-mail: NTSAD@aol.com
www.tay-sachs.org
Rebecca Tantala, Executive Director

8918 **National TaySachs & Allied Diseases**
2001 Beacon Street 617-277-4463
Boston, MA 2135 800-906-8723
Fax: 617-277-0134
e-mail: info@ntsad.org
www.ntsad.org
A mutual support group coordinated by staff and volunteers who are parents of affected children or affected adults. One of several programs supported and sponsored by the association.
Kim Crawford, Member Services Coordinator

Books

8919 **Home Care Book**
National Tay-Sachs and Allied Diseases Association
2001 Beacon Street
Brighton, MA 02135 800-906-8723
Fax: 617-277-0134
e-mail: info@ntsad.org
www.ntsad.org
Written by parents for parents and professionals, the Home Care Book is a guide to caring for children with progressive neurological disorders at home.
John F Crowley MBA, JD, President

8920 **Home-Care Book**
National Tay-Sachs and Allied Diseases Association
2001 Beacon Street
Brookline, MA 02146 800-906-8723
A guide for caring for children with progressive neurological diseases.

8921 **Late Onset Tay-Sachs Disease Medical Bibliography**
National Tay-Sachs and Allied Diseases Association
2001 Beacon Street
Brookline, MA 02146 800-906-8723

8922 **Lifting of Canavan's Carrier Testing Facilities**
National Tay-Sachs and Allied Diseases Association
2001 Beacon Street
Brookline, MA 02146 800-906-8723

8923 **Monograph on Canavan's Disease**
National Tay-Sachs and Allied Diseases Association
2001 Beacon Street
Brookline, MA 02146 800-906-8723

8924 **Tay-Sachs Carrier Testing Directory**
National Tay-Sachs and Allied Diseases Association
2001 Beacon Street
Brookline, MA 02146 800-906-8723

8925 **Tay-Sachs: The Dreaded Inheritance**
National Tay-Sachs and Allied Diseases Assocation
2001 Beacon Street
Brighton, MA 02135 800-906-8723
Fax: 617-277-0134
e-mail: NTSAD-Boston@worldnet.att.net
www.ntsad.org
Descriptive narrative on caring for a child with Tay-Sachs Disease.

8926 **There is Only One Child**
National Tay-Sachs and Allied Diseases Association
2001 Beacon Street
Brookline, MA 02146 800-906-8723

8927 **What Every Family Should Know Sixth Edition**
National Tay-Sachs & Allied Diseases Association
2001 Beacon Street
Brighton, MA 02135 800-906-8723
Fax: 617-277-0134
e-mail: info@ntsad.org
www.ntsad.org
Detailing lysosomal storage and leukodystrophy disorders, with sections on Tay-Sachs, Sandhoff, Niemann-Pick, Gaucher, Canavan, Fabry, Pompe, therapeutic approaches and unique disease table.
50 pages
John F Crowley MBA. JD, President

Newsletters

8928 **Breakthrough**
National Tay-Sachs and Allied Diseases Association
2001 Beacon Street
Boston, MA 02135 800-906-8723
Fax: 617-277-0134
e-mail: info@ntsad.org
www.ntsad.org
Each year NTSAD publishes a newsletter for friends and supporters that focuses on the latest advances in research, profiles of families and individuals helped by NTSAD and disease profiles.
Annual
John F Crowley MBA, JD, President

8929 **Late Onset Community Newsletter**
National Tay-Sachs and Allied Diseases Association
2001 Beacon Street
Brighton, MA 02135 800-906-8723
Fax: 617-277-0134
e-mail: info@ntsad.org
www.ntsad.org
PSG members dealing with chronic forms of the allied diseases receive this newsletter focused specifically on the issues and perspectives unique to adults struggling with long-term disability issues. Public editions of the newsletter are also available.
Bi-Monthly
John F Crowley MBA, JD, President

8930 **Lifeline**
National Tay-Sachs and Allied Diseases Association
2001 Beacon Street
Brighton, MA 02135 800-906-8723
Fax: 617-277-0134
e-mail: info@ntsad.org
www.ntsad.org
The editorial content is wide ranging: symptom management and home health care; new product reviews; guidance in benefits and services advocacy for families and affected individuals of all ages; science and medical research updates; coverage of NTSAD events, fundraising, programs and administrative activities. Members only.
Quarterly
John F Crowley MBA, JD, President

Pamphlets

8931 **Late Onset Tay-Sachs Fact Sheet**
National Tay-Sachs and Allied Diseases Association
2001 Beacon Street
Brighton, MA 02135 800-906-8723
Fax: 617-277-0134
e-mail: info@ntsad.org
www.ntsad.org
This quick reference information sheet on the chronic or late onset form of Tay-Sachs is available for no charge.
John F Crowley MBA, JD, President

8932 **Services to Families**
National Tay-Sachs and Allied Diseases Association
2001 Beacon Street
Brookline, MA 02146 800-906-8723
Offers information on the Association parent peer groups, referrals and advocacy services to families and patients.

8933 **Tay-Sachs Information Sheet**
March of Dimes
233 Park Avenue South 212-353-8353
New York, NY 10003 Fax: 212-254-3518
e-mail: NY639@marchofdimes.com
www.marchofdimes.com
Offers a brief overview of the illness, causes, symptoms and treatments are covered. Availabe electronically on the website: www.marchofdimes.com

8934 **Tay-Sachs is**
National Tay-Sachs and Allied Diseases Association
2001 Beacon Street
Brookline, MA 02146 800-906-8723
Information on the history of the disease, what a victim of the disease should know and what they can do as far as resources and referrals.

8935 **Understanding Lysosomal Storage Diseases**
National Tay-Sachs and Allied Diseases Association
2001 Beacon Street
Brookline, MA 02146 800-906-8723

8936 **What is Canavan Disease?**
National Tay-Sachs and Allied Diseases Association
2001 Beacon Street
Brighton, MA 02135 800-906-8723
Fax: 617-277-0134
e-mail: info@ntsad.org
www.ntsad.org
The educational pamphlet describing Canavan Disease.
John F Crowley MBA, JD, President

8937 **What is Tay-Sachs? Russian Translation**
National Tay-Sachs and Allied Diseases Association
2001 Beacon Street
Brighton, MA 02135 800-906-8723
Fax: 617-277-0134
e-mail: info@ntsad.org
www.ntsad.org
This informative educational pamphlet describing Infantile Tay-Sachs, its inheritance and prevention is available for no charge.
John F Crowley MBA, JD, President

Audio & Video

8938 For My Sister, Elyssa
National Tay-Sachs & Allied Diseases Assocation
2001 Beacon Street
Brighton, MA 02135
800-906-8723
Fax: 617-277-0134
e-mail: NTSAD-Boston@worldnet.att.net
www.ntsad.org

Moving and informative 15 minute presentation told by a teenager who baby siter died from Tay-Sachs Disease. Contains information on Tay-Sachs Disease and simple steps each individual can take to prevent the tragedy of Tay-Sachs.

Web Sites

8939 Healing Well
www.healingwell.com

An online health resource guide to medical news, chat, information and articles, newsgroups and message boards, books, disease-related web sites, medical directories, and more for patients, friends, and family coping with disabling diseases, disorders, or chronic illnesses.

8940 Health Finder
www.healthfinder.gov

Searchable, carefully developed web site offering information on over 1000 topics. Developed by the US Department of Health and Human Services, the site can be used in both English and Spanish.

8941 Healthlink USA
www.healthlinkusa.com

Health information concerning treatment, cures, prevention, diagnosis, risk factors, research, support groups, email lists, personal stories and much more. Updated regularly.

8942 Helios Health
www.helioshealth.com

Online resource for your health information. Detailed information about specific health topics, access to expert advice from our Medical Advisory Board, and up-to-date health news.

8943 MedicineNet
www.medicinenet.com

An online resource for consumers providing easy-to-read, authoritative medical and health information.

8944 Medscape
www.mywebmd.com

Medscape offers specialists, primary care physicians, and other health professionals the Web's most robust and integrated medical information and educational tools.

8945 WebMD
www.webmd.com

Information on Tay-Sachs disease, including articles and resources.

Description

8946 **Thyroid Disease**

Thyroid Disease refers to a number of conditions that affect the thyroid, a small, butterfly-shaped gland located in the middle of the lower neck. Hormones T3 and T4, produced by the thyroid, deliver energy to cells of the body, thus controlling the body's metabolism. Conditions that result from an imbalance of these hormones are Hypothyroidism — not enough hormones that results in the body using energy slower than it should, and Hyperthyroidism — too much hormones that results in the body using energy faser than it should. These conditions can be caused by an inflammation of the thyroid gland, too much or too little iodine (used to produce thyroid hormones), or autoimmune disease, in which antibodies gradually either destroy the thyroid gland or speed up its function. Other thyroid conditions are Goiter — an enlarged thyroid; Thyroid Nodules — cysts, lumps, bumps and tumors that can be cancerous or benign; and Thyroiditis — inflammation of the thyroid gland. More than 20 million Americans have thyroid disease, and it affects many more women than men. Treatment includes synthetic hormone medication to replace missing hormones, radioactive iodine to deactivate the thyroid, and surgery for some goiters and cancerous nodules. Early diagnosis is often the key in prescribing treatment even before the onset of symptoms. Although thyroid disease is a chronic condition, careful disease manangement allows affected individuals to live healthy, normal lives.

National Agencies & Associations

8947 **American Thyroid Association**
6066 Leesburg Pike
Falls Church, VA 22041
703-998-8890
800-479-7634
Fax: 703-998-8893
e-mail: thyroid@thyroid.org
www.thyroid.org
Promotes excellence and innovation in clinical care research education and public policy.
Barbara R. Smith, CAE, Executive Director

8948 **National Women's Health Resource Center**
157 Broad Street
Red Bank, NJ 07701
877-986-9472
877-986-9472
Fax: 732-530-3347
e-mail: snelson@healthwomen.org
www.healthywomen.org
NWHRC develops and distributes up-to-date and objective women's health information based on the latest advances in medical research and practice.
Patricia Gurne, Chairman
Elizabeth Ba Cahill, Executive Director

8949 **Thyroid Federation International**
797 Princess Street
Kingston, Ontario, K7L-1G1
613-544-8364
Fax: 613-544-9731
e-mail: tfi@on.aibn.com
www.thyroid-fed.org
Aims to work for the benefit of those affected by thyroid disorders throughout the world.
Yvonne Andersson, President, Board of Directors
Peter Lakwijk, VP, Board of Directors

8950 **Thyroid Foundation of Canada**
797 Princess Street
Kingston, Ontario, K7L-1G1
613-544-8364
800-267-8822
Fax: 613-544-9731
www.thyroid.ca
Thyroid Foundation of Canada is a registered charity.
Katherine Keen, National Office Coordinator

Books

8951 **Autoimmune Connection: Essential Informati on for Women on Diagnosis, Treatment**
National Women's Health Resource Center
157 Broad Street
Red Bank, NJ 07701
877-986-9472
Fax: 732-530-3347
e-mail: info@healthywomen.org
www.healthywomen.org
Readers learn about the recent groundbreaking discovery of the links between the different autoimmune diseases and why women are more likely to develop them.
Elizabeth Battaglino Cahill, Executive Director

8952 **The Thyroid Gland**
Joel I Hamburger MD & Michael M Kaplan, author
Thyroid Foundation of Canada
797 Princess Street
Kingston, Ontario, K7L-1G1
613-544-8364
800-267-8822
Fax: 613-544-9731
www.thyroid.ca
Provides material for the patient to study at home, and to review at subsequent visits to the physician.

8953 **Thyroid Balance**
National Women's Health Resource Center
157 Broad Street
Red Bank, NJ 07701
877-986-9472
Fax: 732-530-3347
e-mail: info@healthywomen.org
www.healthywomen.org
An authoritative guide to treating thyroid issues-using both traditional and alternative methods.
Elizabeth Battaglino Cahill, Executive Director

8954 **Thyroid Disease: The Facts**
RIS Bayliss & WMG Tunbridge MD, author
Thyroid Foundation of Canada
797 Princess Street
Kingston, Ontario, K7L-1G1
613-544-8364
800-267-8822
Fax: 613-544-9731
www.thyroid.ca
Provides patients, their friends, and relatives with an up-to-date, readable account of disorders of the thyroid and the treatments which are now available.

8955 **Thyroid Power: Ten Steps to Total Health**
Richard Shames & Karilee H Shames, author
National Women's Health Resource Center
157 Broad Street
Red Bank, NJ 07701
877-986-9472
Fax: 732-530-3347
e-mail: snelson@healthwomen.org
www.healthywomen.org
Discusses the labyrinth of diagnostic and treatment issues a patient must endure.

8956 **Thyroid Solution: A Mind-Body Program for Beating Depression and Regaining Health**
National Women's Health Resource Center
157 Broad Street
Red Bank, NJ 07701
877-986-9472
Fax: 732-530-3347
e-mail: info@healthywomen.org
www.healthywomen.org
This book explains the link between stress and thyroid imbalance; how thyroid imbalance affects your emotions, sex life, and relationships; and how to cope with the effects of this imbalance.
Elizabeth Battaglino Cahill, Executive Director

8957 **Thyroid Sourcebook**
Thyroid Foundation of Canada

797 Princess Street
Kingston, Ontario, K7L-1G1
613-544-8364
800-267-8822
Fax: 613-544-9731
www.thyroid.ca

Provides the guidance, reassurance, and important information you need to manage your health and make informed decisions.

8958 Your Thyroid: A Home Reference
Lawrence Wood MD & David S Cooper MD, author
Thyroid Foundation of Canada
797 Princess Street
Kingston, Ontario, K7L-1G1
613-544-8364
800-267-8822
Fax: 613-544-9731
www.thyroid.ca

Explains the latest scientific advances can mean to you.

Magazines

8959 Clinical Thyroidology
American Thyroid Association
6066 Leesburg Pike
Falls Church, VA 12041
703-998-8890
800-849-7634
Fax: 703-998-8893
e-mail: editorclinthy@thyroid.org
www.thyroid.org

An online publication, available monthly, this is a broad-ranging look at clinical and preclinical thyroid literature. The Editor searches the world literature for excellent thyroid studies and then summarizes them along side his expert commentary.
Ernest L. Mazzaferri, MD, Editor

8960 THYROID
American Thyroid Association
6066 Leesburg Pike
Falls Church, VA 12041
703-998-8890
800-849-7643
Fax: 703-998-8893
e-mail: thyroideditor@umassmed.edu
www.thyroid.org

The Associations monthly journal that touches on topics from the molecular biology of the thyroid gland to clinical management of thyroid disorders. All Association members receive a suvscription, and it is available to non-members.

8961 Clinical Thyroidology for Patients
American Thyroid Association
6066 Leesburg Pike
Falls Church, VA 12041
703-998-8890
800-849-7634
Fax: 703-998-8893
e-mail: editorclinthy@thyroid.org
www.thyroid.org

A collection of summaries of recently published articles fromt the medical literature that covers the broad spectrum of thryroid disorders. Notes descxribing published research studies were prepared by THYROID Editor, Ernest Mazzaferri, MD.

Newsletters

8962 SIGNAL
American Thyroid Association
6066 Leesburg Pike
Falls Church, VA 12041
703-998-8890
800-849-7643
Fax: 703-998-8893
e-mail: thyroid@thyroid.org
www.thyroid.org

Covers Association news, meetings, policies, leaders, and important thyroid-related issues.

Pamphlets

8963 Hypothyroidism Web Booklet
American Thyroid Association
6066 Leesburg Pike
Falls Church, VA 12041
703-998-8890
800-489-7643
Fax: 703-998-8893
e-mail: thyroid@thyroid.org
www.thyroid.org

This online booklet introduces the thryoid and hypothyroidism to the reader, explains symptoms, treatments, causes, who's at risk, and more.
2003 25 pages

Web Sites

8964 American Thyroid Association
www.thyroid.com

Promotes excellence and innovation in clinical care, research, education, and public policy.
David S Cooper MD, President
Gregory A Brent MD, Secretary

8965 MedicineNet
www.medicinenet.com

An online resource for consumers providing easy-to-read, authoritative medical and health information.

8966 National Women's Health Resource Center
www.healthywomen.org

NWHRC developes and distributes up-to-date and objective women's health information based on the latest advances in medical research and practice.
Elizabeth Battaglino Cahill, RN, Executive Director
Maria Bushee, Director of Marketing & Communications

8967 Thyroid Federation International
www.thyroid-fed.org

Aims to work for the benefit of those affected by thyroid disorders throughout the world.

8968 Thyroid Foundation of Canada
www.thyroid.ca

Thyroid Foundation of Canada is a registered charity.

Description

8969 **Tick-Borne Disease**

Ticks transmit disease to humans by being carriers for a variety of microorganismns. The most common tick-borne illness is Lyme disease, first recognized and so named in 1975 because of a cluster of cases found in Lyme, Connecticut. It is a bacterial infection spread by the bite of an infected deer tick.The disease in its earliest stages causes an expanding red rash in at least 75 percent of patients. Flu-like symptoms—headaches, fever, fatigue—are common. The rash may be followed by progressive joint pain and swelling. Dysfunction of the heart (8 percent) and nervous system (15 percent) develop weeks to months later. Further progression causes arthritis and more serious neurologic problems.

Although only one third of patients remember a tick bite, greater than 60 percent do develop the tell-tale rash. Diagnosis requires a blood test to confirm the physical symptoms.

Oral antibiotics may be sufficient for the disease caught in the early stages. Long-standing, disseminated disease responds best to intravenous antibiotics.

Rocky Mountain spotted fever, also known as tick fever, is transmitted by a bite from either a dog tick or wood tick, depending on the part of the country. Like Lyme disease, it begin with flu-like symptoms — chills, fever and loss of appetite. A rash of small, reddish bumps, which gives the disease its name, begins on the wrist and ankle and spreads to the rest of the body. Aggressive antibotic treatment should begin as early as possible. If left untreated, Rocky Mountain spotted fever has a mortality rate of 10 to 80 percent.

Prevention of tick-borne disease requires avoidance of tick bites, by using insect repellants and protective clothing, plus daily checks for ticks during periods of exposure. A vaccine may provide partial protection from Lyme disease for those regularly engaged in high-risk activities (i.e. property maintenance), although other conditions may complicate this treatment.

National Agencies & Associations

8970 **Lyme Disease Foundation**
PO Box332 860-870-0070
Tolland, CT 06084-0332 800-886-5963
Fax: 860-870-0080
e-mail: info@lyme.org
www.lyme.org
Provides a wide range of services including information and referral network on Lyme Disease, distribution of educational videos to state libraries, educational materials for public and professionals, national public forums and training for community education.
John F Anderson, Board of Director
Willy Burgdorfer, Board of Director

Libraries & Resource Centers

8971 **California Lyme Disease Association**
PO Box 707
Weaverville, CA 96093 e-mail: info@lymedisease.org
www.lymedisease.org
The California Lyme Disease Association (CALDA) is an affiliate of the Lyme Disease Association, Inc. CALDA, a non-profit organization, was originally founded in 1990 as The Lyme Disease Resource Center (LDRC). We provide services for Lyme disease patients, their families and friends; provide a forum for physicians and health professionals for the exchange of ideas and information about symptoms, diagnosis, and treatment of Lyme disease.
Marilynn Barkley, Board of Directors
Barbara Barsoschinni, Board of Directors

Research Centers

8972 **Ball State University Public Health Entomology Laboratory**
2000 University Avenue 765-289-1241
Muncie, IN 47306 800-382-8540
www.bsu.edu
Offers information on mosquitoes and mosquito-born diseases specializing in Lyme Disease.
Bob Pinger, Director
Jeffrey Clark, Department Chair and Professor

8973 **Centers for Disease Control Division of Vector Borne Infectious Diseases**
US Public Health Service
PO Box 2087 970-221-6400
Fort Collins, CO 80521 Fax: 970-216-76
www.cdc.gov
Research done into lyme disease tularemia bubonic plague and all vector-borne infectious diseases — including west nile virus.
Lyle Petersen, Director

Support Groups & Hotlines

8974 **Advocates 4 Health: Tick-borne Disease Self-Help Group**
PALS
PO Box 1271 805-544-0984
San Luis Obispo, CA 93406 e-mail: advocates4heatlh@yahoo.com
Advocacy and support group increasing awareness, education and understanding of tick-borne disorders and other zoonotic diseases. This group fosters a supportive network between human/animal sufferers, caregivers, health care professionals and the general community.
Sheryl Glidden

8975 **American Lyme Disease Foundation**
PO Box 466
Lyme, CT 06371 e-mail: Inquire@aldf.com
www.aldf.com
Supports research and plays a key role in providing reliable and scientifically accurate information to the public and health care providers.
David L Weld, Executive Director
Jeffery Black, Partner

8976 **Lyme Alliance**
PO Box 454
Concord, MI 49237 517-563-3582
www.lymealliance.org
Lyme Alliance volunteers will address your questions concerning the newsletter, website, or questions about doctor referrals, medical treatment options, or information about Lyme disease.

8977 **Lyme Disease Network**
1613 Hewitt Avenue 651-644-7239
St. Paul, MN 55104 e-mail: olivierlynn@switchboardmail.com
Lynn M Olivier

8978 Lyme Disease Network Support Group of Alabama: Mobile Chapter
Mobile, AL 35758 256-772-6482
e-mail: alabamalyme@usa.com
www.lymnet.org/supportgroups
Support information, and referrals for victims of Lyme disease and their families.
Kara Tyson

8979 Lyme Disease Network of New Jersey
43 Winton Road
East Brunswick, NJ 08816 e-mail: carol@lymenet.org
www.lymenet.org
Support information, and referrals for victims of Lyme disease and their families. Maintains comuter information system.
Bill Stolow, President

8980 Lyme Disease Network of South Carolina
Po Box 6634 803-798-5963
Columbia, SC 29260-6634 e-mail: lyme@sc-lyme.org
www.sc-lyme.org
Sue Fox

8981 National Health Information Center
PO Box 1133 310-565-4167
Washington, DC 20013 800-336-4797
Fax: 301-984-4256
e-mail: info@nhic.org
www.health.gov/nhic
Offers a nationwide information referral service, produces directories and resource guides.

Books

8982 Coping with Lyme Disease: A Practical Guide
Henry Holt & Company
115 W 18th Street 212-886-9200
New York, NY 10011-4113 Fax: 212-633-0748
1993 288 pages Paperback
ISBN: 0-805026-50-9

8983 Ecology & Environment Management of Lyme Disease
Rutgers University Press
109 Church Street 201-932-7762
New Brunswick, NJ 08901-1242
1993 224 pages
ISBN: 0-813519-28-4

8984 Everything You Need to Know About Lyme Disease
John Wiley & Sons Publishing
605 3rd Avenue 212-850-6000
New York, NY 10158-0012 800-225-5945
Fax: 212-850-6088
www.wiley.com
237 pages
ISBN: 0-471160-61-X

8985 Let's Talk About Having Lyme Disease
Rosen Publishing Group's PowerKids Press
29 E 21st Street 212-777-3017
New York, NY 10010 800-237-9932
Fax: 888-436-4643
e-mail: customerservice@rosenpub.com
www.rosenpublishing.com
Kids are taught to take precautions when walking in the woods and how to inspect themselves for ticks. The illness and recovery are also explained.
Grades K-4
ISBN: 0-823950-29-8
Elizabeth Weitzman, Author

Children's Books

8986 Lyme Disease
Franklin Watts Grolier
90 Old Sherman Tpke 203-797-3500
Danbury, CT 06816-0001 800-621-1115
Fax: 203-797-3197
www.grolier.com
This book discusses the symptoms, prevention, treatments and the role of the tick. This source will not only help readers become aware of Lyme Disease, it will help them become informed.
64 pages Grades 5-7
ISBN: 0-531109-31-3

8987 Lyme Disease and Other Pest-Borne Illnesses
Franklin Watts Grolier
90 Old Sherman Turnpike 203-797-3500
Danbury, CT 06816-0001 800-621-1115
Fax: 203-797-3197
www.grolier.com
Scientific, without being technical, this book explains what Lyme Disease is, symptoms, causes and what a person can do if they contract it.
112 pages Grades 7-12
ISBN: 0-531125-23-8

Magazines

8988 Vector Borne & Zoonotic Diseases
Mary Ann Liebert
Two Madison Avenue 914-834-3100
Larchmont, NY 10538-1961 800-654-3238
Fax: 914-834-1388
www.liebertpub.com/vbz
Essential multidisiplinary journal dedicated to all aspects of human diseases that occur as zoonoses or are transmitted by invertibrate vectors.
Quarterly

Newsletters

8989 Lymelight Newsletter
Lyme Disease Foundation
1 Financial Plaza 860-525-2000
Hartford, CT 06103-2608 800-886-5963
Fax: 860-525-8425
Newsletter offering up to date information on Lyme Disease and related disorders, Foundation activities, conference and fund-raising information and resources.
4x Year

Pamphlets

8990 Frequently Asked Questions
Lyme Disease Foundation
1 Financial Plaza 860-525-2000
Hartford, CT 06103-2608 800-886-5963
Fax: 860-525-8425
Overview of testing, treatment, transmission, and pregnancy.

8991 Guide to Lyme Disease
Lyme Disease Foundation
1 Financial Plaza 860-525-2000
Hartford, CT 06103-2608 800-886-5963
Fax: 860-525-8425
Detailed information about Lyme disease and the LDF.

8992 Guide to Tick Spread Diseases
Lyme Disease Foundation
1 Financial Plaza 860-525-2000
Hartford, CT 06103-2608 800-886-5963
Fax: 860-525-8425
www.lyme.org
Symptoms, diagnosis and treatment for a variety of diseases.
16 pages

8993 Guide to Tick-Borne Disorders
Lyme Disease Foundation

1 Financial Plaza — 860-525-2000
Hartford, CT 06103-2608 — 800-886-5963
Fax: 860-525-8425

Symptoms, diagnosis, and treatment for a variety of diseases.

8994 **LD Alert Card**
Lyme Disease Foundation
1 Financial Plaza — 860-525-2000
Hartford, CT 06103-2608 — 800-886-5963
Fax: 860-525-8425

LD symptoms and prevention information.

8995 **LD Awareness Packet**
Lyme Disease Foundation
1 Financial Plaza — 860-525-2000
Hartford, CT 06103-2608 — 800-886-5963
Fax: 860-525-8425

Educational letter-size posters, brochures listed above, case counts, Spanish information, insurance problem information, General Diagnostic poster, & more.

8996 **Lyme Disease & Pets**
Lyme Disease Foundation
1 Financial Plaza — 860-525-2000
Hartford, CT 06103-2608 — 800-886-5963
Fax: 860-525-8425
e-mail: lymefna@aol.com
www.lyme.org

Offers information on Lyme Disease and other tick-borne disorders, through pets and animal transmission.
T Forchaser, Executive Director

8997 **Quick Guide to Lyme Disease**
American Lyme Disease Foundation
293 Route 100 — 914-277-6970
Somers, NY 10589 — Fax: 914-277-6974
e-mail: inquire@aldf.com
www.aldf.com

Epidemiology, the cause of the disease, recognizing the symptoms, what to do if you are bitten, treatment, vaccine and other tick-borne diseases are all covered. One free copy, quantity prices vary.

8998 **Self-Help (S-H) Program**
Lyme Disease Foundation
1 Financial Plaza — 860-525-2000
Hartford, CT 06103-2608 — 800-886-5963
Fax: 860-525-8425

How to establish and conduct a S-H Group. Video, instruction manual, brochure masters, posters, and more.
28 minutes

8999 **Understanding Lyme Disease: Entendiendo Lyme Disease**
American Lyme Disease Foundation
293 Route 100 — 914-277-6970
Somers, NY 10589 — Fax: 914-277-6974
e-mail: inquire@aldf.com
www.aldf.com

Only available in Spanish, this brochure is for children ages 10-15 years old. Includes a basic desription of Lyme disease, symptoms, diagnosis, prevention and proper tick removal. One free copy, quantity prices vary.

9000 **Understanding Ticks and Lyme Disease**
American Lyme Disease Foundation
293 Route 100 — 914-277-6970
Somers, NY 10589 — Fax: 914-277-6974
e-mail: inquire@aldf.com
www.aldf.com

For children 10-15 years old, basic description of Lyme disease, symptoms, diagnosis, prevention and proper tick removal. One free copy, quantity prices vary.

Audio & Video

9001 **Case of the Great Imitator**
American Lyme Disease Foundation
293 Route 100 — 914-277-6970
Somers, NY 10589 — Fax: 914-277-6974
e-mail: inquire@aldf.com
www.aldf.com

For children ages 9-14 years old. Educational video made in cooperation with the Centers for Disease Control and Prevention.

9002 **LD: Diagnosis & Treatment**
Lyme Disease Foundation
1 Financial Plaza — 860-525-2000
Hartford, CT 06103-2608 — 800-886-5963
Fax: 860-525-8425

Physicians discuss the challenges of diagnosing and treating LD.
60 minutes

9003 **LD: Facts for Kids**
Lyme Disease Foundation
1 Financial Plaza — 860-525-2000
Hartford, CT 06103-2608 — 800-886-5963
Fax: 860-525-8425

Targeted toward kindergarten to fourth grade children, these videos educate youngsters about Lyme Disease and ticks.

9004 **Lyme Disease: What You Should Know**
Lyme Disease Foundation
1 Financial Plaza — 860-525-2000
Hartford, CT 06103-2608 — 800-886-5963
Fax: 860-525-8425

Diagnosis, treatment, transmission, prevention, and research. Interviews with patients, doctors, school officials, researchers, and health department officials.
60 minutes

9005 **Tick Talk**
American Lyme Disease Foundation
293 Route 100 — 914-277-6970
Somers, NY 10589 — Fax: 914-277-6974
e-mail: inquire@aldf.com
www.aldf.com

For children ages 5-8 years old. Educational video made in cooperation with the Centers for Disease Control and Prevention.

Web Sites

9006 **America's Doctor Online Consulting**
www.americasdoctor.com

Provides pharmaceutical and biotech companies and contract research organizations an exclusive source for conducting phase II-IV clinical research.

9007 **American Lyme Disease Foundation**
www.aldf.com

Provides a wide range of information, both in English and in Spanish, on the diagnosis, treatment, prevention and control of lyme disease and other tick-borne infections.

9008 **CDC Intro to Lyme Disease**
www.cdc.gov/ncidod/dvbid/lyme/incex.htm

Accurate, evidence based information on symptoms, diagnosis, treatment and prevention of Lyme disease and other tick-borne illnesses. Includes vaccine information, late-braking news, frequently asked questions and related links.

9009 **Healing Well**
www.healingwell.com

An online health resource guide to medical news, chat, information and articles, newsgroups and message boards, books, disease-related web sites, medical directories, and more for patients, friends, and family coping with disabling diseases, disorders, or chronic illnesses.

9010 **Health Finder**
www.healthfinder.gov

Searchable, carefully developed web site offering information on over 1000 topics. Developed by the US Department of Health and Human Services, the site can be used in both English and Spanish.

9011 **Healthlink USA**
www.healthlinkusa.com

Health information concerning treatment, cures, prevention, diagnosis, risk factors, research, support groups, email lists, personal stories and much more. Updated regularly.

9012 **Helios Health**

www.helioshealth.com

Online resource for your health information. Detailed information about specific health topics, access to expert advice from our Medical Advisory Board, and up-to-date health news.

9013 **Lyme Disease Foundation**

www.lyme.org

Provides a wide range of services including information and referral network on Lyme disease.

9014 **MGH Neurology WebForums**

Provides both unmoderated message board and chat rooms for specific neurological disorders including: amyloidosis, asachnoiditis, cerebellar ataxia, congenital fiber type disproportion, CFS leak, DeMorsiers syndrome, erythomelalgia, Lewy body disease, meningitis, meralgia paresthetic, Norrie disease, periodic paralysis, phantom limb pain, Romber disorder, Syndenhams chorea, tethered cord syndrome, and thoracic outlet syndrome.

9015 **MedicineNet**

www.medicinenet.com

An online resource for consumers providing easy-to-read, authoritative medical and health information.

9016 **Medscape**

www.mywebmd.com

Medscape offers specialists, primary care physicians, and other health professionals the Web's most robust and integrated medical information and educational tools.

9017 **Neurology Channel**

www.neurologychannel.com

Find clearly explained, medically accurate information regarding conditions, including an overview, symptoms, causes, diagnostic procedures and treatment options. On this site it is possible to ask questions and get information from a neurologist and connect to people who have similar health interests.

9018 **Pubmed**

www.ncbi.nlm.nih.gov/PubMed

National institutes of Health search engine for published medical and scientific research.

9019 **University of Rhode Island Tick Research Laboratory**

www.riaes.org/resources/ticklab

Pictures of ticks and tick-borne disease information.

9020 **WebMD**

www.webmd.com

Information on Lyme disease, including articles and resources.

Description

9021 **Tourette Syndrome**

Tourette syndrome, TS, is a neurological disorder characterized by tics - involuntary, rapid, sudden movements or vocalizations that occur repeatedly in the same way. Onset of the disorder occurs before 18 years of age, and usually before the age of 12. Roughly one person in 2000 will demonstrate this behavior at some time in his life. Boys are 3 or 4 times as likely as girls to develop TS.

Multiple motor and vocal tics can appear separately or simultaneously as part of the syndrome. Tics may occur many times daily, or intermittently, with periodic changes in their number, frequency, type and location. Sometimes they may disappear for weeks.

Over time, symptoms can range from hand jerking and throat clearing in the syndrome's early stages to jumping and vocalizing socially unacceptable phrases. Movements may also occur in combination with each other.

Although the cause of TS is unknown, researchers have identified factors which may be involved in producing the disease. Persons with TS may show subtle abnormalities in the structure of certain parts of the brain. The disease may reflect abnormal metabolism of a neurotransmitter (a chemical that brain cells use to signal one another) called dopamine; drugs affecting dopamine levels may reduce symptoms. Relatives of affected persons have an increased risk of disease, suggesting a genetic component. Finally, in some cases the brain's function may be affected by antibodies triggered by infection with a bacterium called Group A Strep. Children who are not bothered by their tics should not be treated with drugs. Medications are reserved for those whose tics lead to symptoms which impair behavioral, physiologic or social function. Simple tics respond to benzodiazepines (tranquilizers). For more severe cases, haloperidol, an antipsychotic, may be used, but should be started slowly. Unfortunately, it sometimes causes other movement disorders after prolonged use. Whether drug treatment is used or not, patients and their families may need counseling to deal with the disease's secondary effects, which may include bullying at school or conflict within the family. Fortunately, the condition often becomes much less severe, without any treatment, after 10 or 15 years.

National Agencies & Associations

9022 **American Academy of Neurology: Tourette Syndrome**
1080 Montreal Avenue — 651-695-2717
Saint Paul, MN 55116-2311 — 800-879-1960
Fax: 651-695-2791
e-mail: memberservices@aan.com
www.aan.com

A medical specialty society established to advance the art and science of neurology and thereby promote the best possible care for patients wit neurological disorders.
Catherine Rydell, Executive Director

9023 **National Institute of Neurological Disorders and Stroke**
NIH Neurological Institute — 301-496-5751
Bethesda, MD 20824-5801 — 800-352-9424
Fax: 301-402-2186
TTY: 301-468-5981
www.ninds.nih.gov

Offers a fact sheet on Tourette syndrome and is America's focal point for support of research on brain and nervous system disorders.
Story C Landis PhD, Director
Walter J Koroshetz, Deputy Director

9024 **Tourette Syndrome Association**
42-40 Bell Boulevard — 718-224-2999
Bayside, NY 11361 — 888-486-8738
Fax: 718-279-9596
e-mail: grantadministrator@tsa-usa.org
www.tsa-usa.org

The only national organization exclusively devoted to the research, diagnosis, education and treatments for persons with Tourette Syndrome.
Judit Ungar, President
Sue Levi-Pearl, VP Meical & Scientific Programs

9025 **Tourette Syndrome Foundation of Canada**
#206 194 Jarvis Street — 800-361-3120
Toronto, Ontario, M5B-2B7 — Fax: 416-861-2472
e-mail: tsfc@tourette.ca
www.tourette.ca

National voluntary organization dedicated to improving the quality of life for those with or affected by Tourette Syndrome through programs of education, advocacy, self-help and the promotion of research.
Rosie Wartecker, Executive Director

Research Centers

9026 **Tourette Syndrome Clinic Yale Child Study Center**
Yale Child Study Center
230 S Frontage Road
New Haven, CT 06520 — 203-785-5880
www.medicine.yale.edu

Clinical care center offering research solely into the causes symptoms and treatments for persons with Tourette Syndrome.
Diane B Findley, Associate Research Scientist and Clinic
Robert King, Medical Director

Support Groups & Hotlines

9027 **National Health Information Center**
PO Box 1133 — 310-565-4167
Washington, DC 20013 — 800-336-4797
Fax: 301-984-4256
e-mail: info@nhic.org
www.health.gov/nhic

Offers a nationwide information referral service, produces directories and resource guides.

Books

9028 **Children with Tourette Syndrome**
Woodbine House
6510 Bells Mill Road
Bethesda, MD 20817-1636 — 800-843-7323

This book offers parents information on Tourette Syndrome, causes, symptoms and medications, as well as the other disorders which are commonly linked with it. Other chapters include information on family life, education, advocacy and legal rights.
340 pages Paperback
ISBN: 0-933149-44-1

9029 **Children with Tourette Syndrome: A Parent's Guide**
Adam Ward Seligman, Echolalia Press
35158 Annapolis Road — 707-886-1972
Annapolis, CA 95412-9713 — e-mail: seligman@sonic.net
www.sonic.net/echolaliapress/

9030 Living with Tourette Syndrome
Simon & Schuster
611 W Bay Street
Tampa, FL 33606-2703 800-999-5479
Provides valuable advice for children and adults with TS, their families, co-workers, teachers and friends. Describes the symptoms and related disorders, exposes many myths surrounding the disease, and advises adults on business and personal relationships.
256 pages
ISBN: 0-684811-60-0

9031 Ryan: A Mother's Story of her TS/ADHD Child
Adam Ward Seligman, Echolalia Press
35158 Annapolis Road 707-886-1972
Annapolis, CA 95412-9713
Available in hardcover.
Softcover

9032 Teaching the Tiger: An Educator's Guide to TS/OCD/ADHD
Adam Ward Seligman, Echolalia Press
35158 Annapolis Road 707-886-1972
Annapolis, CA 95412-9713
Workbook

9033 Tourette Syndrome and Human Behavior
Adam Ward Seligman, Echolalia Press
35158 Annapolis Road 707-886-1972
Annapolis, CA 95412-9713
Available in hardcover.
Softcover

9034 Tourette Syndrome: Advances in Neurology
Tourette Syndrome Association
42-40 Bell Boulevard 718-224-2999
Bayside, NY 11361-2861 888-480-8737
Fax: 718-279-9596
In this single-volume reference, more than 90 of the foremost research and clinical leaders in the field review the current state of knowledge about this disorder.
400 pages
Thomas N Chase MD, Editor
Arnold J Friedhoff MD, Editor

9035 What Makes Ryan Tic?
Adam Ward Seligman, Echolalia Press
35158 Annapolis Road 707-886-1972
Annapolis, CA 95412-9713
Softcover

Children's Books

9036 Adam and the Magic Marble
Adam Ward Seligman, Echolalia Press
35158 Annapolis Road 707-886-1972
Annapolis, CA 95412-9713

9037 Hi! I'm Adam!
Adam Ward Seligman, Echolalia Press
35158 Annapolis Road 707-886-1972
Annapolis, CA 95412-9713

9038 Matthew and the Tics
Tourette Syndrome Association
42-40 Bell Boulevard 718-224-2999
Bayside, NY 11361-2861 888-480-8738
Fax: 718-279-9596
A story for young children with TS and their peers.
2 pages

Newsletters

9039 Tourette Syndrome Association Newsletter
42-40 Bell Boulevard 718-224-2999
Bayside, NY 11361 888-480-8738
Fax: 718-279-9596
e-mail: ts@tsa-usa.org
www.tsa-usa.org/
Offers information, articles and news on the latest technology and advancements for persons with Tourette Syndrome.
Quarterly

Pamphlets

9040 Commentary on Alternative Therapies for TS
Tourette Syndrome Association
42-40 Bell Boulevard 718-224-2999
Bayside, NY 11361-2861 888-480-8738
Fax: 718-279-9596
Summarizes physician/patient reports of symptom management through non-pharmacological interventions.
2 pages

9041 Consumer's Guide to TS Medications
Tourette Syndrome Association
42-40 Bell Boulevard 718-224-2999
Bayside, NY 11361-2861 888-480-8738
Fax: 718-279-9596
Covers common medications used for the control of TS motor and vocal tics as well as those traditionally prescribed for associated behaviors.
1992 12 pages

9042 Coping with TS in the Classroom
Tourette Syndrome Association
42-40 Bell Boulevard 718-224-2999
Bayside, NY 11361-2820 Fax: 718-279-9596
Includes practical guidelines for education developed from a study about cognitive effects on learning.
18 pages

9043 Coping with TS, A Parent's Viewpoint
Tourette Syndrome Association
42-40 Bell Boulevard 718-224-2999
Bayside, NY 11361-2861 888-480-8738
Fax: 718-279-9596
An accalaimed medical writer and mother of three children with TS, the author sensitively addresses common concerns and feelings of parents.
1994 23 pages

9044 Coping with Tourette Syndrome in Early Adulthood
Tourette Syndrome Association
42-40 Bell Boulevard 718-224-2999
Bayside, NY 11361-2861 888-480-8738
Fax: 718-279-9596
Focuses on two fundamental challenges facing adults with TS: employment and interpersonal relationships. Provides specific techniques for overcoming barriers.

9045 Current Pharmacology of TS
Tourette Syndrome Association
42-40 Bell Boulevard 718-224-2999
Bayside, NY 11361-2861 888-480-8738
Fax: 718-279-9596
Covers all current medications used to treat TS with specific information about clinical evaluations and diagnosis.
12 pages

9046 Dental Treatment of Patients with Gilles de la Tourette Syndrome
Tourette Syndrome Association
42-40 Bell Boulevard 718-224-2999
Bayside, NY 11361-2861 888-480-8738
Fax: 718-279-9596
Discusses TS movements and possible adverse interactions of dentistry and TS medications.
5 pages

9047 Development of Behavioral and Emotional Problems in TS
Tourette Syndrome Association
42-40 Bell Boulevard 718-224-2999
Bayside, NY 11361-2861 888-480-8738
Fax: 718-279-9596
Using the Child Behavior Checklist, 78 male children were assessed for a variety of behavioral problems. Relation to tic severity covered.
1989 3 pages

9048 **Discipline and the Child with TS**
Tourette Syndrome Association
42-40 Bell Boulevard 718-224-2999
Bayside, NY 11361 888-480-8738
Fax: 718-279-9596

Helps children redirect impulses and compulsions through teaching cause and effect relationships.
15 pages

9049 **Educator's Guide to Tourette Syndrome**
Tourette Syndrome Association
42-40 Bell Boulevard 718-224-2999
Bayside, NY 11361-2861 888-480-8738
Fax: 718-279-9596

Covers symptoms, treatments and techniques for classroom management, attentional, writing and language problems.
16 pages

9050 **Genetics of Tourette's Syndrome: Who it Affects and How it Occurs in Families**
Tourette Syndrome Association
42-40 Bell Boulevard 718-224-2999
Bayside, NY 11361-2861 888-480-8738
Fax: 718-279-9596

10 pages

9051 **Getting Into College: Strategies for the Student with TS**
Tourette Syndrome Association
42-40 Bell Boulevard 718-224-2999
Bayside, NY 11361 888-480-8738
Fax: 718-279-9596

10 pages

9052 **Gift of Hope**
Tourette Syndrome Association
42-40 Bell Boulevard 718-224-2999
Bayside, NY 11361-2861 888-480-8738
Fax: 718-279-9596

TSA Brain Bank Program registration information. Includes donor cards.

9053 **Grandparents Club**
Tourette Syndrome Association
42-40 Bell Boulevard 718-224-2999
Bayside, NY 11361-2861 888-480-8738
Fax: 718-279-9596

A flyer describing how to join with other grandparents to support TS research to benefit future generations.

9054 **Guide to Diagnosis & Treatment**
Tourette Syndrome Association
42-40 Bell Boulevard 718-224-2999
Bayside, NY 11361-2861 888-480-8738
Fax: 718-279-9596

Covers symptoms, pharmacology and clinical assessments.
30 pages

9055 **Guide to Housing for Adults with TS**
Tourette Syndrome Association
42-40 Bell Boulevard 718-224-2999
Bayside, NY 11361-2861 888-480-8738
Fax: 718-279-9596

A guide to finding housing, housing laws that help people with TS and ways to maximize living environments.
1991 16 pages

9056 **Health Insurance & Tourette Syndrome**
Tourette Syndrome Association
42-40 Bell Boulevard 718-224-2999
Bayside, NY 11361-2861 888-480-8738
Fax: 718-279-9596

Detailed, up-to-date packet of medical information for obtaining health insurance as well as information for submission to insurance carriers.

9057 **Helpful Techniques to Aid the Student with TS**
Tourette Syndrome Association
42-40 Bell Boulevard 718-224-2999
Bayside, NY 11361-2861 888-480-8738
Fax: 718-279-9596

Helpful hints for teacher with specific suggestions for test taking, math computation, and note taking.
1 pages

9058 **Learning Problems & the Child with TS**
Tourette Syndrome Association
42-40 Bell Boulevard 718-224-2999
Bayside, NY 11361-2861 888-480-8738
Fax: 718-279-9596

Report on learning problems identified through a study of 200 children with TS.
1 pages

9059 **Need to Know**
Tourette Syndrome Association
42-40 Bell Boulevard 718-224-2999
Bayside, NY 11361-2861 888-480-8738
Fax: 718-279-9596

Recollections of a young woman who was diagnosed with TS in her 20s.
4 pages

9060 **Neuropsychological Performance in Adults with TS**
Tourette Syndrome Association
42-40 Bell Boulevard 718-224-2999
Bayside, NY 11361-2861 888-480-8738
Fax: 718-279-9596

Describes clinical and neuropsychological testing on learning and memory with TS adults.
7 pages

9061 **Peer Problems in Tourette's Disorder**
Tourette Syndrome Association
42-40 Bell Boulevard 718-224-2999
Bayside, NY 11361-2861 888-480-8738
Fax: 718-279-9596

Detailed research findings of peer problems in children with TS. Includes statistical results obtained from these studies.
1991 7 pages

9062 **Pharmacotherapy of TS and Associated Disorders**
Tourette Syndrome Association
42-40 Bell Boulevard 718-224-2999
Bayside, NY 11361-2861 888-480-8738
Fax: 718-279-9596

Overview with emphasis on the complexities of prescribing TS medications.
19 pages

9063 **Problem Behaviors & TS**
Tourette Syndrome Association
42-40 Bell Boulevard 718-224-2999
Bayside, NY 11361-2861 888-480-8738
Fax: 718-279-9596

Describes recent research and what is now known about the relationship of a variety of behaviors and TS.
21 pages

9064 **Recognizing TS in the Classroom**
Tourette Syndrome Association
42-40 Bell Boulevard 718-224-2999
Bayside, NY 11361-2861 888-480-8738
Fax: 718-279-9596

Provides an overview offering detailed symptoms checklist, post-diagnosis advice and covers special education needs.
4 pages

9065 **Risperidone as a Treatment for TS**
Tourette Syndrome Association
42-40 Bell Boulevard 718-224-2999
Bayside, NY 11361-2861 888-480-8738
Fax: 718-279-9596

6 pages

9066 **Specific Classroom Strategies and Techniques for Students with TS**
Tourette Syndrome Association
42-40 Bell Boulevard 718-224-2999
Bayside, NY 11361-2861 888-480-8738
Fax: 718-279-9596

An educator with TS spells out concrete methods for managing students with TS. She outlines many valuable classroom interventions to help youngsters deal with tic symptons, ADHD, visual motor and fine motor integration, and behavioral difficulties.
1994 2 pages

9067 TS and Other Tic Disorders
Tourette Syndrome Association
42-40 Bell Boulevard 718-224-2999
Bayside, NY 11361-2861 888-480-8738
Fax: 718-279-9596
Comprehensive overview of the complexities of TS. Includes tic syndrome classifications, epidemiology, genetics, behavioral aspects, and summary.
17 pages

9068 TS and the School Nurse
Tourette Syndrome Association
42-40 Bell Boulevard 718-224-2999
Bayside, NY 11361-2861 888-480-8738
Fax: 718-279-9596
Comprehensive professional guide to educational, social and medical implications.
19 pages

9069 TS and the School Psychologist
Tourette Syndrome Association
42-40 Bell Boulevard 718-224-2999
Bayside, NY 11361-2861 888-480-8738
Fax: 718-279-9596
The role of the school psychologist is covered including testing procedures, counseling strategies and social implications.
1993 (rev.) 14 pages

9070 TS: A Look at the Interface Between TS & the Law
Tourette Syndrome Association
42-40 Bell Boulevard 718-224-2999
Bayside, NY 11361-2861 888-480-8738
Fax: 718-279-9596
Summarizes important legislation protecting the rights of students with TS. Also covers resources and hints about how to prepare for dealing successfully with educators and school systems.
1 pages

9071 TSA Medical Letters
Tourette Syndrome Association
42-40 Bell Boulevard 718-224-2999
Bayside, NY 11361-2861 888-480-8738
Fax: 718-279-9596
Annual publication of TSA's Medical Committe covering recent, significant findings from scientific articles.
16 pages

9072 Teens and Tourette Syndrome
Tourette Syndrome Association
42-40 Bell Boulevard 718-224-2999
Bayside, NY 11361-2820 Fax: 718-279-9596
e-mail: ts@tsa-usa.org
www.tsa-usa.org/
Covers self esteem, friends, dating, drugs and alcohol, stress, depression, academic and vocational planning, sibling relationships and medication.
16 pages

9073 Tourette Syndrome and the School Nurse
Tourette Syndrome Association
42-40 Bell Boulevard 718-224-2999
Bayside, NY 11361-2820 Fax: 718-279-9596
e-mail: ts@tsa-usa.org
http://tsa-usa.org
Includes symptoms, epidemiology, associated beviors, developmental consequences, causes, treatments, role of the school nurse and additional resources.
20 pages

9074 Tourette: The Man and His Times
Tourette Syndrome Association
42-40 Bell Boulevard 718-224-2999
Bayside, NY 11361-2861 888-480-8738
Fax: 718-279-9596
Rare historical biography of the famous French neurologist G. Gilles De La Tourette.
9 pages

9075 What School Bus Drivers Need to Know About Students with Tourette Syndrome
Tourette Syndrome Association
42-40 Bell Boulevard 718-224-2999
Bayside, NY 11361-2820 Fax: 718-279-9596
e-mail: ts@tsa-usa.org
http://tsa-usa.org
Includes a description of the disorder, as well as related disorders and suggestions as to what school bus drivers can do for students with TS.
1 pages

Audio & Video

9076 A Regular Kid That's Me: Inservice Film for Educators
Tourette Syndrome Association
42-40 Bell Boulevard 718-224-2999
Bayside, NY 11361 888-480-8738
Fax: 718-279-9596
e-mail: ts@tsa-usa.org
http://tsa-usa.org
Nineteen students with TS (ages 7-17) along with several educators are seen interacting in classroom settings. Includes the basic criteria for diagnosis, discussions of common associated behaviors, e.g. ADD with or without hyperactivity, obsessive compulsive symptoms and specific learning disabilities. Professionals describe the impact of having TS on educational placement and specific classroom strategies are presented. 45 minutes. May be purchased as part of a curriculum or separately. #AV-2
VHS 1/2 inch

9077 After the Diagnosis...the Next Steps
42-40 Bell Boulevard 718-224-2999
Bayside, NY 11361 888-480-8738
Fax: 718-279-9596
e-mail: ts@tsa-usa.org
http://tsa-usa.org
When the diagnosis is Tourette Syndrome, what do you do first? How do you sort out the complexities of the disorder? Whose advice do you follow? What steps do you take to lead a normal life? Six people with TS—as different as any six people can be—relate the sometimes difficult, but finally triumphant path each took to lead the rich, fulfilling life they now enjoy. Narrated by Academy Award-winning actor, Richard Dreyfuss, the stories are blends of poignancy, fact and inspiration.

9078 Clinical Counseling: Towards a Better Understanding of TS
Tourette Syndrome Association
42-40 Bell Boulevard 718-224-2999
Bayside, NY 11361 888-480-8738
Fax: 718-279-9596
e-mail: ts@tsa-usa.org
http://tsa-usa.org
Targeted to counselors, social workers, educators, psychologists and families, this video features expert physicians, allied professionals and several families summarizing key issues that can arise when counseling families with TS. 15 minutes. #AV-10A

9079 Complexities of TS Treatment: A Physician's Round Table
Tourette Syndrome Association
42-40 Bell Boulevard 718-224-2999
Bayside, NY 11361 888-480-8738
Fax: 718-279-9596
e-mail: ts@tsa-usa.org
http://tsa-usa.org
Three internationally recognized TS experts provide colleagues with valuable information about the complexities of treating and advising families with TS. Emphasis is on different clinical approaches to patients with a broad range of symptom severity. Co-morbid and associated conditions are covered. 15 minutes. #AV-10

9080 Educator's In-Service Program
Tourette Syndrome Association

42-40 Bell Boulevard 718-224-2999
Bayside, NY 11361 888-480-8738
Fax: 718-279-9596

A curriculum designed to train educators to recognize and understand TS and guide students with TS and associated disorders in a classroom setting. Developed by the Tourette Syndrome Association for the training of all educational personnel. Includes 2 videos, a particpant's guide, a set of 20 transparencies, 2 scripted curriculum modules and a comprehensive teacher's guide. Discounted for members.

9081 **Gift of Hope**
Tourette Syndrome Association
42-40 Bell Boulevard 718-224-2999
Bayside, NY 11361 888-480-8738
Fax: 718-279-9596
e-mail: ts@tsa-usa.org
http://tsa-usa.org

The cause of TS lies in the brain. Because their are no animal models to study this disorder, human brain tissue is of vital importance for progress in research. Increased brain bank registration is a prime objective of the TSA. VHS 1/2 inch. 14 minutes. Available for shipping cost only. #AV- 7

9082 **Guide to Diagnosis**
Tourette Syndrome Association
42-40 Bell Boulevard 718-224-2999
Bayside, NY 11361-2861 888-480-8738
Fax: 718-279-9596

A video and companion guide for interested medical professionals who have not seen a substantial number of TS patients.
30 minutes

9083 **I'm a Person Too**
Tourette Syndrome Association
42-40 Bell Boulevard 718-224-2999
Bayside, NY 11361 888-480-8738
Fax: 718-279-9596
e-mail: ts@tsa-usa.org
http://tsa-usa.org

Narrated by Cliff Robertson, this video features 5 people with TS; 2 elementary school students and 3 adults from diverse social backgrounds. They talk about a broad variety of symptoms and their personal experiences living with the disorder. VHS 1/2 inch. 22 minutes. #AV1

9084 **Panel of Experts**
Tourette Syndrome Association
42-40 Bell Boulevard 718-224-2999
Bayside, NY 11361-2861 888-480-8738
Fax: 718-279-9596

Five leading authorities bring their in-depth knowledge and experience to bear in a wide-ranging discussion that covers current strategies in TS diagnosis, and medication.
30 minutes

9085 **Parent's Perspective: Diplomacy in Action**
Tourette Syndrome Association
42-40 Bell Boulevard 718-224-2999
Bayside, NY 11361-2861 888-480-8738
Fax: 718-279-9596

The child with TS faces a set of special problems in school. The level of achievement reached in large measure is dependent on the attitude of teachers and administrators. Therefore, educating the educators becomes a high priority with the parent.
45 minutes

9086 **Stop It!... I Can't!**
Tourette Syndrome Association
42-40 Bell Boulevard 718-224-2999
Bayside, NY 11361 888-480-8738
Fax: 718-279-9596
e-mail: ts@tsa-usa.org
http://tsa-usa.org

Narrated by William Shatner, this video promotes sensitivity, education, acceptance and confidence for children with TS. Produced in the 1970's, but provides a valuable and classic message. VHS 1/2 inch. 13 minutes.

9087 **TS-The Parent's Perspective: Diplomacy in Action**
Tourette Syndrome Association
42-40 Bell Boulevard 718-224-2999
Bayside, NY 11361 888-480-8738
Fax: 718-279-9596
e-mail: ts@tsa-usa.org
http://tsa-usa.org

The child with TS faces a set of special problems in school. The level of achievement reached in large measure is dependent on the attitude of teachers and administrators. Therefore educating the educators becomes a high priority for the parent. Special education professionals provide firm guidance to famililies on school advocacy issues. Concrete suggestions are offered to smooth the road to success in school for the student with TS. VHS 1/2 inch. 45 minutes. #AV-6

9088 **TS: A Panel of Experts**
Tourette Syndrome Association
42-40 Bell Boulevard 718-224-2999
Bayside, NY 11361 888-480-8738
Fax: 718-279-9596
e-mail: ts@tsa-usa.org
http://tsa-usa.org

Five leading authorities bring their in-depth knowledge and experience to bear in a wide-ranging discussion that covers current strategies in TS diagnosis and medication, behavioral problems, predicted course and other aspects of this disorder. VHS 1/2 inch. 30 minutes. # AV-5

9089 **Talking About Tourette Syndrome**
Tourette Syndrome Association
42-40 Bell Boulevard 718-224-2999
Bayside, NY 11361 888-480-8738
Fax: 718-279-9596
e-mail: ts@tsa-usa.org
http://tsa-usa.org

When the professional is also the patient, a unique perspective emerges. A psychiatrist leads a candid probing discussion with a brother and sister- all have Tourette syndrome. This free-wheeling exchange brings to the viewer many instructive and often surprising observations about TS and obsessive compulsive symptoms. VHS 1/2 inch. 45 minutes. #AV-8

9090 **Tourette Syndrome: Guide to Diagnosis**
Tourette Syndrome Association
42-40 Bell Boulevard 718-224-2999
Bayside, NY 11361 888-480-8738
Fax: 718-279-9596
e-mail: ts@tsa-usa.org
http://tsa-usa.org

Video for interested medical professionals who have not seen substantial numbers of TS patients. Presents 7 patients with TS who exhibit the full range of movements, vocalizations and behavioral patterns associated with the disorder. Descriptions and demonstrations of other movement disorders are also presented for the purpose of differential diagnosis. VHS 1/2 inch. 30 minutes. A 29 page companion piece by Drs. Ruth Brunn, Donald Cohen and James Leckman is available at $6.00/3.50 shipping.#AV4

9091 **Family Life with Tourette Syndrome... Personal Stories: Professor Peter**
Tourette Syndrome Association
42-40 Bell Boulevard 718-224-2999
Bayside, NY 11361 888-480-8738
Fax: 718-279-9596
e-mail: ts@tsa-usa.org
tsa-usa.org

Now a world class scientific research expert and a professor of biology at Harvard and Purdue, Professor Hollenbeck talks about growing up positively with TS, never hesitating to have children, and offering good advice for newly diagnosed families. 7 minutes, 27 seconds. If purchased together, the six videos in this series are $50.00. #AV-11A

9092 **Family Life with Tourette Syndrome... Personal Stories: Reverend Mike**
Tourette Syndrome Association
42-40 Bell Boulevard 718-224-2999
Bayside, NY 11361 888-480-8738
Fax: 718-279-9596
e-mail: ts@tsa-usa.org
tsa-usa.org

Mike Higgins did not receive a diagnosis of TS until he was in the army! Mike overcame significant symptoms and childhood teasing. Reverend Mike talks about the value of strong family life, faith, support groups and acceptance of the person, and not the disorder as a good way to live positively with TS. If purchased together, the six videos in this series are $50.00. #AV-11B

9093 **Family Life with Tourette Syndrome... Personal Stories: Rachel**
Tourette Syndrome Association
42-40 Bell Boulevard 718-224-2999
Bayside, NY 11361 888-480-8738
Fax: 718-279-9596
e-mail: ts@tsa-usa.org
http://tsa-usa.org

Challenged by TS, ADHD and OCD Rachel and her family endured difficult reactions, behavioral episodes, and at times, a great loss of hope. Now seventeen years old, Rachel and family overcame stresses and strains by sticking together through the highs and lows to find Rachel today a confident and happy teen. 10 minutes. If purchased together, the six videos in this series are $50.00. #AV-11C

9094 **Family Life with Tourette Syndrome... Personal Stories: The Turners**
Tourette Syndrome Association
42-40 Bell Boulevard 718-224-2999
Bayside, NY 11361 888-480-8738
Fax: 718-279-9596
e-mail: ts@tsa-usa.org
http://tsa-usa.org

Three of the four Turner daughters have TS in varying degrees. The family wondered how their symptoms came to be, how to dispense attention fairly, what to say to teachers and friends. They learned how to deal with sibling issues and low self esteem among the sisters. This determined family never gave up! 12 minutes. If purchased together, the six videos in this series are $50.00. #AV-11D

9095 **Family Life with Tourette Syndrome... Personal Stories: Ryan**
Tourette Syndrome Association
42-40 Bell Boulevard 718-224-2999
Bayside, NY 11361 888-480-8738
Fax: 718-279-9596
e-mail: ts@tsa-usa.org
http://tsa-usa.org

Ryan's family first thought his behavior was a deliberate way to get attention. A school principal was harshly critical. The family soon learned to educate themselves and others about Ryan's TS. Things turned around as a result. A good teacher took a great interest, friends began to seek him out and Ryan grew into a young man with a positive outlook. 11 minutes, 28 seconds. If purchased together, the six videos in this series are $50.00. #AV-11E

9096 **Family Life with Tourette Syndrome... Personal Stories: Dakota**
Tourette Syndrome Association
42-40 Bell Boulevard 718-224-2999
Bayside, NY 11361 888-480-8738
Fax: 718-279-9596
e-mail: ts@tsa-usa.org
http://tsa-usa.org

A happy 11 year old baseball playing, video game whiz, Dakota was initially diagnosed as having a brain tumor! He was actually affected by TS and AHD. This is a story of a child who developed a strong confidence and a good attitude, learning to believe in himself. He says the love of his grandparents was a special help! 7 minutes, 12 seconds. If purchased together, the 6 videos in this series are $50.00. #AV-11F

Web Sites

9097 **American Academy of Neurology: Tourette Syndrome**
www.aan.com

The American Academy of Neurology (AAN) is a worldwide professional association of more than 17,000 neurologists and neuroscience professionals dedicating to providing the best possible care for patients with neurological disorders.

9098 **Healing Well**
www.healingwell.com

An online health resource guide to medical news, chat, information and articles, newsgroups and message boards, books, disease-related web sites, medical directories, and more for patients, friends, and family coping with disabling diseases, disorders, or chronic illnesses.

9099 **Health Finder**
www.healthfinder.gov

Searchable, carefully developed web site offering information on over 1000 topics. Developed by the US Department of Health and Human Services, the site can be used in both English and Spanish.

9100 **Healthlink USA**
www.healthlinkusa.com

Health information concerning treatment, cures, prevention, diagnosis, risk factors, research, support groups, email lists, personal stories and much more. Updated regularly.

9101 **Helios Health**
www.helioshealth.com

Online resource for your health information. Detailed information about specific health topics, access to expert advice from our Medical Advisory Board, and up-to-date health news.

9102 **MedicineNet**
www.medicinenet.com

An online resource for consumers providing easy-to-read, authoritative medical and health information.

9103 **Medscape**
www.mywebmd.com

Medscape offers specialists, primary care physicians, and other health professionals the Web's most robust and integrated medical information and educational tools.

9104 **National Institute of Neurological Disorders and Stroke**
www.ninds.nih.gov

Offers a fact sheet on Tourette syndrome and is America's focal point for support of research on brain and nervous system disorders.

9105 **WebMD**
www.webmd.com

Information on Tourette Syndrome, including articles and resources.

Description

9106 **Transplant-Related Conditions**

In recent decades, transplantation of solid organs (heart, liver, lung, kidney), bone marrow and stem cells has become an established part of medical care for advanced diseases in many patients who otherwise face end-rgan failure and poor prognosis. While on one hand, transplantation may serve to cure the underlying disease it nonetheless often entails chronic medical therapy that will likely include the use of immunosuppressants, complications from chronic medications, frequent and long-term medical follow-up and diagnostic testing which may be invasive.

A number of clinical management protocols are utilized in the care of post-transplantation patient, and these vary depending on the type of transplant undertaken, the extent of the tissue match between donor and recipient, and the experience of the given transplantation center. In general however, most patients who receive a transplanted organ or cells will require some chronic therapy (short or long-term) with immunosuppressive medications. These can be several or many and are given in an effort to control the patient's own immunologic response to receiving an organ or cells from another person. The body's natural response after recognizing such an exposure is to "fight" thses cells and tissues with its own defense cells, which are designed to attack and kill foreign material. The immunosuppressive medications help modulate this response so that the transplanted organ is not damaged, injured or "rejected" by the recipient who needs the organ or cells to function in a healthier manner. Immunosuppressive therapy and protection of the transplanted organ must be balanced against the adverse creation of an immunocompromised state in the patient placing him at greater risk for contracting infections that can be serious and even life threatning. Given these circumstances, transplant patients require close working relationships with their medical team along with a true commitment to be compliant with these potentially difficult and complicated medical regimens.

In addition to the medical therapy for patients who have received transplants, one must also consider the significant psychological and social aspects of having undergone such procedures. Strong social support systems and close attention to a healthy emotional and psychological status are important for successful management of these patients. Many transplant centers have extensive support services available to patients from which they and their families can benefit.

National Agencies & Associations

9107 **American Society of Transplantation (AST)**
15000 Commerce Parkway
Mount Laurel, NJ 08054
856-439-9986
Fax: 856-439-9982
e-mail: ast@ahint.com
www.a-s-t.org

The American Society of Transplantation is an international organization of transplant professionals dedicated to advancing the field of transplantation through the promotion of research education advocacy and organ donation to improve patient care.
Barbara Murphy, President
Susan J Nelson, Executive Vice President

9108 **Association of Organ Procurement Organizations (AOPO)**
1364 Beverly Road
McLean, VA 22101
703-556-4242
Fax: 703-556-4852
e-mail: aopo@aopo.org
www.aopo.org

Organization involved in helping people find and obtain the organs they need for transplantation.
Bruce A Wilson, Executive Director
Sue Dunn, President/CEO

9109 **Children's Organ Transplant Association (COTA)**
2501 COTA Drive
Bloomington, IN 47403
700-366-2682
800-366-2682
Fax: 812-336-8885
e-mail: cota@cota.org
www.cota.org

Not-for-profit national chairty dedicated to helping families and communities raise the necessary funds for transplant expenses.
Rick Lofgren, President/CEO
Lisa Fulkerson, VP/CFO

9110 **Donate Life America**
700 N Fourth Street
Richmond, VA 23219
804-782-4920
Fax: 804-782-4643
e-mail: coalition@donatelife.net
www.donatelife.net

A not-for-profit alliance of national organizations and local coalitions across the United States that have joined forces to educate the public about organ, eye and tissue donation, correcting misconceptions about donation and creating a greater willingness to donate.
Sara Pace Jones, Chairwoman
Bruce Wilson, Director of Organ Procurement

9111 **Health Resources and Services Administration (HRSA)**
5600 Fishers Lane
Rockville, MD 20857
301-443-7577
e-mail: comments@hrsa.gov
www.hrsa.gov

Envisions optimal health for all, supported by a health care system that assures access to comprehensive, culturally competant, quality care. Provides national leadership, program resources and services needed to improve access to culturally competant, quality health care.
Elizabeth M Duke PhD, Administrator
Dennis P Williams PhD MA, Deputy Administrator

9112 **Jewish Hospital Transplant Center**
200 Abraham Flexner Way
Louisville, KY 40202
502-587-4011
www.jewishhospital.com

An elite group approved to perform five solid organ transplants and has been named a Federally Designated Medicare Heart Lung Kidney Liver and Pancreas Transplant Center.
Robert L Shircliff, President/CEO
Barbara Mackovic, Senior Manager

9113 **National Foundation for Transplants**
5350 Poplar Avenue
Memphis, TN 38119
901-684-1697
800-489-3863
Fax: 901-684-1128
e-mail: info@transplants.org
www.transplants.org

Mission is to reach out to help those who seek a new life through transplantation by providing healthcare and financial support services and patient advocacy for transplant candidates families nationwide.
Jackie D Hancock, President
Connie Gonitzke, Vice President

9114 **National Institute of Allergy and Infectious Diseases (NIAID)**
6610 Rockledge Drive
Bethesda, MD 20892-6612
301-496-2263
www.niaid.nih.gov

Conducts and supports basic and applied research to better understand, treat, and ultimately prevent infectious, immunologic and allergic diseases. Research has led to new therapies, vaccines, di-

agnostic tests, and other technologies that have improved the health of millions of people in the United States and around the world.
Anthony S. Fauci, Director

9115 National Transplant Assistance Fund (NTAF)
150 N Radnor Chester Road
Radnor, PA 19087
610-353-9684
800-642-8399
Fax: 610-353-1616
e-mail: ntaf@transplantfund.org
www.transplantfund.org
Helps to raise funds for transplant and catastrophic injury patients by providing compassionate support education and expertise to them their families and communities.
Lynne Coughl Samson, Executive Director
Judy B Diner, Managing Director

9116 Organ Procurement and Transplantation Network (OPTN)
700 N 4th Street
Richmond, VA 23219
804-782-4800
888-TXI-NFO1
Fax: 804-782-4994
www.optn.org
A unified transplant network established by the United States Congress under the National Organ Transplant Act (NOTA) of 1984. A unique public-private partnership that links all of the professionals involved in the donation and transplantation system.
Robert S Higgins, President
James Wynn, Vice President

9117 United Network for Organ Sharing (UNOS)
700 N 4th Street
Richmond, VA 23218
804-782-4800
Fax: 804-782-4817
www.unos.org
Non-profit scientific and educational organization that administers the nation's only Organ Procurement and Transplantation Network (OPTN). Mission is to advance organ availability and transplantation by uniting and supporting our communities.
Walter K Graham, Executive Director
Marcia D Manning, Director of Community Affairs

9118 United Organ Transplant Association (UOTA)
3405 Arlington Avenue
Riverside, CA 92506
e-mail: pres@uota.org
www.uota.org
Non-profit charitable corporation dedicated to providing educational emotional and financial support to pre- and post- transplant patients.

State Agencies & Associations

Alabama

9119 Alabama Organ Center
500 S 22 Street S
Birmingham, AL 35233
205-731-9200
800-252-3677
Fax: 205-731-9250
e-mail: Rebecca.davis@ccc.uab.edu
alabamaorgancenter.org
A non-profit, independent organ procurement organization (OPO) serving the population of the Southeastern United States.
Demosthenes Lalisan I MBA CPTC, Director
R Alan Hicks MPH CPTC, Associate Director

Arizona

9120 Donor Network of Arizona
201 W Coolidge
Phoenix, AR 85013
602-222-2200
800-94D-ONOR
Fax: 602-222-2202
e-mail: Contact.Us@dnaz.org
www.dnaz.org
Participates in the equitable distribution of organs, tissues, and corneas for transplant. Also offers donor family support services, community and health care education, and presentations.
Sara Pace Jones, Public Education Contact

Arkansas

9121 Arkansas Regional Organ Recovery Agency
1701 Aldersgate Road
Little Rock, AR 72205
501-907-9150
800-727-6726
Fax: 501-372-6279
e-mail: info@arora.org
www.arora.org
Makes every effort to provide organs and tissues for life-saving and life-enhancing transplantation. Goal will be accomplished through continuous hospital involvement which includes hospital training community involvement andpublic education.
Audrey Brown, Director of Community Education
Boyd Ward, Executive Director

California

9122 California Transplant Donor Network
1000 Broadway
Oakland, CA 94607
510-444-8500
888-570-9400
Fax: 510-444-8501
e-mail: info@ctdn.org
www.ctdn.org
Helps patients in Northern and Central California and Northern Nevada receive organ and tissue transplants. Recovers organs from donors and matches them with the more than 6 000 people who are currently waiting for transplants in this region.
Cindy Siljestrom, Chief Executive Officer
Sonia Salloum, Community Outreach Coordinator

9123 Golden State Donor Services
1760 Creekside Oaks Drive
Sacramento, CA 95833
916-567-1600
Fax: 916-567-8300
e-mail: info@gsds.org
www.gsds.org
Support, enhance, and provide for the recovery and allocation of anatomical gifts. Also work to educate the public regarding the critical need for organ and tissue doors.
Katherine Doolittle, Senior Public Education Coordinator
Helen Nelson, Executive Director

9124 LifeSharing Community Organ & Tissue Donation
3465 Camino Del Rio S
San Diego, CA 92108
619-521-1983
Fax: 619-521-2833
e-mail: info@lifesharing.org
www.lifesharing.org
Non-profit unique and creative organ procurement organization that has centers at the University of California at San Diego Medical Center, Green Hospital of Scripps Clinic, Sharp Hospital.
Sharie Shipley, Public Education Contact
Bill Dawson, Chairman of Volunteer Action Committee

9125 One Legacy Transplant Donor Network
221 S Figueroa Street
Los Angeles, CA 90012
213-229-5600
800-786-4077
Fax: 213-229-5601
e-mail: tmone@onelegacy.org
www.onelegacy.org
One Legacy is dedicaated to achieving the donation of life saving and life enhancing organs and tissues for those in need of transplants and to providing a sense of purpose and comfort to those families we serve.
Stephanie Collazo, Director Clinical Education
Thomas Mone, Chief Executive Officer/EVP

Colorado

9126 Donor Alliance
720 S Colorado Boulevard
Denver, CO 80246
303-329-4747
888-868-4747
Fax: 303-321-0366
www.donoralliance.org
In cooperation with others Donor Alliance facilitates the donation and recovery of organs and tissues for people needing transplantation. Donor Alliance is one of 58 not-for-profit organ recovery organizations federally designated by the U.S..
Jennifer Moe, Director of Community Relations/PR
Nancy Williams, Chairman

Connecticut

9127 **New England Organ Bank Connecticut**
One Gateway Center 203-785-4237
Newton, MA 02158 800-446-NEOB
Fax: 617-244-8755
e-mail: info@neob.com
www.neob.org
Non-profit organ procurement organization that the geographical areas covered are New Haven Connecticut Area, Maine, Eastern Massachusetts, New Hampshire, Rhode Island, and Vermont.
Sean Fitzpatrick, Public Education Director

Delaware

9128 **Gift of Life Donor Program Delaware**
401 N. 3rd St. 215-557-8090
Philadelphia, PA 19123 888-366-6771
Fax: 215-963-0587
e-mail: info@donors1.org
www.donors1.org
Formerly (Delaware Valley Transplant Program) is the region's nonprofit organ and tissue donor program serving eastern half of Pennsylvania, southern New Jersey and the state of Delaware. Also, considered a model program in the United States.
John Green, Director of Community Relations

District of Columbia

9129 **Washington Regional Transplant Consortium**
7619 Little River Turnpike 703-641-0100
Annandale, VA 22003 866-232-3666
Fax: 703-658-0711
e-mail: contactwrtc@wrtc.org
www.wrtc.org
WRTC is the official link between organ and tissue donors and the patients who are waiting for transplants.
Sara Idler, Public Education Contact

Florida

9130 **LifeLink of Florida**
409 Bayshore Boulevard 813-253-2640
Tampa, FL 33606 800-262-5775
Fax: 813-348-0634
e-mail: info@lifelinkfound.org
www.lifelinkfound.org
Independent, nonprofit community service organization dedicated to the recovery and transplantation of organs and tissues. Operates under the authority of the Social Security Act, and in accordance with the National Organ Transplant Act passed by Congress.
Dennis F Heinrichs, President
Dana L Shires Jr, Chairman of the Board

9131 **LifeLink of Southwest Florida**
409 Bayshore Boulevard 813-253-2640
Tampa, FL 33906 800-262-5775
Fax: 813-348-0634
e-mail: info@lifelinkfound.org
www.lifelinkfound.org
LifeLink of Southwest Florida and Florida Gulf Coast University joined forces to develop a survey instrument to assss student attitudes and opinions about donation. Worked to conduct and evaluate the impact of the multifaceted education campaign.
Dennis F Heinrichs, President
Dana L Shires Jr, Chairman of the Board

9132 **TransLife/Florida Hospital**
1560 Orange Avenue 407-644-3770
Winter Park, FL 32789 800-443-6667
Fax: 407-303-2473
www.translife.org
Works closely with hospitals and donor families to coordinate the gift of life in Central Florida. Also a critical link between donors and possible recipients.
Carol Rumsey, Public Education Contact

Georgia

9133 **LifeLink of Georgia**
2875 Northwoods Parkway 770-225-5465
Norcross, GA 30071 800-544-6667
e-mail: info@lifelinkfound.org
www.lifelinkfound.org/georgia/ga.html
The Foundation atempts to work in a sensitive diligent and compassionate manner with donor families to facilitate the donation of desperately needed organs and tissues for waiting patients.
Dennis F Heinrichs, President
Dana L Shires, Chairman of the Board

Hawaii

9134 **Organ Donor Center of Hawaii**
1149 Bethel Street 808-599-7630
Honolulu, HI 96813 877-855-0603
Fax: 808-599-7631
e-mail: info@organdonorhawaii.com
www.organdonorhawaii.com
Non-profit organ procurement organization.
Stephen A Kula, Executive Director
Christine L Bogee, Administrative Services Director

Illinois

9135 **Regional Organ Bank of Illinois, Inc.**
800 S. Wells 312-431-3600
Chicago, IL 60607 888-307-3668
Fax: 312-803-7643
e-mail: info@robi.org
www.robi.org
ROBI'S mission is to save and enhance the lives of as many people as possible through organ and tissue donation.
Kim McCullough, Public Education Contact

Indiana

9136 **Indiana Organ Procurement Organization,**
3760 Guion Road 317-685-0389
Indianapolis, IN 46222-1816 888-275-4676
Fax: 317-685-1687
e-mail: info@iopo.org
www.iopo.org
Non-profit organ procurement organization designed to recover and distribute organ and tissues for transplantation.
Sam Davis, Director of Professional Services
Lynn Driver, President and CEO

Iowa

9137 **Iowa Donor Network**
550 Madison Avenue 319-665-3787
N Liberty, IA 52317 800-831-4131
Fax: 319-665-3788
www.iowadonornetwork.org
Iowa Donor Network is dedicated to serving donow families potentialdonors and candidates doe transplantation through identifying potential donorssupporting and respecting donation decisions and maximizing the recovery of transplantable organs and tissues.
Kelly Sorensen, Public Education Contact

Kansas

9138 **Midwest Transplant Network & Organ Bank**
1900 W 47th Place 913-262-1668
Westwood, KS 66205 Fax: 913-262-5130
e-mail: info@mwob.org
www.mwtn.org
Provides quality transplantation related services that will maximize the availability of organs and tissues to the comunities we serve. Provides procurement services for organ and tissue and laboratory services for HLA.
Ray Gable, Public Education Contact
Marcia Schoenfeld, Public Education Contact

Kentucky

9139 **Kentucky Organ Donor Affiliates**
106 E Broadway 502-581-9511
Louisville, KY 40202 800-525-3456
Fax: 502-589-5157
e-mail: info@kyorgandonor.org
www.kyorgandonor.org
Non-profit organ donor center that retrieves and distributes organs to qualified recipients.

Louisiana

9140 **Louisiana Organ Procurement Agency**
4441 N I-10 Service Road 504-837-3355
Metairie, LA 70006-3626 800-521-GIVE
Fax: 504-837-3587
e-mail: info@lopa.org
www.lopa.org
Non-profit organ procurement organization federally-designated to increase the number of transplantable organs by providing families an opportunity to donate organs and tissues to support these families regardless of their decision.
John Egan, Public Education Contact

Maine

9141 **New England Organ Bank Maine**
One Gateway Center 800-870-5230
Newton, MA 02158 800-446-NEOB
Fax: 617-244-8755
e-mail: info@neob.org
www.neob.org
Independent, not-for-profit agency whose mission is to recover, peerve, and distribute human organs and tissues for transplantation. The New England Organ Bank is a federally-designated organ procurement organization for all parts of the six New England states, it serves 177 acute care hospitals and 14 transplant centers.
Sean Fitzpatrick, Public Education Contact

Maryland

9142 **Transplant Resource Center of Maryland**
1730 Twin Springs Road 410-242-7000
Baltimore, MD 21227 800-641-HERO
Fax: 410-242-1871
e-mail: communications@TheLLF.org
www.mdtransplant.org
Provides organ and tissue donation and recovery services hospital donor program development and community education to 42 hospitals and the citizens living in Maryland.
Ann Bromery, Chief Financial Officer
Charles Alexander, President & Chief Executive Officer

9143 **Washington Regional Transplant Consortium**
7619 Little River Turnpike 703-641-0100
Annandale, VA 22003 866-232-3666
Fax: 703-658-0711
e-mail: contactwrtc@wrtc.org
www.wrtc.org
Recently partnered with fellow Mid-Atlantic Coalition on Donation members and a company called Sports America to sponsor the second annual DeMatha Invitational. WRTC is the official link between organ and tissue donors and the patients who are waiting for transplant.
Sara Idler, Public Education Contact

Massachusetts

9144 **New England Organ Bank Massachusetts**
One Gateway Center
Newton, MA 02158 800-446-NEOB
Fax: 617-244-8755
e-mail: info@neob.com
www.neob.org
Independent, not-for-profit agency whose mission is to recover, preserve, and distribute human organs and tissues for transplantation. A federally-designated organ procurement organization for all or part of the six New England states, it serves 177 acute care hospitals and 14 transplant centers.
Sean Fitzpatrick, Public Education Contact

9145 **NorthEast Organ Procurement Organization**
80 Seymour Street 800-874-5215
Hartford, CT 06102-5037 Fax: 860-545-4143
www.harthosp.org/NEOPO/index.html
Assures that comprehensive organ and tissue donation services are provided to the community in an efficient and professional manner.
Ginger Van Nostrand, Public Education Contact

Michigan

9146 **Transplantation Society of Michigan**
3861 Research Park Drive 734-973-1577
Ann Arbor, MI 48108 800-482-4881
Fax: 734-973-3133
e-mail: info@giftoflifemichigan.org
www.giftoflifemichigan.org
Nonprofit independent corporation certified by Medicare and designated by the Centers for Medicare and Medicaid Services as an organ recovery organization for Michigan.
Tammie Harvermahl, Public Education Contact

Minnesota

9147 **LifeSource, Upper Midwest Organ Procurement Organization, Inc.**
2550 University Avenue West 651-603-7800
St. Paul, MN 55114-1904 Fax: 651-603-7801
e-mail: info@life-source.org
www.life-source.org
Nonprofit, federally-designated organ procurement organization for the Upper Midwest, managing all organ donation activities in Minnesota.
Jill Halimi, Donor Family Services

Mississippi

9148 **Mississippi Organ Recovery**
12 River Bend Place 601-933-1000
Flowood, MS 39232 800-690-8878
Fax: 601-933-1006
www.msora.org
Not-for-profit organization coordinates the recovery of human organs for transplantation by working with and providing education to medical professionals donor families and the people of Mississippi.
Kelly Nations, Community Education Coordinator
Kevin Stump, Chief Executive Officer

Missouri

9149 **Mid-America Transplant Services**
1110 Highlands Plaza Drive E 314-735-8200
Saint Louis, MO 63110-3205 Fax: 314-991-2805
e-mail: info@mts-stl.org
www.mts-stl.org
Community based not-for-profit organ procurement organization dedicated to enhancing the quality of human life. Coordinates the procurement of vital organs tissues and eyes in hospitals throughout its service area.
Diane Brockmeier, COO
Dean F Kappel, President and CEO

Nebraska

9150 **Nebraska Organ Retrieval System**
8502 W Center Road 402-733-1800
Omaha, NE 68124 877-633-1800
Fax: 402-733-9312
www.NEdonation.org
Responsible for retrieving the proper organs and distrbuting them to the recipients.
Stephanie Lochmiller, Public Relations Coordinator
Karen Risk, Executive Director

Nevada

9151 **Nevada Donor Network**
2085 E Sahara Avenue 702-796-9600
Las Vegas, NV 89104 Fax: 702-796-4225
e-mail: ksatcher@nvdonor.org
www.nvdonor.org
Improving the quality of human life through the recovery of all available organs and tissues for transplantation education and research while maintaining the dignity of the donors and their families.
Liliana Arredondo, Public Education Coordinator
Ken Richardson, Executive Director

New Hampshire

9152 **New England Organ Bank New Hampshire**
One Gateway Center
Newton, MA 02158 800-446-NEOB
Fax: 617-244-8755
e-mail: info@neob.com
www.neob.org
Non-profit organ procurement organization that the geographical areas covered are New Haven Connecticut Area, Maine, Eastern Massachusetts, New Hampshire, Rhode Island, and Vermont.
Sean Fitzpatrick, Public Education Director

New Jersey

9153 **Gift of Life Donor Program New Jersey**
2000 Hamilton Street 215-557-8090
Philadelphia, PA 19103-3813 888-366-6771
Fax: 215-963-0587
e-mail: info@donors1.org
www.donors1.org
Formerly (Delaware Valley Transplant Program) is the region's nonprofit organ and tissue donor program serving eastern half of Pennsylvania, southern New Jersey and the state of Delaware. Also, considered a model program in the United States.
John Green, Director of Community Relations

9154 **Sharing Network Organ Tissue Donation Services**
841 Mountain Avenue 973-379-4535
Springfield, NJ 07081 800-742-7365
Fax: 973-379-5113
e-mail: tsn@sharenj.org
www.sharenj.org
Federally certified state-approved organ procurement organization responsible for recovering organ and tissue for New Jersey residents currently awaiting transplants.
Melissa Honohan, Director of External Relations
Joseph Roth, President and Chief Executive Officer

New Mexico

9155 **New Mexico Donor Services**
2715 Broadbent Parkway NE 505-843-7672
Albuquerque, NM 87107 800-843-7672
Fax: 505-343-1828
e-mail: info@donatelifenm.org
www.donatelifenm.org
Transplant centers in the service area are: University of New Mexico Hospitals Presbyterian Hospital.
Maria Sanders, Community Services
Patricia Niles, Executive Director

New York

9156 **Center for Donation & Transplantation**
218 Great Oaks Boulevard 518-262-5606
Albany, NY 12203 800-256-7811
Fax: 518-262-5427
e-mail: dfloeser@cdtny.org
www.cdtny.org
Dedicated to increasing organ and tissue donation by following procurement and equitable distribution of medically suitable organs and tissue for transplantation.
Antonio Di Carlo, Assistant Medical Director
David Conti, Board Chairman/Medical Director

9157 **Finger Lakes Donor Recovery Network**
Corporate Woods of Brighton 585-272-4930
Rochester, NY 14623 800-810-5494
Fax: 585-272-4956
e-mail: info@donorrecovery.org
www.donorrecovery.org
Nonprofit organization that covers the Finger Lakes Region Central and Upstate New York for transplant centers.
Richard Padula, Operations Manager
Rob Kochik, Executive Director

9158 **New York Organ Donor Network, Inc**
132 West 31st Street 646-291-4444
New York, NY 10001 Fax: 646-291-4600
www.nyodn.org
The New York Organ Donor Network is dedicated to the recovery of organs and tissues for people in need of life-saving and life-improvving transplants.
Elaine Berg, President/CEO

9159 **Upstate New York Transplant Services, Inc.**
110 Broadway 716-853-6667
Buffalo, NY 14203 800-227-4771
Fax: 716-853-6674
e-mail: info@unyts.org
www.unyts.org
An independent nonprofit organization that encourages and coordinates the donation of human organs and tissue for transplantation.
Sallyann Ieraci, Vice President of Community Relations
Mark J Simon, President/CEO

North Carolina

9160 **Life Share of the Carolinas**
5000 D Airport Center Parkway 704-512-3303
Charlotte, NC 28208 800-932-4483
Fax: 704-512-3056
e-mail: lifeshare@carolinas.org
www.lifesharecarolinas.org
Mission is to improve the quality of human life through the provision of organs and tissues for transplantation and to serve our hospitals and their respective communities by rpoviding educational support services which enhance the donation process.
Debbie Gibbs, Public Relations Manager
Bill Faircloth, Executive Director

Ohio

9161 **Life Connection of Ohio**
3661 Briarfield Boulevard 419-893-1618
Maumee, OH 43537 800-262-5443
Fax: 419-893-1827
e-mail: nellis@lcotro.org
www.lifeconnectionofohio.org
Life Connection of Ohio is committed to serving humanity by ending the wait for organ and tissue transplants in a manner that is beneficial to patients, donor families, and health care professionals.
Nancy Ellis, Director of Community Relations (Toledo)
Cathi Arends, Director of Community Relations (Dayton)

9162 **LifeBanc**
20600 Chaggrin Boulevard 216-752-5433
Cleveland, OH 44122-5343 888-558-LIFE
Fax: 216-751-4204
e-mail: info@lifebanc.org
www.lifebanc.org
Non-profit organization that covers all of Northeast Ohio.
Monica Morgan, Public Education Contact

9163 **Lifeline of Ohio Organ Procurement Agency, Inc.**
770 Kinnear Road 614-291-5667
Columbus, OH 43212 800-525-5667
Fax: 614-291-0660
www.lifelineofohio.org
Lifeline of Ohio (LOOP) is an independent non-profit organization whose purpose is to promote and coordinate the donation of human organs and tissue dor transplantation.
Roger L Walker, Vice-Chair Governing Board of Directors
Marilyn Tomasi, Chair Governing Board of Directors

9164 **Ohio Valley LifeCenter**
2925 Vernon Place 513-558-5555
Cincinnati, OH 45219-2430 800-981-5433
Fax: 513-558-5556
e-mail: info@lifepassiton.org
www.lifecnt.org

Encourages amd coordinates the donation of human organs and tissues in the Greater Cincinnati area. Provides educational and motivational progams to healthcare professionals regarding their important role in the donation of organs and tissues for transplant.
Mark Sommerville, Public Education Contact
Michael Edwards, Chairman

Oklahoma

9165 **Oklahoma Organ Sharing Network**
5801 N Broadway
Oklahoma City, OK 73118 888-580-5680
Fax: 405-840-9748
e-mail: philvs@oosn.org ÿ
www.oosn.org

LifeShare Transplant Donor Services of Oklahoma is committed to providing a better quality of life for those people who require organ or tissue transplantation while respecting and honoring those families who share the gift of life.
Harlan Wright, President

Oregon

9166 **Pacific NW Transplant Bank**
2611 SW 3rd Avenue 503-494-5560
Portland, OR 97201-4952 800-344-8916
Fax: 503-494-4725
e-mail: pntb@ohsu.edu
www.pntb.org

Federally designated nonprofit organ procurement organization serving Oregon southwest Washington and western Idaho.
Jean Shepard, Public Education Contact
Barbara Thompson, Clinical Director

Pennsylvania

9167 **Center for Organ Recovery & Education**
RIDC Park
Pittsburgh, PA 15238 800-366-6777
Fax: 412-963-3563
e-mail: hbulvony@core.org
www.core.org

Continues its efforts to lead the procurement field by becoming a full-service OPO.
Susan A Stuart, President & CEO
Joseph P Weber, Vice President Finance

9168 **Gift of Life Donor Program Pennsylvania**
2000 Hamilton Street 215-557-8090
Philadelphia, PA 19103-3813 888-366-6771
Fax: 215-963-0587
e-mail: info@donors1.org
www.donors1.org

Formerly (Delaware Valley Transplant Program) is the region's nonprofit organ and tissue donor program serving eastern half of Pennsylvania, southern New Jersey and the state of Delaware. Also, considered a model program in the United States.
John Green, Director of Community Relations

Rhode Island

9169 **New England Organ Bank Rhode Island**
One Gateway Center
Newton, MA 02158 800-446-NEOB
Fax: 617-244-8755
e-mail: info@neob.com
www.neob.org

Independent, not-for-profit agency whose mission is to recover, preserve, and distribute human organs and tissues for transplantation. A federally-designated organ procurement organization for all or part of the six New England states, it serves 177 acute care hospitals and 14 transplant centers.
Sean Fitzpatrick, Public Education Contact

South Carolina

9170 **LifePoint**
4200 Faber Place Drive 843-763-7755
Charleston, SC 29405-5711 800-462-0755
Fax: 843-763-6393
e-mail: info@lifepoint-sc.org
www.lifepoint-sc.org

Dedicated to saving and improving lives by providing organ recovery services to hospitals treating potential organ donors and to support donor families.
Peggy Drake, VP Organ Recovery Services
Nancy A Kay, President & CEO

Tennessee

9171 **Mid-South Transplant Foundation, Inc. Tennessee**
910 Madison Avenue 901-328-4438
Memphis, TN 38103 877-228-LIFE
Fax: 901-448-8126
www.midsouthtransplant.org

Mission is to provide the option of donation to all families of potential organ donors and to protect their rights and interest throughout the donation process.
Lisa Peoples, Public Education Contact

9172 **Tennessee Donor Services**
110 KLM Drive 423-915-0808
Gray, TN 37615 888-562-3774
Fax: 901-448-8126
e-mail: info@donatelifetn.org
donatelifetn.org

Mission is to represent the interests of the people of our service area in the formulation of policies procedures and regulations concerning organ donation and transplantation.
Lisa Peoples, Public Education Contact
Jennifer Jenks, Contact

Utah

9173 **Intermountain Donor Services**
230 S 500 E 801-521-1755
Salt Lake City, UT 84102 800-833-6667
Fax: 801-364-8815
e-mail: debbie@idslife.org
www.idslife.org

Provides high quality organ and tissue procurement services to the medical and public communities. Educating medical professionals and the poublic sector on the benefits of organ and tissue donation.
Alex McDonald, Public Education Director
Tracy C Schmidt, Executive Director

Vermont

9174 **New England Organ Bank Vermont**
One Gateway Center 802-656-8454
Newton, MA 02158 800-446-NEOB
Fax: 617-244-8755
e-mail: info@neob.com
www.neob.org

Independent, not-for-profit agency whose mission is to recover, preserve, and distribute human organs and tissues for transplantation. A federally-designated organ procurement organization for all or part of the six New England states, it serves 177 acute care hospitals and 14 transplant centers.
Sean Fitzpatrick, Public Education Contact

Virginia

9175 **LifeNet**
1864 Concert Drive ÿ75- 46- 476
Virginia Beach, VA 23453 800-847-7831
Fax: 757-301-6582
e-mail: lifenet@trans.org
www.lifenet.org

An organ procurement agency and the largest full-service tissue bank in the United States providing musculoskeletal and cardiovascular tissues for transplant on a national and international basis.
Becky Lawson, Public Education Contact

Washington

9176 LifeCenter Northwest
11245 SE 6th Street
Bellevue, WA 98004
425-201-6563
877-275-5269
Fax: 425-688-7641
e-mail: info@lcnw.org
www.lcnw.org

LifeCenter Northwest Organ Donation Network is a nonprofit organization that facilitates organ donation for a population of over 7.5 million people throughout Washington Montana Alasks and Northern Idaho. Our mission is to fund education and outreach programs.
Megan Erwin, Vice President Community Relations
Diana Clark, President & CEO

Wisconsin

9177 University of Wisconsin Organ Procurement Organization
University of Wisconsin Hospital and Clinics
450 Science Drive
Madison, WI 53711-1735
608-265-0356
Fax: 608-262-9099
e-mail: uwhcopo@uwhealth.org
www.uwhcopo.org

Located within a major academic center and is recognized as one of the most successful organ procurement programs in the nation.
Jill Ellefson, Public Education Contact

9178 Wisonsin Donor Network
9200 W Chester Street
Milwaukee, WI 53214
414-805-2024
800-432-5405
Fax: 414-259-8059
e-mail: cjastroc@fmlh.edu
www.wisdonornetwork.org

Recovers organs for transplant as well as provides public and professional education about the tremendous need for organ and tissue donors.
Judy Suchman, Director
Colleen McCarthy, Assistant Director

Wyoming

9179 Donor Alliance
720 S Colorado Boulevard
Denver, CO 80246
303-329-4747
888-868-4747
Fax: 303-321-0366
www.donoralliance.org

Jennifer Moe, Director of Community Relations/PR
Nancy Williams, Chairman

International

9180 Lifelink of Puerto Rico
Digital Plaza, Suite 402
Guaynabo, PR 00968
787-277-0900
800-558-0977
Fax: 787-277-0876
e-mail: lifelink@PPTC.Net
www.lifelinkfound.org

An independent, nonprofit community service organization dedicated to the recovery and transplantation of organs and tissues.
Ruth Duncan Bell, Public Education Contact

Foundations

9181 Musculoskeletal Transplant Foundation
125 May Street
Edison, NJ 08837
732-661-0202
Fax: 732-661-2298
e-mail: information@mtf.org
www.mtf.org

Non-profit service organization dedicated to providing quality tissue through a commitment to excellence in education, research, recovery and care for recipients, donors, and their families.
Bruce W Stroever, President/CEO
George A Oram, EVP Sales/Marketing

Research Centers

9182 Georgetown University Hospital Transplant Institute
3800 Reservoir Road, NW
Washington, DC 20007
202-444-2000
www.georgetownuniversityhospital.org

Founded to promote health through education, research, and patient care.

Books

9183 History of Organ and Cell Transplantation
Imperial College Press
57 Shelton St., Convent Garden
United Kingdom,
e-mail: edit@icpress.co.uk
www.icpress.co.uk

Covers the areas of modern medical literature.
464 pages Hardcover
ISBN: 1-860942-09-1

9184 Legal and Ethical Aspects of Organ Transplantation
David P T Price, author
Cambridge University Press
40 West 20th Street
New York, NY 10011-4221
212-924-3900
Fax: 212-691-3239
www.cambridge.org/us

A comprehensive analysis of existing laws and policies governing transplantation practices around the world. Examines the meaning of death, cadaver organ procurement policies, use of living donors, trading in human organs, experimental transplant procedures and xenotransplantation.
507 pages Hardcover
ISBN: 0-521651-64-6

9185 Organ Procurement and Transplantation:
Intitute of Medicine, author
National Academies Press
500 Fifth Street NW
Washington, DC 20055
202-334-3313
888-624-8373
Fax: 202-334-2451
www.nap.edu

This book assesses the potential impact of the Final Rule on organ transplantation. Prensents new, original data, and assesses medical practices, social and economic observations, and other information.
232 pages Hardcover

9186 Organ Transplants from Executed Prisoners:
Louis J Palmer, author
McFarland & Company
960 NC Hwy 88W
Jefferson, NC 28640
336-246-4460
Fax: 336-246-5018
e-mail: info@mcfarlandpub.com
www.mcfarlandpub.com

A study of the utilitarian creation of "death sentence organ removal statutes" that would make legal the harvesting of transplantable organs from the cadavers of executed capital murders.
156 pages
ISBN: 0-786406-73-9

9187 Transplantation Ethics
Robert M. Veatch, author
Georgetown University Press
3240 Prospect Street, NW
Washington, DC 20007
202-687-5889
Fax: 202-687-6340
e-mail: gupress@georgetown.edu
www.press.georgetown.edu

The first complete and systematic account of the ethical and policy controversies surrounding organ transplants.
2000 448 pages Paperback
ISBN: 0-878408-12-2

9188 Twice Dead: Organ Transplants and the Reinvention of Death
Margaret Lock, author
University of California Press

1445 Lower Ferry Road
Ewing, NJ 08618 800-UCB-OOKS
Fax: 800-999-1958
www.ucpress.edu/index.html

Raises critically important questions about life and death in the modern world.

429 pages Paperback
ISBN: 0-520228-14-6

9189 **US Organ Procurement System: A Prescription for Reform**
David L. Kaserman, A.H. Barnett, author

American Enterprise Institute
1150 Seventeenth St, NW 202-862-5800
Washington, DC 20036 Fax: 202-862-7177
www.aei.org

Isolates the procurement issue from others to make a compelling and persuasive case for markets in cadaveric organs.

177 pages Paperback
ISBN: 0-844741-71-X

Magazines

9190 **Encore: Another Chance for Life**
Chronimed Pharmacy
Po Box 59032
Minneapolis, MN 55459-9686 800-888-5753

Published exclusively for transplant patients, their families, and friends, this publication provides a broad look at many issues surrounding transplantation and encourages personal stories and feedback from readers.

Quarterly

9191 **Renalife**
The American Association of Kidney Patients
100 S. Ashley Drive
Tampa, FL 33260 800-749-2257
e-mail: aakpaz@enet.net

Provides articles, news items, and information of interest to kindey patients and their families, individuals, and organizations in the renal health care field.

3 Year

9192 **Stadtlanders LifeTIMES**
Stadtlanders Pharmacy
600 Penn Center Boulevard
Pittsburgh, PA 15235-5810 800-238-7828
www.statlander.com/transplant/#resource

Designed to be an educational, informative and supportive, focusing on a variety of health-care issues of concern to patients (including transplant patients).

Newsletters

9193 **Advocate**
National Foundation for Transplants
1102 Brookfield Road 901-684-1697
Memphis, TN 38119 800-489-3863
Fax: 901-684-1128
e-mail: info@transplants.org
www.transplants.org

Judy Strickland, Patient Services Coordinator

9194 **Children's Organ Transplant Association (COTA)**
2501 COTA Drive 800-366-2682
Bloomington, IN 47403 Fax: 812-336-8885
e-mail: cota@cota.org
www.cota.org

Provides fundraising assistance to children and young adults needing life-saving transplants and promotes organ, marrow and tissue donation.

Rick Lofgren, President/CEO
Lisa Fulkerson, VP/CFO

9195 **New Start News**
National Transplant Assistance Fund (NTAF)
3475 West Chester Pike 610-353-9684
Newtown Square, PA 19073 800-642-8399
Fax: 610-353-1616
e-mail: ntaf@transplantfund.org
www.transplantfund.org

Sidney P. Constien, Editor
Judy Walker, Editor

Web Sites

9196 **American Society of Transplantation (AST)**
www.a-s-t.org

An organization of transplant professionals dedicated to research, education, advocacy and patient care in transplantation science and medicine.

9197 **Association of Organ Procurement Organizations (AOPO)**
www.aopo.org

Organization involved in helping people find and obtain the organs they may need for transplantation.

9198 **Children's Organ Transplant Association (COTA)**
www.cota.org

Not-for-profit national chairty dedicated to helping families and communities raise the necessary funds for transplant expenses.

9199 **Donate Life America**
www.donatelife.net

A not-for-profit alliance of national organizations and local coalitions across the United States that have joined forces to educate the public about organ, eye and tissue donation, correcting misconceptions about donation and creating a greater willingness to donate.

9200 **Georgetown University Hospital Transplant Institute**
www.georgetownuniversityhospital.org

Founded to promote health through education, research, and patient care.

9201 **Health Resources and Services Administration (HRSA)**
www.hrsa.gov

Envisions optimal health for all, supported by a health care system that assures access to comprehensive, culturally competant, quality care. Provides national leadership, program resources and services needed to improve access to culturally competant, quality health care.

9202 **Jewish Hospital Transplant Center**
www.jewishhospital.com

An elite group approved to perform five solid organ transplants and has been named a Federally Designated Medicare Heart, Lung, Kidney, Liver and Pancreas Transplant Center.

9203 **MedicineNet**
www.medicinenet.com

An online resource for consumers providing easy-to-read, authoritative medical and health information.

9204 **National Foundation for Transplants**
www.transplants.org

Mission is to reach out to help those who seek a new life through transplantation, by providing healthcare and financial support services and patient advocacy for transplant candidates families nationwide.

9205 **National Transplant Assistance Fund (NTAF)**
www.transplantfund.org

Helps to raise funds for transplant and catastrophic injury patients by providing compassionate support, education and expertise to them, their families and communities.

9206 **Organ Procurement and Transplantation Network (OPTN)**
www.optn.org

A unified transplant network established by the United States Congress under the National Organ Transplant Act (NOTA) of 1984. A unique public-prvate partnership that links all of the professionals nvolved in the donation and transplantation system.

9207 **Transweb: All About Transplantation and Donation**
www.transweb.org

Non-profit educational website serving the world transplant community. Features news and events, real peoples experinces, the top 10 myths about donation, a donation quiz, and a large collection of questions and answers, as well as a reference area with everything from articles to videos.

9208 United Network for Organ Sharing (UNOS)

www.unos.org

Mon-profit, scientific and educational organization that administers the nation's only Organ Procurement and Transplantation Network(OPTN). Mission is to advance organ availability and transplantation by uniting and supporting our communities for the benefit of patients through education, technology and policy development.

9209 United Organ Transplant Association (UOTA)

www.uota.org

Non-profit charitable Corporation dedicated to providing educational, emotional and financial support to pre- and post- transplant patients.

Description

9210 Tuberculosis

Tuberculosis, TB, is an infectious disease caused by mycobacteria. It is spread through the air and normally affects the lungs (pulmonary tuberculosis). Extremely common in the United States early in the twentieth century, tuberculosis declined dramatically after 1950. This trend reversed itself after about 1985, due to immigration, the HIV epidemic, and the development of drug resistance by the germ responsible for the disease.

The usual symptoms of TB infection of the lungs include persistent cough, chest pain and coughing up blood. TB infection can cause weight loss, night sweats and fatigue. Left untreated, TB may spread to the spine, causing bone breakdown with deformity, to the lining of the brain, causing tuberculous meningitis, or, in fact, to any organ of the body (extrapulmonary TB).

People who are otherwise healthy, and who are infected with a strain of mycobacterium that is sensitive to standard drugs, can almost always be cured after 6-9 months of therapy. Persons infected with HIV, because of their lowered resistance to disease, have trouble clearing their TB infection, even if they use effective drugs faithfully. Therefore, they should be treated for one year. Regardless of length of treatment, during this time the germ may become resistant to the drug being used. Therefore treatment includes at least 2 drugs, so that a bacterium that develops resistance to one drug will still be killed by another one. Incomplete or interrupted treatment often leads to drug resistance. Germs that are resistant to multiple drugs may be passed to others, and are now a serious public health menace. Unfortunately, the HIV-infected patient is an ideal breeding ground for drug-resistant TB germs.

Persons with drug-sensitive TB who are otherwise healthy and will cooperate with treatment are generally treated by community physicians. Those with complicated medical status (HIV, drug-resistant organisms) or social difficulties (alcoholism, substance abuse, homelessness) generally require specialized public health clinics that can combine medical expertise with nursing and social outreach support.

Many persons who have been infected by TB keep it successfully contained by their own immune systems. There is some risk of the contained germ, however, even years later, overcoming the body's resistance and causing active disease. The tuberculin skin test (PPD) is used to widely screen certain high-risk populations, particularly those who have been exposed to an infectious individual. Prior, adequately treated infection may be diagnosed by a positive PPD, and is sometimes treated with antibiotics to reduce the risk of future disease.

National Agencies & Associations

9211 American Lung Association
1301 Pennsylvania Avenue NW 212-315-8700
Washington, DC 20004 800-LUN-GUSA
www.lungusa.org
The mission of the American Lung Association is to prevent lung disease and promote lung health. Founded in 1904 to fight tuberculosis the American Lung Association today fights disease in all its forms, with special emphasis on asthma and tobacco control.
H James Gooden, Secretary
Stephen J Nolan, Chair

9212 Centers for Disease Control and Prevention National Center for Prevention Services
National Center for Prevention Services
1600 Clifton Road 404-639-8135
Atlanta, GA 30333 800-CDC-INFO
TTY: 888-232-6348
e-mail: cdcinfo@cdc.gov
www.cdc.gov
CDC has been dedicated to protecting health and promoting quality of life through the prevention and control of disease, injury and disability.
Richard E Besser, Acting Director
Ileana Arias, Director Center Injury Prevention

9213 National Institute of Allergy and Infectious Diseases
6610 Rockledge Drive 301-496-5717
Bethesda, MD 20892-6621 866-284-4107
Fax: 301-402-3573
TTY: 800-877-8339
e-mail: afauci@niaid.nih.gov
www.niaid.nih.gov
Conducts and supports basic and applied research to better understand, treat and ultimately prevent infectious, immunologic and allergic diseases.
Anthony S Fauci MD, Director
H Clifford Lane MD, Acting Deputy Director

9214 New Jersey Medical School: National Tuberculosis Center
225 Warren Street 973-972-3270
Newark, NJ 07101-1709 800-482-3627
Fax: 973-972-3268
www.umdnj.edu/ntbcweb/tbsplash.html
Provides expert medical consultation, trains health care providers and other health related professionals, utilize innovative educational methodologies such as standardized patients, develop linkages with health care delivery systems and collaborate with health care professionals.
Lee B Reichman, Executive Director
Reynard J McDonald, Medical Director

9215 Occupational Safety & Health Administration
200 Constitution Avenue Northwest
Washington, DC 20210 800-321-6742
TTY: 877-889-5627
www.osha.gov
OSHA's mission is to assure the safety and health of America's workers by setting and enforcing standards, providing training, outreach and education, establishing partnerships and encouraging continual improvement in workplace safety and health.
Doug Kalinowski, Director

State Agencies & Associations

Alabama

9216 American Lung Association of Alabama
PO Box 3188 205-933-8821
Bessemer, AL 35023 800-LUN-GUSA
Fax: 205-930-1717
e-mail: kperry@alabamalung.org
www.alabamalung.org
Kim Perry, Director of Development

Alaska

9217 **American Lung Association of Alaska**
500 W International Airport Road
Anchorage, AK 99518
907-276-5864
800-LUN-GUSA
Fax: 907-565-5587
e-mail: mlarson@aklung.org
www.aklung.org

Marge Larson, Director

Arizona

9218 **American Lung Association of Arizona/New Mexico**
102 W McDowell Road
Phoenix, AZ 85003-1299
602-258-7505
800-586-4872
Fax: 602-258-7507
www.lungusa.org

9219 **Northern Arizona Branch:Phoenix Area**
102 W McDowell Road
Phoenix, AZ 85003-1299
602-258-7505
800-LUN-GUSA
Fax: 602-258-7507
e-mail: infophoenix@lungaz.org
www.lungarizona.org

Nancy Cohrs, Executive Director
Evelyn Frear, Office Manager

9220 **Southern Arizona Branch: Tucson Area**
2819 E Broadway
Tuscon, AZ 85716
520-323-1812
800-LUN-GUSA
Fax: 520-323-1816
e-mail: infotucson@lungaz.org
www.lungarizona.org

Keith Kaback, Chairman
Heidi Miller, Vice Chairman

Arkansas

9221 **American Lung Association of Arkansas**
1 Castle Rock Cove
Little Rock, AR 72212-1539
501-224-0773
Fax: 866-571-9608
e-mail: wdavenport@breathehealthy.org
www.lungusa2.org/arkansas/index.html

California

9222 **American Lung Association of California**
424 Pendleton Way
Oakland, CA 94621-2189
510-638-LUNG
800-LUN-GUSA
Fax: 510-638-8984
e-mail: contact@californialung.org
www.californialung.org

Trisha Murakawa, Chairman
Laura Keegan Boudreau, Acting CEO

Colorado

9223 **American Lung Association of Colorado**
5600 Greenwood Plaza Boulevard
Greenwood Village, CO 80111-2305
303-388-4327
800-LUN-GUSA
Fax: 303-377-1102
e-mail: cmichael@lungcolorado.org
www.lungcolorado.org

Curt Huber, Executive Director
Connor Michael, Communications Manager

Connecticut

9224 **American Lung Association of Connecticut**
45 Ash Street
E Hartford, CT 06108-3272
860-289-5401
800-992-2263
Fax: 860-289-5405
e-mail: alaofct@alact.org
www.alact.org

Margaret LaCroix, Vice President Communications

Delaware

9225 **American Lung Association of Delaware**
1021 Gilpin Avenue
Wilmington, DE 19806-3280
302-655-7258
Fax: 302-655-8546
www.aladc.org

Peter Shanley, Chairman

District of Columbia

9226 **American Lung Association of the District of Columbia**
530 7th Street SE
Washington, DC 20003-2617
202-682-5864
Fax: 202-682-5607
e-mail: info@aladc.org
www.aladc.org

Jan Morgan, Special Events Director
Phoebe Robinson, Administrative Coordinator

Florida

9227 **American Lung Association of Florida**
6852 Belfort Oaks Place
Jacksonville, FL 32216-5216
904-743-2933
800-940-2933
Fax: 904-743-2916
e-mail: alaf@lungfla.org
www.lungfla.org

Michael Diamond, President
Marilin K Glassberg, President-Elect

Georgia

9228 **American Lung Association of Georgia**
2452 Spring Road
Smyrna, GA 30080
770-434-5864
800-586-4872
Fax: 770-319-0349
e-mail: mail@alaga.org
www.alase.org

Charles J White, Chief Executive Officer
June Deen, VP Public Affairs

Hawaii

9229 **American Lung Association of Hawaii**
680 Iwilei Road
Honolulu, HI 96817
808-537-5966
Fax: 808-537-5971
e-mail: lung@ala-hawaii.org
www.ala-hawaii.org

Karen J Lee, President, Executive Director

Illinois

9230 **American Lung Association of Illinois-Iowa**
3000 Kelly Lane
Springfield, IL 62707
217-787-5864
800-586-4872
Fax: 217-787-5916
e-mail: info@lungil.org
www.lungil.org

Harold Wimmer, CEO
Lori Younker, Manager

Indiana

9231 **American Lung Association of Indiana: State Office & Support Office**
115 W Washington Street
Indianapolis, IN 46204
317-819-1181
800-LUN-GUSA
Fax: 317-819-1187
e-mail: info@lungin.org
www.lungin.org

Dana Pitts, VP Communications/Marketing

Kansas

9232 **American Lung Association of Kansas**
PO Box 8630
Topeka, KS 66618-2419
785-246-0377
Fax: 866-575-1761
e-mail: menisam@kylung.org
www.lungusa.org

Judy Keller, Executive Director

Kentucky

9233 **American Lung Association of Kentucky**
4100 Churchman Avenue
Louisville, KY 40209-0067
502-363-2652
800-LUN-GUSA
Fax: 502-363-0222
e-mail: info@kylung.org
www.kylung.org

Todd Adams, Development Director
Laura Collins, Executive Assistant

Louisiana

9234 **American Lung Association of Louisiana**
2325 Severn Avenue
Metairie, LA 70001-6918
504-828-5864
800-LUN-GUSA
Fax: 504-828-5867
e-mail: info@louisianalung.org
www.louisianalung.org

Aline Palmisano-Vita, Deputy Executive Director
Thomas P Lotz, Chief Executive Officer

Maine

9235 **American Lung Association of Maine**
122 State Street
Augusta, ME 04330
207-622-6394
800-LUN-GUSA
Fax: 639-426-2919
e-mail: info@lungme.org
www.mainelung.org

Lee Scott, President of Health Promotion
Edward Miller, Executive Director/SVP

Maryland

9236 **American Lung Association of Maryland**
11350 McCormick Road
Hunt Valley, MD 21031
410-560-2120
Fax: 410-560-0829
e-mail: info@marylandlung.org
www.marylandlung.org

Melina Davis-Martin, President and CEO
Krista Jennings, Chief Operations Officer

Massachusetts

9237 **American Lung Association of Massachusetts**
460 Totten Pond Road
Waltham, MA 02451
781-890-4262
Fax: 781-890-4280
e-mail: info@lungma.org
www.lungusa.org

Michigan

9238 **American Lung Association of Michigan**
25900 Greenfield Road
Oak Park, MI 48237
248-784-2000
800-543-5864
Fax: 248-784-2008
e-mail: alam@alam.org
www.alam.org

Colette Scholzen, President

Minnesota

9239 **American Lung Association of Minnesota**
490 Concordia Avenue
Saint Paul, MN 55103-2441
651-227-8014
800-LUN-GUSA
Fax: 651-227-5459
e-mail: info@alamn.org
www.alamn.org

Bill Westhoff, President

Mississippi

9240 **American Lung Association of Mississippi**
731 Pear Orchard Road
Ridgeland, MS 39158
601-206-5810
800-586-4872
Fax: 601-206-5813
www.alams.org

Greg Wynne, Chairman
Jennifer Cofer, Deputy Executive Director

Missouri

9241 **American Lung Association of Missouri**
1118 Hampton Avenue
Saint Louis, MO 63139
314-645-5505
Fax: 314-645-7128
e-mail: pickens@lungmo.org
www.lungusa2.org

Lori Pickens, Chief Executive Officer
Barry Freedman, VP Community Initiatives

Montana

9242 **American Lung Association of the Northern Rockies: Montana and Wyoming**
825 Helena Avenue
Helene, MT 59601-3459
406-442-6556
Fax: 406-442-2346
e-mail: ala-nr@ala-nr.org
www.lungusa.org

Nebraska

9243 **American Lung Association of Nebraska**
7101 Newport Avenue
Omaha, NE 68152
402-502-4950
Fax: 402-502-3012
e-mail: jegerton@breathehealthy.org
www.lungusa.org

Nevada

9244 **American Lung Association of Idaho/Nevada**
10615 Double R Boulevard
Reno, NV 89521-7056
775-829-LUNG
800-LUN-GUSA
Fax: 775-829-5850
e-mail: lmartin@lungnevada.org
www.lungnevada.org/Reno

Louise Martin, Executive Director
Gwen Bourne, Development Manager - Events

New Hampshire

9245 **American Lung Association of New Hampshire**
20 Warren Street
Concord, NH 03301
603-369-3977
Fax: 603-369-3978
e-mail: info@nhlung.org
www.lungne.org

Jeff Seyler, President & CEO
David Ales, Senior Vice President

New Jersey

9246 **American Lung Association of New Jersey**
1600 Route 22 E
Union, NJ 07083-3407
908-687-9340
800-LUN-GUSA
Fax: 908-851-2625
e-mail: info@lunginfo.org
www.alanewjersey.org

John A Rutkowski, President

New Mexico

9247 **New Mexico Branch**
7001 Menaul Boulevard NE
Albuquerque, NM 87110
505-265-0732
800-LUN-GUSA
Fax: 505-260-1739
e-mail: ronh@alanm.org
www.lungusa.org

New York

9248 **American Lung Association of Mid New York**
155 Washington Avenue
Albany, NY 12210
518-465-2013
Fax: 518-465-2926
e-mail: info@alany.org
www.alany.org

The mission of the American Lung Association and the American Lung Association of New York State is to prevent lung disease and promote lung health. The American Lung Association is the oldest voluntary health organization in the United States.
Deborah Carioto, President
Michael Seilback, Vice President Public Policy

North Carolina

9249 **American Lung Association of North Carolina**
3801 Lake Boone Trail
Raleigh, NC 27607
919-832-8326
800-892-5650
Fax: 919-856-8530
e-mail: dbryan@lungnc.org
www.lungnc.org
Deborah C. Bryan, President

9250 **American Lung Association of North Dakota**
8300 Health Park
Raleigh, NC 27615
919-832-8326
Fax: 919-856-8530
e-mail: dbryan@lungnc.org
www.lungnc.org
Deborah C Bryan, VP Advocacy & Donor Value
Mendi Nieters, Regional VP Development

North Dakota

9251 **American Lung Association of North Dakota**
212 N 2nd Street
Bismarck, ND 58502-5004
701-223-5613
800-252-6325
Fax: 701-223-5727
e-mail: amerlungnd@gcentral.com
www.lungusa2.org/northdakota
Judy Mourhess, Office Manager

Ohio

9252 **American Lung Association of Ohio**
1950 Arlingate Lane
Columbus, OH 43228
614-279-1700
800-LUN-GUSA
Fax: 614-279-4940
e-mail: alao@ohiolung.org
www.ohiolung.org
Tracy Ross, President / CEO

Oklahoma

9253 **American Lung Association of Oklahoma**
1010 E 8th Street
Tulsa, OK 74120
918-747-3441
Fax: 918-747-4629
www.oklung.org
Sara Dreiling, Chief Executive Officer
Edward C Rosentel, Chief Financial and Operating Officer

Oregon

9254 **American Lung Association of Oregon**
7420 SW Bridgeport Road
Tigard, OR 97224
503-924-4094
Fax: 503-924-4120
e-mail: info@lungoregon.org
www.lungoregon.org
Jan Jensen, President
Dana Kaye, Executive Director

Pennsylvania

9255 **American Lung Association of Pennsylvania**
3001 Old Gettysburg Road
Camp Hill, PA 17011
717-541-5864
800-LUN-GUSA
Fax: 717-541-8828
e-mail: info@lunginfo.org
www.lunginfo.org

South Carolina

9256 **American Lung Association of South Carolina**
1817 Gadsen Street
Columbia, SC 29201-2392
803-779-5864
800-849-5864
Fax: 803-254-2711
e-mail: alasc@lungsc.org
www.lungsc.org

9257 **American Lung Association of South Dakota**
1817 Gadsen Street
Columbia, SC 29201
803-779-5864
Fax: 803-254-2711
e-mail: shelps@alasc.org
www.alasc.org
Amanda Strickland, Regional Manager Special Events
Sharon Helps, Regional Manager Programs

South Dakota

9258 **American Lung Association of South Dakota**
108 E 38th Street
Sioux Falls, SD 57105
605-336-7222
800-873-5864
Fax: 605-336-7227
e-mail: lung@americanlungsd.org
www.lungusa2.org/southdakota

Tennessee

9259 **American Lung Association of Tennesse**
One Vantage Way
Nashville, TN 37228
615-329-1151
800-LUN-GUSA
Fax: 615-329-1723
e-mail: alastaff@alatn.org
www.alatn.org

Texas

9260 **American Lung Association of Texas**
5926 Balcones Drive
Austin, TX 78731-0460
512-467-6753
800-252-5864
Fax: 512-467-7621
e-mail: info@texaslung.org
www.texaslung.org
Phillip J Hanson, Senior VP Resource Development
Margaret Crump, Senior VP Community Initiatives

Utah

9261 **American Lung Association of Utah**
1930 S 1100 E
Salt Lake City, UT 84106-2317
801-484-4456
Fax: 801-484-5461
e-mail: info@utahlung.org
www.lungusa2.org/utah

Vermont

9262 **American Lung Association of Vermont**
372 Hurricane Lane
Williston, VT 05495-6196
802-876-6500
Fax: 802-876-6505
e-mail: info@vtlung.org
www.lungne.org
Erin Hickey, Senior Manager Development
Margaret LaCroix, VP Marketing\Communications

Virginia

9263 **American Lung Association of Virginia**
9221 Forest Hill Avenue
Richmond, VA 23235
804-267-1900
Fax: 804-267-5634
e-mail: mdavismartin@lungva.org
www.lungva.org
Melina Davis-Martin, President and CEO
Krista Jennings, Chief Operating Officer

Washington

9264 **American Lung Association of Washington**
2625 Third Avenue 206-441-5100
Seattle, WA 98121 800-732-9339
Fax: 206-441-3277
e-mail: alaw@alaw.org
www.alaw.org
Vivian Echavarria, Chair
Rick Weems, Secretary

West Virginia

9265 **American Lung Association of West Virginia**
415 Dickinson Street 304-342-6600
Charleston, WV 25301-3980 Fax: 304-342-6096
e-mail: cfields@lunginfo.org
www.lungusa.org
Sara Crickenberger, Executive Director

Wisconsin

9266 **American Lung Association of Wisconsin**
13100 W Lisbon Road 262-703-4200
Brookfield, WI 53005-2508 800-586-4872
Fax: 262-781-5180
e-mail: amlung@lungwi.org
www.lungwi.org
Susan Gloede Swan, Executive Director
Dona Wininsky, Director of Public Policy

Research Centers

9267 **University of Illinois at Chicago Lions**
833 S Wood Street 312-355-1715
Chicago, IL 60612 Fax: 312-355-2693
www.uic.edu/pharmacy/research/itr
The Institute for Tuberculosis Research is comprised of approximately 30 individuals: biologists chemists pharmacologists and support staff -ÿ all working towards a single goal - the discovery of new drugs for tuberculosis.
Scott Franzblau, Director
Lorna Haubrich, ITR General Information

9268 **University of Illinois at Chicago: Institute for Tuberculosis Research**
833 S. Wood Street 312-355-1715
Chicago, IL 60612-7631 Fax: 312-355-2693
www.uic.edu/pharmacy/research/itr
Scott Franzblau, Director

Support Groups & Hotlines

9269 **National Health Information Center**
PO Box 1133 310-565-4167
Washington, DC 20013 800-336-4797
Fax: 301-984-4256
e-mail: info@nhic.org
www.health.gov/nhic
Offers a nationwide information referral service, produces directories and resource guides.

Pamphlets

9270 **Classification of Tuberculosis and Other Mycobacterial Diseases**
American Lung Association
1740 Broadway 212-315-8700
New York, NY 10019-4315
Chart listing different classes of tuberculosis and other mycobacterial diseases.

9271 **Facts About Tuberculosis**
American Lung Association
1740 Broadway 212-315-8700
New York, NY 10019-4315
Primary public information leaflet on TB as well as on its impact and treatment.
8 pages

9272 **TB Skin Test**
American Lung Association
1740 Broadway 212-315-8700
New York, NY 10019-4315
Primary public information leaflet on the TB skin test.
8 pages

9273 **TB: What You Should Know**
American Lung Association of Connecticut
45 Ash Street 860-289-5401
East Hartford, CT 06108-3294 800-586-4872
Fax: 860-289-5405
www.alact.org
Offers a brief overview of tuberculosis, how transmission is possible, and TB skin testing.
John E Zinn, President/CEO

9274 **This is Mr. TB Germ**
American Lung Association
1740 Broadway 212-315-8700
New York, NY 10019-4315
Lively booklet of drawings and very brief text giving a basic description of TB and its treatments.
20 pages

Web Sites

9275 **American Lung Association**
www.americanlungusa.org
Offers research, medical updates, fund-raising, educational materials and public awareness campaigns relating to lung disease and related disorders.

9276 **Healing Well**
www.healingwell.org
An online health resource guide to medical news, chat, information and articles, newsgroups and message boards, books, disease-related web sites, medical directories, and more for patients, friends, and family coping with disabling diseases, disorders, or chronic illnesses.

9277 **Health Finder**
www.healthfinder.gov
Searchable, carefully developed web site offering information on over 1000 topics. Developed by the US Department of Health and Human Services, the site can be used in both English and Spanish.

9278 **Healthlink USA**
www.healthlinkusa.com
Health information concerning treatment, cures, prevention, diagnosis, risk factors, research, support groups, email lists, personal stories and much more. Updated regularly.

9279 **Helios Health**
www.helioshealth.com
Online resource for your health information. Detailed information about specific health topics, access to expert advice from our Medical Advisory Board, and up-to-date health news.

9280 **MedicineNet**
www.medicinenet.com
An online resource for consumers providing easy-to-read, authoritative medical and health information.

9281 **Medscape**
www.mywebmd.com
Medscape offers specialists, primary care physicians, and other health professionals the Web's most robust and integrated medical information and educational tools.

9282 **National Institute of Allergy & Inf. Dis.**
www.niaid.nih.gov
NAID is composed of four extramural divisions: the Division of AIDS; the Division of Allergy, Immunology and Transplantation; the Division of Microbology and Infectious Diseases; and the Division of Extramural Activities. In addition, NIAID scientists con-

duct intramural research in laboratories located in Bethesda, Rockville and Frederick, Maryland, and in Hamilton, Montana.

9283 **WebMD**

www.webmd.com

Information on Tuberculosis, including articles and resources.

Description

9284 **Tuberous Sclerosis**

Tuberous sclerosis is a genetic disorder that causes benign, (non-cancerous) tumors to form in different locations - primarily in the brain, skin, kidneys, heart, lungs and even eyes. The name is derived from tuber-like growths on the brain that become hard. It usually shows itself in infancy or early childhood, and may cause seizures and/or mental retardation. It is inherited through chromosome 9 or 16. Disease severity is highly variable, even within the same family. Those with tuberous sclerosis can have mental retardation as well as seizures.

There are various skin abnormalities that may provide a clue to the diagnosis when an infant or young child exhibits seizures or delayed development. The first is an area of decreased skin pigmentation, called an ash-leaf spot because of its shape. Multiple ash-leaf spots may appear on the trunk and limbs during infancy. At age 3 or 4, tiny red bumps, adenoma sebaceum, resembling acne may appear on the nose and cheeks. Finally, a roughened spot with the consistency of orange peel, shagren patch, may appear over the lower spine.

There is no cure so treatment is based on symptoms and can include anti-epileptic drugs for seizures, removal of skin lesions, treatment of high blood pressure caused by kidney problems, special education and, in some instances, surgery to remove growing tumors.

National Agencies & Associations

9285 **National Tuberous Sclerosis Association**
801 Roeder Road
Sliver Spring, MD 20910
301-562-9890
800-225-6872
Fax: 301-562-9870
e-mail: info@tsalliance.org
www.ntsa.org

A voluntary nonprofit organization that is dedicated to fostering and supporting tuberous sclerosis research; to provide education of the public educators and health care professionals; and to providing support of individuals with tuberous sclerosis.
Kari Luther Carlson, President & Chief Executive Officer
Gail Alexander, Senior Manager of Operations

Support Groups & Hotlines

9286 **National Health Information Center**
PO Box 1133
Washington, DC 20013
310-565-4167
800-336-4797
Fax: 301-984-4256
e-mail: info@nhic.org
www.health.gov/nhic

Offers a nationwide information referral service, produces directories and resource guides.

Books

9287 **Tuberous Sclerosis**
Oxford University Press
2001 Evans Road
Cary, NC 27513
800-451-7556
Fax: 919-677-1303
www.oup-usa.org

A revision offering up-to-date medical information to families, researchers, and professionals on TS.

ISBN: 0-195122-10-0

Newsletters

9288 **NTSA Perspective**
National Tuberous Sclerosis Association
8181 Professional Place
Landover, MD 20785-2226
301-459-9888
800-225-6872
Fax: 301-459-0394
e-mail: ntsa@ntsa.org
www.ntsa.org

Offers the latest research and medical information on tuberous sclerosis to physicians and health care professionals.
Quarterly

Web Sites

9289 **Healing Well**
www.healingwell.com

An online health resource guide to medical news, chat, information and articles, newsgroups and message boards, books, disease-related web sites, medical directories, and more for patients, friends, and family coping with disabling diseases, disorders, or chronic illnesses.

9290 **Health Finder**
www.healthfinder.gov

Searchable, carefully developed web site offering information on over 1000 topics. Developed by the US Department of Health and Human Services, the site can be used in both English and Spanish.

9291 **Healthlink USA**
www.healthlinkusa.com

Health information concerning treatment, cures, prevention, diagnosis, risk factors, research, support groups, email lists, personal stories and much more. Updated regularly.

9292 **Helios Health**
www.helioshealth.com

Online resource for your health information. Detailed information about specific health topics, access to expert advice from our Medical Advisory Board, and up-to-date health news.

9293 **MedicineNet**
www.medicinenet.com

An online resource for consumers providing easy-to-read, authoritative medical and health information.

9294 **Medscape**
www.mywebmd.com

Medscape offers specialists, primary care physicians, and other health professionals the Web's most robust and integrated medical information and educational tools.

9295 **National Tuberous Sclerosis Association**
www.ntsa.org

NTSA provides information to individuals and families through its family support network, quarterly newsletters, brochures and other printed materials.

9296 **WebMD**
www.webmd.com

Information on Tuberous Sclerosis, including articles and resources.

Description

9297 **Turner Syndrome**

Turner syndrome is a genetic disorder that occurs in 1 in 2,500 to 10,000 live female births. It only affects females because, rather than having two female sex (X) chromosomes, Turner syndrome patients have only one. The disease usually hinders sexual development and produces small stature and varying degrees of mental retardation. There may be associated anomalies such as webbed neck and defects of the heart or aorta, which may occur in up to 25 percent of individuals.

Turner syndrome cannot be cured, but hormonal treatment may give the patient a more normal life. Growth hormone injections can help the patient reach a taller adult height, and estrogen replacement can encourage breast development and other sex characteristics. A few patients will develop menstrual periods spontaneously, and a few have become pregnant; most, however, are infertile. Psychological support for the patient and her family is important.

National Agencies & Associations

9298 **Human Growth Foundation: Turner Syndrome Division**
997 Glen Cove Avenue
Glen Head, NY 11545-1554
800-451-6434
Fax: 516-671-4055
e-mail: hgf1@hgfound.org
www.hgfound.org

A nonprofit, national organization committed to expanding and accelerating research into growth and growth disorders, provides education and support to those affected by growth disorders and their families and fosters the exchange of information.
Frank Diamond, President
Emily Germain-Lee, Vice President

9299 **MAGIC Foundation for Children's Growth: Turner's Syndrome Division**
6645 W N Avenue
Oak Park, IL 60302-1376
708-383-0808
800-362-4423
Fax: 708-383-0899
e-mail: dianne@magicfoundation.org
www.magicfoundation.org

A national nonprofit organization created to provide support services for the families of children afflicted with a wide variety of chronic and/or critical disorders that affect a child's growth.
James Andrews, Director/Co- Founder
Mary Andrews, CEO

9300 **Turner's Syndrome Society of Canada**
323 Chapel Street
Ottawa, K1N
613-321-2267
800-465-6744
Fax: 613-321-2268
e-mail: tssincan@web.net
www.turnersyndrome.ca

International society providing support services, educational information and activities to persons with Turner's Syndrome, their families and the professionals who work with them.

9301 **Turner's Syndrome Society of the United States**
10960 Millridge N Drive
Houston, TX 77070
832-249-9988
800-365-9944
Fax: 832-912-6446
e-mail: tssus@turner-syndrome-us.org
www.turnersyndrome.org

Through this society members have available a host of informational and support services including consultation services a resource center offering access to the most recently published articles on Turner's Syndrome conferences and advocacy.
Catherine Ward, President
Melissa Carlucci, Medical Advisor

State Agencies & Associations

California

9302 **Bay Area Turner Syndrome Society**
Moraga, CA 94556
925-846-0608
e-mail: jenakiko@aol.com
www.turnersyndrome.org
Jennifer Saito, Contact

9303 **Turner's Syndrome Society**
10960 Millridge N Drive
Houston, TX 77070
832-912-6006
800-365-9944
Fax: 832-912-6446
e-mail: tssus@turnersyndrome.org
www.turnersyndrome.org
Catherine Ward, President
Deanna Swanson, Secretary

Colorado

9304 **Turner's Syndrome Society of Rocky Mountain**
Longmount, CO 80501
303-774-0720
e-mail: bpblick@earthlink.net
www.turnersyndrome.org
Brian Blick, President

Florida

9305 **Florida Southwest Turner Syndrome Society**
Orlando, FL 33919
407-859-3131
e-mail: cjubelt@affirmativemanagement.com
www.turnersyndrome.org
Lauren Jubelt, Leader

9306 **Turner's Syndrome Society of South Florida**
5215 N Dixie Highway
Oakland Park, FL 33334
945-815-9100
e-mail: tigger3927@aol.com
www.turnersyndrome.org
Rachel Nowak, Leader

Georgia

9307 **Georgia Atlanta Turner Syndrome Society**
10635 Jones Bridge Road
Alpharetta, GA 30022
770-918-3120
e-mail: jbrownlee@rockdale.org
www.turnersyndrome.org
Judy Brownlee, Contact

Illinois

9308 **Metro Chicago Turner Syndrome Society**
5467 S Ingleside #3E
Chicago, IL 60615
773-667-1364
e-mail: sgfhoff@sbcglobal.net
www.turnersyndrome.org
Susan Hoffman, President

9309 **St. Louis Turner Syndrome Society**
14450 TC Jester
Houston, TX 77014
832-689-3901
800-365-9944
Fax: 832-249-9987
e-mail: heatherandben@earthlink.net
www.turnersyndrome.org

Turner Syndrome is a chromosomal condition that describes girls and women with common features that are caused by complete or partial absence of the second sex chromosome.
Heather Derousse, Contact

Indiana

9310 Indiana Chapter Turner Syndrome Society
2030 S Odell Street
Brownsburg, IN 46112
317-858-9398
e-mail: candjgarland@yahoo.com
www.turnersyndrome.org
Connie Garland, Contact

Iowa

9311 Turner's Syndrome Society of Iowa
2615 Meadow Glen Road
Ames, IA 50014-8238
515-292-2757
e-mail: mkepolashek@msn.com
www.turnersyndrome.org
Mary Kay Polashek, Leader

Louisiana

9312 Southeast Louisiana Turner Syndrome Society
14450 TC Jester
Houston, TX 77014
832-249-9988
Fax: 832-249-9987
e-mail: cajungirl302003@yahoo.com
www.turnersyndrome.org
The Turner Syndrome Society of the United States creates awareness promotes research and provides support for all persons touched by Turner Syndrome.
Delaine Reed, Contact

Massachusetts

9313 Southern New England Turner Syndrome Society
1034 Maple Street
Mansfield, MA 02048
401-732-2136
e-mail: deb_pomerantz@hotmail.com
www.turnersyndrome.org
Deborah Pomerantz, Leader

Michigan

9314 Michigan Chapter: Southeast
146 Meadow Lane Circle
Rochester Hills, MI 48307
248-608-6127
e-mail: ksemrau@aol.com
www.turnersyndrome.org
Kim Semrau, President

9315 Michigan West Turner Syndrome Society
PO Box 307
Nashville, MI 49073
517-852-9593
e-mail: r-m-ohler4@triton.net
www.turnersyndrome.org
Mary Ohler, Contact

Minnesota

9316 Turner's Syndrome Society of Minnesota
3732 Tonkawood Road
Minnetonkaie, MN 55345
612-869-0394
e-mail: jleon101@hotmail.com
www.turnersyndrome.org
Julie Leon, Contact

Missouri

9317 Kansas/Missouri- Turner Syndrome Society
Chapter Headquarters
6721 E 127th Street
Grandview, MO 64030
816-763-9550
Fax: 816-763-8884
e-mail: tsskc@hotmail.com
www.tsskc.com
Dennis McKenzie, Co-President
Carolyn McKenzie, Vice-President

9318 Missouri/St. Louis Turner Syndrome Society
8831 Madge
Brentwood, MO 63144
314-963-0565
e-mail: loch5@juno.com
www.turnersyndrome.org
Mary Jo Lochmoeller, Co-President

9319 Turner's Syndrome Society of St. Louis/West Illinois
8831 Madge
Brentwood, MO 63144
314-963-0565
e-mail: loch5@juno.com
www.turner-syndrome-us.org
Mary Jo Lochmoeller, President

New Hampshire

9320 Northern New England Turner Society
38 Beaman Street
Laconia, NH 03246
603-524-6011
e-mail: tssnnepa@hotmail.com
www.turnersyndrome.org
Lori Ann Pawlowski, Leader

New Jersey

9321 New Jersey Metroplitan Turner Syndrome Society Association
107 Crabapple Lane
Franklin Park, NJ 08823
732-217-3021
e-mail: tssusnj@turnersyndromenj.com
www.turnersyndrome.org
Laura Fasciano, Contact

New York

9322 Turner Syndrome Support Group of Central N Y
476 Ford Hill Road
Berkshire, NY 13736
607-223-4142
e-mail: tlkwwjd@frontiernet.net
www.turnersyndrome.org
Tammy Kozak, President

9323 Turner's Syndrome Society New York - Metro
215 E 95th Street #24M
New York, NY 10128
607-223-4142
e-mail: tlkwwjd@frontiernet.net
www.turnersyndrome.org
Tammy Kozak, Contact

North Carolina

9324 North Carolina Turner Syndrome Society
1223 Pine Springs Drive
Hendersonville, NC 28739
828-699-1088
e-mail: inmydna@charter.net
www.turnersyndrome.org
Cheryl Tuttle, Contact

Ohio

9325 Turner Syndrome Chapter of Ohio
3333 Burnet Avenue ML 5006
Cincinnati, OH 45229
513-697-0941
e-mail: lwestcott@fuse.net
www.turnersyndrome.org
Leslie Westcott, Contact

9326 Turner Syndrome Chapter of Oklahoma
5904 E Lattimer
Tulsa, OK 74115-6728
918-838-7355
www.turnersyndrome.org
Jean Radtke, Contact

Pennsylvania

9327 Philadelphia Turner Syndrom Society
169 Trappe Lane
Langhorne, PA 19047
215-752-4405
e-mail: wolfepac5@comcast.net
www.turnersyndrome.org
This society covers the 5 surrounding counties of Philadelphia, along with Eastern Pennsylvania, Delaware and Southern New Jersey.
Eileen Wolfe, President

9328 SW Pennsylvania Turner Syndrome Support Gr oup
3110 Westchester
Pittsburgh, PA 15238
412-767-4321
e-mail: fay_larkin@pghcorning.com
www.turnersyndrome.org
Fay Larkin, Contact

Rhode Island

9329 Rhode Island Turner Syndrome Society
24 Turner Street
Warwick, RI 02886
401-732-2136
e-mail: deb_pomerantz@hotmail.com
www.turnersyndrome.org
Debbie Pomerantz, Contact

South Carolina

9330 **South Carolina Palmetto Turner Syndrome So ciety**
153 Gannet Point Road
Beaufort, SC 29902
843-521-4461
e-mail: auntrobin74@yahoo.com
www.turnersyndrome.org
Robin Butler, Contact

9331 **Turner's Syndrome Society: Palmetto Area**
Drachman Hall 1295 N Martin
Tucson, AZ 85721
843-521-4461
888-285-3410
e-mail: auntrobin74@yahoo.com
www.turnersyndrome.org
Teratology Information Services are comprehensive and multidisciplinary resources for medical consultation on prenatal exposures. TIS interpret information regarding known and potential reproductive risks into risk assessments.
Robin Butler, Leader

Texas

9332 **Houston/South Texas Turner Syndrome Society**
Houston, TX
832-689-3901
e-mail: heatherandben@earthlink.net
www.turnersyndrome.org
Heather Derousse, Contact

9333 **Turner's Syndrome Society of North Texas**
5633 Cork Lane
N Richland Hills, TX 76180
817-485-1684
e-mail: bright165@cs.com
www.turnersyndrome.org
Hollye Bright, Leader

Utah

9334 **Utah Turner Syndrome Society**
American Fork, UT 84003
801-754-1792
e-mail: abclaker@aol.com
www.turnersyndrome.org
Angela Dawn Laker, Contact

Washington

9335 **Washington Puget Sound Turner Syndrome Society**
12321 22nd Street NE
Seattle, WA 98125
206-417-6776
e-mail: pugetsoundtss@gmail.com
www.turnersyndrome.org
Larin Amos, President

Libraries & Resource Centers

9336 **Turner Syndrome Society Resource Center**
Turner Syndrome Society of the United States
14450 TC Jester
Houston, TX 77014
832-249-9988
800-365-9944
Fax: 832-249-9987
e-mail: tssus@tuRNersyndromeus.org
www.turnersyndrome.org
The Turner Syndrome Society of the US creates awareness, promotes research, and provides support for all persons touched by Turner Syndrome.
Barbara Flink, President
Dr Catherine Ward, President Elect

Support Groups & Hotlines

9337 **National Health Information Center**
PO Box 1133
Washington, DC 20013
310-565-4167
800-336-4797
Fax: 301-984-4256
e-mail: info@nhic.org
www.health.gov/nhic
Offers a nationwide information referral service, produces directories and resource guides.

Newsletters

9338 **Turner's Syndrome News**
Turner's Syndrome Society of the United States
1313 5th Street SE
Minneapolis, MN 55414-4509
800-365-9944
Fax: 612-379-3619
www.turner-syndrome-us.org
Includes articles addressing current issues in Turner's Syndrome, updates on national and local activities and letters from girls and women with Turner's syndrome and their families.
Quarterly

Pamphlets

9339 **Answers to Some Commonly Asked Questions**
Turner's Syndrome Society of the United States
1313 5th Street SE
Minneapolis, MN 55414-4509
800-365-9944
Fax: 612-379-3619
www.turner-syndrome-us.org
Offers information on the Society's activities and the role they play in supporting people with Turner's syndrome.

9340 **Facing the Challenges of Turner's Syndrome Together**
Turner's Syndrome Society of the United States
1313 5th Street SE
Minneapolis, MN 55414-4509
800-365-9944
Fax: 612-379-3619
www.turner-syndrome-us.org
A brochure offering information on Turner's syndrome, statistics on how widespread the disease is and the Society's role in conquering this disease and supporting their members.

9341 **Facts About Turner's Syndrome**
Turner's Syndrome Society of the United States
1313 5th Street SE
Minneapolis, MN 55414-4509
800-365-9944
Fax: 612-379-3619
www.turner-syndrome-us.org
Offers statistical and factual information on the disease of Turner's syndrome, causes, symptoms, prevention and treatment.

9342 **How to Start a Turner's Syndrome Support Group**
Turner's Syndrome Society of the United States
1313 5th Street SE
Minneapolis, MN 55414-4509
800-365-9944
Fax: 612-379-3619
www.turner-syndrome-us.org
Offers information to the lay person on how to obtain material from medical professionals, publicity aspects and funding aspects in pertaining to starting a support group.

9343 **Turner's Syndrome Society Resource Bibliographies**
Turner's Syndrome Society of the United States
1313 5th Street SE
Minneapolis, MN 55414-4509
800-365-9944
Fax: 612-379-3619
www.turner-syndrome-us.org
These fact sheets offer information on books, videos and other resources available on Turner's syndrome.

9344 **Turner's Syndrome: A Guide for Families**
Turner's Syndrome Society of the United States
1313 5th Street SE
Minneapolis, MN 55414-4509
800-365-9944
Fax: 612-379-3619
www.turner-syndrome-us.org
Offers information to parents on the causes, symptoms, diagnosis and prognosis of Turner' syndrome, includes resources of where to go for help and support.

9345 **Turner's Syndrome: A Personal Perspective**
Turner's Syndrome Society of the United States
1313 5th Street SE
Minneapolis, MN 55414-4509
800-365-9944
Fax: 612-379-3619
www.turner-syndrome-us.org

A reprint from the Adolescent and Pediatric Gynecology Journal offering a personal account of a woman with Turner's syndrome and her experiences.

9346 Turner's Syndrome: Hows and Whys of the Missing X Chromosome
Human Growth Foundation
977 Glen Cove Avenue 516-671-4041
Glen Head, NY 11545-1554 800-451-6434
Fax: 516-671-4055
e-mail: hgf1@hgfound.org
www.hgfound.org
Provides a brief overview for parents about Turner's Syndrome.
Patricia D Costa, Executive Director

Web Sites

9347 Healing Well
www.healingwell.com
An online health resource guide to medical news, chat, information and articles, newsgroups and message boards, books, disease-related web sites, medical directories, and more for patients, friends, and family coping with disabling diseases, disorders, or chronic illnesses.

9348 Health Finder
www.healthfinder.gov
Searchable, carefully developed web site offering information on over 1000 topics. Developed by the US Department of Health and Human Services, the site can be used in both English and Spanish.

9349 Healthlink USA
www.healthlinkusa.com
Health information concerning treatment, cures, prevention, diagnosis, risk factors, research, support groups, email lists, personal stories and much more. Updated regularly.

9350 Helios Health
www.helioshealth.com
Online resource for your health information. Detailed information about specific health topics, access to expert advice from our Medical Advisory Board, and up-to-date health news.

9351 Human Growth Foundation
www.genetic.org
National organization committed to expanding and accelerating research into growth and growth disorders, provides education and support to those affected by growth disorders and their families, and fosters the exchange of information with the medical community.

9352 MAGIC Foundation for Children's Growth: Turner's Syndrome Division
www.magicfoundation.org
National organization created to provide support services for the families of children afflicted with a wide variety of chronic and/or critical disorders that affect a child's growth.

9353 MedicineNet
www.medicinenet.com
An online resource for consumers providing easy-to-read, authoritative medical and health information.

9354 Medscape
www.mywebmd.com
Medscape offers specialists, primary care physicians, and other health professionals the Web's most robust and integrated medical information and educational tools.

9355 Turner's Syndrome Society of the United States
www.turner-syndrome-us.org
Through this society, members have available a host of informational and support services including consultation services, a resource center offering access to the most recently published articles on Turner's syndrome, conferences, advocacy, information and referral services and public relations activities.

9356 WebMD
www.webmd.com
Information on Turner's syndrome, including articles and resources.

Description

9357 **Ulcerative Colitis**

Ulcerative colitis is an inflammatory condition of the large bowel, or colon. The cause is unknown, but there is a strong genetic association. First degree relatives have a 3 to 9 percent lifetime risk of the disease, and the illness is much more common in certain racial groups.

Inflammation of the wall of the bowel leads to ulcerations of its surface. Symptoms include weight loss, fatigue, abdominal pain, and diarrhea, which may be bloody. Ulcerative colitis in patients who have a specific antibody in their system (HLA-B27) has a strong association with an arthritis called ankylosing spondylitis. Several kinds of liver and biliary tract disease, inflammation of the eye, and certain characteristic skin rashes may occur.

Treatment depends on the severity of symptoms. Mild cases may respond to simple anti-diarrheal medicines. More severe cases are treated with either rectal or oral forms of 5-ASA, marketed under several trade names. Corticosteroids are sometimes necessary. Disease confined to the rectum can generally be managed with steroid enemas. Extensive disease requires oral steroid medication. Immunosuppressive drugs like azathioprine and 6-mercaptopurine are sometimes given if the disease is resistant to steroids or if steroid side effects are unacceptable. Twenty percent of patients will eventually have their entire colon removed, which cures the disease.

After many years of active ulcerative there is an increased risk of colon cancer. It is usually preceded by warning signs visible on colonoscopy, so physicians generally begin an aggressive surveillance program after 8 to 10 years of disease.

National Agencies & Associations

9358 **American Gastroenterological Association**
4930 Del Ray Avenue 301-654-2055
Bethesda, MD 20814 Fax: 301-654-5920
e-mail: member@gastro.org
www.gastro.org
Dedicated to the mission of advancing the science and practice of gastroenterology. As the oldest specialty medical society in the United States the membership includes physicians and scientists who research diagnose and treat disorders.
Robert B Greenberg JD, Executive Vice President
Michael H Stolar PhD, Senior VP

9359 **Crohn's & Colitis Foundation of America**
386 Park Avenue S 212-685-3440
New York, NY 10016-8804 800-932-2423
Fax: 212-779-4098
e-mail: info@ccfa.org
www.ccfa.org
Supports basic and clinical research into a cure and prevent Crohn's disease and ulcerative colitis; conducts professional and patient education activities; produces public service programs and a wide variety of literature about inflammatory bowel disease.
Richard S Blumberg MD, Chairperson

9360 **National Institute of Diabetes and Digestive Disorders**
5 Information Way
31 Center Drive MSC 2560 301-496-3583
Bethesda, MD 20892-3568 800-860-8747
www2.niddk.nih.gov
Offers information and referrals to persons afflicted with ulcerative colitis.
Dora Abankwah, Staff
Adil Abdalla, Staff

9361 **Reach Out for Youth with Ileitis and Colitis**
84 Northgate Circle 631-293-3102
Melville, NY 11747 e-mail: info@reachourforyouth.org
www.reachoutforyouth.org
Provides educational seminars and individual and group support to patients and their families. Fundraising efforts support the Center's programs clinical and laboratory research and purchase of state-of-the-art equipment.
Irwin Maltz, President

9362 **United Ostomy Association**
PO Box 66 949-660-8624
Fairview, TN 37062 800-826-0826
Fax: 949-660-9262
e-mail: info@uoaa.org
www.uoa.org
Volunteer based health organization dedicated to providing education information support and advocacy for those who have or will have an intestinal or urinary diversion. We provide patient visiting services, 800 number referral and information services.
Ken Aukett, President
Kristin Knipp, President-Elect

Support Groups & Hotlines

9363 **National Health Information Center**
PO Box 1133 310-565-4167
Washington, DC 20013 800-336-4797
Fax: 301-984-4256
e-mail: info@nhic.org
www.health.gov/nhic
Offers a nationwide information referral service, produces directories and resource guides.

Books

9364 **Alive and Kicking**
Rolf Benirschke Enterprises
PO Box 9922
Rancho Santa Fe, CA 92067-4922 800-571-4770
Football star writes of his struggle with ulcerative colitis.

9365 **Ask Audrey**
7466 Pebble Lane 248-626-6960
West Bloomfield, MI 48322-3521
A compilation of material and the personal story of a medical psychotherapist who has inflammatory bowel disease. Includes practical tips on issues such as handling diarrhea, sexuality, relationships, traveling, coping with hospital stays, ostomies, and TPN.

9366 **IBD Nutrition Book**
John Wiley & Sons
1 Wiley Drive
Somerset, NJ 08873-1222 800-225-5945
Clinical dietitian/nutritionist's overview of the role of diet in IBD, including recipes and meal plans.

9367 **Inflammatory Bowel Disease**
Williams & Wilkins
351 W Camden Street 301-528-4000
Baltimore, MD 21201-7912 800-638-0672
Detailed information on every aspect of IBD. Topics include medical and surgical management, epidemiology, fertility and pregnancy, psychosocial factors, and diagnostic techniques. Written for medical professionals and laypersons who are comfortable with medical terminology.

9368 Treating IBD: A Patient's Guide to the Medical and Surgical Management
Crohn's and Colitis Foundation of America
386 Park Avenue S
New York, NY 10016-8804
212-685-3440
800-932-2423
Fax: 212-779-4098
e-mail: info@ccfa.org
www.ccfa.org

Children's Books

9369 You're Bigger Than it
Hotel Dieu Hospital
Ontario, Canada,
613-544-3310
This cartoon book offers a lively, brief introduction to the basics of living with IBD. Contact can be reached at extension 2400.

Newsletters

9370 Inner Circle
Reach Out for Youth with Ileitis and Colitis
84 Northgate Circle
Melville, NY 11747
631-293-3102
e-mail: reachoutforyouth@reachoutforyouth.org
www.reachoutforyouth.org
Newsletter for youth with ileitis and colitis.
Irwin Maltz, President

Pamphlets

9371 Bleeding in the Digestive Tract
Nat'l Digestive Diseases Information Clearinghouse
9000 Rockville Pike
Bethesda, MD 20892-0001
301-496-3583
Informational fact sheet.

9372 Inside Story
Reach Out for Youth with Ileitis and Colitis
84 Northgate Circle
Melville, NY 11747
631-293-2102
e-mail: reachoutforyouth@reachoutforyouth.org
www.reachoutforyouth.org
Educational brochure for youth with illeitis and colitis.
Irwin Maltz, President

9373 Ulcerative Colitis
National Organization For Rare Disorders
PO Box 8923
New Fairfield, CT 06812-8923
203-746-6518
e-mail: orphan@rarediseases.org
www.rarediseases.org
Informational fact sheet.

Web Sites

9374 Crohn's & Colitis Foundation of America
www.ccfa.org
Supports basic and clinical research into a cure and prevent Crohn's disease and ulcerative colitis; conducts professional and patient education activities; produces public service programs and a wide variety of literature about inflammatory bowel disease for patients and their families, professionals and the public; and sponsors chapters nationwide.

9375 Healing Well
www.healingwell.com
An online health resource guide to medical news, chat, information and articles, newsgroups and message boards, books, disease-related web sites, medical directories, and more for patients, friends, and family coping with disabling diseases, disorders, or chronic illnesses.

9376 Health Finder
www.healthfinder.gov
Searchable, carefully developed web site offering information on over 1000 topics. Developed by the US Department of Health and Human Services, the site can be used in both English and Spanish.

9377 Healthlink USA
www.healthlinkusa.com
Health information concerning treatment, cures, prevention, diagnosis, risk factors, research, support groups, email lists, personal stories and much more. Updated regularly.

9378 Helios Health
www.helioshealth.com
Online resource for your health information. Detailed information about specific health topics, access to expert advice from our Medical Advisory Board, and up-to-date health news.

9379 MedicineNet
www.medicinenet.com
An online resource for consumers providing easy-to-read, authoritative medical and health information.

9380 Medscape
www.mywebmd.com
Medscape offers specialists, primary care physicians, and other health professionals the Web's most robust and integrated medical information and educational tools.

9381 United Ostomy Association
www.uoa.org
Extensive information about ostomy surgery, support, products and advocacy for Medicaid/Insurance reimbursement. Interactive discussion board to post and answer questions, weekly updates on ostomy-related news items.

9382 WebMD
www.webmd.com
Information on Ulcerative Colitis, including articles and resources.

Description

9383 Visual Impairment

Visual impairment encompasses a wide variety of disorders of the eye. It includes damage to the cornea or retina (macular degeneration or secondary to diabetes), cataracts, glaucoma, muscular imbalance, infections, congenital disorders and those associated with premature birth. Occasionally visual impairment reflects a disease behind the eye, involving some part of the brain that receives and processes images from the eyes.

Visual impairment covers a continuum from decreased visual acuity correctible by refractive means (glasses and contact lenses) to legal blindness, indicating less than 20/200 vision in the better eye, or an extremely limited field of vision. Totally blind represents the complete loss of sight.

Many health problems and eye injuries lead to visual impairment. Half a million Americans are visually impaired, and an additional 50,000 lose their sight each year. Cataracts account for one third of all visual impairments and cause 16 persons to lose their sight every day. Glaucoma causes vision impairment in 2 million persons. One thousand eye injuries resulting in some level of vision impairment occur in the workplace or home each day. Diabetic retinopathy is one of the leading causes of the new cases of blindness. Retinitis pigmentosa, a degeneration of the light-sensing tissue at the back of the eye, also causes vision (especially night vision) deterioration.

Depending on the cause of vision loss, the condition may be fully or partially correctible through surgery or visual aids. Sometimes treatment will not reverse prior losses, but will slow the progression of vision loss. When the visual loss cannot be reversed, a variety of supportive devices and services, improved over the past twenty years, can greatly enhance the person's functional status and quality of life.

Technology has played an increasing role in helping the visually impaired function in their daily lives. Recently, doctors implanted the first artificial retina, and relatively new laser technology allows eye specialists to surgically treat extreme degrees of nearsightedness and astigmatism(blurredvision caused by uneven curvature of the eye).

National Agencies & Associations

9384 **ACB Radio Amateurs**
2200 Wilson Boulevard
Arlington, VA 22201
202-467-5081
800-424-8666
Fax: 703- 46- 508
e-mail: info@acb.org
www.acb.org

A radio amateur network of blind, visually impaired and sighted members who gather and share common problems and solutions to help members improve radio amateurs in getting started, provides access to educational materials in special media and publishes a newsletter.
Mitch Pomerantz, President
Kim Charlson, First Vice President

9385 **Alliance for Aging Research**
2021 K Street NW
Washington, DC 20006
202-293-2856
Fax: 202-785-8574
e-mail: info@agingresearch.org
www.agingresearch.org

Alliance for Aging Research is the nation's leading citizen advocacy organization for improving the health and independence of Americans as they age. It was founded to promote medical and behavioral research into the aging process.
Daniel P Perry, Executive Director
Sarah Rhyne, Executive Coordinator

9386 **American Academy of Ophthalmology**
PO Box 7424
San Francisco, CA 94120-7424
415-561-8500
Fax: 415-561-8533
e-mail: customer_service@aao.org
www.aao.org

Sponsors National Eye Care Project that gives free eye care to the elderly.

9387 **American Association of the Deaf-Blind**
8630 Fenton Street
Silver Spring, MD 20910-4500
301-495-4403
Fax: 301-495-4404
TTY: 301-495-4402
e-mail: AADB-Info@aadb.org
www.aadb.org

Promotes better opportunities and services for deaf-blind people. The mission of this organization is to assure that a comprehensive coordinated system of services is accessible to all deaf-blind people, enabling them to achieve their maximum potential.
35-50 pages 600 Members
Jamie McNama Pope, Executive Director
Elizabeth Spiers, Director of Information Services

9388 **American Coucnil of the Blind Impairment**
1155 15th Street NW Suite 1004
Washington, DC 20005
202-467-5081
800-424-8666
Fax: 202-467-5085
e-mail: cindybur@comcast.net
www.acb.org

A network of blind or visually impaired people that offers support and outreach, shares experiences and exchanges information.
Cindy Burgett, President

9389 **American Council of Blind Lions**
148 Vernon Avenue
Louisville, KY 40206
502-897-1472
Fax: 502-721-9929
e-mail: adam148@bellsouth.net
www.acb.org/acbl

The American Council of Blind Lions (ACBL) is a specially chartered Lions club. The goal of this club is to assist other Lions clubs in understanding the issues surrounding people who are blind or visually impaired.
Adam Ruschival, President

9390 **American Council of the Blind**
2200 Wilson Boulevard
Arlington, VA 22201-2706
202-467-5081
800-424-8666
Fax: 703-465-5085
e-mail: info@acb.org
www.acb.org

A national membership organization whose members are visually impaired and fully sighted individuals who are concerned about dignity and well-being of blind people throughout America. Formed in 1961, the Council has become the largest organization of blind individuals.
Mitch Pomerantz, President

9391 **American Foundation for the Blind**
11 Penn Plaza
New York, NY 10001
212-502-7600
800-232-5463
Fax: 212-502-7777
e-mail: afbinfo@afb.net
www.afb.org

AFB is the cause and organization to which Helen Keller dedicated more than 40 years of her life. In addition to being a national information consultative and advocacy resource engaged in a wide variety of initiatives AFB is home to the Helen Keller Arch.
Carl R Augusto, President/CEO
Richard J O'Brien, Chair

9392 American Foundation for the Blind: National Employment Center
11 Penn Plaza 212-502-7600
New York, NY 10001 Fax: 212-502-7777
e-mail: afbinfo@afb.net
www.afb.org
Leads initiatives in the area of employment. Nationally offers consultation, technical assistance and support and undertakes local and national efforts such as training programs and public education in the area of employment. Responds to inquiries from blind and visually impaired people and thier families, service providers and the general public in the region and nationally.
Richard J O'Brien, Chair
John T Bourger, Vice Chair

9393 American Foundation for the Blind: SE National Literacy Center
100 Peachtree Street 404-525-2303
Atlanta, GA 30303 Fax: 404-659-6957
e-mail: iteracy@afb.net
www.afb.org
Leads initiatives in the area of literacy. Offers consultation technical assistance and support and undertakes local and national efforts such as training programs and public education in the area of literacy. Offers training and in-service opportunities.

9394 American Optometric Association
243 N Lindbergh Boulevard 314-991-4100
Saint Louis, MO 63141-7881 800-365-2219
Fax: 314-991-4101
e-mail: PHKehoe@aoa.org
www.aoanet.org
The AOA and affiliates work to provide the public with quality vision and eye care. It sets professional standards helping its members conduct patient care efficiently and effectively. It also lobbies government and other organizations on behalf of the visually impaired population.
Peter H Kehoe, President
Joe E Ellis, Vice President

9395 American Printing House for the Blind
1839 Frankfort Avenue 502-895-2405
Louisville, KY 40206-0085 800-223-1839
Fax: 502-899-2274
e-mail: info@aph.org
www.aph.org
The oldest nonprofit organization of its kind in the US that creates education, workplace and lifestyle products for visually impaired people. This organization promotes the independence of blind persons by providing special media, tools and materials.
Tuck Tinsley III, President
Bob Brasher, Vice President Advisory Services

9396 Assoc. for Education & Rehabilitation of the Blind & Visually Impaired
1703 N Beauregard Street 703-671-4500
Alexandria, VA 22311 877-492-2708
Fax: 703-671-6391
e-mail: jkellyinom@msn.com
www.aerbvi.org
The only professional membership organization dedicated to the advancement of education and rehabilitation of blind and visually impaired children and adults.
Jim Gandorf, Executive Director
Bette Anne Preston, Director of Affiliate Affairs

9397 Associated Services for the Blind
919 Walnut Street 215-627-0600
Philadelphia, PA 19107-5237 Fax: 215-922-0692
e-mail: asbinfo@asb.org
www.asb.org
Limited funding is available to assist aspiring visually impaired users in the purchase of helpful high tech equipment.
Patricia C Johnson, President/CEO
Victor Difelice, Director Strategic Analysis & Planning

9398 Association for Macular Diseases
210 E 64th Street 212-605-3719
New York, NY 10065-7480 Fax: 212-605-3795
e-mail: association@retinal-research.org
www.macula.org
A nonprofit corporation to promote education and research in this scarcely-explored field. A nationwide support group for individuals and their families to adjust to the restrictions and changes brought about by macular disease.
Lawrence A Yannuzzi, President
Yale L Fisher, VP

9399 Blinded Veterans Association
477 H Street NW 202-371-8880
Washington, DC 20001-2694 800-669-7079
Fax: 202-371-8258
e-mail: bva@bva.org
www.bva.org
The organization seeks and identifies legally blind veterans who need services linking them to appropriate benefits training and opportunities in both the public and the private sectors. It represents blinded veterans before congress.
Paperback
Thomas H Miller, Executive Director
Brigitte Jones, Administrative Director

9400 Braille Institute of America Library
741 North Vermont Avenue 323-663-1111
Los Angeles, CA 90029-3594 800-272-4553
e-mail: info@brailleinstitute.org
www.brailleinstitute.org
Discs, cassettes, braille, Optacon, home visits, braille writer, reference materials on blindness and other handicaps. Closed-circuit TV, Optacon, braille writer, and large print copier also available. Home visits and cassette books are part of special services offered.
Adama Dyoniziak, Regional Program Director

9401 Canine Companions for Independence National Offices
National Offices
PO Box 446 707-528-0830
Santa Rosa, CA 95402-0446 800-572-2275
Fax: 866-224-3647
www.caninecompanions.org
A nonprofit organization that provides loyal canine partners for people with disabilities helping them to achieve greater independence and live happier and more fulfilling lives.
Corey Hudson, CEO
Anne Gittinger, Interim Chair

9402 Canine Helpers for the Disabled
5699 Ridge Road 716-433-4035
Lockport, NY 14094 e-mail: chhdogs@aol.com
ww.caninehelpers.org
A non-profit organization devoted to training dogs to assist people with disabilities to lead more independent, secure lives.

9403 Catholic Guild for the Blind Catholic Charities of the Archdiocese of
Catholic Charities of the Archdiocese of New York
180 N Michigan Avenue 312-236-8569
Chicago, IL 60601-7463 Fax: 312-236-8128
e-mail: info@guildfortheblind.org
www.guildfortheblind.org
A nonprofit organization under the sponsorship of the Catholic Charities of the Archdiocese of New York. Daily living skills, orientation and mobility training, communication skills and bilingual preparation for high school equivalency diplomas are among things covered.
Kathy Austin, Coordinator of Adult Rehabilitation
Lauri Dishman, Manager of Career Services

9404 Council for Exceptional Children
1110 N Glebe Road
Arlington, VA 22201
703-620-3660
888-232-7733
Fax: 703-264-9494
TTY: 866-915-5000
e-mail: service@cec.sped.org
www.cec.sped.org

Advocates appropriate policies standards and development for individuals with special needs. Provides professional development for special educators.
Bruce Ramirez, Executive Director
Joan Melner, Assistant Executive Director

9405 Council of Citizens with Low Vision International
1155 15th Street NW
Washington, DC 20005
714-630-8098
800-733-2258
www.cclvi.org

Affiliated with American Council of the Blind. Promotes the concept that persons with partial sight/low vision are not blind and should have every right to maximize the use of their residual vision.
John Horst, President
Richard Rueda, 1st Vice President

9406 Fidelco Guide Dog Foundation
103 Old Iron Ore Road
Bloomfield, CT 06002-0142
860-243-5200
Fax: 860-243-7215
e-mail: info@fidelco.org
www.fidelco.org

Fidelco breeds raises trains and places German shepherd guide dogs with men and women who are visually impaired primarily in the Northeast. The pioneer of in-community training in this country the visually impaired individual can remain independent.
Roberta C Kaman, Chairman
George J Salpietro, Executive Director

9407 Fight for Sight
381 Park Avenue S
New York, NY 10016
212-679-6060
Fax: 212-679-4466
e-mail: info@fightforsight.com
www.fightforsight.com

Voluntary health organization that works to conquer defective sight and blindness. Provides grants to accredited medical colleges and institutions to help supply equipment technical assistance and materials for research projects.
Mary Prudden, Executive Director
Kenneth R Barasch MD, President

9408 Foundation Fighting Blindness
11435 Cronhill Drive
Owings Mills, MD 21117-2220
410-568-0150
800-683-5555
TTY: 800-683-5551
TDD: 800-683-5551
e-mail: info@FightBlindness.org
www.blindness.org

FFB offers information and referral services for affected individuals and their families as well as for doctors and eye care professionals. The Foundation also provides comprehensive information kits on retinitis pigmentosa.
William T Schmidt, CEO
Gordon Gund, Chairman

9409 Foundation for Glaucoma Research
251 Post Street
San Francisco, CA 94108
415-986-3162
800-826-6693
Fax: 415-986-3763
e-mail: question@glaucoma.org
www.glaucoma.org

A national organization dedicated to protecting the sight of people with glaucoma through research and education. The Foundation conducts and supports research that contributes to improved patient care and a better understanding of the disease process.
Andrew Jackson, Director of Communications
Thomas M Brunner, President and CEO

9410 Foundation for the Advancement of the Blind
4058 Moore Street
Los Angeles, CA 90066-5118
310-301-0344

Helps blind people attain and retain employment.

9411 Friends-In-Art
2331 Poincianna Street
Huntsville, AL 35801
202-467-5081
800-424-8666
Fax: 202-467-5085
e-mail: nansong@knology.net
www.friendsinart.com

Aims to enlarge the art experience of blind people encourages blind people to visit museums galleries concerts the theater etc. offers consultation to program planners in establishing accessible art and museum exhibits.
Nancy Pendegraph, President
Gordon Kent, Board Member

9412 Guide Dog Users
14311 Astrodome Drive
Silver Spring, MD 20906-2245
866-799-8436
e-mail: beckyb@cloud9.net
www.gdui.org

Promotes the acceptance of blind people and their dogs works for enforcement and expansion of laws admitting guide dogs into public places advocates for quality training and follow-up services.
Elizabeth Barnes, President
Rebecca Floyd-Collin, First Vice President

9413 Guide Dogs for the Blind
PO Box 151200
San Rafael, CA 94915-1200
650-499-4000
800-298-4050
e-mail: information@guidedogs.com
www.guidedogs.com

Offers educational materials transportation seminars and newsletters for the blind providing 2 field offices.
Edward Schaefer, Board Chair
Morgan Watkins, First Vice Chair

9414 Helen Keller National Center's National Parent Network
141 Middle Neck Road
Sands Point, NY 11050-1218
516-944-8900
Fax: 516-944-7302
TTY: 516-944-8637
e-mail: hkncinfo@hknc.org
www.hknc.org

Establishes a coalition of state parent organizations to promote the exchange of information among parents of deaf-blind youth. Provides training to parents to develop their legislative advocacy skills, empowers parents and their families to obtain needed services.
Kathy Mezack, Coordinator of Vocational Services

9415 Independent Visually Impaired Enterprises
230 Robinhood Lane
McMurray, PA 15317
e-mail: lengual@concentric.net
www.acb.org

Strives to broaden vocational opportunities in business for the visually impaired. Works to improve rehabilitation facilities for all types of business enterprises and publicizes the capabilities of blind and visually impaired business persons.
Carla Hayes, President

9416 International Agency for the Prevention of Blindness
National Eye Institute
2020 Vision Place
Bethesda, MD 20892-3655
301-496-5248
www.nei.nih.gov

Ophthalmic societies and committees for the prevention of blindness whose members include ophthalmologists public health officers nutritionists geneticists and other health workers. Coordinates international research into the causes of impaired vision.
Carl Kupfer, Volunteer
Paul A Sieving, Director

9417 Library Users of America
2200 Wilson Boulevard
Arlington, VA 22201
202-467-5081
800-424-8666
Fax: 703-465-5085
e-mail: info@acb.org
www.acb.org

Provides for chapters in states through the US to encourage the development acquisition and use of technology which enables blind

and visually impaired persons to use printed material independently in library settings and elsewhere.
Barry Levine, President

9418 **Lighthouse International Headquarters**
111 E 59th Street
New York, NY 10022-1202
212-821-9200
800-821-0500
Fax: 212-821-9707
TTY: 212-821-9713
e-mail: info@lighthouse.org
www.lighthouse.org
A leading resource worldwide on vision impairment and vision rehabilitation. Pioneer in vision rehabilitation services, education, research and advocacy enabling people of all ages who are blind or partially sighted to lead independent and productive lives.
Roger O Goldman, Chairman
Tara A Cortes, President/CEO

9419 **Lions World Services for the Blind Lions Clubs International**
Lions Clubs International
2811 Fair Park Boulevard
Little Rock, AR 72204
501-664-7100
800-248-0734
Fax: 501-664-2743
e-mail: training@lwsb.org
www.lwsb.org
Lions World Services for the Blind was founded in 1947 to serve people who are blind and visually impaired who needed to learn independent living skills or job training skills that considered the special requirements of their individual visual impairments.
Ramona Sangalli, President and Chief Executive Officer
Larry Morgan, Vice President for Development

9420 **Macular Degeneration Foundation**
PO Box 515
Northampton, MA 01061-0515
413-268-7660
888-622-8527
e-mail: amdf@macular.org
www.macular.org
The American Macular Degeneration Foundation is committed to the prevention and cure of macular degeneration and offers hope and support to those afflicted and their families.
Chip Goehring, President and Trustee
Mark E Torrey, Vice President and Trustee

9421 **National Alliance of Blind Students**
2200 Wilson Boulevard
Arlington, VA 22201
202-467-5081
800-424-8666
Fax: 703-465-5085
e-mail: info@acb.org
www.acb.org
Works to facilitate progress toward full accessibility of college programs and facilities provides opportunities for discussion of issues important to students and assists with National Student Seminars.
Rebecca Bridges, President

9422 **National Association for Parents of the Visually Impaired**
PO Box 317
Watertown, MA 02471-0317
617-972-7441
800-562-6265
Fax: 781-972-7444
e-mail: napvi@perkins.org
www.napvi.org
The only national organization that strives to serve families of children of all ages and ranges with visual loss. It is a community based organization whose members include parents parent organizations agencies and other persons with common objectives.
Susan LaVenture, Executive Director
Doug Halverson, President

9423 **National Association for Visually Handicapped**
22 West 21st Street
New York, NY 10010
212-889-3141
888-205-5951
Fax: 212-727-2931
e-mail: navh@navh.org
www.navh.org
NAVH ensures that those with limited vision do not lead limited lives. We offer emotional support; training in the use of and access to a wide variety of optical aids and lighting; a large print, nationwide, free-by-mail loan library; large print educational materials; quarterly newsletter; referrals; self-help groups and educational outreach.
Cesar Gomez, Executive Director

9424 **National Association for Visually Hand.**
22 W 21st Street
New York, NY 10010
212-889-3141
Fax: 212-727-2931
e-mail: navh@navh.org
www.navh.org
NAVH ensures that those with limited vision do not lead limited lives. We offer emotional support; training in the use of and access to a wide variety of optical aids and lighting and a large print, nationwide, free-by-mail loan library.
Lorraine H Marchi, Founder & CEO
Miriam Rosen, Executive Director

9425 **National Association of Blind Educators Sheila Koenig**
Sheila Koenig
2214 Emerson Avenue S
Minneapolis, MN 55401
612-375-1625
e-mail: jsanders.nfb@comcast.net
www.nfb.org
Membership organization of blind teachers professors and instructors in all levels of education. Provides support and information regarding professional responsibilities classroom techniques national testing methods and career obstacles.
Judy Sanders, President

9426 **National Association of Blind Lawyers Scott LaBarre**
Scott LaBarre
1660 S Albion Street
Denver, CO 80222-4046
303-504-5979
Fax: 303-757-3640
e-mail: slabarre@labarrelaw.com
www.nfb.org
Membership organization of blind attorneys law students judges and others in the law field. Provides support and information regarding employment techniques used by the blind, advocacy, laws affecting the blind and current information about the American legal system.
Scott LaBarre, President

9427 **National Association of Blind Musicians Linda Mentink**
Linda Mentink
1865 42nd Avenue
Columbus, NE 68601-0952
402-563-8138
e-mail: mentink@frontiernet.net
www.nfb.org
Blind persons dedicated to advancing employment and entertainment opportunities in various music fields. Offers support and information regarding copyright publishing promotion and other career details.
Linda Mentik, Chairperson

9428 **National Association of Blind Office Professionals**
Lisa Hall
7001ÿHamilton Avenue
Cincinnati, OH 45231-6104
513-931-7070
e-mail: Lhall007@cinci.rr.com
www.nfb.org
Membership organization of blind secretaries and transcribers at all levels including medical and paralegal transcription office workers customer-service personnel and many other similar fields. Addresses issues such as technology, accommodation and caregivers.
Lisa Hall, President

9429 **National Association of Blind Students Angela Wolf**
Angela Wolf
3106 Barrett Place
Wichita Falls, TX 76308-1803
512-417-8190
e-mail: nabs.president@gmail.com
www.nfb.org
For over 30 years this national organization of blind students has provided support information and encouragement to blind college and university students. Leads the way in offering resources in issues such as national testing and accessible textbooks.
Terri Rupp, President

9430 **National Association of Guide Dog Users Priscilla Ferris**
Priscilla Ferris
1003 Papaya Drive
Tampa, FL 33619-3714
813-626-2789
800-558-8261
e-mail: president@nfb-nagdu.org
www.nfb-nagdu.org

Provides information and support for guide dog users and works to secure high standards in guide dog training. Addresses issues of discrimination of guide dog users and offers public education about guide dog use.
Marion Gwizdala, President

9431 **National Association to Promote the Use of Braille**
Nadine Jacobson
5805 Kellogg Avenue
Edina, MN 55424-1819
952-927-7694
e-mail: nadine.jacobson@visi.com
www.nfb.org
Dedicated to securing improved Braille instruction increasing the number of Braille materials available to the blind and providing information about the importance of Braille in securing independence education and employment for the blind.
Nadine Jacobson, President

9432 **National Braille Association**
95 Allens Creek Road
Rochester, NY 14618-2513
585-427-8260
Fax: 585-427-0263
e-mail: nbaoffice@nationalbraille.org
www.nationalbraille.org
Provides transcription service for and maintains a depository of braille books.
Diane Spence, President
Jan Carroll, Vice President

9433 **National Braille Press**
88 Saint Stephen Street
Boston, MA 02115-4302
617-266-6160
888-965-8965
Fax: 617-437-0456
www.nbp.org
The guiding purposes of National Braille Press are to promote the literacy of blind children through braille and to provide access to information that empowers blind people to actively engage in work family and community affairs.
Paul Parravano, Chair
Gayle L Yarnall, Clerk

9434 **National Center for Vision and Aging Lighthouse**
Lighthouse
111 E 59th Street
New York, NY 10022-1202
212-821-9200
800-829-0500
Fax: 212-821-9707
TTY: 212-821-9713
TDD: 212-821-9713
e-mail: info@lighthouse.org
www.lighthouse.org
The National Center for Vision and Aging provides information on eye conditions and visual impairment of all ages resources education and professionally prepared multimedia and print material for community education lectures.
Roger O Goldman, Chairman
Tara A Cortes, President and Chief Executive Officer

9435 **National Center for Vision and Child Development**
Lighthouse
111 E 59th Street
New York, NY 10022
212-821-9200
800-829-0500
Fax: 212-821-9707
TTY: 212-821-9713
e-mail: info@lighthouse.org
www.lighthouse.org
Our mission is to overcome vision impairment for people of all ages through worldwide leadership in rehabilitation services education research prevention and advocacy.
Roger O Goldman, Chairman
Tara A Cortes PhD RN, President and Chief Executive Officer

9436 **National Diabetes Action Network for the Blind**
National Federation of the Blind
1800 Johnson Street
Baltimore, MD 21230-7337
410-659-9314
Fax: 410-685-5653
e-mail: nfb@nfb.org
www.nfb.org
Leading support and information organization of persons losing vision due to diabetes. Provides personal contact and resource information with other blind diabetics about non-visual techniques of independently managing diabetes and monitoring glucose levels.
Marc Maurer, President
Fredric Schroeder, First Vice President

9437 **National Eye Institute National Institutes of Health**
National Institutes of Health
2020 Vision Place
Bethesda, MD 20892-3655
301-496-5248
www.nei.nih.gov
Mission is to discover safe and effective methods to prevent diagnose and treat diseases and disorders of the visual system. In this way the Institute helps to prevent reduce and possibly eliminate blindness and visual impairment.
Paul A Sieving, Director
Carl Kupfer, Volunteer

9438 **National Federation of the Blind**
1800 Johnson Street
Baltimore, MD 21230
410-659-9314
Fax: 410-685-5653
e-mail: pmaurer@nfb.org
www.nfb.org
The largest consumer membership organization for the blind founded in 1940 it has 50 000 members nationwide in 52 affiliates and over 700 local chapters. Provides public education about blindness, support services to the newly blinded and scholarships.
50M Members
Marc Maurer, President
Fredric Schroeder, First Vice President

9439 **National Federation of the Blind in Computer Science**
Curtis Chong
3000 Grand Avenue
Des Moines, IA 50312-4256
515-277-1288
Fax: 515-281-1361
e-mail: curtischong@earthlink.net
www.nfb.org
National organization of blind persons knowledgeable in the computer science and technology fields. Works to develop new technologies, to secure access to current technology and to develop new ways of using current or new technologies by the blind.
Curtis Chong, President

9440 **National Federation of the Blind: Blind/Deaf Division**
Robert Eschbach
1186 North Verbena Place
Casa Grande, AZ 85222-5440
520-836-3689
e-mail: Resch@earthlink.net
www.nfb-db.org
Deaf-blind persons working nationally to improve services, training and independence for the deaf-blind. Offers personal contact with other deaf-blind individuals knowledgeable in advocacy, education, employment, technology, discrimination and other issues surrounding deaf-blindness.
Robert Eschbach, President

9441 **National Federation of the Blind: Blind Industrial Workers of America**
National Federation of the Blind
1800 Johnson Street
Baltimore, MD 21230-4998
410-659-9314
Fax: 410-685-5653
e-mail: nfb@nfb.org
www.nfb.org
Membership organization of blind persons employed in industrial and manufacturing work or in government job programs for the blind. Dedicated to protecting the rights of blind workers in salary, job stability, advancement and labor issues.
Ken Staley, President

9442 **National Federation of the Blind: Human Services Division**
Melissa Riccobono
1026 E 36th Street
Baltimore, MD 21218
410-235-3073
e-mail: maricco@uwalumni.com
www.nfb.org
Membership organization of blind persons working in counseling personnel psychology social work psychiatry rehabilitation and other social science and human resource fields. Dedicated to improving employment opportunities and advancement for blind persons.
Melissa Riccobono, President

9443 National Federation of the Blind: Masonic Square Club
Fred Flowers
46 Powderock Place
Baltimore, MD 21236-4766 410-598-0155
www.nfb.org
Blind individuals committed to sharing of Masonic experiences goals and history.
Fred Flowers, President

9444 National Federation of the Blind: Public Employees Division
Ivan Weich
4301 Clogston Avenue NE 360-782-9575
Bremerton, WA 98310-3009 e-mail: IEWeich@comcast.net
www.nfb.org
Organization of blind persons holding local state or federal jobs. Focuses on issues such as changes in governmental hiring and retention practices new job skills needed for the future, government employment downsizing, new electronic means of finding employment and more.
Ivan Weich, President

9445 National Federation of the Blind: Science and Engineering Division
John Miller
10955 Deering Street 858-527-1727
San Diego, CA 92126-1920 e-mail: j8miller@soe.ucsd.edu
www.nfb.org
Blind persons with expertise and experience in fields such as genetics, telecommunications, biology, chemistry, physics and nuclear physics or mechanical electronic and chemical engineering. This is a strong support group to encourage blind persons to excel in science and engineering.
John Miller, President

9446 National Federation of the Blind: Writers Division
Tom Stevens
504 S 57th Street 402-556-3216
Omaha, NE 68106-0809 e-mail: newmanrl@cox.net
www.nfb-writers-division.org
Blind writers in all styles including poetry short story fiction non-fiction magazine writing and theatrical work offer encouragement and support to blind writers and authors. Issues cover various aspects of this business including selling your work.
Robert L Newman, President

9447 National Industries for the Blind
1310 Braddock Place 703-310-0500
Alexandria, VA 22314-1727 Fax: 703-998-8268
e-mail: communications@nib.org
www.nib.org
A nonprofit organization that represents over 100 associated industries serving people who are blind in thirty-six states. These agencies serve people who are blind or visually impaired and help them to reach their full potential.
Kevin Lynch, President/CEO
Steve Brice, Vice President/CFO

9448 National Library Service for the Blind and Physically Handicapped
Library of Congress
1291 Taylor Street NW 202-707-5100
Washington, DC 20011 888-657-7323
TTY: 202-707-0744
TDD: 202-707-0744
e-mail: nls@loc.gov
www.loc.gov/nls
Administers a national library service that provides braille and recorded books and magazines on free loan to anyone who cannot read standard print because of visual or physical disabilities who are eligible residents of the United States.
12 pages Quarterly
Frank Kurt Cylke, Director
Michael M Moodie, Research and Development Officer

9449 National Organization of Parents of Blind Children
Barbara Cheadle
1152 106th Lane NE 763-784-8590
Minneapolis, MD 55434-4998 Fax: 410-685-5653
e-mail: carrie.gilmer@gmail.com
www.nfb.org/nfb/Parents_and_Teachers.asp
Support information and advocacy organization of parents of blind or visually impaired children. Addresses issues ranging from help to parents of a newborn blind infant, mobility and Braille instruction, education, social and community participation.
Carrie Gilmer, President

9450 New Eyes for the Needy
549 Milburn Avenue 973-376-4903
Short Hills, NJ 07078 Fax: 973-376-3807
e-mail: neweyesfortheneedy@yahoo.com
www.neweyesfortheneedy.org
Provides new glasses for those with low vision who may not be able to afford them.

9451 Prevent Blindess America
211 W Wacker Drive
Chicago, IL 60606-5624 800-331-2020
e-mail: info@preventblindness.org
www.preventblindness.org
Information and referral services provided on specific eye disorders. Publishes literature and supports community screening and testing programs.
Hugh R Parry, President/CEO

9452 Randolph-Sheppard Vendors of America
1808 Faith Place 504-368-7785
Terrytown, LA 70056-4104 800-467-5299
Fax: 504-368-7739
e-mail: rsva@juno.com
www.acb.org/rsva
Protects the interests of blind vendors seeks proper implementation of the Randolph-Sheppard Act and encourages facility locations in more visible and profitable areas.
Charles Glaser, President
John Gordon, First Vice President

9453 Recording for the Blind and Dyslexic
20 Roszel Road
Princeton, NJ 08540-6294 866-RFB-D585
www.rfbd.org
Provides materials for all people who cannot effectively read standard print because of a visual perceptual or other physical disability.

9454 Research to Prevent Blindness
645 Madison Avenue 212-752-4333
New York, NY 10022-1010 800-621-0026
e-mail: inforequest@rpbusa.org
www.rpbusa.org
National voluntary health foundation supported by foundations corporations and voluntary gifts and bequests from individuals. Established to stimulate basic and applied research into the causes prevention and treatment of blinding eye diseases.
David Weeks, Chairman
Diane S Swift, President

9455 Seeing Eye
PO Box 375 973-539-4425
Morristown, NJ 07963-0375 Fax: 973-539-0922
e-mail: info@seeingeye.org
www.seeingeye.org
A training school for dogs to guide qualified blind persons.
James A Kutsch, President and Chief Executive Officer

9456 Smith-Kettlewell Eye Research Foundation
2318 Fillmore Street 415-345-2000
San Francisco, CA 94115 Fax: 415-345-8455
www.ski.org
Dedicated to research on human vision founded to encourage a productive collaboration between the medical clinic and the scientific laboratories.

9457 Taping for the Blind
3935 Essex Lane 713-622-2767
Houston, TX 77027-5113 Fax: 713-622-2772
www.tapingfortheblind.org
Records reading material on audiotape copied onto cassettes for use by blind and physically handicapped persons. Promotes in-

creased interest in and use of free audio materials. Books textbooks and technical manuals are recorded and sent to libraries.
Cynthia Franzetti, Executive Director
Ginger Gish, Volunteer Coordinator

9458 **United States Association for Blind Athletes**
33 N Institute Street
Colorado Springs, CO 80903-3508
719-630-0422
Fax: 719-630-0616
e-mail: mlucas@usaba.org
www.usaba.org
Athletic association for blind athletes this association is the national governing body for the United States visually impaired athletes.
Mark Lucas, Executive Director
Nicole Jomantas, Communications Director

9459 **Vision World Wide**
5707 Brockton Drive
Indianapolis, IN 46220-5481
317-254-1332
800-431-1739
Fax: 317-251-6588
e-mail: info@visionenhancement.org
www.visionww.org
Believing there is hope when vision fails. It disseminates relevant information on a variety of topics through its information and referral helpline website e-mail announce list and journal Vision Enhancement all designed to encourage and support individuals with vision impairments.
Patricia Price, Editor-In-Chief
William Corbin, Board Chairman

9460 **Washington Ear**
12061 Tech Road
Silver Spring, MD 20904-2437
301-681-6636
Fax: 301-625-1986
e-mail: information@washear.org
www.washear.org
A nonprofit organization providing reading and information services for the blind visually impaired and physically disabled persons who cannot effectively read print see plays watch television programs or view museum exhibits.
Margaret Pfanstiehl, President
George Long, Vice President

9461 **National Federation of the Blind: Blind Merchants Division**
Kevin Worley
1223 Lake Plaza Drive
Colorado Springs, CO 80906-3591
719-527-0488
866-543-6808
Fax: 303-695-1828
e-mail: kevinworley@blindmerchants.org
www.blindmerchants.org
Membership organization of blind persons employed in either self-employment work or the Randolph-Sheppard vending program. Provides information regarding rehabilitation social security tax and other issues which directly affect blind merchants.
Kevin Worley, President

State Agencies & Associations

Alabama

9462 **Alabama Council of the Blind**
1018 E Street S
Talladega, AL 35160
256-362-5649
e-mail: dart1018@charter.net
www.acbalabama.org
David Trott, President

9463 **National Federation of the Blind: Alabama**
4905 Brooke Court
Mobile, AL 36618-2708
251-344-7960
e-mail: mwkoger21@bellsouth.net
www.nfbofalabama.org
Minnie K Walker, President

Alaska

9464 **National Federation of the Blind: Alaska**
700 Hollywood
Anchorage, AK 99501
907-339-9578
e-mail: priddle@gci.net
www.nfb.org
Steven Priddle, President

Arizona

9465 **Arizona Center for the Blind and Visually Impaired**
3100 E Roosevelt Street
Phoenix, AZ 85008-5036
602-273-7411
Fax: 602-273-7410
e-mail: jlamay@acbvi.org
www.acbvi.org
Provides services for individuals to enhance the quality of life of people who are blind or otherwise visually impaired. Services are available to adults who are either legally blind or visually impaired as well as those who have a degenerative eye condition.
Jim LaMay, Executive Director
Diana Miladin, Director of Communications/Development

9466 **Arizona Industries for the Blind**
515 N 51st Avenue
Phoenix, AZ 85043
602-771-9100
Fax: 602-353-5703
e-mail: LHudspeth@azdes.gov
www.azdes.gov/aib
Arizona Industries for the Blind was established in 1952 to provide employment and training opportunities for Arizonans who are legally blind.
Lorraine Hudspeth, Controller
Letty Cerpa, Senior Accountant

9467 **National Federation of the Blind: Arizona**
9014 E Bellevue Street
Tucson, AZ 85715-5652
520-733-5894
e-mail: krezguy@cox.net
www.nfbarizona.com
Bob Kresmer, President
Vicki Hodges, 1st Vice President

9468 **Region 6 of the National Association for Parents of the Visually Impaired**
Walnut Creek, CA 85282-5724
602-730-8282
e-mail: mebphillips@comcast.net
www.spedex.com/napvi
Mary Beth Phillips, NAPVI Region 6 Representative

Arkansas

9469 **Arkansas Lighthouse for the Blind**
6818 Murray Street
Little Rock, AR 72209-2666
510-562-2222
Fax: 501-568-5275
e-mail: bjohnson@arkansaslighthouse.org
www.arkansaslighthouse.org
Bill Johnson, CEO
Lyn Cossey, Director of Operations

9470 **National Federation of the Blind: Arkansas**
608 Cedar Ridge
Paragould, AR 72450-2304
870-565-4484
e-mail: nfbofarkansas@yahoo.com
www.nfb.org
Jerree Harris, President

California

9471 **Helen Keller National Center: South Region**
9939 Hibert Street
San Diego, CA 92131
858-578-1600
Fax: 858-578-3800
TTY: 858-578-1600
e-mail: Ckirscher@att.net
www.hknc.org
Cathy Kirscher, Regional Representative

9472 **Lighthouse for the Blind and Visually Impaired**
Lighthouse Industries
214 Van Ness Avenue
San Francisco, CA 94102
415-431-1481
Fax: 415-863-7568
TTY: 415-431-4572
e-mail: info@lighthouse-sf.org
www.lighthouse-sf.org
The LightHouse promotes the independence, equality and self-reliance of people who are blind or visually impaired through rehabilitation training and relevant services, such as access to employment, education, government, information, recreation and transportation.
Chuck Godwin, Executive Support
Anthony Fletcher, Associate Executive Director and COO

9473 **National Federation of the Blind: California**
5530 Corbin Avenue 818-342-6524
Tarzana, CA 91356 877-558-6524
Fax: 818-344-7930
e-mail: nfbcal@sbcglobal.net
http://www.nfbcal.org/
Robert Stigile, President

9474 **Northwest Regional Training Center: Canine Companions for Independence**
2965 Dutton Avenue 707-577-1791
Santa Rosa, CA 95407-0446 800-572-2275
TTY: 707-577-1756
e-mail: kpierson@cci.org
www.cci.org
Canine Companions for Independence is a non-profit organization that enhances the lives of people with disabilities by providing highly trained assistance dogs and ongoing support to ensure quality partnerships.
Kathy Pierson, Executive Director
Daniel Y Harris, Development Director

9475 **Southwest Regional Training Center: Canine Companions for Independence**
124 Rancho del Oro Drive 760-901-4300
Oceanside, CA 92057 800-572-2275
Fax: 760-901-4350
TTY: 760-901-4326
TDD: 760-901-4350
www.cci.org
Canine Companions for Independence is a non-profit organization that enhances the lives of people with disabilities by providing highly trained assistance dogs and ongoing support to ensure quality partnerships.
Linda Valliant, Executive Director
Chuck Contreras, Director of Development

Colorado

9476 **National Federation of the Blind: Colorado**
2233 W Shepperd Avenue 303-778-1130
Littleton, CO 80120 800-401-4NFB
e-mail: slabarre@labarrelaw.com
www.nfbco.org
Scott LaBarre, President
Kevan Worley, 1st Vice President

9477 **Rocky Mountain Region: Helen Keller National Center**
1880 S Pierce Street 303-934-9037
Lakewood, CO 80232 Fax: 303-934-2939
TTY: 303-934-9037
e-mail: maureen.mcgowan@hknc.org
www.hknc.org
Maureen McGowan, Regional Representative

Connecticut

9478 **BESB Industries**
184 Windsor Avenue 860-602-4000
Windsor, CT 06095-4536 800-842-4510
Fax: 860-602-4220
TTY: 860-602-4221
e-mail: besb@ct.gov
www.ct.gov/besb
Brian S Sigman, Executive Director

9479 **National Federation of the Blind: Connecticut**
580 Burnside Avenue 860-289-1971
East Hartford, CT 06108-3579 e-mail: aldelucia@nfbct.org
http://www.nfbct.org/
Alfonse DeLucia, President

9480 **Prevent Blindness Tri-State**
101 Whitney Avenue
New Haven, CT 06510 800-850-2020
e-mail: info@preventblindnesstristate.org
www.preventblindness.org/tristate
Kathryn Garre-Ayars, President & CEO
Maria Giarratana, Grants Manager

9481 **Region 1 of the National Association for Parents of the Visually Impaired**
Hudson, MA 06016-9560 860-623-4129
e-mail: sue.rawley@verizon.net
www.spedex.com/napvi
Sue Rawley, NAPVI Region 1 Representative

Delaware

9482 **Delaware Assocation for the Blind Department of Health & Social Services**
Department of Health & Social Services
800 W Street 302-655-2111
Wilmington, DE 19801-1526 888-777-3925
Fax: 302-655-1442
e-mail: contact@dabdel.org
www.dabdel.org

9483 **National Federation of the Blind: DC**
627 Dahlia Street NW 202-882-8090
Washington, DC 20012-1841 e-mail: dnj.galloway@starpower.net
www.nfb.org
Don Galloway, President

District of Columbia

9484 **American Foundation for the Blind: Governmental Relations**
820 1st Street NE 202-408-0200
Washington, DC 20002 Fax: 202-289-7880
e-mail: afbgov@afb.net
www.afb.org
Advocates on behalf of people who are blind or visually impaired before Congress and Executive Branch offices, and participates in advocacy-related coalitions and initiatives nationwide.
Paul W Schroeder, Vice President, Governmental Relations
Barbara Jackson LeMoine, Legislative Assistant

9485 **Columbia Lighthouse for the Blind**
1825 K Street NW 202-454-6400
Washington, DC 20006 877-324-5252
Fax: 202-454-6401
e-mail: info@clb.org
www.clb.org
Columbia Lighthouse for the blind offers programs and services that enable individuals who are blind or visually impaired to obtain and maintain independence at home, school and in the community.
Anthony Cancelosi, President/CEO

9486 **National Federation of the Blind: Delaware**
3618 Kiamensi Street 302-999-7242
Wilmington, DE 19808-2646 e-mail: rhbennett.nfb@comcast.net
www.nfb.org
Richard Bennett, President

Florida

9487 **Goodwill Industries-Suncoast Goodwill Industries-Suncoast**
Goodwill Industries-Suncoast
10596 Gandy Boulevard 727-523-1512
Saint Petersburg, FL 33702 888-279-1988
Fax: 727-579-0850
TTY: 727-579-1068
e-mail: gw.marketing@goodwill-suncoast.com
www.goodwill-suncoast.org
A non-profit community based organization whose purpose is to improve the quality of life for people who are disabled, disadvantaged and/or aged. This mission is accomplished through a staff of over 1,200 employees providing independent living skills.
R Lee Waits, President/Chief Executive Officer
Chris Ward, Marketing and Media Relations Manager

9488 **National Federation of the Blind: Florida**
121 Deer Lake Circle 386-677-6886
Ormond Beach, FL 32174-4266 888-282-5972
e-mail: kdavisnfbf@cfl.rr.com
www.nfbflorida.org
Kathy Davis, President

9489 **Southeast Regional Center: Canine Companions for Independence**
Anheuser-Busch/SeaWorld Campus
8150 Clarcona Ocoee Road 407-522-3300
Orlando, FL 32818-0388 Fax: 407-522-3347
e-mail: mager@cci.org
www.cci.org

Canine Companions for Independence is a non-profit organization that enhances the lives of people with disabilities by providing highly trained assistance dogs and ongoing support to ensure quality partnerships.
Margaret S Ager, Executive Director
Nancy Baumann, President

9490 **Tampa Lighthouse for the Blind**
1106 W Platt Street 813-251-2407
Tampa, FL 33606-2142 866-251-2407
Fax: 813-254-4305
e-mail: TLH@tampalighthouse.org
www.tampalighthouse.org

Tampa Lighthouse for the Blind provides comprehensive rehabilitation programs for persons who are blind or visually impaired.
Cliff Olstrom, Executive Director

Georgia

9491 **Georgia Industries for the Blind**
700 Faceville Highway
Bainbridge, GA 39818-0218 229-248-2666
www.vocrehabga.org

The primary mission of the Georgia Industries for the Blind (GIB) is to provide employment opportunities for people who are visually impaired or blind.

9492 **National Federation of the Blind: Georgia**
315 Ponce de Leon Avenue 404-371-1000
Decatur, GA 30030 Fax: 404-371-1002
e-mail: alewis@nfbga.org
www.nfb.org

Anil Lewis, President

9493 **Southeastern Region: Helen Keller National Center**
1003 Virginia Avenue 404-766-9625
Atlanta, GA 30354-1365 Fax: 404-766-3447
TTY: 404-766-2820
e-mail: bc4hknc@aol.com
www.hknc.org

Barbara Chandler, Regional Representative

Hawaii

9494 **Division of Vocational Rehabilitation and Services for the Blind**
Department of Human Services
601 Kamokila Boulevard 808-692-7715
Kapolei, HI 96707 Fax: 808-692-7727
TTY: 808-692-7715
e-mail: info@hawaiivr.org
www.hawaiivr.org

The American Macular Degeneration Foundation is committed to the prevention and cure of macular degeneration and offers hope and support to those afflicted and their families. The Foundation is a major voice in establishing national research.
Joe Cordova, Administrator

9495 **Ho'opono Workshop for the Blind**
1901 Bachelor Street 808-586-5286
Honolulu, HI 96817 Fax: 808-586-5288
TTY: 808-586-5269
e-mail: hoopono@hawaiivr.org
www.hawaiivr.org

Dave Eveland, Administrator

9496 **National Federation of the Blind: Hawaii**
PO Box 4482 808-391-1214
Honolulu, HI 96812 e-mail: nanifife@aol.com
hawaii.nfb.org

Nani Fife, President
Charlene Ota, Vice-President

Idaho

9497 **National Federation of the Blind: Idaho**
300 Willard Avenue 208-377-9825
Pocatello, ID 83201 Fax: 208-232-5416
e-mail: ElsieLamp@yahoo.com
www.nfbidaho.org

Elsie H Lamp, President

Illinois

9498 **AFB Midwest: American Foundation for the Blind**
949 Third Avenue 304-523-8651
Huntington, WV 25701 e-mail: muslan@afb.net
www.afb.org

Leads initiatives in the area of technology. Nationally offers consultation technical assistance and support and undertakes local and national efforts such as training programs in the area of technology. Responds to inquiries from blind and visually impaired.
Mark Uslan, Director
Darren Burton, National Program Associate

9499 **Aid to the Aged, Blind or Disabled**
Department of Human Services
100 South Grand Avenue, East
Springfield, IL 62762 800-252-8635
TTY: 800-447-6404
www.macular.org/stagency/state_il.html

The American Macular Degeneration Foundation is committed to the prevention and cure of macular degeneration and offers hope and support to those afflicted and their families. The Foundation will be a major voice in establishing the national research agenda for macular degeneration through promoting an alliance among the scientific community, government, and victims of the disease and their families to ensure the prevention and cure of the disease.

9500 **Chicago Lighthouse for People Who are Blind and Visually Impaired**
1850 W Roosevelt Road 312-666-1331
Chicago, IL 60608-1298 Fax: 312-243-8539
TTY: 312-666-8874
TDD: 312-666-8874
e-mail: helpdesk@chicagolighthouse.org
www.thechicagolighthouse.org

The Chicago Lighthouse is a comprehensive private rehabilitation and educational facility dedicated exclusively to assisting children youth and adults who are blind visually impaired or multi-disabled.
Janet P Szlyk, Executive Director
William L Conaghan, Chairman

9501 **Helen Keller National Center Regional Representatives**
485 Avenue of the Cities 309-755-0018
E Moline, IL 61244 Fax: 309-755-0025
TTY: 309-755-0018
TDD: 309-755-0021
e-mail: HKNC5LJT@aol.com
www.hknc.org

Laura J Thomas, Regional Representative

9502 **National Federation of the Blind: Illinois**
6919 W Berwyn Avenue 773-307-6440
Chicago, IL 60656-2040 e-mail: president@nbfofillinois.org
www.nfbofillinois.org

Patti Gregory-Chang, President
Deborah Kent Stein, First Vice-President

9503 **Region 3 of the National Association for Parents of the Visually Impaired**
Highland Park, IL 60047-7711 847-438-0705
e-mail: wizoz4@aol.com
www.spedex.com/napvi

Pam Stern, NAPVI Region 3 Representative

Indiana

9504 **Bosma Industries for the Blind**
8020 Zionsville Road 317-684-0600
Indianapolis, IN 46268-3876 800-362-5463
Fax: 317-684-1946
e-mail: info@bosma.org
www.bosma.org
It is the mission of Bosma Industries for the Blind to enhance opportunities for individuals who are blind or visually impaired to achieve their potential in vocational, economic, social and personal independence.
Lou Moneymaker, CEO
Connie F Campbell, CFO/COO

9505 **National Federation of the Blind: Indiana**
6010 Winnpeny Lane 317-205-9226
Indianapolis, IN 46220-5253 e-mail: rb15@iquest.net
www.nfb.org
Ron Brown, President

Iowa

9506 **National Federation of the Blind: Iowa**
2721 34th Street 515-771-8348
Des Moines, IA 50310 e-mail: m.barber@mchsi.com
www.nfbi.org
Michael D Barber, President
April Enderton, First Vice-President

Kansas

9507 **Great Plains Region: Helen Keller National Center**
4330 Shawhee Mission Parkway 913-677-4562
Shawnee Mission, KS 66205 Fax: 913-677-1544
TTY: 913-677-4562
e-mail: hknc7bj@aol.com
www.helenkeller.org
Services are free and offer client advocacy consultation and technical assistance to schools and agencies; assistance in developing local services information and referral; public education and awareness; maintenance of the National Registry.
Beth Jordan, Regional Representative
Jody Searing, Administrative Assistant

9508 **Kansas Industries for the Blind**
425 MacVicar Street 785-296-3211
Topeka, KS 66606 Fax: 785-296-0728

9509 **National Federation of the Blind: Kansas**
11405 W Grant 913-339-9341
Wichita, KS 67209-3621 e-mail: donnajwood@cox.net
www.nfbks.org
Donna Wood, President
Susan L Stanzel, First Vice President

Kentucky

9510 **Kentucky Industries for the Blind**
1900 Brownsboro Road 502-893-0211
Louisville, KY 40206-2102 Fax: 502-893-3885

9511 **National Federation of the Blind: Kentucky**
210 Cambridge Drive 502-366-2317
Louisville, KY 40214-2809 e-mail: cathyj@iglou.com
www.nfbky.org
Cathy Jackson, President
Pamela Roark-Glisson, Vice President

Louisiana

9512 **Industries for the Blind and Visually Impaired of Louisiana**
PO Box 366 318-878-8171
Delhi, LA 71232-0366

9513 **Louisiana Association for the Blind**
1750 Claiborne Avenue 318-635-6471
Shreveport, LA 71103 877-913-6471
Fax: 318-635-8902
e-mail: labstore@lablind.com
www.lablind.com
LAB employs people who are blind in manufacturing administrative training and a variety of job positions that match an individual's goals and potential.
Shelly Taylor, President/CEO
William G Rogers, Vice President Administration

9514 **National Federation of the Blind: Louisana**
605 University Boulevard 318-251-1511
Ruston, LA 71270-4862 800-234-4166
e-mail: pallenp@lcb-ruston.com
www.nfbla.org
Pam Allen, President

Maine

9515 **Maine Center for the Blind and Visually Impaired**
189 Park Avenue 207-774-6273
Portland, ME 04102-2909 Fax: 207-774-0679
e-mail: info@theiris.org
www.theiris.org
Phipps, Executive Director
Retta Choate, Executive Assistant

9516 **National Federation of the Blind: Maine**
13 Whispering Pines Drive 207-221-6710
Limington, ME 04049-9707 e-mail: sallylaughlin@earthlink.net
www.nfb.org
Sally Laughlin, President

Maryland

9517 **Blind Industries and Services of Maryland**
3345 Washington Boulevard 410-737-2600
Baltimore, MD 21227 888-322-4567
Fax: 410-737-2665
www.bism.org
Blind Industries and Services of Maryland provides innovative rehabilitation services training and stable employment opportunities to our state's citizens who are blind or visually impaired.
Don Morris, Chairperson
Walter Brown, Vice-Chairperson

9518 **East Central Region: Hellen Keller National Center**
9320 Annapolis Road 301-459-5474
Lanham, MD 20706 Fax: 301-459-5070
TTY: 301-459-5433
TDD: 301-459-5433
e-mail: hkncreg3cl@aol.com
www.helenkeller.org
The Helen Keller National Center for Deaf- Blind Youths& Adu;ts offers intensive and comprehensive rehabilitation raining to individuals who are deaf- blind.
Cynthia L Ingraham, Regional Representative
Jackie Greenfield, Administrative Assistant

9519 **National Federation of the Blind: Maryland**
1026 E 36th Street 410-235-3073
Baltimore, MD 21218 e-mail: president@nfbmd.org
www.nfbmd.org/
Melissa Riccobono, President
Debbie Brown, First Vice President

Massachusetts

9520 **Carroll Center for the Blind**
770 Centre Street 617-969-6200
Newton, MA 02458-2597 800-852-3131
Fax: 617-969-6204
TTY: 617-969-6204
e-mail: info at carroll dot org
www.carroll.org
Assists blind and visually impaired adults and adolescents to adjust to loss of vision. The goal of this dynamic program is to en-

courage independence, restore self-confidence, prepare for employment and improve the quality of life.
Dina Rosenbaum, Vice President of Marketing
Rachel Rosenbaum, President

9521 **Ferguson Industries for the Blind**
One Highland Avenue 617-727-9840
Malden, MA 02148 Fax: 781-324-3111
www.state.ma.us/mcb/ferguson.html

9522 **Massachusetts Commission for the Blind**
48 Boylston Street 617-727-5550
Boston, MA 2116—4718 800-392-6450
Fax: 617-626-7685
TTY: 800-392-6556
TDD: 800-392-6556
e-mail: cheryl.standley@state.ma.us
www.state.ma.us/mcb
Provides services to blind citizens of Massachusetts, enabling them to lead more fulfilling and independent lives. Offers vocational rehabilitation, independent living, social services, home care and respite assistance, radio reading programs and print resources.
Cheryl Standley, Contact
Janet LaBreck, Commissioner

9523 **National Federation of the Blind: Massachusetts**
140 Wood Street 508-679-8543
Somerset, MA 02726-5225 e-mail: nfbmass@earthlink.net
http://www.nfbmass.org/
Priscilla Ferris, President

9524 **New England Region: Helen Keller National Center**
152 Lincoln Road 781-259-7100
Lincoln, MA 01773 Fax: 781-259-4014
e-mail: hknc1mcb@comcast.net
www.hknc.org
Mary Ellen Barbiasz, Regional Representative
Peg Ouellette, Administrative Assistant

Michigan

9525 **Association for the Blind & Visually Impaired**
456 Cherry Southeast 616-458-1187
Grand Rapids, MI 49503 800-466-8084
Fax: 616-458-7113
e-mail: blindser@abvimichigan.org
www.abvimichigan.org
To advance the independence of people who are visually impaired and to promote the prevention of blindness.
Richard A Stevens, Executive Director
George Kremer, Director of Rehabilitation Services

9526 **Greater Detroit Agency for the Blind and Visually Impaired**
16625 Grand River Avenue 313-272-3900
Detroit, MI 48227-1419 Fax: 313-272-6893
e-mail: information@gdabvi.org
www.gdabvi.org
We are a non-profit organization dedicated to preventing blindness reducing the impact of blindness and advocating for those with severe vision loss.
Gail L McEntee, President & CEO
Christina Schlitt, Administrative Manager

9527 **National Federation of the Blind: Michigan**
1212 N Foster Avenue 517-482-1800
Lansing, MI 48912-3309 e-mail: f.wurtzel@comcast.net
www.nfbmi.org
Fred Wurtzel, President
Mary Ann Rojek, State Braille Coin Project Coordinator

Minnesota

9528 **Duluth Lighthouse for the Blind**
4505 W Superior Street 218-624-4828
Duluth, MN 55807-2728 800-422-0833
Fax: 218-624-4479
e-mail: info@lighthousefortheblind-duluth.org
www.lighthousefortheblind-duluth.org
The LightHouse for the blind is a sheltered facility providing employment for blind and visually-impaired individuals.
Georgia G, Executive Director
Julaine Netzel, Intervenor/Service Support Person

9529 **National Federation of the Blind: Minnesota**
5132 Queen Avenue South 612-872-9363
Minneapolis, MN 55410-2217 e-mail: joyce.scanlan@earthlink.net
http://www.nfbmn.org/
Joyce Scanlan, President

Mississippi

9530 **Mississippi Industries for the Blind**
2501 N W Street 601-984-3200
Jackson, MS 39296-4417 866-859-4461
Fax: 601-987-3892
e-mail: bcoy@msblind.org
www.msblind.org
The Mississippi Industries for the Blind seeks to provide jobs for the blind and visually-impaired.
Michael Chew, Executive Director
Bob Coy, Sales Manager

9531 **National Federation of the Blind: Mississippi**
268 Lexington Avenue 601-969-3352
Jackson, MI 39209-5431 e-mail: samgleese@earthlink.net
Sam Gleese, President

Missouri

9532 **Alphapointe Association for the Blind**
7501 Prospect 816-421-5848
Kansas City, MO 64132 Fax: 816-237-2019
e-mail: sliptak@alphapointe.org.
www.alphapointe.org
The Alphapointe Association for the Blind has a Braille library a Senior Adult Services Program and a dedication to finding employment for the blind and visually-impaired.
Reinhard Mabry, President/CEO
James E Van Winkle, VP Administration/CFO

9533 **Kansas City Association for the Blind**
1844 Broadway Street 816-333-2173
Kansas City, MO 64108-2007

9534 **National Federation of the Blind: Missouri**
3910 Tropical Lane 573-874-1774
Columbia, MO 65202-6205 e-mail: info@nfbmo.org
www.nfbmo.org
Gary Wunder, President
Shelia Wright, First Vice President

Montana

9535 **National Federation of the Blind: Montana**
408 W Sussex Avenue 406-546-8546
Missoula, MT 59801 e-mail: burk.dall@gmail.com
www.mt-blind.org
Daniel Burke, President
Dick Howse, 1st Vice President

Nebraska

9536 **National Federation of the Blind: Nebraska**
1033 O Street 402-477-7711
Lincoln, NE 68508-2468 866-254-6347
e-mail: amy.buresh@ncbvi.ne.gov
nfbn.inebraska.com
Amy Buresh, President
Jeff Altman, First Vice President

Nevada

9537 **National Federation of the Blind: Nevada**
8455 W Sahara Avenue 702-639-9072
Las Vegas, NV 89117 e-mail: terri.rupp@gmail.com
ww.nfb.org
Terri Rupp, President

9538 **Southern Nevada Sightless**
1001 N Bruce Street
Las Vegas, NV 89101-1247
702-642-6000
Fax: 702-649-6739
e-mail: info@blindcenter.org
www.blindcenter.org
Neal Marek, Chairman
Veronica Wilson, President/CEO

New Hampshire

9539 **National Federation of the Blind: New Hampshire**
11 Springfield Street
Concord, NH 03301
603-225-7917
e-mail: jomar2000@comcast.net
Marie Johnson, President

New Jersey

9540 **Bestwork Industries for the Blind**
801 E Clements Bridge Road
Runnemede, NJ 08078
856-939-5220
800-370-9560
Fax: 856-939-5022
e-mail: bestwork@bestworkindustries.org
www.bestworkindustries.org
Bestwork Industries for the Blind is dedicated to providing employment opportunities for those with visual impairments.
James Varsaci, Founder

9541 **National Federation of the Blind: New Jersey**
254 Spruce Street
Bloomfield, NJ 07003
973-743-0075
e-mail: nfbnj@yahoo.com
http://www.nfbnj.org/
Joe Ruffalo, President

New Mexico

9542 **National Federation of the Blind: New Mexico**
1331 Park Avenue Southwest
Albuquerque, NM 87102
505-243-6165
e-mail: blindart@myfreedombox.com
http://www.nfbnm.org/
Arthur Schreiber, President

9543 **New Mexico Industries for the Blind**
2200 Yale Boulevard SE
Albuquerque, NM 87106-4212
505-841-8844
888-513-7958
Fax: 505-841-8850
e-mail: Greg.Trapp@state.nm.us
www.state.nm.us/cftb
Greg Trapp, Executive Director
Dallas Allen, Commissioner

9544 **Region 5 of the National Association for Parents of the Visually Impaired**
PO Box 1337
Alamogordo, NM 88311-1337
505-682-2693
ww.spedex.com/napvi

9545 **State of New Mexico Commission for the Blind**
2905 Rodeo Park Drive E
Santa Fe, NM 87505
505-476-4479
888-513-7968
e-mail: Greg.Trapp@state.nm.us
www.state.nm.us/cftb
The mission of the New Mexico Commission for the Blind is to encourage and enable blind citizens to achieve vocational economic and social equality. It provides career preparation and training in the skills of blindness.
Greg Trapp, Executive Director
Arthur A Schreiber, Chairman

New York

9546 **Association for the Blind & Visually Impaired of Greater Rochester**
422 South Clinton Avenue
Rochester, NY 14620-1198
585-232-1111
www.raen.org
Our mission is to assist people who are blind or visually impaired to achieve their highest level of independence in all aspects of their lives.
A Gidget Hopf, EdD, President/CEO

9547 **Blind Association of Western New York**
1170 Main Street
Buffalo, NY 14209-2331
716-882-1025
e-mail: guildcarebuffalo@jgb.org
www.olmstedcenter.org
Ronald Maier, President
Milissa Acquard, Chief Operations Officer/CFO

9548 **Blind Work Association**
55 Washington Street
Binghamton, NY 13901-3770
607-724-2428
Fax: 607-771-8045
e-mail: bobh@clarityconnect.com
www.co.tompkins.ny.us

9549 **Central Association for the Blind and Visually Impaired**
507 Kent Street
Utica, NY 13501-2317
315-797-2233
877-719-9996
Fax: 315-797-2244
e-mail: info@cabui.org
www.cabvi.org
Paul Drejza, Chairman
Peter Emery Sr, Vice Chairman

9550 **National Federation of the Blind: New York**
PO Box 09-0363
Brooklyn, NY 11209-4617
718-567-7821
Fax: 718-765-1843
e-mail: office@nfbny.org
www.nfbny.org
Carl Jacobsen, President
Mindy Fliegelman, Vice President

9551 **Northeast Regional Training Center: Canine Companions for Independence**
SUNY Farmingdale
PO Box 205
Farmingdale, NY 11735-0205
631-694-6938
800-572-2275
TTY: 631-694-6938
e-mail: jdiamond@caninecompanions.org
www.caninecompanions.org
Canine Companions for Independence is a non-profit organization that enhances the lives of people with disabilities by providing highly trained assistance dogs and ongoing support to ensure quality partnerships.
Alan Feinne, CFO
Corey Hudson, CEO

9552 **Northeastern Association of the Blind of Albany**
301 Washington Avenue
Albany, NY 12206-3012
518-463-1211
Fax: 518-463-5883
e-mail: info@naba-vision.org
www.naba-vision.org
NABA offers a wide range of services to those with visual impairments from its free vision screening service for children to training and placing legally blind adults in professional employment. Also provides rehabilitation services to seniors with age-related conditions.
Christopher Burke, Interim Executive Director
Larry N Volk, Chair

9553 **Southern Tier Association for the Visually Impaired**
719 Lake Street
Elmira, NY 14901-2538
607-734-1554
Fax: 607-734-9467
e-mail: info@st-avi.org
www.st-avi.org
Timothy Hertlein, Executive Director
Cindy Young, Fiscal Administrator

North Carolina

9554 **Lions Industries for the Blind**
4126 Berkeley Avenue
Kinston, NC 28504-8321
252-523-1019
Fax: 252-523-7090
e-mail: ray_amyette@lionsindustries.org
www.lionsindustries.com
The Lions Industries for the Blind provides employment opportunities for the blind and visually-impaired.
Bob Smith, Executive Director
Danny Rice, Chairman

9555 **National Federation of the Blind: North Carolina**
128 Summerlea Drive
Charlotte, NC 28214-1324
704-491-1486
Fax: 704-391-3204
e-mail: tjnc2@carolina.rr.com
http://www.nfbofnc.org/
Tim Jones, President

9556 **Winston-Salem Industries for the Blind**
7730 N Point Drive
Winston-Salem, NC 27106-3310
336-759-0551
800-242-7726
Fax: 336-759-0990
e-mail: info@wsifb.com
www.wsifb.com
The Winston-Salem Industries for the Blind provides employment opportunities for the blind and visually-impaired.
Daniel J Boucher, Executive Chairman
Ann Johnston, Chairman

North Dakota

9557 **National Federation of the Blind: North Dakota**
2581 Villa Drive S
Fargo, ND 58103
701-298-2963
e-mail: jcbichler@msn.com
www.nfb.org
Jennelle Bichler, President

Ohio

9558 **Cincinnati Association for the Blind**
2045 Gilbert Avenue
Cincinnati, OH 45202-1490
513-221-8558
888-687-3935
Fax: 513-221-2995
e-mail: info@cincyblind.org
www.cincyblind.org
Persons who are blind visually impaired or print impaired may choose from a wide range of services to help them live more independently. Our services are provided by qualified certified instructors and staff with highly specialized skills.

9559 **Cleveland Sight Center**
1909 E 101st Street
Cleveland, OH 44106-8696
216-791-8118
Fax: 216-791-1101
e-mail: sfriedman@clevelandsightcenter.org
www.clevelandsightcenter.org
Mission is to enable people with vision impairment to reach their full potential and assure that adequate services are available to make a normal life possible.
Stanley E Wertheim, Chair
Steven M Friedman, President/CEO

9560 **Cleveland Skilled Industries**
2239 E 55th Street
Cleveland, OH 44103-4451
216-431-8085
Fax: 216-431-5123

9561 **National Federation of the Blind: Ohio**
237 Oak Street
Oberlin, OH 44074-1517
440-775-2216
e-mail: bbpierce@pobox.com
www.nfbohio.org
J Webster Smith, President
Barbara Pierce, President Emerita

9562 **North Central Regional Training Center: Canine Companions for Independence**
4989 State Route 37 E
Delaware, OH 43015-9682
740-548-4447
800-572-2275
Fax: 740-363-0555
TTY: 740-548-4447
www.caninecompanions.org
Canine Companions for Independence is a non-profit organization that enriches the lives of people with disabilities by providing highly trained assistance dogs and ongoing support to ensure quality partnerships.
Corey Hudson, CEO
Alan Feinne, CFO

9563 **Region 2 of the National Association for Parents of the Visually Impaired**
5786 Arlyne Lane
Medina, OH 44256-3825
330-722-6609
www.spedex.com/napvi
Victoria Gor Miller
Rachel Miller, President

9564 **Society of the Blind: Akron Center**
325 E Market Street
Akron, OH 44304-1340
330-253-2555
Fax: 330-996-4088

Oklahoma

9565 **National Federation of the Blind: Oklahoma**
242 E 35th Street
Tulsa, OK 74105
918-850-6751
e-mail: selena.j.sundling@irs.gov
www.nfb.org
Selena Sundling-Craw, President

9566 **Oklahoma League for the Blind**
501 N Douglas Avenue
Oklahoma City, OK 73106
405-232-4644
Fax: 405-236-5438
e-mail: info@olb.org
www.olb.org
The mission of the Oklahoma League for the Blind is to facilitate independence and improve the quality of life for people who are blind or vision impaired by providing employment opportunities and services.
Lauren White, President/CEO
Carol Campbell, Executive Assistant

Oregon

9567 **Blind Enterprises of Oregon**
6540 SE Foster Road
Portland, OR 97206
503-774-6387
Fax: 503-774-0585
e-mail: blindent@aol.com
www.blindenterprises.com
Jennifer Williams, Operations Manager
Tami Foss, Executive Director

9568 **National Federation of the Blind: Oregon**
1616 5th Street NE
Salem, OR 97301
503-585-4318
800-422-7093
e-mail: artds55@comcast.net
www.nfb.org
Art Stevenson, President

Pennsylvania

9569 **Association for the Blind & Visually Impaired of Lehigh County**
845 Wyoming Street
Allentown, PA 18103-2199
610-433-6018
Fax: 610-433-4856
e-mail: info@abvi.org
www.abvi.org
The ABVI mission is to strive to be our community's foremost provider and coordinator of preventative, educational, social and rehabilitative programs concerning vision loss. Our goal is to assist each individual and his/her family to achieve their greatest potential.
Kathleen Meckes, Executive Director

9570 **Beaver County Association for the Blind**
616 Fourth Street
Beaver Falls, PA 15010
724-843-1111
Fax: 724-843-8886
e-mail: bcab@forcomm.net
bcab2.tripoid.com
The Beaver County Association for the Blind conducts educational programs about blindness or vision problems by request and provides opportunities to learn experience share and celebrate in the lives of the blind and visually impaired in Beaver County.
Fay Lentz, Executive Director
Linda Borghi, Controller/Business Manager

9571 **Cambria County Association for the Blind and Handicapped**
211 Central Avenue
Johnstown, PA 15902
814-536-3531
Fax: 814-539-3270
e-mail: ccabh@ccabh.com
www.ccabh.com

The mission of the Cambria County Association for the Blind and Handicapped is to develop and support an environment for persons with disabilities which promotes vocational and employment training, independence and community involvement through rehabilitative programs.
Richard C Bosserman, President

9572 Chester County Association for the Blind
71 S First Avenue 610-384-2767
Coatesville, PA 19320 Fax: 610-384-8005
e-mail: info@chescoblind.org
www.chescoblind.org
Anita Cavuto, Executive Director
John W Esworthy, President

9573 Chester County Branch of the Pennsylvania Association for the Blind
71 S First Avenue 610-384-2767
Coatesville, PA 19320-3461 Fax: 610-384-8005
e-mail: info@chescoblind.org
www.chescoblind.org
John W Esworthy, President
Anita Cavuto, Executive Director

9574 DELCO Blind/Sight Center
100 W Fifteenth Street 610-874-1476
Chester, PA 19013 Fax: 610-874-6454
e-mail: info@delcoblind.org
www.delcoblind.org
This agency is dedicated to helping individuals in the greater Delaware Valley area to prevent, prepare for and adapt to vision loss in order to achieve independence. Our goal is to help those with blindness or vision loss to lead well adjusted, independent lives.
Robert M Nelson, Executive Director

9575 Delaware County Branch of the Pennsylvania Association for the Blind
100-106 W 15th Street 610-874-1476
Chester, PA 19013 Fax: 610-874-6454
e-mail: delcosce@liberty.org
www.libertynet.org

9576 Greater Wilkes-Barre Association for the Blind
1825 Wyoming Avenue 570-693-3555
Exeter, PA 18643 877-693-3555
Fax: 570-823-4841
e-mail: info@wilkesbarreblind.com
www.wilkesbarreblind.com
Our mission is to address the needs of those with limited vision and we also take an active role in the prevention of blindness.
Ronald V Petrilla, Executive Director
Denise Culver, Office Manager

9577 Indiana County Association for the Blind
31 S 10th Street 724-465-5549
Indiana, PA 15701-2649

9578 Keystone Blind Association
1230 Stambaugh Avenue 724-347-5501
Sharon, PA 16146 800-837-4122
Fax: 724-347-2204
e-mail: kba@keystoneblind.org
www.keystoneblind.org
The Keystone Blind Association is dedicated to maintaining and improving the quality of life for blind and/or visually impaired persons preventing blindness and providing employment opportunities and advocacy for persons who are disabled.
Jonathan G Fister, President/CEO
Perry Templeton, Vice President of Operations

9579 Lancaster County Association for the Blind
244 N Queen Street
Lancaster, PA 17603-3512 717-291-5951
www.sabvi.com
Dennis L Steiner, President/CEO
Kay L Macsi, VP Rehabilitation and Education

9580 Montgomery County Association for the Blind
212 N Main Street 215-661-9800
North Wales, PA 19454-3117 Fax: 215-661-9888
e-mail: mcab@mcab.org
www.mcab.org
MCAB's mission is to enhance the quality of life and independence of people coping with blindness and vision impairment through rehabilitation education support and advocacy.
Douglas Yingling, Executive Director
Sharon Zislis, Director of Development

9581 National Federation of the Blind: Pennsylvania
42 South 15th Street 215-988-0888
Philadelphia, PA 19102-2206 e-mail: nfbofpa@att.net
http://www.nfbp.org/
James Antonacci, President

9582 North Central Sight Services
2121 Reach Road 570-323-9401
Williamsport, PA 17704-0292 866-320-2580
Fax: 570-323-8194
e-mail: ncss@ncsight.org
www.ncsight.org
Our agency philosophy focuses on helping people help themselves and emphasizes the abilities and capabilities of the blind and visually impaired people we serve.
Robert B Garrett, President/CEO
Barbara Snauffer, Administrative Assistant

9583 Pennsylvania Association for the Blind
90 E Shady Lane 717-234-3261
Enola, PA 17025 Fax: 717-234-4733
e-mail: neal.carrigan@pablind.org
www.pablind.org
Neal J Carrigan, President/CEO
Willard D Brown, Vice-President for Finance

9584 Pittsburgh Branch for the Pennsylvania Association for the Blind
1800 W Street 412-368-4400
Homestead, PA 15120-3707 800-706-5050
Fax: 412-368-4090
TTY: 412-368-4095
e-mail: info&ref@pghvis.org
ww.pghvis.org
Stephen S Barrett, President
James Baumgartner, Vice President of Finance

9585 Pittsburgh Vision Services
1800 W Street 412-368-4400
Homestead, PA 15120 800-706-5050
Fax: 412-368-4090
TTY: 412-368-4095
e-mail: info&ref@pghvis.org
www.pghvis.org
Pittsburgh Vision Services is a private non-profit United Way agency whose mission is to reduce the limitations that may result from loss of vision.
Stephen S Barrett, President
James Baumgartner, Vice President of Finance

9586 Somerset County Blind Center
748 S Center Avenue 814-445-1310
Somerset, PA 15501 Fax: 814-445-3184
e-mail: rob@somersetblind.org
www.somersetblind.org
The Somerset Blind Center offers a number of services to those who are blind or visually impaired, including work opportunities, eyeglass prescription programs, free vision screenings, and training facilities.
Rob Stemple, Executive Director
Anna Hope, Finance Manager

9587 Tri-County Association for the Blind
1130 S 19th Street 717-238-2531
Harrisburg, PA 17102-2200 Fax: 717-238-0710
e-mail: info@tricountyblind.org
www.tricountyblind.org
The Tri-County Association for the Blind works to improve the quality of life for people who are visually-impaired in the

Tri-County region, by helping each person achieve his or her full potential and maximum independence.
Danette Blank, Executive Director
Laurie Thompson, Public Relations/Development Director

9588 **VIABL Services of Northampton County**
260 E Broad Street
Bethlehem, PA 18018
610-866-8049
Fax: 610-866-8730
e-mail: viabl@viablservices.org
www.viablservices.org
Our mission is to promote the social economic and physical self-sufficiency of blind deaf-blind and visually impaired individuals by providing them with the resources and skills needed to live rewarding productive and independent lives.
Jan Leon, Executive Director

9589 **Washington-Greene County Branch for the Pennsylvania Association for Blind**
566 E Maiden Street
Washington, PA 15301-3720
412-228-0770
Fax: 412-228-6617
e-mail: washgreene@verizon.net
www.pablind.org
Elaine R Welch, President/CEO
Willard D Brown, Vice-President for Finance

9590 **York Industries for the Blind: Division of York County Blind Center**
A Division of York County Blind Center
1380 Spahn Avenue
York, PA 17403-5711
717-848-1690
Fax: 717-845-3889
www.forsight.org
William H Rhinesmith, President

Rhode Island

9591 **IN-SIGHT**
43 Jefferson Boulevard
Warwick, RI 02888
401-941-3322
Fax: 401-941-3356
e-mail: insightri@gmail.com
www.in-sight.org
IN-SIGHT is a private non-profit agency which has been serving the blind and visually impaired since 1925.
Gerard Goulet, President
Eleanor Acton, Director of Communications

9592 **National Federation of the Blind: Rhode Island**
PO Box 154564
Riverside, RI 02915
401-433-2606
Fax: 877-383-3682
e-mail: info@nfbri.org
www.nfbri.org
Richard Gaffney, President

South Carolina

9593 **National Federation of the Blind: South Carolina**
1293 Professional Drive
Myrtle Beach, SC 29577
803-254-3777
e-mail: parnell@sccoast.net
http://www.nfbsc.net/
Parnell Diggs, President

9594 **Region 4 of the National Association for Parents of the Visually Impaired**
1032 Trail Road
Belton, SC 29627-7926
864-338-9593
www.spedex.com/napvi

South Dakota

9595 **National Federation of the Blind: South Dakota**
903 Fulton Street
Rapid City, SD 57701
605-791-3939
e-mail: President@nfb-south-dakota.org
www.nfb-south-dakota.org
Kenneth Rollman, President

Tennessee

9596 **Ed Lindsey Industries of the Blind**
4110 Charlotte Avenue
Nashville, TN 37209-3749
615-741-2251
Fax: 615-741-5024

9597 **National Federation of the Blind: Tennessee**
1226 Goodman Circle West
Memphis, TN 38111-6524
901-452-6596
e-mail: michael.seay@ssa.gov
http://www.nfb-tennessee.org/
Michael Seay, President

9598 **West Tennessee Lions Blind Industries**
PO Box 2175
Memphis, TN 38101-2175
901-767-5466

Texas

9599 **American Foundation for the Blind**
11030 Ables Lane
Dallas, TX 75229
214-352-7222
Fax: 214-352-3214
e-mail: dallas@afb.net
www.afb.org
Leads initiatives in the areas of aging and education. Nationally offers consultation, technical assistance and support and undertakes local and national efforts such as training programs, public education and coalition building in the areas of aging and elder care.

9600 **American Foundation for the Blind: National Aging Center**
11030 Ables Lane
Dallas, TX 75229
214-352-7222
Fax: 214-352-3214
e-mail: dallas@afb.net
www.afb.org
Leads initiatives in the areas of aging and education. Nationally offers consultaion, technical assistance and support and undertakes local and national efforts such as training programs, public education and coalition building in the areas of aging and education. Responds to inquiries from blind and visually impaired people and their families, service providers and the general public in the region and nationally.

9601 **Beacon Lighthouse**
300 7th Street
Wichita Falls, TX 76301-1699
940-767-0888
800-262-6412
Fax: 817-767-0893
e-mail: jkoszarek@beaconwf.com
www.beaconwf.com

9602 **Dallas Lighthouse for the Blind**
4245 Office Parkway
Dallas, TX 75204
214-821-2375
Fax: 214-824-4612
www.dallaslighthouse.org
The Dallas Lighthouse for the Blind provides work opportunities for the blind and visually impaired.
Michael Orfinik, Chief Executive Officer
Nancy J Perkins, President

9603 **East Texas Lighthouse for the Blind**
500 N Bois D'Arc
Tyler, TX 75702
903-595-3444
888-595-3444
Fax: 903-595-3447
e-mail: customerservice@horizonind.com
www.horizonind.com

9604 **El Paso Lighthouse for the Blind**
200 Washington Street
El Paso, TX 79905
915-532-4495
Fax: 915-532-6338
e-mail: htyler@elp.rr.com
www.lighthouse-elpaso.com
Lighthouse is guided by the unwavering belief that its rehabilitative and employment services can help any person overcome his or her disability and enable them to reach their fullest potential for self-sufficiency and independence.
Harry Tyler, President/CEO
Rusty Hooten, CFO

9605 **Lighthouse for the Blind of Houston**
3602 W Dallas
Houston, TX 77019-0435
713-527-9561
Fax: 713-284-8451
e-mail: houstonlighthouse@houstonlighthouse.org
ww.houstonlighthouse.org
Founded in 1839 the Lighthouse of Houston is a private nonprofit rehabilitation center dedicated to helping blind and visually impaired people live independently.
Gibson M DuTerroil, President

9606 Lighthouse of the Blind of Fort Worth
912 W Broadway Street 817-332-3341
Fort Worth, TX 76104 Fax: 817-332-3456
e-mail: plattallen@lighthousefw.org.
www.lighthousefw.org
The Lighthouse of the Blind of Fort Worth offers many services including skills assessment orientation and mobilty training assisted employment and senior services.
Platt Allen, President
Steve Peglar, Chairman

9607 National Federation of the Blind: Texas
314 E Highland Mall Boulevard 512-323-5444
Austin, TX 78752-3123 866-636-3289
Fax: 512-420-8160
e-mail: tccraig@earthlink.net
www.nfb-texas.org
Tommy Craig, President

9608 South Central Region: Helen Keller National Center
12160 Abrams Road 972-490-9677
Dallas, TX 75243-5903 Fax: 972-490-6042
TTY: 972-490-9677
e-mail: ccfutbol@aol.com
www.hknc.org
C C Davis, Regional Representative

9609 South Texas Lighthouse for the Blind
PO Box 9697 361-883-6553
Corpus Christi, TX 78469 888-255-8011
Fax: 361-883-1041
e-mail: Regisb@stlb.net
www.stlb.net
Regis Barber, President/CEO
Nicky Ooi, VP/COO

9610 Texas Association of Retinitis Pigmentosa
PO Box 8388 361-852-8515
Corpus Christi, TX 78468-8388 Fax: 361-852-8515
e-mail: tarpmail@homebiz101.com
www.geocities.com/HotSprings/7815
A nonprofit organization based in Texas serving as a national information-sharing center to provide human services to persons with progressive vision loss from retinitis pigmentosa and other retinal degenerative disorders.
Dorothy H Stiefel, Executive Director

9611 Travis Association for the Blind
2307 Business Center Drive 512-442-2329
Austin, TX 78764-3297 Fax: 512-442-5498
e-mail: info@austinlighthouse.org
www.austinlighthouse.org
Travis Association for the Blind (aka Austin Lighthouse) is a service oriented non-profit organization with the mission to assist people who are blind or vision impaired to attain the skills they need to become gainfully employed in the community.
Jerry A Mayfield, Executive Director
Benny Galloway, Chief Financial Officer

9612 West Texas Lighthouse for the Blind
2001 Austin Street 325-653-4231
San Angelo, TX 76903-8705 Fax: 325-657-9367
e-mail: d.wells@lighthousefortheblind.org
www.lighthousefortheblind.org
The West Texas Lighthouse for the Blind is a sheltered facility providing employment for blind and visually impaired individuals.
David Wells, Executive Director
Stephen Horton, Operations Manager

Utah

9613 National Federation of the Blind: Utah
161 W 600 S 801-292-3000
Salt Lake City, UT 84010-7634 888-292-3007
Fax: 801-294-6000
e-mail: president@nfbutah.org
www.nfbutah.org
Ron Gardner, President
Cheralyn Bra Creer, First Vice President

9614 Utah Industries for the Blind
PO Box 258 801-533-9689
Salt Lake Cty, UT 84110-1258

Vermont

9615 National Federation of the Blind: Vermont
1 Mechanic Street 802-229-0748
Montpelier, VT 5602 e-mail: fshiner@verizon.net
www.nfbvt.org
Franklin Shiner, President

Virginia

9616 National Federation of the Blind: Virginia
9522 Lagersfield Circle 703-319-9226
Vienna, VA 22181 e-mail: fschroeder@sks.com
www.nfbv.org
Fredric K Schroeder, President
Seville Allen, First Vice President

9617 Virginia Industries for the Blind
1102 Monticello Road 434-295-5168
Charlottesville, VA 22902 Fax: 434-977-0122
e-mail: Robert.Berrang@dbvi.virginia.gov
www.vdbvi.org/vib
Our mission is to be a self-sufficient and self-supporting industry enhance the quality of life for blind and visually impaired individuals through providing gainful employment; and provide opportunities in career development and employment related services.
Robert C Berrang, Deputy Commissioner
Richard C Bohrer, Plant Manager

Washington

9618 Lighthouse for the Blind of Washington
PO Box 14119 206-322-4200
Seattle, WA 98114 Fax: 206-329-3397

9619 National Federation of the Blind: Washington
101 NE 83rd Street 360-576-5965
Vancouver, WA 98665-7900 e-mail: k7uij@panix.com
Mike Freeman, President

9620 Northwestern Region: Helen Keller National Center
1620 18th Avenue 206-324-9120
Seattle, WA 98122-6501 Fax: 206-324-9159
TTY: 206-324-1133
e-mail: nwhknc@juno.com
www.hknc.org
Dorothy Walt, Regional Representative

9621 Washington State Department of Services for the Blind
402 Legion Way 360-725-3830
Olympia, WA 98504-0933 800-552-7103
Fax: 360-407-0679
e-mail: information@dsb.wa.gov
www.dsb.wa.gov
The Washington State Department of Services for the Blind (DSB) is a state rehabilitation agency that offers assistance to persons who are blind or visually impaired. We also provide various services for employers interested in accomodating or hiring workers with visual impairments.
Bill Palmer, Director

West Virginia

9622 AFB Technology & Employment Center
949 Third Avenue 304-523-8651
Huntington, WV 25701 800-824-2184
Fax: 304-523-8656
e-mail: AFBTECH@afb.net
www.afb.org
AFB Technology runs AFB's CareerConnect and the AFB TECH Product Evaluation Laboratory. Nationally offers consultation, technical assistance and support and undertakes local and national efforts in employment and technology.
Brad Hodges, National Technology Associate

9623 National Federation of the Blind: West Virginia
220 Buena Vista Avenue 304-622-0626
Clarksburg, WV 26301 e-mail: cs.nfbwv@verizon.net
www.nfbwv.org

Charlene Smyth, President

Wisconsin

9624 National Federation of the Blind: Wisconsin
27824 Nuthatch Road 608-758-4800
Kendall, WI 54638 e-mail: johnfritz@centurytel.net
http://www.nfbwis.org/

John Fritz, President

9625 National Federation of the Blind: Writers
27824 Nuthatch Road 608-758-4800
Kendall, WI 54638 e-mail: johnfritz@centurytel.net
www.nfbwis.org

John Fritz, President

9626 Wiscraft: Wisconsin Enterprises for the Blind
5316 W State Street 414-778-5800
Milwaukee, WI 53208-2686 Fax: 414-778-5805
e-mail: sales@wiscraft.com
www.wiscraft.com

Wiscraft provides long-term supportive employment for people who are blind. It is a manufacturing company that operates as a non-profit with the clear mission of employing people who are blind by sellng blind-made products and services.
Jim Kerlin, President
Ron Hutchinson, Chair

Wyoming

9627 National Federation of the Blind: Wyoming
PO Box 347
Sheridan, WY 82801-0347 307-672-1821
www.nfb.org

Max Aguilar, President

Foundations

9628 Foundation Fighting Blindness
11435 Cronhill Drive 410-568-0150
Owings Mills, MD 21117-2220 800-683-5555
TDD: 800-683-5551
e-mail: info@FightBlindness.org
www.fightblindness.org

For a $25.00 annual membership fee, FFB offers information and referral services for affected individuals and their families as well as for doctors and eye care professionals. The Foundation also provides comprehensive information kits on retinitis pigmentosa, macular degeneration, and usher syndrome. Their newsletter, InFocus, and their e-newsletter, InSight, present articles on coping research updates, and Foundation news. A national conference is usually held every other year.
Gordon Gund, Chairman
Edward H. Gollob, President

9629 Glaucoma Research Foundation
251 Post Street 415-986-3162
San Francisco, CA 94108 800-826-6693
Fax: 415-986-3763
e-mail: info@glaucoma.org
www.glaucoma.org

The Glaucoma Research Foundation is a nationa nonprofit dedicated to curing glaucoma. We receive no government funding. Your contribution is tax-deductible as allowed by law.
Thomas M Brunner, President/CEO

Libraries & Resource Centers

9630 District of Columbia Public Library Librarian for the Deaf Community
901 G Street North West
Washington, DC 20001 202-727-1111
www.dclibrary.org

Offers reference services through TDD, portable TDD for public use at pay phone, signers for library programs, sign language classes, information about deafness, print and non-print materials for persons who are deaf.
John W Hill, Jr, President
James W Lewis, Vice President

Alabama

9631 Alabama Radio Reading Service Network
WBHM
650 11th Street South 205-934-6576
Birmingham, AL 35294-4530 800-444-9246
Fax: 205-934-5075
e-mail: philip@wbhm.org
www.wbhm.org/ARRS

Services and readings are relayed over the radio to three-quarters of Alabama for the benefit of the visually impaired.
Philip Habeeb, Program Director

9632 Alabama Regional Library for the Blind and Physically Handicapped
Alabama Public Library Service
6030 Monticello Drive 334-213-3906
Montgomery, AL 36130-6000 800-392-5671
Fax: 334-213-3993
e-mail: fzaleski@apls.state.al.us
www.apls.state.al.us

To promote and support equitable access to library and information resources and services to enable all Alabamians to satisfy their educational, working, cultural, and leisure-time interests. These resources and services will be provided through APLS's statewide programs and through direct grants and assistance to libraries and library systems to meet user's needs.
Fara Zaleski, Division
Rebecca Mitchell, Director

9633 Houston Love Memorial Library
212 West Burdeshaw Street 334-793-9767
Dothan, AL 36303 e-mail: bforbus@yahoo.com
www.houstonlovelibrary.org

Offers magnifiers, summer reading programs and more for the blind and physically handicapped. Scanner, software and jaws for windows.
Bettye Forbus, President

9634 Huntsville Subregional Library for the Blind and Physically Handicapped
P.O. Box 443 256-532-5980
Huntsville, AL 35804 Fax: 256-532-5994
e-mail: bphdept@hpl.lib.al.us
www.hpl.lib.al.us/departments/bph

The Subregional Library for the Blind and Physically Handicapped is located in the Main branch of the Huntsville-Madison County Public Library. It is also part of a Library of Congress administered nationwide network of libraries serving persons who cannot use conventional printed materials.
Joyce Welch, Librarian

9635 Library and Resource Center for the Blind and Physically Handicapped
Alabama Institute for Deaf and Blind
705 South Street 256-761-3237
Talladega, AL 35161 800-848-4722
Fax: 256-761-3561
e-mail: lacy.teresa@aidb.state.al.us
http://www.aidb.org

Using federal and state funds, the Resource Center purchases or produces braille textbooks and other necessary materials for students. The Resource Center also loans equipment, like braillewriters, to help students learn alternative methods of communication.
Teresa Lacy, Director

9636 Tuscaloosa Subregional Library for the Blind & Physically Handicapped
1801 Jack Warner Parkway 205-345-5820
Tuscaloosa, AL 35401 Fax: 205-752-8300
e-mail: bjordan@tuscaloosa-library.org
www.tuscaloosa-library.org

Provide talking books to patrons who are unable to use standard print because of a visual or physical limitation. Deliver playback equipment to qualified patrons. Provides reference and referral service to this special population also.
Barbara Jordan, Librarian

Alaska

9637 **Alaska State Library Talking Book Center**
National Library Services
344 W 3rd Avenue
Anchorage, AK 99501-2337
907-269-6575
800-776-6566
Fax: 907-269-6580
TDD: 907-269-6575
e-mail: tbc@eed.state.ak.us
www.library.state.ak.us
The Alaska State Library Talking Book Center is a cooperative effort between the National Library Service and the Alaska State Library to provide print handicapped Alaskans with talking book and Braille service.
Bev Griffin, Library Assistant II
Rachel Garner, Administrative Clerk I

Arizona

9638 **Arizona State Braille and Talking Book Library**
1030 N 32nd Street
Phoenix, AZ 85008-5108
602-255-5578
800-255-5578
Fax: 602-255-4312
e-mail: btbl@lib.az.us
www.lib.az.us
Closed-circuit TV, summer reading programs, volunteer-produced cassette books, braille writer, films, large-print photocopier and more.
Linda Montgomery, Division Director

9639 **Flagstaff City Coconino County Public Library**
300 W Aspen Avenue
Flagstaff, AZ 86001-5304
520-779-7670
www.flagstaffpubliclibrary.org
Reference materials on blindness and other handicaps, braille writer, magnifiers and large-print photocopier.

9640 **Phoenix Public Library: Special Needs Section**
Burton Barr Central Library
1221 North Central Avenue
Phoenix, AZ 85004
602-262-4636
TDD: 602-254-8205
e-mail: specialneeds@phxlib.org
www.phoenixpubliclibrary.org
The Special Needs Center is designed to make the services and resources of the Phoenix Public Library accessible to people with disabilities.
Toni Garvey, City Librarian

Arkansas

9641 **Arkansas Regional Library for the Blind and Physically Handicapped**
One Capitol Mall
Little Rock, AR 72201-1049
501-682-1155
866-660-0885
Fax: 501-682-1529
TDD: 501-682-1002
e-mail: nlsbooks@asl.lib.ar.us
www.asl.lib.ar.us
Public library books in recorded or braille format. Popular fiction and nonfiction books for all ages, books and players are on free loan, sent to patrons by mail and may be returned postage free. Anyone who cannot see well enough to read regular print with glasses on or who has a disability that makes it difficult to hold a book or turn the pages is eligible.
John D Hall, Coordinator

9642 **Library for the Blind and Handicapped, Southwest**
Columbia County Library
220 East Main Street
Magnolia, AR 71754
870-234-0399
866-234-8273
Fax: 870-234-5077
e-mail: lbph@hotmail.com
www.youseemore.com/columbia
The mission of the Columbia County Library is to help the people of our community in their pursuits of information and education , as well as vocational and recreational endeavors, by providing current materials, services, and programs. Our inviting public libraries are the cornerstone of our diverse communities where all people, regardless of age, race, or socio-economic circumstances can experience personal enrichment and literary growth.
Dana Thornton, Interim Director
Sandra Grissom, Librarian

California

9643 **Blind Childrens Center**
4120 Marathon Street
Los Angeles, CA 90029-3584
323-664-2153
Fax: 323-665-3828
www.blindchildrenscenter.org
The Blind Childrens Center is a family-centered agency which serves children with visual impairments from birth to school-age. The center-based and home-based programs and services help the children acquire skills and build their independence. The Center utilizes its expertise and experience to serve families and professionals worldwide through support services, education, and research.
Midge Horton, Executive Director
Muriel Scharf, Director Development

9644 **Braille Institute Library Services**
741 North Vermont Avenue
Los Angeles, CA 90029-3594
323-663-1111
800-808-2555
Fax: 323-662-2440
TDD: 323-660-3880
e-mail: dls@braillelibrary.org
www.braillelibrary.org
The Braille Institute is a non-profit organization whose mission is to eliminate barriers to a fulfilling life caused by blindness and severe sight loss. The Institute provides an environment of hope and encouragement for people who are blind and visually impaired through integrated educational, social and recreational services and programs.
Henry C. Chang, Librarian

9645 **California State Library Braille and Talking Book Library**
National Library Service
PO Box 942837
Sacramento, CA 94237-0001
916-654-0640
800-952-5666
Fax: 916-654-1119
e-mail: btbl@library.ca.gov
www.library.ca.gov
Library services in braille and recorded formats. Free to residents of Northern California who are unable to read ordinary print on hold a printed book.
Michael Marlin, Manager
Mary Jane Kayes, Outreach Coordinator

9646 **Fresno County Public Library: Talking Book Library for the Blind**
770 North San Pablo Avenue
Fresno, CA 93728-3640
559-488-3217
800-742-1011
Fax: 559-488-1971
TDD: 559-488-1642
e-mail: wendy.eisenberg@fresnolibrary.org
www.fresnolibrary.org/tblb
We provide books and magazines on cassette tape and in Braille to people of all ages who are blind, visually impaired, or have physical disabilities preventing the reading of standard print.
Karen Bosch Cobb, County Librarian
Wendy Eisenberg, Librarian

9647 **San Francisco Public Library for the Blind and Print Disabled**
100 Larkin Street
San Francisco, CA 94102-4733
415-557-4253
TTY: 415-557-4433
e-mail: citylibrarian@sfpl.org
www.sfpl.lib.ca.us
Foreign-language books on cassette, children's books on cassettes and more.
Luis Herrera, City Librarian
Marcia Schneider, Chief, Communications/Adult Services

9648 **San Jose State University Library**
1 Washington Square
San Jose, CA 95192-0001 408-924-1000
www.library.sjsu.edu
Information on physical disabilities, accessibility and learning disabilities.

Colorado

9649 **Boulder Public Library**
1000 Canyon Boulevard 303-441-3100
Boulder, CO 80302-1326 Fax: 303-442-1808
e-mail: ask@boulder.lib.co.us
www.boulder.lib.co.us
Offers braille books, cassettes, talking books, large print photocopier, large print books and more for the visually impaired.
Tony Tallent, Library & Arts Director

9650 **Colorado Talking Book Library**
180 Sheridan Boulevard 303-727-9277
Denver, CO 80226-8101 800-685-2136
Fax: 303-727-9281
e-mail: ctbl.info@cde.state.co.us
www.cde.state.co.us
Take advantage of the services offered by the Colorado Talking Book Library (CTBL). CTBL provides postage-free recorded, braille, and large print library materials to eligible residents in Colorado.
Debbi MacLeod, Director

Connecticut

9651 **Connecticut State Library for the Blind and Physically Handicapped**
198 W Street 860-721-2020
Rocky Hill, CT 06067-3554 800-842-4516
Fax: 860-721-2056
e-mail: lbph@cslib.org
www.cslib.org/lbph.htm
Free audio cassettes and braille books and magazines along with reference materials on blindness and other handicaps. Necessary playback equipment for eligible residents of Connecticut.
Carol Taylor, Director

Delaware

9652 **Delaware Division of Libraries: Library for the Blind and Physically Handicapped**
43 South DuPont Highway 302-739-4748
Dover, DE 19901 800-282-8676
Fax: 302-739-6787
TDD: 302-739-4847
e-mail: john.phillos@state.de.us
www.state.lib.de.us
Since 1971, the Delaware Library for the Blind and Physically Handicapped has provided books in Braille and audio books on record and cassette for the blind and physically handicapped residents of Delaware.
John Phillos, Librarian

District of Columbia

9653 **Council of Families with Visual Impairment**
American Council of the Blind
1155 15th Street NW 202-467-5081
Washington, DC 20005 800-424-8666
Fax: 202-467-5085
e-mail: info@acb.org
www.acb.org
Members are sighted parents of blind or visually impaired children. Offers a forum for support and outreach, sharing of experiences in parent-child relationships, and educational and cultural information about child development. Monitors developments in technical and legislative arenas.
Melanie Brunson, Executive Director

9654 **DC Public Library Adaptive Services Division**
901 G Street NW, Room 215 202-727-2142
Washington, DC 20001 Fax: 202-727-1129
TTY: 202-727-2255
TDD: 202-727-1129
e-mail: lbph.dcpl@dc.gov
www.dclibrary.org
The DC Public Library has a special Adaptive Technology Program to help older adults, the deaf, and those with visual and physical disabilities use library materials and resources.
Venetia V. Demson, Librarian

9655 **National Library Service for the Blind and Physically Handicapped**
Library of Congress 202-707-9261
Washington, DC 20542 Fax: 202-707-0712
TDD: 202-707-0744
e-mail: raj@loc.gov
www.loc.gov/nls
The NLS, Library of Congress, administers the free programs that loans recorded and braille books and magazines, music scores in braille and large print, and specially designed playback equipment to residents of the United States who are unable to read or use standard print materials due to visual or physical impairment.
Yealuri Rathan Raj, Librarian

Florida

9656 **Brevard County Libraries: Talking Books Library**
308 Forrest Avenue 321-633-1810
Cocoa, FL 32922-7781 Fax: 321-633-1838
e-mail: dmartin@brev.org
www.brev.org
The Talking Books/Homebound Services has many devices and special materials to assist blind, physically handicapped and/or homebound citizens to access library services.
Debra A. Martin, Librarian

9657 **Broward County Talking Book Library**
100 S Andrews Avenue 954-357-7555
Fort Lauderdale, FL 33301-1830 Fax: 954-577-20
e-mail: talkingbooks@browardlibrary.org
www.broward.org/library/talkingbooks
Reference materials on blindness and other handicaps, closed-circuit TV, Talking Book cassettes, print/Braille and descriptive videos.
William Forbes, Librarian

9658 **Florida Bureau of Braille and Talking Book Library Services**
421 Platt Street 386-239-6000
Daytona Beach, FL 32114-2803 800-226-6075
Fax: 386-239-6069
e-mail: mike.gunde@dbs.fldoe.org
dbs.myflorida.com/library/index.php
The Florida Bureau of Braille and Talking Book Library Services provides information and reading materials needed by Florida residents who are unable to use standard print as the result of visual, physical, or reading disabilities.
Michael Gunde, Librarian

9659 **Hillsborough County Talking Book Library**
Jan Kaminis Platt Regional Library
3910 South Manahattan Avenue 813-272-6024
Tampa, FL 33611-1214 Fax: 813-272-6072
TDD: 813-272-6305
e-mail: talkingbooks@hillsboroughounty.org
hcplc.org/hcplc/liblocales/tbl
This free program provides recorded and braille books and magazines to people who are blind, visually impaired or physically handicapped.
Ann Palmer, Librarian

9660 **Jacksonville Public Library**
303 North Laura Street
Jacksonville, FL 32202 904-630-2665
http//jpl.coj.net
Discs, cassettes, reference materials on blindness and other handicaps and children's books on cassettes.
Mark S. Wood, Chairperson
Bill E. Scheu, Vice Chair

9661 **Lee County Talking Books Library**
13240 North Cleveland Avenue, #5-6 239-995-2665
North Ft. Myers, FL 33903-4855 800-854-8195
Fax: 239-995-1681
TDD: 2399952665
e-mail: talkingbooks@leegov.com
www.lee-county.com/library

Talking Books are books and magazines that are recorded for people who need to "hear" their reading. The books are played on special players provided free by the National Library Service for the Blind and Physically Handicapped.
Sheldon Kaye, Librarian

9662 **Miami Dade Talking Book Library**
Miami Dade Public Library System
2455 North West 183rd Street 305-751-8687
Miami, FL 33056 800-451-9544
Fax: 305-757-8401
TDD: 305-474-7258
e-mail: talkingbooks@mdpls.org
www.mdpls.org

The Talking Books Library loans books and magazines on cassette tapes or in Braille FREE by mail to persons who have difficulty seeing or using standard small print.
Barbara Moyer, Librarian

9663 **Orange County Library System: Orlando Public Library**
101 E Central Boulevard 407-835-7323
Orlando, FL 32801-2462 Fax: 407-425-6779
www.ocls.info

The library's collection consists of a wide variety of print materials, including fiction, nonfiction, world languages, genealogy, and special materials that comprise the Florida and Disney collections. The library also has audiovisual materials and electronic resources to meet customer needs.
Mary Anne Hodel, Library Director/CEO

9664 **Palm Beach County Library Annex: Talking Books**
Mil-Lake Plaza
4639 Lake Worth Road 561-649-5500
Lake Worth, FL 33463 888-780-5151
Fax: 561-649-5402
e-mail: talkingbooks@pbclibrary.org
www.pbclibrary.org

The Talking Books Library is a special service of the Palm Beach County Library and a part of the Library of Congress National Library Service for the Blind and Physically Handicapped.
Pat Mistretta, Librarian

9665 **Pinellas Talking Book Library for the Blind and Physically Handicapped**
1330 Cleveland Street 727-441-9958
Clearwater, FL 33755-5103 Fax: 727-441-9068
TDD: 727-441-3168
www.pplc.us/tbl/

The Pinellas Talking Book Library's mission is to encourage and support reading by providing free library services to Pinellas County residents for whom conventional print is a barrier. The Pinellas Talking Book Library is part of a nationwide network of cooperating libraries serving people who have difficulty using or reading regular print.
Marilyn Stevenson, Access Services Librarian

9666 **Sub Regional Talking Book Library**
1755 Edgewood Avenue West 904-765-5588
Jacksonville, FL 32208-7206 Fax: 904-768-7822
TDD: 904-768-7822
e-mail: jerryco@j.net

Susan V Arthur, Librarian
Laurie Baumgardner, Librarian

9667 **West Florida Public Library: Talking Book Library**
200 West Gregory Street 850-436-5065
Pensacola, FL 32502-4822 Fax: 850-436-5039
e-mail: talkingbooks@ci.pensacola.fl.us
www.cityofpensacola.com/library

As a subregional Talking Book Library, the Pensacola Public Library offers free service by mail to blind and physically handicapped adults and children who have difficulty reading ordinary print or holding or turning the pages of a book.
Susan C. Voss, Librarian

Georgia

9668 **Albany Library for the Blind and Physically Handicapped**
Dougherty County Public Library
300 Pine Avenue 229-420-3220
Albany, GA 31701 800-337-6251
Fax: 229-420-3240
e-mail: lbph@docolib.org
www.docolib.org/libblind.html

The Library for the Blind and Physically Handicapped provides resources to individuals who are blind, visually impaired, physically handicapped or learning disabled in a thirteen-county area.
Kathryn Sinquefield, Librarian

9669 **Atlanta Metro Subregional Library**
1150 Murphy Avenue, SW 404-756-4619
Atlanta, GA 30310 800-248-6701
Fax: 404-756-4618
e-mail: glass@georgialibraries.org
www.georgialibraries.org/public.glass

Through Georgia's Regional Library for the Blind and Physically Handicapped and cooperating local libraries, Georgians have access to a free national library program that offers books and magazines on cassette tape and in Braille.

9670 **Augusta Regional Library Talking Book Center**
425 James Brown Boulevard 706-821-2625
Augusta, GA 30901 Fax: 706-724-5403
e-mail: talkbook@ecgrl.org
www.ecgrl.public.lib.ga.ua/lbph.htm

Through the Georgia Library for Accessible Services, Georgians have access to a free national library program that offers books and magazines on cassette tape and in Braille.
Gary Swint, Librarian

9671 **Bainbridge Subregional Library for the Blind and Physically Handicapped**
Southwest Georgia Regional Library
301 South Monroe Street 229-248-2680
Bainbridge, GA 39819-4029 800-795-2680
Fax: 229-248-2670
TDD: 229-248-2665
e-mail: lbph@swgrl.org
www.swgrl.org

The library houses a large collection of recorded materials as well as reference materials.
Susan S. Whittle, Director

9672 **Columbus Library for Accessible Services (CLASS)**
The Columbus Public Library
3000 Macon Road 706-243-2686
Columbus, GA 31906-2201 800-652-0782
Fax: 706-243-2710
e-mail: sbarnes@cvrls.net
www.thecolumbuslibrary.org

CLASS serves as one of the Georgia subregional distribution centers for books and magazines on audiocassettes published by the National Library Service for the Blind and Physically Handicapped.
Suzanne Barnes, Librarian

9673 **Georgia Library for Accessible Services (GLASS)**
1150 Murphy Avenue SW 404-756-4619
Atlanta, GA 30310-3803 800-248-6701
Fax: 404-756-4618
e-mail: glass@georgialibraries.org
www.georgialibraries.org

Georgians have access to a free national library program that offers books and magazines on cassette tape and in Braille. These materials are provided by the Library of Congress, National Library Service for the Blind & Physically Handicapped (NLS),), to eligible persons with a visual or physical disability. All reading material and playback equipment is sent to borrowers and returned by postage-free mail.
Linda B Stetson, Director

9674 **Hall County Library System: East Hall Branch and Special Needs Library**
2434 Old Cornelia Highway
Gainesville, GA 30507
770-532-3311
Fax: 770-531-2502
TDD: 770-531-2530
e-mail: kevans@hallcountylibrary.org
www.hallcountylibrary.org/ehmap.htm
The East Hall Branch and Special Needs Library goal is to provide excellent service to those with disabilities including the blind, handicapped, mobility impaired and deaf.
Kathy Evans, Branch Manager

9675 **Middle Georgia Subregional Library for the Blind and Physically Handicapped**
Washington Memorial Library
1180 Washington Avenue
Macon, GA 31201-1790
478-744-0877
800-805-7613
Fax: 478-744-0840
e-mail: harringj@bibblib.org
www.co.bibb.ga.us/library/TBC.htm
Books, magazines, newspapers, radio programs and various publications are available. Assistive technology equipment is also available at the library.
Judy T. Harrington, Librarian

9676 **Oconee Regional Library for the Blind and Physically Handicapped**
801 Bellevue Avenue
Dublin, GA 31040
478-275-5382
800-453-5541
Fax: 478-275-3821
e-mail: wdaniel@ocrl.org
www.laurens.public.lib.ga.us
Through the Georgia Library for Accessible Services and cooperating local libraries, Georgians have access to a free national library program which offers braille and recorded materials.
Wanda Daniel, Librarian

9677 **Rome Subregional Library for People with Disabilities**
205 Riverside Parkway NE
Rome, GA 30161-2911
706-236-4618
888-263-0769
Fax: 706-236-4631
TDD: 706-236-4618
e-mail: dhickman@rome-lpd.org
www.rome-lpd.org
Provides free library service to the disabled in eleven counties of Northwest Georgia.
Delana Hickman, Coordinator

9678 **Special Needs Library of Northeast Georgia**
Athens-Clarke County Regional Library
2025 Baxter Street
Athens, GA 30606-6331
706-613-3655
800-531-2063
Fax: 706-613-3660
TDD: 706-613-3655
e-mail: specialneedslibrary@athenslibrary.org
www.clarke.public.lib.ga.us/specneeds
The Special Needs Library of Northeast Georgia provides free library services for patrons with visual, physical, and reading disabilities.
Claudia L. Markov, Librarian

9679 **Subregional Library for the Blind and Physically Handicapped**
Live Oak Public Libraries, Thunderbolt Branch
2708 Mechanics Avenue
Savannah, GA 31404
912-354-5864
800-342-4455
Fax: 912-354-5534
e-mail: stokesl@liveoakpl.org
www.liveoakpl.org
Library for the blind and physically handicapped.
LaTrelle Mobley, Manager

9680 **Three Rivers Regional Library**
Brunswick-Glynn County Regional Library
208 Gloucester Street
Brunswick, GA 31520-5324
912-267-1212
866-833-2878
Fax: 912-267-9597
e-mail: bransom@trrl.org
www.trrl.org
The Talking Book Center serves 12 counties with over 1200 patrons. The center provides talking books which are recorded at a slower speed which requires the use of a special player.
Betty D. Ransom, Librarian

9681 **Valdosta Talking Book Library**
South Georgia Regional Library
300 Woodrow Wilson Drive
Valdosta, GA 31602-2592
229-333-7658
800-246-6515
Fax: 229-333-0774
e-mail: djernigan@sgrl.org
www.sgrl.org
The Talking Book Center is available to blind persons with visual difficulty or physical handicaps which prevent them from using printed material.
Diane Jernigan, Librarian

Hawaii

9682 **Hawaii State Library for the Blind and Physically Handicapped**
402 Kapahulu Avenue
Honolulu, HI 96815
808-733-8444
800-559-4096
Fax: 808-733-8449
TDD: 808-733-8444
e-mail: olbcirc@librarieshawaii.org
www.librarieshawaii.org
The Library for the Blind and Physically Handicapped serves as the regional library and machine lending agency for the blind and physically disabled throughout the state and the outlying Pacific Islands in cooperation with the Library of Congress and the National Library Service for the Blind and Physically Handicapped.
Fusako Miyashiro, Librarian

Idaho

9683 **Idaho Commission for Libraries Talking Book Service**
325 West State Street
Boise, ID 83702-6072
208-334-2150
800-458-3271
Fax: 208-334-4016
TDD: 800-377-1363
e-mail: talkingbooks@libraries.idaho.gov
http://libraries.idaho.gov/tbs
The Idaho Talking Book Service provides books and magazines in cassette format for individuals who are unable to read standard print.
Sue Walker, Librarian

Illinois

9684 **Catholic Guild for the Blind**
180 N Michigan Avenue
Chicago, IL 60601
312-236-8569
Fax: 312-236-8128
e-mail: info@guildfortheblind.org
www.guildfortheblind.org
The Guild's adult rehabilitation services include a program geared towards seniors experiencing new vision loss called New Visions. This program promotes independence within the home and community by providing participants with the information, techniques, and tools they need to successfully adjust to their new lives with impaired sight. Two workshop series are available to beginners or to those ready for more advanced topics.
David J Tabak, Executive Director
Polly Abbott, Manager Adult Rehabilitation Services

9685 **Illinois State Library Talking Book and Braille Service**
401 East Washington
Springfield, IL 62701-1207
217-782-9435
800-665-5576
Fax: 217-558-4723
TDD: 888-261-7863
The Illinois State Library Talking Book and Braille Service plays a supporting rols for the Illinois Network of Libraries Serving the Blind and Physically Handicapped.

9686 **Mid-Illinois Talking Book Center**
600 Highpoint Lane
East Peoria, IL 61611
217-224-6619
800-426-0709
Fax: 217-224-9818
e-mail: info@mitbc.org
www.mitbc.org

We provide free library service for anyone unable to read regular print because of low vision, blindness, or a physical disability. We provide recorded and Braille books and popular magazines. There are over 60,000 titles available including popular fiction and non-fiction, bestsellers, classics, history, biographies, children's books and more.
Karen Bershe, Director
Valerie Brandon, PR/Outreach Coordinator

9687 **Shawnee Library System: Southern Illinois Talking Book Center**
607 South Greenbriar Road 618-985-8375
Carterville, IL 62918 800-445-2665
Fax: 618-985-4211
TDD: 618-985-8375
www.shawls.lib.il.us/talkingbooks
The Talking Book Program is a free library service for anyone who has difficulty reading print or holding books and turning pages due to any visual or physical limitation or medically diagnosed reading disability. Participants are loaned cassette players along with unabridged books and magazines on tape and in Braille.
Diana Brawley Sussman, Director/Librarian

9688 **Skokie Accessible Library Services**
Skokie Public Library
5215 Oakton Street 847-673-7774
Skokie, IL 60077-3634 Fax: 847-673-7797
e-mail: anthe@skokie.library.info
www.skokie.lib.il.us
Library services for people with disabilities, including electronic aids, materials in special formats, programs and special services, and access to the North Suburban Library System.
Carolyn A Anthony, Director

9689 **Voices of Vision Talking Book Center**
127 S First Street 630-208-0398
Geneva, IL 60134 800-227-0625
Fax: 630-208-0399
e-mail: kodean@dupagels.lib.il.us
www.vovtbc.org
Voices of Vision is part of a statewide and national network of libraries which provide the talking book and braille service. We provide free library service to persons unable to read or use conventional print material due to a visual or physical disability. There is no cost to eligible readers.
Karen Odean, Director

Indiana

9690 **Bartholomew County Public Library**
National Library Services
536 Fifth Street 812-379-1277
Columbus, IN 47201 800-685-0524
Fax: 812-791-75
e-mail: talkingbooks@barth.lib.in.us
www.barth.lib.in.us
Talking Books for the Blind and Physically Handicapped is a free library service for visually or physically challenged persons of all ages. Anyone who is unable to use regular printed materials as the result of a temporary or permanent visual or physical limitation is eligible.
Sharon Thompson, Librarian

9691 **Evansville-Vanderburgh County Public Library**
200 SE Martin Luther King Jr Blvd 812-428-8200
Evansville, IN 47713 Fax: 812-428-8397
www.evcpl.lib.in.us
The Evansville-Vanderburgh County Public Library, an essential provider of shared information and a core community service, promotes reading, lifelong learning, and economic vitality through its resources, services and programs to the residents of Vanderburgh County.
Mike Russ, President
Brenda Schiedler, Vice President

9692 **Indiana Talking Book & Braille Library**
140 North Senate Avenue 317-232-3684
Indianapolis, IN 46204 800-622-4970
e-mail: lbph@statelib.lib.in.us
www.in.gov/library/tbbl.htm
The TBBL provides large print books, braille books, and books on tape to Indiana residents who are unable to read regular print.
Roberta L Brooker, Interim Director

9693 **Lake County Public Library**
1919 W 81st Street 219-769-3541
Merrillville, IN 46410 Fax: 219-769-0690
www.lakeco.lib.in.us
Talking books provides cassette books, descriptive videos, magazines and large print books to people who are blind and physically handicapped. Materials are sent through the mail and the service is free to those who qualify.
Renee Lewis, Director

Iowa

9694 **Iowa Department for the Blind**
524 Fourth Street 515-281-1333
Des Moines, IA 50309-2364 800-362-2587
Fax: 515-281-1263
TTY: 515-281-1355
e-mail: information@blind.state.ia.us
www.blind.state.ia.us/Library/
Our program offers the specialized, integrated services that blind and severely visually impaired Iowans need to live independently and work competitively.
Allen Harris, Director

Kansas

9695 **CKLS Headquarters**
1409 Williams Street 620-792-4865
Great Bend, KS 67530-4090 800-362-2642
Fax: 620-793-7270
e-mail: jswan@ckls.org
www.ckls.org
Offers direct services to rural residents and those who need special services because of disability.
James Swan, Administrator
Joanita Doll-Masden, Department Head

9696 **Manhattan Subregional Library of the Kansas Talking Books Service**
629 Poyntz Avenue 785-776-4741
Manhattan, KS 66502-6006 800-432-2796
Fax: 785-776-1545
e-mail: annp@manhattan.lib.ks.us
www.manhattan.lib.ks.us
Books and magazines in braille and recorded format and playback equipment are provided to any Kansas citizen residing in the twelve county area of the North Central Kansas Libraries System who is unable to use standard print as a result of temporary or permanent visual or physical impairments.
Ann Pearce, Department Manager
Wandean Rivers, Assistive Technology Center Instructor

9697 **Northwest Kansas Library System**
Northwest Kansas Library System
2 Washington Square 785-877-5148
Norton, KS 67654 800-432-2858
Fax: 785-877-5697
www.skyways.lib.ks.us
The Kansas Library Network for the Blind and Physically Handicapped, in cooperation with the Library of Congress, National Library Service for the Blind and Physically Handicapped, provides library services and materials to Kansans unable to use conventional print.
Leslie Bell, Director
Clarice Howard, BPH Librarian

9698 **South Central Kansas Library System**
321A North Main Street
South Hutchinson, KS 67505 800-234-0529
Fax: 313-663-9797
e-mail: phawkins@sckls.info
www.sckls.info/
Summer reading programs, braille writer, magnifiers, closed-circuit TV, large-print photocopier, cassette books and magazines,

children's books on cassette, home visits and other reference materials on blindness and other handicaps.
Paul Hawkins, Director

9699 **Talking Books Service**
Topeka and Shawnee County Public Library
1515 SW 10th Avenue
Topeka, KS 66604-1304
785-580-4530
800-432-2925
Fax: 785-580-4530
e-mail: tbooks@tscpl.lib.ks.us
www.tscpl.org/services/talkingbooks
Summer reading programs, braille writer, magnifiers, closed-circuit TV, large-print photocopier, cassette books and magazines, children's books on cassette, home visits and other reference materials on blindness and other handicaps.
Suzanne Bundy, Librarian

9700 **Wichita Public Library**
223 S Main
Wichita, KS 67202
316-261-8500
Fax: 316-262-4540
TDD: 316-262-3972
www.wichita.lib.ks.us
Talking books provides cassette books, descriptive videos, magazines adn large print books to people who are blind and physically handicapped. Materials are sent through the mail and the service is free to those who qualify.
Brad Reha, Talking Books Manager

Kentucky

9701 **Kentucky Talking Book Library**
PO Box 537
Frankfort, KY 40602-0537
502-564-8300
800-372-2968
Fax: 502-564-5773
e-mail: Wendy.Hatfield@ky.gov
www.kdla.ky.gov
Our mission is to provide library service to individuals who have a visual or physical disability that prevents them from using standard print materials. We send books on tape and Braille books through the mail at no cost to our patrons.
Wendy Hatfield, Librarian, Talking Books

9702 **Louisville Talking Book Library for the Blind and Physically Handicapped**
301 York Street
Louisville, KY 40203-2205
502-574-1625
www.lfpl.org/tbl
The Louisville Talking Book Library offers recorded books and other materials to eligible visually and physically handicapped Jefferson County, KY residents. All recorded books & equipment may be sent to borrowers and returned by postage-free mail.
Linda Atzinger, Supervisor Accessibility Services

9703 **Northern Kentucky Talking Book Library**
502 Scott Boulevard
Covington, KY 41011
859-962-4095
866-491-7610
Fax: 859-962-4096
www.kenton.lib.ky.us
Our library provides books and magazines on specially recorded cassettes for people who are visually impaired and/or physically handicapped and live in Boone, Campbell, Carroll, Gallatin, Grant, Kenton, Owen and Pendleton counties.
Dave Schroeder, Director

Louisiana

9704 **State Library of Louisiana**
701 N 4th Street
Baton Rouge, LA 70802
225-342-4943
Fax: 225-219-4804
e-mail: admin@state.lib.la.us
www.state.lib.la.us
Talking books provides cassette books, descriptive videos, magazines and large print books to people who are blind and physically handicapped. Materials are sent through the mail and the service is free to those who qualify.

Maine

9705 **Bangor Public Library**
145 Harlow Street
Bangor, ME 04401-4900
207-947-8336
Fax: 207-945-6694
e-mail: bplill@bpl.lib.me.us
www.bpl.lib.me.us
Summer reading programs, braille writer, magnifiers, closed-circuit TV, large-print photocopier, cassette books and magazines, children's books on cassette, home visits and other reference materials on blindness and other handicaps.
Barbara McDade, Director

9706 **Cary Library**
107 Main Street
Houlton, ME 04730-2196
207-532-1302
Fax: 207-532-4350
www.cary.lib.me.us
Summer reading programs, braille writer, magnifiers, closed-circuit TV, large-print photocopier, cassette books and magazines, children's books on cassette, home visits and other reference materials on blindness and other handicaps.
Linda Faucher, Librarian

9707 **Lewiston Public Library**
200 Lisbon Street
Lewiston, ME 04240-7203
207-784-0135
Fax: 207-784-3011
TTY: 207-784-3123
e-mail: lplweb@lplonline.org
www.lplonline.org
Summer reading programs, braille writer, magnifiers, closed-circuit TV, large-print photocopier, cassette books and magazines, children's books on cassette, home visits and other reference materials on blindness and other handicaps.

9708 **Maine State Library**
64 State House Station
Augusta, ME 04333-0064
207-287-5650
800-452-8793
Fax: 207-287-5624
www.state.me.us/msl
Large Print Books is a service through Outreach Services for residents of Maine who are certified as visually impaired and public libraries who serve the visually impaired.
J Gary Nichols, Librarian

9709 **Portland Public Library**
5 Monument Square
Portland, ME 04101-4072
207-871-1700
Fax: 207-871-1715
e-mail: reference@portland.lib.me.us
www.portlandlibrary.com
Portland Public Library's Outreach Services brings library resources to those who are unable to visit the library in person. For people living in nursing homes or assisted living facilities, or for those confined to home due to illness or disability, the library will deliver print and audio books right to your doorstep.
Stephen J Podgajny, Director

9710 **Waterville Public Library**
73 Elm Street
Waterville, ME 04901-6027
207-872-5433
Fax: 207-873-4779
www.waterville.lib.me.us
Summer reading programs, braille writer, magnifiers, closed-circuit TV, large-print photocopier, cassette books and magazines, children's books on cassette, home visits and other reference materials on blindness and other handicaps.
Sarah Sugden, Director

Maryland

9711 **American Action Fund for Blind Children and Adults**
1800 Johnson Street, Suite 100
Baltimore, MD 21230
410-659-9315
e-mail: actionfund@actionfund.org
www.actionfund.org
Our mission is to assist blind persons in securing reading matter, to educate the public about blindness, to give aid to the deaf-blind, to provide specialized aids and appliances to the blind, to give consultation to governmental and private agencies serving the blind, to offer assistance to older blind persons, to offer services to blind

children and their parents, and to do any other lawful thing which it can to improve the quality of life for blind persons.
Barbara Loos, President
Ramona Walhof, First Vice President

9712 Disability Resource Center of Montgomery County Public Libraries
Rockville Library
21 Maryland Avenue 240-777-0140
Rockville, MD 20850 TTY: 240-777-0902
e-mail: drcinfo@montgomerycountymd.gov
www.montgomerycountymd.gov
The Disability Resource Center (DRC) is the focal point within the Montgomery County Public Libraries (MCPL) for library and literacy services to people with disabilities, their families, caretakers and professionals.
Kay Bowman, Agency Manager

9713 International Braille and Technology Center for the Blind
National Federation of the Blind
1800 Johnson Street 410-659-9314
Baltimore, MD 21230-4998 Fax: 410-685-5653
e-mail: ataylor@nfb.org
www.nfb.org
A comprehensive and complete evaluation and demonstration center for assistive technology used by the blind worldwide. Includes all Braille, synthetic speech, print-to-speech scanning, internet and portable devices and programs. Available for tours by appointment to blind persons, employers, technology manufacturers, teachers, parents and those working in the assistive technology field.
Ann Taylor, Director Technology

9714 Maryland State Library for the Blind and Physically Handicapped
415 Park Avenue 410-230-2424
Baltimore, MD 21201 800-964-9209
Fax: 410-333-2095
TTY: 800-934-2541
www.lbph.lib.md/us
The basic mission of the Maryland State Library for the Blind and Physically Handicapped is to provide comprehensive library services to the eligible blind and physically handicapped residents of the State of Maryland.
Jill Lewis, Director

9715 Prince George's County Memorial Library: Talking Book Center
6532 Adelphi Road
Hyattsville, MD 20782-2098 301-699-3500
www.prge.lib.md.us
Talking books provides cassette books, descriptive videos, magazines and large print books to people who are blind and physically handicapped. Materials are sent through the mail and the services are free to those who qualify.
Maralita Freeny, Director

Massachusetts

9716 Caption Center
125 Western Avenue 617-492-9225
Allston, MA 02134-1008 Fax: 617-562-0590
Provides closed captioning for videos, including training, safety, instructional and educational films. Maintains a consumer information service for overcoming communications barriers in the workplace.
Lori Kay, Co-Director
Tom Apone, Co-Director

9717 Laboure College Library
2120 Dorchester Avenue 617-296-8300
Boston, MA 02124-5617 e-mail: library@laboure.edu
www.laboure.edu
Offers information on physical disabilities, independent living, peer counseling and advocacy.
Maryann O'Toole, Director

9718 Perkins Braille and Talking Book Library
175 N Beacon Street 617-972-7240
Watertown, MA 02472-2751 800-852-3133
Fax: 617-972-7363
TTY: 617-972-7690
e-mail: library@perkins.org
www.perkins.org
The Perkins Braille & Talking Book Library, funded in part by the Massachusetts Board of Library Commissioners, provides free services to Massachusetts residents of any age who are unable to read traditional print materials due to a visual or physical disability.
Kim Charlson, Director

9719 Talking Book Library at Worcester Public Library
3 Salem Square 508-799-1730
Worcester, MA 1608-2074 800-762-0085
Fax: 508-799-1676
e-mail: talkbook@cwmars.org/talkingbook
www.cwmars.org/talkingbook
Adapted computers, braille embosser, magnifiers, closed circuit TV, large print books, cassette books and magazines, children's books on cassette, reference materials on blindness and other disabilities. Summer reading programs.
James L Izatt, Librarian

Michigan

9720 Detroit Subregional Library for the Blind and Physically Handicapped
Detroit Public Library
3666 Grand River Avenue 313-833-5494
Detroit, MI 48208 Fax: 313-325-97
TDD: 313-833-5492
e-mail: dmiddle@detroitpubliclibrary.org
www.detroit.lib.mi.us
Talking books along with talking book machines are available to eligible residents who live in a 14 ZIP code area of Detroit and Highland Park. Loans of the books and machines are made to individuals and to institutions such as schools, nursing homes and senior residences. Over 45,000 books are available. Magazines available in recorded format include Ebony, Good Housekeeping, and Sports Illustrated.
Dori V. Middleton, LBPH Specialist

9721 Grand Traverse Area Library for the Blind and Physically Handicapped
322 6th Street 616-935-6520
Traverse City, MI 49684-2414 Fax: 616-922-0904
TDD: 616-922-0901
Evelyn Welty

9722 Kent County Library for the Blind
775 Ball Avenue NE 616-336-3250
Grand Rapids, MI 49503-1397 Fax: 616-336-3256
e-mail: kdlem@lakeland.lib.mi.us
Summer reading programs, braille writer, magnifiers, closed-circuit TV, large-print photocopier, cassette books and magazines, children's books on cassette, home visits and other reference materials on blindness and other handicaps.
Claudya Muller, Librarian

9723 Library of Michigan Service for the Blind
PO Box 30007 517-373-5614
Lansing, MI 48909-7507 Fax: 517-735-65
e-mail: sbph@michigan.gov
www.michigan.gov/sbth
Braille writer, magnifiers, closed circuit TV, large print photocopier, cassette books and magazines, children's books on cassette, reference materials on blindness and other handicaps. Books on cassette and braille books and cassette players will be loaned and sent through the mail at no charge. For blind and those physically unable to read standard print or turn the pages.
Susan Thinault, Manager

9724 **Macomb Library for the Blind and Physically Handicapped**
16480 Hall Road
Clinton Township, MI 48038-1132
810-286-1580
Fax: 810-286-0634
TDD: 8102869940
e-mail: macbld@libcoop.net
www.macomb.lib.mi.us/macspe
Summer reading programs, braille writer, closed-circuit TV, cassette books and magazines, children's books on cassette, reference materials on blindness and other handicaps.
Beverlee Babcock, Librarian

9725 **Midwestern Michigan Library Cooperative**
G4195 West Pasadena Avenue
Flint, MI 48504
810-732-1120
Fax: 810-321-15
www.mideasteRN.lib.mi.us
Roger Mendell, Director

9726 **Muskegon County Library for the Blind**
635 Ottawa Street
Muskegon, MI 49442-1016
616-724-6248
Fax: 616-724-6675
TDD: 616-722-4103
Summer reading programs, braille typewriter, magnifiers, closed-circuit TV, large-print photocopier, cassette books and magazines, children's books on cassette, home visits and other reference materials on blindness and other handicaps, The Reading Edge, Perkins Brailler and large print books.
Linda Clapp, Librarian

9727 **Northland Library Cooperative**
316 E Chisholm Street
Alpena, MI 49707-2892
517-356-1622
Fax: 517-354-3939
e-mail: nlc.lib.mi.us/lbph.htm
Summer reading programs, braille writer, magnifiers, closed-circuit TV, large-print photocopier, cassette books and magazines, children's books on cassette, home visits and other reference materials on blindness and other handicaps.
Catherine Glomski, Librarian

9728 **Oakland County Library for the Visually and Physically Impaired**
1200 N Telegraph Road
Pontiac, MI 48341-1032
248-858-5050
800-774-4542
Fax: 248-858-9313
e-mail: lVPi@co.oakland..mi.us
www.co.oakland.mi.us/lVPi
Free cassette book service to eligible visually or physically impaired Oakland County residents; demonstrations, CCTV and hand held magnifiers and a large print collection.
David Conklin, Head Librarian

9729 **St. Clark County Library for the Blind and Physically Handicapped**
210 McMorran Boulevard
Port Huron, MI 48060-4014
810-987-7323
Fax: 810-987-7327
Offers library services to the blind and visually impaired.
Jackie Skinner, Librarian

9730 **Upper Peninsula Library for the Blind and Physically Handicapped**
1615 Presque Isle Avenue
Marquette, MI 49855-2811
906-228-7697
Fax: 906-285-27
e-mail: uproc.lib.mi.us
www.michigan.gov/sbth
Summer reading programs, braille writer, magnifiers, closed-circuit TV, large-print photocopier, cassette books and magazines, children's books on cassette, home visits and other reference materials on blindness and other handicaps.
Susan Thinault, Manager

9731 **Washtenaw County Library for the Blind and Physically Disabled**
PO Box 8645
Ann Arbor, MI 48107-8645
734-971-6059
Fax: 734-971-3892
e-mail: lbpd@co.washtennaw.mi.us
comnet.org/cgi-bin/helpnet/viewitem?290+
Book lovers club.adaptive technology,cassette equipment, cassette books and magazines, described videos, low vision aids reference and referral services.
Margaret Wolfe, Cordinator

9732 **Wayne County Regional Library for the Blind and Physically Handicapped**
30555 Michigan Avenue
Westland, MI 48186-5310
734-727-7300
888-968-2737
Fax: 734-727-7333
TDD: 313-326-3008
e-mail: werlbph@tln.lib.mi.us
www.tln.lib.mi.us
Summer reading programs, braille writer, magnifiers, closed-circuit TV, large-print photocopier, cassette books and magazines, children's books on cassette, home visits and other reference materials on blindness and other handicaps.
Pat Klemans, Librarian

Minnesota

9733 **Duluth Public Library**
City of Duluth Department
520 W Superior Street
Duluth, MN 55802-1578
218-723-3800
Fax: 218-233-15
e-mail: webmail@duluth.li.mn.us
www.duluth.lib.mn.us
Adapted access to Apple computer, adapted toys and adapted library equipment.
Randall Deth Kelly, Director

9734 **Minnesota Library for the Blind**
388 South East 6 Avenue
Faribault, MN 55021
507-333-4828
800-722-0550
Fax: 507-333-4832
e-mail: mn.lbph@state.mn.us
www.education.state.mn.us
Summer reading programs, braille writer, magnifiers, closed-circuit TV, large-print photocopier, cassette books and magazines, children's books on cassette, home visits and other reference materials on blindness and other handicaps.
Catherine Durivage, Director

Mississippi

9735 **Mississippi Library Commission**
1221 Ellis Avenue
Jackson, MS 39209-7328
601-961-4111
800-647-7542
Fax: 601-961-4113
TDD: 601-354-6411
e-mail: mslib@mic.lib.ms.us
www.mlc.lib.ms.us
Summer reading programs, braille writer, magnifiers, closed-circuit TV, large-print photocopier, cassette books and magazines, children's books on cassette, home visits and other reference materials on blindness and other handicaps.
Larry Mc Millan, Director

Missouri

9736 **Adriene Resource Center for Blind Children**
Assembly of God Center for Blind
1445 Boonville Avenue
Springfield, MO 65802
417-831-1964
Fax: 417-625-20
e-mail: blind@ag.org
www.blind.ag.org
Offers braille and cassette lending library, braille and cassette Sunday school materials for all ages, braille and cassette periodicals and resource assistance, and resources for blind children and children of blind parents.
Paul Weingariner, Director
Caryl Weingariner, Co-Director

9737 **Assemblies of God National Center for the Blind**
1445 Boonville Avenue
Springfield, MO 65802
417-831-1964
Fax: 417-627-66
e-mail: blind@ag.org
Offers braille and cassette lending library, braille and cassette Sunday school materials for all ages, braille and cassette periodicals and resource assistance, and resources for blind children and children of blind parents.
Paul Weingariner, Director

9738 **Church of the Nazarene**
Nazarene Publishing House
PO Box 419527 816-931-1900
Kansas City, MO 64141-6527 800-877-0700
e-mail: NPH@direct.nph.com
www.nph.com
Offers braille and large print books. Also offers a lending library and cassettes for the blind.

9739 **Lutheran Library for the Blind**
Lutheran Church - Missouri Synod
1333 S Kirkwood Road 314-965-9000
Saint Louis, MO 63122-7295 800-843-5267
Fax: 314-996-1016
e-mail: infocenter@lcms.org
www.lcms.org
Offers braille and large print books and cassettes for the blind and visually impaired.

9740 **Whitney Library for the Blind: Assemblies of God**
1445 N Boonville Avenue 417-862-2781
Springfield, MO 65802-1894 Fax: 417-863-7566
www.gospelpublishing.com
Offers braille and cassette lending library, braille and cassette Sunday school materials for all ages, braille and cassette periodicals and resource assistance.
Paul Weingariner, Librarian

9741 **Wolfner Memorial Library for the Blind**
PO Box 387 573-751-8720
Jefferson City, MO 65102-387 800-392-2614
Fax: 573-526-2985
TDD: 800-347-1379
e-mail: wolfner@sos.mo.gov
www.sos.mo.gov/wolfner
Summer reading programs, braille writer, closed circuit TV, large print photocopier, cassette books and magazines, children's books on cassette, home visits and other reference materials on blindness and other handicaps.
Richard J Smith, Director Wolfner Library
Debbie Musselman, Administrative Program Coordinator

Montana

9742 **Montana State Library**
1515 E 6th Avenue 406-444-3009
Helena, MT 59620-1800 Fax: 406-444-5612
Summer reading programs, braille writer, magnifiers, closed-circuit TV, large-print photocopier, cassette books and magazines, children's books on cassette, home visits and other reference materials on blindness and other handicaps.
Darlene Staffeldt, Director

Nebraska

9743 **Nebraska Library Commission Talking Book and Braille Services**
1200 N Street, Suite 120 402-471-4038
Lincoln, NE 68508-2023 800-742-7691
e-mail: doertli@nlc.state.ne.us
www.nlc.state.ne.us/tbbs/tbbs
Free loan of books and magazines on cassette and in Braille, including children's materials, along with specially designed playback equipment. Summer reading program for children, Braille embossing, closed circuit TV, large-print copier. Reference materials on blindness and other disabilities.
David Oertli, Director
Kay Goehring, Reader Services Coordinator

9744 **North Platte Public Library**
120 W 4th Street 308-535-8036
North Platte, NE 69101-3901 Fax: 308-535-8296
e-mail: library@ci.north-platte.ne.us
www.ci.north-platte.ne.us/library
Summer reading programs, braille writer, magnifiers, closed-circuit TV, large-print photocopier, cassette books and magazines, children's books on cassette, home visits and other reference materials on blindness and other handicaps.
Cecelia Lawrence, Library Director

Nevada

9745 **Las Vegas Clark County Library District**
833 Las Vegas Boulevard N
Las Vegas, NV 89101-5256 702-734-7323
www.lvccld.org
Summer reading programs, braille writer, magnifiers, closed circuit TV, large-print photocopier, cassette books and magazines, children's books on cassette, home visits and other reference materials on blindness and other handicaps.
Daniel Walters, Executive Directors

9746 **Nevada State Library and Archives**
100 North Stewart Street 775-684-3360
Carson City, NV 89701-4285 800-922-2880
Fax: 775-684-3330
TDD: 775-687-8338
e-mail: nslref@clan.lib.nv.us
dmla.clan.lib.nv.us/
Summer reading programs, braille writer, magnifiers, closed-circuit TV, large-print photocopier, cassette books and magazines, children's books on cassette, home visits and other reference materials on blindness and other handicaps.
Kevin E Putnam, Librarian

New Hampshire

9747 **New Hampshire State Library**
117 Pleasant Street 603-271-3429
Concord, NH 03301-3852 Fax: 603-271-8370
e-mail: talking@lilac.nhsh.lib.nh.us
www.state.nh.us
Summer reading programs, braille writer, magnifiers, closed-circuit TV, large-print photocopier, cassette books and magazines, children's books on cassette, home visits and other reference materials on blindness and other handicaps.
Eileen Keim, Librarian

9748 **Voices for the Blind**
PO Box 781 603-332-9355
Barrington, NH 3825
Tape library and depository for people with visual and learning disabilities. Recording services available by request.
Connie Hindman, Director

New Jersey

9749 **New Jersey Library for the Blind and Handicapped**
2300 Stuyvesant Avenue 609-530-4000
Trenton, NJ 08618-3226 800-792-8322
Fax: 609-530-6384
TDD: 877-882-5593
e-mail: nglbh@njstatelib.org
www2.njstatelib.org/lbh/index.htm
Summer reading programs, large print, cassette, braille books and magazines, children's books on cassette and brailles and other reference materials on blindness and other handicaps.
Deborah Toomey, Director

New Mexico

9750 **New Mexico State Library for the Blind and Physically Handicapped**
National Library Services
1209 Camino Carlos Rey 505-476-9770
Santa Fe, NM 87507 800-456-5515
Fax: 505-476-9776
e-mail: lbph@stlib.state.nm.us
www.stlib.state.nm.us
Summer reading programs, braille writer, magnifiers, closed-circuit TV, large-print photocopier, cassette books and magazines, children's books on cassette, home visits and other reference materials on blindness and other handicaps.
John Mugford, Library Manager

New York

9751 **Choice Magazine Listening**
85 Channel Drive
Port Washington, NY 11050-2216
516-883-8280
888-724-6423
Fax: 516-944-6849
e-mail: choicemag@aol.com
www.choicemagazinelistening.org
A free recorded spoken word magazine anthology for anyone college level and older unable to read large print because of visual or physical handicaps. Produced on special speed cassette format, playable on free library of congress player.
Sondra Mochson, Editor

9752 **JGB Cassette Library International**
Jewish Guild for the Blind
15 W 65th Street
New York, NY 10023-6601
212-769-6331
Fax: 212-769-6266
e-mail: bemass@aol.com
Summer reading programs, braille writer, magnifiers, closed-circuit TV, large-print photocopier, cassette books and magazines, children's books on cassette, home visits and other reference materials on blindness and other handicaps.
Bruce Massis

9753 **Nassau Library System**
900 Jerusalem Avenue
Uniondale, NY 11553-3039
516-292-8920
Fax: 516-481-4777
e-mail: nls@lilrc.org
Summer reading programs, braille writer, magnifiers, closed-circuit TV, large-print photocopier, cassette books and magazines, children's books on cassette, home visits and other reference materials on blindness and other handicaps.
Dorothy Pruyear, Librarian

9754 **New York State Talking Book & Braille Library, New York State Library, DOE**
Empire State Plaza, CEC
Albany, NY 12230-0001
518-474-5935
800-342-3688
Fax: 518-486-1957
e-mail: tbbl@mail.nysed.gov
www.nysl.nysed.gov/tbbl/
Books on audio cassette, cassette players, braille books, summer reading programs, braille writer, magnifiers, closed-circuit TV, large-print photocopier, cassette books and magazines, children's books on cassette, reference materials on blindness and other disabilities. Library is part of the National Service Network serving those with print disabilities. Available: audio and braille books sent post-free by mail, euipment loans, services to schools and institutions. Serves 55 New York counties.
Sharon B. Phillips, Program Director

9755 **Suffolk Cooperative Library System**
627 N Sunrise Service Road
Bellport, NY 11713-9000
631-286-1600
Fax: 631-286-1647
scls.suffolk.lib.ny.us
Talking books services.
Julie Klauber, Adjunt Professor

9756 **Xavier Society for the Blind**
154 E 23rd Street
New York, NY 10010-4501
212-473-7800
800-637-9193
Fax: 212-473-7801
e-mail: xaviersocietyfortheblind@yahoo.com
www.xaviersociety.com
Provides spiritual and inspirational reading material to visually impaired persons in suitable format: Braille, large print and cassette, throughout the USA and Canada. Services provided by way of regular periodicals which are non-returnable, and through our lending library where books are returned. All services are provided free of charge, and interested persons can write or phone.
Alfred Caruana, Executive Director
Margie Montenegro, Client Services Representative

North Carolina

9757 **North Carolina Library for the Blind**
Library of Congress Washington DC
1811 Capital Boulevard
Raleigh, NC 27635-1
919-733-4376
888-388-2460
Fax: 919-733-6910
TDD: 919-733-1462
e-mail: nclbth@ncmail.net
www.htdt//statelibrary.tcr.state.nt.us/l
A general interest library offering books and magazines at no cost in large print, in braille and on audio cassette for anyone who cannot use regular print in North Carolina due to physical or visual disability. Summer reading programs, braille writer, magnifiers, closed circuit TV, large print photocopier, cassette books and magazines, children's books on cassette, home visits and other reference materials on blindness and other handicaps.
Francine Martin, Director

North Dakota

9758 **North Dakota State Library Services for the Disabled**
North Dakota State Library
604 E Boulevard Avenue
Bismarck, ND 58505-800
701-328-1408
800-843-9948
Fax: 701-328-2040
TDD: 800-892-8622
e-mail: tbooks@state.nd.us
ndsl.lib.state.nd.us
Stella Cone, Regional Librarian

9759 **North Dakota State Library Talking Book Services**
604 E Boulevard Avenue
Bismarck, ND 58505-0800
701-328-1408
800-843-9948
Fax: 701-328-2040
TDD: 800-892-8622
e-mail: twilhelm@state.nd.us
ndsl.lib.state.nd.us
Terria Wilhelm, Talking Book Manager

9760 **Services for the Visually Impaired**
8720 Georgia Avenue
Silver, MD 20910
301-589-0894
Fax: 301-589-7281
www.servicesvi.org
Eligible readers of North Dakota receive library service from the regional library in Pierre, South Dakota.
Betty Bender

Ohio

9761 **Case Western Reserve University**
10900 Euclid Avenue
Cleveland, OH 44117-2620
216-368-2000
www.cwru.edu
Research in electrical stimulation and rehabilitation technology.
Jeanne O'Malley Teeter, Manager

9762 **Ohio Regional Library for the Blind and Physically Handicapped**
800 Vine Street
Cincinnati, OH 45202
513-369-6999
800-528-0335
Fax: 513-369-3111
TDD: 513-369-6072
www.cincinatilibrary.org/main/lb.asp
Summer reading programs, braille writer, magnifiers, closed-circuit TV, large-print photocopier, cassette books and magazines, children's books on cassette, home visits and other reference materials on blindness and other handicaps.
Donna Foust, Librarian

9763 **State Library of Ohio Talking Book Program**
274 E First Avenue
Columbus, OH 43201-3673
614-644-6895
800-686-1531
Fax: 614-995-2186
winslo.state.oh.us/services
A machine-lending agency for the visually impaired.
Roger Verney, Head Supervisor

Oklahoma

9764 **Oklahoma Library for the Blind and Physically Handicapped**
300 NE 18th Street
Oklahoma City, OK 73105-3212
405-521-3514
Fax: 405-214-82
www.state.ok.us/~library

Summer reading programs, braille writer, magnifiers, closed-circuit TV, large-print photocopier, cassette books and magazines, children's books on cassette, home visits and other reference materials on blindness and other handicaps.
Geraldine Adams, Director

9765 **Tulsa City: County Library System**
400 Civic Center 918-596-7977
Tulsa, OK 74103-3830 Fax: 918-596-7990
www.tulsalibrary.org
Summer reading programs, braille writer, magnifiers, closed-circuit TV, large-print photocopier, cassette books and magazines, children's books on cassette, home visits and other reference materials on blindness and other handicaps.
Ellen Ontko, Librarian

Oregon

9766 **Oregon State Library**
250 Winter Street NE 503-378-4243
Salem, OR 97301-3950 800-452-0292
Fax: 503-588-7119
TDD: 503-378-4276
www.oregon.gov/osl
Summer reading programs, braille writer, magnifiers, closed-circuit TV, large-print photocopier, cassette books and magazines, children's books on cassette, home visits and other reference materials on blindness and other handicaps.
Jim Scheppke, Head Librarian

Pennsylvania

9767 **Carnegie Library of Pittsburgh**
4724 Baum Boulevard 412-687-2440
Pittsburgh, PA 15213-1321 800-242-0586
Fax: 412-687-2442
e-mail: lbph@carneigelibrary.org
www.clpgh.org/clp/LBPH
Provides on loan recorded books and magazines, large print books, and described videos to Western Pennsylvannia residents unable to use standard printed materials due to visual, physical, or physically-based reading disabilities. Also loans special cassette and disc machines; does not loan equipment to play described videos. Information about disabilities and related agencies is also available.
Sue Murdock, Director
Kathleen Kappel, Assistant Director

9768 **Free Library of Philadelphia**
919 Walnut Street 215-925-3213
Philadelphia, PA 19107-5237 Fax: 215-928-0856
e-mail: flpblind@library.phila.gov
Summer reading programs, braille writer, magnifiers, closed-circuit TV, large-print photocopier, cassette books and magazines, children's books on cassette, home visits and other reference materials on blindness and other handicaps.
Vickie Lange Collins, Librarian

Rhode Island

9769 **Rhode Island Department of State Library for the Blind and Physically Handicapped**
1 Capitol Hl 401-277-2726
Providence, RI 02908-5803 Fax: 401-277-4195
e-mail: richard@dsl.rhilinet.gov
Offers information and services for the visually impaired including reference materials, braille printers, braille writers, large-print books and more.
Richard Ledue, Librarian

South Carolina

9770 **South Carolina State Library**
PO Box 11469 803-734-8666
Columbia, SC 29202-0821 Fax: 803-734-8676
TDD: 803-734-7298
e-mail: guynell@leo.scsl.state.sc.us
www.state.sc.us/scsl
Summer reading programs, braille writer, magnifiers, closed-circuit TV, large-print photocopier, cassette books and magazines, children's books on cassette, home visits and other reference materials on blindness and other handicaps.
Guynell Williams, Librarian

South Dakota

9771 **South Dakota State Library**
800 Governors Drive 605-773-3131
Pierre, SD 57501-2235 Fax: 605-734-50
TDD: 605-773-4950
e-mail: daRN@stlib.state.sd.us
www.sdstatelibrary.com
Summer reading programs, braille writer, magnifiers, closed-circuit TV, large-print photocopier, cassette books and magazines, children's books on cassette, home visits and other reference materials on blindness and other handicaps.
Daniel Boyd, Librarian

Tennessee

9772 **LRC for Students with Disabilities**
MSU Library Reference Department
Memphis State University 901-678-2208
Memphis, TN 38152-0001 800-669-2267
Fax: 901-678-3070
www.memphis.edu
Information on physical disabilities, blindness and visual impairments.
Ross Johnson, Reference Librarian

9773 **Tennessee Library for the Blind and Physically Handicapped**
National Library Services
403 7th Avenue N 615-741-3915
Nashville, TN 37243-1409 800-342-3308
Fax: 615-532-8856
e-mail: tlbph@mail.state.tn/sos/statelib/LBPH/
www.state.tn.us
Offers free public library services to those unable to hold, read, or turn the pages of books and magazines due to physical or visual impairment. Collections include books and magazines in large print, braille and audio format. Players loaned for the audio books and magazines. All items are delivered and returned via the US Postal Service free matter mailing.
Ruth Hemphill, Director
Janie Murphee, Assistant Director

Texas

9774 **Christian Resource for People Who Are Blind**
Care Ministries Inc
PO Box 1830 662-323-4999
Starkville, MS 39760-1830 800-366-2232
e-mail: care@careministries.org
www.careministries.org
Offers braille and large print books and cassettes for the visually impaired.
B J LeJeune, Director

9775 **Houston Public Library Access Center**
500 McKinney Street 832-393-1313
Houston, TX 77002-2534 Fax: 832-931-83
e-mail: website@hpl.lib.tx.us
www.houstonlibrary.org
Offers Kurzweil Reading Machine 400, closed-circuit TV, braille writer, reference materials on visual impairments and other handicaps.
Heidi Miller, Supervisor

9776 **Texas State Library**
PO Box 12927 512-463-5460
Austin, TX 78711-2927 Fax: 512-635-36
TDD: 512-463-5449
e-mail: dale.propp@tsl.state.tx.us
Summer reading programs, braille writer, magnifiers, closed-circuit TV, large-print photocopier, cassette books and magazines,

children's books on cassette, home visits and other reference materials on blindness and other handicaps.
Dale Propp, Librarian

9777 **Texas State Library: Talking Book Program**
1201 Brazos Street 512-463-5458
Austin, TX 78711-2927 800-252-9605
Fax: 512-936-0685
e-mail: tbp.services@tsl.state.tx.us
www.texastalkingbooks.org
Part of the free National Library Services. Provides equipment and books in alternate formats to qualified individuals who cannot read standard print. Certified applications required. Disabilities and information referral services available.
Ava Smith, Librarian
Dina Abramson, Disabilities/Information Referral

Utah

9778 **Utah State Library Division**
Program for the Blind and Disabled
250 North 1950 West, Suite A 801-715-6789
Salt Lake City, UT 84116-7901 800-662-5540
Fax: 801-715-6767
TDD: 801-715-6721
e-mail: blind@utah.gov
http://blindlibrary.utah.gov
Library providing services to individuals with visual impairments who cannot read standard print.
Bessie Y. Oakes, Director

Vermont

9779 **Vermont Department of Libraries Special Services Unit**
578 Paine Turnpike North 802-828-3273
Berlin, VT 05602 800-479-1711
Fax: 802-828-2199
e-mail: ssu@mail.dol.state.vt.us
dol.state.vt.us
Summer reading programs, braille writer, magnifiers, closed-circuit TV, large-print photocopier, cassette books and magazines, children's books on cassette, home visits and other reference materials on blindness and other handicaps.
Theresa Faust, Librarian

Virginia

9780 **Arlington County Department of Libraries**
1015 N Quincy Street 703-228-5959
Arlington, VA 22201-4603 Fax: 703-358-5962
TDD: 703-358-6320
Summer reading programs, braille writer, magnifiers, closed-circuit TV, large-print photocopier, cassette books and magazines, children's books on cassette, home visits and other reference materials on blindness and other handicaps.
Roxanne Barnes, Librarian

9781 **Central Rappahannock Regional Library**
1201 Caroline Street 540-372-1144
Fredericksburg, VA 22401-3701 Fax: 540-373-9411
TDD: 540-371-9165
e-mail: nschiff@hq.crrl.org
Offers reference materials on blindness and other disabilities.
Nancy Schiff, Librarian

9782 **Division for the Visually Handicapped**
1110 N Glebe Road 703-620-3660
Arlington, VA 22201 888-232-7733
Fax: 703-264-9494
e-mail: service@cec.sped.org
www.cec.sped.org
Members are teachers, college faculty members, administrators, supervisors and others concerned with the education and welfare of visually handicapped and blind children and youth. This is a division of the Council For Exceptional Children.

9783 **Fairfax County Public Library**
12000 Government Center Parkway 703-660-6943
Fairfax, VA 22035-0012 Fax: 703-765-5893
TDD: 703-660-8524
e-mail: sjapikse@leo.vsla.edu
www.co.fairfax.va.us.
Summer reading programs, braille writer, magnifiers, closed-circuit TV, large-print photocopier, cassette books and magazines, children's books on cassette, home visits and other reference materials on blindness and other handicaps.
Jeanette Studley, Librarian

9784 **Hampton Subregional Library for the Blind**
1 South Malory Street 757-727-1900
Hampton, VA 23663-4243 800-552-7015
www.hamptonpubliclibrary.org
Summer reading programs, braille writer, magnifiers, closed-circuit TV, large-print photocopier, cassette books and magazines, children's books on cassette, home visits and other reference materials on blindness and other handicaps.
Douglas Perry, Director

9785 **Newport News Public Library System**
110 Main Street 757-591-4858
Newport News, VA 23601-4105 Fax: 757-591-7425
e-mail: shalswin@leo.vsla.edu
www.newport-news.va.us
Summer reading programs, braille writer, magnifiers, closed-circuit TV, large-print photocopier, cassette books and magazines, children's books on cassette, home visits and other reference materials on blindness and other handicaps.
Sue Balswin, Librarian

9786 **Roanoke City Public Library System**
2607 Salem Tpke NW 540-853-2648
Roanoke, VA 24017-5333 Fax: 540-853-1030
Summer reading programs, braille writer, magnifiers, closed-circuit TV, large-print photocopier, cassette books and magazines, children's books on cassette, home visits and other reference materials on blindness and other handicaps.
Rebecca Cooper, Librarian

9787 **Staunton Public Library: Talking Book Center**
1 Churchville Avenue 540-885-6215
Staunton, VA 24401-3229 800-995-6215
Fax: 540-332-3906
e-mail: talkingbook@ci.staunton.via.us
www.loc.gov/nls
Sub-regional library for those who are unable to use standard print materials due to visual, physical, or reading disability.
Oakley Pearson, Librarian

9788 **University Library Services**
Virginia Commonwealth University
901 Park Avenue 804-828-1105
Richmond, VA 23284-2033 Fax: 804-828-0150
www.ucu.edu
Library services for the visually disabled.
Sally Jacobs, Reference Librarian

9789 **Virginia Beach Public Library**
936 Independence Boulevard 757-460-7518
Virginia Beach, VA 23455-6006 Fax: 757-460-6741
vbgov.com/libraries
Summer reading programs, braille writer, magnifiers, closed-circuit TV, large-print photocopier, cassette books and magazines, children's books on cassette, home visits and other reference materials on blindness and other handicaps.
Susan Head, Librarian

Washington

9790 **Washington Library for the Blind and Physically Handicapped**
2021 9th Avenue 206-615-0400
Seattle, WA 98121 Fax: 206-615-0437
e-mail: wtbbl@spl.lib.wa.us
www.wtbbl.org
Summer reading programs, braille writer, magnifiers, closed-circuit TV, large-print photocopier, cassette books and magazines,

children's books on cassette, home visits and other reference materials on blindness and other handicaps.
Jan Ames, Librarian

West Virginia

9791 Cabell County Public Library
455 9th Street 304-528-5700
Huntington, WV 25701-1417 Fax: 304-285-01
e-mail: tbooks@cabell.libwv.us
www.cabell.lib.wv.us
Summer reading programs, braille writer, magnifiers, Arkenstone reader/scanner, cassette books and magazines, children's books on cassette, home visits and other reference materials on blindness and other handicaps.
Vicky Woods, Talking Books Coordinator
Kurle K Judy, Director

9792 Kanawha County Public Library
123 Capitol Street 304-343-4646
Charleston, WV 25301-2609 Fax: 304-348-6530
kanawha.lib.wv.us
Summer reading programs, braille writer, magnifiers, closed-circuit TV, large-print photocopier, cassette books and magazines, children's books on cassette, home visits and other reference materials on blindness and other handicaps.
Dixie Smith, Librarian

9793 Ohio County Public Library Services for the Blind and Physically Handicapped
52 16th Street 304-232-0244
Wheeling, WV 26003-3671 Fax: 304-232-6848
e-mail: llnicholson@hotmail.com
Lori Nicholson, Subregional Librarian BIPH

9794 Parkersburg and Wood County Public Library
3100 Emerson Avenue 304-420-4587
Parkersburg, WV 26104-2414 800-642-8674
Fax: 304-420-4589
e-mail: raitzb@hp9k.park.lib.wv.us
parkersburg.lib.wv.us
Services for the bind and physically handicapped.
Michael Hickman

9795 West Virginia Library Commission
1900 Kanawha Boulevard E 304-558-2041
Charleston, WV 25305-0009 800-642-9021
Fax: 304-558-2044
e-mail: web_one@wvlc.lib.wv.us
librarycommission.lib.wv.us
Summer reading programs, braille writer, magnifiers, closed-circuit TV, large-print photocopier, cassette books and magazines, children's books on cassette, home visits and other reference materials on blindness and other handicaps.
Francis Fesenmainer, Librarian

9796 West Virginia School for the Blind
301 E Main Street 304-822-4800
Romney, WV 26757-1828 Fax: 304-822-3377
e-mail: cjohn@access.mountain.net
Summer reading programs, braille writer, magnifiers, closed-circuit TV, large-print photocopier, cassette books and magazines, children's books on cassette, home visits and other reference materials on blindness and other handicaps.
Cynthia Johnson, Librarian

Wisconsin

9797 Brown County Library
515 Pine Street 920-448-4400
Green Bay, WI 54301-5194 Fax: 920-448-4376
www.co.brown.wi.us
Summer reading programs, braille writer, magnifiers, closed-circuit TV, large-print photocopier, cassette books and magazines, children's books on cassette, home visits and other reference materials on blindness and other handicaps.
Lynn Stainbrook, Director

9798 Wisconsin Regional Library for the Blind Talking Book Program
813 W Wells Street 414-286-3045
Milwaukee, WI 53233-1436 800-242-8822
Fax: 414-286-3102
TDD: 414-286-3548
e-mail: mvalne@mpl.org
www.regionallibrary.wi.gov
Circulates recorded materials, playback equipment and braille materials to print-handicapped Wisconsin residents.
Marsha Valance, Regional Librarian

Wyoming

9799 Wyoming Services for the Visually Disabled
State Department of Education
2300 Capitol Avenue Hathaway Buildi 307-777-7690
Cheyenne, WY 82002-50 Fax: 307-776-34
http//www.k12.wy.us
Eligible readers of Wyoming receive library service from the regional library in Salt Lake City, Utah.
Duane Edmonds, Chairman
Ruby Calvert, Vice Chairman

Research Centers

9800 Baylor College of Medicine: Cullen Eye Institute
6565 Fannin 713-798-6100
Houston, TX 77030-2703 800-229-5676
Fax: 713-798-4231
e-mail: ophthalmology@bcm.edu
www.bcm.edu/eye
Research activities focus on restoring vision and preventing blindness through a better understanding of the disease.
Dan B Jones, Professor and Chair
Milton Boniuk, Professor

9801 BermanGund Laboratory for the Study of Retinal Degenerations
Massachusetts Eye & Eye Infirmary
243 Charles Street 617-523-7900
Boston, MA 02114-3002 Fax: 617-733-44
e-mail: directors@meei.harvard.edu
www.meei.harvard.edu
We strive to offer you the highest quality care from our physicians nurses and clinical staff who are world-leaders in their specialties.ÿFrom the moment you arrive at Mass. Eye and Ear through the completion of your visit we hope that you will feel confident you are in the best hands for care of your eyes ears nose throat head and neck.ÿ
John Fernandez, President
Javier Balloffet, VP-Ophthalmology

9802 Braille Institute Desert Center
70251 Ramon Road 760-321-1111
Rancho Mirage, CA 92270-5203 800-212-4533
Fax: 760-321-9715
e-mail: dc@brailleinstitute.org
www.brailleinstitute.org
Dedicated to providing blind and visually impaired men women and children with the training programs and services they need to enjoy productive lives. Services offered include child development youth programs library services and adult education.
Leslie E Stocker Jr, President
Sally H Jameson, VP of Programs and Services

9803 Braille Institute Orange County Center
527 N Dale Avenue 714-821-5000
Anaheim, CA 92801-4899 Fax: 714-527-7621
e-mail: oc@brailleinstitute.org
www.brailleinstitute.org
Offers services publications information and programs to blind and visually impaired persons.
Sheila F Daily, Orange County Regional Director
Gene Mathiowetz, Assistant Regional Director

9804 Braille Institute Santa Barbara Center Braille Institute of Los Angeles
Braille Institute of Los Angeles

2031 De La Vina Street
Santa Barbara, CA 93105-3895
805-682-6222
800-272-4553
Fax: 805-687-6141
e-mail: sb@brailleinstitute.org
www.brailleinstitute.org

Offers classes type library services and information for persons with visual impairments.

Angela Nowlin, Assistant Regional Director
Michael Lazarovits, Santa Barbara Regional Director

9805 **Braille Institute Sight Center**
741 N Vermont Avenue
Los Angeles, CA 90029
323-663-1111
800-272-4553
Fax: 323-663-0867
e-mail: la@brailleinstitute.org
www.brailleinstitute.org/los_angeles

Offers help programs services and information to the blind and visually impaired children and adults.

Dr Henry C Chang, Director of Library Services
Anita Wright, Los Angeles Regional Program Director

9806 **Braille Institute Youth Center**
3450 Cahuenga Boulevard W
Los Angeles, CA 90068-1381
800-272-4553
Fax: 323-851-6961
www.brailleinstitute.org

Offers various youth programs and services for the blind and visually impaired youngster.

Leslie E Stocker Jr, President
Sally H Jameson, Vice President of Programs and Services

9807 **Braille Textbook Assignment Service National Braille Association**
National Braille Association
95 Allens Creek Road
Rochester, NY 14618-2537
585-427-8260
Fax: 585-427-0263
e-mail: nbaoffice@nationalbraille.org
www.nationalbraille.org

Certified braillists provide readers with technical and nontechnical materials by transcribing for this service.

Diane Spence, President
David W Shaffer, Executive Director

9808 **Carroll Center for the Blind**
770 Centre Street
Newton, MA 02458-2597
617-969-6200
800-852-3131
Fax: 617-969-6204
TTY: 617-969-6204
e-mail: info@carroll.org
www.carroll.org

Assists blind and visually impaired adults and adolescents to adjust to loss of vision. The goal of this dynamic program is to help the person become more independent to restore self-confidence prepare for employment and improve the quality of life. Programs of individual counseling are offered as part of the program.

Dina Rosenbaum, Director of Marketing
Heather Platt, Mobility Instructor

9809 **Clearinghouse for Specialized Media and Technology**
California Department of Education/CSMT
1430 N Street
Sacramento, CA 95814
916-319-0800
Fax: 916-323-9732
TTY: 916-445-4556
e-mail: rbrawleye@cde.ca.gov
www.cde.ca.gov/re/pn/sm

Assists schools and students in the identification and acquisition of textbooks reference books and study materials in aural media braille large print and electronic media access technology.

Rod Brawley, Director

9810 **Clovernook Center for the Blind and Visually Impaired**
7000 Hamilton Avenue
Cincinnati, OH 45231-5240
513-522-3860
888-234-7156
Fax: 513-728-3946
www.clovernook.org

Information and resources for the blind and visually impaired as well as rehabilitation services for youth to mature adults braille production and manufacturing of paper products.

Robin L Usalis, President
Jacqueline L Conner, VP of Multi-State Center East

9811 **Dean A McGee Eye Institute**
608 Stanton L Young Boulevard
Oklahoma City, OK 73104-5065
405-271-6060
800-787-9012
Fax: 405-271-4442
www.dmei.org

Basic and clinical investigations in visual sciences.

David W Parke II, President
Jean Ann Vickery, Director Contact Lens Services

9812 **Department of Ophthalmology/Eye and Ear Infirmary**
1855 W Taylor Street
Chicago, IL 60612-7242
312-996-6590
Fax: 312-996-7770
e-mail: eyeweb@uic.edu
www.uic.edu/com/eye

Offers help support information and research for persons with vision problems including Retinitis Pigmentosa.

Timothy McMahon, Director of Contact Lens Service
Elmer Tu, Director of Cornea Service

9813 **Emory University: Laboratory for Ophthalmic Research**
1365-B Clifton Road NE
Atlanta, GA 30322-1013
404-778-2020
www.eyecenter.emory.edu

Various studies into the aspects of blindness.

Henry F Edelhauser, Director

9814 **Eye Institute of New Jersey New Jersey Medical School**
New Jersey Medical School
PO Box 1709
Newark, NJ 07101-2425
973-972-2036
Fax: 973-723-94
njms.umdnj.edu

Ophthamology including research into cornea retina and neuro-ophthamalogy.

Marco A Zarbin, Chair

9815 **Florida Ophthalmic Institute**
7106 NW 11th Pl
Gainesville, FL 32605-3157
352-331-2020
Fax: 352-331-2019

Nonprofit organization that understands and treats ocular diseases including glaucoma.

Norman S Levy MD, Director

9816 **Foundation for Glaucoma Research**
251 Post Street
San Francisco, CA 94108
415-986-3162
800-826-6693
Fax: 415-986-3763
e-mail: info@glaucoma.org
www.glaucoma.org

Clinical and laboratory studies of glaucoma.

Thomas M Brunner, Chief Executive Officer/President
Andrew Jackson, Director of Communications

9817 **Glaucoma Laser Trabeculoplasty Study Sinai Hospital of Detroit**
Sinai Hospital of Detroit
6767 W Outer Drive
Detroit, MI 48235-2899
313-966-3256
Fax: 313-966-4296

Examines the effectiveness and safety of the treatments of glaucoma.

Hugh Beckman, Chairman

9818 **Harvard University Howe Laboratory of Ophthalmology**
Massachusetts Eye & Ear Infirmary
243 Charles Street
Boston, MA 02114-3002
617-523-7900
www.masseyeandear.org

Development ophthalmology and eye research.

John Fernandez, President
Javier Balloffet, VP Ophthalmology

9819 **Helen Keller International**
352 Park Avenue S
New York, NY 10010
212-532-0544
877-535-5374
Fax: 212-532-6014
e-mail: info@hki.org
www.hki.org

Nonprofit organization for the blind.

Kathy Spahn, President/CEO
Shawn K Baker, VP/Regional Director-Africa

9820 **Helen Keller National Center for Deaf/Blind Youths and Adults**
141 Middle Neck Road 516-944-8900
Sands Point, NY 11050-1299 Fax: 516-944-7302
TTY: 516-944-8637
e-mail: hkncinfo@hknc.org
www.hknc.org
We enable all those who are deaf-blind to live and work in the community of their choice. We provide comprehensive vocational rehabilitation training at our headquarters in NY and assistance with job and residential placements when training is completed.
Joseph McNulty, Executive Director

9821 **Institute for Visual Sciences**
1 E 71st Street 212-305-2919
New York, NY 10021-4102
Ophthalmology with emphasis on the development of care for the eye.
Melissa Mount, Executive Director

9822 **Jerusalem Center for Multi-Handicapped Blind Children**
350 7th Avenue 212-279-4070
New York, NY 10001-7903 Fax: 212-279-4043
e-mail: info@keren-or.org
keren-or.org
Maintains the Keren-Or Center for the Multiply Handicapped Blind Child in Jerusalem for rehabilitation and training. Funds acquired through contributions bequests and legacies.
Madelyn Cohen, Executive Director
Tamara Silberberg, Director Keren-Or Center

9823 **Johns Hopkins University: Dana Center for Preventive Ophthalmology**
Wilmer Ophthalmology Institute
600 N Wolfe Street
Baltimore, MD 21287-0001 410-955-2777
www.hopkinsmedicine.org/wilmer/danacente
Research at the Dana Center focuses on national and international public health prevention of blinding eye disease.
Harry A Quigley, Director

9824 **New Beginnings: The Blind Children's Center**
4120 Marathon Street 213-664-2153
Los Angeles, CA 90029-3505 800-222-3566
The purpose of the Center is to turn initial fears into hope. Helps children and their families become independent by creating a climate of safety and trust. Children learn to develop self confidence and to master a wide range of skills. Services include an infant stimulation program, educational preschool, interdisciplinary assessment services, family services, correspondence program, toll free national hotline and a publication and research service.

9825 **New Beginnings: The Blind Children's Cente**
4120 Marathon Street 323-664-2153
Los Angeles, CA 90029 800-222-3566
Fax: 323-665-3828
www.blindchildrenscenter.org
The purpose of the Center is to turn initial fears into hope. Helps children and their families become independent by creating a climate of safety and trust. Children learn to develop self confidence and to master a wide range of skills. Services include an infant stimulation program educational preschool interdisciplinary assessment services family services correspondence program toll free national hotline and a publication and research service.

9826 **Oregon Health Sciences University: Elk's Children's Eye Clinic**
Casey Eye Institute
3375 SW Terwilliger Boulevard 503-494-3000
Portland, OR 97239-4197 Fax: 503-494-5347
www.ohsucasey.com
Our mission at the Casey Eye Institute is to provide excellent eye care in a quality cost-effective environment that combines education research clinical leadership and service to the community.
Earl Palmer, Director

9827 **Reader-Transcriber Registry National Braille Association**
National Braille Association
3 Townline Circle 716-427-8260
Rochester, NY 14623-2537
Certified braillists fill requests for college textbooks and other technical works through this service of the National Braille Association.

9828 **Smith-Kettlewell Eye Research Institute**
2318 Fillmore Street 415-345-2000
San Francisco, CA 94115-1821 Fax: 415-345-8455
www.ski.org
Dedicated to research on human vision. The Institute was founded to encourage a productive collaboration between the medical clinic and scientific laboratory. Research is conducted with clinical studies which relate directly to the diagnosis and treatment of eye diseases the development of devices and vocational programs to aid the partially sighted and basic research to understand how the eye and brain work for both the clinical and rehabilitation programs.
Arthur Jampolsky, Executive Director
Ruth S Poole, COO

9829 **University of Illinois at Chicago Lions of Illinois Eye Research Institute**
UIC Eye Center
1905 W Taylor Street 312-996-1466
Chicago, IL 60612-7245 Fax: 312-355-4248
www.uic.edu/com/eye/Lions
Visual impairments and blindness research including glaucoma studies.
Janet Szlyk, Presidentÿ
Julie Daraska, Secretaryÿ

9830 **University of Miami: Bascom Palmer Eye Institute**
Department of Ophthalmalogy
900 NW 17th Street 305-326-6000
Miami, FL 33136-1015 800-329-7000
Fax: 305-326-6306
www.bpei.med.miami.edu/site/default.asp
Clinical and basic research into blindness and visual impairments.
John G Clarkson, Dean Emeritus

9831 **Visually Impaired Center**
1422 W Court Street 810-767-4014
Flint, MI 48503 Fax: 810-767-0020
e-mail: info@vicflint.org
www.vicflint.org
A private non-profit agency which offers special programs and some very practical help to people who are blind or partially sighted. Offers rehabilitation low vision aids orientation and mobility vocational training reading and information recreation counseling services volunteer services and community awareness.
Fharon Reigle, Director

9832 **Warren Grant Magnuson Clinical Center National Institute of Health**
National Institute of Health
9000 Rockville Pike 301-496-4000
Bethesda, MD 20892 800-411-1222
Fax: 301-480-9793
TTY: 866-411-1010
e-mail: prpl@mail.cc.nih.gov
www.cc.nih.gov
Established in 1953 as the research hospital of the National Institutes of Health. Designed so that patient care facilities are close to research laboratories so new findings of basic and clinical scientists can be quickly applied to the treatment of patients. Upon referral by physicians patients are admitted to NIH clinical studies.
John I Gallin, Director
David Henderson, Deputy Director for Clinical Care

9833 **Yale University: Vision Research Center**
330 Cedar Street 203-785-5687
New Haven, CT 06510-3218 800-395-7949
Fax: 203-785-7401
e-mail: sarah.gelo@yale.edu
visionresearch.med.yale.edu
Vision including studies on growth and development.
Bruce Shields, Chair
Sarah Gelo, Administrator

Kansas

9834 **Kansas Services for the Blind and Visually Impaired**
Social Rehabilitation Services
915 SW Harrison 785-368-7471
Topeka, KS 66612-2445 800-547-5789
Fax: 785-368-7467
TTY: 785-368-7478
e-mail: rehab@srs.ks.gov
www.srskansas.org/rehab/text/SBVI.htm
Instructional employment oriented services for blind adults.
Laura Howard, Deputy Secretary and Chief Financial Off
Theresa Addington, Accounting and Administrative Operations

Support Groups & Hotlines

9835 **1-800-BRAILLE**
Braille Institute
741 N Vermont Avenue 323-663-1111
Los Angeles, CA 90029-3594 800-272-4553
www.brailleinstitute.org
A toll free information and referral service where callers can obtain information about community programs and referrals to organizations serving the blind in their local areas.
Carol Mora, Director

9836 **AFB Toll-Free Hotline**
American Foundation for the Blind
11 Penn Plaza 212-502-7600
New York, NY 10001-2018 800-232-5463
Fax: 212-502-7777
e-mail: afbinfo@afb.net
www.afb.org
Supplies information on visual impairment and blindness, answers queries regarding AFB services, products, publications, technology, the Careers and Technology Information Bank (a national data bank) and much more.
Richard J. O'Brien, Chair

9837 **American Foundation for the Blind Information Center**
11 Penn Plaza 212-502-7600
New York, NY 10001 800-232-5463
Fax: 212-502-7777
e-mail: afbinfo@afb.net
www.afb.org
Nationally recognized information clearinghouse on blindness and visual impairment. Serves people who are blind or visually impaired, professionals in the field of blindness and visual impairment — including the staff at AFB, business and government organizations and the general public. Provides a toll-free information line available 24 hours a day, online information and referral services, professional library and archival services.

9838 **Aurora of Central New York**
518 James Street 315-422-7263
Syracuse, NY 13203 Fax: 315-422-4792
TTY: 315-422-9746
TDD: 315-422-9746
e-mail: auroracny@auroraofcny.org
www.auroraofcny.org/
Professional counseling services to assist individuals and their families deal with the trauma of hearing or vision loss.
Earleen Foulk, President Board of Directors
Debra Chaiken, Executive Director

9839 **Carroll Center for the Blind**
770 Centre Street 617-969-6200
Newton, MA 2458-2597 800-852-3131
Fax: 617-969-6204
e-mail: dloux@seeingeye.org
www.carroll.org
Rehabilition and educational facility for persons with vision loss.
Dina Rosenbaum, VP Marketing

9840 **Department of Ophthalmology Information Line**
Illinois Eye & Ear Infirmary
1855 W Taylor Street m/c 648 312-996-6500
Chicago, IL 60612-7242 Fax: 312-996-7770
e-mail: eyeweb@uic.edu
www.uic.edu/com/eye/
Offers eye clinic and physician referrals to persons suffering from vision disorders as well as offers emergency information.
Dimitri Azar, Director

9841 **Glaucoma Support Network**
490 Post Street 415-986-3162
San Francisco, CA 94102-1409 800-826-6693
Fax: 415-986-3763
e-mail: info@glaucoma.org
www.glaucoma.org
A peer support service for glaucoma patients and their families. The Network provides meaningful, helpful answers to questions from individuals concerned about vision and glaucoma.
Thomas Brunner, President
Rita Loskill, Executive Director

9842 **Job Opportunities for the Blind**
National Federation of the Blind
1800 Johnson Street 410-659-9314
Baltimore, MD 21230-4998 Fax: 410-685-5653
e-mail: nfb@nfb.org
www.nfb.org
A specialized service that provides free support, resources and information to blind persons seeking employment and to employers interested in hiring the blind. A partnership program with the US Department of Labor, this is the most successful program of it's kind in helping blind persons find competitive work.
Anthony Cobb, Dircetor

9843 **National Association for Parents of the Visually Impaired**
Watertown, MA 2471 617-972-7441
800-562-6265
Fax: 617-972-7444
e-mail: napvi@perkins.org
www.napvi.org
Susan Laventure, Executive Director

9844 **National Center for Sight**
National Society to Prevent Blindness
211 Wacker Drive 312-363-6001
Chicago, IL 60606 800-331-2020
Fax: 312-363-6052
A toll-free line offering information on a broad range of vision, eye health and safety topics including sports eye safety, lazy eye, diabetic retinopathy, glaucoma, cataracts, children's eye disorders, and more.

9845 **National Eye Health Education Program**
1855 W Taylor Street 312-996-6590
Chicago, IL 60612-7242 800-786-3937
Fax: 312-996-9967
www.uic.edu
Offers information and support for persons with vision disorders, including Retinitis Pigmentosa.
Mary Go, Supervisor

9846 **National Health Information Center**
PO Box 1133 310-565-4167
Washington, DC 20013 800-336-4797
Fax: 301-984-4256
e-mail: info@nhic.org
www.health.gov/nhic
Offers a nationwide information referral service, produces directories and resource guides.

9847 **National Service Dog Center**
Delta society
875 124th Avenue, NE 425-226-7357
Bellevue, WA 98005 Fax: 425-235-1076
e-mail: info@deltasociety.org
www.deltasociety.org
A service of the Delta Society, provides information about the selection, training, stewardship, and roles of service dogs; referral to service dog training programs and related resources; education to businesses, health care professionals, and the general public regarding service dog issues; research assistance athrough a re-

source library and network of professional esperts; and advocacy on behalf of people with service dogs.
Linda M Hines, Director
Susan Duncan, Contact

9848 PXE International
4301 Connecticut Avenue, NW 202-362-9599
Washington, DC 20008-2369 Fax: 202-966-8553
e-mail: info@pxe.org
www.pxe.org
Offers vital services to those with pseudoxanthoma elasticum, a connective tissue disorder causing calcification of connective tissue in various places throughout the body, often affecting the membrane behind the eye.
Patrick Terry, President

9849 Recorded Periodicals
Associated Services for the Blind
919 Walnut Street 215-627-0600
Philadelphia, PA 19107-5237 Fax: 215-220-92
e-mail: asbinfo@asb.org
www.asb.org
A subscription service of Associated Services for the Blind, these periodicals provide 21 magazines through this subscription service. A magazine list can be sent, in both large print and on audio cassette.
Patricia C Johnson, President/Chief Executive Officer

9850 Recording for the Blind Helpline
20 Roszel Road 609-452-0606
Princeton, NJ 08540-6294 800-221-4792
e-mail: audioaccesssupport@rfbd.org
www.rfbd.org
An organization dedicated to helping people with print disabilities.
Jay Haggith, Director of Communications

9851 Vision Use in Employment
Carroll Center for the Blind
770 Centre Street 617-969-6200
Newton, MA 02458-2597 800-852-3131
Fax: 617-969-6204
www.carroll.org
VUE provides engineering solutions plus training to help people keep jobs despite their vision loss.
Rachel Rosenbaum, President

9852 Washington Connection
American Council of the Blind
1155 15th Street NW 202-467-5081
Washington, DC 20005-2706 800-424-8666
Fax: 202-467-5085
e-mail: info@acb.org
www.acb.org
Coverage of issues affecting blind people via legislative information, participates in law-making, legislative training seminars and networking of support resources across the US.
Melanie Brunson, Executive Director

Books

9853 AFB Directory of Services for Blind/Vis. Impaired Persons in the US & Canada
AFB Press: American Foundation for the Blind
11 Penn Plaza 212-502-7600
New York, NY 10001 800-232-3044
Fax: 212-502-7774
e-mail: afbdirectory@afb.net
www.afb.org/store
Provides the most comprehensive collection of information available on services for blind and visually impaired individuals. Over 800 pages of revised and updated information on more than 1,500 agencies and 45 new indexes. Includes complete descriptions of services offered by organizations and web sites and e-mail addresses. Available online on a subscription basis.

9854 APH Catalog of Accessible Books for People Who are Visually Impaired
American Printing House for the Blind
1839 Frankfort Avenue 502-895-2405
Louisville, KY 40206-3148 800-223-1839
Fax: 502-895-1509
e-mail: info@aph.org
Offers thousands of selections and publishers of large type and braille books for persons with visual impairments.

9855 Access to Mass Transit for Blind & Visually Impaired Travelers
AFB Press: American Foundation for the Blind
11 Penn Plaza 212-502-7600
New York, NY 10001 800-232-3044
Fax: 212-502-7774
www.afb.org/store
Addresses several travel issues vital to the independence of blind and visually impaired persons from serveral perspectives — those of the blind and visually impaired persons who use mass transit, orientation and mobility instructors and transportation professionals. Focusing on national and international issues, this information filled manual covers approaches to making mass transit available in several cities in the US and Canada, the United Kingdom and Japan.
192 pages Paperback
ISBN: 0-891281-66-5

9856 An Orientation and Mobility Primer for Families and Young Children
American Foundation for the Blind
11 Penn Plaza 212-502-7600
New York, NY 10001-2018 800-232-5463
Fax: 212-502-7777
Practical information for helping a child learn about his or her environment right from the start. Covers sensory training, concept development and orientation skills.
48 pages Papbperback
ISBN: 0-891281-57-6

9857 Art Beyond Sight: Resource Guide to Art, Creativity and Visual Impairment
AFB Press: American Foundation for the Blind
11 Penn Plaza 212-502-7600
New York, NY 10001 800-232-3044
Fax: 212-502-7774
www.afb.org/store
AFB and Art Education for the Blind have joined together to co-publish this one-of-a-kind resource that provides vital information on all aspects of exploring art and creativity by people who are blind or visually impaired. Includes a section of reproducible pages for classroom or workshop activities.
504 pages Paperback
ISBN: 0-891288-50-3

9858 Art and Science of Teaching Orientation to the Visually Impaired
AFB Press: American Foundation for the Blind
11 Penn Plaza 212-502-7600
New York, NY 10001 800-232-3044
Fax: 212-502-7774
www.afb.org/store
Updated and comprehensive description of the techniques of teaching orientation and mobility, presented along with strategies for sensitive and effective teaching. Such factors as individual needs, environmental features and ethical issues are discussed in this important text.
200 pages Paperback
ISBN: 0-891282-59-9

9859 Beginning with Braille: Balanced Approach to Literacy
AFB Press: American Foundation for the Blind
11 Penn Plaza 212-502-7600
New York, NY 10001 800-232-3044
Fax: 212-502-7774
www.afb.org/store
Exciting resource from a skilled practitioner, this book provides a wealth of effective activitoes for promoting literacy at the early stages of braille instruction. The text includes creative and practical strategies for designing and delivering quality braille instruction and offers teacher-friendly suggestions for many areas, such as reading aloud to young children, selecting and making early tac-

tile books and teaching tactile and hand movement skills. Tips on lessons and worksheets.

ISBN: 0-891283-23-4

9860 **Behavioral Vision Approaches for Persons with Physical Disabilities**

William V. Padula, author

Optometric Extension Program Foundation
1921 E. Carnegie Ave., Suite 3-L 949-250-8070
Santa Ana, CA 92705-5510 Fax: 949-250-8175
e-mail: smc.oep@worldnet.att.net
www.oepf.org

A discussion of the behavioral vision/neuro-motor approach to providing directions for prescriptive and therapeutic services for the visually handicapped child or adult.
197 pages
ISBN: 0-943599-04-0
Beverly Roberts, President
Gregory Kitchener, O.D., Vice President

9861 **Blindness and Early Childhood Development**
AFB Press: American Foundation for the Blind
11 Penn Plaza 212-502-7600
New York, NY 10001 800-232-3044
Fax: 212-502-7774
www.afb.org/store

Reviews knowledge of motor and locomotor development, language and cognitive processes and social, emotional and personality development. It is a classic resource for teachers and those who work with children who are blind or visually impaired.
384 pages Paperback
ISBN: 0-891281-23-1

9862 **Braille Book Bank: Music Catalog**
National Braille Association
95 Allens Creek Road, 1-202 585-427-8260
Rochester, NY 14618 Fax: 585-427-0263
e-mail: NBAOffice@nationalbraille.org
www.nationalbraille.org

Offers hundreds of musical titles in print form, braille and on cassette.
62 pages

9863 **Building Blocks: Foundations for Learning for Young Blind & Vis. Impaired Children**
AFB Press: American Foundation for the Blind
11 Penn Plaza 212-502-7600
New York, NY 10001 800-232-3044
Fax: 212-502-7774
www.afb.org/store

Available in English and Spanish, this work presents the essential components of a successful early intervention program, including collaboration with family members, positive relationships between parents and professionals, public education, and attention to important programming components such as space exploration, braille readiness, orientation and mobility, play, cooking and music. VHS video also available.
149 pages Paperback
ISBN: 0-891281-87-8

9864 **Burns Braille Transcription Dictionary**
AFB Press: American Foundation for the Blind
11 Penn Plaza 212-502-7600
New York, NY 10001 800-232-3044
Fax: 212-502-7774
www.afb.org/store

A handy, portable guide that is a quick reference for anyone who needs to check print-to-braille and braille-to-print meanings and symbols. This easy-to-use listing provides readers with the essential alphabet, contractions, punctuation and signs and symbols for braille, as well as brief descriptions of rules for thier use. Organized into four clear sections aimed at providing information at a glance, this valuable tool is an ideal reference for teachers, rehabilitation professionals and others.
96 pages Paperback
ISBN: 0-891292-32-7

9865 **Business Owners Who Are Blind or Visually Impaired**
AFB Press: American Foundation for the Blind
11 Penn Plaza 212-502-7600
New York, NY 10001 800-232-3044
Fax: 212-502-7774
www.afb.org/store

Demonstrates the wide range of careers and talents that can be pursued by persons with visual impairments. Each profile features a successful individual who has accomplised his or her dream of business ownership and who shares important insights. Available in paperback, audio cassette or ASCII disk.
148 pages
ISBN: 0-891283-24-2

9866 **Career Perspectives: Interviews with Blind & Visually Impaired Professionals**
AFB Press: American Foundation for the Blind
11 Penn Plaza 212-502-7600
New York, NY 10001 800-232-3044
Fax: 212-502-7774
www.afb.org/store

Profiles of 20 successful archivers who describe in their own words what it takes to pursue and attain professional success in a sighted world. From all around the country and representing a wide range of professions, including law, science, journalism, management and medicine, the blind and visually impaired individuals featured serve as role models for others who wnat to follow career paths.
96 pages Paperback
ISBN: 0-891281-70-3

9867 **Childhood Glaucoma: A Reference Guide for Families**
NAPVI
PO Box 317 617-972-7441
Watertown, MA 02471-0317 800-562-6265
Fax: 617-972-7444
e-mail: napvi@perkins.org
www.napvi.org

Susan LaVenture, Executive Director

9868 **Communication Skills for Visually Impaired**
Charles C Thomas Publisher
2600 S 1st Street 217-789-8980
Springfield, IL 62704-4730 Fax: 217-789-9130
e-mail: books@ccthomas.com
www.ccthomas.com

322 pages
ISBN: 0-398066-92-2

9869 **Concept Development for Visually Impaired Children: Resource Guide**
AFB Press: American Foundation for the Blind
11 Penn Plaza 212-502-7600
New York, NY 10001 800-232-3044
Fax: 212-502-7774
www.afb.org/store

Program for integrating such concepts as body imagery, gross motor movement, posture and tactile discrimination into the curriculum from kindergarten on.
80 pages Paperback
ISBN: 0-891280-18-9

9870 **Coping with Vision Loss**

Bill Chapman, EdD, author

Hunter House Publishing
PO Box 2914 510-865-5282
Alameda, CA 94501 800-266-5592
Fax: 510-865-4295
e-mail: ordering@hunterhouse.com
www.hunterhouse.com

Maximizing what you can see and do. The Author explains the five leading causes of vision loss, and how to use new skills and vision aids.
2001 304 pages Paperback
Cristina Sverdrup, Customer Service Manager

9871 **Development of Social Skills by Blind and Visually Impaired Students**
AFB Press: American Foundation for the Blind

11 Penn Plaza 212-502-7600
New York, NY 10001 800-532-3044
Fax: 212-502-7774
www.afb.org/store

Examination of the social interactions of children with visual impairments, theory and research are combined to explore how these children can be helped to succeed socially. Innovative practical strategies are provided for educators, researchers and families on how to assist children in the development of social skills. Qualitative ethnographic approaches demonstrate how classroom teachers can work effectively with individual children and present valuable insights about children's interactions.
232 pages Paperback
ISBN: 0-891282-17-3

9872 Early Focus: Working with Young Children Who Are Blind or Visually Impaired
AFB Press: American Foundation for the Blind
11 Penn Plaza 212-502-7600
New York, NY 10001 Fax: 212-502-7777
www.afb.org/store

Early intervention has increasingly been recognized as critical in the development and growth of children with visual impairments and other disabilities. Federal regulations have mandated early indentifacation and assesment, underscoring its importance for children's well being. This revised and updated edition of Early Focus provides the important information you need to know including serving culturally diverse families with children who have multiple disabilities and practical tips.
376 pages Paperback
ISBN: 0-891282-15-7

9873 Encyclopedia of Blindness and Vision Impairment
Facts on File
11 Penn Plaza 212-967-8800
New York, NY 10001 800-322-8755
Fax: 800-678-3633

Designed to provide both laymen and professionals with concise, practical information on the second most common disability in the US.
340 pages Hardcover

9874 Equals in Partnership: Basic Rights for Families of Children with Blindness
NAPVI
PO Box 317 617-972-7441
Watertown, MA 02471-0317 800-562-6265
Fax: 617-972-7444
e-mail: napvi@perkins.org
www.napvi.org

Susan LaVenture, Executive Director

9875 Essential Elements in Early Intervention: Visual Impairment & Multiple Disability
AFB Press: American Foundation for the Blind
11 Penn Plaza 212-502-7600
New York, NY 10001 800-232-3044
Fax: 212-502-7774
www.afb.org/store

Latest comprehensive resource from an outstanding early childhood specialist, this guide provides a range of information on effective early intervention with young children who are visually impaired and have other disabilities.
503 pages Paperback
ISBN: 0-891283-05-6

9876 Eye and Your Vision
Dr Lorrain H Marchi, author
National Association for Visually Handicapped
22 W 21st Street 212-889-3141
New York, NY 10010-6904 Fax: 212-727-2931
e-mail: navh@navh.org
www.navh.org

A large booklet offering information, with illustrations, on the eye. Includes information on protection of eyesight, how the eye works and vision disorders.
19 pages $5.00 n/members
Lorraine Marchi LHD, Founder/CEO
Cesar Gomez, Executive Director

9877 First Steps
Blind Children's Center
4120 Marathon Street 213-664-2153
Los Angeles, CA 90029-3584 Fax: 213-665-3828
e-mail: info@blindcntr.org
www.blindcntr.org

A handbook for teaching young children who are visually impaired. Designed to assist students, professionals and parents working with children who are visually impaired.
203 pages

9878 Foundations of Education
AFB Press: American Foundation for the Blind
11 Penn Plaza 212-502-7600
New York, NY 10001 800-232-3044
Fax: 212-502-7774
www.afb.org/store

Complete revision of landmark text. Comprehensive compilation of state-of-the-art information is the essential resource on educating visually impaired students, the essential theory forming the knowledge base, and methodology of teaching visually impaired students in all areas.
2000
ISBN: 0-891283-49-8

9879 Foundations of Orientation and Mobility
AFB Press: American Foundation for the Blind
11 Penn Plaza 212-502-7600
New York, NY 10001 800-232-3044
Fax: 212-502-7774
www.afb.org

Updated and revised, this new edition of the field's founding classics includes current research fom a variety of disiplines, an international perspective, and expanded contents on low vision, aging, multiple disabilities, accessibility, program design and adaptive technology from more than 30 eminent subject experts. Divided into four main sections, the book explores every of Orientation and Mobility learning and instruction.
800 pages Hardcover
ISBN: 0-891289-46-1

9880 Foundations of Rehabilitation Counseling with Persons Who Are Blind/Visually Imp.
AFB Press: American Foundation for the Blind
11 Penn Plaza 212-502-7600
New York, NY 10001 800-232-3044
Fax: 212-502-7774
www.afb.org/store

Rehabilitation professionals have long recognized that the needs of people who are blind or visually impaired are unique and require a special knowledge and expertise for the provision and coordination of effective rehabilitation services. Contributions to this text from more than 25 experts provide essential information on subjects as functional, medical, vocational and phychological assessments, demographic and cultural issues, pacement and employment issues, and the rehabilitation team.
464 pages Hardcover
ISBN: 0-891289-45-3

9881 Get a Wiggle On
American Alliance For Health, Phys. Ed. & Dance
1900 Association Drive 703-476-3400
Reston, VA 20191-1598 800-213-7193
www.aahperd.org/

Gives teachers and parents practical suggestions for helping blind and visually impaired infants grow and learn like other children.
80 pages
ISBN: 0-883140-77-2

9882 Guide to Independence for the Visually Impaired and Their Families
Demos Medical Publishing
386 Park Avenue S 212-683-0072
New York, NY 10016-8804 800-532-8663
Fax: 212-683-0118
e-mail: orderdept@demopub.com
www.demosmedpub.com

This first comprehensive, hands-on book for the newly visually impaired and their families presents detailed instructions to deal with emotional reactions and fioght depression; contact organiza-

tions and get information; obtain federal and other types of financial aid; use the other senses more effectively; adapt their homes and do household chores; handle paperwork and become socially active.
248 pages Paperback
ISBN: 0-939957-61-2
Dr. Diana M Schneider, President

9883 **Guidelines and Games for Teaching Efficient Braille Reading**
AFB Press: American Foundation for the Blind
11 Penn Plaza 212-502-7600
New York, NY 10001 800-232-3044
Fax: 212-502-7774
www.afb.org/store
Based on research in the areas of rapid reading and precision teaching, these effective guidelines and games represent a unique adaptation of a general reading program to the needs of braille readers.
116 pages Paperback
ISBN: 0-891281-05-3

9884 **Hammond Large Type World Atlas**
American Map-Langensceidt Publishing Group
15 Tyger River Drive 864-486-0214
Duncan, SC 29334 800-432-6277
Fax: 888-773-7979
www.hammondmap.com
100 maps.

ISBN: 0-816159-11-4

9885 **Handbook for Itinerant and Resource Teachers of Blind Students**
National Federation of the Blind
1800 Johnson Street 410-659-9314
Baltimore, MD 21230-4998 Fax: 410-685-5653
e-mail: subscribe@diabetes.nfb.org
www.nfb.org
The Handbook provides help to teachers, school administrators or other school personnel that have experience with blind or visually impaired students. The Handbook devotes 45 pages to Braille and how to teach Braille for parents and teachers; other chapters iclude law, physical education, fitting in socially, testing and evaluation, home economics, daily living skills and more.
533 pages Softcover
Eileen Ley, Director of Publishing
Elizabeth Lunt, Editor

9886 **Health Care Professionals Who are Blind or Visually Impaired**
AFB Press: American Foundation for the Blind
11 Penn Plaza 212-502-7600
New York, NY 10001 800-232-3044
Fax: 212-502-7774
www.afb.org/store
Exciting career possibilities for people who are visually impaired as well as those who are sighted. Inspirational profiles of 15 sucessful role models. Written in an accesible, easy-to-read style, this book documents the stories and stategies of professionals ranging from a forensic psychiatrist to a radiology dark room technician. Information on technology and tactics that are used to perform demanding jobs are also included. Available in paperback, audio casette, or ASCII disk.
2001 166 pages
ISBN: 0-891283-88-9

9887 **I Keep Five Pairs of Glasses in a Flower Pot**
Henrietta Levner, author
National Association for Visually Handicapped
22 W 21st Street 212-889-3141
New York, NY 10010-6904 Fax: 212-727-2931
e-mail: navh@navh.org
www.navh.org
A short story, printed in 18 point type, is the saga of one womans struggle with low vision.
Lorraine Marchi LHD, Founder/CEO
Cesar Gomez, Executive Director

9888 **If Blindness Comes**
National Federation of the Blind
1800 Johnson Street 410-659-9314
Baltimore, MD 21230-4998 Fax: 410-685-5653
e-mail: subscribe@diabetes.nfb.org
www.nfb.org
An introduction to issues relating to vision loss and provides a positive, supportive philosophy about blindness. It is a general information book which includes answers to many common questions about blindness, information about services and programs for the blind and resource listings.
Eileen Ley, Director of Publishing
Elizabeth Lunt, Editor

9889 **Independence Without Sight or Sound: Suggestions for Practitioners**
AFB Press: American Foundation for the Blind
11 Penn Plaza 212-502-7600
New York, NY 10001 800-232-3044
Fax: 212-502-7774
www.afb.org/store
Written in a personal and informal style, this practical guidebook covers the essential aspects of communicating and working with deaf-blind persons. Full of valuable information on subjects such as how to talk with deaf-blind people, adapt orientation and mobility techniques for deaf-blind travelers, and interact with deaf-blind individuals socially, this useful manual also contains a substantial resource section detailing sources of information and adapted equipment. Also available in braille.
193 pages Paperback
ISBN: 0-891282-46-7

9890 **Jewish Heritage for the Blind**
1655 E 24th Street 718-338-4999
Brooklyn, NY 11229-2401 800-995-1888
Offers large print traditional prayer books for the High Holy days, festivals, fast days and daily rituals for those finding it difficult or impossible to read small print.

9891 **Kernel Book Series**
National Federation of the Blind
1800 Johnson Street 410-659-9314
Baltimore, MD 21230-4998 Fax: 410-685-5653
e-mail: subscribe@diabetes.nfb.org
www.nfb.org
A series of books written by the blind themselves. Each book is a collection of articles and stories about the real life experiences of blind persons. These books help educate the blind and the sighted alike about a positive philosophy regarding blindness.
Eileen Ley, Director of Publishing
Elizabeth Lunt, Editor

9892 **King James Bible: Large Print**
Science Products
PO Box 888
Southeastern, PA 19399-0888 800-888-7400
24 point type easily seen with 20/200 acuity. Makes bible reading for children easier too.

9893 **Knotholes are for Seeing: Therapy Through Poetry, Prose & Other Writings**
Business of Living Publications
PO Box 8388 512-852-8515
Corpus Christi, TX 78468-8388

ISBN: 1-879518-08-2

9894 **Large Print American Heritage Dictionary**
Houghton Mifflin Harcourt
222 Berkeley Street 617-351-5000
Boston, MA 02116 800-888-7400
www.hmco.com
More than 35,000 easy to read entries for those who prefer large type.

ISBN: 0-395929-32-6

9895 **Legislative Handbook for Parents**
NAPVI

PO Box 317 617-972-7441
Watertown, MA 02471-0317 800-562-6265
Fax: 617-972-7444
e-mail: napvi@perkins.org
www.spedex.com

Written by parents for parents in dealing with legislative processes that ultimately affect their children's lives.
Susan LaVenture, Executive Director

9896 **Library Resources for the Blind and Physically Handicapped**
National Library Service for the Blind
1291 Taylor Street NW 202-707-5100
Washington, DC 20542-0002 Fax: 202-707-0712
www.loc.gov/nls

9897 **Low Vision: Reflections of the Past, Issues for the Future**
AFB Press: American Foundation for the Blind
11 Penn Plaza 212-502-7600
New York, NY 10001 800-232-3044
Fax: 212-502-7774
www.afb.org/store

Research report based on a multiphase survey of professionals. Identifies important trends that will shape the field of low vision services into the next century. Designed for administrators, policy planners and university instructors, as well as for direct service providers, Low Vision includes overview papers by six eminent leaders in the low vision field.
181 pages Paperback
ISBN: 0-891282-18-1

9898 **Madness of Usher's: Coping with Vision & Hearing Loss**
Richard A. Lewis, Dorothy H. Stiefel, author
Business of Living Publications
PO Box 8388 512-852-8515
Corpus Christi, TX 78468-8388
Paperback
ISBN: 1-879518-06-6
Dorothy H Stiefel, Author

9899 **Mainstreaming & the American Dream: Soc. Logical Perspectives on Parental Coping**
AFB Press: American Foundation for the Blind
11 Penn Plaza 212-502-7600
New York, NY 10001 800-232-3044
Fax: 212-502-7774
www.afb.org/store

Based on in-depth interviews with parents and professionals, this research monograph presents a sociological framework for looking at the needs and aspirations of parents of blind and visually impaired children.
256 pages Paperback
ISBN: 0-891281-91-6

9900 **Mainstreaming the Visually Impaired Child**
NAPVI
PO Box 317 617-972-7441
Watertown, MA 02471-0317 800-562-6265
Fax: 617-972-7444
e-mail: napvi@perkins.org
www.napvi.org

A unique, informative guide for teachers and educational professionals that work with the visually impaired.
Susan LaVenture, Executive Director

9901 **Making Life More Livable: Adaptations for Living at Home After Vision Loss**
AFB Press: American Foundation of the Blind
11 Penn Plaza 212-502-7600
New York, NY 10001 800-232-3044
Fax: 212-502-7774
www.afb.org/store

Essential guide for adults experiencing vision loss and an invaluable resource for their family and friends. Full of practical tips and illustrated by numerous photographs, this easy-to-use resource shows how people who are visually impaired can continue living independent, productive lives at home on their own. Useful general guidelines and room-by-room specifics provide simple and effective solutions for making homes accessible and everyday activities doable for visually impaired individuals.
132 pages Cassette avail.
ISBN: 0-891281-15-0

9902 **Occupational Therapy Practice Guidelines for Adults with Low Vision**
American Occupational Therapy Association
4720 Montgomery Lane 301-652-2682
Bethesda, MD 20824-1220 Fax: 301-652-7711
TDD: 800-377-8555
www.aota.org

25 pages
ISBN: 1-569001-50-2

9903 **Perkins Activity and Resource Guide: A Handbook for Teachers**
Perkins School for the Blind Publications
175 N Beacon Street 617-924-3434
Watertown, MA 02472-2790 Fax: 917-926-2027

This is a comprehensive, two volume guide with over 1,000 pages of activities, resources and instructional strategies for teachers and parents of students with visual and multiple disabilities.

9904 **Preschool Learning Activities for the Visually Impaired Child**
NAPVI
PO Box 317 617-972-7441
Watertown, MA 02471-0317 800-562-6265
Fax: 617-972-7444
e-mail: napvi@perkins.org
www.napvi.org

This guide for parents offers games and activities to keep visually impaired children active during the preschool years.
Susan LaVenture, Executive Director

9905 **Prescriptions for Independence: Working with Older People Who Are Visually Imp.**
AFB Press: American Foundation for the Blind
11 Penn Plaza 212-502-7600
New York, NY 10001 800-232-3044
Fax: 212-502-7774
www.afb.org/store

Easy-to-read manual on how older persons with visual impairments can pursue their interests and activities in community residences, senior centers, long-term care facilities and other community settings. Topics covered include signs of vision loss, recreation, personal care, orientation and mobility and modifications in the environment.
87 pages Paperback
ISBN: 0-891282-44-0

9906 **Providing Services for People with Vision Loss: Multidisciplinary Perspective**
Resources For Rehabilitation
22 Bonad Road 781-368-9094
Winchester, MA 01890 Fax: 781-368-9096
e-mail: info@rfr.org
www.rfr.org

A collection of articles by ophthalmologists and rehabilitation professionals, including chapters on operating a low vision service, starting self-help programs, mental health services, aids and techniques that help people with vision loss.
136 pages
ISBN: 0-929718-02-X

9907 **Psychoeducational Assessment of Visually Impaired Students**
Pro-Ed, Inc.
8700 Shoal Creek Boulevard 512-451-3246
Austin, TX 78757-6897 800-897-3202
Fax: 800-397-7633
e-mail: info@proedinc.com
www.proedinc.com

Professional reference book that addresses the problems specific to assessment of visually impaired children. Of particular value to the practitioner are the extensive reviews of available tests, including ways to adapt those not designed for use with the visually handicapped.
140 pages Paperback
Lindy Jordaan, Marketing Coordinator

9908 **Resources Family Centered Intervention for Infants, Toddlers & Preschoolers**
Hope
1856 N 1200 E 435-245-2888
North Logan, UT 84341 Fax: 435-245-2888
Describes children with vision impairment in terms of characteristics, needs, and parent concerns.
Hardcover

9909 **Show Me How: Manual for Parents Preschool Visually Impaired & Blind Children**
AFB Press: American Foundation for the Blind
11 Penn Plaza 212-502-7600
New York, NY 10001 800-232-3044
Fax: 212-502-7774
www.afb.org/store
Practical guide for parents, teachers and others who help preschool children attain age-related goals. Includes activities for growing and learning, building self-concept, moving around, playing, perfecting daily living skills and developing sensory awareness. It also covers such issues as observing safety precautions, choosing appropriate toys and facilitating relationships with playmates.
56 pages Paperback
ISBN: 0-891281-13-4

9910 **Starting Points**
Blind Children's Center
4120 Marathon Street 213-664-2153
Los Angeles, CA 90029-3584 Fax: 213-665-3828
Basic information for the clasroom teacher of 3 to 8 year olds whose multiple disabilities include visual impairment.
160 pages

9911 **Tactile Graphics**
AFB Press: American Foundation for the Blind
11 Penn Plaza 212-502-7600
New York, NY 10001 800-232-3044
Fax: 212-502-7774
www.afb.org/store
Easy-to-read encyclopedia handbook on translating visual information into a three-dimensional form that the blind and visually impaired persons can understand. This heavily illustrated guide covers therory, techniques, materials and step-by-step instructions for educators, rehabilitators, graphic artists, museum and busines personnel, employers and anyone involved in producing tactile material for visually impaired persons.
544 pages Paperback
ISBN: 0-891281-94-0

9912 **Teachers Who Are Blind or Visually Impaired**
AFB Press: American Foundation for the Blind
11 Penn Plaza 212-502-7600
New York, NY 10001 800-232-3044
Fax: 212-502-7774
www.afb.org/store
First volume in the Jobs That Matter series, this book profiles 18 visually impaired individuals who have successfully fulfilled their dreams of becoming teachers. These engaging individuals demonstrate how visually impaired teachers can be effective in their jobs and achieve classroom sucess and satisfaction. Available in paperback, audio cassette or braille.
1998 176 pages
ISBN: 0-891283-06-4

9913 **Textbook Catalog**
National Braille Association
95 Allens Creek Road 1-202 585-427-8260
Rochester, NY 14618 Fax: 585-427-0263
www.nationalbraille.org
Lists hundreds of scholarly, college and professional textbooks offered in large print, braille or on cassette for visually impaired readers.
80 pages

9914 **To Love This Life: Quotations by Helen Keller**
AFB Press: American Foundation for the Blind
11 Penn Plaza 212-502-7600
New York, NY 10001 800-232-3044
Fax: 212-502-7774
www.afb.org/store
Beautiful and moving souvenir of one of the world's most admired women. This memorable collection of quotations from Helen Keller brings words of wisdom, courage and inspiration from a remarkable individual who above all wanted to make a difference in the lives of her fellow men and women. The thought captured here — many from unpublished letters and speeches — offer profound statements on the meaning of being human and on life in all its complexity. Available in hardcover and audio cassette.
2000 118 pages
ISBN: 0-891283-47-1

9915 **Unseen Minority: Social History of Blindness in the US**
Frances A. Koestler, author
David McKay Company/AFB Press, Distributor
11 Penn Plaza 412-741-1398
New York, NY 10001 800-232-3044
Fax: 412-741-0609
e-mail: afborder@abdintl.com
www.afb.org
Lively narrative, peppered with anecdotes, recounts how the blind overcame discrimination to gain full participation in the social, educational, economic and legislative spheres. Here are the gripping stories: Why it took a century for braille to become a universal medium in English, how america's first school for the blind began with a chance encounter on a Boston street, and how the talking book came into existence.
573 pages Hardcover
ISBN: 0-679505-39-3

9916 **Vision and Aging: Crossroads for Service Delivery**
AFB Press: American Foundation for the Blind
11 Penn Plaza 212-502-7600
New York, NY 10001 800-232-3044
Fax: 212-502-7774
www.afb.org/store
This overview of the service delivery systems in the aging and blindness fields covers the essential issues concerning vision loss among older persons in this country, the growth of visual impairment among the increasing number of elderly people in the US, and the policy and service questions that will demand national attention throughout this and the coming decades.
392 pages Paperback
ISBN: 0-891282-16-5

9917 **Visual Aids and Informational Material**
National Association for Visually Handicapped
22 W 21st Street 212-889-3141
New York, NY 10010-6904 Fax: 212-727-2931
e-mail: navh@navh.org
www.navh.org
A large reference guide offering a list of visual aids and resources for persons with visual impairments.
65 pages
Lorraine Marchi LHD, Founder/CEO
Cesar Gomez, Executive Director

9918 **Visual Handicaps and Learning**
Pro-Ed, Inc.
8700 Shoal Creek Boulevard 512-451-3246
Austin, TX 78757-6897 800-897-3202
Fax: 800-397-7633
e-mail: info@proedinc.com
www.proedinc.com
This text covers a range of topics associated with visual impairment, from past practices to up-to-date research, and from legal responsibilities to personal beliefs, without losing sight of the individual child.
180 pages
ISBN: 0-890795-15-0
Lindy Jordaan, Marketing Coordinator

9919 **Visual Impairment: An Overview**
AFB Press: American Foundation for the Blind
11 Penn Plaza 212-502-7600
New York, NY 10001 800-232-3044
Fax: 212-502-7774
www.afb.org/store
Down-to-earth look at the common forms of vision loss and their impact on the individual. Explains the different aspects of visual

impairment, describes adaptive techniques and devices and provides information on available resources and services in a concise and easy-to-understand manner for professionals and visually impaired people and their families.
56 pages Paperback
ISBN: 0-891281-74-6

9920 Walking Alone and Marching Together
Floyd Matson, author
National Federation of the Blind
1800 Johnson Street 410-659-9314
Baltimore, MD 21230-4998 Fax: 410-685-5653
e-mail: subscribe@diabetes.nfb.org
www.nfb.org
The history of the organized blind movement, this book spans more than 50 years of civil rights, social issues, attitudes and experiences of the blind. Published in 1990, it has been read by thousands of blind and sighted persons and is used in colleges, libraries and programs across the country as an important tool in understanding blindness and it's impact on both personal lives and the society at large.
1100 pages
Eileen Ley, Director of Publishing
Elizabeth Lunt, Editor

9921 Webster Large Print Dictionary
Random House
1745 Broadway, 15-3 212-782-9000
New York, NY 10019 800-888-7400
www.randomhouse.com
Ten point type, more than 60,000 word entries and illustrations.
880 pages
ISBN: 0-375722-32-7

9922 What Museum Guides Need to Know: Access for Blind & Visually Impaired Visitors
AFB Press: American Foundation for the Blind
11 Penn Plaza 212-502-7600
New York, NY 10001 800-232-3044
Fax: 212-502-7774
www.afb.org/store
Provides practical, easy-to-use guidelines on how to greet and help blind and visually impaired museum goers. With numerous photographs taken at the High School Museum of Art and the Atlanta Historical Society, this handbook also covers aesthetics and visual impairment, legal requirements for accessibility, resources, a training outline for museum requirements for accessibility, a bibliography on art and museum access for blind and visually impaired persons, and guidelines for preparing media.
64 pages Paperback
ISBN: 0-891281-58-4

Children's Books

9923 Belonging
Dial Books
375 Hudson Street
New York, NY 10014-3658 212-366-2000
www.penguingroup.com
Meg attended special schools for the blind until she was ready for high school. She decided that she wanted to go to a regular high school. She and her mother practiced her walks to school and studied the layout of the building prior to school starting, but Meg was unprepared for the trip when there were 1,500 students. She adjusted quickly to the crowds and the pace of the new school.
200 pages Hardcover
ISBN: 0-803705-30-1

9924 Beside Me
Leader Dogs For The Blind
1039 S. Rochester Road 248-651-9011
Rochester Hills, MI 48307 888-777-5332
Fax: 248-651-5812
TTY: 248-651-3713
e-mail: leaderdog@leaderdog.org
www.leaderdog.org
Marion became blind as an adult. She was totally dependent on her parents to move around and go places she wanted to be. Marion decided to go to the leader-dog program and learn to use a leader dog. Particularly she wanted the independence she would need to go to college. Marion enrolled at the Leader-Dog-For-The-Blind Program in Rochester, Michigan. After weeks of training she was given a German Shepherd named Heidi. Marion and Heidi trained together until they were a team and ready.
Films

9925 Guide Dog Goes to School
William Morrow and Company
105 Madison Avenue 212-889-3050
New York, NY 10016-7418 800-843-9389
william-morrow-co.1.searchbook.net
Cinderena is a golden retriever. As a puppy Cindy is outgoing and not afraid of things in her environment. This disposition is ideal for a guide dog to the blind, and Cindy is selected to be in a program for guide dogs. Follow Cindy as we focus on the guide dog training.
51 pages Hardcover
ISBN: 0-688068-44-8

9926 How Do You Kiss a Blind Girl?
Charles C Thomas Publisher
2600 S First Street 217-789-8980
Springfield, IL 62704-4730 Fax: 217-789-9130
e-mail: books@ccthomas.com
www.ccthomas.com
Focuses, in a humorous way, on the attitudes toward persons with visual impairments.
126 pages
ISBN: 0-398052-62-X

9927 Living with Blindness
Franklin Watts Grolier
90 Old Sherman Tpke 203-797-3500
Danbury, CT 06816-0001 800-621-1115
Fax: 203-797-3197
www.grolier.com
Shows how persons with visual impairments and blindness can overcome their disability and lead productive lives.
32 pages Grades 5-7
ISBN: 0-531108-43-0

9928 Man Who Sang in the Dark
Eth Clifford, author
Houghton, Mifflin & Company
1 Beacon Street 617-725-5000
Boston, MA 02108-3107
The story of a girl and a man who is blind and how they both come to an understanding about certain prejudices.
Grades 3-5

9929 Out of the Corner of My Eye
American Foundation for the Blind
15 W 16th Street 212-502-7600
New York, NY 10011-6301 Fax: 212-502-7777
A personal account of students' vision loss and subsequent adjustment that is full of practical advice and cheerful encouragement, told by an 87 year old retired college teacher who has maintained her independence and zest for life.

ISBN: 0-891281-93-2

9930 She'll Never Walk Alone
Leader Dog For The Blind
1964 Park Street 306-565-8211
Regina, SK, S4P 3G4,
Leader dogs for the blind require many weeks of training before they are ready to work with the blind individual. Two courses, basic and advanced, are provided for each dog.
Films

Magazines

9931 Access World: Technology and People with Visual Impairments
AFB Press: American Foundation for the Blind

11 Penn Plaza
New York, NY 10001
212-502-7600
800-232-3044
Fax: 212-502-7774
e-mail: afbdirectory@afb.net
www.afb.org/store

Comprehensive and reader friendly online magazine covering every aspect of assistive technology and visual impairment.
Bimonthly

9932 **Blind Educator**
National Federation of the Blind
1800 Johnson Street
Baltimore, MD 21230-4998
410-659-9314
Fax: 410-685-5653
e-mail: subscribe@diabetes.nfb.org
www.nfb.org

The articles in this newsletter are written by people who are blind. Blind people can teach. In fact, this newsletter captures a glimpse of the range of subjects and grade levels in which blind people are engaged.
Eileen Ley, Director of Publishing
Elizabeth Lunt, Editor

9933 **Braille Forum**
Penny Reeder, author
American Council of the Blind
1155 15th Street NW
Washington, DC 20005-2706
202-467-5081
800-424-8666
Fax: 202-467-5085
e-mail: info@acb.org
www.acb.org

Offered in large print, braille, half speed cassette, via email and on the website.
32 pages 10x/year
Sharon Lovering, Editor

9934 **Braille Monitor**
National Federation of the Blind
1800 Johnson Street
Baltimore, MD 21230-4998
410-659-9314
Fax: 410-685-5653
e-mail: subscribe@diabetes.nfb.org
www.nfb.org

The leading publication in the blindness field, with a circulation of 30,000, this publication addresses issues of concern to the blind and the philosophy and activities of the National Federation of the Blind.
100 pages Monthly
Eileen Leyrce, Director of Publishing
Elizabeth Lunt, Editor

9935 **Dialogue Magazine**
Blindskills
PO Box 5181
Salem, OR 97304-0181
503-581-4224
800-860-4224
Fax: 503-518-0178
e-mail: blindsici@teleport.com
www.teleport.com

Publishes quarterly magazine in braille, large-type, cassette and disk of news items, fiction and articles of special interest.
Quarterly

9936 **Future Reflections**
Barbara Cheadler, author
National Federation of the Blind
1800 Johnson Street
Baltimore, MD 21230-4998
410-659-9314
Fax: 410-685-5653
e-mail: subscribe@diabetes.nfb.org
www.nfb.org

National magazine written specifically for parents and educators of blind children. Each issue addresses various topics important to blind children, their families and to school personnel.
Quarterly
Eileen Ley, Director of Publishing
Elizabeth Lunt, Editor

9937 **Illinois Braille Messenger**
Illinois Council of the Blind
PO Box 1336
Springfield, IL 62705-1336
217-523-4967
888-698-1862
Fax: 217-523-4302
e-mail: icb@fgi.net

Quarterly
Laura Booker, Editor

9938 **Journal of Vision Rehabilitation**
Media Productions & Marketing
2440 O Street
Lincoln, NE 68510-1125
402-474-2676

Multidisciplinary journal containing articles and papers dealing with low vision, its evaluation, instrumentation and rehabilitation.

9939 **Journal of Visual Impairment & Blindness**
AFB Press: American Foundation for the Blind
11 Penn Plaza
New York, NY 10001
212-502-7600
800-232-3044
Fax: 212-502-7774
www.afb.org/store

Peer-reviewed journal reporting on the cutting-edge research, innovative practice and news on all aspects of visual impairment. Available online, on cassette and ASCII disk.
10 Issues

9940 **Recorded Periodicals**
Associated Services for the Blind
919 Walnut Street
Philadelphia, PA 19107-5237
215-627-0600
Fax: 215-922-0692
e-mail: asbinfo@asb.org
www.asb.org

A subscription service of Associated Services for the Blind, this service provides 26 recorded magazines for blind and visually impaired individuals.
Audio Cassette
Patricia C Johnson, President/CEO

9941 **Review**
AER
206 N Washington Street
Alexandria, VA 22314-2528
703-823-9690
Fax: 703-823-9695

The Association's practice-oriented journal.

9942 **Tactic**
Clovernook Ctr. for the Blind & Visually Impaired
7000 Hamilton Avenue
Cincinnati, OH 45231-5240
513-522-3860
888-224-7156
Fax: 513-728-3946
www.clovernook.org

Quarterly
Jeffrey D Brasie, President

9943 **Vision Enhancement Journal**
Vision World Wide
5707 Brockton Drive
Indianapolis, IN 46220-5481
317-254-1332
800-733-2258
Fax: 317-251-6588
e-mail: info@visionww.org
www.visionww.org

Leading International publication providing information and resources for people with vision loss. Journal is available in large print, audio cassette and computer disk.
68-78 pages Quarterly
Patricia Price, President/Managing Editor

9944 **Vision World Wide**
5707 Brockton Drive
Indianapolis, IN 46220-5481
317-254-1332
800-733-2258
Fax: 317-251-6588
e-mail: info@visionww.org
www.visionww.org

Believing there is hope when vision fails. It disseminates relevant information on a variety of topics through its information and referral helpline, website, e-mail announce list and journal Vision Enhancement, all designed to encourage and support individuals with vision loss, family memebers, professionals who serve them. Aims to enhance everyday living so as to maintain an independent

lifestyle. It also serves as a consumer protection against misrepresentation and fraud.
72-78 pages Quarterly
Patricia Price, President/Managing Editor

9945 Voice of the Diabetic
National Federation of the Blind
1800 Johnson Street 410-659-9314
Baltimore, MD 21230-4998 Fax: 410-685-5653
e-mail: subscribe@diabetes.nfb.org
www.nfb.org
The leading publication in the diabetes field. Each issue addresses the problems and concerns of diabetes, with a special emphasis for those who have lost vision due to diabetes. Available in print and on cassette.
30 pages Quarterly
Eileen Ley, Director of Publishing
Elizabeth Lunt, Editor

Newsletters

9946 ACB Reports
American Council of the Blind
1155 15th Street NW 202-467-5081
Washington, DC 20005-2706 800-424-8666
Fax: 202-467-5085
e-mail: info@acb.org
www.acb.org
Radio news feature program for radio information services.
Monthly
Melanie Brunson, Executive Director

9947 AER Report
AER
4600 Duke Street 703-823-9690
Alexandria, VA 22304 877-492-2708
Fax: 703-823-9695
www.aerbvi.org
Contains organizational news, conference dates and information concerning services to visually impaired people.
28 pages BiMonthly
Jackie Fairbarns, Assistant Director

9948 AFB News
American Foundation for the Blind
11 Penn Plaza 212-502-7600
New York, NY 10001-2018 800-232-5463
Fax: 212-502-7777
National newsletter for general readership about blindness and visual impairments featuring people, programs, services and activities.
12 pages Quarterly

9949 Aging and Vision News
National Center for Vision and Aging
800 2nd Avenue 212-808-0077
New York, NY 10017 800-334-5497
3x Year

9950 Awareness
NAPVI
PO Box 317 617-972-7441
Watertown, MA 02471-0317 800-562-6265
Fax: 617-972-7444
e-mail: napvi@perkins.org
www.napvi.org
Newsletter offering regional news, sports and activities, conferences, camps, legislative updates, book reviews, audio reviews, professional question and answer column and more for the visually impaired and their families.
Quarterly
Susan LaVenture, Executive Director

9951 Braille Book Review
National Library Service for the Blind
1291 Taylor Street NW 202-707-5100
Washington, DC 20542-0002 Fax: 202-707-0712
www.loc.gov/nls
New braille books and product news.
BiMonthly

9952 Bulletin
National Association for Visually Handicapped
22 W 21st Street 212-889-3141
New York, NY 10010-6904 Fax: 212-727-2931
e-mail: navh@navh.org
www.navh.org
Annual report offering information on association activities and events, conferences, vision aids and resources for the visually impaired.
Lorraine Marchi LHD, Founder/CEO
Cesar Gomez, Executive Director

9953 DVH Quarterly
University of Arkansas At Little Rock
2801 S University Avenue 501-296-1815
Little Rock, AR 72204-1000 Fax: 501-663-3536
Offers information on upcoming events, conferences and workshops on and for visual disabilities. Book reviews, information on the newest resources and technology, educational programs, want ads and more.
Quarterly
Bob Brasher, Editor

9954 Focus
Visually Impaired Center
1422 West Court Street 810-767-4014
Flint, MI 48503 Fax: 810-767-0020
e-mail: info@vicflint.org
www.vicflint.org
Newsletter offering information for the visually impaired person in the forms of legislative and law updates, ADA information, support groups, hotlines, and articles on the newest technology in the field.
Quarterly
Laurie MacArthur, Executive Director

9955 Gleams Newsletter
Glaucoma Research Foundation
251 Post Street 415-986-3162
San Francisco, CA 94108 800-826-6693
Fax: 415-986-3763
e-mail: question@glaucoma.org
www.glaucoma.org
It includes information about glaucoma, new treatments, updates on research findings, and more.
3x/year
Thomas M Brunner, President/CEO
Andrew Jackson, Director Communications

9956 Guide Dog Foundation for the Blind Newsletter
371 E Jericho Turnpike 631-265-2121
Smithtown, NY 11787-2976 800-548-4337
Fax: 631-361-5192
e-mail: info@guidedog.org
www.guidedog.org
This organization relies on voluntary public contributions to provide persons with blindness the gift of second sight through the eyes of a guide dog. This nonprofit organization furnishes guide dogs, free of charge, to qualified people who seek independence, mobility and companionship.
Wells B Jones CAE CFRE, CEO
Michelle Lavitt, Marketing Manager

9957 Guideway
Guide Dog Foundation for the Blind
371 E Jericho Turnpike 631-265-2121
Smithtown, NY 11787-2976 800-548-4337
Fax: 631-361-5192
e-mail: info@guidedog.org
www.guidedog.org
Offers updates and information on the foundation's activities and guide dog programs. In print form but is also available on cassette.
6 pages Monthly
Wells B Jones CAE CFRE, CEO
Michelle Lavitt, Marketing Manager

9958 **Hearsay**
Radio Information Service
600 Forbes Avenue
Pittsburgh, PA 15282
412-488-3944
Fax: 412-488-3953
e-mail: info@readingservice.org
www.readingservice.org
Newsletter for persons interested in radio reading services.
Quarterly

9959 **Hub**
SPOKES Unlimited
415 Main Street
Klamath Falls, OR 97601
541-883-7547
Fax: 541-885-2469
www.spokesunlimited.org
Newsletter on rehabilitation, peer counseling, blindness, visual impairments, information and referral.
Meg Graf, Resource Librarian

9960 **InSight**
Foundation Fighting Blindness
11435 Cronhill Drive
Owings Mill, MD 21117-2220
410-568-0150
800-683-5555
Fax: 410-363-2393
TDD: 410-363-7139
e-mail: info@fightblindness.org
www.fightblindness.org
The Foundation Fighting Blindness newsletter, delivered to members monthly. The major emphasis is to report on research and science news, and FDA approved clinical trials around retinal degenerative dieseases.
20 pages 3 per year
William T. Schmidt, CEO

9961 **Lion**
Lions Clubs International
300 W 22nd Street
Oak Brook, IL 60523-8815
312-571-5466
Publication for the blind.

9962 **Listen Up**
Recording for the Blind & Dyslexic (RFB&D)
20 Roszel Road
Princeton, NJ 08540-6294
609-452-0606
800-221-4792
Fax: 609-987-8116
e-mail: custserv@rfbd.org
www.rfbd.org
RFB&D's bi-monthly newsletter for members.

9963 **Long Cane News**
American Foundation for the Blind
15 W 16th Street
New York, NY 10011-6301
212-502-7600
800-232-5463
Fax: 212-502-7777
Semiannual

9964 **Musical Mainstream**
National Library Service for the Blind
1291 Taylor Street NW
Washington, DC 20542-0002
202-707-5100
Fax: 202-707-0712
Articles selected from print music magazines.
Quarterly

9965 **NAVH UPDATE**
National Association for Visually Handicapped
22 W 21st Street
New York, NY 10010-6904
212-889-3141
Fax: 212-727-2931
e-mail: navh@navh.org
www.navh.org
This newsletter offers vision news, medical updates, assistive device information, resources and more for the visually impaired.
4 pages Quarterly
Lorraine Marchi LHD, Founder/CEO
Cesar Gomez, Executive Director

9966 **NLS News**
National Library Service for the Blind
1291 Taylor Street NW
Washington, DC 20542-0002
202-707-5100
Fax: 202-707-0712
Newsletter on current program developments.
Quarterly

9967 **NLS Update**
National Library Service for the Blind
1291 Taylor Street NW
Washington, DC 20542-0002
202-707-5100
Fax: 202-707-0712
Newsletter on the services volunteer activities.
Quarterly

9968 **NOAH News**
National Organization for Albinism
PO Box 959
E. Hampsted, NH 03826-0959
603-887-2310
800-473-2310
Fax: 603-887-2310
www.albinism.org
BiAnnually

9969 **Newsline for the Blind**
National Federation of the Blind
1800 Johnson Street
Baltimore, MD 21230-4998
410-659-9314
Fax: 410-685-5653
e-mail: subscribe@diabetes.nfb.org
www.nfb.org
Nation's only digital talking newspaper service for the blind. Allows the blind to read the full text of leading national and local newspapers by using a touch-tone telephone. Service is free of charge and available 24 hours a day, 7 days per week.
Eileen Ley, Director of Publishing
Elizabeth Lunt, Editor

9970 **Open Windows**
Sunday School Board of the Southern Baptists
127 9th Avenue N
Nashville, TN 37234-0001
800-458-2772
Guide for personal devotions on audio cassette tape, using Bible references, devotional readings, and prayer calendar of popular Open Windows devotional guide for visually handicapped adults.
Quarterly

9971 **Personal Reader Update**
Personal Reader Department
9 Centennial Drive
Peabody, MA 01960-7906
978-977-2000
800-343-0311
Fax: 978-977-2437
Offers information on new services, assistive devices and technology for the blind.

9972 **Prevent Blindness America News**
Prevent Blindness America
211 West Wacker Drive, Suite 1700
Chicago, IL 60606
847-843-2020
800-331-2020
www.preventblindness.org
Offers information and articles on eye safety, programs, and services of the Society.
Quarterly

9973 **RP Messenger**
Texas Association of Retinitis Pigmentosa
PO Box 8388
Corpus Christi, TX 78468-8388
361-852-8515
Fax: 361-852-8515
A bi-annual newsletter offering information on Retinitis Pigmentosa.
BiAnnual

9974 **Raised Dot Computing Newsletter**
Raised Dot Computing
211 S Paterson Street
Madison, WI 53703-3789
608-257-9595
Discusses braille computer techniques and devices for blind persons.

9975 **SCENE**
Braille Institute
741 N Vermont Avenue
Los Angeles, CA 90029-3594
213-663-1111
800-272-4553
www.brailleinstitute.org

Offers information on the organization, question and answer column, articles on the newest technology and more for visually impaired persons.
Paul J Porelli, Managing Editor

9976 Smith-Kettlewell Technical File
Smith-Kettlewell Eye Research Foundation
2232 Webster Street 415-561-1619
San Francisco, CA 94115-1821 Fax: 415-561-1610
Quarterly

9977 Student Advocate
National Alliance of Blind Students
1155 15th Street NW, Suite 1004 202-467-5081
Washington, DC 20005 800-424-8666
e-mail: president@acbstudents.org
www.acbstudents.org
A communication forum covering issues of concern to postsecondary students who are blind.

Cammie Vloedman, President
Olivia Norman, First Vice President

9978 Talking Book Topics
National Library Services For The Blind
1291 Taylor Street NW 202-707-5100
Washington, DC 20542-0002 Fax: 202-707-0712
Offers hundreds of listings of books, fiction and nonfiction, for adults and children on cassette. Also offers listings on foreign language books on cassette, talking magazines and reviews.
Bimonthly

9979 The Macula Foundation Manhattan Eye, Ear & Throat Hospital
American Macular Degeneration Foundation
8th Floor 210 East 64th St. 212-605-3777
New York, NY 10021-0515 Fax: 212-605-3795
e-mail: foundation@retinal-research.org
www.macular.org/spotlite.html
Newsletter of the American Macular Degeneration Foundation, a nationwide support group for individuals and their families to adjust to the restrictions and changes brought about by macular disease.
Quarterly
Nikolai Stevenson, President
Walter Ross, VP

9980 The Pioneer Projects and Programs Periodic al
TelecomPioneers
930 15th St. 12th Floor
Denver, CO 80202 303-571-1200
www.pioneersvolunteer.org
Monthly

9981 Viva Vital News
5016 Silk Oak Drive 941-371-2153
Sarasota, FL 34232-5410
Membership service organization offering information for veterans and is an affiliate of the American Council of the Blind.

9982 Voice of Vision
GW Micro
310 Racquet Drive 219-483-3625
Fort Wayne, IN 46825-4229 Fax: 219-489-2608
e-mail: webmaster@gwmicro.com
www.gwmicro.com
Offers product reviews, product announcements, tips for making systems or applications more accessible, or explanations of concepts of interest to any computer user or would-be computer user. This association newsletter is available in braille, in large print, on audio cassette and on 3.5 or 5.25 IBM format diskette.
Quarterly

9983 What's Line
Alabama Regional Library for the Blind
6030 Monticello Drive 334-213-3906
Montgomery, AL 36130-6000 800-392-5671
Fax: 334-213-3993
e-mail: fzaleski@apls.state.al.us
www.apls.state.al.us
Recreational reading in special format for persons unable to use standard print. Reference materials offered include materials on blindness and other handicaps, films, local subjects and authors.
4 pages Quarterly
Fara Zaleski, Division
Rebecca Mitchell, Director

Pamphlets

9984 About Children's Vision: Guide for Parents
National Association for Visually Handicapped
22 W 21st Street 212-889-3141
New York, NY 10010-6904 Fax: 212-727-2931
e-mail: navh@navh.org
www.navh.org
Offers a better understanding of the normal and possible abnormal development of a childs eyesight.
Lorraine Marchi LHD, Founder/CEO
Cesar Gomez, Executive Director

9985 Age Related Macular Degeneration
National Association for Visually Handicapped
22 W 21st Street 212-889-3141
New York, NY 10010-6904 Fax: 212-727-2931
e-mail: navh@navh.org
www.navh.org
Describes various conditions which affect the macular area and how to best maximize the use of residual peripheral vision.
Lorraine Marchi LHD, Founder/CEO
Cesar Gomez, Executive Director

9986 Are You Looking for a Few Good Workers?
AFB Press: American Foundation for the Blind
11 Penn Plaza 212-502-7600
New York, NY 10001 800-232-3044
Fax: 212-502-7774
www.afb.org/store
Helpful pamphlet explores both the importance and the advantage of hiring workers who are blind or visually impaired. Designed for human resource and other professionals responsible for hiring, it answers critical questions about hiring blind or visually impaired applicants. This enlightening guide to employment practices relating to these individuals offers insights on interviewing, job performance, tax incentives for businesses, insurance issues and more.
7 pages Pack of 20
ISBN: 0-891283-60-9

9987 BVA Bulletin
Blinded Veterans Association
477 H Street NW 202-371-8880
Washington, DC 20001-2694 800-669-7079
Fax: 202-371-8258
e-mail: bva@bva.org
www.bva.org
The Bulletin informs blinded veterans, their families, and those of the general public with an interest in BVA issues, about the organization. The publication includes current information relating to technology for the blind, legislation affecting blinded veterans, and news about the people who have overcome the challenges of blindness and are doing amazing work in their lives.
32 pages Quarterly
Thomas Miller, Executive Director
Stuart Nelson, Coordinator Public Relations

9988 Books are Fun for Everyone
National Library Service for the Blind
1291 Taylor Street NW 202-707-5100
Washington, DC 20542 Fax: 202-707-0712

9989 Braille Alphabet and Numbers
AFB Press: American Foundation for the Blind
11 Penn Plaza 212-502-7600
New York, NY 10001 800-232-3044
Fax: 212-502-7774
www.afb.org/store

Embossed with the braille alphabet and numbers, this 9 x 4 inch display card includes an explanation of braille and a short history of its development.
Pack of 25
ISBN: 0-891281-98-3

9990 Braille Literacy: Blind Persons, Families, Prof. & Producers of Braille
AFB Press: American Foundation for the Blind
11 Penn Plaza
New York, NY 10001
212-502-7600
800-232-3044
Fax: 212-502-7774
www.afb.org/store
Vigorous defece of the use of braille and an explanation of the importance of positive attitudes toward it that states: Braille is an assertion of equality between blind and sighted persons with respect to written communication. For everyone who uses or teaches braille and is interested in its future.
12 pages Pack of 25
ISBN: 0-891289-28-3

9991 Braille: An Extraordinary Volunteer Opportunity
National Library Service for the Blind
1291 Taylor Street NW
Washington, DC 20542-0002
202-707-5100
Fax: 202-707-0712

9992 Cataracts
National Eye Institute, Information Office
31 Center Drive MSC 2510
Bethesda, MD 20892-2510
301-496-5248
e-mail: 2020@nei.nih.gov
www.nei.nih.gov
Provides information about this common condition and its treatment.

9993 Classification of Impaired Vision
National Association for Visually Handicapped
22 W 21st Street
New York, NY 10010-6904
212-889-3141
Fax: 212-727-2931
e-mail: navh@navh.org
www.navh.org
Describes various degrees of impaired vision.
Lorraine Marchi LHD, Founder/CEO
Cesar Gomez, Executive Director

9994 Communicating with People Who Have Trouble Hearing & Seeing: A Primer
National Association for Visually Handicapped
22 W 21st Street
New York, NY 10010-6904
212-889-3141
Fax: 212-727-2931
e-mail: navh@navh.org
www.navh.org
Line drawings that depict problems for those with both deficiencies.
Lorraine Marchi LHD, Founder/CEO
Cesar Gomez, Executive Director

9995 Dancing Cheek to Cheek
Blind Children's Center
4120 Marathon Street
Los Angeles, CA 90029-3584
213-664-2153
Fax: 213-665-3828
Discusses beginning social, play and language interactions.
33 pages

9996 Diabetes, Vision Impairment and Blindness
AFB Press: American Foundation for the Blind
11 Penn Plaza
New York, NY 10001
212-502-7600
800-232-3044
Fax: 212-502-7777
www.afb.org/store
Presentation of how chronic diabetes affects vision and how diabetes can be managed at home by blind and visually impaired individuals.
32 pages
ISBN: 0-891289-02-0

9997 Diabetic Retinopathy
National Association for Visually Handicapped
22 W 21st Street
New York, NY 10010-6904
212-889-3141
Fax: 212-727-2931
e-mail: navh@navh.org
www.navh.org
Describes types of this disease and methods of treatment.
Lorraine Marchi LHD, Founder/CEO
Cesar Gomez, Executive Director

9998 Directory of Radio Reading Services
Radio Information Service
600 Forbes Avenue
Pittsburgh, PA 15282
412-488-3944
Fax: 412-488-3953
e-mail: info@readingservice.org
www.readingservice.org
Annually

9999 Don't Lose Sight of Age-Related Macular Degeneration
National Eye Institute, Information Office
31 Center Drive MSC 2510
Bethesda, MD 20892-2510
301-496-5248
e-mail: 2020@nei.nih.gov
www.nei.nih.gov

10000 Don't Lose Sight of Cataracts
National Eye Institute, Information Office
31 Center Drive MSC 2510
Bethesda, MD 20892-2510
301-496-5248
e-mail: 2020@nei.nih.gov
www.nei.nih.gov

10001 Don't Lose Sight of Glaucoma
National Eye Institute, Information Office
31 Center Drive MSC 2510
Bethesda, MD 20892-2510
301-496-5248
e-mail: 2020@nei.nih.gov
www.nei.nih.gov

10002 Eye-Q Test
National Association for Visually Handicapped
22 W 21st Street
New York, NY 10010-6904
212-889-3141
Fax: 212-727-2931
e-mail: navh@navh.org
www.navh.org
Five questions and answers to assist in knowing more about vision.
Lorraine Marchi LHD, Founder/CEO
Cesar Gomez, Executive Director

10003 Facts: Books for Blind and Physically Handicapped Individuals
National Library Service for the Blind
1291 Taylor Street NW
Washington, DC 20542-0002
202-707-5100
Fax: 202-707-0712
www.loc.gov
Annual

10004 Facts: Music for Blind and Physically Handicapped Individuals
National Library Service for the Blind
1291 Taylor Street NW
Washington, DC 20542-0002
202-707-5100
Fax: 202-707-0712
www.loc.gov
Annual

10005 Facts: Playback Machines and Accessories Provided on Free Loan
National Library Service for the Blind
1291 Taylor Street NW
Washington, DC 20542-0002
202-707-5100
Fax: 202-707-0712
www.loc.gov

10006 Facts: Sources for Purchase of Cassette & Disc Players From NLS
National Library Service for the Blind
1291 Taylor Street NW
Washington, DC 20542-0002
202-707-5100
Fax: 202-707-0712
www.lov.gov

10007 Family Guide to Vision Care
American Optometric Association
243 N Lindbergh Boulevard
Saint Louis, MO 63141-7881
314-991-4100
Fax: 314-991-4101
www.aoanet.org
Offers information on the early developmental years of your vision, finding a family optometrist and how to take care of your eyesight through the learning years, the working years and the mature years.

10008 Family Guide: Growth & Development of the Partially Seeing Child
National Association for Visually Handicapped

22 W 21st Street 212-889-3141
New York, NY 10010-6904 Fax: 212-727-2931
e-mail: navh@navh.org
www.navh.org
Offers information for parents and guidelines in raising a partially seeing child.
Lorraine Marchi LHD, Founder/CEO
Cesar Gomez, Executive Director

10009 **General Facts and Figures on Blindness**
National Society to Prevent Blindness
500 Remington Road
Schaumburg, IL 60173-5624 800-331-2020

10010 **General Interest Catalog**
National Braille Association
3 Townline Circle 716-427-8260
Rochester, NY 14623-2537
Lists hundreds of titles of fiction and non-fiction books offered in large print, braille or on cassette to visually impaired readers.
19 pages

10011 **Glaucoma**
Foundation For Glaucoma Research
490 Post Street 415-986-3162
San Francisco, CA 94102-1409
Offers information on what glaucoma is, the causes, treatments, types of glaucoma, eye exams and prevention.

10012 **Glaucoma: Sneak Thief of Sight**
National Association for Visually Handicapped
22 W 21st Street 212-889-3141
New York, NY 10010-6904 Fax: 212-727-2931
e-mail: navh@navh.org
www.navh.org
A pamphlet describing the disease, treatment and medications.
Lorraine Marchi LHD, Founder/CEO
Cesar Gomez, Executive Director

10013 **Guide Dog Foundation Flyer**
Guide Dog Foundation for the Blind
371 E Jericho Turnpike 631-265-2121
Smithtown, NY 11787-2976 800-548-4337
Fax: 631-361-5192
e-mail: info@guidedog.org
www.guidedog.org
Offers information on the programs and services provided by the foundation.
Wells B Jones CAE CFRE, CEO
Michelle Lavitt, Marketing Manager

10014 **Guidelines for Comprehensive Low Vision Care**
National Association for Visually Handicapped
22 W 21st Street 212-889-3141
New York, NY 10010-6904 Fax: 212-727-2931
e-mail: navh@navh.org
www.navh.org
A description of the proper method to conduct a low vision evaluation.
Lorraine Marchi LHD, Founder/CEO
Cesar Gomez, Executive Director

10015 **Guidelines for Helping Deaf/Blind Persons**
Helen Keller National Center for Deaf/Blind
111 Middle Neck Road 516-944-8900
Sands Point, NY 11050-1299 Fax: 516-944-7302
TTY: 516-944-8637
e-mail: hkncinfo@rcn.com
www.hknc.org
Pamphlet offering information on how persons should interact with deaf/blind individuals. Includes drawings of the one hand manual alphabet.
Joseph McNulty, Executive Director

10016 **Heart to Heart**
Blind Children's Center
4120 Marathon Street 213-664-2153
Los Angeles, CA 90029-3584 Fax: 213-665-3828
Parents of blind and partially sighted children talk about their feelings.
12 pages

10017 **Heartbreak of Being a Little Bit Blind**
National Association for Visually Handicapped
22 W 21st Street 212-889-3141
New York, NY 10010-6904 Fax: 212-727-2931
e-mail: nvah@navh.org
www.navh.org
Summary of what it means to have impaired vision with illustrations. Free for members.
Lorraine Marchi LHD, Founder/CEO
Cesar Gomez, Executive Director

10018 **Helen Keller**
AFB Press: American Foundation for the Blind
11 Penn Plaza 212-502-7600
New York, NY 10001 800-232-3044
Fax: 212-502-7774
www.afb.org/store
Brief biography that focuses on the major events of Helen Keller's life, from her birth in Tuscumbia, Alabama on June 27, 1880 to her death in Connecticut on June 1, 1968.
6 pages Pack of 25
ISBN: 0-891282-03-3

10019 **How Does a Blind Person Get Around?**
AFB Press: American Foundation for the Blind
11 Penn Plaza 212-502-7600
New York, NY 10001 800-232-3044
Fax: 212-502-7774
www.afb.org/store
Offers information on daily living as a blind person.

10020 **How to Develop a Self-Help Group for Elders Losing Eyesight**
National Association for Visually Handicapped
22 W 21st Street 212-889-3141
New York, NY 10010-6904 Fax: 212-727-2931
e-mail: navh@navh.org
www.navh.org
The pioneer for development of self-help groups, using the NAVH model, this publication is designed to help start and facilitate self-help groups.
Lorraine Marchi LHD, Founder/CEO
Cesar Gomez, Executive Director

10021 **How to Use Your Low Vision Glasses**
National Association for Visually Handicapped
22 W 21st Street 212-889-3141
New York, NY 10010-6904 Fax: 212-727-2931
e-mail: navh@navh.org
www.navh.org
A line drawing showing the correct way to benefit from low vision glasses.
Lorraine Marchi LHD, Founder/CEO
Cesar Gomez, Executive Director

10022 **Information on Glaucoma**
Foundation for Glaucoma Research
490 Post Street 415-986-3162
San Francisco, CA 94102-1409

10023 **Information on Macular Degeneration**
American Council of the Blind
1155 15th Street NW 202-467-5081
Washington, DC 20005-2706 800-424-8666
Fax: 202-467-5085
e-mail: info@acb.org
www.acb.org
Melanie Brunson, Executive Director

10024 **It's All Right to Be Angry**
National Association for Visually Handicapped
22 W 21st Street 212-889-3141
New York, NY 10010-6904 Fax: 212-727-2931
e-mail: navh@navh.org
www.navh.org
A helpful pamphlet describing reactions to learning to live with vision impairment.
Lorraine Marchi LHD, Founder/CEO
Cesar Gomez, Executive Director

10025 **Large Print Loan Library Catalog**
National Association for Visually Handicapped

22 W 21st Street
New York, NY 10010-6904
212-889-3141
Fax: 212-727-2931
e-mail: navh@navh.org
www.navh.org

Listing of over 9,000 commercially published and NAVH large print books available through NAVH on a loan basis. Includes a limited selection of titles available for purchase.
Lorraine Marchi LHD, Founder/CEO
Cesar Gomez, Executive Director

10026 Learning to Play
Blind Children's Center
4120 Marathon Street
Los Angeles, CA 90029-3584
213-664-2153
Fax: 213-665-3828
Discusses how to present play activities to the visually impaired preschool child.
12 pages

10027 Let's Eat
Blind Children's Center
4120 Marathon Street
Los Angeles, CA 90029-3584
213-664-2153
Fax: 213-665-3828
Teaches competent feeding skills to children with visual impairments.
28 pages

10028 Low Vision Questions and Answers
AFB Press: American Foundation for the Blind
11 Penn Plaza
New York, NY 10001
212-502-7600
800-232-3044
Fax: 212-502-7774
www.afb.org/store
What does low vision mean? What do low vision services cost? What diseases cause low vision? Answers to these and other questions are presented in a straightforward yet comprehensive format. Photographs show how objects appear to people with low vision, what low vision devices look like, and how they are used.
21 pages Pack of 25
ISBN: 0-891281-96-7

10029 Magnifier
Macular Degeneration Foundation
PO Box 9752
San Jose, CA 95157-0752
408-260-1335
888-633-3937
www.eyesight.org
Large-font publication.

10030 Magnifier Highlights
Independent Living Aids
200 Robbins Lane
Jericho, NY 11753-2341
800-537-2118
Fax: 516-752-3135
e-mail: indlivaids@aol.com
www.independentliving.com
Full line of magnifiers, ranging from high-powered vision aids to instruments and accessories
Marvin Sandler, President

10031 Move with Me
Blind Children's Center
4120 Marathon Street
Los Angeles, CA 90029-3584
213-664-2153
Fax: 213-665-3828
A parent's guide to movement development for visually impaired babies.
12 pages

10032 Music Is for Everyone
National Library Service for the Blind
1291 Taylor Street NW
Washington, DC 20542-0002
202-707-5100
Fax: 202-707-0712

10033 Parenting Preschoolers: Raising Young Blind & Visually Impaired Child
AFB Press: American Foundation for the Blind
11 Penn Plaza
New York, NY 10001
212-502-7600
800-232-3044
Fax: 212-502-7774
www.afb.org/store
Why is my baby so quiet? Why does my child seem slower than other children? What will happen when my child goes to school? This primer provides practical answers to the questions most freqently asked by parents and gives advice on what to expect, how to adapt to the child's situation and needs, and what to look for in early education programs.
28 pages Pack of 25
ISBN: 0-891289-98-4

10034 Patient's Guide to Visual Aids and Illumination
National Association for Visually Handicapped
22 W 21st Street
New York, NY 10010-6904
212-889-3141
Fax: 212-727-2931
e-mail: navh@navh.org
www.navh.org
A reference booklet offering information on aids for the visually impaired.
Lorraine Marchi LHD, Founder/CEO
Cesar Gomez, Executive Director

10035 Puppy Walker Brochure
Guide Dog Foundation for the Blind
371 E Jericho Turnpike
Smithtown, NY 11787-2976
631-265-2121
800-548-4337
Fax: 631-361-5192
e-mail: info@guidedog.org
www.guidedog.org
Offers information on being a volunteer puppy walker family.
Wells B Jones CAE CFRE, CEO
Michelle Lavitt, Marketing Manager

10036 Reaching, Crawling, Walking-Let's Get Moving
Blind Children's Center
4120 Marathon Street
Los Angeles, CA 90029-3584
213-664-2153
Fax: 213-665-3828
Orientation and mobility for visually impaired preschool children.
24 pages

10037 Reading is for Everyone
National Library Service for the Blind
1291 Taylor Street NW
Washington, DC 20542-0002
202-707-5100
Fax: 202-707-0712

10038 Reading with Low Vision
National Library Service for the Blind
1291 Taylor Street NW
Washington, DC 20542-0002
202-707-5100
Fax: 202-707-0712

10039 Reference and Information Services from NLS
National Library Service for the Blind
1291 Taylor Street NW
Washington, DC 20542-0002
202-707-5100
Fax: 202-707-0712

10040 Resource List for Persons with Low Vision
American Council of the Blind
1155 15th Street NW
Washington, DC 20005-2706
202-467-5081
800-424-8666
Fax: 202-467-5085
e-mail: info@acb.org
www.acb.org
Melanie Brunson, Executive Director

10041 Seeing Eye to Eye: An Administrator's Guide
AFB Press: American Foundation for the Blind
11 Penn Plaza
New York, NY 10001
212-502-7600
800-232-3044
Fax: 212-502-7774
www.afb.org/store
Visual impairment often has a profound impact on a child's ability to learn language and basic communication concepts. This easy-to-read booklet explains the student's needs and the practical services essential for helping them become literate and successful. An ideal tool for administrators and educators, it includes clear explanations of common terminology, the impact of visual impairment on learning, specialized services for visually impaired students, and in-service training for teachers.
72 pages Pack of 10
ISBN: 0-891283-59-5

10042 Selecting a Program
Blind Children's Center
4120 Marathon Street
Los Angeles, CA 90029-3584
213-664-2153
Fax: 213-665-3828

A guide for parents of infants and preschoolers with visual impairments.
28 pages

10043 Standing on My Own Two Feet
Blind Children's Center
4120 Marathon Street 213-664-2153
Los Angeles, CA 90029-3584 Fax: 213-665-3828
A step-by-step guide to designing and constructing simple, individually tailored adaptive mobility devices for preschool-age children who are visually impaired.
36 pages

10044 Talk to Me
Blind Children's Center
4120 Marathon Street 213-664-2153
Los Angeles, CA 90029-3584 Fax: 213-665-3828
A language guide for parents of deaf children.
11 pages

10045 Talk to Me II
Blind Children's Center
4120 Marathon Street 213-664-2153
Los Angeles, CA 90029-3584 Fax: 213-665-3828
A sequel to Talk To Me, available in English and Spanish.
15 pages

10046 Talking Books for Senior Adults
National Library Service for the Blind
1291 Taylor Street NW 202-707-5100
Washington, DC 20542-0002 Fax: 202-707-0712

10047 Touch the Baby: Blind & Visually Impaired Children as Patients
American Foundation for the Blind
11 Penn Plaza 212-502-7600
New York, NY 10001-2018 800-232-3044
Fax: 212-502-7774
www.afb.org/store
How-to manual for health care professionals working in hospitals, clinics and doctors' offices that teaches the special communication and touch-related techniques needed to prevent blind and visually impaired patients from withdrawing from healthcare staff and the outside world. includes how to talk to infants and how to signal to children that a procedure may cause discomfort.
13 pages Pack of 25
ISBN: 0-891281-97-5

10048 Volunteer at Your Braille and Talking Book Library
National Library Service for the Blind
1291 Taylor Street NW 202-707-5100
Washington, DC 20542-0002 Fax: 202-707-0712
Brochure

10049 What Do You Do When You See a Blind Person — and What Don't You Do?
AFB Press: American Foundation for the Blind
11 Penn Plaza 212-502-7600
New York, NY 10001 800-232-3044
Fax: 212-502-7774
www.afb.org/store
Examples of real-life situations that teach sighted persons how to interact effectively with blind persons. Topics covered include how to help someone across the street, how not to distract a guide dog and how to take leave of a blind person.
8 pages Pack of 25
ISBN: 0-891281-95-9

10050 Wings for the Future
American Printing House for the Blind
1839 Frankfort Avenue 502-895-2405
Louisville, KY 40206-3148 800-223-1839
Fax: 502-895-1509
e-mail: info@ahp.org
This booklet offers an introduction to the American Printing House For The Blind's programs, services, tools, aids and more.
13 pages

10051 Without Sight and Sound
Helen Keller National Center for Deaf/Blind
111 Middle Neck Road 516-944-8900
Sands Point, NY 11050-1299 Fax: 516-944-7302
TTY: 516-944-8637
e-mail: hkncinfo@rcn.com
www.hknc.org
Pamphlet offering facts, causes, types and descriptions of deaf/blindness.
Joseph McNulty, Executive Director

10052 You Seem Like a Regular Kid to Me
AFB Press: American Foundation for the Blind
11 Penn Plaza 212-502-7600
New York, NY 10001 800-232-3044
Fax: 212-502-7774
www.afb.org/store
An interview with Jane, a blind child, allows other children to understand what it's like to be blind. Jane explains how she gets around, takes care of herself, does her school work, spends her leisure time and even pays for things when she can't see money. Photographs show Jane engaged in various activities.
16 pages Pack of 25
ISBN: 0-891289-21-6

Audio & Video

10053 Adult Bible Study
Sunday School Board of the Southern Baptists
127 9th Avenue N
Nashville, TN 37234-0001 800-458-2772
Unabridged Sunday School lessons recorded on audio cassette as printed in Adult Bible Study.
Quarterly

10054 Aging and Vision: Declarations of Independence
AFB Press: American Foundation for the Blind
11 Penn Plaza 212-502-7600
New York, NY 10001 800-232-3044
Fax: 212-502-7774
www.afb.org/store
Very personal look at five older people who have successfully coped with visual impairment and continue to lead active, satisfying lives. Their stories are not only inspirational, they also provide paractical, down-to-earth suggestions for adapting to vision loss later in life.
18 Minutes VHS
ISBN: 0-891282-20-3

10055 Bible Alliance
PO Box 621 941-748-3031
Bradenton, FL 34206-0621 e-mail: aurora@auroraministries.org
www.careministries.org
Offers the Christian bible on cassettes in over 52 languages for those finding it impossible to read small print.

10056 Blindness: A Family Matter
AFB Press: American Foundation for the Blind
11 Penn Plaza 212-502-7600
New York, NY 10001 800-232-3044
Fax: 212-502-7774
www.afb.org/store
Frank exploration of the effects of an individual's visual impairment on other members of the family and how family members can play a positive role in the rehabilitation process. Features three families whose success stories provide advice and encouragement, as well as interviews with newly blinded adults currently involved in a rehabilitation program. Also available in PAL.
23 Minutes VHS
ISBN: 0-891282-22-X

10057 Braille Documents
Metrolina Sight Services
704 Louise Avenue 704-372-3870
Charlotte, NC 28204-2128 e-mail: braille@charlotte.infi.net
www.careministries.org
This production shop creates Braille and large-print documents.

10058 Brief Encounters of the Right Kind: How to Make Your Point in 10 Minutes or Less
AFB Press: American Foundation for the Blind

11 Penn Plaza
New York, NY 10001
212-502-7600
800-232-3044
Fax: 212-502-7774
www.afb.org/store

Humorous and instructional tour through the do's and don'ts of lobbying at the local, state and national levels. Three seasoned lobbyists discuss how professionals, families, consumers and volunteer advocates can use their expert knowledge to influence public policy. A Toolkit for Advocates, the accompanying manual, complements the video by providing a summary of the legislative process and key points on how to meet successfully with legislators.
VHS & PAL
ISBN: 0-891282-83-1

10059 Destination Unlimited
Leader Dog For The Blind
1964 Park Street
306-565-8211
Regina, SK, S4P 3G4,

This is a documentary about Leader-Dog-For-The-Blind Program. The needs of various people and how their dog fulfills their needs are shown. In addition, the overall leader-dog program is reviewed. This training program would be of interest to many teenagers.
Films

10060 Employed Ability: Blind Persons on the Job
AFB Press: American Foundation for the Blind
11 Penn Plaza
New York, NY 10001
212-502-7600
800-232-3044
Fax: 212-502-7774
www.afb.org/store

Blind and visually impaired people from a wide variety of occupations talk about career opportunities and their experiences in the workplace. Employers and coworkers are also interviewed and speak openly about supervising and working alongside visually impaired employees.
14 Minutes VHS
ISBN: 0-891282-24-6

10061 Focused On: Importance and Need for Skills
AFB Press: American Foundation for the Blind
11 Penn Plaza
New York, NY 10001
212-502-7600
800-232-3044
Fax: 212-502-7774
www.afb.org/store

Provides an overview of the importance of social competence and details the course of social skills development in children in general and in children who are blind or visually impaired in particular. This study guide examines both the development of social skills in general and how this process applies to children who are blind or who have visual impairments.
VHS & PAL
ISBN: 0-891283-25-0

10062 Hand in Hand: It Can Be Done
AFB Press: American Foundation for the Blind
11 Penn Plaza
New York, NY 10001
212-502-7600
800-232-3044
Fax: 212-502-7774
www.afb.org/store

One hour introduction to working effectively with individuals who are deaf-blind. Designed as both an overview and a reinforcer of the self-study text, this video can be used as a whole or in sections for parents and regular educators, as well as in the community. Includes a discussion guide. Available in audioscribed or open captioned VHS and PAL.

ISBN: 0-891283-25-0

10063 Heart to Heart
Blind Children's Center
4120 Marathon Street
Los Angeles, CA 90029-3584
213-664-2153
Fax: 213-665-3828

Parents of blind and partially sighted children talk about their feelings.
Videotape

10064 Helen Keller in Her Story
AFB Press: American Foundation for the Blind
11 Penn Plaza
New York, NY 10001
212-502-7600
800-232-3044
Fax: 212-502-7774
www.afb.org/store

Patty Duke, who portrayed the young Helen Keller on stage and on screen in The Miracle Worker, introduces this Oscar-winning documentary about the extraordinary lives of Ms. Keller, her teacher Anne Sullivan Macy and her friend and companion Polly Thompson. Includes vintage still photographs as well as early movie footage and newsreel footage.
VHS & PAL
ISBN: 0-891282-25-4

10065 Let's Eat
Blind Children's Center
4120 Marathon Street
Los Angeles, CA 90029-3584
213-664-2153
Fax: 213-665-3828

Teaches competent feeding skills to children with visual impairments.
Videotape

10066 Making the Most of Early Communication: Strategies for Supporting Communication
AFB Press: American Foundation for the Blind
11 Penn Plaza
New York, NY 10001
212-502-7600
800-232-3044
Fax: 212-502-7774
www.afb.org/store

Demonstrates selected interventions to assist infants and toddlers with multiple disabilities, including vision and hearing loss, in developing early communication and other skills. Emphasizing the critical importance of early intervention, this video is designed to help service providers and families create effective communication straegies that encourage cognitive development and funtional abilities in young children with multiple disabilities and those who are deaf-blind. 37 minutes.
VHS & PAL
ISBN: 0-891282-96-3

10067 New What Do You Do When You See a Blind Person?
AFB Press: American Foundation for the Blind
11 Penn Plaza
New York, NY 10001
212-502-7600
800-232-3044
Fax: 212-502-7774
www.afb.org/store

Engaging remake of the 1971 classic brings a fresh perspective on how to interact comfortably with someone who is visually impaired. The entertaining experiences of Mark Johnson, a computer programmer who is blind, and Dave Simon, a computer salesman who is not, show the simple ways to provide assistance, if it is needed, to someone who is blind or visually impaired. 16 minutes.
VHS & PAL
ISBN: 0-891283-13-7

10068 Oh, I See
AFB Press: American Foundation for the Blind
11 Penn Plaza
New York, NY 10001
212-502-7600
800-232-3044
Fax: 212-502-7774
www.afb.org/store

Lively and entertaining video provides practical suggestions on helping students who are blind and visually impaired adapt to the mainstream classroom. The modifacations shown can easily be used by teachers, students, or anyone working with blind and visually impaired students. Seven minutes.
VHS & PAL
ISBN: 0-891282-52-1

10069 Out of Left Field
AFB Press: American Foundation for the Blind
11 Penn Plaza
New York, NY 10001
212-502-7600
800-232-3044
Fax: 212-502-7774
www.afb.org/store

Illustrates how youngsters who are blind or visually impaired are integrated with their sighted peers in a variety of recreational and athletic activites. 17 minutes.
VHS & PAL
ISBN: 0-891282-28-9

10070 **Profiles in Aging and Vision**
AFB Press: American Foundation for the Blind
11 Penn Plaza 212-502-7600
New York, NY 10001 800-232-3044
Fax: 212-502-7774
www.afb.org/store
Can be used on its own or in conjunction with the text, this is an informative overview of the common eye conditions that affect older people, with a detailed description of the vision-related services that help older people who are visually impaired continue to lead independent lives. Experienced professionals provide valuable information on crucial issues, and older visually impaired persons offering their own revealing perspectives. 33 minutes.
VHS
ISBN: 0-891289-48-8

10071 **Reaching Out: A Creative Access Guide for Designing Exhibits & Cultural Programs**
AFB Press: American Foundation for the Blind
11 Penn Plaza 212-502-7600
New York, NY 10001 800-232-3044
Fax: 212-502-7774
www.afb.org/store
Video and accompanying manual are a creative package for making information on cultural programs and facilities accessable to people who are blind or visually impaired. Created especially for libraries, museums, historical societies, outdoor cultural facilities, corporations and everyone whose mission involves providing information to the community, this video offers practical design and program solutions. 22 minutes.
VHS & PAL
ISBN: 0-891289-49-6

10072 **Seven Minute Lesson**
AFB Press: American Foundation for the Blind
11 Penn Plaza 212-502-7600
New York, NY 10001 800-232-3044
Fax: 212-502-7774
www.afb.org/store
Introduction to the basic techniques used when acting as a sighted guide for a person who is blind or visually impaired.
VHS & PAL
ISBN: 0-891282-29-7

10073 **Solutions for Everyday Living for Older People with Visual Impairments**
AFB Press: American Foundation for the Blind
11 Penn Plaza 212-502-7600
New York, NY 10001 800-232-3044
Fax: 212-502-7774
www.afb.org/store
Presents a positive and helpful view of how older people who have lost some or all of their vision can continue to lead satisfying lives within supportive environments. This engaging video shows how staff members in continuing care communities and other living settings for older people can help residents function as independently as possible.Different types of vision loss are explained, and simple solutions are offered for carrying out everyday activities. 34 minutes.
VHS & PAL
ISBN: 0-891288-52-X

10074 **Strategies for Community Access: Braille & Raised Large Print Facility Signs**
AFB Press: American Foundation for the Blind
11 Penn Plaza 212-502-7600
New York, NY 10001 800-232-3044
Fax: 212-502-7774
www.afb.org/store
Brief and effective advocacy tool that can be used to educate architects, planners, facility managers, sign makers and consumers about the value of accessible signs. Topics covered include ADA requirements for accessible signs, samples of signs designed to be compatible with an organization's interior design, demonstrations of how blind and print signs are a cost-effective way to provide access. Reproducible fact sheets on ADA signage guidelines are enclosed. Seven minutes.
VHS & PAL
ISBN: 0-891282-56-4

10075 **Understanding Braille Literacy**
AFB Press: American Foundation for the Blind
11 Penn Plaza 212-502-7600
New York, NY 10001 800-232-3044
Fax: 212-502-7774
www.afb.org/store
Motovational and intructional video covers all aspects of a successful braille education program. Teachers and students demonstate how braille is learned and used from preschool through high school and describes how braille skills contribute to literacy, independence, mastry of academic skills and successful education experiences in the regular classroom. Parents, classroom teachers and school administrators also speak out about the importance of braille. 25 minutes.
VHS & PAL
ISBN: 0-891282-61-0

10076 **We Can Do it Together: Mobility for Students with Multiple Disabilities**
AFB Press: American Foundation for the Blind
11 Penn Plaza 212-502-7600
New York, NY 10001 800-232-3044
Fax: 212-502-7774
www.afb.org/store
Illustrates a transdisiplinary team approach to teaching orientation and mobility to students with severe visual and multiple impairments, covering both adapted communication systems that are used to teach mobility skills and basic indoor mobility in the school. For mobility instructors, administrators, teachers of visually impaired and severely disabled students, occupational, physical and speech therapists and parents. Discussion guide included, 13 minutes.
VHS & PAL
ISBN: 0-891282-13-0

10077 **What Can Baby See? Vision Tests & Intervention Strategies for Infants**
AFB Press: American Foundation for the Blind
11 Penn Plaza 212-502-7600
New York, NY 10001 800-232-3044
Fax: 212-502-7774
www.afb.org/store
Presents common vision tests and methods of gathering information that can be used with infants and very young children to help indentify visual impairments that require early intervention services. Effective ways of working with families and early intervention strategies for encouraging infants with multiple disabilities to use their vision in functional ways are demonstrated to help families and service providers contribute to children's growth and development.
VHS & PAL
ISBN: 0-891282-99-8

Web Sites

10078 **ACB Government Employees**
www.acb.org
Concerns of the organization include recruitment, placement and advancement of blind and visually impaired employees.

10079 **ACB Radio Amateurs**
www.acb.org
A radio amateur network of blind, visually impaired and sighted members who gather and share common problems and solutions to help members improve radio amateurs in getting started, provides access to educational materials in special media and publishes a directory for the visually impaired.

10080 **ACB Social Service Providers**
www.acb.org
Information on blind and visually impaired social workers, social service professionals, students pursuing careers in social work, and other interested persons.

10081 **American Blind Lawyers Association**
www.acb.org
Information on law school admission tests and bar exams, private sector and government employment relations and specialized work techniques for the blind and visually impaired.

10082 American Council of Blind Lions

www.acb.org

Information concerning Club activities in the field of work for the blind and encourages blind people to join Lions Clubs and other civic activities.

10083 American Council of the Blind

www.acb.org

Information for the visually impaired and fully sighted individuals who are concerned about the dignity and well-being of blind people throughout America.

10084 American Foundation for the Blind

www.afb.org

Our web site unique in that it combines state-of-the-art features, an attractive visual environment and an accessible design for people with all types of disabilities. Features include a searchable database of vision services nationwide, community message boards and the largest collection of Helen Keller memorbilia on the web. It meets the stringent AAA guidelines of the Web Accessibility Initiative of the World Wide Web Consortium, established to help organizations build accessible websites.

10085 American Printing House for the Blind

www.aph.org

This organization promotes the independence of blind persons by providing special media, tools and materials needed for education and life.

10086 Blinded Veterans Association

www.bva.org

Offers two main service programs without cost to blinded veterans. Field service program provides counseling to veterans and families, and information on benefits and rehabilitation.

10087 Braille Revival League

www.acb.org

Information for people to read and write in braille, advocates for mandatory braille instruction in educational facilities for the blind, strives to make available a supply of braille materials from libraries and printing houses and more.

10088 Council of Families with Visual Impairment

www.acb.org

Offers support and outreach, shares experiences in parent/child relationships, exchanges educational, cultural and medical information about child development and more.

10089 Fidelco Guide Dog Foundation

www.fidelco.org

Fidelco breeds, raises, trains, and places German shepherd guide dogs with men and women who are visually impaired, primarily in the Northeast.

10090 Friends-In-Art

www.acb.org

Offers consultation to program planners in establishing accessible art and museum exhibits and presents Performing Arts Showcases.

10091 Guide Dog Foundation for the Blind

www.guidedog.org

Furnishes guide dogs, free of charge, to qualified people who seek independence, mobility and companionship.

10092 Guide Dog Users

www.acb.org

Promotes the acceptance of blind people and their dogs, works for enforcement and expansion of laws admitting guide dogs into public places, advocates for quality training and follow-up services.

10093 Healing Well

www.healingwell.com

An online health resource guide to medical news, chat, information and articles, newsgroups and message boards, books, disease-related web sites, medical directories, and more for patients, friends, and family coping with disabling diseases, disorders, or chronic illnesses.

10094 Health Finder

www.healthfinder.gov

Searchable, carefully developed web site offering information on over 1000 topics. Developed by the US Department of Health and Human Services, the site can be used in both English and Spanish.

10095 Healthlink USA

www.healthlinkusa.com

Health information concerning treatment, cures, prevention, diagnosis, risk factors, research, support groups, email lists, personal stories and much more. Updated regularly.

10096 Helios Health

www.helioshealth.com

Online resource for your health information. Detailed information about specific health topics, access to expert advice from our Medical Advisory Board, and up-to-date health news.

10097 Independent Visually Impaired Enterprises

www.acb.org

Information on rehabilitation facilities for all types of business enterprises and publicizes the capabilities of blind and visually impaired business persons.

10098 Library Users of America

www.acb.org

Provides for chapters in states through the US to encourage the development, acquisition and use of technology which enables blind and visually impaired persons to use printed material independently in library settings and elsewhere.

10099 Lighthouse International

www.lighthouse .org

Offers information about vision impairment and vision rehabilitation, and provides referrals to services and support groups nationwide.

10100 MedicineNet

www.medicinenet.com

An online resource for consumers providing easy-to-read, authoritative medical and health information.

10101 Medscape

www.mywebmd.com

Medscape offers specialists, primary care physicians, and other health professionals the Web's most robust and integrated medical information and educational tools.

10102 National Alliance of Blind Students

www.acb.org

Works to facilitate progress toward full accessibility of college programs and facilities, provides opportunities for discussion of issues important to students and assists with National Student Seminars.

10103 National Association for Visually Hand.

www.navh.org

NAVH ensures that those with limited vision do not lead limited lives. We offer emotional support; training in the use of and access to a wide variety of optical aids and lighting; a large print, nationwide, free-by-mail loan library; large print educational materials; quarterly newsletter; referrals; self-help groups and educational outreach.

10104 National Association of Blind Educators

www.nfb.org

Provides support and information regarding professional responsibilities, classroom techniques, national testing methods and career obstacles. Publishes The Blind Educator, national magazine specifically for blind educators.

10105 National Association of Blind Lawyers

www.nfb.org

Provides support and information regarding employment, techniques used by the blind, advocacy, laws affecting the blind, current information about the American Bar Association and other issues for blind lawyers.

10106 National Association of Blind Secretaries and Transcribers

www.nfb.org

Addresses issues such as technology, accomodation, career planning and job training.

10107 National Association of Blind Students

www.nfb.org

Provides support, information and encouragement to blind college and university students.

10108 National Association of Blind Teachers

www.acb.org

Works to advance the teaching profession for blind and visually impaired people, protects the interest of teachers, presents discussions and solutions for special problems encountered by blind teachers and publishes a directory of blind teachers in the US.

10109 National Association of Guide Dog Users

www.nfb.org

Provides information and support for guide dog users and works to secure high standards in guide dog training. Addresses issues of discrimination of guide dog users and offers public education about guide dog use.

10110 National Association to Promote the Use of Braille

www.nfb.org

Provides information about the importance of Braille in securing independence, education and employment for the blind.

10111 National Braille Association

www.nationalbraille.org/

Provides transciption service for, and maintains a depository of, braille books.

10112 National Federation of the Blind: Blind/Deaf Division

www.nfb.org

Offers personal contact with other deaf-blind individuals knowledgeable in advocacy, education, employment, technology, discrimination and other issues surrounding deaf-blindness.

10113 National Federation of the Blind

www.nfb.org

Provides public education about blindness, support services to the newly blinded, scholarships, publications about blindness, adaptive equipment for the blind, advocacy services, Newsline for the Blind, assistive technology information and Job Opportunities for the Blind.

10114 National Federation of the Blind in Computer Science

www.nfb.org

New technologies, to secure access to current technology and to develop new ways of using current or new technologies by the blind.

10115 National Federation of the Blind: Blind Merchants Division

www.nfb.org

Provides information regarding rehabilitation, social security, tax and other issues which directly affect blind merchants. Serves as advocacy and support group.

10116 National Federation of the Blind: Human Services Division

www.nfb.org

Organization of blind persons working in counseling, personnel, psychology, social work, psychiatry, rehabilitation and other social science and human resource fields. Provides resources regarding blindness-related techniques and methods used in these fields.

10117 National Federation of the Blind: Masonic Square Club

www.nfb.org

Blind individuals committed to sharing of Masonic experiences, goals and history.

10118 National Federation of the Blind: Music Division

www.nfb.org

Offers support and information regarding copyright, publishing, promotion and other career details.

10119 National Federation of the Blind: Public Employees Division

www.nfb.org

Focuses on issues such as changes in governmental hiring and retention practices, new job skills needed for the future, government employment downsizing, new electronic means of finding public sector jobs, self-advocacy and career planning strategies.

10120 National Federation of the Blind: Science and Engineering Division

www.nfb.org

This is a strong support group to encourage blind persons in pursuit of these careers, many of which have been considered not possible for the blind in the past.

10121 National Federation of the Blind: Writers Division

www.nfb.org

Covers various aspects of this business, including selling your work, publishing, technology, motivation and discovering writing and publishing resources.

10122 National Library Service for the Blind

www.loc.gov/nls

Administers a national library service that provides braille and recorded books and magazines on free loan to anyone who cannot read standard print because of visual or physical disabilities who are eligible residents of the United States or American citizens living abroad.

10123 National Organization of Parents of Blind Children

www.nfb.org

Addresses issues ranging from help to parents of a newborn blind infant, mobility and Braille instruction, education, social and community participation, development of self-confidence and other vital factors involved in the growth of a blind child.

10124 National Organization of the Senior Blind

www.nfb.org

Provides support and information to other blind seniors. Issues include concerns such as remaining active in community and social life, maintaining private homes or living in retirement communities or nursing homes, learning the techniques used by the blind, independently caring for oneself and maintaining a positive approach to vision loss.

10125 Randolph-Sheppard Vendors of America

www.acb.org

Protects the interests of blind vendors, seeks proper implementation of the Randolph-Sheppard Act and encourages facility locations in more visible and profitable areas.

10126 Vision World Wide

www.visionww.org

Aims is to enhance everyday living so as to maintain an independent lifestyle. It also serves as a consumer protection against misrepresentation and fraud.

10127 Visually Impaired Data Processors International

www.acb.org

Provides for the exchange of work technique ideas and works with agencies to increase the availability of braille and recorded materials.

10128 Visually Impaired Piano Tuners International

www.acb.org

Works to preserve, advance and enrich the skilled professional piano tuning for competent, well-trained blind and visually impaired persons.

10129 Visually Impaired Veterans of America

www.acb.org

Promotes the rights of visually impaired veterans to receive all benefits, encourages research and development of new products for blind people.

10130 WebMD

www.webmd.com

Information on Blindness and Visual Impairments, including articles and resources.

Description

10131 **War Syndromes**

War syndromes have plagued soldiers for centuries. Though symptoms may vary, soldiers may become affected by various postulated physiological diseases as well as psychological illnesses. Agent Orange and the Gulf War Syndrome are two of the conditions still prevelant today.

Agent Orange is the common name for a mix of chemicals developed by the military. It was first used during the Vietnam War to destroy vegetation that concealed the enemy. During the war, soldiers were exposed heavily to this chemical; years later, many of them contracted a variety of conditions. There has been an intense controversy about whether Agent Orange caused these conditions, with medical scientists, patients, politicians and advocacy groups all involved.

Among the conditions sometimes attributed to Agent Orange exposure are a variety of cancers, an acne-like skin condition called chloracne, neurological diseases, repeated infections, sterility, and birth defects in the children of exposed persons.

To further understand this condition, the Department of Veterans Affairs has been established a registry of Vietnam veterans concerned that they may have been exposed to Agent Orange. Veterans who suspect their symptoms are related to this exposure can contact the Department's Medical Administrative Services to request the Agent Orange Registry Examination, a complete health evaluation. The Department offers service-connected compensation for those veterans who develop a condition believed to be related to exposure to Agent Orange.

Gulf War Syndrome, GWS, or Persian Gulf War Syndrome is a constellation of illnesses experienced by 5,000 to 80,000 US veterans after returning from the Persian Gulf Wars in the 1990's and 2000's. Symptoms are predominately neurologic and consist of impaired cognition, with problems of attention, memory, reasoning, insomnia, depression and headaches. Complaints of muscle and joint pain, gastrointestinal difficulties, vertigo and weakness are also common. As veterans resumed family life, various birth defects were added to the list. The cause of GWS is unknown.

A 1997 study funded by the Centers for Disease Control shows that Gulf War personnel are more likely than others to report depression, syptoms similar to post-traumatic stress disorder, chronic fatigue, cognitive difficulties, bronchitis, asthma, fibromyalgia, alcohol abuse, anxiety and sexual dysfunction.

Many causes of GWS have been suggested, but none have been definately identified or eliminated. These include: effects of chemical and/or biological weapons; exposure to pesticides; smoke from oil well fires; airborne contamination from munitions plants destroyed in Iraq, exposure to depleted uranium used as a material in some US munitions and exposure to volatile solvents used in the normal course of equipment maintenance. None of these exposures have been convincingly linked to a cause of the illness.

Given the range of reported GWS effects, treatment is highly individualized and symptomatic. A number of specialized support groups and websites have been established by members of the Persian Gulf War Community.

National Agencies & Associations

10132 **Advocacy for the Gulf War Children**
1692 6th Road 308-795-2319
St Libory, NE 68872 e-mail: Firefly@mail.hamilton.net
Gives listings of names and addresses of families with children with gulf war syndrome.

10133 **Agent Orange Registry Department of Veterans Affairs**
Department of Veterans Affairs
810 Vermont Avenue NW 202-233-4000
Washington, DC 20420 800-827-1000
www.va.gov
Offers a computerized index of examinations of Vietnam veterans who were worried that they may have been exposed to chemical herbicides which might be causing a variety of ill effects. Services available to any veteran, male or female, who had active military service.

10134 **Centers for Disease Control**
1600 Clifton Road 404-639-3311
Atlanta, GA 30333 800-232-4636
Fax: 404-639-3435
TTY: 888-232-6348
e-mail: cdcinfo@cdc.gov
www.cdc.gov
Offers reprints from the CDC Health Status of Vietnam veterans and the Journal of the American Medical Association. Also offers reports from the Centers for Disease Control Vietnam Experience Study, which was a multidimensional assessment of the health of Vietnam War veterans.
William H Gimson, Chief Operating Officer
John Tibbs, Director

10135 **National Veterans Services Fund**
PO Box 2465 203-656-0003
Darien, CT 06820-0465 800-521-0198
Fax: 203-656-1957
e-mail: philvet@NVSF.org
www.nvsf.org
Supports and informs those who were exposed to the defoliant Agent Orange or dioxin while serving the US in the conflict in Vietnam. The organization has developed a detailed exposure survey form to collect information on exposed veterans.
Phil Kraft, President Treasurer
Cathie Green Stansell, Vice President

10136 **VA Data Processing Center**
1615 E Woodward Street 512-389-5380
Austin, TX 78772-0001
Helps veterans register after receiving the Agent Orange examination.

State Agencies & Associations

Alabama

10137 **Gulf War Veterans of Alabama**
2344 Glendale Avenue 205-265-7723
Montgomery, AL 36107 e-mail: 76163 1323@compuserve.com
Don Reeves
Shannon Reeves

10138 Veterans Administration Medical Center: Alabama
3701 Loop Road E — 205-554-2000
Tuscaloosa, AL 35404 — Fax: 205-554-2034
www2.va.gov/directory

10139 Veterans Association Medical Center
700 S 19th Street — 205-933-8101
Birmingham, AL 35233 — 866-487-4243
Fax: 205-933-4484
www2.va.gov/directory

Alaska

10140 Alaska Gulf War Syndrome Referral Coordinator
23740 Sunny Glen Drive — 907-696-8688
Eagle River, AK 99577 — Fax: 907-696-8688
e-mail: mcclure@alaska.net
Larry McClure

10141 Veterans Adm. Medical Center: Anchorage Outpatient Clinic
Outpatient Clinic
2925 DeBarr Road — 907-257-4700
Anchorage, AK 99508 — 888-383-7574
Fax: 907-257-6774
www2.va.gov/directory

Arizona

10142 Veterans Adm. Medical Center: Arizona Carl T. Hayden VA Medical Center
Carl T. Hayden VA Medical Center
650 E Indian School Road — 602-277-5551
Phoenix, AZ 85012 — 800-554-7174
www.phoenix.med.va.gov
Renee Stover, VA Employees Association President
Paula Pedene, Public Affairs Officer

10143 Veterans Adm. Medical Center: Tucson Southern Arizona VA Health Care System
Southern Arizona VA Health Care System
3601 S 6th Avenue — 520-792-1450
Tucson, AZ 85723 — 800-470-8262
Fax: 520-629-1818
www2.va.gov/directory
Jonathan Gardner, Chief Executive Officer

Arkansas

10144 Central Arkansas Veterans Healthcare Syste Eugene J. Towbin Healthcare Center
Eugene J. Towbin Healthcare Center
2200 Fort Roots Drive
North Little Rock, AR 72114-1706 — 501-257-1000
www2.va.gov/directory

10145 Gulf War Veterans of Arkansas
11127 Eglia Valley Drive — 501-225-9347
Little Rock, AR 72212
Lydia Pace

10146 Veterans Adm. Medical Center: Fayetville
1100 N College Avenue — 479-443-4301
Fayetteville, AR 72703 — 800-691-8387
www2.va.gov/directory

10147 Veterans Adm. Medical Center: Little Rock
4300 W 7th Street
Little Rock, AR 72205-5484 — 501-257-1000
www2.va.gov/directory

California

10148 California Association of Persian Gulf Veterans
PO Box 3661 — 408-476-6684
Santa Cruz, CA 95063 — Fax: 415-227-0848
e-mail: CAGulfVets@aol.com
Erika Lundholm

10149 Northern California Association of Persian Gulf Veterans
9141 East Stockton Boulevard — 916-684-1693
Elk Grove, CA 95624 — Fax: 916-684-1693
e-mail: NCAPGV@aol.com
Debbie Judd

10150 Sacramento Veterans Center
1111 Howe Avenue — 916-566-7430
Sacramento, CA 95825 — Fax: 916-566-7433
www2.va.gov/directory
Michael Miracle, Team Leader
Edna Gabaldon, Counselor

10151 Sepulveda Ambulatory Care Center
16111 Plummer Street — 818-891-7711
North Hills, CA 91343 — 800-516-4567
Fax: 818-895-9559
www2.va.gov/directory

10152 VA Northern California Health Care System
10535 Hospital Way — 916-843-7000
Mather, CA 95655 — 800-382-8387
Fax: 916-843-9001
www2.va.gov/directory
Lawrence Sandler, Disabilities Committee Chair

10153 Veterans Adm. Medical Center: Livermore
4951 Arroyo Road — 925-373-4700
Livermore, CA 94550 — 800-455-0057
www2.va.gov/directory

10154 Veterans Adm. Medical Center: Long Beach
5901 E 7th Street — 562-826-8000
Long Beach, CA 90822 — Fax: 562-826-5972
www.long-beach.med.va.gov

10155 Veterans Adm. Medical Center: Los Angeles
11301 Willshire Boulevard — 310-478-3711
Los Angeles, CA 90073 — Fax: 310-268-3494
www.losangeles.va.gov

10156 Veterans Adm. Medical Center: Martinez
150 Muir Road — 916-366-5366
Martinez, CA 94553 — 800-382-8387
Fax: 925-372-2020
www2.va.gov/directory

10157 Veterans Adm. Medical Center: Palo Alto
3801 Miranda Avenue — 650-493-5000
Palo Alto, CA 94304 — 800-455-0057
Fax: 650-852-3228
www.palo-alto.med.va.gov/
John Didty, Director
Jeanette Hsu, Director of Training

10158 Veterans Adm. Medical Center: Salem
4150 Clement Street — 415-221-4810
San Francisco, CA 94121 — Fax: 415-750-2185
www.sanfrancisco.va.gov
Sheila M Cullen, Director
C Diana Nicoll, Chief of Staff

10159 Veterans Adm. Medical Center: San Francisco
4150 Clement Street — 415-221-4810
San Francisco, CA 94121 — Fax: 415-750-2185
Sheila M Cullen, Director
C Diana Nicoll, Chief of Staff

10160 Veterans Administration Medical Center: Fresno
3636 N 1st Street — 559-487-5660
Fresno, CA 93726 — Fax: 559-487-5399
www2.va.gov/directory
Herman Barretto, Counselor
Mary Jordan-Church, Counselor

10161 Veterans Affairs Medical Center: Loma Linda
11201 Benton Street — 909-825-7084
Loma Linda, CA 92357 — 800-741-8387
Fax: 909-422-3106
www.lom.med.va.gov/
Annie Tuttle, Public Affairs Director

Colorado

10162 Persian Gulf Veterans of Colorado
405 Cody
Wheat Ridge, CO 80033
303-424-6235
Fax: 303-422-2962
e-mail: GJMF90B@prodigy.com
Denise Nichols

10163 Veterans Adm. Medical Center: Denver
300 S Jackson Street
Denver, CO 80206
303-331-7500
800-733-8387
Fax: 303-331-7800
e-mail: hac.inq@med.va.gov
www.va.gov/hac/
Ralph Charlip, Director

10164 Veterans Adm. Medical Center: Grand Junction
2121 N Avenue
Grand Junction, CO 81501
970-242-0731
866-206-6415
Fax: 970-244-1303
www1.va.gov/directory

Connecticut

10165 Gulf War Veterans of Connecticut: New England Chapter
8 Frances Lane
Windsor Locks, CT 6096
860-623-1456
Fax: 860-292-1849
e-mail: DIANEDULKA@aol.com
Diane Dulka

Delaware

10166 Veterans Adm. Medical Center: Wilmington Wilmington VA Medical Center
Wilmington VA Medical Center
1601 Kirkwood Highway
Wilmington, DE 19805
302-994-2511
Fax: 302-633-5591
www2.va.gov/directory

District of Columbia

10167 Disabled American Veterans National Service Headquarters
807 Maine Avenue SW
Washington, DC 20024
202-554-3501
Fax: 202-554-3581
www.dav.org

Serves America's disabled veterans and their families. Direct services include legislative advocacy professional counseling about compensation pension educational and job training programs and VA health care. Also offers assistance in applying for those programs.
Arthur H Wilson, National Adjutant
David G Gorman, Executive Director

10168 US Veteran's Administration
810 Vermont Avenue NW
Washington, DC 20420
202-273-5400
Fax: 202-273-4877
www2.va.gov/directory

Provides a wide range of services for those who have been in the military and their dependents as well as offering information on driver assessment and education programs.
Louise R Van Diepen MS CGP, Chief of Staff
Patricia Van MHA BS, Assistant Deputy Policy/Planning

10169 Veterans Adm. Medical Center: Washington
50 Irving Street NW
Washington, DC 20422
202-745-8000
Fax: 202-754-8530
www.washington.med.va.gov
Sanford M Garfunkel, Medical Center Director
Ross D Fletcher, Chief of Staff

Florida

10170 Desert Storm Justice Foundation: Florida
10 Marlow Road
Frostproof, FL 33843-9321
813-635-3261
Fax: 813-635-3261
e-mail: BillCarpenter@cjewel.com
William Carpenter

10171 Desert Storm Veterans of Florida
PO Box 6081
Titusville, FL 32782
407-269-3453
e-mail: GulfVet@Metrolink.net
Kevin Knight

10172 Veterans Adm. Medical Center: Bay Pines
10000 Bay Pines Boulevard
Bay Pines, FL 33744
727-398-6661
Fax: 727-398-9442
www.va.gov/visn8/baypines
Wallace M Hopkins, Medical Center Director
George F Van Buskirk MD, Chief of Staff

10173 Veterans Adm. Medical Center: Gainesville
1601 SW Archer Road
Gainesville, FL 32608-1197
352-376-1611
Fax: 352-374-6113
www2.va.gov/directory
Frederick L Malphurs, Director
Bradley S Bender MD, Chief of Staff

10174 Veterans Adm. Medical Center: Lake City
Lake City Veterans Administration Medical Center
619 S Marion Avenue
Lake City, FL 32025-5808
386-755-3016
800-308-8387
Fax: 386-758-3209
www2.va.gov/directory

10175 Veterans Adm. Medical Center: Miami
1201 NW 16th Street
Miami, FL 33125
305-575-7000
888-276-1785
Fax: 305-575-3232
www.va.gov/visn8/miami
Stephen M Lucas, Director
John R Vara MD, Chief of Staff

10176 Veterans Adm. Medical Center: St. Petersburg
Bay Pines VA Medical Center
10000 Bay Pines Boulevard
Saint Petersburg, FL 33744
727-398-6661
888-820-0230
Fax: 727-322-1248
www2.va.gov/directory

10177 Veterans Adm. Medical Center: Tampa
Tampa Veterans Administration Medical Center
13000 Bruce B Downs Boulevard
Tampa, FL 33612
813-972-2000
Fax: 813-972-7673
www.va.gov/visn8/tampa
Richard A Silver, Medical Center Director
Thomas E Bowen, Chief of Staff

10178 Vietnam Veterans of Brevard The Vietnam And All Veterans Of Brevard
The Vietnam And All Veterans Of Brevard
1125 W King Street
Cocoa, FL 32922-0929
321-690-0805
Fax: 321-690-0106
e-mail: BVagianos@cfl.rr.com
www.vietnamandallveteransofbrevard.com
Bill Vagianos, President
Don Wassmer, Vice President

10179 West Palm Beach VA Medical Center
7305 N Military Trail
West Palm Beach, FL 33410-6400
561-422-8262
800-972-8262
Fax: 561-422-8613
www.westpalmbeach.va.gov
Edward H Seiler, Medical Center Director
Darin Rubin, Chief of Staff

Georgia

10180 Gulf War Veterans of Georgia
307 Adair Street
Decatur, GA 30030
404-373-3741
Fax: 404-377-3741
e-mail: 70711 3174@compuserve.com
Paul Sullivan

10181 VA Southeast Network: Georgia
3700 Crestwood Parkway NW
Duluth, GA 30096-5585
678-924-5700
Fax: 678-924-5757
www2.va.gov/directory

10182 Veterans Adm. Medical Center: Augusta
One Freedom Way
Augusta, GA 30904
706-733-0188
800-836-5561
Fax: 706-823-3934
www1.va.gov/augustaga

10183 Veterans Adm. Medical Center: Decatur Atlanta VA Medical Center
Atlanta VA Medical Center
1670 Clairmont Road
Decatur, GA 30033
404-321-6111
Fax: 404-728-7733
www.va.gov/atlanta

Thomas Cappello, Director
David J Bower, Chief of Staff

10184 Veterans Adm. Medical Center: Dublin Carl Vinson VA Medical Center
Carl Vinson VA Medical Center
1826 Veterans Boulevard
Dublin, GA 31021
912-272-1210
800-595-5229
Fax: 912-277-2717
www2.va.gov/directory

Hawaii

10185 Veterans Adm. Medical Centery: Honolulu VA Pacific Islands Health Care System
VA Pacific Islands Health Care System
459 Patterson Road
Honolulu, HI 96819-1522
808-433-0600
Fax: 808-433-0390
www.va.gov/hawaii

Idaho

10186 Idaho Persian Gulf Veterans
2055 Sotuh Colorado Street
Boise, ID 83706
208-344-3028
Vaughn Kidwell

10187 Veterans Adm. Medical Center: Boise Boise VA Medical Center
Boise VA Medical Center
500 W Fort Street
Boise, ID 83702
208-422-1000
866-437-5093
Fax: 208-422-1326
www2.va.gov/directory

Wayne Tippets, Director

Illinois

10188 Desert Storm Justice Foundation: Illinois
Rural Route 4
Carbondale, IL 62901
618-457-2621
Shan Now

10189 Edward J Hines Jr VA Hospital
5th & Roosevelt Road
Hines, IL 60141
708-202-8387
Fax: 708-202-7998
www2.va.gov/directory

10190 Great Lakes Health Care System
PO Box 5000
Hines, IL 60141-5000
708-202-8400
Fax: 708-202-8424
www.visn12.va.gov

10191 Jesse Brown VA Medical Center
820 S Damen Avenue
Chicago, IL 60612
312-569-8387
www.chicago.va.gov

10192 VA Illinois Health Care System
1900 E Main Street
Danville, IL 61832-5198
217-554-3000
Fax: 217-554-4552
www2.va.gov/directory

10193 Veterans Adm. Medical Center: Marion Marion VA Medical Center
Marion VA Medical Center
2401 W Main Street
Marion, IL 62959
618-997-5311
www2.va.gov/directory

10194 Veterans Adm. Medical Center: North Chicago
North Chicago VA Medical Center
3001 Green Bay Road
North Chicago, IL 60064
847-688-1900
Fax: 847-578-3806
www.vision12.med.va.gov/northchicag

10195 Veterans Adm. Medical Center: Northport North Chicago VA Medical Center
3001 Green Bay Road
North Chicago, IL 60064
847-688-1900
Fax: 847-578-3806
www.northchicago.va.gov

10196 Veterans Administration West Side Medical Center
820 S Damen Avenue
Chicago, IL 60612
312-569-8387
Fax: 312-569-6188
www2.va.gov/directory

Stan Johnson, Director
DeAnn Dietrich, Deputy Director

Indiana

10197 VA Northern Indiana Health Care System Marion Campus
1700 E 38th Street
Marion, IN 46953-4589
765-674-3321
800-360-8387
Fax: 765-677-3124
www2.va.gov/directory

10198 Veterans Adm. Medical Center: Fort Wayne
2121 Lake Avenue
Fort Wayne, IN 46805
260-426-5431
800-360-8387
Fax: 260-460-1336
www2.va.gov/directory

10199 Veterans Adm. Medical Center: Indianapolis
1481 W Tenth Street
Indianapolis, IN 46202
317-554-0000
888-878-6889
Fax: 317-554-0127
www2.va.gov/directory

Iowa

10200 Cedar Rapids Persian Gulf Veterans, Spouses and Children
909-28th Street Southeast 1
Cedar Rapids, IA 52403
319-366-0756
Mary Shears

10201 Des Moines Division: VA Central Iowa Health Care System
3600 30th Street
Des Moines, IA 50310-5774
515-699-5999
800-294-8387
Fax: 515-699-5862
www2.va.gov/directory

10202 Knoxville Division: VA Central Iowa Health Care System
1515 W Pleasant Street
Knoxville, IA 50138
641-842-3101
800-816-8878
Fax: 515-699-5862
www2.va.gov/directory

10203 Veterans Adm. Medical Center: Iowa City
601 Highway 6 W
Iowa City, IA 52246-2208
319-338-0581
800-637-0128
Fax: 319-339-7171
www2.va.gov/directory

Kansas

10204 Veterans Adm. Medical Center: Leavenwoth Dwight D. Eisenhower VA Medical Center
Dwight D. Eisenhower VA Medical Center
4101 S 4th Street
Leavenworth, KS 66048-5055
913-682-2000
800-952-8387
Fax: 913-758-4149
www2.va.gov/directory

10205 Veterans Adm. Medical Center: Topeka Colmery O'Neil VA Medical Center
Colmery O'Neil VA Medical Center
2200 SW Gage Boulevard
Topeka, KS 66622
785-350-3111
800-574-8387
Fax: 785-350-4336
www2.va.gov/directory

10206 Veterans Adm. Medical Center: Wichita Robert J. Dole Department Of VA Medical
Robert J. Dole Department Of VA Medical Center
5500 E Kellogg
Wichita, KS 67218
316-685-2221
888-878-6881
Fax: 316-651-3666
www2.va.gov/directory

Kentucky

10207 Carol and Dr. James W Stutts
108 Whispering Hills Drive
Berea, KY 40403
606-986-3267
e-mail: cstutts@kih.net

10208 National Association of State Directors of Veterans Affairs
Kentucky Department of Veteran Affairs
1111 Louisville Road
Frankfort, KY 40601
502-564-9203
Fax: 502-564-9240
e-mail: les.beavers@ky.gov
www.nasdva.net

Provides a medium for the exchange of ideas and information; facilitates reciprocal state services; fosters a better understanding of the national veterans' problems; and secures uniformity and equality of services in all states and territories.
Leslie Beavers, Commissioner
Terry Schow, Senior Vice President

10209 Veterans Adm. Medical Center: Lexington Lexington VA Medical Center
Lexington VA Medical Center
1101 Veterans Drive
Lexington, KY 40502
859-233-4511
www2.va.gov/directory

10210 Veterans Adm. Medical Center: Louisville Louisville VA Medical Center
Louisville VA Medical Center
800 Zorn Avenue
Louisville, KY 40206
502-287-4000
800-376-8387
Fax: 502-287-6225
www2.va.gov/directory

10211 Veterans Adm. Regional Office: Louisville Louisville Regional Office
Louisville Regional Office
1347 S 3rd Street
Louisville, KY 40208
502-634-1916
Fax: 502-625-7082
www2.va.gov/directory
Phillip Goudeau, Team Leader
Carolyn Beisler, Counselor

Louisiana

10212 Mission Project
PO Box 92574
Lafayette, LA 70509-2574
318-236-3599
e-mail: mission@linknet.net
Carol Picou
Tony Picou

10213 Veterans Adm. Medical Center: Alexandria Alexandria VA Medical Center
Alexandria VA Medical Center
PO Box 69004
Alexandria, LA 71360
318-473-0010
800-375-8387
Fax: 318-483-5029
www2.va.gov/directory
Barbara C Watkins, Medical Center Director
Hollis Reed MD, Chief of Staff

10214 Veterans Adm. Medical Center: New Orleans New Orleans VA Medical Center
New Orleans VA Medical Center
1601 Perdido Street
New Orleans, LA 70146
504-568-0811
Fax: 504-589-5210
www1.va.gov

10215 Veterans Adm. Medical Center: Shreveport Overton Brooks VA Medical Center
Overton Brooks VA Medical Center
510 E Stoner Avenue
Shreveport, LA 7110
318-221-8411
800-863-7441
Fax: 318-424-6156
www2.va.gov/directory

Maine

10216 Veterans Adm. Medical Center: Augusta Togus VA Medical Center
Togus VA Medical Center
1 VA Center
Augusta, ME 4330
207-623-8411
866-590-2976
Fax: 207-623-5792
TTY: 800-829-4833
TDD: 800-829-4833
e-mail: togus.query@vba.va.gov
www2.va.gov/directory
Dale Denners, Regional Office Director

Maryland

10217 Baltimore VA Rehabilitation and Extended Care Center (BRECC)
3900 Loch Raven Boulevard
Baltimore, MD 21218
410-605-7000
Fax: 410-605-7900
www2.va.gov/directory

10218 Fort Howard VA Outpatient Clinic
9600 N Point Road
Fort Howard, MD 21052
410-477-1800
800-351-8387
Fax: 410-477-7177
www.maryland.va.gov/facilities/Fort_Howa
Dennis H Smith, Director

10219 Maryland Group
8725 Fairhaven Place
Jessup, MD 20794
301-725-4269
Nancy Kaplan

10220 VA Capitol Health Care Network
849 International Drive
Linthicum, MD 21090
410-691-1131
Fax: 410-684-3189
www.va.gov/visn5
Sanford M Garfunkel, Network Director

10221 VA Maryland Health Care System Perry Point VA Medical Center
Perry Point VA Medical Center
Perry Point, MD 21902
410-642-2411
800-949-1003
Fax: 410-642-1161
www.maryland.va.gov/facilities/Perry_Poi
Dennis H Smith, Director
Dorothy M Snow, Chief of Staff

10222 Veterans Adm. Medical Center: Baltimore
10 N Greene Street
Baltimore, MD 21201
410-605-7000
800-463-6295
Fax: 410-605-7901
www.maryland.va.gov/facilities/Baltimore
Carol Nizzardini, Chief Nurse Executive
Dennis H Smith, Director

Massachusetts

10223 New England Health Care System
200 Springs Road
Bedford, MA 01730
781-687-4821
Fax: 781-687-3470
www.newengland.va.gov
Michael F Mayo-Smith, Network Director
Christine Croteau, Deputy Network Director

10224 Northhampton VA Medical Center
421 N Main Street
Leeds, MA 01053-9764
413-584-4040
800-893-1522
Fax: 413-582-3121
www.northampton.va.gov
Mary A Dowling, Director
George Fuller, Chief of Staff

10225 **Persian Gulf Era Veterans**
24 Beacon Street
Boston, MA 02133
617-329-8149
e-mail: jagmedic@pgev.org
www.pgev.org

VenusVal Hammack, Executive Director

10226 **VA Boston Healthcare System: Jamaica Plain Jamaica Plain Campus**
Jamaica Plain Campus
150 S Huntington Avenue
Jamaica Plain, MA 02130
617-232-9500
Fax: 617-278-4508
www.boston.va.gov

Michael M Lawson, Director
Michael E Charness, Chief of Staff

10227 **VA Boston Healthcare System: West Roxbury West Roxbury Campus**
West Roxbury Campus
1400 VFW Parkway
W Roxbury, MA 02132
617-323-7700
www.boston.va.gov

Michael M Lawson, Director
Susan MacKenzie, Associate Director

10228 **Veterans Adm. Medical Center: Bedford Edith Nourse Rogers Memorial Veterans Ho**
Edith Nourse Rogers Memorial Veterans Hospital
200 Springs Road
Bedford, MA 01730
781-687-2000
800-VET-MED1
Fax: 781-687-2101
www.bedford.va.gov

Tammy A Follensbee, Hospital Director
Gregory Binus, Chief Medical Officer

10229 **Veterans Adm. Medical Center: Brockton Brockton Campus**
Brockton Campus
940 Belmont Street
Brockton, MA 02301
508-583-4500
800-865-3384
Fax: 700-885-1000
www.boston.va.gov

Michael M Lawson, Director
Michael E Charness MD, Chief of Staff

Michigan

10230 **Detroit VA Medical Center John D. Dingell VA Medical Center**
John D. Dingell VA Medical Center
4646 John R
Detroit, MI 48201
313-576-1000
800-511-8056
Fax: 313-576-1025
www.detroit.va.gov

Pamela J Reeves, Director
Basim Dubaybo, Chief of Staff

10231 **International Advocacy for Gulf War Syndrome**
2297 Westfield Drive
Niles, MI 49102
616-684-5903
e-mail: DSVETERAN1@juno.com
Brian Martin

10232 **Veterans Adm. Medical Center: Ann Arbor Ann Arbor Healthcare System**
Ann Arbor Healthcare System
2215 Fuller Road
Ann Arbor, MI 48105
734-769-7100
800-361-8387
Fax: 734-845-3245
www.annarbor.va.gov

Eric W Young, Acting Director
Stacey Breedveld, Associate Director Patient Care

10233 **Veterans Adm. Medical Center: Bath Battle Creek VA Medical Center**
5500 Armostrong Road
Battle Creek, MI 49015
269-966-5600
Fax: 269-966-5483
www.battlecreek.va.gov

Denise Deitzen, Acting Director
Alan Sooho, Chief of Staff

10234 **Veterans Adm. Medical Center: Battle Creek**
Battle Creek VA Medical Center
5500 Armostrong Road
Battle Creek, MI 49016
269-966-5600
Fax: 269-966-5483
www.va.gov

10235 **Veterans Adm. Medical Center: Iron Mountain**
Iron Mountain VA Medical Center
325 E H Street
Iron Mountain, MI 49801
906-774-3300
800-215-8262
Fax: 906-779-3188
www.ironmountain.va.gov

Michael J Murphy, Director
Craig L Holmes, Chief of Staff

10236 **Veterans Adm. Medical Center: Saginaw Aleda E. Lutz VA Medical Center**
Aleda E. Lutz VA Medical Center
1500 Wiess Street
Saginaw, MI 48602
989-497-2500
800-406-5143
Fax: 989-321-4903
www.saginaw.va.gov

Gabriel Perez, Director
Gregory Movsesian, Acting Chief of Staff

10237 **Veterans In Partnership**
PO Box 134002
Ann Arbor, MI 48113-4002
734-222-4300
888-838-6446
Fax: 734-222-4340
www.visn11.va.gov

Minnesota

10238 **Desert Storm Justice Foundation: Minnesota**
PO Box 186
Buhl, MN 55713
218-258-3685
Jeff Zakula

10239 **Desert Storm Justice Foundation: Virginia**
PO Box 186
Buhl, MN 55713
218-258-3685
Jeff Zakula

10240 **Veterans Adm. Medical Center: Minneapolis Minneapolis VA Medical Center**
Minneapolis VA Medical Center
1 Veterans Drive
Minneapolis, MN 55417
612-725-2000
866-414-5058
Fax: 612-725-2049
www1.va.gov/minneapolis

Steven P Kleinglass, Director
John J Drucker, Chief of Staff

10241 **Veterans Adm. Regional Office: St. Paul**
1 Federal Drive Fort Snelling
Saint Paul, MN 55111
612-644-4022
800-827-1000
Fax: 612-970-5415
e-mail: VBCINQ@VBA.VA.GOV
www1.va.gov

Mississippi

10242 **Gulf War Babies**
PO Box 198
Clara, MS 39324
601-735-9206
Aimee West

10243 **South Central VA Health Care Network**
1600 E Woodrow Wilson
Jackson, MS 39216
601-364-7900
800-639-5137
Fax: 601-364-7996
www.visn16.med.va.gov

George Gray, Network Director
Gregg Parker, Chief Medical Officer

10244 **VA Gulf Coast Veterans Health Care System**
400 Veterans Avenue
Biloxi, MS 39531
228-523-5000
800-296-8872
Fax: 228-523-5719
www.biloxi.va.gov

Charles Sepich, Director
Ana Mello, Chief of Staff

10245 **Veterans Adm. Medical Center: Jackson**
1500 E Woodrow Wilson Drive 601-362-4471
Jackson, MS 39216 800-949-1009
Fax: 601-364-1359
www.jackson.va.gov

Linda F Watson, Director
Kent A Kirchner, Chief of Staff

10246 **Veterans Adm. Regional Office: Jackson**
1600 E Woodrow Wilson Avenue 601-364-7000
Jackson, MS 32916 800-827-1000
Fax: 601-364-7007
www.vba.va.gov/ro/south/jacks/JacksonInt

Missouri

10247 **VA Heartland Network**
1201 Walnut Street 816-701-3000
Kansas City, MO 64106 Fax: 816-221-0930
www.visn15.med.va.gov

10248 **Veterans Adm. Medical Center: Columbia Harry S. Truman Memorial**
Harry S. Truman Memorial
800 Hospital Drive 573-814-6000
Columbia, MO 65202-5297 800-349-8262
Fax: 573-814-6600
www.columbiamo.va.gov

10249 **Veterans Adm. Medical Center: Kansas City Kansas City VA Medical Center**
Kansas City VA Medical Center
4801 Linwood Boulevard 816-861-4700
Kansas City, MO 64128 800-525-1483
Fax: 816-922-3303
www.va.gov

10250 **Veterans Adm. Medical Center: Poplar Bluff**
John J. Pershing VA Medical Center
1500 N Westwood Boulevard 573-686-4151
Poplar Bluff, MO 63901 888-557-8262
Fax: 573-778-4559
www.poplarbluff.va.gov

Judy K McKee, Acting Director
Vijayachandr Nair, Chief of Staff

10251 **Veterans Adm. Regional Office: St. Louis John Cochran Division**
John Cochran Division
915 N Grand Boulevard 314-652-4100
Saint Louis, MO 63125 800-228-5459
Fax: 314-289-6557
www.stlouis.va.gov

Glen E Struchtemeyer, Director
Nathan Ravi, Chief of Staff

Montana

10252 **Veterans Adm. Medical Center: Fort Harrison**
VA Montana Health Care System
William Street 406-442-6410
Fort Harrison, MT 59636 800-827-1000
Fax: 406-477-7916
www.va.gov

10253 **Veterans Adm. Medical Center: Miles City**
210 S Winchester 406-874-5600
Miles City, MT 59301 877-468-8387
Fax: 406-232-8298
www1.va.gov

Nebraska

10254 **Veterans Adm. Medical Center: Grand Island**
2201 N Broadwell Avenue 308-382-3660
Grand Island, NE 68803-2196 866-580-1810
Fax: 308-389-5113
www.nebraska.va.gov

10255 **Veterans Adm. Medical Center: Lincoln**
600 S 70th Street 402-489-3802
Lincoln, NE 68510 866-851-6052
Fax: 402-486-7840
www.nebraska.va.gov

10256 **Veterans Adm. Medical Center: Omaha Western Iowa Health Care System**
Western Iowa Health Care System
4101 Woolworth Avenue 402-346-8800
Omaha, NE 68105 800-451-5796
Fax: 402-449-0684
www.nebraska.va.gov

Al Washko, Director
Thomas Lynch, Acting Chief of Staff

Nevada

10257 **Veterans Adm. Medical Center: Las Vegas VA Southern Nevada Healthcare System (VA**
VA Southern Nevada Healthcare System (VASNHS)
901 Rancho Lane 702-636-3000
Las Vegas, NV 89106 877-252-4866
Fax: 702-636-3027
www.lasvegas.va.gov

John B Bright, Director
Ramu Komanduri, Chief of Staff

10258 **Veterans Adm. Medical Center: Reno VA Sierra Nevada Health Care System**
VA Sierra Nevada Health Care System
1000 Locust Street 775-786-7200
Reno, NV 89502 888-838-6256
Fax: 775-328-1464
www.reno.va.gov

Kurt W Schlegelmilch, Director
Steven E Brilliant, Chief of Staff

New Hampshire

10259 **Veterans Adm. Medical Center: Manchester Manchester VA Medical Center**
Manchester VA Medical Center
718 Smyth Road 603-624-4366
Manchester, NH 03104 800-892-8384
Fax: 603-626-6579
www.manchester.va.gov

Marc F Levenson MD, Director
Andrew Breuder, Chief of Staff

New Jersey

10260 **Veterans Adm. Medical Center: East Orange East Orange Campus**
East Orange Campus
385 Tremont Avenue 973-676-1000
E Orange, NJ 07018 Fax: 973-676-4226
www.eastorange.va.gov

Kenneth H Mizrach, Director
Steven L Lieberman, Chief of Staff

10261 **Veterans Adm. Medical Center: Lyons Lyons Campus**
Lyons Campus
151 Knollcroft Road 908-647-0180
Lyons, NJ 07939 Fax: 908-647-3452
www.lyons.va.gov

Kenneth H Mizrach, Director
Steven L Lieberman, Chief of Staff

New Mexico

10262 **Veterans Adm. Medical Center: Albuquerque New Mexico VA Health Care System**
New Mexico VA Health Care System
1501 San Pedro Drive SE 505-265-1711
Albuquerque, NM 87108-5153 800-465-8262
Fax: 505-256-2855
www.albuquerque.va.gov

George Marnell, Director
Meghan Gerety, Chief of Staff

New York

10263 Gulf War Veterans of Long Island, NY
100 Robinson
E Patchogue, NY 11772
516-289-1580
Fax: 516-447-5871
e-mail: DStormMom@aol.com
Jackie Olsen

10264 Persian Gulf Veterans
212 Garfield Avenue
E Rochester, NY 14445-1314
716-385-4097
Fax: 716-924-2161
Beverly Place

10265 VA Helathcare Network: Upstate New York
PO Box 8980
Albany, NY 12208-8980
518-626-7300
Fax: 518-626-7333
www.visn2.va.gov
Stephen L Lemons, Network Director
Lawrence H Flesh, Chief Medical Officer

10266 VA NY/NJ Veterans Healthcare Network
130 W Kingsbridge Road
Bronx, NY 10468
718-584-9000
Fax: 718-579-1671
www1.va.gov//visn03
Michael A Sabo, Network Director

10267 Veterans Adm. Medical Center: Albany Samuel S. Stratton: VA Medical Center
Samuel S. Stratton: VA Medical Center
113 Holland Avenue
Albany, NY 12208
518-626-5000
Fax: 518-626-5500
www.albany.va.gov
Mary-Ellen Pich,, Director
Lourdes Irizarry, Chief of Staff

10268 Veterans Adm. Medical Center: Batavia VA Western New York Healthcare System
VA Western New York Healthcare System at Batavia
222 Richmond Avenue
Batavia, NY 14020
585-297-1000
Fax: 716-344-3305
www.buffalo.va.gov/batavia.asp
David J West, Interim Director
Miguel Rainstein, Chief of Staff

10269 Veterans Adm. Medical Center: Bath Bath VA Medical Center
Bath VA Medical Center
76 Veterans Avenue
Bath, NY 14810
607-664-4000
877-845-3247
Fax: 607-664-4511
www.bath.va.gov
Thomas W Sharpe, Acting Medical Center Director
Steven Speroni, Acting Chief of Staff

10270 Veterans Adm. Medical Center: Brooklyn Brooklyn Campus
Brooklyn Campus
800 Poly Place
Brooklyn, NY 11209
718-836-6600
Fax: 718-630-2840
www.brooklyn.va.gov
John J Donnellan Jr, Director

10271 Veterans Adm. Medical Center: Buffalo
3495 Bailey Avenue
Buffalo, NY 14215
716-834-9200
800-532-8387
Fax: 716-862-8759
www.buffalo.va.gov
David J West, Interim Director
Miguel Rainstein, Chief of Staff

10272 Veterans Adm. Medical Center: Montrose Franklin Delano Roosevelt Campus
Franklin Delano Roosevelt Campus
2094 Albany Post Road
Montrose, NY 10548
914-737-4400
800-269-8749
Fax: 914-788-4244
www.hudsonvalley.va.gov
Gerald F Culliton, Director
Joanne Malina, Chief of Staff

10273 Veterans Adm. Medical Center: New York New York Campus
New York Campus
423 E 23rd Street
New York, NY 10010
212-686-7500
Fax: 718-567-4082
www.manhattan.va.gov
John J Donnellan Jr, Director

10274 Veterans Adm. Medical Center: Northport Northport VA Medical Center
Northport VA Medical Center
79 Middleville Road
Northport, NY 11768
516-261-4400
800-551-3996
Fax: 631-754-7933
www.northport.va.gov
Philip C Moschitta, Director
Edward Mack, Chief of Staff

10275 Veterans Adm. Medical Center: Syracuse Syracuse VA Medical Center
Syracuse VA Medical Center
800 Irving Avenue
Syracuse, NY 13210
315-425-4400
800-792-4334
Fax: 315-425-4375
www.syracuse.va.gov
James Cody, Director
William H Marx, Chief of Staff

10276 Veterans Affairs Medical Center Canandaigua
Canadaigua VA Medical Center
400 Fort Hill Avenue
Canandaigua, NY 14424
716-394-2000
Fax: 716-393-8328
www.va.gov/visns/visn02
Sally Martin, Geriatrics/Extended Care Line Co-Manager
Diane West, Geriatrics/Extended Care Line Co-Manager

North Carolina

10277 Desert Storm Veterans of North Carolina
739 E Haggard Avenue
Ellon College, NC 27224
910-584-5038
Kevin Treiber

10278 Veterans Adm. Medical Center: Asheville Asheville VA Medical Center
Asheville VA Medical Center
1100 Tunnel Road
Asheville, NC 28805
828-298-7911
800-932-6408
Fax: 828-299-2502
www.asheville.va.gov
Susan Pendergrass, Director
Mary Ann Curl, Chief of Staff

10279 Veterans Adm. Medical Center: Durham Durham VA Medical Center
Durham VA Medical Center
508 Fulton Street
Durham, NC 27705
919-286-0411
888-878-6890
Fax: 919-286-6825
www.durham.va.gov
Ralph T Gigliotti, Director
John D Shelburne, Chief of Staff

10280 Veterans Adm. Medical Center: Fayetville Fayettville VA Medical Center
Fayettville VA Medical Center
2300 Ramsey Street
Fayetteville, NC 28301
910-488-2120
800-771-6106
Fax: 910-822-7093
www.fayettevillenc.va.gov
Bruce C Triplett, Director
Kanan Chatterjee, Interim Chief of Staff

10281 Veterans Adm. Medical Center: Salisbury W.G. Hefner VA Medical Center
W.G. Hefner VA Medical Center
1601 Brenner Avenue
Salisbury, NC 28144
704-683-9000
800-469-8262
Fax: 704-638-3395
www.salisbury.va.gov
Carolyn L Adams, Director
Miguel H LaPuz, Chief of Staff

North Dakota

10282 Veterans Adm. Regional Office: Fargo Regional Office Center
Fargo VA Medical.Regional Office Center
2101 N Elm Street
Fargo, ND 58102
701-232-3241
800-410-9723
Fax: 701-239-3705
www.fargo.va.gov
Robert P McDivitt, Director
Lavonne Liversage, Associate Medical Director

Ohio

10283 Persian Gulf War Veterans of Western Pennsylvania, W Virginia and NE Ohio
600 North Market Street
East Palestine, OH 44413
216-426-3203
Fax: 216-426-3309
Barry M Walker

10284 VA Healthcare System Of Ohio
11500 Northlake Drive
Cincinnati, OH 45249
513-247-4621
Fax: 513-247-4620
e-mail: visn10webmaster@med.va.gov
www.visn10.va.gov

10285 Veterans Adm. Medical Center: Chillicothe Chillicothe VA Medical Center
Chillicothe VA Medical Center
17273 State Route 104
Chillicothe, OH 45601
740-773-1141
800-358-8262
Fax: 740-773-1141
www.chillicothe.va.gov
Jeffrey T Gering, Director
Deborah M Meesig, Chief of Staff

10286 Veterans Adm. Medical Center: Cincinnati Cincinnati VA Medical Center
Cincinnati VA Medical Center
3200 Vine Street
Cincinnati, OH 45220
513-861-3100
888-267-7873
Fax: 513-475-6500
www.cincinnati.va.gov
Linda D Smith, Director
Sidney R Steinberg, Chief of Staff

10287 Veterans Adm. Medical Center: Cleveland Louis Stokes VA Medical Center
Louis Stokes VA Medical Center
10701 E Boulevard
Cleveland, OH 44106
216-791-3800
Fax: 216-421-3217
www.cleveland.va.gov
William Montague, Director
Murray D Altose, Chief of Staff

10288 Veterans Adm. Medical Center: Columbus Chalmers P. Wylie Outpatient Clinic
Chalmers P. Wylie Outpatient Clinic
420 N James Road
Columbus, OH 43219-1278
614-257-5200
888-615-9448
Fax: 614-257-5460
www.columbus.va.gov
Lilian T Thome, Director
Miguel LaPuz, Chief of Staff

10289 Veterans Adm. Medical Center: Dayton Dayton VA Medical Center
Dayton VA Medical Center
4100 W 3rd Street
Dayton, OH 45428
937-268-6511
800-368-8262
Fax: 937-262-2179
TTY: 800-829-4833
www.dayton.va.gov
Guy B Richardson, Medical Center Director
Terry E Taylor, Associate Director

10290 Veterans and Families Support Network Ohio
5488 State Route 7
New Waterford, OH 44445
216-457-0641
Fax: 216-457-1923
e-mail: VFSN@delphi.com
Gina Brown

Oklahoma

10291 American Veterans Justice Foundation
3908 NW Santa Fe
Lawton, OK 73505
405-355-3811
e-mail: dwolf@sirinet.net
Dannie Wolf

10292 Veterans Adm. Medical Center: Muskogee Dayton VA Medical Center
Dayton VA Medical Center
1011 Honor Heights Drive
Muskogee, OK 74401
918-577-3000
888-397-8387
Fax: 918-680-3648
www.muskogee.va.gov
Adam C Walmus, Director
A Rudy Klopfer, Associate Director

10293 Veterans Adm. Medical Center: Oklahoma City
Oklahoma City VA Medical Center
921 NE 13th Street
Oklahoma City, OK 73104
405-456-1000
866-835-5273
Fax: 405-270-1560
www.oklahoma.va.gov
David P Wood, Director
Anne Kreutzer, Associate Director

Oregon

10294 Northwest Network
PO Box 1035
Portland, OR 97207
360-619-5925
Fax: 360-737-1405
www.visn20.med.va.gov

10295 Northwest Vets for Peace
811 E Burnside Street
Portland, OR 97214
503-656-9785
e-mail: NWVP@teleport.com
Marvin Simmons

10296 Veterans Adm. Medical Center: Roseburg VA Roseburg Healthcare System
VA Roseburg Healthcare System
913 NW Garden Valley Boulevard
Roseburg, OR 97470
541-440-1000
800-549-8387
Fax: 541-440-1225
www.visn20.med.va.gov/roseburg
Susan Yeager, Acting Director
Stephen J Broskey, Associate Director

10297 Veterans Adm. Medical Center: White City VA S Oregon Rehabilitation Center
VA Southern Oregonrehabilitation Center & Clinics
8495 Crater Lake Highway
White City, OR 97503
541-826-2111
800-809-8725
Fax: 541-830-3500
www.visn20.med.va.gov/Southern-Oregon
Pam Harris, Human Resources Assistant

10298 Veterans Adm. Regional Office: Portland Portland VA Medical Center
Portland VA Medical Center
3710 SW US Veterans Hospital Road
Portland, OR 97239
503-220-8262
800-949-1004
Fax: 503-273-5319
www.visn20.med.va.gov
James Tuchschmidt, Director
John D Dryden, Chief of Staff

10299 Veterans Administration Domicillary
8495 Crater Lake Highway
White City, OR 97503
541-826-2111
Fax: 541-830-3519
e-mail: David.Schwing@med.va.gov
www1.va.gov/domiciliary

Pennsylvania

10300 Erie VA Medical Center
135 E 38th Street
Erie, PA 16504
814-868-8661
800-274-8387
Fax: 814-860-2120
www1.va.gov/erie

Michael D Adelman MD, Director
Melissa Sundin, Associate Director

10301 Pennsylvania Gulf War Veterans
RR 3
Clarion, PA 16214
814-226-4084
e-mail: kjsmith@penn.com
Kenneth J Smith, President
Daniel J Meck, VP

10302 VA Pittsburgh Healthcare System: University Drive Division
University Drive
Pittsburgh, PA 15240
866-482-7488
Fax: 412-688-6121
www.va.gov/pittsburgh

Terry Gerigk Wolf, Director
Rajiv Jain MD, Chief of Staff

10303 VA Stars & Stripes Healthcare Network
1010 Delafield Road
Pittsburgh, PA 15240
412-688-6000
866-482-7488
Fax: 412-784-3724
www.visn4.va.gov

Michael E Moreland FACHE, Network Director
Bradley P Shelton, Deputy Network Director

10304 Veterans Adm. Medical Center: Philadelphia
Philadelphia VA Medical Center
University & Woodland Avenues
Philadelphia, PA 19104
215-823-5800
877-626-2500
Fax: 215-823-6007
www.va.gov

10305 Veterans Adm. Medical Center: Altoona Coatesville VA Medical Center
James E. Van Zandt VA Medical Center
1400 Black Horse Hill Road
Coatesville, PA 19320-4377
610-384-7711
877-626-2500
Fax: 610-383-0207
e-mail: Coatesville.Query@med.va.gov
www.coatesville.med.va.gov

Gary W Devansky, Director
Donald R Means, Associate Director

10306 Veterans Adm. Medical Center: Coatesville
Coatesville VA Medical Center
1400 Black Horse Hill Road
Coatesville, PA 19320
610-384-7711
e-mail: coatesville.query@med.va.gov
www.coatesville.med.va.gov

10307 Veterans Adm. Medical Center: Lebanon Lebanon VA Medical Center
Lebanon VA Medical Center
1700 S Lincoln Avenue
Lebanon, PA 17042
717-272-6621
800-409-8771
Fax: 717-228-5907
e-mail: Norman.Faas@va.gov
www.lebanon.va.gov

Robert W Callahan Jr, Director
William H Mills, Associate Director

10308 Veterans Adm. Medical Center: Pittsburg VA Pittsburgh Healthcare System
VA Pittsburgh Healthcare System
7180 Highland Drive
Pittsburg, PA 15206
412-365-4900
866-482-7488
Fax: 412-365-4213
e-mail: VHAPTHwebteam@va.gov
www.pittsburgh.va.gov

Terry Gerigk Wolf, Director
Rajiv Jain MD, Chief of Staff

10309 Wilkes-Barre VA Medical Center
1111 E End Boulevard
Wilkes-Barre, PA 18711
570-824-3521
877-928-2621
Fax: 570-821-7278
www.wilkes-barre.va.gov

anice M Boss MS CHE, Director
C Gene Molino, Associate Director

Rhode Island

10310 Veterans Adm. Medical Center: Providence Providence VA Medical Center
Providence VA Medical Center
830 Chalkstone Avenue
Providence, RI 02908-4799
401-273-7100
866-590-2976
Fax: 401-457-3370
www.providence.va.gov

Vincent Ng, Director
William J Burney, Associate Director

South Carolina

10311 Ralph H. Johnson VA Medical Center
109 Bee Street
Charleston, SC 29401-5799
843-577-5011
Fax: 843-937-6100
www2.va.gov

10312 William Jennings Bryan Dorn VA Medical Center
6439 Garners Ferry Road
Columbia, SC 29209
803-776-4000
800-293-8262
Fax: 803-695-6739
www.va.gov/columbiasc

Falea Maney, Program Manager

South Dakota

10313 Department of Veterans Affairs Medical Center: Sioux Falls
2501 W 22nd Street
Sioux Falls, SD 57117-5046
605-336-3230
800-316-8387
Fax: 605-333-6878
www.visn23.med.va.gov

Healthcare for eligible veterans.

10314 VA Black Hills Health Care System- Fort Meade Campus
113 Comanche Road
Fort Meade, SD 57741
605-347-2511
800-743-1070
Fax: 605-347-7171
e-mail: Jeffrey.Honeycutt@med.va.gov
www2.va.gov

Jeffrey Honeycutt

10315 VA Black Hills Health Care System- Hot Springs Campus
500 N 5th Street
Hot Springs, SD 57747
605-745-2000
800-764-5370
Fax: 605-745-2091
www2.va.gov

Tennessee

10316 Mountain Home VA Medical Center
PO Box 4000
Mountain Home, TN 37684
423-926-1171
877-573-3529
Fax: 423-979-3519
www2.va.gov

Carl J Gerber MD PhD, Director
John W McFadden, Associate Director

10317 Persian Gulf Information Network
PO Box 10160
Clarksville, TN 37042
931-674-1518
Fax: 615-431-5222
e-mail: pgin@knightwave.com
home.att.net/~vetcenter/vetgrps.htm

Paul Lyons

10318 Tennessee Valley Healthcare System- Nashville Campus
1310 24th Avenue, South
Nashville, TN 37212-2637
615-327-4751
Fax: 615-321-6350

10319 **Tennessee Valley Healthcare System- Alvin C. York (Murfreesboro) Campus**
3400 Lebanon Pike
Murfreesboro, TN 37129
615-867-6000
800-876-7093
Fax: 615-225-4901
www2.va.gov

10320 **VISN 9: VA Mid South Healthcare Network**
1801 W End Avenue
Nashville, TN 37203
615-695-2200
Fax: 615-695-2210
www.visn9.va.gov

10321 **Veterans Adm. Medical Center: Murfreesboro**
3400 Lebanon Road
Murfreesboro, TN 37130
615-893-1360
Fax: 615-898-4872

10322 **Veterans Adm. Medical Center: Memphis**
1030 Jefferson Avenue
Memphis, TN 38104
901-523-8990
800-636-8262
www.memphis.va.gov

10323 **Veterans Adm. Medical Center: Muskogee**
3400 Lebanon Pike
Murfreesboro, TN 37129
615-867-6000
Fax: 615-225-4901
www.tennesseevalley.va.gov

10324 **Veterans Adm. Medical Center: Nashville**
1310 24th Avenue S
Nashville, TN 37212
615-327-4751
800-228-4973
Fax: 901-577-7306
www.memphis.va.gov

10325 **Veterans Affairs Medical Center**
1030 Jefferson Avenue
Memphis, TN 38104
901-523-8990
800-636-8262
Fax: 901-577-7251
www.memphis.va.gov

10326 **Veterans Affairs Medical Center, Memphis, Tennessee**
1030 Jefferson Avenue
Memphis, TN 38104
901-523-8990
Fax: 901-577-7251

Texas

10327 **Amarillo VA Health Care System**
6010 Amarillo Boulevard W
Amarillo, TX 79106
806-355-9703
800-687-8262
Fax: 806-354-7860
www.amarillo.va.gov

10328 **Austin Outpatient Clinic**
2901 Montopolis Drive
Austin, TX 78741
512-389-1010
Fax: 512-389-6545
www2.va.gov

10329 **Central Texas Veterans Health Care System**
1901 Veterans Memorial Drive
Temple, TX 76504
254-778-4811
800-423-2111
www.centraltexas.va.gov
Bruce A Gordon, Director
Karen Spada MSN MPH MHA FN, Associate Director Nursing Services

10330 **El Paso VA Health Care Center**
5001 N Piedras
El Paso, TX 79930-4211
915-564-6100
800-672-3782
Fax: 915-564-7920
www.elpaso.va.gov

10331 **Michael E. DeBakey VA Medical Center**
2002 Holcombe Boulevard
Houston, TX 77030-4298
713-791-1414
800-639-5137
Fax: 713-794-7218
www.houston.med.va.gov

10332 **Operation Desert Shield/Desert Storm**
PO Box 1712
Odessa, TX 79760
915-368-4667
Fax: 915-580-7451
Vic Sylvester

10333 **Persian Gulf Veterans of America**
PO Box 190222
San Antonio, TX 78280
210-666-4409
e-mail: KathyPGVA@aol.com
Kathy Hughes

10334 **South Texas Veterans Health Care System**
7400 Merton Minter
San Antonio, TX 78229
210-617-5300
877-469-5300
www.south-texas.med.va.gov

10335 **Thomas T. Connally Medical Center Marlin,T X**

10336 **VA Heart of Texas Health Care Network Dallas VA Medical Center**, TX 76661
Dallas VA Medical Center
4500 S Lancaster Road
Dallas, TX 75216
214-742-8387
800-849-3597
Fax: 214-857-1171
www.northtexas.va.gov

10337 **VISN 17: VA Heart of Texas Health Care Network**
2301 E Lamar Boulevard
Arlington, TX 76006
817-652-1111
Fax: 817-385-3700
www.heartoftexas.va.gov

10338 **Veterans Adm. Medical Center: Big Spring**
300 Veterans Boulevard
Big Spring, TX 79720-5500
432-263-7361
800-472-1365
Fax: 432-264-4834
www2.va.gov

10339 **Veterans Adm. Medical Center: Dallas**
4500 S Lancaster Road
Dallas, TX 75216
214-742-8387
800-849-8387
Fax: 214-857-1171
www2.va.gov

10340 **Veterans Adm. Medical Center: Kerrville**
3600 Memorial Boulevard
Kerrville, TX 78028
830-896-2020
www2.va.gov

10341 **Veterans Adm. Medical Center: Marlin**
1016 Ward Street
Marlin, TX 76661
254-883-3511
Fax: 254-883-9240

10342 **Veterans Adm. Medical Center: San Antonio**
7400 Merton Minter Boulevard
San Antonio, TX 78284
210-617-5300
www.va.gov

10343 **Veterans Adm. Medical Center: Temple**
1901 Veterans Memorial Drive
Temple, TX 76504
254-778-4811
800-423-2111
Fax: 254-771-4588
www2.va.gov

10344 **Waco VA Medical Center**
4800 Memorial Drive
Waco, TX 76711
254-752-6581
800-423-2111
www2.va.gov

10345 **West Texas VA Health Care System**
300 Veterans Boulevard
Big Spring, TX 79720
432-263-7361
800-472-1365
Fax: 432-264-4834
www2.va.gov

Utah

10346 **VA Salt Lake City Health Care System**
500 Foothill Drive
Salt Lake City, UT 84148
801-582-1565
800-613-4012
Fax: 801-584-1289
www.va.gov

Vermont

10347 **White River Junction VA Medical Center**
215 N Main Street
White River Junction, VT 05009
802-295-9363
866-687-8387
Fax: 802-296-6354
www.va.gov

Virginia

10348 **Desert Storm Justice Foundation: Virginia**
PO Box 6812 703-550-1346
Alexandria, VA 22309 Fax: 703-550-1346
Diane St Julian

10349 **Gulf War Veterans of Virginia**
PO Box 3124 757-988-3PGW
Chesapeake, VA 23320
Ted Myers, President

10350 **Veterans Adm. Medical Center: Hampton Hampton VA Medical Center**
Hampton VA Medical Center
100 Emancipation Drive 757-722-9961
Hampton, VA 23667 888-869-6060
Fax: 757-723-6620
www.hampton.va.gov

10351 **Veterans Adm. Medical Center: Richmond Hunter Holmes McGuire VA Medical Center**
Hunter Holmes McGuire VA Medical Center
1201 Broad Rock Boulevard 804-675-5000
Richmond, VA 23249 800-784-8381
Fax: 804-675-5581
www.va.gov

10352 **Veterans Adm. Medical Center: Roanoke Roanoke Vet Center**
Roanoke Vet Center
350 Albemarle Avenue SW 540-342-9726
Roanoke, VA 24016 Fax: 540-857-2405
www.va.gov
Lynn McGhee, Team Leader
John Whitlock, Counselor

10353 **Veterans Adm. Medical Center: Salem Salem VA Medical Center**
Salem VA Medical Center
1970 Roanoke Boulevard 540-982-2463
Salem, VA 24153 888-982-2463
Fax: 540-983-1096
www.va.gov

Washington

10354 **Persian Gulf Veterans of Washington**
13523 202nd Street E 360-893-2480
Graham, WA 98338 Fax: 360-893-3998
e-mail: amehl@ix.netcom.com
Alyssa Mehl

10355 **VA Puget Sound Health Care System**
1660 S Columbian Way 206-762-1010
Seattle, WA 98108-1597 800-329-8387
Fax: 206-764-2224
www.va.gov/pugetsound

10356 **Veterans Adm. Medical Center: Seattle**
1660 S Columbian Way 206-762-1010
Seattle, WA 98108 800-329-8387
Fax: 206-764-2224
www2.va.gov

10357 **Veterans Adm. Medical Center: Spokane Spokane VA Medical Center**
Spokane VA Medical Center
4815 N Assembly Street 509-434-7000
Spokane, WA 99205-6197 Fax: 509-434-7119
www.va.gov

10358 **Veterans Adm. Medical Center: Tacoma Tacoma Vet Center**
Tacoma Vet Center
4916 Center Street 253-565-7038
Tacoma, WA 98409 Fax: 253-565-4981
www.va.gov
Robert Ramsey, Team Leader
George Rippon, Counselor

10359 **Veterans Adm. Medical Center: Walla Walla Johnathan M. Wainwright Memorial VA MC**
Johnathan M. Wainwright Memorial VA Medical Center
77 Wainwright Drive 509-525-5200
Walla Walla, WA 99362 888-687-8863
Fax: 509-527-3452
www.va.gov

West Virginia

10360 **Veterans Adm. Medical Center: Beckley Beckley VA Medical Center**
Beckley VA Medical Center
200 Veterans Avenue 304-255-2121
Beckley, WV 25801 877-902-5142
Fax: 304-255-2431
www.va.gov

10361 **Veterans Adm. Medical Center: Clarksburg Louis A. Johnson VA Medical Center**
Louis A. Johnson VA Medical Center
One Medical Center Drive 304-623-3461
Clarksburg, WV 26301 800-733-0512
Fax: 304-626-7026
www.va.gov

10362 **Veterans Adm. Medical Center: Huntington**
1540 Spring Valley Drive 304-429-6741
Huntington, WV 25704 800-827-8244
Fax: 304-429-6713
www.va.gov

10363 **Veterans Affairs Medical Center: Martinsburg**
900 Winchester Avenue 304-263-6776
Martinsburg, WV 25401 800-817-3807
Fax: 304-262-7448
www.va.gov
Robert Hogue, Counselor
Cindy Hughes, Counselor

Wisconsin

10364 **Clement J. Zablocki Veterans Affairs Medical Center**
5000 W National Avenue 414-382-5300
Milwaukee, WI 53295-1000 Fax: 414-382-5321
www.va.gov

10365 **Gulf War Veterans of Wisconsin**
33 University Square 608-250-9645
Madison, WI 53715 e-mail: gulfwarwisc@geocities.com
Anthony Hardie

10366 **MidWest Gulf War Veterans Association**
PO Box 108 414-695-8694
Pewaukee, WI 53072 Fax: 414-695-8694
e-mail: mrlbrty@execpc.com
Robert Schramm

10367 **Veterans Adm. Medical Center: Tomah**
500 E Veterans Street 608-372-3971
Tomah, WI 54660 800-872-8662
www.va.gov

10368 **William S. Middleton Memorial Veterans Hospital**
2500 Overlook Terrace 608-256-1901
Madison, WI 53705-2286 Fax: 608-280-7096
www.va.gov

Wyoming

10369 **Veterans Adm. Medical Center: Cheyenne**
2360 E Pershing Boulevard 307-778-7550
Cheyenne, WY 82001 888-483-9127
Fax: 307-778-7336
www.va.gov

10370 **Veterans Adm. Medical Center: Sheridan**
1898 Fort Road 307-672-3473
Sheridan, WY 82801 866-822-6714
Fax: 307-672-1900
www.va.gov

Libraries & Resource Centers

10371 **ARCH Training Center**
2427 Martin Luther King Jr Avenue — 202-889-6344
Washington, DC

10372 **American GI Forum NVOP**
219 Tampico Street — 210-212-4088
San Antonio, TX 78207

10373 **COPIN Foundation**
2644 North Avenue — 716-283-5622
Niagara Falls, NY 14305 — Fax: 716-283-5721

10374 **Kennedy-Krieger Institute**
707 N Broadway — 443-923-9200
Baltimore, MD 21205 — 800-873-3377
Fax: 443-923-9405
www.kennedykrieger.org

10375 **Shriver Center University Affiliated Program**
Eunice Kennedy Shriver Center
200 Trapelo Road — 781-642-0001
Waltham, MA 02452-6319 — e-mail: shriver.center@umassmed.edu
www.shriver.org

10376 **Veterans Benefits Clearinghouse**
38 Dudley Street — 617-541-8846
Roxbury, MA 02119-1707

Support Groups & Hotlines

10377 **National Health Information Center**
PO Box 1133 — 310-565-4167
Washington, DC 20013 — 800-336-4797
Fax: 301-984-4256
e-mail: info@nhic.org
www.health.gov/nhic
Offers a nationwide information referral service, produces directories and resource guides.

10378 **National Veterans Services Fund**
PO Box 2465 — 203-656-0003
Darien, CT 06820-0465 — 800-521-0198
Fax: 203-656-1957
e-mail: NatVetSvc@aol.com
www.nvsf.org
Agent Orange informational hotline.
Phil Kraft, President

Books

10379 **An Assessment of Technical Issues Raised in RW Haley's Critique of Health Studies**
Gus Haggstrom, author
Rand Corporation
1776 Main Street — 310-393-0411
Santa Monica, CA 90407-2138 — Fax: 310-393-4818

ISBN: 0-833027-52-2

10380 **Gulf War and Health**
National Academy Press
500 5th Street NW — 202-334-3313
Washington, DC 20055 — 888-624-8373
Fax: 202-334-2793
e-mail: zjones@nas.edu

Lyla M Hernandez, Editor
Merwyn R Greenlick, Editor

10381 **Natural Attenuation for Groundwater Remediation**
National Academy Press
500 5th Street NW — 202-334-3313
Washington, DC 20055 — 888-624-8373
Fax: 202-334-2793
e-mail: zjones@nas.edu

10382 **Yes, You Can**
Demos Medical Publishing
386 Park Avenue S — 212-683-0072
New York, NY 10016 — Fax: 212-683-0118
e-mail: orderdept@demospub.com
www.demosmedpub.com

112 pages
ISBN: 1-888799-48-x
Dr. Diana M Schneider

Newsletters

10383 **Agent Orange Briefs**
Department of Veterans Affairs
810 Vermont Avenue NW — 202-233-4000
Washington, DC 20420-0002
Designed to answer questions regarding Agent Orange and related matters. This fact sheet series is prepared and updated annually.
Monthly

10384 **Agent Orange Review**
Department of Veterans Affairs
810 Vermont Avenue NW — 202-233-4000
Washington, DC 20420-0002
Published periodically to provide information on Agent Orange to concerned veterans and their families. The most recent issues include updated information about Federal government studies and activities related to Agent Orange and the Vietnam experience.

Pamphlets

10385 **Agent Orange Anxiety: The Human Response to Possable Oncogenicity and Mutagencity**
National Veterans Services Fund
PO Box 2465 — 203-656-0003
Darien, CT 06820-0465 — 800-521-0198
Fax: 203-656-1957
e-mail: NatVetSvc@optonline.net
www.angelfire.com/ct2/natvetsvc

10386 **Agent Orange Fact Sheet: A Historical Perspective**
Veterans Of The Vietnam War
805 South Township Boulevard — 570-603-9740
Pittston, PA 18640-3327 — Fax: 570-603-9741
www.vvnw.org
Fact sheet designed to bring an awareness of Agent Orange and related herbicides to the American public, includes a bibliography for the professional.
10 pages

10387 **Agent Orange and Birth Defects**
Veterans Health Adminstration
810 Vermont Avenue Northwest — 202-273-8580
Washington, DC 20420-3517 — Fax: 202-273-9080
www.tpromo2.com/usvi/index2.htm
Letters to the editor, New England Journal of Medicine articles.

10388 **Agent Orange and Chloracme**
National Veterans Services Fund
PO Box 2465 — 203-656-0003
Darien, CT 06820-0465 — 800-521-0198
Fax: 203-656-1957
e-mail: NatVetSvc@optonline.net
www.angelfire.com/ct2/natvetsvc

10389 **Agent Orange and Hodgkin's Disease**
Veterans Health Administration
810 Vermont Avenue Northwest — 203-273-8580
Washington, DC 20420-3517 — Fax: 203-273-9080
www.tpromo2.com/usvi/index2.htm

10390 **Agent Orange and Mutiple Myeloma**
National Veterans Services Fund
PO Box 2465 — 203-656-0003
Darien, CT 06820-0465 — 800-521-0198
Fax: 203-656-1957
e-mail: NatVetSvc@optonline.net
www.angelfire.com/ct2/natvetsvc

10391 Agent Orange and Non-Hodgkin's Lymphoma
Veterans Health Administration
810 Vermont Avenue 203-273-8580
Washington, DC 20420-3517 Fax: 203-273-9080
www.tpromo2.com/usvi/index2.htm

10392 Agent Orange and Peripheral Neuropathy
Veterans Health Administration
810 Vermont Avenue 203-273-8580
Washington, DC 20420-3517 Fax: 203-273-9080
www.tpromo2.com/usvi/index2.htm

10393 Agent Orange and Porphyria Cutanea Tarda
National Veterans Services Fund
PO Box 2465 203-656-0003
Darien, CT 06820-0465 800-521-0198
Fax: 203-656-1957
e-mail: NatVetSvc@optonline.net
www.angelfire.com/ct2/natvetsvc

10394 Agent Orange and Prostate Cancer
National Veterans Services Fund
PO Box 2465 203-656-0003
Darien, CT 06820-0465 800-521-0198
Fax: 203-656-1957
e-mail: NatVetSvc@optonline.net
www.angelfire.com/ct2/natvetsvc

10395 Agent Orange and Respiratory Cancers
National Veterans Services Fund
PO Box 2465 203-656-0003
Darien, CT 06820-0465 800-521-0198
Fax: 203-656-1957
e-mail: NatVetSvc@optonline.net
www.angelfire.com/ct2/natvetsvc

10396 Agent Orange and Soft Tissue Sarcomas
National Veterans Services Fund
PO Box 2465 203-656-0003
Darien, CT 06820-0465 800-521-0198
Fax: 203-656-1957
e-mail: NatVetSvc@optonline.net
www.angelfire.com/ct2/natvetsvc

10397 Agent Orange and Spina Bifida
National Veterans Services Fund
PO Box 2465 203-656-0003
Darien, CT 06820-0465 800-521-0198
Fax: 203-656-1957
e-mail: NatVetSvc@optonline.net
www.angelfire.com/ct2/natvetsvc

10398 Agent Orange: It is Part of Your Life
National Veterans Services Fund
PO Box 2465 203-656-0003
Darien, CT 06820-0465 800-521-0198
Fax: 203-656-1957
e-mail: NatVetSvc@optonline.net
www.angelfire.com/ct2/natvetsvc

10399 Brief History of the Agent Orange Lawsuit
National Veterans Services Fund
PO Box 2465 203-656-0003
Darien, CT 06820-0465 800-521-0198
Fax: 203-656-1957
e-mail: NatVetSvc@optonline.net
www.angelfire.com/ct2/natvetsvc

10400 Case Control Study: Soft-Tissue Sarcomas and Exposure to Phenoxyacetic Acids
National Veterans Services Fund
PO Box 2465 203-656-0003
Darien, CT 06820-0465 800-521-0198
Fax: 203-656-1957
e-mail: NatVetSvc@optonline.net
www.angelfire.com/ct2/natvetsvc
Case control study: soft-tissue sarcoma and exposure to phenoxyacetic acids or chlorophenols.

10401 Children of Vietnam Veterans: Complex Concerns and Innovative Solutions
National Veterans Services Fund
PO Box 2465 203-656-0003
Darien, CT 06820-0465 800-521-0198
Fax: 203-656-1957
e-mail: NatVetsvc@optonline.net
www.angelfire.com/ct2/natvetsvc
7 pages

10402 Dioxin, A Case in Point
National Veterans Services Fund
PO Box 2465 203-656-0003
Darien, CT 06820-0465 800-521-0198
Fax: 203-656-1957
e-mail: NatVetSvc@optonline.net
www.angelfire.com/ct2/natvetsvc

10403 Enviromental Chloracne
National Veterans Services Fund
PO Box 2465 203-656-0003
Darien, CT 06820-0465 800-521-0198
Fax: 203-656-1957
e-mail: NatVetSvc@optonline.net
www.angelfire.com/ct2/natvetsvc

10404 History of the Agent Orange Litigation
National Veterans Services Fund
PO Box 2465 203-656-0003
Darien, CT 06820-0465 800-521-0198
Fax: 203-656-1957
e-mail: NatVetsvc@optonline.net
www.angelfire.com/ct2/natvetsvc

10405 List of Agent Orange-Related Illnesses Recognized By the VA
National Veterans Services Fund
PO Box 2465 203-656-0003
Darien, CT 06820-0465 800-521-0198
Fax: 203-656-1957
e-mail: NatVetsvc@optonline.net
www.angelfire.com/ct2/natvetsvc

10406 List of Diseases Accepted by the VA for Presumptive Service-Connection
National Veterans Services Fund
PO Box 2465 203-656-0003
Darien, CT 06820-0465 800-521-0198
Fax: 203-656-1957
e-mail: NatVetSvc@optonline.net
www.angelfire.com/ct2/natvetsvc
List of diseases accepted by the VA for presumptive service-connection that are associated with exposure to certain herbicide agents including Agent Orange.

10407 Relation of Soft-Tissue Sarcome, Malignant Lymphoma & Colon Cancer
National Veterans Services Fund
PO Box 2465 203-656-0003
Darien, CT 06820-0465 800-521-0198
Fax: 203-656-1957
e-mail: NatVetSvc@optonline.net
www.angelfire.com/ct2/natvetsvc
Relation to soft-tissue sarcomas, malignant lymphoma and colon cancer to phenoxy acids, chlorphenois and other agents.

10408 Spina Bifida Benefits Guide
National Veterans Services Fund
PO Box 2465 203-656-0003
Darien, CT 06820-0465 800-521-0198
Fax: 203-656-1957
e-mail: NatVetsvc@optonline.net
www.angelfire.com/ct2/natvetsvc
4 pages

Audio & Video

10409 Agent Orange Videotapes
Regional Learning Resources Service
915 N. Grand Boulevard 314-652-4100
St. Louis, MO 63106
Produces several Agent Orange videotape programs that explain what Agent Orange is, where, when and how it was used, why persons are concerned about exposure to it and what VA and other de-

partments and agencies are doing in response to these concerns. These videotapes are maintained at all VA medical centers across the country.

Web Sites

10410 Gulf War Syndrome Database

www.louisville.edu/library/ekstrom

This is a substantial database of relevant documents and studies kept by University of Louisville, Ekstrom Library.

10411 Gulf War Veteran Resource Pages

www.gulfweb.org

This page is administered by Gulf War veterans and provides a great range of information on a variety of Gulf War-related items, including GWS. The site includes many links to other groups interested in GWS and to GWS studies.

10412 Healing Well

www.healingwell.com

An online health resource guide to medical news, chat, information and articles, newsgroups and message boards, books, disease-related web sites, medical directories, and more for patients, friends, and family coping with disabling diseases, disorders, or chronic illnesses.

10413 Health Finder

www.healthfinder.gov

Searchable, carefully developed web site offering information on over 1000 topics. Developed by the US Department of Health and Human Services, the site can be used in both English and Spanish.

10414 Healthlink USA

www.healthlinkusa.com

Health information concerning treatment, cures, prevention, diagnosis, risk factors, research, support groups, email lists, personal stories and much more. Updated regularly.

10415 Heatlhcentral.com

www.healthcentral.com

The HealthCentral Network has a collection of owned and operated web sites and multimedia affiliate properties providing timely, in-depth, trusted medical information, personalized tools and resources for people seeking to manage and improve their health.

10416 Helios Health

www.helioshealth.com

Online resource for your health information. Detailed information about specific health topics, access to expert advice from our Medical Advisory Board, and up-to-date health news.

10417 InteliHealth

www.intelihealth.com

InteliHealth's mission is to empower people with treusted solutions for healthier lives. They accomplish this by providing credible information fromt he most trusted sources.
Brian Berkenstock, Writer/Editor

10418 MedicineNet

www.medicinenet.com

Medicine Net is an online healthcare media publishing company. It provides easy-to-read, in-depth, authoritative medical information for consumers via its robust, user-friendly, interactive web site.

10419 Medscape

www.mywebmd.com

Medscape offers specialists, primary care physicians, and other health professionals the Web's most robust and integrated medical information and educational tools.

10420 National Veterans Services Fund

www.nvsf.org

Supports and informs those who were exposed to the defoliant Agent Orange, or dioxin, while serving the US in the conflict in Vietnam.

10421 Office of the Special Assistant for Gulf War Illnesses

www.gulflink.osd.mil

This is a page sponsored by the Defense Department's Special Assistant for Gulf War Illnesses. It provides information on and linkes to Federal and State-funded studies of Gulf War Illnesses.

10422 WebMD

www.webmd.com

Information on Agent Orange related injuries, including articles and resources.

Description

10423 **Wilson's Disease**

Wilson's disease is a rare genetic disorder that results from an inability to adequately excrete copper. In the United States, approximately one person in 40,000 has this condition. The resulting accumulation of copper in the body's tissues and organs leads to disease of the brain and liver, and to a lesser extent, the kidney and red blood cells. The disease is genetic; if two carriers have children, the disease would have a 1 in 4 chance of being passed on.

Build-up of copper in the liver causes a hepatitis-like illness with loss of appetite, low grade fever, abdominal discomfort and jaundice. If not detected and treated, this process can lead to cirrhosis and fatal liver failure. In 40 to 50 percent of patients, the illness affects the brain and can include unsteadiness, tremors, slurred speech and intellectual deterioration. Copper rings may appear in the eye in up to 10 percent of patients. Although they do not cause any symptoms, their appearance may help establish the diagnosis.

In untreated Wilson's, the disease is fatal, generally before the age of 30. Continual, lifelong treatment is mandatory for any patient with confirmed Wilson's disease, whether symptomatic or not. The critical therapy is to administer a drug that helps the body release its copper stores. D-penicillamine is the most common such drug. Some patients have required liver transplantation.

National Agencies & Associations

10424 **American Liver Foundation**
75 Maiden Lane
New York, NY 00038
212-668-1000
800-465-4837
Fax: 212-483-8179
e-mail: info@liverfoundation.org
www.liverfoundation.org
The only national voluntary health group dedicated to fighting all liver diseases through research education and patient self-help groups.
Rick Smith, President/CEO
Newton Guerin, COO

10425 **United Liver Foundation**
11646 W Pico Boulevard
Los Angeles, CA 90064
213-445-4204
Foundation offering information public awareness materials support and medical research for persons suffering from liver diseases.

10426 **Wilson's Disease Association**
1802 Brookside Drive
Wooster, OH 44691
330-264-1450
888-264-1450
Fax: 330-264-0974
e-mail: info@wilsonsdisease.org
www.wilsonsdisease.org
Serves as a communications support network for individuals affected by Wilson's disease; distributes information to professionals and the public; makes referrals; and holds meetings.
8 pages
Kimberly Symonds, Executive Director

Foundations

10427 **Hepatitis B Foundation**
3805 Old Easton Road
Doylestown, PA 18902
215-489-4900
Fax: 215-489-4313
e-mail: info@hepb.org
www.hepb.org
We are dedicated to finding a cure and improving the quality of life for those affected by hepatitis B worldwide. Our commitment includes funding focused research, promoting disease awareness, supporting immunization and treatment initiatives, and serving as the primary source of information for patients and their families, the medical and scientific community, and the general public.

Molli Conti, Chair
Timothy Block, PhD, Founder/President

Support Groups & Hotlines

10428 **National Health Information Center**
PO Box 1133
Washington, DC 20013
310-565-4167
800-336-4797
Fax: 301-984-4256
e-mail: info@nhic.org
www.health.gov/nhic
Offers a nationwide information referral service, produces directories and resource guides.

Pamphlets

10429 **Wilson's Disease**
American Liver Foundation
1425 Pompton Avenue
Cedar Grove, NJ 07009
800-465-4837
Fax: 973-256-3214
e-mail: info@liverfoundation.org
www.liverfoundation.org
A brochure offering information on the causes, symptoms and treatments of Wilson's Disease.
Rick Smith, President & CEO

Web Sites

10430 **Healing Well**
e-mail: webmaster@healingwell.com
www.healingwell.com
An online health resource guide to medical news, chat, information and articles, newsgroups and message boards, books, disease-related web sites, medical directories, and more for patients, friends, and family coping with disabling diseases, disorders, or chronic illnesses.
Peter Waite, MS, MA, Founder/Editor

10431 **Health Finder**
PO Box 1133
Washington, DC 20013-1133
e-mail: healthfinder@nhic.org
www.healthfinder.gov
Searchable, carefully developed web site offering information on over 1000 topics. Developed by the US Department of Health and Human Services, the site can be used in both English and Spanish.

10432 **Healthlink USA**
www.healthlinkusa.com
Health information concerning treatment, cures, prevention, diagnosis, risk factors, research, support groups, email lists, personal stories and much more. Updated regularly.

10433 **Helios Health**
www.helioshealth.com
Online resource for your health information. Detailed information about specific health topics, access to expert advice from our Medical Advisory Board, and up-to-date health news.

10434 **MedicineNet**
www.medicinenet.com

An online resource for consumers providing easy-to-read, authoritative medical and health information.

10435 **Medscape**
Corporate Headquarters
76 Ninth Avenue, Suite 719
New York, NY 10011
212-624-3700
www.mywebmd.com
Medscape offers specialists, primary care physicians, and other health professionals the Web's most robust and integrated medical information and educational tools.
Kevin M Cameron, CEO
Tony G Holcombe, President

10436 **WebMD**
www.webmd.com
Information on Wilson's disease, including articles and resources.

National Agencies & Associations

10437 **ABLEDATA**
8630 Fenton Street
Silver Spring, MD 20910
301-608-8998
800-227-0216
Fax: 301-608-8958
TTY: 301-608-8912
e-mail: abledata@macrointernational.com
www.abledata.com
An information and referral service that uses computer listings and a large file system to answer requests related to assistive devices. Houses a large file system library and contacts with other sources which enables them to answer just about any question.
Katherine Belknap, Project Director
Steve Lowe, Associate Project Manager and Webmaster

10438 **ABLEDATA-REHAB DATA Alliance for Technology Access (ATA)**
8630 Fenton Street
Silver Spring, MD 20910
301-608-8998
800-227-0216
Fax: 301-608-8958
TTY: 301-608-8912
e-mail: abledata@macrointernational.com
www.abledata.com
National organization dedicated to providing access to technology for people with disabilities through its coalition of 45 community-based resource centers in 34 states and the Virgin Islands. Each center provides information, awareness and training.
Katherine Belknap, Project Director
Juanita Hardy, Information Specialist

10439 **Access Unlimited**
570 Hance Road
Binghamton, NY 13903
607-669-4822
800-849-2143
Fax: 607-669-4595
e-mail: tom@accessunlimited.com
www.accessunlimited.com
Assists educators health care providers and parents in discovering lift and transfer aids help children and adults with disabilities compensate for some of the barriers imposed by their conditions. Access Unlimited markets and offers technical support.
Tom Egan, Owner
Tom Cole, Contact

10440 **American Academy of Pediatrics**
141 NW Point Boulevard
Elk Grove Village, IL 60007-1019
847-434-4000
Fax: 847-434-8000
www.aap.org
Offers information referrals treatment and services to children and youth.
Errol R Alden MD, Executive Director
David T Tayloe, President

10441 **American Association for the Advancement of Science**
1200 New York Avenue NW
Washington, DC 20005
202-326-6400
Fax: 202-789-0455
e-mail: webmaster@aaas.org
www.aaas.org
Addresses the concerns of scientists and engineers with disabilities and offers suggestions about improving accessibility of science programs for students with disabilities and offers 5 different fellowships.
Dr Allan I Leshner, AAAS CEO
Dr Peter C Agre, President

10442 **American Association of People with Disabilities**
1629 K Street NW
Washington, DC 20006
202-457-0046
800-840-8844
Fax: 202-457-0473
TTY: 202-457-0046
e-mail: AAPD@aol.com
www.aapd-dc.org
Promotes the economic and political empowerment of all 56 million children and adults with disabilities including their family friends and supporters and to be a national voice for change in implementing the goals of the Americans with Disabilities Act.
Quarterly
Andrew Imtarato, President

10443 **American Autoimmune Related Diseases Association**
22100 Gratiot Avenue
Eastpointe, MI 48021
586-776-3900
800-598-4668
Fax: 586-776-3903
e-mail: aarda@aarda.org
www.aarda.org
Awareness education referrals for patients with any type of autoimmune disease.
Virginia T Ladd, President/Executive Director
Stanley M Finger, Chairman

10444 **American Bar Association Commission on Mental and Physical Disability Law**
740 15th Street NW
Washington, DC 20005-1019
202-662-1000
Fax: 202-662-1032
e-mail: askaba@abanet.org
www.abanet.org/disability
The Commission's mission is to promote the ABA's commitment to justice and the rule of law for persons with mental physical and sensory disabilities and to promote their full and equal participation in the legal profession.
William C Hubbard, Chair
John W Parry, Director

10445 **American Camp Association**
5000 State Road 67 N
Martinsville, IN 46151-7902
765-342-8456
800-428-2267
Fax: 765-349-6357
e-mail: bookstore@acacamps.org
www.acacamps.org
Formerly the American Camping Association, the American Camp Association works to preserve, promote and improve the camp experience.
Peg Smith, Chief Executive Officer
Rhonda Begley, Chief Financial Officer

10446 **American Counseling Association**
5999 Stevenson Avenue
Alexandria, VA 22304-3302
800-347-6647
Fax: 800-473-2329
www.counseling.org
The American Counseling Association is a non-profit professional and educational organization that is dedicated to the growth and enhancement of the counseling profession. Founded in 1952, ACA is the world's largest association of its kind.
Colleen R Logan, President
Richard Yep, Executive Director

10447 **American Foundation for The Blind**
11 Penn Plaza
New York, NY 10001
212-502-7600
800-232-5463
Fax: 212-502-7777
e-mail: afbinfo@afb.net
www.afb.org
AFB's priorities include broadening access to technology; elevating the quality of information and tools for the professionals who serve people with vision loss; and promoting independent and healthy living for people with vision loss.
Carl R Augusto, President/CEO
Richard J O'Brien, Chair

10448 **American Institute for Preventive Medicine**
30445 NW Highway
Farmington Hills, MI 48334-3107
248-539-1800
Fax: 248-539-1808
e-mail: aipm@healthy.net
www.healthylife.com/
The institute provides health promotion programs, disease management guides and self-care publications to hospitals, HMOs, corporations and government agencies. Programs are designed to lower health care costs, decrease absenteeism, improve productivity and increase visibility.
Don R Powell PhD, Founder/President
Susan Jackson, VP

10449 **American Institute for Preventive Medicine**
30445 NW Highway
Farmington Hills, MI 48334
248-539-1800
800-345-2476
Fax: 248-539-1808
e-mail: aipm@healthylife.com
www.healthylife.com

The institute provides health promotion programs disease management guides and self-care publications to hospitals HMOs corporations and government agencies. Programs are designed to lower health care costs, decrease absenteeism and improve productivity.
Don R Powell PhD, President and CEO
Larry Chapman, Senior Vice President

10450 American Organ Transplant Association
21175 Tomball Parkway 713-344-2402
Houston, TX 77070 Fax: 713-344-9422
www.aotaonline.org
Helps defray out-of-pocket expenses for liver heart lung and pancreas transplant recipients.
Pamela H Terry, Board President
David Hileman, Board Vice President

10451 American Red Cross National Headquarters
2025 E Street NW 202-303-5000
Washington, DC 20006 800-733-2767
e-mail: info@usa.redcross.org
www.redcross.org
Offers seminars conferences and newsletters with 2 889 local chapters.
Gail J McGovern, President/CEO
Bonnie McElveen-Hunt, Chairman

10452 American Rehabilitation Counseling Association
5999 Stevenson Avenue
Alexandria, VA 22304-3300 800-347-6647
Fax: 800-473-2329
TTY: 703-823-6862
TDD: 7038236862
e-mail: webmaster@counseling.org
www.counseling.org
Mission of ARCA is to enhance the development of persons with disabilities throughout their life span and to promote excellence in the rehabilitation counseling professional.
Colleen Logan, President
Richard Yep, Executive Office

10453 American Society of Dermatology
411 Hamilton Boulevard 309-676-4074
Peoria, IL 61602-1104 Fax: 309-676-3522
e-mail: mcraig@asd.org
www.asd.org
The mission of this organization is to facilitate optimal dermatologic care being available to all citizens of this country by preserving promoting and enhancing the private practice of deratlogy.
M John Hanni Jr, Executive Director
Monica L Craig, Assistant

10454 Americas Association for the Care of Children
P.O. Box 2154
Boulder, CO 80306-2154 303-527-2742
www.aacchildren.net
An international multidisciplinary organization which promotes the emotional, developmental, and psychosocial well-being of children and families in all health care settings.

Laurene Philips, President
Douglas Johnson, Vice President

10455 Asbestos Information Association/North America
1745 Jefferson Davis Highway 703-412-1150
Arlington, VA 22202 Fax: 703-412-1586
e-mail: aiabjpigg@aol.com
Founded to represent the interests of the asbestos industry and to collect and disseminate information about asbestos and asbestos products with emphasis on safety health and environmental issues.

10456 Beach Center on Families and Disability University of Kansas
University of Kansas
1200 Sunnyside Avenue 785-864-7600
Lawrence, KS 66045 Fax: 786-864-3434
e-mail: beachcenter@ku.edu
www.beachcenter.org
A federally funded center that conducts research and training in the factors that contribute to the successful functioning of families with members who have disabilities.
Wayne Sailor, Associate Director

10457 Breaking New Ground Resource Center
Purdue University ABE Building 765-494-1191
W Lafayette, IN 47907 800-825-4264
e-mail: field@ecn.purdue.edu
A resource center devoted to helping farmers and ranchers with physical disabilities. Several resource materials related to rural assistive technology are available at low cost and a free newsletter are available to anyone.
William E Field, Professor

10458 Center for Children with Chronic Illness and Disability
University of Minnesota School of Public Health
2525 Chicago Avenue
Minneapolis, MN 55404 612-813-6000
www.childrensmn.org
Dr Joan Patterson, Director

10459 Center for Chronic Disease Prevention and Health Promotion
Centers for Disease Control
1600 Clifton Rd 404-639-3311
Atlanta, GA 30333 800-232-4636
TTY: 800-232-6348
e-mail: cdcinfo@cdc.gov
www.cdc.gov/
The mission of the CDC is to promote health and quality of life by preventing and controlling disease, injury and disability.
Richard Besser, MD, Acting Director
Tanja Popovic, MD, Chief Science Officer

10460 Center for Chronic Disease Prevention and Centers for Disease Control
1600 Clifton Road 404-639-3311
Atlanta, GA 30333 800-232-4636
TTY: 888-232-6348
e-mail: cdcinfo@cdc.gov
www.cdc.gov
Chronic diseases such as heart disease cancer and diabetes are the leading causes of death and disability in the United States. These diseases account for 7 of every 10 deaths and affect the quality of life of 90 million Americans.
Richard E Besser, Director

10461 Center for Developmental Disabilities University of South Carolina
8301 Farrow Road 803-935-5231
Columbia, SC 29208 Fax: 803-935-5059
uscm.med.sc.edu/cdrhome
The vision of The Center for Developmental Disabilities is to work as a team to create a quality environment in which the following values are embraced: Everyone is treated with dignity and respect. Individual strengths and abilities are recognized.

10462 Center for Disability Resources Resources
University of South Carolina
8301 Farrow Road 803-935-5231
Columbia, SC 29208 Fax: 803-935-5059
uscm.med.sc.edu/cdrhome
The vision of The Center for Developmental Disabilities is to work as a team to create a quality environment in which the following values are embraced: Everyone is teated with dignity and respect. Individual strengths and abilities are recognized.
Jerry Junkins, Project Director

10463 Center for Health Research
3800 N Interstate Avenue 503-335-2400
Portland, OR 97227 e-mail: information@kpchr.org
www.kpchr.org
Produces eight videotapes accompanying printed materials and a videotaped public services announcement to serve as training and resource materials for use by daycare centers.
Mary L Durham PhD, Director

10464 Center for Medical Consumers
239 Thompson Street 212-674-7105
New York, NY 10012 Fax: 212-674-7100
e-mail: medconsumers@earthlink.net
www.medicalconsumers.org
A non-profit organization which acts as an independent source of information to enable consumers to critically evaluate information they receive from health professionals.
Arthur Aaron Levin MPH, Director
Maryann Napoli, Associate Director/Writer of Healthfacts

10465 Center for Universal Design North Carolina State University
North Carolina State University
Campus Box 7701 919-513-2022
Raleigh, NC 27695-8613 800-647-6777
Fax: 919-515-8951
e-mail: nilda_cosco@ncsu.edu
www.design.ncsu.edu
National research information and technical assistance center that evaluates develops and promotes accessible and universal design in housing buildings outdoor and urban environments and related products.
Nilda Cosco PhD, Education Specialist
Leslie Young, Director of Design

10466 Child Center
3995 Marcola Road 541-726-1465
Springfield, OR 97477 Fax: 541-726-5085
e-mail: info@thechildcenter.org
www.thechildcenter.org
Non-profit human services agency that has been offering a continuum of psychiatric and special education programs throughout Lane County since 1971.
Scott Diehl, President
Dennis Konrady, Vice President

10467 Children's Hospice International
1101 King Street 703-684-0330
Alexandria, VA 22314 800-24C-HILD
Fax: 703-684-0226
e-mail: info@chionline.org
www.chionline.org
This organization was founded to provide a network of support and care for children with life threatening conditions and their families. The hospice is a team effort which provides medical psychological social and spiritual expertise in the US and abroad.
Ann Armstrong-Dailey, Founding Director/CEO
Rebecca Brant, Director

10468 Children's National Medical Center
111 Michigan Avenue NW 202-749-5000
Washington, DC 20010-2916 Fax: 202-939-4449
e-mail: webteam@cnmc.org
www.dcchildrens.com
Offers diagnosis treatment follow-up services outpatient services and medical services to children in need of medical care.
Edwin K Zechman Jr, President and Chief Executive Officer

10469 Christian Horizons
PO Box 3381
Grand Rapids, MI 49501 616-965-7063
www.christian-horizons.org
A Christian organization dedicated to enriching the lives of people with mental impairments. We provide day programs, camping ministries, and Bible studies. We assist churches in identifying persons with special needs and add support to parents of those whose children have special needs.
Camping Charges
Ed Sider, CEO
Stan Cox, Chair

10470 Clearinghouse on Disability Information Office of Special Education & Rehab Svcs
US Department of Education
550 12th Street SW 202-245-7307
Washington, DC 20202-2550 Fax: 202-245-7636
TTY: 202-205-5637
TDD: 2022055637
www.ed.gov
Provides information to people with disabilities or anyone requesting information by doing research and providing documents in response to inquiries. Information provided includes areas of federal funding for disability-related programs.
Carolyn Corlett, Contact

10471 Council for Learning Disabilities (CLD)
11184 Antioch Road 913-491-1011
Overland Park, KS 66210 Fax: 913-491-1012
e-mail: CLDInfo@ie-events.com
www.cldinternational.org
National professional organization dedicated solely to professionals working with individuals who have learning disabilities. Committed to enhancing the education and life span development of those individuals.
Dan Boudah, President
Christina Curran, President Elect

10472 Developmental Disability Councils
225 Reinekers Lane 703-739-4400
Alexandria, VA 22314 Fax: 703-739-6030
e-mail: info@nacdd.org
www.nacdd.org
Councils in each state provide training and technical assistance to local and state agencies employers and the public on improving services to people with developmental disabilities.
Karen Flippo, Executive Director
Phyllis Guinivan, Council Services Liaison

10473 Disabled & Alone: Life Services for the Handicapped
61 Broadway 212-532-6740
New York, NY 10006-1709 800-995-0066
Fax: 212-532-3588
e-mail: info@disabledandalone.org
www.disabledandalone.org
National nonprofit organization providing services to handicapped persons their families and organizations serving them by helping parents of a handicapped child plan for when they will no longer be here, providing an alternative service program.
Leslie D Park, Chairman
Lee Alan Ackerman, Executive Director

10474 Disabled Outdoors
2213 Tallahassee Drive 850-668-7323
Tallahassee, FL 32308 Fax: 850-894-0875
e-mail: davidjones@fdoa.org
Besides publishing the magazine, this organization acts as a clearinghouse for people with disabilities who request information on accessible facilities adaptive products and service providers across the nation and in Canada. Also provides research.
John Kopchik
Carolyn Dohme

10475 Distance Education and Training Council
1601 18th Street NW 202-234-5100
Washington, DC 20009-2529 Fax: 202-332-1386
e-mail: Karen@detc.org
www.detc.org
Advocates quality correspondence education in America. Serves as a clearinghouse of information about the home study field and sponsors a nationally recognized accrediting agency.
Michael P Lambert, Executive Director
Karen Black, Information Specialist

10476 Educational Equity Center at The Academy f or Educational Development
100 Fifth Avenue 212-243-1110
New York, NY 10011 Fax: 212-627-0407
e-mail: lcolon@aed.org
www.edequity.org
Provides information resources and referrals. Publishes a national directory which lists organizations that serve women and girls (a program of educational concepts). Publishes curriculum on teasing and bullying science and issues of disability.
Merle Froschl, Co-Founder/Co-Director
Barbara Sprung, Co-Founder/Co-Director

10477 Equal Opportunity Employment Commission
1801 L Street NE
Washington, DC 20507-0001
202-663-4903
800-669-4000
www.eeoc.org
This agency is responsible for drafting and implementing the regulations of Title I of the ADA.

10478 Estate Planning for the Disabled
2232 W Avenue 133
San Leandro, CA 94577-1050
510-352-4127
Fax: 510-352-4127
e-mail: EFM@EFMOODY.com
www.efmoody.com
Counsels and assists parents of children with special needs to develop viable estate plans, letters of intent, wills and special needs trusts. EPD will work with the appropriate professionals and agencies to help put together an effective comprehensive plan.

10479 Extensions for Independence
555 Saturn Boulevard
San Diego, CA 92154
866-632-7149
e-mail: info@mouthstick.net
www.mouthstick.net
Develops manufactures and markets for the physically handicapped vocational equipment such as: mouthsticks turntable desks motorized easels etc.
Arthur Heyer, President

10480 Favarh
225 Commerce Drive
Canton, CT 06019-1099
860-693-6662
Fax: 860-693-8662
www.favarh.org
Provides a variety of programs and services to adults with developmental, physical or mental disabilities and their families, throughout the Farmington Valley communities of Avon, Burlington and more.
Stephen Morr MPA, Executive Director

10481 Federation for Children with Special Needs
1135 Tremont Street
Boston, MA 02120
617-482-2915
800-331-0688
Fax: 617-572-2094
e-mail: fcsninfo@fcsn.org
fcsn.org
A center for parents and parent organizations to work together on behalf of children with special needs and their families.
Richard J Robison, Executive Director
Peter Brenna CPA, Board of Director

10482 Goodwill Industries International
15810 Indianola Drive
Rockville, MD 20855
301-530-6500
800-741-0186
Fax: 301-530-1516
TTY: 301-530-9759
e-mail: contactus@goodwill.org
www.goodwill.org
Strives to achieve the full participation in society of disabled persons and other individuals with special needs by expanding their opportunities and occupational capabilities through a network of 179 autonomous, nonprofit, community-based organizations.
George A Kessinger, President/CEO
Jarret Lobb, Chair Board of Directors

10483 HEATH Resource Center
2134 G Street NW
Washington, DC 20052-1132
202-939-9329
800-544-3284
Fax: 202-994-3365
e-mail: AskHEATH@gwu.edu
www.heath.gwu.edu
National clearinghouse for information about education after high school for people with disabilities. Also serves as an information exchange about educational support services, policies, procedures, adaptations and opportunities on American campuses.
Rhona Hartman

10484 Health Care For All
30 Winter Street, 10th Floor
Boston, MA 02108
617-350-7279
Fax: 617-451-5838
TTY: 617-350-0974
www.hcfa.org
HCFA seeks to create a consumer-centered health care system that provides comprehensive, affordable, accessible, culturally competent, high quality care and consumer education for everyone, especially the most vulnerable.
Amy Whitcomb Slemmer, Executive Director

10485 International Association for the Study of Pain
111 Queen Anne Avenue N
Seattle, WA 98109-4955
206-283-0311
Fax: 206-283-9403
e-mail: iaspdesk@iasp-pain.org
www.iasp-pain.org
The International Association for the Study of Pain is the leading professional forum for science practice and education in the field of pain.
Gerald F Gebhart PhD, President
Kathy Kreiter, Executive Director

10486 International Council on Disability
1710 Rhode Island Avenue NW
Washington, DC 20036
202-207-0338
Fax: 202-207-0341
e-mail: usicd@ncil.org
www.usicd.org
Enlists the cooperation of the UN and specified agencies to develop a well coordinated international program for the rehabilitation of disabled people; to serve as a permanent liaison body to develop cooperation between nongovernmental organizations.
Tony Coelho, Chair

10487 LAUNCH Department of Special Education
Department of Special Education
Commerce, TX 75428
903-886-5932
Provides resources for learning disabled individuals coordinates efforts of other local state and national LD organizations acts as a communication channel for people with learning disabilities through a monthly newsletter and provides programs.

10488 Learning Disabilities Association of America
4156 Library Road
Pittsburgh, PA 15234-1349
412-341-1515
888-300-6710
Fax: 412-344-0224
e-mail: info@ldaamerica.org
www.ldaamerica.org
An information and referral center for parents and professionals dealing with learning disabilities.
Sheila Buckley, Executive Director
Andrea Turkheimer, Director Resource/Referral/Education

10489 Learning How
1583 Sulphur Spring Road
Baltimore, MD 21227-5481
410-242-7100
Fax: 410-242-5246
www.learninghow.com
Strives to build self-esteem and confidence among disabled persons and encourages volunteer involvement. Seeks to train the disabled for leadership positions and to serve as a support group for disabled persons.
Deborah McKeithan, Founder

10490 Life Development Institute
18001 N 79th Avenue
Glendale, AZ 85308
623-773-2774
Fax: 623-773-2788
e-mail: info@life-development-inst.org
www.life-development-inst.org
LDI's mission to inspire individuals to experience success while optimizing their potential for an enhanced quality of life in a challenging and supportive learning environment. LDI is a nonprofit private organization based in Glendale Arizona.
Veronica Lie (Crawford), President
Rob Crawford, CEO

10491 Lions Quest
300 W 22nd Street
Oak Brook, IL 60523
630-571-5466
Fax: 630-571-5735
e-mail: Jayne.Westerlund@lionsclubs.org
www.lions-quest.org
School based comprehensive positive youth development and prevention programs that unite the home, school and community to cultivate capable and healthy young people of strong character through life skills, character education, SEL, civic values and drug awareness.
Jayne Westerlund, Manager

10492 Lymphatic Research Foundation
40 Garvies Point Road 516-625-9675
Glen Cove, NY 11542 Fax: 516-625-9410
e-mail: lrf@lymphaticresearch.org
www.lymphaticresearch.org
An internationally recognized not-for-profit organization with the goal of promoting significant advances in research to find effective treatments and ultimately a cure.
Jaqueline Reinhard, Executive Director
Wendy Chaite, Esq., Founder & President

10493 MedEscort International ABE International Airport
ABE International Airport
PO Box 8766 610-792-3111
Allentown, PA 18105-8766 800-255-7182
Fax: 610-791-9189
e-mail: medescort@fast.net
www.medescort.com
Offers specially trained escorts for individuals who cannot travel alone due to age or disability.
David M Stein DO, Medical Director
Sherry L Sefcik RN/BSN, Senior Flight Nurse

10494 Medic Alert Foundation International
2323 Colorado Avenue 209-668-3333
Turlock, CA 95382-2018 888-633-4298
Fax: 209-669-2450
e-mail: customer_service@medicalert.org
www.medicalert.org
Organization offering persons with medical problems descriptive warning bracelets or neck chains to alert emergency personnel.
Martin Kabat, President/CEO
Kenton Whitefield, CFO

10495 Mental Health Services Training Collaborative
University of Maryland
685 W Baltimore Street 410-706-6669
Baltimore, MD 21201-1549 Fax: 410-706-0022
e-mail: hgoldman@erols.com
Provides technical assistance to local mental health authorities on the development operation and financing supports for mentally ill persons.
Catherine Z Bailey JD, Program Director

10496 National Center for Family-Centered Care
695 Park Avenue 212-772-4000
New York, NY 10021 Fax: 212-452-7475
e-mail: gmallon@hunter.cuny.edu
www.hunter.cuny.edu/socwork/nrcfcpp//tra
Goals are to promote implementation of a family-centered care approach for children with special health care needs.
Karen Lawrence

10497 National Chronic Pain Outreach Association
PO Box 274 540-862-9437
Millboro, VA 24460 Fax: 540-862-9485
e-mail: ncpoa@cfw.com
www.chronicpain.org
An information and referral service for patients dealing with chronic pain due to any cause. They offer numerous educational materials, support groups, health professional referrals and a newsletter.

10498 National Clearinghouse of Rehabilitation Training Materials
Utah State University
6524 Old Main Hill
Logan, UT 84322-6524 866-821-5355
Fax: 435-797-7537
e-mail: ncrtm@cc.usu.edu
www.nchrtm.okstate.edu
Offers reference materials on rehabilitation for professionals and the disabled.

10499 National Council on Disability
1331 F Street NW 202-272-2004
Washington, DC 20004 Fax: 202-272-2022
TTY: 202-272-2074
e-mail: ncd@ncd.gov
www.ncd.gov
The National Council on Disability is an independent federal agency that works with the President and Congress to increase the inclusion independence and empowerment of Americans with disabilities. They are involved in policy making issues.
John R Vaughn, Chairperson

10500 National Council on Independent Living
1710 Rhode Island Avenue NW 202-207-0334
Washington, DC 20036 877-525-3400
Fax: 202-207-0341
TTY: 202-207-0340
e-mail: ncil@ncil.org
www.ncil.org
Offers information referrals advocacy and guides for the disabled regarding living independently.
John Lancaster, Executive Director
Justin Chappel, Development and Communications Advisor

10501 National Digestive Diseases Information Clearinghouse
Two Information Way
Bethesda, MD 20892-3570 800-891-5389
Fax: 703-738-4929
TTY: 866-569-1162
e-mail: nddic@info.niddk.nih.gov
www.digestive.niddk.nih.gov
Offers various educational information public resources and reprints public awareness materials and more on digestive disorders.
Griffin P Rodgers MD MACP, Director

10502 National Dissemination Center for Children
PO Box 1492 202-884-8200
Washington, DC 20013 800-695-0285
Fax: 202-884-8441
TTY: 202-884-8200
e-mail: nichcy@aed.org
www.nichcy.org
Publishes free fact filled newsletters. Arranges workshops. Advises parents on the laws entitling children with disabilities to special education and other services.
Dr Suzanne Ripley, Executive Director
Stephen D Luke EdD, Director of Research

10503 National Endowment for the Arts: Office for Accessability
1100 Pennsylvania Avenue NW 202-682-5400
Washington, DC 20506-0001 Fax: 202-682-5715
TTY: 202-682-5496
e-mail: webmgr@arts.endow.gov
www.nea.gov
Offers disabled and elderly persons advocacy programs to make the arts accessible to everyone. Offers information, referrals and technical assistance.
Paula Terry, Accessibility Specialist

10504 National Institute for People with Disabil ities
460 W 34th Street
New York, NY 10001-2382 212-273-6100
www.yai.org
A nonprofit professional organization serving developmentally disabled children and adults in many programs throughout the New York metropolitan area. Provides over 50 program sites for thousands of participants.
Joel M Levy DSW, CEO
Philip H Levy PhD, President/COO

10505 National Institute of Child Health and Human Development
31 Center Drive 301-496-5133
Bethesda, MD 20892 800-370-2943
Fax: 301-496-7101
TTY: 888-320-6942
e-mail: mcgrathj@mail.nih.gov
www.nichd.nih.gov
NICHD conducts and supports research on topics related to the health of children, adults, families and populations. Some of these topics include: reducing infant deaths; improving the health of women, men and families; and understanding reproductive health.
Duane Alexan MD, Director
John McGrath, Coordinator

10506 National Institute of Disability and Rehabilitation Research
US Department of Education

400 Maryland Avenue SW
Washington, DC 20202-0004
202-245-7640
Fax: 202-245-7643
TTY: 202-245-7640
www.ed.gov/offices/OSERS/NIDRR

Provides funding for three major programs to assist ADA compliance: ADA Regional Disability and Business Technical Assistance; Materials Development Projects and Peer Training Projects. Also funds research projects that provide information on assistive technology.

10507 National Job Accommodation Network
PO Box 6080
Morgantown, WV 26506-6080
304-293-7186
800-526-7234
Fax: 304-293-5407
TTY: 877-293-7186
e-mail: jan@jan.wvu.edu
www.jan.wvu.edu

The JAN is an international information service for people with disabilities and their employers. They have information about implementation of workplace accommodations as well as resources to promote an awareness of functional limitations.
Anne Hirsh, Co-Director
Louis Orslene, Co-Director

10508 National Legal Center for the Medically Dependent & Disabled
50 S Meridian Street
Indianapolis, IN 46204-3537
317-632-6245
Fax: 317-632-6542

Committed to defending the rights of vulnerable persons threatened by infanticide, euthanasia, assisted suicide, non-voluntary withdrawal/withholding of essential medical treatment and care and discrimination in health care financing.
Marilyn Bove, President

10509 National Network of Learning Disabled Adults
808 N 82nd Street
Scottsdale, AZ 85257
602-941-5112

Provides information and referral for LD adults involved with or in search of support groups and networking opportunities.

10510 National Organization for Rare Disorders
55 Kenosia Avenue
Danbury, CT 06813-1968
203-744-0100
800-999-6673
Fax: 203-798-2291
TTY: 203-797-9590
TDD: 203-797-9590
e-mail: orphan@rarediseases.org
www.rarediseases.org

The National Organization for Rare Disorders(NORD) a 501(c)3 organization is a unique federation of voluntary health organizations dedicated to helping people with rare orphan diseases and assisting the organizations that serve them.
Carolyn Asbu PhD, Chair
Frank Sasinowski, Vice Chair

10511 National Organization on Disability
888 Sixteenth Street NW
Washington, DC 20006
202-293-5960
Fax: 202-293-7999
TTY: 202-293-5968
e-mail: ability@nod.org
www.nod.org

The purpose is to increase the acceptance and participation in all aspects of life of all men women and children with physical or mental disabilities offering programs such as: Community Partnership Program; National Organization; and Business Partner Program.
Tom Ridge, Chairman
Carol Glazer, President

10512 National Parent Network on Disabilities
1130 17th Street NW
Washington, DC 20036
202-434-8686
Fax: 202-638-7299
www.npnd.org

Established to provide a presence and national voice for parents of children youth and adults with special needs. The organization shares information and resources in order to promote parents influence on policy issues concerning the needs of people with disabilities.

10513 National Rehabilitation Information Center
8201 Corporate Drive
Landover, MD 20785
301-459-5900
Fax: 301-459-4263
TTY: 301-459-5984
e-mail: naricinfo@heitechservices.com
www.naric.com/

One of the three components of the office of Special Education and Rehabilitative Services. Operates in concert with the Rehabilitation Services Administration and the Office of Special Education Programs.
Mark Odum, Director

10514 North American Society for Pediatric Gastroenterology and Nutrition
PO Box 6
Flourtown, PA 19031
215-233-0808
Fax: 215-233-3918
e-mail: naspghan@naspghan.org
www.naspghan.org

Promotes research and provides a forum for professionals in the areas of pediatric GI liver disease gastroenterology and nutrition. Associated with fellow organizations in Europe and Australia (ESPGAN AUSPGAN).
Margaret K Stallings, Executive Director
B Li MD, President

10515 Office of Policy Planning and Legislation
200 Independence Avenue SW
Washington, DC 20201-0004
202-619-0257
877-696-6775
www.hhs.gov/about/referlst.html

Administers grants to the states for social services under Title XX of the Social Security Act to welfare recipients and others likely to become welfare recipients.
G Barry Nielsen, Director

10516 Office of Special Education Programs: Department of Education
400 Maryland Avenue SW
Washington, DC 20202
202-401-1576
800-872-5327
Fax: 202-401-0689
TTY: 800-437-0833
www.ed.gov/offices/OSERS/OSEP

Administers the Education of the Handicapped Act and related programs for the education of handicapped children including grants to institutions of higher learning and fellowships to train educational personnel. Grants to states for the education of handicapped individuals.
Madeline Will, Assistant Secretary

10517 Office on Smoking and Health: Centers for Disease Control and Prevention
1600 Clifton Road
Atlanta, GA 30333
404-639-3311
800-232-4636
TTY: 888-232-6348
www.cdc.gov/netinfo.htm

This office is a division of the Center for Disease Control and Prevention. Among its many functions, OSH develops and distributes the annual Surgeon general's report on smoking and health and coordinates a national public information and education program.

10518 Option Istitute Learning and Training Center
2080 S. Undermountain Road
Sheffield, MA 01257
413-229-2100
800-714-2779
Fax: 413-229-8931
e-mail: happiness@option.org
www.option.org

As the worldwide teaching center for the Option Process(R). The Option Institute offers empowering personal growth programs and seminars using life-changing experiential learning techniques that help people overcome adversity, maximize their success and happiness and greatly improve their health, career, relationships and quality of life.
Zoe

10519 Pediatric Neurology Georgetown University Hospital
Georgetown University Hospital
3800 Reservoir Road NW
Washington, DC 20007-2196
202-444-8785
Fax: 202-444-7161
www.georgetownuniversityhospital.org

Offers infants and children to age 21 with neurological problems diagnosis consultation recommendations for therapy and more services.

10520 **People-to-People Committee for the Handicapped**
PO Box 18131 301-774-7446
Washington, DC 20036-8131
Individuals concerned about the circumstances of handicapped people throughout the world. Disseminates information acts as a consultant in promoting exchange activities coordinates special assistance projects in developing countries and more.
David Brigham, Chairman

10521 **President's Committee on the Employment of People with Disabilities**
200 Constitution Avenue NW 202-693-6000
Washington, DC 20210 Fax: 202-693-7888
TTY: 877-889-5627
e-mail: webmaster@dol.gov
www.dol.gov
Independent federal agency to facilitate the communication coordination and promotion of public and private efforts to empower Americans with disabilities through employment.
John Davey, Deputy Assistant Secretary

10522 **Rehabilitation International**
25 E 21st Street 212-420-1500
New York, NY 10010-6298 Fax: 212-505-0871
e-mail: ri@riglobal.org
www.riglobal.org
A federation of 120 disability organizations in 80 countries working together to promote the prevention of disability the rehabilitation of disabled people and the equalization of opportunities within society on behalf of disabled people and their families.
Venus Ilagan, Secretary General
Shantha Rau Barriga, Senior Program Manager

10523 **Rehabilitation Services Administration**
400 Maryland Avenue SW
Washington, DC 20202-2800 202-245-7488
www.ed.gov/about/offices/list/osers/rsa
Offers information law/legislation resources referrals and more to the disabled and rehabilitation professionals.
Edward Anthony, Deputy Commissioner
Mary Lovley, Director of Program Support Staff

10524 **Social Security Administration Office of Public Inquiries**
Office of Public Inquiries
Windsor Park Building
Baltimore, MD 21235 800-772-1213
TTY: 800-325-0778
www.ssa.gov
Administers old age survivors and disability insurance programs under Title II of the Social Security Act. Also administers the federal income maintenance program under Title XVI of the Social Security Act. Maintains networks of local/regional offices.
Michael J Astrue, Commissioner
James A Winn, Chief of Staff

10525 **US Department of Education: Office of Civil Rights**
400 Maryland Avenue SW
Washington, DC 20202-1100 800-421-3481
Fax: 202-245-6840
TTY: 877-521-2172
e-mail: ocr@ed.gov
www.ed.gov/offices/OCR
Prohibits discrimination on the basis of disability in programs and activities funded by the Department of Education. Investigates complaints and provides technical assistance to individuals and entities with rights and responsibilities under Section 504.
Sandra Battle, Director of the Program Legal Group
Lester Slayton, Resource Management Group Director

10526 **US Department of Justice**
950 Pennsylvania Avenue NW 202-514-2000
Washington, DC 20530-0001 e-mail: askdoj@usdoj.gov
www.usdoj.gov
Coordinates the implementation by federal agencies of section 504 of the Rehabilitation Act of 1973 as amended which prohibits discrimination on the basis of handicap in federally assisted programs and in programs and activities conducted by federal executives.
Eric Holder, Attorney General
David Ogden, Deputy Attorney General

10527 **US Department of Transportation**
1200 New Jersey Avenue SE 202-366-4000
Washington, DC 20590 866-377-8642
TTY: 800-877-8339
e-mail: dot.comments@dot.gov
www.dot.gov
Enforces ADA provisions that require nondiscrimination in public and private mass transportation systems and services.
Ray LaHood, Secretary of Transportation
Joan DeBoer, Chief of Staff

10528 **US Office of Personnel Management**
1900 E Street NW 202-606-1800
Washington, DC 20415 TTY: 202-606-2532
e-mail: General@opm.gov
www.opm.gov
Establishes policies for employment of the handicapped within the federal service. Administers a merit system for the federal employment that includes recruiting, examining, training and promoting people on the basis of knowledge and skills.
Kathie Ann Whipple, Acting Director
Richard B Lowe, Chief of Staff/External Affairs Director

10529 **VSA Arts**
818 Connecticut Avenue NW 202-628-2800
Washington, DC 20006 800-933-8721
Fax: 202-429-0868
TTY: 202-737-0645
e-mail: info@vsarts.org
www.vsarts.org
VSA arts is an international nonprofit organization founded in 1974 by Ambassador Jean Kennedy Smith to create a society where all people with disabilities learn through participate in and enjoy the arts.
Soula Antoniou, President
Jean Kennedy Smith, Founder

10530 **World Institute on Disability**
510 16th Street 510-763-4100
Oakland, CA 94612-1520 Fax: 510-763-4109
TTY: 510-208-9493
e-mail: wid@wid.org
www.wid.org
A public policy center that is run by persons with disabilities. Research public education training and model program development as means to create a more accessible and supportive society for all people - disabled and nondisabled alike.
Kathy Martinez, Executive Director
Rebecca Palmer, Executive Assistant

State Agencies & Associations

Alabama

10531 **Division of Rehabilitation: Montgomery**
PO Box 11586 334-281-8780
Montgomery, AL 36111-0586
Marilyn Bove, President

Alaska

10532 **CAP ASSIST**
2900 Boniface Parkway 907-333-2211
Anchorage, AK 99504-3132 Fax: 907-333-1186
e-mail: akcap@alaska.com
www.adap.net
Angie Allen, Case Advocate
Nancy Anderson, Senior Staff Attorney

Arizona

10533 **HPV Support Groups: Arizona**
7331 E Osborn Drive 602-994-8330
Scottsdale, AZ 85251-6422 800-223-2159
e-mail: sthf@home.com

Arkansas

10534 Advocacy Services of Little Rock
1100 N University
Little Rock, AR 72207
501-296-1775
Fax: 501-296-1779
e-mail: panda@advocacyservices.org
www.advocacyservices.org

Marilyn Bove, President

California

10535 Client Assistance Program: California
PO Box 944222
Sacramento, CA 94244-3510
916-558-5390
800-952-5544
Fax: 916-263-7464
TTY: 916-558-5392
TDD: 800-598-3273
e-mail: apinfo@dor.ca.gov
www.dor.ca.gov

State wide program providing advocacy services to consumers and applicants. Federal Rehabilitation Act funded programs, projects and facilities.
Sheila Conlo Mentkowski, Chief

Colorado

10536 Disability Careers
5760 E Evans Avenue
Denver, CO 80222-5305
303-757-3070
Fax: 303-757-3392

This is a non profit corporation that provides employee and employer services. Founder and Executive Director Ted Pavakis is a former commercial real estate broker with multiple sclerosis.

10537 Legal Center for People with Disabilities and Older People
455 Sherman Street
Denver, CO 80203
303-722-0300
800-288-1376
Fax: 303-722-0720
TTY: 303-722-3619
e-mail: tlcmail@thelegalcenter.org
www.thelegalcenter.org

Mary Anne Harvey, Executive Director
Randy Chapman, Director Legal Services

Connecticut

10538 Office of Protection & Advocacy for the Handicapped
60 Weston Street
Hartford, CT 06120-1551
860-297-4300
Marilyn Bove, President

Delaware

10539 Client Assistance Program: Delaware
13 SW Front Street
Milford, DE 19963-1900
302-422-6744
Marilyn Bove, President

District of Columbia

10540 Client Assistance Program: District of Columbia
Rehabilitation Services Administration
605 G Street NW
Washington, DC 20001-3705
202-727-0977
Jim Tolbert, Director

10541 Information Protection & Advocacy Center for Handicapped Individuals
Center for Handicapped Individuals
4455 Connecticut Avenue NW
Washington, DC 20008-2328
202-966-8081
Marilyn Bove, President

Florida

10542 Advocacy Center for Persons with Disabilities
2671 Executive Center Circle West
2728 Centerview Drive
Tallahassee, FL 32301-5092
850-488-9071
800-342-0823
Fax: 850-488-8640
TTY: 800-346-4127
e-mail: info@advocacycenter.org
www.advocacycenter.org

The Advocacy Center for Persons with Disabilities is a non-profit organization providing protection and advocacy services in the State of Florida. The Center's mission is to advance the dignity, equality, self-determination and expressed choices of people with disabilities.
Marilyn Bove, President

10543 North Florida: HPV Support Group
126 Salem Court
Tallahassee, FL 32301-2810
850-877-3183

Georgia

10544 Division of Rehabilitation Service
148 Andrew Young International Boul
Atlanta, GA 30303-4469
404-232-3910
www.vocrehabga.org

Marilyn Bove, President

Hawaii

10545 Protection & Advocacy Agency
900 Fort Street Mall
Honolulu, HI 96813-9607
808-949-2922
800-882-1057
Fax: 808-949-2928
TTY: 808-949-2922
e-mail: info@hawaiidisabilityrights.org
www.hawaiidisabilityrights.org

Gary L Smith, Executive Director

Idaho

10546 Co-Ad
4477 Emerald
900 Fort Street Mall, 90 900 F-2017
208-336-5353
800-632-5125
Fax: 208-336-5396
TTY: 208-336-5353
e-mail: coadinc@cableone.net
users.moscow.com

Marilyn Bove, President

Illinois

10547 Illinois Client Assistance Program
100 N 1st Street
Springfield, IL 62702-5011
217-782-5374
www.state.il.us

Marilyn Bove, President

Indiana

10548 Indiana Advocacy Services
4701 N Keystone Avenue
Indianapolis, IN 46205
317-722-5555
TTY: 800-838-1131
e-mail: info@ipas.state.in.us
www.in.gov/ipas

Karen Pedevilla, President
Karen Pedevilla, Education and Training Director

Iowa

10549 Client Assistance Program: Iowa Division on Persons with Disabilities
Division on Persons with Disabilities
Lucas State Office Building
Des Moines, IA 50310
515-281-3656
800-652-4298
Fax: 515-242-6119
TTY: 800-652-4298
e-mail: jackie.wipperman@iowa.gov
www.icdri.org

Marilyn Bove, President

Kansas

10550 Client Assistance Program: Kansas
635 SW Harrison
Topeka, KS 66603
785-273-9661
877-776-1541
Fax: 785-273-9414
e-mail: rocky@drckansas.org
www.icdri.org

Marilyn Bove, President

Kentucky

10551 Client Assistance Program: Kentucky
209 Saint Clair Street
Frankfort, KY 40601
502-564-8035
800-633-6283
Fax: 502-564-2951
e-mail: VickiL.Staggs@ky.gov
www.icdri.org

Marilyn Bove, President

Louisiana

10552 Advocacy Center for the Elderly and Disabled
1010 Common Street
New Orleans, LA 70112-1821
504-522-2337
800-960-7705
Fax: 504-522-5507
e-mail: AdvocacyCenter@AdvocacyLA.org
www.advocacyla.org

Elizabeth Dalferes, Board Member
Patti DeMichele, Vice President

Maine

10553 Maine Advocacy Services
PO Box 2007
Augusta, ME 04338-2007
207-626-2774
Fax: 207-621-1419
e-mail: advocate@disabilityrightsctr.org

Marilyn Bove, President

Maryland

10554 Client Assistance Program: Maryland State Department of Education
Division of Vocational Rehabilitation
Baltimore, MD 21218-2308
410-554-9362
800-638-6243
e-mail: cap@dors.state.md.us
www.govoter.org

Beth Lash, President

Massachusetts

10555 Massachusetts Office on Disability Client Assistance Program
Client Assistance Program
250 Washington Street
Boston, MA 02108-1518
617-624-5463
800-322-2020
Fax: 617-624-5075
e-mail: Olga.Higuera@state.ma.us
www.mass.gov

Marilyn Bove, President

10556 Merrimack Valley HPV Support Group Holy Family Hospital
Holy Family Hospital
70 E Street
Methuen, MA 01844-4597
978-687-0156

10557 Neurosurgical Service at Massachusetts Gen eral Hospital
Massachusetts General Hospital, Wang ACC-835
MGH Neurogenetics Unit
Boston, MA 02114
617-726-5732
Fax: 617-726-9620
e-mail: sims@helix.mgh.harvard.edu
neurosurgery.mgh.harvard.edu

Multidisciplinary management of inherited neurologic syndromes including neurologic tuberous sclerosis and van Hippel-lindau disease. Members of the unit are also active in research into the genetic basis of, and treatments for a variety of inherited neurologic conditions.
Katherine B Sims MD, Director

Michigan

10558 Client Assistance Program: Michigan Department of Rehabilitation Services
Department of Rehabilitation Services
4095 Legacy Parkway
Lansing, MI 48911-7508
517-487-1755
800-292-5896
e-mail: molson@mpas.org
www.icdri.org

Marilyn Bove, President

10559 Commission for the Blind
201 N Washington Square
Lansing, MI 48909-7515
517-373-6425
www.mrs.state.mi.us/cs/agencies

Marilyn Bove, President

Minnesota

10560 Minnesota Disability Law Center
300 Kickernick Building
2324 University Avenue W
Saint Paul, MN 55114-1742
651-228-9105
800-292-4150
Fax: 651-222-0745
e-mail: statesupport@mnlegalservices.org
www.mnlegalservices.org

Maureen O'Connell, State Support Director
Jessie Spire Carlson, Supervising Attorney

Mississippi

10561 Client Assistance Program: Mississippi Easter Seal Society
Easter Seal Society
226 N State Street
Jackson, MS 39296-4005
601-362-2585
Fax: 601-982-1951
TTY: 800-962-2400
e-mail: pposey8803@aol.com
www.icdri.org

Marilyn Bove, President

Missouri

10562 Missouri Protection and Advocacy Services
925 S Country Club Drive
Jefferson City, MO 65109-4510
573-893-3333
866-777-7199
Fax: 573-893-4231
TTY: 8007352966
TDD: 8007352966
e-mail: mopasjc@embarqmail.com
moadvocacy.org

Protection and advocacy for individuals with disabilities, providing information, referral, training, direct advocacy and legal services.
Shawn de Loyola, Executive Director

Montana

10563 Montana Advocacy Program
1022 Chestnut Street
Helena, MT 59601
406-449-2344
800-245-4743
Fax: 406-449-2418
TTY: 406-449-2344
e-mail: advocate@disabilityrightsmt.org
www.disabilityrightsmt.org

Susie McIntyre, Board President
Sylvia Danforth, Board Vice-President

Nebraska

10564 Client Assistance Program: Nebraska Division of Rehabilitative Services
Division of Rehabilitative Services
301 Centennial Mall S
Lincoln, NE 68509
402-471-3656
800-742-7594
e-mail: victoria.rasmussen@cap.ne.gov
www.cap.state.ne.us

The Nebraska Client Assistance Program is a free service to help you find solutions if you are having problems with any of the following programs: Vocational Rehabilitation, Nebraska Commis-

sion for the Blind and Visually Impaired or Centers for Independent Living.
Marilyn Bove, President

10565 Omaha HPV Support Group: PP of Omaha
Planned Parenthood
4610 Dodge Street
Omaha, NE 68132-3234
402-397-2739
www.aad.org

Nevada

10566 Client Assistance Program: Nevada
2800 E Saint Louis Avenue
Las Vegas, NV 89104-3689
702-486-6688
800-633-9879
Fax: 702-486-6691
e-mail: detrcap@nvdetr.org
www.icdri.org
Marilyn Bove, President

New Hampshire

10567 Client Assistance Program: NH Governor's Commission for the Handicapped
Governor's Commission for the Handicapped
57 Regional Drive
Concord, NH 03301
271-277-
Fax: 603-271-2837
TTY: 603-271-2774
e-mail: bhagy@gov.state.nh.us
www.icdri.org
Marilyn Bove, President

New Jersey

10568 Client Assistance Program: New Jersey Depa artment of Public Advocacy
New Jersey Department of the Public Advocate
210 S Broad Street
Trenton, NJ 08608
609-292-9742
www.icdri.org
Marilyn Bove, President

New Mexico

10569 Protection and Advocacy System of Alburque rque
1720 Louisiana Boulevard NE
Albuquerque, NM 87110-7070
505-256-3100
Fax: 505-256-3184
www.protectionandadvocacy.com
Marilyn Bove, President

New York

10570 Client Assistance Program: NY State Commission of Quality of Care
Advocacy Bureau
99 Washington Avenue
Albany, NY 12210-2810
518-473-4057
800-624-4143
Fax: 518-473-6296
e-mail: hn5344@handsnet.org
Marilyn Bove, President

10571 March of Dimes Foundation
1275 Mamaroneck Avenue
White Plains, NY 10605-5298
914-997-4488
www.marchofdimes.com
Volunteers and professionals providing leadership in the treatment and prevention of birth defects and prematurity.
Ann Umemoto MPH MPA, Associate Director

North Carolina

10572 Client Assistance Program: NC Division of Vocation Rehabilitation Services
NC Division of Vocation Rehabilitation Services
2806 Mail Service Center
Raleigh, NC 27699-1275
919-855-3600
Fax: 919-715-2456
e-mail: NCCAP@ncmail.net
www.icdri.org
Marilyn Bove, President

North Dakota

10573 Client Assistance Program: North Dakota
1237 W Divide Avenue
Bismarck, ND 58501-4038
701-328-8947
800-207-6122
Fax: 701-328-8969
TTY: 701-328-8968
e-mail: cap@state.nd.us
www.icdri.org
Marilyn Bove, President

Ohio

10574 Cincinnati HPV Support Group: PP of Cincin nati
Planned Parenthood
PO Box 12407
Cincinnati, OH 45212-0407
513-357-7300
www.dermconsultants.com

10575 Client Assistance Program: Ohio Governor's Office for People with Disabilities
Governor's Office for People with Disabilities
50 W Broad Street
Columbus, OH 43215-2541
614-466-7264
Fax: 614-644-1888
TTY: 614-728-2553
e-mail: CKnight@olrs.state.oh.us
www.icdri.org
Marilyn Bove, President

10576 Richland County HPV Support Group
PO Box 3881
Mansfield, OH 44907-3881
419-525-3075
www.skinpatient.com

10577 Technology Resource Center
2140 Arbor Boulevard
Dayton, OH 45439
937-294-8086

Oklahoma

10578 Client Assistance Program: Oklahoma Office of Handicapped Concerns
Oklahoma Office of Handicapped Concerns
2401 NW 23rd
Oklahoma City, OK 73107-5106
405-521-3756
Fax: 405-522-6695
e-mail: Marilyn.Burr@ohc.state.ok.us
www.icdri.org
Marilyn Bove, President

10579 Oklahoma City HPV Support Group: PP of Cen tral Oklahoma
Planned Parenthood of Central Oklahoma
Oklahoma City, OK 73103-1415
405-528-0221
www.aad.org

Oregon

10580 Oregon Disabilities Commission
676 Church Street NE
Salem, OR 97310-1211
503-373-7605
800-358-3117
Fax: 503-373-1133
TTY: 800-521-9615
www.odc.state.or.us
Lori Nelson, Manager
Jeff Brownson, Communications Coordinator

Pennsylvania

10581 Client Assistance Program: Medical Center East
Medical Center East
4200 Forbes Boulevard
Lanham, MD 20706
301-459-2742
Fax: 215-557-7602
TTY: 301-459-5984
The Advocacy Center for Persons with Disabilities is a non-profit organization providing protection and advocacy services. Its mission is to advance the dignity, equality, self-determination and expressed choices of individuals with disabilities.
Marilyn Bove, President

10582 Client Assistance Program: Philadelphia
1617 JFK Boulevard
Philadelphia, PA 19103
215-557-7112
888-745-2357
Fax: 215-557-7602
TTY: 215-557-7112
e-mail: info@equalemployment.org
www.equalemployment.org
Marilyn Bove, President

Rhode Island

10583 Rhode Island Disability Law Center
275 Westminster Street
Providence, RI 02903
401-831-3150
Fax: 401-274-5568
TTY: 401-831-5335
e-mail: info@ridlc.org
www.ridlc.org

To assist people with differing abilities in their efforts to achieve full inclusion in society and to exercise their civil and human rights through the provision of legal advocacy. Rhode Island Disability Law Center was formerly Rhode Island Protection and Advocacy System.
Marilyn Bove, President

South Carolina

10584 South Carolina Protection & Advocacy System for the Handicapped
3710 Landmark Drive
Columbia, SC 29204-4034
803-782-0639
800-922-5225
Marilyn Bove, President

10585 Tri County HPV Support Group
PO Box 1997
Mt Pleasant, SC 29465-1997
843-884-7333
www.aad.org

South Dakota

10586 South Dakota Advocacy Services
221 S Central Avenue
Pierre, SD 57501-2428
605-224-8294
800-658-4782
Fax: 605-224-5125
TTY: 800-658-4782
e-mail: sdas@sdadvocacy.com
www.icdri.org
Marilyn Bove, President

Tennessee

10587 Tennessee Protection & Advocacy
PO Box 121257
Nashville, TN 37212-1257
615-298-1080
800-342-1660
Marilyn Bove, President

Texas

10588 Advocacy Program of Austin
7800 Shoal Creek Boulevard
Austin, TX 78757-1097
512-454-4816
Fax: 512-323-0902
TTY: 800-252-9108
www.advocacyinc.org
Marilyn Bove, President

10589 Dallas/Ft.Worth Metroplex HPV Support Group
8215 Westchester Drive
Dallas, TX 75225-6116
214-363-6733

Utah

10590 Legal Center for People with Disabilities
455 E 400 S
Salt Lake City, UT 84111-3076
801-363-1347
800-662-9080
Marilyn Bove, President

Vermont

10591 Citizen Advocacy of Burlington
Chase Mill 1 Mill Street
Burlington, VT 05401
802-655-0329
Marilyn Bove, President

10592 Client Assistance Program: Vermont Ladd Hall
Ladd Hall
57 N Main Street
Rutland, VT 05701-8409
802-775-0021
800-769-7459
Fax: 802-775-0022
e-mail: nbreiden@vtlegalaid.org
www.icdri.org
Marilyn Bove, President

Virginia

10593 Department for Rights of Virginians with Disabilities
1910 Byrd Avenue
Richmond, VA 23230-3684
804-225-2042
800-552-3962
Fax: 804-225-3221
e-mail: general.vopa@vopa.virginia.gov
www.icdri.org/legal/VirginiaPADD.htm

Disability Resources on the Internet is a non-profit center based in the United States and designated as a entity. ICDRI's mission is to collect a global knowledge base of quality disability resources and best practices and to provide education and outreach.
Marilyn Bove, President

10594 Richmond HPV Support Group: Fan Free Clini c
Fan Free Clinic
PO Box 5669
Richmond, VA 23220-0669
804-358-6343
www.ashastd.org

Washington

10595 Client Assistance Program: Washington Stat e
2531 Rainer Avenue S
Seattle, WA 98144-9510
206-721-5999
800-544-2121
Fax: 206-721-4537
TTY: 206-721-6072
e-mail: caprogram@qwest.net
www.icdri.org
Marilyn Bove, President

10596 Seattle HPV Support Group
PO Box 31171
Seattle, WA 98103-1171
425-619-7190
www.aad.org

West Virginia

10597 Northcentral West Virginia HPV Support Group
Monongalia County Health Department
453 Van Voorhis Road
Morgantown, WV 26505-3408
304-598-5100

10598 West Virginia Advocates
1207 Quarrier Street
Charleston, WV 25301-2413
304-346-0847
800-950-5250
Fax: 304-346-0867
e-mail: wvainfo@wvadvocates.org
www.wvadvocates.org
Ted Johnson, President & PAIMI Representative
Jamie Bailey, President-Elect

Wisconsin

10599 Governor's Commission for People with Disabilities
1 W Wilson Street Room 558
Madison, WI 53702-0007
608-267-4896
Fax: 608-264-9832
Marilyn Bove, President

Wyoming

10600 Wyoming Protection & Advocacy System
320 W 25th Street
Cheyenne, WY 82001-3075
307-632-3496
800-821-3091
Fax: 307-638-0815
e-mail: wypanda@wypanda.com
www.wypanda.com
Marilyn Bove, President

Libraries & Resource Centers

Alabama

10601 Horizon Program: University of Alabama
2018 15th Avenue South
Birmingham, AL 35205
205-322-6606
800-822-6242
Fax: 205-322-6605
www.horizonsschool.org
College-based, nondegree program for students with specific learning disabilities and other mild learning problems. This specially-designed, two-year program prepares students aged 18-26 for successful transitions to the community.
Jade Carter, Director
Marie McElheny, Assistant Director

Arizona

10602 Life Development Institute
18001 N 79th Avenue, Bldg. E-71
Glendale, AZ 85308
623-773-2774
Fax: 623-773-2788
e-mail: info@life-development-inst.org
www.life-development-inst.org
LDI'S mission is to inspire individuals to experience success while optimizing their potential for an enhanced quality of life in a challenging and supportive learning environment. LDI is a non-profit, private organization based in Glendale, Arizona, and provides a supportive residential community that gives individuals the education, skills and training they need to live independently.
Rob Crawford, Chief Executive Officer
Veronica Lieb (Crawford), President

California

10603 Center for Adaptive Learning
3227 Clayton Road
Concord, CA 94519-2840
925-827-3863
Fax: 925-274-80
e-mail: info@centerforadaptiveleaRNing.org
www.centerforadaptiveleaRNing.org
Adults 18-40 years of age learn the essentials of independent living in a program that offers residential living, social skills training, sensory motor training, counseling, roommate peer counseling, cognitive retraining, and job placement. Students either work or attend local community colleges, and job coaching and tutoring are available. Apartments in the community are avabilable and most are clients of Vocational Rehabilitation.
Genevieve Stolarz, Executive Director
Paula Groesbeck, Assistant Director

10604 Independence Center
3640 S Sepulveda Boulevard
Los Angeles, CA 90034-6840
310-202-7102
Fax: 310-398-3776
Provides a supportive program in which young adults with learning disabilities learn the skills necessary to live independently. These include job skills, apartment care, social skills, and adult decision making. Vocational training is accomplished through apprenticeships and/or enrollment in vocational school or community college programs.

Connecticut

10605 Chapel Haven
1040 Whalley Avenue
New Haven, CT 6515
203-397-1714
Fax: 203-923-89
www.chapelhaven.org
Chapel Haven is a not-for-profit independent living skills program that provides a continuum of support services to adults with a cognitive disabilities. We offer training in life skills, employment, education, and recreation both intensively in an apartment style residential setting and on an individualized basis.
Betsey Parlato, President/ Chief Executive Officer
Judy Lefkowitz, Vice President Admissions

Georgia

10606 Creative Community Services (CCS)
1543 Lilbur Stone Mountain Road
Stone, GA 30087
770-469-6226
Fax: 770-696-10
www.ccsgeorgia.org
Serving young adults 20-35 years of age, this organization creates living arrangements for people with a range of learning disabilities who want to lead adult lifestyles but still need some support and assistance. CCS helps locate housing; provides a live-in counselor, if needed; helps develop a plan for each participant's future development; provides one-to-one training in necessary areas; and offers ongoing support for participants and their families.
Sally Dbufhanan, Executive Director

Massachusetts

10607 Berkshire Center
18 Park Street
Lee, MA 01238-1702
413-243-2576
Fax: 413-243-3351
www.berkshirecenter.org
A postsecondary program for young adults with learning disabilities ages 18-26. Half the students attend Berkshire Community College part-time while others go directly into the world of work. Services include: Vocational/Adacademic preparation, tutoring, college liason, life skills instruction, driver's education, money management, psychotherapy, and more. The program is year-round with two years being the average stay.
Michael McManmon, Director

Minnesota

10608 National Resource Library on Youth with Disabilities
University of Minnesota
Box 721-UMHC
Minneapolis, MN 55455
612-626-3087
800-276-8642
Fax: 612-626-2134
TTY: 612-624-3939
e-mail: kdwb-var@umn.edu
www.peds.umn.edu
Offers comprehensive sources of information related to adolescents, disability and transition. The database contains bibliographic, programs, training/education and technical assistance files for the medical community, families, parents and children with chronic illnesses.
Peggy Mann Reinhart, Director
Elizabeth Latts, Resource Coordinator

New Hampshire

10609 Camp Allen
56 Camp Allen Road
Bedford, NH 03110-6606
603-622-8471
Fax: 603-626-4295
e-mail: mary@campallennh.orgg
www.campallennh.org
A summer camp for individuals with disabilities.
Mary Constances, Director

New Jersey

10610 National Women's Health Resource Center
157 Broad Street, Suite 106
Red Bank, NJ 07701
877-986-9472
Fax: 732-530-3347
e-mail: info@healthywomen.org
www.healthywomen.org
The National Women's Health Resource Center is credited with providing women with in-depth, objective and physician-approved information on a broad range of women's health issues. Through nationwide public education campaigns and personal assistance, NWHRC has helped women be informed health care consumers.
Elizabeth Battaglino Cahill, RN, Executive Director
Maria Bushee, Director of Marketing & Communications

New York

10611 Center for Medical Consumers
239 Thompson Street 212-674-7105
New York, NY 10012-1017 Fax: 212-674-7100
e-mail: medconsumers@earthlink.net
www.medicalconsumers.org
Free medical and health reading library designed for consumers containing over 1,200 books and periodicals, including medical texts and journals.
Arthur Aaron Levin MPH, Director
Maryann Napoli, Associate Director

Virginia

10612 ERIC Clearinghouse on Disabilities and Gifted Education
ERIC Project
C/O Computer Sciences Corporation
Washington, DC 20008 800-538-3742
Fax: 703-620-4334
TTY: 703-264-9449
www.eric.ed.gov
The ERIC mission is to provide a comprehensive, easy-to-use, searchable, Internet-based bibliographic and full-text database of education research and information. The simple version of that is that it provides an enormous amount of print materials online, for easy access to important research and journal materials.
Cheryl Racey, Director

Support Groups & Hotlines

10613 Alliance of Genetic Support Groups
4301 Connecticut Avenue NW 202-966-5557
Washington, DC 20008-2369 800-336-4363
Fax: 202-966-8553
e-mail: info@geneticalliance.org
www.geneticalliance.org
A nonprofit coalition of support groups, consumers and professionals dedicated to promoting the common interests of children, adults and families with, or at risk for, genetic disorders. Deals with not only childhood disorders, but mental illness, all types of genetic conditions, including adult onset, more common conditions, disabilities and chronic illness.
Michelle S. Brown, Director of Communications

10614 Behavioral Pediatrics Program
KDWP Variety Family Center
200 Oak Street SE 612-626-4260
Minneapolis, MN 55455-2002 800-276-8642
Fax: 612-624-0997
TTY: 612-624-3939
www.peds.umn.edu/pedsadol
Behavioral Pediatrics Staff help children, teen and their families with a wide variety of behavioral concerns including adjustment to coping with chronic illness. Treatments vary depending on the age, developmental state and needs of each child and family. Often, children are taught to self-regulate their behavior.
Daniel Kohen MD, Director

10615 Childrens Hospice International
901 N Pitt Street 703-684-0330
Alexandria, VA 22314 800-242-4453
Fax: 703-684-0226
e-mail: info@chionline.org
www.chionline.org
This nonprofit organization works to improve hospice care for children. Free services include information and referral service for child care, counseling, support groups, pain management, professional education and research. This is a membership group, with a membership fee for other services.
Ann Armstrong Dailey, Founding Director/CEO

10616 Fetal Alcohol Network
KDWP Variety Family Center
200 Oak Street SE 612-626-4260
Minneapolis, MN 55455-2002 800-276-8642
Fax: 612-624-0997
TTY: 612-624-3939
e-mail: kdwb-var@umn.edu
www.peds.umn.edu/peds-adol
Staff provide assessment, intervention and consultation regarding the physical, developmental learning, behavioral and emotional well-being of children and individuals affected by prenatal exposure to alcohol and drugs.
Daniel Kohen MD, Director

10617 Foundation for Hospice and Homecare
323 Payntz Avenue 785-537-0688
Manhattan, KS 66502 800-748-7474
Fax: 785-537-1309
www.homecarehospice.org
The foundation for Hospice and Homecare has several publications available for home health care providers. They also have a directory of approved and accredited homecare agencies.

10618 Friends Health Connection
PO Box 114 732-418-1811
New Brunswick, NJ 08903 800-483-7436
Fax: 732-249-9897
e-mail: Info@friendshealthconnection.org
www.friendshealthconnection.org
Nonprofit organization that connects people who are currently experiencing or have overcome the same disease, illness, handicap, or injury in order to communicate for mutual support.
Roxanne Black-Weisheit, Executive Director

10619 KDWB Family Resource Center
200 Oak Street SE 612-626-3087
Minneapolis, MN 55455-2002 800-276-8642
Fax: 612-624-0997
TTY: 612-624-3939
e-mail: kdwb-var@umn.edu
www.peds.umn.edu/peds-adol
A place families can visit to learn about their child's chronic illness or disability, identify psychological and developmental issues, and link-up with program and community resources. Information will be available by telephone and via the web site.
Elizabeth Latts, Resource Coordinator

10620 KDWB Variety Family Canter
200 Oak Street SE 612-626-3087
Minneapolis, MN 55455-2002 800-276-8642
Fax: 612-624-0997
TTY: 612-624-3939
e-mail: kdwbvar@umn.edu
www.peds.umn.edu/pedsadol/
University-Community pertnership that provides family-centered services that promote physical, emotional, psychological and social health and well being for children and youth at risk, including children and youth with disabilities. The Center is dedicated to teaching, research, outreach, and community services.
Peggy Mann Reinhart, Director
Elizabeth Latts, Resource Coordinator

10621 National Association for Home Care
228 7th Street SE 202-547-7424
Washington, DC 20003-4306 Fax: 202-547-3540
www.nahc.org
This is a trade association representing various home care, hospice and health aid orgainizations.

10622 National Family Caregivers Association
10400 Connecticut Avenue 301-942-6430
Kensington, MD 20895-3104 800-896-3650
Fax: 301-942-2302
e-mail: info@thefamilycaregiver.org
www.thefamilycaregiver.org
Provides information and support for caregivers, which include a quarterly newletter and also advocates about caregiving issues.
Suzanne Mintz, President

10623 National Health Information Center
PO Box 1133
Washington, DC 20013
310-565-4167
800-336-4797
Fax: 301-984-4256
e-mail: info@nhic.org
www.health.gov/nhic

Offers a nationwide information referral service, produces directories and resource guides.

10624 National Parent to Parent Support and Information System
PO Box 907
Blue Ridge, GA 30513
706-632-8822
800-651-1151
Fax: 706-632-8830
e-mail: judd103w@wonder.em.cdc.gov
www.iser.com/NPPSIS-GA.html

NPPSIS is a nonprofit organization established to support, strengthen, and empower families through one-on-one parent contacts. They link families nationally whose children have special health care needs and rare disorders. They provide parents with heath care information, resources and referrals to allow them to identify appropriate services.

10625 Okizu Foundation Camps
16 Digital Drive
Novato, CA 94949-6115
415-382-9083
Fax: 415-382-8384
e-mail: info@okizu.org
www.okizu.org

This foundation runs family camp programs for children who have cancer and their families, and for children who have or had a parent with cancer.
Suzanne Randall, Executive Director

10626 Parent to Parent of New York State
500 Balltown Road
Schenectady, NY 12304-2247
518-381-4350
800-305-8817
Fax: 518-393-9607
e-mail: p2pnys@adelphia.net
www.parenttoparentnys.org

Parent to Parent programs provide informatonal and emotional support to parents who have a child, adolescent or adult family member with special needs. Offers an important connection for a parent who is seeking support for special disability issues, by matching him or her with a trained veteran parent who has already been there. Because the two parents share so many common concerns and interests, the support given and received is often uniquely meaningful. Also helps families locate information.
Janice Fitzgerald, Executive Director

10627 Pediatric Psychology
KDWP Variety Family Center
200 Oak Street SE
Minneapolis, MN 55455-2002
612-626-4260
800-276-8642
Fax: 612-624-0997
TTY: 612-624-3939
e-mail: kdwbvar@umn.edu
www.peds.umn.edu/pedsadol

Staff provide assessment, intervention and consultation regarding the physical, developmental, learning, behavioral and emotional well-being of children and individuals affected by prenatal exposure to alcohol and drugs.
Daniel Kohen MD, Director

10628 STAR Center for Family Health
KDWB Variety Family Center
200 Oak Street SE
Minneapolis, MN 55455-2002
612-626-4260
800-276-8642
Fax: 612-624-0997
TTY: 6126243939
e-mail: kdwb-var@umn.edu
www.peds.umn.edu/peds-adol/

Helps children, youth and families develop new and enhanced ways of coping with stress, learn strategies for adjusting to living with a chronic illness, and discover new ways of finding health, balance and well-being.

10629 U Special Kids
KDWB Variety Family Center
200 Oak Street SE
Minneapolis, MN 55455-2002
612-626-3081
800-276-8642
Fax: 612-624-0997
TTY: 6126243939
e-mail: uspclkid@umn.edu
www.peds.umn.edu/peds-adol/

A program that provides care coordinators for children with complex medical conditions. A team of health care providers advocates for children and their families within the health care system.
Anne Kelly MD, Director

10630 Visiting Nurse Association of America
390 Grant Street
Denver, CO 80203
303-698-2121
Fax: 303-986-71
www.vnaacolorado.org

This agency represents independent VNA units across the United States. Each VNA unit may vary in their services, but most provide skilled nursing, physical therapy, occupational therapy, speech therapy, and home health aid services.
Laura Reilly, Director

10631 Well Spouse Association
63 W Main Street
Freehold, NJ 7728
732-577-8899
800-838-0879
Fax: 732-577-8644
e-mail: info@wellspouse.org
www.wellspouse.org

This association is a nonprofit national self-help organization serving the well spouse of the chronically ill. Members help each other develop coping and survival skills through local support groups (including bereavement), letter and telephone networks, and personal outreach and a quarterly newsletter.

Books

10632 A History of Childhood and Disability
Philip Safford and Elizabeth Safford, author
Teachers College Press
1234 Amsterdam Avenue
New York, NY 10027
212-678-3929
Fax: 212-678-4149
e-mail: tcpress@tc.columbia.edu
www.teacherscollegepress.com

This book presents an interdisciplinary perspective on children considered exceptional and how services have evolved in reponse to their diverse neeeds.
1996 352 pages
ISBN: 0-807734-85-3

10633 Art of Getting Well
David Spero, RN, author
Hunter House Publishing
PO Box 2914
Alameda, CA 94501
510-865-5282
800-266-5592
Fax: 510-865-4295
e-mail: ordering@hunterhouse.com
www.hunterhouse.com

A five step plan for maximazing health when you have a chronic illness.
224 pages Paperback
Cristina Sverdrup, Customer Service Manager

10634 Assisstive Technology for Young Children: A Guide to Family-Centered Services
Sharon Lesar Judge and Howard P Parette, author
Brookline Books
PO Box 1209
Brookline, MA 02445
617-734-6772
800-666-2665
Fax: 617-734-3952
www.brooklinebooks.com

Explores the wide range of considerations involved in evaluating children's needs, selecting and prescribing devices, and training children, families, and teachers to use the technology.
1998 Softcover
ISBN: 1-571290-51-6

10635 Awaking to Disability
Volcano Press

PO Box 270
Volcano, CA 95689-0270
209-296-3445
800-879-9636
Fax: 209-296-4995
e-mail: sales@volcanopress.com
www.volcanopress.com

From the disability activist whose columns have been avidly followed by readers of the Albuquerque Journal and Miami Herald comes this revealing compedium of her thoughts. It offers a perspective for parents of children with disabilites, or for newly disabled people.

1997 288 pages
ISBN: 1-884244-14-9

10636 Blood Pressure Book: How to Get it Down & Keep it Down
Bull Publishing
PO Box 1377
Boulder, CO 80306
800-676-2855
Fax: 303-545-6354
www.bullpub.com

Provides basic information on the causes and treatment of high blood pressure includes check up charts and illustrations that will help readers find out where they stand and lead them to practical advice tailored to their own needs.

1996 136 pages
ISBN: 0-923521-97-6

10637 Building Partnerships in Hospital Care
Bull Publishing
PO Box 1377
Boulder, CO 80306
800-676-2855
Fax: 303-545-6354
www.bullpub.com

Aims to desensetize patients and families to their fears of illness, hospital machinery and authority figures at the same time resensitize institution weary professionals to the feelings, instincts and emotions that brought them into the field in the first place.

304 pages
ISBN: 0-923521-07-0

10638 Child of Mine: Feeding with Love and Good Sense
Bull Publishing
PO Box 1377
Boulder, CO 80306
800-676-2855
Fax: 303-545-6354
www.bullpub.com

Parents need to learn how to provide a nutritionally wholesome diet, but they also need to know how to feed in a way that nurtures a child's senses of autonomy and trust in themselves and their bodies.

470 pages
ISBN: 0-923521-51-8

10639 Childhood Emergencies: What to Do A Quick Refrence Guide
Bull Publishing
PO Box 1377
Boulder, CO 80306
800-676-2855
Fax: 303-545-6354
www.bullpub.com

Handy book contains clear and quick referance for most common injuries including cuts and wounds, broken bones, abdominal pain, burns, toothaches, convulsion, eye and ear injuries, abrasions, bites insect and animal, bleeding, choking, seizures, freezing and frostbite, CPR, etc.

44 pages
ISBN: 0-923521-62-3

10640 Chiropractor's Self-Help Back and Body Book
Samuel Homola, DC, author
Hunter House Publishers
PO Box 2914
Alameda, CA 94501
510-865-5282
800-266-5592
Fax: 510-865-4295
e-mail: ordering@hunterhouse.com
www.hunterhouse.com

How to relieve common aches and pains at home and on the job.

2002 320 pages Paperback
Cristina Sverdrup, Customer Service Manager

10641 Choose the Right Long Term Care
NOLO
950 Parker Street
Berkeley, CA 94710
510-549-1976
800-955-4775
Fax: 510-548-5902
www.nolo.com

You can use this book to figure out how to choose a nursing home, or find a viable alternative. Covers how to get the most out of Medicare and other benefit programs.

336 pages
ISBN: 0-873375-15-7
Maira Dizgalvis, Trade Customer Service Manager
Susan McConnell, Directorf Sales

10642 Chronic Physical Illness
S. Newman, E. Steed, K. Mulligan, author
McGraw-Hill Companies
Returns Department
Dubuque, IA 52002
877-833-5524
Fax: 609-308-4484
e-mail: pbg.ecommerce_custserv@mcgraw-hill.com
www.mcgraw-hill.com

Provides an overview of self-management in chronic physical illness, theoretical and conceptual background, and examines issues related to the delivery of self-management. Discussion of a range of chronic conditions including: asthma, coronary artery disease, heart failure, COPD, hypertension, diabetes and rheumatoid arthritis. Authored by a number of leading international experts in the diseases they discuss. Hardcover also available for $136.95.

2008 240 pages
ISBN: 0-335217-86-9

10643 Directory of Health Grants
Research Grant Guides
PO Box 1214
Loxahatchee, FL 33470-1214
561-795-6129
Fax: 561-795-7794

1000 foundation profiles.

Second edition
ISBN: 0-945078-19-6

10644 Directory of Social Service Grants
Research Grant Guides
PO Box 1214
Loxahatchee, FL 33470-1214
561-795-6129
Fax: 561-795-7794

1100 foundation profiles.

Second edition
ISBN: 0-945078-18-8

10645 Family Interventions Throughout Chronic Illness and Disability
Springer Publishing Company
536 Broadway
New York, NY 10012-3955
212-431-4370
Fax: 212-941-7842
e-mail: marketing@springerpub.com
www.springerpub.com

This book provides usable methods for professionals to help families deal with the reality of chronic illness of disability of a family member. Included at the end of each section are study questions and suggested activities for those working with the disabled, as well as for students.

336 pages Hardcover
ISBN: 0-826155-80-1
Annette Imperati, Marketing Director

10646 Get Fit While You Sit: Easy Workouts From Your Chair
Hunter House Publishing
PO Box 2914
Alameda, CA 94501
510-865-5282
800-266-5592
Fax: 510-865-4295
e-mail: ordering@hunterhouse.com
www.hunterhouse.com

Three total body workout programs that can be done right from your chair, anywhere. Spiral Bound - $17.95.

160 pages Paperback
Cristina Sverdrup, Customer Service Manager

10647 Good Bones: Complete Guide to Building and Maintaining the Healthiest Bones
Barbara Luke, author
Bull Publishing

PO Box 1377
Boulder, CO 80306
800-676-2855
Fax: 303-545-6354
www.bullpub.com

Examines 17 major risks in bone health with women. Author offers nutrional advice and preventative nutritional advice and prevenative measures in this comprehensive and scientifically sound guide for woman of all ages.
192 pages
ISBN: 0-923521-44-5

10648 Grants for Organizations Serving People with Disabilities
Research Grant Guides
PO Box 1214
Loxahatchee, FL 33470-1214
Fax: 561-795-7794

800 foundation profiles, including funding for all types of nonprofits. Also two key articles on winning grant strategies.
Tenth edition
ISBN: 0-945078-17-X

10649 Habits Not Diets: Secret to Lifetime Weight Control
Bull Publishing
PO Box 1377
Boulder, CO 80306
800-676-2855
Fax: 303-545-6354
www.bullpub.com

This sensible approach puts the emphasis on how to eat rather than what. Uses the cognitive aspects of weight management including thinking skills, stress management and problem solving to help analyze individual eating habits , break undesirable patterns and establish new ones.
2003 352 pages
ISBN: 0-923521-70-4

10650 Health
Sage Publications
2455 Teller Road
Thousand Oaks, CA 91320
805-499-9774
800-818-7243
Fax: 805-499-0871
e-mail: journals@sagepub.com
www.sagepublications.com

A interdisciplinary and international journal committed to the social and cultural study of health, illness and medicine with a particular focus on the changing place of health matters in modern society and in public onsciousness.
Quarterly

10651 I Can't Chew Cookbook
J Randy Wilson, author
Hunter House Publishing
PO Box 2914
Alameda, CA 94501
510-865-5282
800-266-5592
Fax: 510-865-4295
e-mail: ordering@hunterhouse.com
www.hunterhouse.com

Delicious soft-diet recipes for people with chewing, swallowing and Dry-Mouth Disorders. Spiral Bound - $22.95.
2003 224 pages Paperback
Cristina Sverdrup, Customer Service Manager

10652 Informed Woman's Guide to Breast Health
Bull Publishing
PO Box 1377
Boulder, CO 80306
800-676-2855
Fax: 303-545-6354
www.bullpub.com

A manual designed for every woman who has questions regarding their breasts, diseases concerned with and both self and medical exam. Answers the questions in an easy to read manner.
156 pages
ISBN: 0-923521-61-5

10653 Insider's Guide to HMOs
Penguin Putnam
PO Box 999
Bergenfield, NJ 07621-0903
800-526-0275
Fax: 800-227-9604

ISBN: 0-452276-91-8

10654 Journel to Pain Relief
Phyllis Berger, author
Hunter House Publishing
PO Box 2194
Alameda, CA 94501
510-865-5282
800-266-5592
Fax: 510-865-4295
e-mail: ordering@hunterhouse.com
www.hunterhouse.com

Hands-on guide to breakthroughs in pain treatment.
2007 288 pages Paperback
Cristina Sverdrup, Customer Service Manager

10655 Joy of Laziness
Peter Axt, PhD, author
Hunter House Publishing
PO Box 2914
Alameda, CA 94501
510-865-5282
800-266-5592
Fax: 510-865-4295
e-mail: ordering@hunterhouse.com
www.hunterhouse.com

Why life is better slower-and how to get there.
2003 160 pages Paperback
Cristina Sverdrup, Customer Service Manager

10656 Just Like Everyone Else
World Institute on Disability
510 16th Street, Suite 100
Oakland, CA 94612-1520
510-763-4100
Fax: 510-763-4109
TTY: 510-208-9493
e-mail: wid@wid.org
www.wid.org

Provides perspective, inspiration and information about the Independent Living Movement and the Americans with Disabilities Act.
16 pages
Kathy Martinez, Executive Director

10657 Laurel's Kitchen Caring: Recipes for Everyday Home Caregiving
Ten Speed Press
PO Box 7123
Berkeley, CA 94707-0123
510-559-1600
800-841-2665
Fax: 510-524-4588
e-mail: order@tenspeed.com
www.tenspeed.com

A cookbook tailored to the nutritional needs of recovering patients as well as morale booster, caregiving primer, and resource book.
1997 158 pages
ISBN: 0-898159-51-2

10658 Living a Healthy Life with Chronic Conditions
Bull Publishing
PO Box 1377
Boulder, CO 80306
800-676-2855
Fax: 303-545-6354
www.bullpub.com

A complete self managing guide for people with chronic diseases. Features coverage of emotional aspects of living with chronic disease and offers suggestions for planning for the future.
292 pages
ISBN: 1-933503-01-7

10659 Maximize Your Body Potential
Bull Publishing
PO Box 1377
Boulder, CO 80306
800-676-2855
Fax: 303-545-6354
www.bullpub.com

Informs readers everything that they need to know about being successful in managing body weight. Provides self-tests, checklists, paper and pencil exercises for creating a personalized program, diet exercise, behavior patterns and the psychological components of successful weight management.
640 pages
ISBN: 0-923521-71-2

10660 Menopause Without Medicine
Linda Ojeda, author
Hunter House Publishing

PO Box 2194 510-865-5282
Alameda, CA 94501 800-266-5592
Fax: 510-865-4295
e-mail: ordering@hunterhouse.com
www.hunterhouse.com

Menopause Without Medicine, 5th Edition. Non medical approach to menopause. Covers Heart Disease, mood swings, cognitive decline, osteoporosis, weight control, insomnia.
2003 400 pages Paperback
Cristina Sverdrup, Customer Service Manager

10661 **Mother to Be: A Guide to Pregnancy and Birth for Women with Disabilities**
Demos Vermande
386 Park Avenue S 212-683-0072
New York, NY 10016-8804 800-532-8663
Fax: 212-683-0118
e-mail: orderdept@demospub.com
www.demospub.com

An in-depth look at every aspect of pregnancy from the disabled woman's perspective, including how to find the best medical care, exercise, nutrition, body changes, fetal development, recognizing the onset of labor, delivery, Caesarean birth, postpartum issues.
424 pages
ISBN: 0-939957-29-9
Dr. Diana M Schneider, President

10662 **Nolo's Guide to Soc. Security Disability: Getting and Keeping Your Benefits**
NOLO
950 Parker Street 510-549-1976
Berkeley, CA 94710 800-955-4775
Fax: 510-548-5902
www.nolo.com

Not many bureaucratic programs are as large, and as confusing, as Social Security disability. This book shows you the ins and outs of the system.
350 pages
ISBN: 0-873375-74-2
Maira Dizgalvis, Trade Customer Service Manager
Susan McConnell, Director Sales

10663 **Ostomy Book: Living Comfortably with Colostomies, Ileostomies and Urostomies**
Bull Publishing
PO Box 1377
Boulder, CO 80306 800-676-2855
Fax: 303-545-6354
www.bullpub.com

Provides a complete, in depth look at the information regarding everything from the surgeries to the appliances.
256 pages
ISBN: 0-923521-12-7

10664 **Psychological Management of Chronic Pain: A Treatment Manual**
Springer Publishing Company
536 Broadway 212-431-4370
New York, NY 10012-3955 Fax: 212-941-7842

This volume provides the clinician with a practical guide to help clients manage and alleviate problems associated with chronic pain and places an emphasis on the cognitive components of treatment. The manual illustrates a time-limited, therapist-guide/self-management program.
1996 80 pages Softcover
ISBN: 0-826161-12-X

10665 **Self Help: Your Strategy for Living with COPD**
Bull Publishing
PO Box 1377
Boulder, CO 80306 800-676-2855
Fax: 303-545-6354
www.bullpub.com

Contains vital information for patients suffering from asthma, emphysema, or chronic bronchitis. Colorful charts, graphs and illustrations highlight major concepts and help make the booklet user friendly.
1997 32 pages
ISBN: 0-923521-40-2

10666 **ShapeWalking**
Marilyn Bach, PhD, author
Hunter House Publishing
PO Box 2194 510-865-5282
Alameda, CA 94501 800-266-5592
Fax: 510-865-4295
e-mail: ordering@hunterhouse.com
www.hunterhouse.com

ShapeWalking, 2nd Edition. Six easy steps to your best body.
2002 144 pages Paperback

10667 **Social Security, Medicare and Government Pensions**
NOLO
950 Parker Street 510-549-1976
Berkeley, CA 94710 800-955-4775
Fax: 510-548-5902
www.nolo.com

A plain English guide explaining the ins and outs of the Social Security system: retirement, disability and benefits for dependents and survivors.
320 pages
ISBN: 0-873374-87-8
Maira Dizgalvis, Trade Customer Service Manager
Susan McConnell, Director Sales

10668 **Strength Training for Seniors**
Michael Fekete, CSCS; ACE, author
Hunter House Publishing
PO Box 2194 510-865-5282
Alameda, CA 94501 800-266-5592
Fax: 510-865-4295
e-mail: ordering@hunterhouse.com
www.hunterhouse.com

How to rewind your biological clock. Reduce a person's biological age by 10-20 years.
2006 160 pages Paperback
Cristina Sverdrup, Customer Service Manager

10669 **Succeeding Against the Odds: Strategies and Insights from the Learning Disabled**
Jeremy P Tarcher
5858 Wilshire Boulevard 213-935-9980
Los Angeles, CA 90036-4521

Filled with information on adults with learning disabilities, including the hidden handicaps, the definition of learning disabilities, and characteristics of individuals with learning disabilities. The book also looks at the responsibility of preparing for adulthood, and includes information for parents and teachers.
Lex Frieden, Program Director

10670 **Taking Care of Caregivers**
Bull Publishing
PO Box 1377
Boulder, CO 80306 800-676-2855
Fax: 303-545-6354
www.bullpub.com

Provides an in depth look at the problems facing caregivers: the needs of caregivers, feelings and how to deal with them, stress management techniques, communicating with people who have progressive dementia, grief, sharing and support.
184 pages
ISBN: 0-923521-09-7

10671 **Tax Options and Strategies for People with Disabilities**
Demos Vermande
386 Park Avenue S 212-683-0072
New York, NY 10016-8804 800-532-8663
Fax: 212-683-0118
e-mail: info@demospub.com

1996 288 pages
ISBN: 0-939957-85-

10672 **Teens Face to Face with Chronic Illness**
Asthma and Allergy Foundation of America
1233 20th Street NW 202-466-7643
Washington, DC 20036-2330 800-727-8462
Fax: 202-466-8940
www.aafa.org

Young people easily relate to this book, which uses anecdotes from teens dealing with chronic illness. Teens address issues such as peer pressure and feeling different.
129 pages Paperback

10673 The Personal Care Attendant Guide: The Art of Finding, Keeping, or Being One
Katie Rodriguez Banister, author
Program Development Associates
5620 Business Avenue 315-452-0643
Cicero, NY 13039-9576 800-543-2119
Fax: 315-452-0710
e-mail: info@disabilitytraining.com
www.disabilitytraining.com/pcgb.html
To live independently, many people with chronic illness and/or disabilitiy hire a personal attendant to assist with day-to-day tasks. Finding a qualified caregiver can be challenging, but not impossible. The Guide teaches readers how to find a competent caregiver, and gives prospective attendants vital information and real-life examples to help them succeed. Includes easy-to-use forms and worksheets to make the search easy and organized, anecdotes, and resources.
2007 160 pages

10674 Time for Healing: Relaxation for Mind and Body
Bull Publishing
PO Box 1377
Boulder, CO 80306 800-676-2855
Fax: 303-545-6354
www.bullpub.com
Helps and guides listeners release tension and acheive deep muscular relaxation, heightened self-awareness and total relaxation.

10675 Understanding Addiction
University Press of Mississippi
3825 Ridgewood Road 601-432-6205
Jackson, MS 39211-6492 Fax: 601-432-6217
e-mail: kburgess@ihl.state.ms.us
www.upress.state.ms.us
A concise overview of this complex affiction for all those affected by addiction - addicts, family members, and even employers.
2001 224 pages Paperback
ISBN: 1-578062-40-3
Kathy Burgess, Advertising/Marketing Services Manager

10676 Understanding Anemia
Ed Uthman, MD, author
University Press of Mississippi
3825 Ridgewood Road 601-432-6205
Jackson, MS 39211-6492 Fax: 601-432-6217
e-mail: kburgess@ihl.state.ms.us
www.upress.state.ms.us
Medicine for the lay reader, a book detailing causes and treatments of the various forms of anemia.
1998 160 pages Paperback
ISBN: 1-578060-38-9
Kathy Burgess, Advertising/Marketing Services Manager

10677 Understanding Child Sexual Abuse
Edward L Rowan, MD, author
University Press of Mississippi
3825 Ridgewood Road 601-432-6205
Jackson, MS 39211-6492 Fax: 601-432-6217
e-mail: kburgess@ihl.state.ms.us
www.upress.state.ms.us
For those looking to comrephend and to prevent child sexual abuse, a succinct guidebook of advice and resources.
2006 96 pages Paperback
ISBN: 1-578068-07-X
Kathy Burgess, Advertising/Marketing Services Manager

10678 Understanding Cosmetic Laser Surgery
Robert Langdon, MD, author
University Press of Mississippi
3825 Ridgewood Road 601-432-6205
Jackson, MS 39211-6492 Fax: 601-432-6217
e-mail: kburgess@ihl.state.ms.us
www.upress.state.ms.us
A description of the processes and procedures available in cosmetic laser surgery.
2004 112 pages
ISBN: 1-578065-87-9
Kathy Burgess, Advertising/Marketing Services Manager

10679 Understanding Dental Health
Francis G Serio, DMD; MS, author
University Press of Mississippi
3825 Ridgewood Road 601-432-6205
Jackson, MS 39211-6492 Fax: 601-432-6217
e-mail: kburgess@ihl.state.ms.us
www.upress.state.ms.us
A user-friendly manual on the basics of dental health.
1998 128 pages Paperback
ISBN: 1-578060-10-9
Kathy Burgess, Advertising/Marketing Services Manager

10680 Understanding Dietary Supplements
Jenna Hollenstein, author
University Press of Mississippi
3825 Ridgewood Road 601-432-6205
Jackson, MS 39211-6492 Fax: 601-432-6217
e-mail: kburgess@ihl.state.ms.us
www.upress.state.ms.us
A handy guide to the evaluation and use of vitamins, minerals, herbs, botanicals, and more.
96 pages Paperback
ISBN: 1-578069-81-5
Kathy Burgess, Advertising/Marketing Services Manager

10681 Understanding Stuttering
Nathan Lavid, MD, author
University Press of Mississippi
3825 Ridgewood Road 601-432-6205
Jackson, MS 39211-6492 Fax: 601-432-6217
e-mail: kburgess@ihl.state.ms.us
www.upress.state.ms.us
Insight into an ailment that impairs more than sixty million in the world population.
2004 112 pages Paperback
ISBN: 1-578065-73-9
Kathy Burgess, Advertising/Marketing Services Manager

10682 Understanding Your Learning Disability
Cheri Warner, author
Ohio State University at Newark
1179 University Drive
Newark, OH 43055 740-366-3321
newark.osu.edu
Provides tips for students based on the author's experience as a Learning Disability Specialist. Offers definitions, characteristics, and suggestions related to reading, math, note taking, test taking, social interactions, and organizational strategies.

10683 Writing from Within
Bernard Selling, author
Hunter House Publishers
PO Box 2194 510-865-5282
Alameda, CA 94501 800-266-5592
Fax: 510-865-4295
e-mail: ordering@hunterhouse.com
www.hunterhouse.com
Writing from Within, 3rd Edition. A guide to creativity and life story writing.
320 pages Paperback
Cristina Sverdrup, Customer Service Manager

10684 Yes, You Can!: Go Beyond Physical Adversity and Live Life to Its Fullest
Demos Medical Publishing

386 Park Avenue S
New York, NY 10016
212-683-0072
Fax: 212-683-0118
e-mail: orderdept@demospub.com
www.demosmedpub.com

120 pages Paperback
ISBN: 1-888799-48-x
Dr Diana M Schneider, President/Publisher

Children's Books

10685 **Are You Tired Again?...I Understand: An Activities Workbook for Children**
Western Psychological Services
12031 Wilshire Boulevard
Los Angeles, CA 90025-1201
310-478-2061
800-648-8857
Fax: 310-478-7838
e-mail: custserv@wpspublish.com
www.wpspublish.com
Reassuring activity and coloring book for children with a chronically ill parent. Gives these youngsters the tools they need to work through their feelings, while gently explaining why mom isn't getting better, and how the family can still enjoy life and function as a family. Can be used with individuals or support groups. Net effect is to help children and patients- by relieving stress in the family and reassuring parents who are worried about how their condition is affecting their children.
Susan Madden, Marketing Director

10686 **In the Hospital**
Peter Alsop, Bill Harley, author
Compassion Books
7036 State Highway 80 S
Burnsville, NC 28714-7569
828-675-5909
800-970-4220
Fax: 828-675-9687
e-mail: heal2grow@aol.com
www.compassionbooks.com
Wonderful songs and entertaining stories dealing with being sick, being different, being scared and finding strength and hope.
Audiotape/Book
Bruce Greene, Director

10687 **Zink the Zebra**
Gareth Stevens, Inc
330 West Olive Street
Milwaukee, WI 53212-3952
414-332-3520
800-542-2595
Fax: 414-336-0156
e-mail: info@gspub.com
www.garethstevens.com
Zink is a zebra with spots instead of stripes. Here is an inspiring and touching tale about being different in ways that don't matter and shouldn't get in the way when it comes to making friends and enjoying companionship and respect. Written by 11-year-old Kelly Weil in the last year of a battle she bravely fought, but ultimately lost, against cancer.
1997
ISBN: 0-836816-26-9

Magazines

10688 **Advance: for Directors in Rehabilitation**
Merion Publications
2900 Horizon Drive
King of Prussia, PA 19406-2651
215-265-7812
800-355-5627
rehabilitation-director.advanceweb.com
An informational magazine designed to provide a balance of material concerning all aspects of a rehabilitation manager's job.
Scott Huelskamp, Editor
Johnathan Bassett, Senior Associate Editor

10689 **Exceptional Parent Magazine**
209 Harvard Street
Brookline, MA 02446-5005
617-730-5800
800-852-2884
Fax: 617-730-8742

Lex Frieden, Program Director

Newsletters

10690 **Asbestos Watch**
PO Box 1483
Baltimore, MD 21203-1483
301-243-5864
Fax: 301-243-5234
A national nonprofit organization dedicated to the education of the public to the hazards of asbestos exposure. The association developed programs of public education and consults with victims of asbestos exposure, school boards, building owners, government agencies, and others interested in identifying asbestos hazards and developing control programs.
Annual

10691 **Chronic Pain Letter**
Dolak
Old Chelsea Station
New York, NY 10011
718-797-0015
Brings current information on the management of chronic pain to the sufferer and the health professional.

Dorothy Fabian, Circulation Manager

10692 **Closing the Gap**
526 Main Street
Henderson, MN 56044-0068
507-248-3294
Fax: 507-248-3810
e-mail: info@closingthegap.com
www.closingthegap.com
Provides in-depth coverage of computers and disabilities for basic education. Annual subscription.
BiMonthly
Lex Frieden, Program Director

10693 **Health Facts**
Center for Medical Consumers
237 Thompson Street
New York, NY 10012-1017
212-674-7105
Fax: 212-674-7100
www.medicalconsumers.org
Analyses of topics such as cancer, nutrition, depression, exercise, prescription drugs and nonmedical therapies.
6 pages Monthly

10694 **In Confidence**
American Health Information Management Association
233 N Michigan Avenue, 21st Floor
Chicago, IL 60601
312-233-1100
800-621-6828
Fax: 312-233-1090
e-mail: info@ahima.org
www.ahima.org
Provides medical, legal and other professionals with a forum to exchange ideas and share knowledge about the confidentiality of health information and people's rights to privacy.
12 pages BiMonthly
Linda Kloss, Chief Executive Officer
Becky Perry, Executive Vice President & CFO

10695 **Johns Hopkins Health Insider**
Intelihealth
960C Harvest Drive
Blue Bell, PA 19422
800-988-1127
Fax: 800-676-3299
e-mail: service@jhinsider.com
www.jhinsider.com
Expert advice and information from America's leading health institution. The most authoritative, cutting-edge health information available today, straight from the leading specialists and experts.
David B Hellmann MD, Associate Editor
Linda A Lewandowski PhD, RN, Associate Editor

10696 **Lifelines**
Leslie Park, author
Disabled & Alone/Life Services for the Handicapped
61 Broadway
New York, NY 10006
212-532-6740
800-995-0066
Fax: 212-532-3588
e-mail: info@disabledandalone.org
www.disabledandalone.org

A newsletter published by Disabled and Alone/Life Services for the Handicapped.
8 pages Quarterly
Leslie D Park, Chairman
Lee Ackerman, Executive Director

10697 Lymphatic Research Matters
Lymphatic Research Foundation
40 Garvies Point Road
Glen Cove, NY 11542
516-625-9675
Fax: 516-625-9410
e-mail: lrf@lymphaticresearch.org
www.lymphaticresearch.org
Reporting information about LRF activities and current research. The newsletters are sent to registrants in our data base: patients, their families, the scientific community and health care providers.
Bi-Annual
Jacqueline Reinhard, Executive Director
Wendy Chaite, Esq., Founder & President

10698 Mainstay
Well Spouse Association
63 W Main Street
Freehold, NJ 7728
732-577-8899
800-838-0879
Fax: 732-577-8644
e-mail: info@wellspouse.org
www.wellspouse.org
The Well Spouse Association quarterly newsletter featuring articles written by WSA members.

10699 NHF Head Lines
National Headache Foundation
820 N Orleans
Chicago, IL 60610-3132
312-640-5399
888-643-5552
Fax: 312-640-9049
e-mail: nhf1970@headaches.org
www.headaches.org

10700 National Networker
National Network of Learning Disabled Adults
808 N 82nd Street
Scottsdale, AZ 85257-3850
602-941-5112
For adults with learning disabilities.
Quarterly
Lex Frieden, Program Director

10701 Orphan Disease Update
National Organization for Rare Disorders
PO Box 8923
New Fairfield, CT 06812-8923
203-746-6518
800-999-6673
Fax: 203-756-6481
e-mail: orphan@rarediseases.org
www.rarediseases.org
Information about rare disorders for families with similar disorders.

10702 VSA Arts
JFK Center for the Performing Arts
1300 Connecticut Avenue NW
Washington, DC 20036-1715
202-628-2600
800-933-8721
Fax: 202-737-0725
TDD: 202-737-0645
e-mail: info@vsarts.org
www.vsarts.org
VSA arts is an international, nonprofit organization dedicated to promoting artistic excellence and providing educational opportunities through the arts for children and adults with disabilities. The Creative Spirit is a quarterly newsletter that features VSA arts special events throughout the world, interviews with artistd and articles relating to disability and the arts.
8 pages
D Dixon, CEO
S Datton-Kumins, Writer/Research Coordinator

10703 Wheel Life News
University of Virginia, Rehab Engineering Centers
3363 University Station
Charlottesville, VA 22903
804-924-0311
Features tie downs and other adaptive technology for persons with disabilities.

10704 Worklife: A Publication of Employment and People with Disabilities
Office of Disability Employment Policy
200 Constitution Avenue NW
Washington, DC 20210
202-693-7880
Fax: 202-693-7888
TDD: 202-376-6205
Quarterly

Pamphlets

10705 Campus Opportunities for Students with Learning Differences
Judith & Stephen Crooker, author
Octameron Associates
PO Box 2748
Alexandria, VA 22301
703-836-5480
Fax: 703-836-5650
e-mail: octameron@aol.com
www.octameron.com
Addresses high school students with learning disabilities and their parents as they take the necessary steps in secondary school to be ready to apply for college.
Anna Leider, Publisher

10706 Issues in Independent Living
Independent Living Research Utilization
2323 S Shepherd Drive
Houston, TX 77019-7024
713-520-0232
Fax: 713-520-5785
This booklet is a report of the National Study Group on the Implications of Health Care Reform for Americans with Disabilities and Chronic Health Conditions.
30 pages
Lex Frieden, Program Director

10707 OSERS News in Print: Office of Special Education & Rehabilitative Services
US Department of Education
400 Maryland Avenue SW
Washington, DC 20202-0001
202-205-8241
800-872-5327
www.ed.gov
Provides information, research, and resources in the area of special learning needs.
Quarterly
Lex Frieden, Program Director

Audio & Video

10708 Assisting Parents Through the Mourning Process
Hope
55 E 100 N
Logan, UT 84321-4648
435-752-9533
Fax: 435-752-9533
Describes the mourning process experienced by some parents of children with disabilities and ways in which the professional can help them through the process.
20 minutes

10709 No Fears, No Tears
Leora Kuttner, PhD, author
Fanlight Productions
4196 Washington Street
Boston, MA 02131-1731
617-469-4999
800-937-4113
Fax: 617-469-3379
e-mail: fanlight@fanlight.com
www.fanlight.com
Dr. Leora Kuttner explores the effects of childrens pain management.
1985 28 Minutes

10710 No Fears, No Tears: 13 Years Later
Leora Kuttner, PhD, author
Fanlight Productions
4196 Washington Street
Boston, MA 02131-1731
617-469-4999
800-937-4113
Fax: 617-469-3379
e-mail: fanlight@fanlight.com
www.fanlight.com

Dr. Leora Kutner explores the effects of childrens pain management therapies 13 years after their use.
1998 47 Minutes
ISBN: 1-572952-77-6

Web Sites

10711 Access Unlimited
www.accessunlimited.com
Assists educators, health care providers and parents in discovering how personal computers help children and adults with disabilities compensate for some of the barriers imposed by their conditions.

10712 American Academy of Pediatrics
www.aap.org
Offers information, referrals, treatment and services to children and youth.

10713 American Association for the Advancement of Science
www.aaas.org
Addresses the concerns of scientists and engineers with disabilities, and offers suggestions about improving accessibility of science programs for students with disabilities.

10714 American Bar Association Commission
www.abanet.org/disability

10715 American Camp Association
www.acacamps.org
Formerly the American Camping Association, the ACA works to preserve, promote and improve the camp experience.

10716 American Counseling Association
www.counseling.org
This association was organized to enhance human development throughout the life span and to promote the counseling profession.

10717 American Institute for Preventive Medicine
www.healthylife.com
The Institute provides health promotion programs and self-care publications to hospitals, HMOs, corporations and governments agencies. Programs are designed to lower health care costs, decrease absenteeism, improve morale and increase visibility.

10718 American Organ Transplant Association
www.aotaonline.org
Helps defray out-of-pocket expenses for liver, heart, lung and pancreas transplant recipients.

10719 American Red Cross
www.redcross.org
Offers seminars, conferences and newsletters with 2,889 local chapters.

10720 American Self-Help Group Clearinghouse
www.selfhelpgroups.org
A clearinghouse that makes referrals to self-help groups throughout the nation. Publishes a variety of materials that are helpful to professionals and consumers who would like to start self-help groups.

10721 American Society of Dermatology
www.asd.org
The purpose of this organization is to make optimal care available to all citizens of this country by preserving, promoting, and enhancing the practice of dermatology.

10722 Americas Association for the Care of the Children
www.aacchildren.net
An international multidisciplinary organization which promotes the emotional, developmental, and psychosocial well-being of children and families in all health care settings.

10723 Beach Center on Families and Disability
www.beachcenter.org
A federally funded center that conducts research and training in the factors that contribute to the successful functioning of families with members who have disabilities.

10724 Center for Chronic Disease Prevention and Health Promotion
www.cdc.gov/nccdphp
The Center for Disease Control and Prevention (CDC) is recognized as the lead federal agency for protecting the health and safety of people - at home and abroad - providing credible information to enhance health decisions, and promoting health through strong partnerships. CDC serves as the national focus for developing and applying disease prevention and control, environmental health, and health promotion and education activities designed to improve the health of the people of the United States.

10725 Center for Developmental Disabilities
www.centerfor.com
The Center for Developmental Disabilities is committed to help children and adults with differing abilities achieve their dreams by overcoming barriers to living, learning, working and recreating in the community of their choice.

10726 ChiroWeb.com
www.chiroweb.com
Chiropractic news source for chiropractors, students, patients and health care professionals. Over 7,000 articles are available.

10727 Commission on Accreditation of Rehabilitation Services
www.carf.org
CARF reviews and grants accreditation services nationally and internationally on request of a facility or program. Their standards are rigorous, so those services that meet them are among the best available.

10728 Disabled & Alone: Life Services
www.disabledandalone.org
Provides services to handicapped persons, their families and organizations.

10729 Discovery Health
www.health.discovery.com
A large website covering various health topics; such as male and female health, senior health, children's health, mental health, alternative medicine, nutrition, fitness, and more.

10730 Educational Equity Center at AED
www.edequity.org
EEC at AED is an outgrowth of Educational Equity Concepts, a national not-for-profit organization with a 22-year history of promoting educational excellence for all children.

10731 Federation for Children with Special Needs
www.fcsn.org
A center for parents and parent organizations to work together on behalf of children with special needs and their families.

10732 Healing Well
www.healingwell.com
An online health resource guide to medical news, chat, information and articles, newsgroups and message boards, books, disease-related web sites, medical directories, and more for patients, friends, and family coping with disabling diseases, disorders, or chronic illnesses.

10733 Health Care For All
www.hcfa.org
HCFA seeks to create a consumer-centered health care system that provides comprehensive, affordable, accessible, culturally competent, high quality care and consumer education for everyone, especially the most vulnerable.

10734 Health Finder
www.healthfinder.gov
Searchable, carefully developed web site offering information on over 1000 topics. Developed by the US Department of Health and Human Services, the site can be used in both English and Spanish.

10735 Health on the Net Foundation
www.hon.ch
One of the world's leading certifiers of the reliability and authority on health-related information on the Internet. Offers individuals suffering from a specific illness or disability access to relevant information and links to support communities. Features a full listing of health information and support community sources, together with testimonials.

10736 Healthcentral.com
www.healthcentral.com

The HealthCentral Network offers timely, in-depth and reliable medical information. It has a collection of owned and operated web sites and multimedia affiliate properties providing personalized tools and resources for people seeking to manage and improve their health.

10737 Healthlink USA

www.healthlinkusa.com

Health information concerning treatment, cures, prevention, diagnosis, risk factors, research, support groups, email lists, personal stories and much more. Updated regularly.

10738 Helios Health

www.helioshealth.com

Online resource for your health information. Detailed information about specific health topics, access to expert advice from our Medical Advisory Board, and up-to-date health news.

10739 Life Development Institute

www.life-development-inst.org

Serves older adolescents and adults with learning disabilities and related disorders. Conducts programs to assist individuals to achieve careers/employment commensurate with capabilities to achieve an independent status.

10740 MedicineNet

www.medicinenet.com

An online resource for consumers providing easy-to-read, authoritative medical and health information.

10741 Medscape

www.mywebmd.com

Medscape offers specialists, primary care physicians, and other health professionals the Web's most robust and integrated medical information and educational tools.

10742 Medtronic

www.medtronic.com

Medtronic is changing the face of chronic disease. By working closely with physicians around the world, they create therapies to help patients do things they never thought were possible.

10743 National Clearinghouse of Rehabilitation Training Materials

www.nchrtm.okstate.edu

The mission of the NCRTM is to advocate for the advancement of best practice in rehabilitation counseling through the development, collection, dissemination, and utilization of professional knowledge, information and skill.

10744 National Council on Disability

www.ncd.gov

The National Council on Disability is an independent federal agency that works with the President and Congress to increase the inclusion, independence and empowerment of Americans with disabilities.

10745 National Organization for Rare Disorders (NORD)

www.rarediseases.org

Serves as a clearinghouse for information about rare disorders and brings together families with similar disorders for mutual support; fosters communication among rare disease voluntary agencies, Government agencies, industry, scientific researchers, academic institutions, and concerned individuals; and encourages and promotes research and education on rare disorders and orphan drugs.

10746 Office of Special Education and Rehabilitative Services

www.ed.gov/offices

The Office of Special Education and Rehabilitative Servics (OSERS) is committed to improving the results and outcomes for people with disabilities of all ages.

10747 WebMD

www.webmd.com

General information, including articles.

10748 World Institute on Disability

www.wid.org

A public policy center that is run by persons with disabilities. Research, public education, training and model program development as means to create a more accessible and supportive society for all people - disabled and nondisabled alike.

National Agencies & Associations

10749 A Wish with Wings
917 W Sanford 817-469-9474
Arlington, TX 76012 Fax: 817-275-6005
e-mail: wish@awishwithwings.org
www.awishwithwings.org
Grants the wishes of Texas children with life-threatening diseases.
Pat Skaggs, Founder
Greg Morse, President

10750 Adventures for Wish Kids
8595 Beechmont Avenue 513-232-5104
Cincinnati, OH 45255 800-543-9735
Fax: 513-474-2324
e-mail: customerservice@afwkids.org
www.akidagain.org
Enrich the lives of children with life threatening illnesses and their families by providing year round fun-filled group activities and destination events fostering joy laughter normalcy and supportive networking opportunities.
Hap Durkin, Executive Director
Kathy Wagoner, Director Volunteers/Program Services

10751 BASE Camp Children's Cancer Foundation
140 N Orlando Avenue 407-673-5060
Winter Park, FL 32789-9061 Fax: 407-673-5095
e-mail: email@basecamp.org
www.basecamp.org
Does not grant wishes but does help obtain free or reduced price tickets to Walt Disney World Universal Studios etc for children with a hematology/oncology disease and their immediate family. Children must be on-treatment when the application is received.
Terri Jones, President/Founder
Jackie Ellis, Executive Director

10752 Believe In Tomorrow National Children's Fo undation
6601 Frederick Road 410-744-1032
Baltimore, MD 21228 800-933-5470
Fax: 410-744-1984
e-mail: info@believeintomorrow.org
www.believeintomorrow.org
Formerly Grant-A-Wish Foundation, this Foundation provides exceptional hospital and retreat housing services to critically ill children and their families. The Foundation also believes that keeping families together during a child's medical crisis, and that the gentle caring environment is crucial.
Brian R Morrison, Founder
Richard E McCready, Chairman

10753 Children's Hopes and Dreams Foundation
138 Cloudland Road 706-482-2248
Dahlonega, GA 30533 800-437-3262
Fax: 706-482-2289
www.helpingnow.org
Fulfills dreams of children with life-threatening illnesses.
Vick Franklin, President

10754 Children's Wish Foundation International
8615 Roswell Road 770-393-9474
Atlanta, GA 30350-7526 800-323-9474
Fax: 770-393-0683
e-mail: arthurs@childrenswish.org
www.childrenswish.org
Committed to bringing joy and happiness to seriously ill children throughout the world and this dedication has created special experiences for children around the globe. Our commitment is also developing hospital enrichment programs.
Arthur Stein, President/CEO
Linda Dozoretz, Executive Director

10755 Cure Our Children Foundation
711 S Carson Street 310-355-6046
Carson City, NV 89701 Fax: 310-454-9592
e-mail: barry@cureourchildren.org
www.cureourchildren.org
Support medical approaches to treatment of Ewings Sarcoma. Alternate and complimentary treatment information is provided only for use in conjunction with traditional approaches.
Barry Sugarman, President

10756 Dream Come True
PO Box 21167 610-865-3475
Lehigh Valley, PA 18002 Fax: 610-865-4710
e-mail: RVasko@aol.com
www.dreamcometrue.org
Seeks to fulfill the dreams of children who are seriously chronically and terminally ill and reside in the greater Lehigh Valley area.
Kostas Kalogeropoulo, Founder/President
David Yanoshik, First Vice President

10757 Dream Factory National Headquarters
National Headquarters
200 W Broadway 502-361-3001
Louisville, KY 40202 800-456-7556
Fax: 502-561-3004
e-mail: info@dreamfactoryinc.com
www.dreamfactoryinc.org
Grants wishes for chronically or seriously ill children.
AP Bunger, National Director/CEO
Elizabeth Wayne, Program Services Coordinator

10758 Dream Foundation
1528 Chapala Street 805-564-2131
Santa Barbara, CA 93101 Fax: 805-564-7002
www.dreamfoundation.org
Enhance the quality of life for individuals and families battling terminal illnesses ages 18 and over.
Thomas Rollerson, Founder/President
Carol Brown, Chief Operating Officer

10759 Fairygodmother Foundation
550 W Webster Avenue 773-388-1160
Chicago, IL 60614 Fax: 773-883-3656
e-mail: info@fairygodmother.org
www.fairygodmother.org
Our wish granting program brings joy to the lives of adults (18 and older) and loved ones in their time of greatest need by turning dreams into reality. In the process of fulfilling wishes, we create an opportunity for peace, closure and a sense of belonging.
Lena Clement, Program Director

10760 Friends of Karen
118 Tactics Road 914-277-4547
Purdys, NY 10578 Fax: 914-277-4967
e-mail: info@friendsofkaren.org
www.friendsofkaren.org
Dedicated to helping terminally and catastrophically ill children and their families in the New York metropolitan area only. They provide assistance with payments for physicians, hospitals and medications, help with extra expenses beyond medical bills.
Judith Factor, Executive Director
Rhonda Ryan, Director of Social Work

10761 Give Kids the World
210 S Bass Road 407-396-1114
Kissimmee, FL 34746 800-995-KIDS
Fax: 407-396-1207
e-mail: dream@gktw.org
www.gktw.org
A 70-acre non-profit resort in Central Florida that creates magical memories for children with life- threatening illnesses and their families. GKTW provides accommodations at its whimsical resort, donated attractions, tickets, meals and more for a week-long stay.
Henri Landwirth, Founder
Pamela Landwirth, President

10762 High Hopes Foundation
416 K Daniel Webster Highway 603-429-1010
Merrimack, NH 03054 800-639-6804
Fax: 603-429-0037
e-mail: info@highhopesnh.net
www.highhopesnh.org
Helps families and friends of seriously ill children ages 3-18 by funding and facilitating the fulfillment of the last or fondest wishes.
Jacque Yinger, Founder
Pam Shuddle, President

10763 Kidd's Kids
220 E Las Colinas Boulevard
Irving, TX 75039
972-432-8595
866-541-5437
Fax: 214-853-5212
e-mail: derrick@kiddlive.com
www.kiddskids.com
Founded by nationally syndicated morning show personality Kidd Kraddick. Provides chronically ill and/or physically challenged children between the ages of 5 to 12 with an unforgettable adventure.
Derrick M Brown, Executive Director
Brenda Adriance, President

10764 Kids Incorporated
9300 Old Keene Mill Road
Burke, VA 22015-4277
703-455-5437
Fax: 703-440-9208
www.jcambellinc.com
Grants wishes to gravely ill children 16 years and younger. Children older than 16 are sometimes eligible depending on child's situation and the availability of resources.
John Campbell, President

10765 Kids Wish Network
4060 Louis Avenue
Holiday, FL 34691
727-937-3600
888-918-9004
Fax: 727-937-3688
e-mail: info@kidswishnetwork.org
www.kidswishnetwork.org
A nationally recognized charitable organization dedicated to infusing hope creating happy memories and improving the quality of life for children. The Network also fulfills the wishes of children ages 3 to 18 with life threatening medical conditions.
Shelley Breiner, Founder
Mark Breiner, Founder

10766 Magic Moments c/o Children's Hospital
c/o Children's Hospital
1600 7th Avenue S
Birmingham, AL 35233
205-939-9372
Fax: 205-939-6717
e-mail: info@magicmoments.org
www.magicmoments.org
Grants wishes to children 4 to 19 living or being treated in Alabama who have chronic life-threatening diseases or who have severe trauma (burn spinal cord head trauma).
Pam Jones, Executive Director
Julie Ellis, Wish Coordinator

10767 Make-A-Wish Foundation
3550 N Central Avenue
Phoenix, AZ 85012-2127
602-279-9474
800-722-9474
Fax: 602-279-0855
e-mail: mawfa@wish.org
www.wish.org
A national organization that grants wishes for children with terminally or life threatening diseases and who are 18 years of age or younger.
David Williams, President/CEO
Robert J Bigler, Board and Executive Committee Chair

10768 Marty Lyons Foundation
326 W 48th Street
New York, NY 10036
212-977-9474
Fax: 212-977-1752
e-mail: maryannc@martylyonsfoundation.org
www.martylyonsfoundation.org
A national organization that grants wishes of children between the ages of three and seventeen who have life-threatening diseases or terminal illnesses. Those interested can submit applications for their wish fulfillment.
Mary Ann Canapi, Executive Director
Pamel Pfarr, Program Services Manager

10769 New Hope for Kids
205 E SR 436
Fern Park, FL 32730
407-331-3059
Fax: 407-331-3063
e-mail: dave@newhopeforkids.org
www.newhopeforkids.org
An Orlando-based organization granting wishes to children aged under one who have life-threatening illnesses. Focuses primarily on children living in Florida but has also granted withes to children from other parts of the US Canada England and Russia.
Dave Joswick, Executive Director
Tamari C Miller, Grief Program Director

10770 Rainbow Connection
621 W University
Rochester, MI 48307
248-601-9474
877-649-4743
Fax: 248-601-0086
e-mail: info@rainbowconnection.org
www.rainbowwishconnection.org
Make the special wishes of children with life-threatening or terminal illnesses come true.
L Brooks Patterson, Founder
Jeff Hauswirth, President

10771 Special Wish Foundation
1250 Memory Lane
Columbus, OH 43209
614-258-3186
800-486-9474
Fax: 614-258-3518
e-mail: info@spwish.org
www.spwish.org
A Special Wish Foundation Inc. is a non-profit charitable organization dedicated to granting the wishes of children under the age of 21 who have been diagnosed with a life-threatening disorder.
Laura Marchetta, Contact/Chicago Chapter
Patti Piening, Contact/Cincinnati

10772 Starlight Foundation
5757 Wilshire Boulevard
Los Angeles, CA 90036-1035
310-479-1212
800-274-7827
www.starlight.org
A non-profit organization dedicated to brightening the lives of seriously ill children and their families.
Steven Spielberg, Chairman Emeritus
Peter Samuelson, Co-Founder

10773 Sunshine Foundation National Headquarters
National Headquarters
1041 Mill Creek Drive
Feasterville, PA 19053
215-396-4770
Fax: 215-396-4774
e-mail: philly@sunshinefoundation.org
www.sunshinefoundation.org
Answers the dreams of seriously ill physically challenged and abused children aged three to eighteen whose families cannot fulfill their requests due to financial strain that the child's illness may cause.
Bill Sample, President/Founder
Kate Sample, Administrator

10774 Teddi Project Camp Good Days & Special Times
Camp Good Days & Special Times
1332 Pittsford-Mendon Road
Mendon, NY 14506
585-624-5555
800-785-2135
Fax: 585-624-5799
www.campgooddays.org
A non-profit organization that provides a camping experience and more for children and adults facing the toughest challenges of life. Accepts the wishes of terminal ill children through age eighteen.
Gary Mervis, Founder/Chairman

10775 Vision Foundation
8901 Strafford Circle
Knoxville, TN 37923-1567
865-357-4603
Fax: 865-690-9322
e-mail: gordon@visionfoundation.net
www.visionfoundation.net
Offers counseling support groups seminars and transportation for the blind providing 600 members.
Gordon Adams, Executive Director/President
Hank Brink, Vice President

10776 Wish Upon A Star
PO Box 4000
Visalia, CA 93278
559-733-7753
800-821-6805
Fax: 559-733-0962
e-mail: info@wishuponastar.org
www.wishuponastar.org

A non-profit law enforcement effort designed to grant the wishes of children afflicted with high-risk and life threatening illnesses.
Keith Gomes, President
Carmen Perez, Executive Director

10777 Wishing Star Foundation
139 S Sherman
Spokane, WA 99202
509-744-3411
Fax: 509-744-3414
e-mail: paulan@wishingstar.org
www.wishingstar.org
Grants wishes to children with life threatening illnesses. Ages 3-21 in Eastern Washington and all of Idaho.
Paula Nordga MEd MSW, Executive Director
Donna Halvorson, Development Director

10778 Wishing Well Foundation
3000 W Esplanade Avenue
Metairie, LA 70002
504-841-0001
888-663-9474
e-mail: wellfoundation@bellsouth.net
www.wishingwellusa.org
To bring joy to children with life threatening illnesses by providing them with their fondest wish for life.
Elwin Lebeau, President

State Agencies & Associations

Connecticut

10779 Dream Come True of Western Connecticut
PO Box 2415
Danbury, CT 06813
203-790-7333
www.dreamcometruect.org
Marilyn Arents, Chair
Betsy Delaney, Vice President

Illinois

10780 Central Illinois Dream Factory
PO Box 1431
Pekin, IL 61554
30- 35- 730
Fax: 309-353-7311
e-mail: cidreamfactory@yahoo.com
www.dreamfactoryci.com
Victoria Buckley, Area Coordinator

Kansas

10781 Dream Factory of Greater Kansas City
PO Box 26185
Shawnee Mission, KS 66225-6185
913-905-2900
e-mail: info@kcdreamfactory.org
www.kcdream.org
Gavin Steketee, President/Board of Directors
Ralph Apel, Vice President

Maryland

10782 Adventures for Wish Kids: Metropolitan DC Chapter
6863 Oak Creek Drive
Columbus, OH 43229
614-797-9500
800-543-9735
Fax: 614-797-9600
e-mail: customerservice@afwkids.org
www.akidagain.org
Jeffrey D Damron CFRE, CEO
Vicki L Poliseno, Director of Operations

Ohio

10783 Adventures for Wish Kids: Columbus Chapter
6863 Oak Creek Drive
Columbus, OH 43229
614-797-9500
800-543-9735
Fax: 614-797-9600
e-mail: customerservice@afwkids.org
www.akidagain.org
Jeffrey D Damron CFRE, CEO
Vicki L Poliseno, Director of Operations

10784 Adventures for Wish Kids: Dayton Chapter
2850 Presidential Drive
Fairborn, OH 45324
937-427-8700
Fax: 937-427-8775
e-mail: dsamic@akidagain.org
www.akidagain.org
Deborah Samic, Executive Director

Wisconsin

10785 Make-A-Wish Foundation of Wisconsin
13195 W Hampton Avenue
Butler, WI 53007
262-781-4445
800-236-9474
Fax: 262-781-3736
e-mail: info@wisconsin.wish.org
www.wisconsin.wish.org
Grants the wishes of children with life-threatening medical conditions to enrich the human experience with hope, strength and joy.
Patty Gorsky, President
Kathy Ehnert, Director of Finance & Operations

10786 Make-A-Wish Foundation of Wisconsin: North eastern Chapter
200 N Durkee Street
Appleton, WI 54911
920-993-9994
Fax: 920-993-9996
e-mail: jvervoort@wisconsin.wish.org
www.wisconsin.wish.org
Patty Gorsky, President
Kathy Ehnert, Director of Finance & Operations

Foundations

10787 Angelwish
PO Box 186
Rutherford, NJ 07070
201-672-0722
Fax: 440-699-4337
e-mail: info@angelwish.org
www.angelwish.org
Provides the public with an easy way to grant wishes to the millions of children that are living with HIV/AIDS around the world. Infected or affected by the disease, their opportunities for a normal childhood are virtually impossible. By harnessing the power of the Internet, Angelwish helps donors add a ray of hope to their lives.
Shimmy Mehta, Founder/CEO
Jim Brinksma, Director

10788 Chef David's Kids
1100 E Oakland Park Boulevard
Fort Lauderdale, FL 33334
954-594-1024
e-mail: chefdavidmitchell@gmail.com
www.chefdavidskids.org
Helps children afflicted with any form of terminal illness such as cancer, leukemia, and pediatric HIV. Also helps neglected and abused children.
Chef David Mitchell, Founder/Director of Operations
Laurie Amber, National Hospital Events Director

10789 Children's Wish Foundation of Canada
350-1101 Kingston Road
Pickering, Ontario, L1V-1B5
905-839-8882
800-700-4437
Fax: 905-839-3745
e-mail: linda.marco@childrenswish.ca
www.childrenswish.ca
Works with the community to provide children living with high risk life threatening illnesses the opportunity to realize their most heartfelt wish.
Chris Kotsopoulos, Director
Linda Marco, Communications/Development Nat'l Manager

10790 Dreams Come True
6803 Southpoint Parkway
Jacksonville, FL 32216
904-296-3030
Fax: 904-296-4244
e-mail: postmaster@dreamscometrue.org
www.dreamscometrue.org
In over 22 years, more than 1,950 dreams already have come true for children battling life-threatening illnesses in Northeast Florida and Southeast Georgia.
Suzanne G Crittenden, Executive Director
Brandi Cook, Director of Dreams

10791 **Jason's Dreams for Kids**
20 Monmouth Street 732-758-0060
Red Bank, NJ 07701 Fax: 732-758-0070
e-mail: jasonsdreams@comcast.net
www.jasonsdreamsforkids.com
Devoted to granting wishes to children diagnosed with life-threatening illnesses. Holds a variety of fundraising events to meet the cost of fulfilling these childrens' wishes.

10792 **Little Star Foundation**
256 Rancho Milagro Way 970-925-9540
Hesperus, CO 81326 800-543-6565
e-mail: info@littlestar.org
www.littlestar.org
Provides lifetime opportunities for children with cancer to enhance the quality of their lives.
Andrea Jaeger, Co-Founder & President

10793 **Make-A-Wish-Foundation of Canada**
4211 Yonge Street 416-224-9474
Toronto, Ontario, M2P-2A9 888-822-9474
Fax: 416-224-8795
e-mail: nationaloffice@makeawish.ca
www.makeawish.ca
Grants the wishes of children with life-threatening illnesses to enrich the human experience with hope, strength and joy.
Brigitte Tschinkel, Corporate Development Director
Trish River, Administrative Coordinator

10794 **Starlight Starbright Children's Foundation**
5757 Whilshire Boulevard 310-479-1212
Los Angeles, CA 90036 800-315-2580
Fax: 310-479-1235
e-mail: info@starlight.org
www.starlight.org
Helps seriously ill children and their families cope with their pain, fear and isolation through entertainment, education and family activities.
Paula Van Ness, CEO
Rafe Pery, COO/VP, Operations

10795 **Sunshine Dreams for Kids**
495 Richmond Street, Suite 400 519-642-0990
London, Ontario, N6A-5A9 800-461-7935
Fax: 800-461-7475
e-mail: info@sunshine.ca
www.sunshine.ca
Grants dreams to children who are between the ages of 3 and 19 who are challenged by severephysical disabilities or life threatening illnesses.
Michael Barr, HBA, President
Jon Osier, CA, Vice-President

10796 **United Special Sportsman Alliance**
7864 Shotwell Road 715-884-2256
Pittsville, WI 54466 800-518-8019
Fax: 715-884-7388
www.childwish.com
A dream wish granting charity that specializes in sending critically ill and disabled youth on the outdoor adventure of their dreams.
Brigid O'Donoghue, President/Founder
Annette Johnson, Communications Director

National Agencies & Associations

10797 Children's Hospice International
901 N Pitt Street
Alexandria, VA 22314
703-684-0330
800-24C-HILD
Fax: 703-684-0226
e-mail: info@chionline.org
www.chionline.org

This organization was founded to provide a network of support and care for children with life threatening conditions and their families. The hospice is a team effort which provides medical, psychological, social and spiritual expertise in the US and abroad.
Ann Armstrong-Dailey, Founding Director/CEO
Rebecca Brant, Director

10798 Compassionate Friends
PO Box 3696
Oak Brook, IL 60522-3696
630-990-0010
877-969-0010
Fax: 630-990-0246
e-mail: nationaloffice@compassionatefriends.org
www.compassionatefriends.org

A national organization that offers 470 local chapters that give support to people who have experienced the death of a child. Offers monthly support meetings to get through the difficult times and learn how to cope.
Patricia Loder, Executive Director
Terry Novy, Chapter Services Coordinator

10799 HOSPICELINK Hospice Education Institute
Hospice Education Institute
3 Unity Square
Machiasport, MA 04655-0098
207-255-8800
800-331-1620
Fax: 207-255-8008
e-mail: info@hospiceworld.org
www.hospiceworld.org

Provides educational and informational services to health professionals and the public on subjects such as hospice care death and dying and bereavement counseling.
Michal Galazka, Executive Director
Jodi Sprague, Administrator

10800 Helping Other Parents in Normal Grieving Underwood Memorial Hospital
Underwood Memorial Hospital
509 N Broad Street
Woodbury, NJ 08096
856-845-0100
www.umhospital.org

Offers support to newly bereaved parents through trained parents who have suffered a similar loss and resolved their grief. Promotes community education regarding the effects that a miscarriage stillbirth of neonatal death has on parents.
Carolyn R Wickman, Coordinator

10801 Hospice Association of America
228 7th Street SE
Washington, DC 20003-4306
202-546-4759
Fax: 202-547-9559
e-mail: ads@nahc.org
www.nahc.org/haa

Promotes the concepts of hospice a philosophy of health care which is expressed through the provision of a variety of medical and nonmedical services to terminally ill patients and their families.
Janet E Neigh, Executive Director

10802 National Hospice & Palliative Care Organization
1700 Diagonal Road
Alexandria, VA 22314
703-837-1500
800-658-8898
Fax: 703-525-5762
e-mail: nhpcoinfo@nhpco.org
www.nhpco.org

The nation's only advocate for terminally ill patients and their families. Founded in 1978, the NHPCO is the only organization devoted to hospice in the United States. Support is included from state hospice organizations, patients, families, communities, provider program members and professional/volunteer members. Represents hospice care interests to Congress, regulatory agencies, courts, voluntary organizations and the public.

10803 National Hospice & Palliative Care Organiz ation
1731 King Street
Alexandria, VA 22314
703-837-1500
800-658-8898
Fax: 703-837-1233
e-mail: nhpco_info@nhpco.org
www.nhpco.org

The nation's only advocate for terminally ill patients and their families. Founded in 1978, the NHPCO is the only organization devoted to hospice in the United States. Support is included from state hospice organizations, patients, families and communities.
J Donald Schumacher, President/CEO
Galen Miller, Executive Vice President

10804 National Institute for Jewish Hospice
732 University Street
N Woodmere, NY 11581
516-791-9888
800-446-4448
Fax: 516-791-6999
e-mail: mlamm@nijh.org
www.nijh.org

Serves as a resource center that seeks to help terminal patients and their families deal with their grief by providing information on traditional Jewish views on death dying and managing the loss of a loved one.
Shirley Lamm, Executive Director
Maurice Lamm, Founder/President

10805 Pregnancy and Infant Loss Center
1421 E Wayzata Boulevard
Wayzata, MN 55391
612-473-9372
www.babycenter.com

Offers studies information statistics help and support to parents who have suffered the loss of a child.

10806 Wrap Myself in a Rainbow Compassion Books
Compassion Books
7036 State Highway 80 S
Burnsville, NC 28714-7569
828-675-5909
800-970-4220
Fax: 828-675-9687
e-mail: bruce@compassionbooks.com
www.compassionbooks.com

This is a collection of poignant songs and sensitive guided images that validates and transforms loss with hope. Side I is guided meditation Side II delivers powerful performances of Over The Rainbow, Rainbow Connection and Bring Rainbows to Children.
Audio Cassette
Bruce Greene, Director
Karen Walker, Staff

Support Groups & Hotlines

10807 Bereavement Group for Children
Corstone Center
33 Buchanan Drive
Sausalito, CA 94965-2535
415-331-6161
Fax: 415-331-4545
e-mail: info@corstone.org
www.corstone.org

For children who have suffered the loss of a close loved one. Parent group meets separately at the same time.
Steve Leventhal, Executive Director
Richard Cuadra, MS, Program Director

10808 Grief & Loss Support Group
First Love Outreach Ministries
PO Box 06204
Milwaukee, WI 53206
414-263-1323
Fax: 414-263-1148
e-mail: zelodius@aol.com
www.firstlovelifecoaching.com

Pr Zelodius Morton, CEO

10809 National Hospice Helpline
1700 Diaganal Road
Alexandria, VA 22314
703-837-1500
800-658-8898
Fax: 703-525-5762
e-mail: nhpcoinfo@nhpco.org
www.nhpco.org

Offers more information on hospice in general and offers referrals to a hospice program in your area.
Scott Vickers, Manager Consumer Resources
John Radulovic, Vice President of Communications

10810 **Rainbows for All God's Children**
2100 Gold Road, Suite 370
Rolling Meadows, IL 60008
847-952-1770
Fax: 847-952-1774
e-mail: info@rainbows.org
www.rainbows.org
A support program for children who have suffered a significant loss in their lives due to death, divorce or any other painful transition.
Suzy Yehl Marta, Founder & President

Books

10811 **A Good Death: Conversations with East Londoners**
Lesley Cullen and Michael Young, author
Routledge
270 Madison Avenue
New York, NY 10016
212-216-7800
Fax: 212-563-2269
www.routledge.com
Based on a survey in East London and provides a wide range of fascinating and helpful insights into all aspects of experiencing death and surviving grief. The voices in the book are those of people who have managed to cope despite being under the shadow of impending death. Their experience could be a comfort to antbody in a similar situation. A Good Death is intended for people who are dying, for thier lay and professional careers and for student doctors, nurses, and social workers.

ISBN: 0-415137-96-9

10812 **Anatomy of Bereavement**
Jason Aronson
PO Box 15100
York, PA 17405-7100
800-782-0015
Fax: 201-840-7242
www.aronson.com
In this comprehensive book, Dr. Raphael describes all the stages of mourning and healing.
454 pages Softcover
ISBN: 1-568212-70-4

10813 **Bereaved Parent**
Harriet Sarnoff Schiff, author
Penguin USA
375 Hudson Street
New York, NY 10014
212-366-2372
Fax: 212-366-2933
www.penguingroup.com
Very understanding book especially useful to parents who may not have a strong religious faith.
146 pages
ISBN: 0-140050-43-4

10814 **Concerning Death: A Practical Guide for the Living**
Earl A. Grollman, author
Beacon Press
25 Beacon Street
Boston, MA 02108-2824
617-742-2110
Fax: 617-723-3097
www.beacon.org
A guide for people to learn how to cope with death and dying, and the many decisions involved in the process.
265 pages
ISBN: 0-807027-65-0

10815 **Conversations At Midnight**
William Morrow & Company/Order Department
39 Plymouth Street
Fairfield, NJ 07004-1633
973-227-7200
800-821-1513
Herbert Kramer is dying of cancer. For him, as for everyone someday, death is now an unavoidable companion. This book tells how Herb learns to acknowledge this presence and come to terms with human mortality. This book is a powerful way to look at death and to deal with losing a loved one.
256 pages Hardcover
ISBN: 0-688120-84-9

10816 **Death and the Quest for Meaning**
Stephen Strack & Herman Feifel, author
Rowman & Littlefield Publishers, Inc.
4501 Forbes Blvd., Suite 200
Lanham, MD 20706
301-459-3366
Fax: 301-429-5748
www.rowmanlittlefield.com
This work covers all aspects of the study of death and dying and the care of the bereaved.
Hardcover
ISBN: 0-765700-14-x

10817 **Death: The Final Stage of Growth**
Elisabeth Kubler-Ross, author
Simon & Schuster
15 Columbus Circle
New York, NY 10023-7707
212-373-8000
www.prenhall.com
This books shows readers how to come to terms with death as a part of human development, and how death can provide us with a key meaning of human existence.

10818 **Difference in the Family**
Penguin Putnam
PO Box 999
Bergenfield, NJ 07621-0903
201-387-0600
800-526-0275
Fax: 800-227-9604
A frank chronicle of the grief, rage and guilt everyone in a family suffers after a death, and the adjustments each make to cope.
Helen Featherstone, Editor

10819 **Dying and Disabled Children**
Haworth Press
10 Alice Street
Binghamton, NY 13904-1580
607-722-5857
800-429-6784
Fax: 607-722-0012
www.haworthpress.com
In this sensitive and compassionate look at terminally ill and disabled children, professionals from the medical community examine the stresses faced by their parents and siblings. They address crucial element of communication in dealing with a child's serious illness. Ethical decision making, learning to recognize the child's suffering, and talking to children about death are honestly and clearly discussed.
153 pages Hardcover
ISBN: 0-866567-59-0

10820 **Explaining Death to Children**
Earl A. Grollman, author
Beacon Press
25 Beacon Street
Boston, MA 02108-2824
617-742-2110
Fax: 617-723-3097
www.beacon.org
A book about explaining death to your children.

10821 **For Those Who Live: Helping Children Cope with Death of a Brother or Sister**
Centering Corporation
7230 Maple Street
Omaha, NE 68134
402-553-1200
866-218-0101
Fax: 402-553-0507
e-mail: danni@centeringcorp.com
www.centering.org
Deals with the grieving family as a whole and offers references for further help.
122 pages
Kathy LaTour, Editor

10822 **Grief, Dying and Death: Clinical Intervention for Caregivers**
Research Press
2612 N Mattis Avenue
Champaign, IL 61822-1053
217-352-3273
800-519-2707
Fax: 217-352-1221
e-mail: rp@researchpress.com
www.researchpress.com
In this comprehensive manual, the author provides both the theoretical background and the practical treatment interventions necessary for working with those who are bereaved or dying. Important topics such as anticipatory grief, postdeath mourning and the stress of grief are described in detail. Grief reactions, both normal and abnormal, as well as their causes are analyzed. Special attention is

given to grief caused by death of a child or spouse, death by suicide, and children's grief.
488 pages Softcover
ISBN: 0-878222-32-4

10823 Helper's Journey
Research Press
2612 N Mattis Avenue 217-352-3273
Champaign, IL 61822-1053 800-519-2707
Fax: 217-352-1221
e-mail: rp@researchpress.com
www.researchpress.com
This groundbreaking work, written for both professional and volunteer caregivers, provides exercises, activities and specific strategies for more successful caregiving, increased personal growth and effective stress management. In this thoughtfully written book, Dr. Larson explores the theory and practice of helping. He includes numerous case examples and verbatim disclosures of fellow caregivers that powerfully convey the joys and sorrows of the helpers journey.
292 pages Softcover
ISBN: 0-878223-44-4

10824 On Children and Death
MacMillan Publishing Company
175 Fifth Avenue 646-307-5151
New York, NY 10010
A touching work about how children and their parents can and do cope with death.
277 pages Paperback

10825 On Death and Dying
MacMillan Publishing Company
175 Fifth Avenue 646-307-5151
New York, NY 10010
A wonderful book offering information on how to deal and cope with death and dying.
Paperback

10826 Recovery from Bereavement
Jason Aronson
PO Box 15100
York, PA 17405-7100 800-782-0015
Fax: 201-840-7242
www.aronson.com
Outstanding authorities on loss and bereavement discuss the factors that play a role in successful recovery.
344 pages Softcover
ISBN: 1-568213-61-1

10827 Talking About Death
Beacon Press
25 Beacon Street 617-742-2110
Boston, MA 02108-2824 Fax: 617-723-3097
www.beacon.org

10828 Treatment of Complicated Mourning
Research Press
2612 N Mattis Avenue 217-352-3273
Champaign, IL 61822-1053 800-519-2707
Fax: 217-352-1221
e-mail: rp@researchpress.com
www.researchpress.com
This is the first book to focus specifically on complicated mourning, often referred to as pathological, unresolved, or abnormal grief. It provides caregivers with practical therapeutic strategies with and specific interventions that are necessary when traditional grief counseling is insufficient. The author provides critically important information on the prediction, identification, assessment, classification and treatment of complicated mourning.
768 pages Hardcover
ISBN: 0-878223-29-0

10829 What Helped Me When My Loved One Died
Beacon Press
25 Beacon Street 617-742-2110
Boston, MA 02108-2824 Fax: 617-723-3097
www.beacon.org

Children's Books

10830 Aarvy Aardvark Finds Hope
Donna O'Toole, author
Centering Corporation
7230 Maple Street
Omaha, NE 68134 866-218-0101
Fax: 402-553-0507
www.centering.org
A best selling illustrated read-aloud story of the pain and sadness of loss and the hope of grief recovery.
80 pages Paperback
Bruce Greene, Director

10831 Badger's Parting Gifts
Susan Varley, author
Compassion Books
7036 State Highway 80 S 828-675-5909
Burnsville, NC 28714-7569 800-970-4220
Fax: 828-675-9687
e-mail: heal2grow@aol.com
www.compassionbooks.com
A story of the death of old Badger. As the animals talk about Badger they remember the gift of skills and kindnesses he taught them.
23 pages Paperback
Bruce Greene, Director

10832 Compassion Books
7036 State Highway 80 S 828-675-5909
Burnsville, NC 28714-7569 800-970-4220
Fax: 828-675-9687
e-mail: heal2grow@aol.com
www.compassionbooks.com
Hand picked resources to help people through loss, grief and changes of all kinds. Carry over 400 books and videos on death and dying, bereavement and change, comfort and healing, hope and much more.
Bruce Greene, VP

10833 Fire in My Heart: Ice in My Veins
Enid Samuel Traisman, author
Compassion Books
7036 State Highway 80 S 828-675-5909
Burnsville, NC 28714-7569 800-970-4220
Fax: 828-675-9687
e-mail: heal2grow@aol.com
www.compassionbooks.com
A fill in scrapbook/journal to help teenagers experiencing a loss express feelings, sort out their thoughts and gather memories.
70 pages Paperback
Bruce Greene, Director

10834 Gentle Willow: A Story for Children About Dying
Joyce C. Mills, PhD, author
Magination Press (American Psychological Assoc.)
750 First Street NE 202-336-5510
Washington, DC 20002-4242 800-374-2721
Fax: 202-336-5502
TDD: 202-336-6123
e-mail: magination@apa.org
www.apamaginationpress.apa.org
This book is written for children who may not survive their own illness or for children who know them. This tender and touching tale helps address feelings of disbelief, anger, and sadness, along with love and compassion.
2003 32 pages Hardcover
ISBN: 1-591470-71-7

10835 Great Change
Compassion Books
7036 State Highway 80 S 828-675-5909
Burnsville, NC 28714-7569 800-970-4220
Fax: 828-675-9687
e-mail: heal2grow@aol.com
www.compassionbooks.com

In this deeply moving Native American story, grandmother uses nature to explain death, the great change, to a grieving granddaughter.
32 pages Hardcover
Bruce Greene, Director

10836 Let's Talk About When A Parent Dies
Rosen Publishing Group's PowerKids Press
29 E 21st Street
New York, NY 10010
212-777-3017
800-237-9932
Fax: 888-436-4643
e-mail: customerservice@rosenpub.com
www.rosenpublishing.com
This book guides children through the grieving process in a language they can understand. Recommended for grades K-4.

ISBN: 0-823923-09-6
Elizabeth Weitzman, Author

10837 Nana Upstairs and Nana Downstairs
Compassion Books
7036 State Highway 80 S
Burnsville, NC 28714-7569
828-675-5909
800-970-4220
Fax: 828-675-9687
e-mail: heal2grow@aol.com
www.compassionbooks.com
This charming picture book recognizes that even after a family member dies the love connections continue in heart and home.
32 pages Paperback
Bruce Greene, Director

Magazines

10838 Compassion Books Catalog
Compassion Books
7036 State Highway 80 S
Burnsville, NC 28714-7569
828-675-5909
800-970-4220
Fax: 828-675-9687
e-mail: heal2grow@aol.com
www.compassionbooks.com
More than 400 books and videos to help with serious illness, death and dying, and losses of all kinds.
32 pages
Bruce Greene, Director

Pamphlets

10839 Approaching Grief
Children's Hospice International
901 N Pitt Street
Alexandria, VA 22314
703-684-0330
800-242-4453
Fax: 703-684-0226
e-mail: info@cionline.org
www.chionline.org
Delves into the different stages of grief, guilt, depression, fear, anger, other symptoms. Also tells how children approach grief and ways in which to help your children get past the sorrow.
Ann Armstrong-Dailey, Founding Director/CEO

10840 Pregnancy After a Loss
Abbott Northwestern Hospital Parent Education
800 E 28th Street-Chicago Avenue
Minneapolis, MN 55407
612-863-4000
This booklet is written by a group of parents that have experienced a pregnancy after a loss, sensitively written with suggestions for coping with the fears and anxieties of the new pregnancy.

10841 Pregnancy Heartbreak: Unfulfilled Promises
Abbott Northwestern Hospital Parent Education
800 E 28th Street-Chicago Avenue
Minneapolis, MN 55407
612-863-4000
This handbook is written for parents who had to face the reality of the diagnosis and birth of a baby with life-threatening conditions.

Audio & Video

10842 Encounters with Grief
Fanlight Productions
4196 Washington Street
Boston, MA 02131-1731
617-469-4999
800-937-4113
Fax: 617-469-3379
e-mail: fanlight@fanlight.com
www.fanlight.com
A mother who lost her teenage son, a woman widowed in her sixties and a man whose wife died at fifty-two discuss the emotional upheaval that followed and their moving perspectives on the process of recovery.
1992 13 Minutes
ISBN: 1-572950-91-9

10843 Grave Words: Tools for Discussing End of Life Choices
Maren Monson, MD, author
Fanlight Productions
4196 Washington Street
Boston, MA 02131-1731
617-469-4999
800-937-4113
Fax: 617-469-3379
e-mail: fanlight@fanlight.com
www.fanlight.com
Blends humor, music and insightful interviews to confront the issues that arise in discussions between physicians and healthcare providers and patients about end-of-life care decisions.
1996 25 Minutes
ISBN: 1-572952-24-5

10844 Pitch of Grief
Eric Strange, author
Fanlight Productions
4196 Washington Street
Boston, MA 02131-1731
617-469-4999
800-937-4113
Fax: 617-469-3379
e-mail: fanlight@fanlight.com
www.fanlight.com
Explores the process of grieving through interviews with four bereaved men and women, young and old.
1985 28 Minutes
ISBN: 1-572950-18-8

10845 There Was a Child
Fred Simon, author
Fanlight Productions
4196 Washington Street
Boston, MA 02131-1731
617-469-4999
800-937-4113
Fax: 617-469-3379
e-mail: fanlight@fanlight.com
www.fanlight.com
Demonstrates the impact that losing a pregnancy, or the birth of a stillborn child, has had on three mothers and a father. Validates the emotions of parents who feel alone with their loss, while helping health care workers and families to give appropriate, meaningful support.
1991 32 Minutes
ISBN: 1-572950-48-X

10846 We Will Remember
Compassion Books
7036 State Highway 80 S
Burnsville, NC 28714-7569
828-675-5909
800-970-4220
Fax: 828-675-9687
e-mail: heal2grow@aol.com
www.compassionbooks.com
A video meditation that uses the beauty of natural photography, soothing music and gentle words to give permission and encouragement in using the memories of the past for healing in the present.
11 minutes
Bruce Greene, Director

10847 When the Bough Breaks
Fanlight Productions

4196 Washington Street
Boston, MA 02131-1731
617-469-4999
800-937-4113
Fax: 617-469-3379
e-mail: fanlight@fanlight.com
www.fanlight.com

Based on the real story of a patient who experienced a stillbirth, these ten vignettes dramatically recreate her interactions with health care providers during the final weeks of pregnancy. Study guide included.

1992 71 Minutes

ISBN: 1-572951-08-7

Web Sites

10848 Compassionate Friends

www.compassionatefriends.org/

Organization that offers 470 local chapters that give support to people who have experienced the death of a child.

10849 Hospice Association of America

www.nahc.org/hospice

Promotes the concepts of hospice, a philosophy of health care which is expressed through the provision of a variety of medical and nonmedical services to terminally ill patients and their families.

10850 National Hospice & Palliative Care Org.

www.nhpco.org

The nation's only advocate for terminally ill patients and their families. Founded in 1978, the NHPCO is the only organization devoted to hospice in the United States. Support is included from state hospice organizations, patients, families, communities, provider program members and professional/volunteer members. Represents hospice care interests to Congress, regulatory agencies, courts, voluntary organizations and the public.

10851 Pregnancy and Infant Loss Center

www.babycenter.com

Offers studies, information, statistics, help and support to parents who have suffered the loss of a child.

A

B

C

D

E

F

G

H

I

J

K

L

M

N

O

P

Q

R

S

T

U

V

W

X

Y

Z

Alabama

Alaska

Arizona

Arkansas

California

Canada

Colorado

Connecticut

Delaware

District of Columbia

Florida

Georgia

Hawaii

Idaho

Illinois

Indiana

Iowa

Kansas

Kentucky

Louisiana

Maine

Maryland

Massachusetts

Michigan

Minnesota

Mississippi

Missouri

Montana

Nebraska

Nevada

New Hampshire

New Jersey

New Mexico

New York

North Carolina

North Dakota

Ohio

Oklahoma

Oregon

PR

Pennsylvania

Rhode Island

South Carolina

South Dakota

Tennessee

Texas

Utah

VI

Vermont

Virginia

Washington

West Virginia

Wisconsin

Wyoming

G.O.L.D.

Grey House OnLine Databases

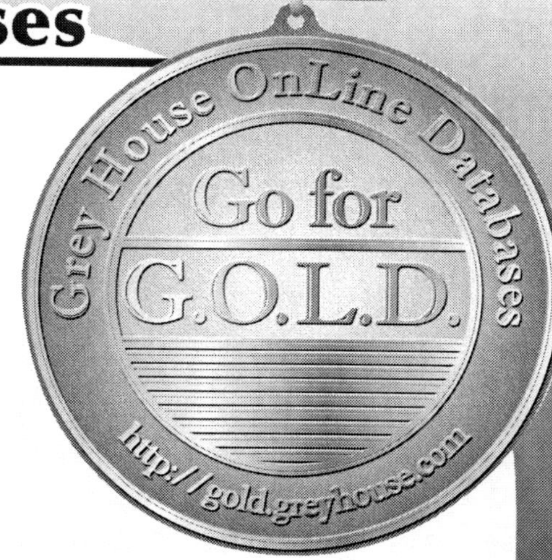

Brand New OnLine Database Platform

- Easy-To-Use Keyword & Quick Searches
- Organization Type & Subject Searches
- Cross-Database Searching
- Search by Area Code or Zip Code Ranges
- Search by Company Size & Geographic Area
- Search by Contact Name or Title
- Hotlinks to Websites & Email Addresses
- Combine Multiple Search Criteria with our Expert Search Page
- Sort Search Results by City, Company Name, Area Code & more
- Save Searches for Quick Lookups
- Create & Save Your Own Search Results Lists
- Download Search Results in TXT, CSV or DOC Formats

Quick Search

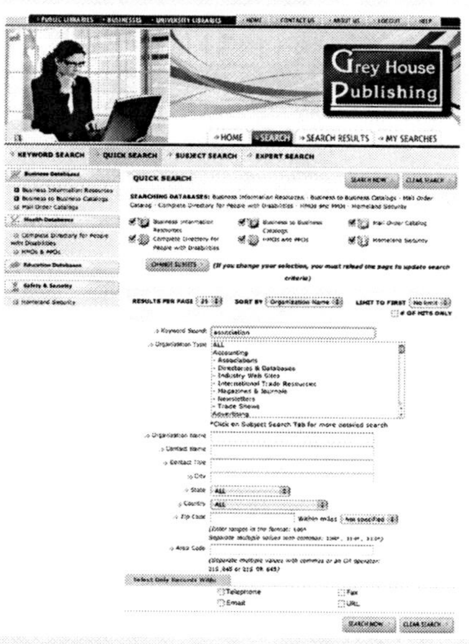

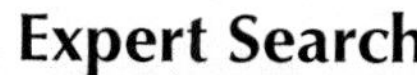

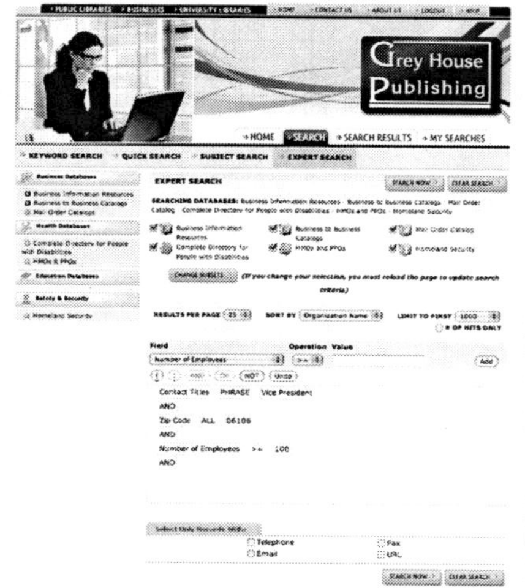

Subject Search

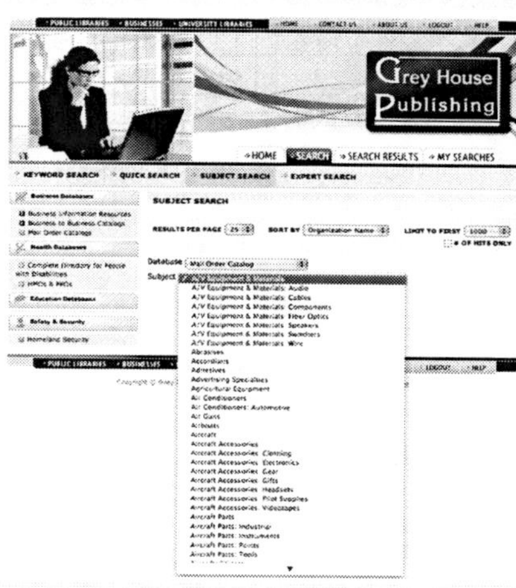

New Databases for 2008

Business

Business Information Resources
Directory of Mail Order & Business to Business Catalogs
Directory of Venture Capital & Private Equity Firms
Environmental Resource Handbook
Food & Beverage Market Place
Homeland Security Directory
Hudson's Washington News Media Contacts Directory
New York State Directory
Performing Arts Directory
Sports Market Place Directory
Washington Associations Contacts Directory

Health

Complete Directory for Pediatric Disorders
Complete Directory for People with Chronic Illness
Complete Directory for People with Disabilities
Complete Learning Disabilities Directory
Complete Mental Health Directory
Directory of Health Care Group Purchasing Organizations
Directory of Hospital Personnel
HMO/PPO Directory
Older Americans Information Directory

Grey House Publishing | PO Box 860 | 185 Millerton Road Millerton, NY 12546
(800) 562-2139 | (518) 789-8700 | FAX (518) 789-0556
www.greyhouse.com | e-mail: books@greyhouse.com

Call (800) 562-2139 for a free trial of the new G.O.L.D. OnLine Database Platform or visit http://gold.greyhouse.com for more information!

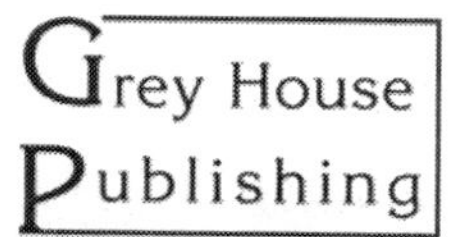

The Directory of Business Information Resources, 2009

With 100% verification, over 1,000 new listings and more than 12,000 updates, *The Directory of Business Information Resources* is the most up-to-date source for contacts in over 98 business areas – from advertising and agriculture to utilities and wholesalers. This carefully researched volume details: the Associations representing each industry; the Newsletters that keep members current; the Magazines and Journals - with their "Special Issues" - that are important to the trade, the Conventions that are "must attends," Databases, Directories and Industry Web Sites that provide access to must-have marketing resources. Includes contact names, phone & fax numbers, web sites and e-mail addresses. This one-volume resource is a gold mine of information and would be a welcome addition to any reference collection.

"This is a most useful and easy-to-use addition to any researcher's library." –The Information Professionals Institute

Softcover ISBN 978-1-59237-399-4, 2,500 pages, $195.00 | Online Database: http://gold.greyhouse.com Call (800) 562-2139 for quote

Hudson's Washington News Media Contacts Directory, 2009

With 100% verification of data, *Hudson's Washington News Media Contacts Directory* is the most accurate, most up-to-date source for media contacts in our nation's capital. With the largest concentration of news media in the world, having access to Washington's news media will get your message heard by these key media outlets. Published for over 40 years, Hudson's Washington News Media Contacts Directory brings you immediate access to: News Services & Newspapers, News Service Syndicates, DC Newspapers, Foreign Newspapers, Radio & TV, Magazines & Newsletters, and Freelance Writers & Photographers. The easy-to-read entries include contact names, phone & fax numbers, web sites and e-mail and more. For easy navigation, Hudson's Washington News Media Contacts Directory contains two indexes: Entry Index and Executive Index. This kind of comprehensive and up-to-date information would cost thousands of dollars to replicate or countless hours of searching to find. Don't miss this opportunity to have this important resource in your collection, and start saving time and money today. Hudson's Washington News Media Contacts Directory is the perfect research tool for Public Relations, Marketing, Networking and so much more. This resource is a gold mine of information and would be a welcome addition to any reference collection.

Softcover ISBN 978-1-59237-407-6, 800 pages, $289.00 | Online Database: http://gold.greyhouse.com Call (800) 562-2139 for quote

Nations of the World, 2009 A Political, Economic and Business Handbook

This completely revised edition covers all the nations of the world in an easy-to-use, single volume. Each nation is profiled in a single chapter that includes Key Facts, Political & Economic Issues, a Country Profile and Business Information. In this fast-changing world, it is extremely important to make sure that the most up-to-date information is included in your reference collection. This edition is just the answer. Each of the 200+ country chapters have been carefully reviewed by a political expert to make sure that the text reflects the most current information on Politics, Travel Advisories, Economics and more. You'll find such vital information as a Country Map, Population Characteristics, Inflation, Agricultural Production, Foreign Debt, Political History, Foreign Policy, Regional Insecurity, Economics, Trade & Tourism, Historical Profile, Political Systems, Ethnicity, Languages, Media, Climate, Hotels, Chambers of Commerce, Banking, Travel Information and more. Five Regional Chapters follow the main text and include a Regional Map, an Introductory Article, Key Indicators and Currencies for the Region. As an added bonus, an all-inclusive CD-ROM is available as a companion to the printed text. Noted for its sophisticated, up-to-date and reliable compilation of political, economic and business information, this brand new edition will be an important acquisition to any public, academic or special library reference collection.

"A useful addition to both general reference collections and business collections." –RUSQ

Softcover ISBN 978-1-59237-273-7, 1,700 pages, $180.00

The Directory of Venture Capital & Private Equity Firms, 2009

This edition has been extensively updated and broadly expanded to offer direct access to over 2,800 Domestic and International Venture Capital Firms, including address, phone & fax numbers, e-mail addresses and web sites for both primary and branch locations. Entries include details on the firm's Mission Statement, Industry Group Preferences, Geographic Preferences, Average and Minimum Investments and Investment Criteria. You'll also find details that are available nowhere else, including the Firm's Portfolio Companies and extensive information on each of the firm's Managing Partners, such as Education, Professional Background and Directorships held, along with the Partner's E-mail Address. *The Directory of Venture Capital & Private Equity Firms* offers five important indexes: Geographic Index, Executive Name Index, Portfolio Company Index, Industry Preference Index and College & University Index. With its comprehensive coverage and detailed, extensive information on each company, The Directory of Venture Capital & Private Equity Firms is an important addition to any finance collection.

"The sheer number of listings, the descriptive information and the outstanding indexing make this directory a better value than ...Pratt's Guide to Venture Capital Sources. Recommended for business collections in large public, academic and business libraries." –Choice

Softcover ISBN 978-1-59237-398-7, 1,300 pages, $565/$450 Lib | Online DB: http://gold.greyhouse.com Call (800) 562-2139 for quote

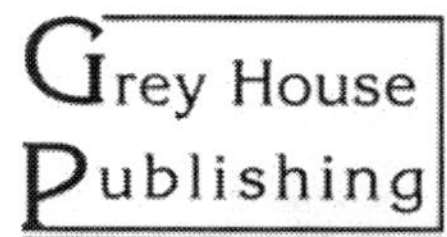

The Encyclopedia of Emerging Industries

*Published under an exclusive license from the Gale Group, Inc.

The fifth edition of the *Encyclopedia of Emerging Industries* details the inception, emergence, and current status of nearly 120 flourishing U.S. industries and industry segments. These focused essays unearth for users a wealth of relevant, current, factual data previously accessible only through a diverse variety of sources. This volume provides broad-based, highly-readable, industry information under such headings as Industry Snapshot, Organization & Structure, Background & Development, Industry Leaders, Current Conditions, America and the World, Pioneers, and Research & Technology. Essays in this new edition, arranged alphabetically for easy use, have been completely revised, with updated statistics and the most current information on industry trends and developments. In addition, there are new essays on some of the most interesting and influential new business fields, including Application Service Providers, Concierge Services, Entrepreneurial Training, Fuel Cells, Logistics Outsourcing Services, Pharmacogenomics, and Tissue Engineering. Two indexes, General and Industry, provide immediate access to this wealth of information. Plus, two conversion tables for SIC and NAICS codes, along with Suggested Further Readings, are provided to aid the user. *The Encyclopedia of Emerging Industries* pinpoints emerging industries while they are still in the spotlight. This important resource will be an important acquisition to any business reference collection.

"This well-designed source…should become another standard business source, nicely complementing Standard & Poor's Industry Surveys. It contains more information on each industry than Hoover's Handbook of Emerging Companies, is broader in scope than The Almanac of American Employers 1998-1999, but is less expansive than the Encyclopedia of Careers & Vocational Guidance. Highly recommended for all academic libraries and specialized business collections." –Library Journal

Hardcover ISBN 978-1-59237-242-3, 1,400 pages, $495.00

Encyclopedia of American Industries

*Published under an exclusive license from the Gale Group, Inc.

The Encyclopedia of American Industries is a major business reference tool that provides detailed, comprehensive information on a wide range of industries in every realm of American business. A two volume set, Volume I provides separate coverage of nearly 500 manufacturing industries, while Volume II presents nearly 600 essays covering the vast array of services and other non-manufacturing industries in the United States. Combined, these two volumes provide individual essays on every industry recognized by the U.S. Standard Industrial Classification (SIC) system. Both volumes are arranged numerically by SIC code, for easy use. Additionally, each entry includes the corresponding NAICS code(s). The *Encyclopedia's* business coverage includes information on historical events of consequence, as well as current trends and statistics. Essays include an Industry Snapshot, Organization & Structure, Background & Development, Current Conditions, Industry Leaders, Workforce, America and the World, Research & Technology along with Suggested Further Readings. Both SIC and NAICS code conversion tables and an all-encompassing Subject Index, with cross-references, complete the text. With its detailed, comprehensive information on a wide range of industries, this resource will be an important tool for both the industry newcomer and the seasoned professional.

"Encyclopedia of American Industries contains detailed, signed essays on virtually every industry in contemporary society. ... Highly recommended for all but the smallest libraries." -American Reference Books Annual

Two Volumes, Hardcover ISBN 978-1-59237-244-7, 3,000 pages, $650.00

Encyclopedia of Global Industries

*Published under an exclusive license from the Gale Group, Inc.

This fourth edition of the acclaimed *Encyclopedia of Global Industries* presents a thoroughly revised and expanded look at more than 125 business sectors of global significance. Detailed, insightful articles discuss the origins, development, trends, key statistics and current international character of the world's most lucrative, dynamic and widely researched industries – including hundreds of profiles of leading international corporations. Beginning researchers will gain from this book a solid understanding of how each industry operates and which countries and companies are significant participants, while experienced researchers will glean current and historical figures for comparison and analysis. The industries profiled in previous editions have been updated, and in some cases, expanded to reflect recent industry trends. Additionally, this edition provides both SIC and NAICS codes for all industries profiled. As in the original volumes, *The Encyclopedia of Global Industries* offers thorough studies of some of the biggest and most frequently researched industry sectors, including Aircraft, Biotechnology, Computers, Internet Services, Motor Vehicles, Pharmaceuticals, Semiconductors, Software and Telecommunications. An SIC and NAICS conversion table and an all-encompassing Subject Index, with cross-references, are provided to ensure easy access to this wealth of information. These and many others make the *Encyclopedia of Global Industries* the authoritative reference for studies of international industries.

"Provides detailed coverage of the history, development, and current status of 115 of "the world's most lucrative and high-profile industries." It far surpasses the Department of Commerce's U.S. Global Trade Outlook 1995-2000 (GPO, 1995) in scope and coverage. Recommended for comprehensive public and academic library business collections." -Booklist

Hardcover ISBN 978-1-59237-243-0, 1,400 pages, $495.00

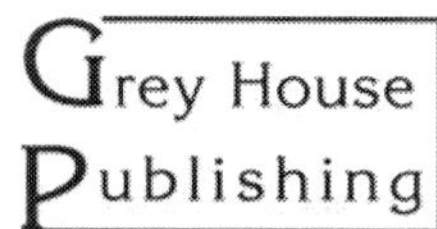
Grey House
Publishing

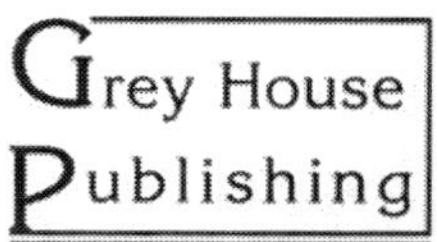

The Environmental Resource Handbook, 2009/10

The Environmental Resource Handbook is the most up-to-date and comprehensive source for Environmental Resources and Statistics. Section I: Resources provides detailed contact information for thousands of information sources, including Associations & Organizations, Awards & Honors, Conferences, Foundations & Grants, Environmental Health, Government Agencies, National Parks & Wildlife Refuges, Publications, Research Centers, Educational Programs, Green Product Catalogs, Consultants and much more. Section II: Statistics, provides statistics and rankings on hundreds of important topics, including Children's Environmental Index, Municipal Finances, Toxic Chemicals, Recycling, Climate, Air & Water Quality and more. This kind of up-to-date environmental data, all in one place, is not available anywhere else on the market place today. This vast compilation of resources and statistics is a must-have for all public and academic libraries as well as any organization with a primary focus on the environment.

"...the intrinsic value of the information make it worth consideration by libraries with environmental collections and environmentally concerned users." –Booklist

Softcover ISBN 978-1-59237-433-5, 1,000 pages, $155.00 | Online Database: http://gold.greyhouse.com Call (800) 562-2139 for quote

New York State Directory, 2009/10

The New York State Directory, published annually since 1983, is a comprehensive and easy-to-use guide to accessing public officials and private sector organizations and individuals who influence public policy in the state of New York. *The New York State Directory* includes important information on all New York state legislators and congressional representatives, including biographies and key committee assignments. It also includes staff rosters for all branches of New York state government and for federal agencies and departments that impact the state policy process. Following the state government section are 25 chapters covering policy areas from agriculture through veterans' affairs. Each chapter identifies the state, local and federal agencies and officials that formulate or implement policy. In addition, each chapter contains a roster of private sector experts and advocates who influence the policy process. The directory also offers appendices that include statewide party officials; chambers of commerce; lobbying organizations; public and private universities and colleges; television, radio and print media; and local government agencies and officials.

"This comprehensive directory covers not only New York State government offices and key personnel but pertinent U.S. government agencies and non-governmental entities. This directory is all encompassing... recommended." -Choice

New York State Directory - Softcover ISBN 978-1-59237-420-5, 800 pages, $145.00
Online Database: http://gold.greyhouse.com Call (800) 562-2139 for quote
New York State Directory with *Profiles of New York* – 2 Volumes, Softcover ISBN 978-1-59237-421-2, 1,600 pages, $225.00

The Grey House Homeland Security Directory, 2010

This updated edition features the latest contact information for government and private organizations involved with Homeland Security along with the latest product information and provides detailed profiles of nearly 1,000 Federal & State Organizations & Agencies and over 3,000 Officials and Key Executives involved with Homeland Security. These listings are incredibly detailed and include Mailing Address, Phone & Fax Numbers, Email Addresses & Web Sites, a complete Description of the Agency and a complete list of the Officials and Key Executives associated with the Agency. Next, *The Grey House Homeland Security Directory* provides the go-to source for Homeland Security Products & Services. This section features over 2,000 Companies that provide Consulting, Products or Services. With this Buyer's Guide at their fingertips, users can locate suppliers of everything from Training Materials to Access Controls, from Perimeter Security to BioTerrorism Countermeasures and everything in between – complete with contact information and product descriptions. A handy Product Locator Index is provided to quickly and easily locate suppliers of a particular product. This comprehensive, information-packed resource will be a welcome tool for any company or agency that is in need of Homeland Security information and will be a necessary acquisition for the reference collection of all public libraries and large school districts.

"Compiles this information in one place and is discerning in content. A useful purchase for public and academic libraries." –Booklist

Softcover ISBN 978-1-59237-365-9, 800 pages, $195.00 | Online Database: http://gold.greyhouse.com Call (800) 562-2139 for quote

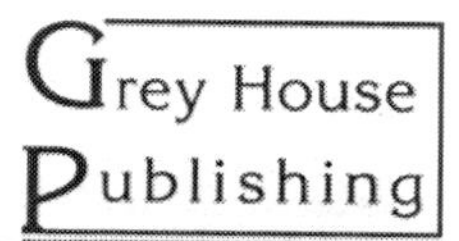

The Grey House Safety & Security Directory, 2009

The Grey House Safety & Security Directory is the most comprehensive reference tool and buyer's guide for the safety and security industry. Arranged by safety topic, each chapter begins with OSHA regulations for the topic, followed by Training Articles written by top professionals in the field and Self-Inspection Checklists. Next, each topic contains Buyer's Guide sections that feature related products and services. Topics include Administration, Insurance, Loss Control & Consulting, Protective Equipment & Apparel, Noise & Vibration, Facilities Monitoring & Maintenance, Employee Health Maintenance & Ergonomics, Retail Food Services, Machine Guards, Process Guidelines & Tool Handling, Ordinary Materials Handling, Hazardous Materials Handling, Workplace Preparation & Maintenance, Electrical Lighting & Safety, Fire & Rescue and Security. Six important indexes make finding information and product manufacturers quick and easy: Geographical Index of Manufacturers and Distributors, Company Profile Index, Brand Name Index, Product Index, Index of Web Sites and Index of Advertisers. This comprehensive, up-to-date reference will provide every tool necessary to make sure a business is in compliance with OSHA regulations and locate the products and services needed to meet those regulations.

"Presents industrial safety information for engineers, plant managers, risk managers, and construction site supervisors..." –Choice

Softcover ISBN 978-1-59237-375-8, 1,500 pages, $165.00

The Grey House Transportation Security Directory & Handbook

This is the only reference of its kind that brings together current data on Transportation Security. With information on everything from Regulatory Authorities to Security Equipment, this top-flight database brings together the relevant information necessary for creating and maintaining a security plan for a wide range of transportation facilities. With this current, comprehensive directory at the ready you'll have immediate access to: Regulatory Authorities & Legislation; Information Resources; Sample Security Plans & Checklists; Contact Data for Major Airports, Seaports, Railroads, Trucking Companies and Oil Pipelines; Security Service Providers; Recommended Equipment & Product Information and more. Using the *Grey House Transportation Security Directory & Handbook*, managers will be able to quickly and easily assess their current security plans; develop contacts to create and maintain new security procedures; and source the products and services necessary to adequately maintain a secure environment. This valuable resource is a must for all Security Managers at Airports, Seaports, Railroads, Trucking Companies and Oil Pipelines.

"Highly recommended. Library collections that support all levels of readers, including professionals/practitioners; and schools/organizations offering education and training in transportation security." -Choice

Softcover ISBN 978-1-59237-075-7, 800 pages, $195.00

The Grey House Biometric Information Directory

This edition offers a complete, current overview of biometric companies and products – one of the fastest growing industries in today's economy. Detailed profiles of manufacturers of the latest biometric technology, including Finger, Voice, Face, Hand, Signature, Iris, Vein and Palm Identification systems. Data on the companies include key executives, company size and a detailed, indexed description of their product line. Information in the directory includes: Editorial on Advancements in Biometrics; Profiles of 700+ companies listed with contact information; Organizations, Trade & Educational Associations, Publications, Conferences, Trade Shows and Expositions Worldwide; Web Site Index; Biometric & Vendors Services Index by Types of Biometrics; and a Glossary of Biometric Terms. This resource will be an important source for anyone who is considering the use of a biometric product, investing in the development of biometric technology, support existing marketing and sales efforts and will be an important acquisition for the business reference collection for large public and business libraries.

"This book should prove useful to agencies or businesses seeking companies that deal with biometric technology. Summing Up: Recommended. Specialized collections serving researchers/faculty and professionals/practitioners." -Choice

Softcover ISBN 978-1-59237-121-1, 800 pages, $225.00

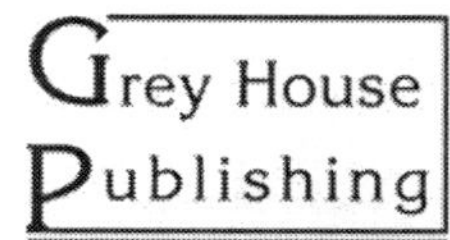

The Rauch Guide to the US Adhesives & Sealants, Cosmetics & Toiletries, Ink, Paint, Plastics, Pulp & Paper and Rubber Industries

The Rauch Guides save time and money by organizing widely scattered information and providing estimates for important business decisions, some of which are available nowhere else. Within each Guide, after a brief introduction, the ECONOMICS section provides data on industry shipments; long-term growth and forecasts; prices; company performance; employment, expenditures, and productivity; transportation and geographical patterns; packaging; foreign trade; and government regulations. Next, TECHNOLOGY & RAW MATERIALS provide market, technical, and raw material information for chemicals, equipment and related materials, including market size and leading suppliers, prices, end uses, and trends. PRODUCTS & MARKETS provide information for each major industry product, including market size and historical trends, leading suppliers, five-year forecasts, industry structure, and major end uses. Next, the COMPANY DIRECTORY profiles major industry companies, both public and private. Information includes complete contact information, web address, estimated total and domestic sales, product description, and recent mergers and acquisitions. *The Rauch Guides* will prove to be an invaluable source of market information, company data, trends and forecasts that anyone in these fast-paced industries.

"An invaluable and affordable publication. The comprehensive nature of the data and text offers considerable insights into the industry, market sizes, company activities, and applications of the products of the industry. The additions that have been made have certainly enhanced the value of the Guide." –Adhesives & Sealants Newsletter of the Rauch Guide to the US Adhesives & Sealants Industry

Paint Industry: Softcover ISBN 978-1-59237-428-1 $595 | Plastics Industry: Softcover ISBN 978-1-59237-445-8 $595 | Adhesives and Sealants Industry: Softcover ISBN 978-1-59237-440-3 $595 | Ink Industry: Softcover ISBN 978-1-59237-126-6 $595 | Rubber Industry: Softcover ISBN 978-1-59237-130-3 $595 | Pulp and Paper Industry: Softcover ISBN 978-1-59237-131-0 $595 | Cosmetic & Toiletries Industry: Softcover ISBN 978-1-59237-132-7 $895

Research Services Directory: Commercial & Corporate Research Centers

This ninth edition provides access to well over 8,000 independent Commercial Research Firms, Corporate Research Centers and Laboratories offering contract services for hands-on, basic or applied research. Research Services Directory covers the thousands of types of research companies, including Biotechnology & Pharmaceutical Developers, Consumer Product Research, Defense Contractors, Electronics & Software Engineers, Think Tanks, Forensic Investigators, Independent Commercial Laboratories, Information Brokers, Market & Survey Research Companies, Medical Diagnostic Facilities, Product Research & Development Firms and more. Each entry provides the company's name, mailing address, phone & fax numbers, key contacts, web site, e-mail address, as well as a company description and research and technical fields served. Four indexes provide immediate access to this wealth of information: Research Firms Index, Geographic Index, Personnel Name Index and Subject Index.

"An important source for organizations in need of information about laboratories, individuals and other facilities." –ARBA

Softcover ISBN 978-1-59237-003-0, 1,400 pages, $465.00

International Business and Trade Directories

Completely updated, the Third Edition of *International Business and Trade Directories* now contains more than 10,000 entries, over 2,000 more than the last edition, making this directory the most comprehensive resource of the worlds business and trade directories. Entries include content descriptions, price, publisher's name and address, web site and e-mail addresses, phone and fax numbers and editorial staff. Organized by industry group, and then by region, this resource puts over 10,000 industry-specific business and trade directories at the reader's fingertips. Three indexes are included for quick access to information: Geographic Index, Publisher Index and Title Index. Public, college and corporate libraries, as well as individuals and corporations seeking critical market information will want to add this directory to their marketing collection.

"Reasonably priced for a work of this type, this directory should appeal to larger academic, public and corporate libraries with an international focus." –Library Journal

Softcover ISBN 978-1-930956-63-6, 1,800 pages, $225.00

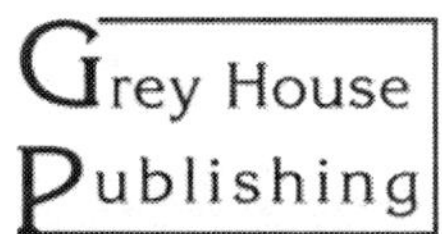

TheStreet.com Ratings Guide to Health Insurers

TheStreet.com Ratings Guide to Health Insurers is the first and only source to cover the financial stability of the nation's health care system, rating the financial safety of more than 6,000 health insurance providers, health maintenance organizations (HMOs) and all of the Blue Cross Blue Shield plans – updated quarterly to ensure the most accurate information. The Guide also provides a complete listing of all the major health insurers, including all Long-Term Care and Medigap insurers. Our *Guide to Health Insurers* includes comprehensive, timely coverage on the financial stability of HMOs and health insurers; the most accurate insurance company ratings available–the same quality ratings heralded by the U.S. General Accounting Office; separate listings for those companies offering Medigap and long-term care policies; the number of serious consumer complaints filed against most HMOs so you can see who is actually providing the best (or worst) service and more. The easy-to-use layout gives you a one-line summary analysis for each company that we track, followed by an in-depth, detailed analysis of all HMOs and the largest health insurers. The guide also includes a list of TheStreet.com Ratings Recommended Companies with information on how to contact them, and the reasoning behind any rating upgrades or downgrades.

"With 20 years behind its insurance-advocacy research [the rating guide] continues to offer a wealth of information that helps consumers weigh their healthcare options now and in the future." -Today's Librarian

Issues published quarterly, Softcover, 550 pages, $499.00 for four quarterly issues, $249.00 for a single issue

TheStreet.com Ratings Guide to Life & Annuity Insurers

TheStreet.com Safety Ratings are the most reliable source for evaluating an insurer's financial solvency risk. Consequently, policyholders have come to rely on TheStreet.com's flagship publication, *TheStreet.com Ratings Guide to Life & Annuity Insurers*, to help them identify the safest companies to do business with. Each easy-to-use edition delivers TheStreet.com's independent ratings and analyses on more than 1,100 insurers, updated every quarter. Plus, your patrons will find a complete list of TheStreet.com Recommended Companies, including contact information, and the reasoning behind any rating upgrades or downgrades. This guide is perfect for those who are considering the purchase of a life insurance policy, placing money in an annuity, or advising clients about insurance and annuities. A life or health insurance policy or annuity is only as secure as the insurance company issuing it. Therefore, make sure your patrons have what they need to periodically monitor the financial condition of the companies with whom they have an investment. The TheStreet.com Ratings product line is designed to help them in their evaluations.

"Weiss has an excellent reputation and this title is held by hundreds of libraries. This guide is recommended for public and academic libraries." -ARBA

Issues published quarterly, Softcover, 360 pages, $499.00 for four quarterly issues, $249.00 for a single issue

TheStreet.com Ratings Guide to Property & Casualty Insurers

TheStreet.com Ratings Guide to Property and Casualty Insurers provides the most extensive coverage of insurers writing policies, helping consumers and businesses avoid financial headaches. Updated quarterly, this easy-to-use publication delivers the independent, unbiased TheStreet.com Safety Ratings and supporting analyses on more than 2,800 U.S. insurance companies, offering auto & homeowners insurance, business insurance, worker's compensation insurance, product liability insurance, medical malpractice and other professional liability insurance. Each edition includes a list of TheStreet.com Recommended Companies by type of insurance, including a contact number, plus helpful information about the coverage provided by the State Guarantee Associations.

"In contrast to the other major insurance rating agencies...Weiss does not have a financial relationship worth the companies it rates. A GAO study found that Weiss identified financial vulnerability earlier than the other rating agencies." -ARBA

Issues published quarterly, Softcover, 455 pages, $499.00 for four quarterly issues, $249.00 for a single issue

TheStreet.com Ratings Consumer Box Set

Deliver the critical information your patrons need to safeguard their personal finances with *TheStreet.com Ratings' Consumer Guide Box Set*. Each of the eight guides is packed with accurate, unbiased information and recommendations to help your patrons make sound financial decisions. TheStreet.com Ratings Consumer Guide Box Set provides your patrons with easy to understand guidance on important personal finance topics, including: *Consumer Guide to Variable Annuities, Consumer Guide to Medicare Supplement Insurance, Consumer Guide to Elder Care Choices, Consumer Guide to Automobile Insurance, Consumer Guide to Long-Term Care Insurance, Consumer Guide to Homeowners Insurance, Consumer Guide to Term Life Insurance, and Consumer Guide to Medicare Prescription Drug Coverage*. Each guide provides an easy-to-read overview of the topic, what to look out for when selecting a company or insurance plan to do business with, who are the recommended companies to work with and how to navigate through these often-times difficult decisions. Custom worksheets and step-by-step directions make these resources accessible to all types of users. Packaged in a handy custom display box, these helpful guides will prove to be a much-used addition to any reference collection.

Issues published twice per year, Softcover, 600 pages, $499.00 for two biennial issues

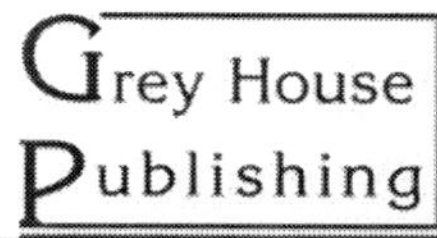

TheStreet.com Ratings Guide to Stock Mutual Funds

TheStreet.com Ratings Guide to Stock Mutual Funds offers ratings and analyses on more than 8,800 equity mutual funds – more than any other publication. The exclusive TheStreet.com Investment Ratings combine an objective evaluation of each fund's performance and risk to provide a single, user-friendly, composite rating, giving your patrons a better handle on a mutual fund's risk-adjusted performance. Each edition identifies the top-performing mutual funds based on risk category, type of fund, and overall risk-adjusted performance. TheStreet.com's unique investment rating system makes it easy to see exactly which stocks are on the rise and which ones should be avoided. For those investors looking to tailor their mutual fund selections based on age, income, and tolerance for risk, we've also assigned two component ratings to each fund: a performance rating and a risk rating. With these, you can identify those funds that are best suited to meet your - or your client's – individual needs and goals. Plus, we include a handy Risk Profile Quiz to help you assess your personal tolerance for risk. So whether you're an investing novice or professional, the *Guide to Stock Mutual Funds* gives you everything you need to find a mutual fund that is right for you.

"There is tremendous need for information such as that provided by this Weiss publication. This reasonably priced guide is recommended for public and academic libraries serving investors." -ARBA

Issues published quarterly, Softcover, 655 pages, $499 for four quarterly issues, $249 for a single issue

TheStreet.com Ratings Guide to Exchange-Traded Funds

TheStreet.com Ratings editors analyze hundreds of mutual funds each quarter, condensing all of the available data into a single composite opinion of each fund's risk-adjusted performance. The intuitive, consumer-friendly ratings allow investors to instantly identify those funds that have historically done well and those that have under-performed the market. Each quarterly edition identifies the top-performing exchange-traded funds based on risk category, type of fund, and overall risk-adjusted performance. The rating scale, A through F, gives you a better handle on an exchange-traded fund's risk-adjusted performance. Other features include Top & Bottom 200 Exchange-Traded Funds; Performance and Risk: 100 Best and Worst Exchange- Traded Funds; Investor Profile Quiz; Performance Benchmarks and Fund Type Descriptions. With the growing popularity of mutual fund investing, consumers need a reliable source to help them track and evaluate the performance of their mutual fund holdings. Plus, they need a way of identifying and monitoring other funds as potential new investments. Unfortunately, the hundreds of performance and risk measures available, multiplied by the vast number of mutual fund investments on the market today, can make this a daunting task for even the most sophisticated investor. This Guide will serve as a useful tool for both the first-time and seasoned investor.

Editions published quarterly, Softcover, 440 pages, $499.00 for four quarterly issues, $249.00 for a single issue

TheStreet.com Ratings Guide to Bond & Money Market Mutual Funds

TheStreet.com Ratings Guide to Bond & Money Market Mutual Funds has everything your patrons need to easily identify the top-performing fixed income funds on the market today. Each quarterly edition contains TheStreet.com's independent ratings and analyses on more than 4,600 fixed income funds – more than any other publication, including corporate bond funds, high-yield bond funds, municipal bond funds, mortgage security funds, money market funds, global bond funds and government bond funds. In addition, the fund's risk rating is combined with its three-year performance rating to get an overall picture of the fund's risk-adjusted performance. The resulting TheStreet.com Investment Rating gives a single, user-friendly, objective evaluation that makes it easy to compare one fund to another and select the right fund based on the level of risk tolerance. Most investors think of fixed income mutual funds as "safe" investments. That's not always the case, however, depending on the credit risk, interest rate risk, and prepayment risk of the securities owned by the fund. TheStreet.com Ratings assesses each of these risks and assigns each fund a risk rating to help investors quickly evaluate the fund's risk component. Plus, we include a handy Risk Profile Quiz to help you assess your personal tolerance for risk. So whether you're an investing novice or professional, the *Guide to Bond and Money Market Mutual Funds* gives you everything you need to find a mutual fund that is right for you.

"Comprehensive... It is easy to use and consumer-oriented, and can be recommended for larger public and academic libraries." -ARBA

Issues published quarterly, Softcover, 470 pages, $499.00 for four quarterly issues, $249.00 for a single issue

TheStreet.com Ratings Guide to Banks & Thrifts

Updated quarterly, for the most up-to-date information, *TheStreet.com Ratings Guide to Banks and Thrifts* offers accurate, intuitive safety ratings your patrons can trust; supporting ratios and analyses that show an institution's strong & weak points; identification of the TheStreet.com Recommended Companies with branches in your area; a complete list of institutions receiving upgrades/downgrades; and comprehensive coverage of every bank and thrift in the nation – more than 9,000. TheStreet.com Safety Ratings are then based on the analysts' review of publicly available information collected by the federal banking regulators. The easy-to-use layout gives you: the institution's TheStreet.com Safety Rating for the last 3 years; the five key indexes used to evaluate each institution; along with the primary ratios and statistics used in determining the company's rating. *TheStreet.com Ratings Guide to Banks & Thrifts* will be a must for individuals who are concerned about the safety of their CD or savings account; need to be sure that an existing line of credit will be there when they need it; or simply want to avoid the hassles of dealing with a failing or troubled institution.

"Large public and academic libraries most definitely need to acquire the work. Likewise, special libraries in large corporations will find this title indispensable." -ARBA

Issues published quarterly, Softcover, 370 pages, $499.00 for four quarterly issues, $249.00 for a single issue

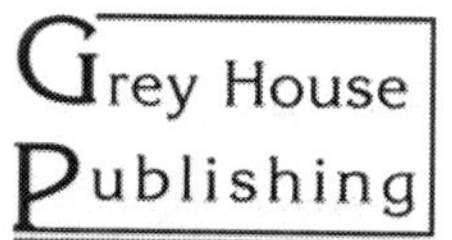

TheStreet.com Ratings Guide to Common Stocks

TheStreet.com Ratings Guide to Common Stocks gives your patrons reliable insight into the risk-adjusted performance of common stocks listed on the NYSE, AMEX, and Nasdaq – over 5,800 stocks in all – more than any other publication. TheStreet.com's unique investment rating system makes it easy to see exactly which stocks are on the rise and which ones should be avoided. In addition, your patrons also get supporting analysis showing growth trends, profitability, debt levels, valuation levels, the top-rated stocks within each industry, and more. Plus, each stock is ranked with the easy-to-use buy-hold-sell equivalents commonly used by Wall Street. Whether they're selecting their own investments or checking up on a broker's recommendation, TheStreet.com Ratings can help them in their evaluations.

"Users... will find the information succinct and the explanations readable, easy to understand, and helpful to a novice." -Library Journal

Issues published quarterly, Softcover, 440 pages, $499.00 for four quarterly issues, $249.00 for a single issue

TheStreet.com Ratings Ultimate Guided Tour of Stock Investing

This important reference guide from TheStreet.com Ratings is just what librarians around the country have asked for: a step-by-step introduction to stock investing for the beginning to intermediate investor. This easy-to-navigate guide explores the basics of stock investing and includes the intuitive TheStreet.com Investment Rating on more than 5,800 stocks, complete with real-world investing information that can be put to use immediately with stocks that fit the concepts discussed in the guide; informative charts, graphs and worksheets; easy-to-understand explanations on topics like P/E, compound interest, marked indices, diversifications, brokers, and much more; along with financial safety ratings for every stock on the NYSE, American Stock Exchange and the Nasdaq. This consumer-friendly guide offers complete how-to information on stock investing that can be put to use right away; a friendly format complete with our "Wise Guide" who leads the reader on a safari to learn about the investing jungle; helpful charts, graphs and simple worksheets; the intuitive TheStreet.com Investment rating on over 6,000 stocks — every stock found on the NYSE, American Stock Exchange and the NASDAQ; and much more.

"Provides investors with an alternative to stock broker recommendations, which recently have been tarnished by conflicts of interest. In summary, the guide serves as a welcome addition for all public library collections." -ARBA

Issues published quarterly, Softcover, 370 pages, $499.00 for four quarterly issues, $249.00 for a single issue

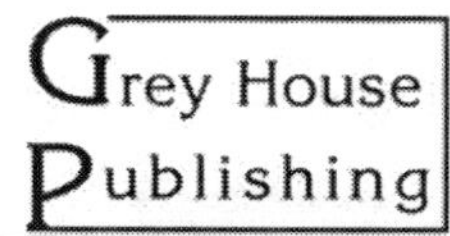

The Value of a Dollar 1860-2009, Fourth Edition

A guide to practical economy, *The Value of a Dollar* records the actual prices of thousands of items that consumers purchased from the Civil War to the present, along with facts about investment options and income opportunities. This brand new Third Edition boasts a brand new addition to each five-year chapter, a section on Trends. This informative section charts the change in price over time and provides added detail on the reasons prices changed within the time period, including industry developments, changes in consumer attitudes and important historical facts. Plus, a brand new chapter for 2005-2009 has been added. Each 5-year chapter includes a Historical Snapshot, Consumer Expenditures, Investments, Selected Income, Income/Standard Jobs, Food Basket, Standard Prices and Miscellany. This interesting and useful publication will be widely used in any reference collection.

"Business historians, reporters, writers and students will find this source... very helpful for historical research. Libraries will want to purchase it." –ARBA

Hardcover ISBN 978-1-59237-403-8, 600 pages, $145.00 | Ebook ISBN 978-1-59237-173-0 www.greyhouse.com/ebooks.htm

The Value of a Dollar 1600-1859, The Colonial Era to The Civil War

Following the format of the widely acclaimed, *The Value of a Dollar, 1860-2004*, *The Value of a Dollar 1600-1859, The Colonial Era to The Civil War* records the actual prices of thousands of items that consumers purchased from the Colonial Era to the Civil War. Our editorial department had been flooded with requests from users of our *Value of a Dollar* for the same type of information, just from an earlier time period. This new volume is just the answer – with pricing data from 1600 to 1859. Arranged into five-year chapters, each 5-year chapter includes a Historical Snapshot, Consumer Expenditures, Investments, Selected Income, Income/Standard Jobs, Food Basket, Standard Prices and Miscellany. There is also a section on Trends. This informative section charts the change in price over time and provides added detail on the reasons prices changed within the time period, including industry developments, changes in consumer attitudes and important historical facts. This fascinating survey will serve a wide range of research needs and will be useful in all high school, public and academic library reference collections.

"The Value of a Dollar: Colonial Era to the Civil War, 1600-1865 will find a happy audience among students, researchers, and general browsers. It offers a fascinating and detailed look at early American history from the viewpoint of everyday people trying to make ends meet. This title and the earlier publication, The Value of a Dollar, 1860-2004, complement each other very well, and readers will appreciate finding them side-by-side on the shelf." -Booklist

Hardcover ISBN 978-1-59237-094-8, 600 pages, $145.00 | Ebook ISBN 978-1-59237-169-3 www.greyhouse.com/ebooks.htm

Working Americans 1880-1999
Volume I: The Working Class, Volume II: The Middle Class, Volume III: The Upper Class

Each of the volumes in the *Working Americans* series focuses on a particular class of Americans, The Working Class, The Middle Class and The Upper Class over the last 120 years. Chapters in each volume focus on one decade and profile three to five families. Family Profiles include real data on Income & Job Descriptions, Selected Prices of the Times, Annual Income, Annual Budgets, Family Finances, Life at Work, Life at Home, Life in the Community, Working Conditions, Cost of Living, Amusements and much more. Each chapter also contains an Economic Profile with Average Wages of other Professions, a selection of Typical Pricing, Key Events & Inventions, News Profiles, Articles from Local Media and Illustrations. The *Working Americans* series captures the lifestyles of each of the classes from the last twelve decades, covers a vast array of occupations and ethnic backgrounds and travels the entire nation. These interesting and useful compilations of portraits of the American Working, Middle and Upper Classes during the last 120 years will be an important addition to any high school, public or academic library reference collection.

"These interesting, unique compilations of economic and social facts, figures and graphs will support multiple research needs. They will engage and enlighten patrons in high school, public and academic library collections." –Booklist

Volume I: The Working Class Hardcover ISBN 978-1-891482-81-6, 558 pages, $150.00 | Volume II: The Middle Class Hardcover ISBN 978-1-891482-72-4, 591 pages, $150.00 | Volume III: The Upper Class Hardcover ISBN 978-1-930956-38-4, 567 pages, $150.00 | www.greyhouse.com/ebooks.htm

Working Americans 1880-1999 Volume IV: Their Children

This Fourth Volume in the highly successful *Working Americans* series focuses on American children, decade by decade from 1880 to 1999. This interesting and useful volume introduces the reader to three children in each decade, one from each of the Working, Middle and Upper classes. Like the first three volumes in the series, the individual profiles are created from interviews, diaries, statistical studies, biographies and news reports. Profiles cover a broad range of ethnic backgrounds, geographic area and lifestyles – everything from an orphan in Memphis in 1882, following the Yellow Fever epidemic of 1878 to an eleven-year-old nephew of a beer baron and owner of the New York Yankees in New York City in 1921. Chapters also contain important supplementary materials including News Features as well as information on everything from Schools to Parks, Infectious Diseases to Childhood Fears along with Entertainment, Family Life and much more to provide an informative overview of the lifestyles of children from each decade. This interesting account of what life was like for Children in the Working, Middle and Upper Classes will be a welcome addition to the reference collection of any high school, public or academic library.

Hardcover ISBN 978-1-930956-35-3, 600 pages, $150.00 | Ebook ISBN 978-1-59237-166-2 www.greyhouse.com/ebooks.htm

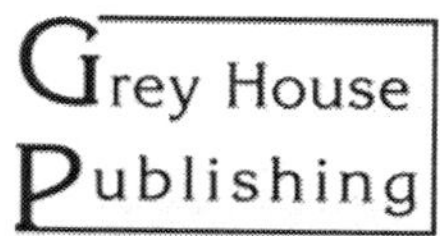

Working Americans 1880-2003 Volume V: Americans At War

Working Americans 1880-2003 Volume V: Americans At War is divided into 11 chapters, each covering a decade from 1880-2003 and examines the lives of Americans during the time of war, including declared conflicts, one-time military actions, protests, and preparations for war. Each decade includes several personal profiles, whether on the battlefield or on the homefront, that tell the stories of civilians, soldiers, and officers during the decade. The profiles examine: Life at Home; Life at Work; and Life in the Community. Each decade also includes an Economic Profile with statistical comparisons, a Historical Snapshot, News Profiles, local News Articles, and Illustrations that provide a solid historical background to the decade being examined. Profiles range widely not only geographically, but also emotionally, from that of a girl whose leg was torn off in a blast during WWI, to the boredom of being stationed in the Dakotas as the Indian Wars were drawing to a close. As in previous volumes of the *Working Americans* series, information is presented in narrative form, but hard facts and real-life situations back up each story. The basis of the profiles come from diaries, private print books, personal interviews, family histories, estate documents and magazine articles. For easy reference, *Working Americans 1880-2003 Volume V: Americans At War* includes an in-depth Subject Index. The Working Americans series has become an important reference for public libraries, academic libraries and high school libraries. This fifth volume will be a welcome addition to all of these types of reference collections.

Hardcover ISBN 978-1-59237-024-5, 600 pages, $150.00 | Ebook ISBN 978-1-59237-167-9 www.greyhouse.com/ebooks.htm

Working Americans 1880-2005 Volume VI: Women at Work

Unlike any other volume in the *Working Americans* series, this Sixth Volume, is the first to focus on a particular gender of Americans. *Volume VI: Women at Work*, traces what life was like for working women from the 1860's to the present time. Beginning with the life of a maid in 1890 and a store clerk in 1900 and ending with the life and times of the modern working women, this text captures the struggle, strengths and changing perception of the American woman at work. Each chapter focuses on one decade and profiles three to five women with real data on Income & Job Descriptions, Selected Prices of the Times, Annual Income, Annual Budgets, Family Finances, Life at Work, Life at Home, Life in the Community, Working Conditions, Cost of Living, Amusements and much more. For even broader access to the events, economics and attitude towards women throughout the past 130 years, each chapter is supplemented with News Profiles, Articles from Local Media, Illustrations, Economic Profiles, Typical Pricing, Key Events, Inventions and more. This important volume illustrates what life was like for working women over time and allows the reader to develop an understanding of the changing role of women at work. These interesting and useful compilations of portraits of women at work will be an important addition to any high school, public or academic library reference collection.

Hardcover ISBN 978-1-59237-063-4, 600 pages, $145.00 | Ebook ISBN 978-1-59237-168-6 www.greyhouse.com/ebooks.htm

Working Americans 1880-2005 Volume VII: Social Movements

Working Americans series, Volume VII: Social Movements explores how Americans sought and fought for change from the 1880s to the present time. Following the format of previous volumes in the Working Americans series, the text examines the lives of 34 individuals who have worked -- often behind the scenes --- to bring about change. Issues include topics as diverse as the Anti-smoking movement of 1901 to efforts by Native Americans to reassert their long lost rights. Along the way, the book will profile individuals brave enough to demand suffrage for Kansas women in 1912 or demand an end to lynching during a March on Washington in 1923. Each profile is enriched with real data on Income & Job Descriptions, Selected Prices of the Times, Annual Incomes & Budgets, Life at Work, Life at Home, Life in the Community, along with News Features, Key Events, and Illustrations. The depth of information contained in each profile allow the user to explore the private, financial and public lives of these subjects, deepening our understanding of how calls for change took place in our society. A must-purchase for the reference collections of high school libraries, public libraries and academic libraries.

Hardcover ISBN 978-1-59237-101-3, 600 pages, $145.00 | Ebook ISBN 978-1-59237-174-7 www.greyhouse.com/ebooks.htm

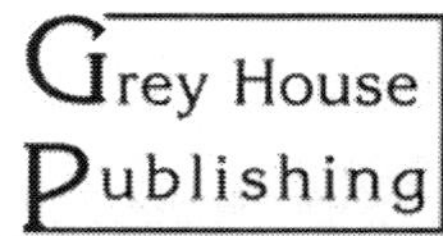

Working Americans 1880-2005 Volume VIII: Immigrants

Working Americans 1880-2007 Volume VIII: Immigrants illustrates what life was like for families leaving their homeland and creating a new life in the United States. Each chapter covers one decade and introduces the reader to three immigrant families. Family profiles cover what life was like in their homeland, in their community in the United States, their home life, working conditions and so much more. As the reader moves through these pages, the families and individuals come to life, painting a picture of why they left their homeland, their experiences in setting roots in a new country, their struggles and triumphs, stretching from the 1800s to the present time. Profiles include a seven-year-old Swedish girl who meets her father for the first time at Ellis Island; a Chinese photographer's assistant; an Armenian who flees the genocide of his country to build Ford automobiles in Detroit; a 38-year-old German bachelor cigar maker who settles in Newark NJ, but contemplates tobacco farming in Virginia; a 19-year-old Irish domestic servant who is amazed at the easy life of American dogs; a 19-year-old Filipino who came to Hawaii against his parent's wishes to farm sugar cane; a French-Canadian who finds success as a boxer in Maine and many more. As in previous volumes, information is presented in narrative form, but hard facts and real-life situations back up each story. With the topic of immigration being so hotly debated in this country, this timely resource will prove to be a useful source for students, researchers, historians and library patrons to discover the issues facing immigrants in the United States. This title will be a useful addition to reference collections of public libraries, university libraries and high schools.

Hardcover ISBN 978-1-59237-197-6, 600 pages, $145.00 | Ebook ISBN 978-1-59237-232-4 www.greyhouse.com/ebooks.htm

Working Americans 1770-1896 Volume IX: From the Revolutionary War to the Civil War

Working Americans 1770-1869: From the Revolutionary War to the Civil War examines what life was like for the earliest of Americans. Like previous volumes in the successful Working Americans series, each chapter introduces the reader to three individuals or families. These profiles illustrate what life was like for that individual, at home, in the community and at work. The profiles are supplemented with information on current events, community issues, pricing of the times and news articles to give the reader a broader understanding of what was happening in that individual's world and how it shaped their life. Profiles extend through all walks of life, from farmers to merchants, the rich and poor, men, women and children. In these information-packed, fun-to-explore pages, the reader will be introduced to Ezra Stiles, a preacher and college president from 1776; Colonel Israel Angell, a continental officer from 1778; Thomas Vernon, a loyalist in 1776, Anna Green Winslow, a school girl in 1771; Sarah Pierce, a school teacher in 1792; Edward Hooker, an attorney in 1805; Jeremiah Greenman, a common soldier in 1775 and many others. Using these information-filled profiles, the reader can develop an understanding of what life was like for all types of Americans in these interesting and changing times. This new edition will be an important acquisition for high school, public and academic libraries as well as history reference collections.

Hardcover ISBN 978-1-59237-371-0, 660 pages, $145.00

Working Americans 1880-2009 Volume X: Sports & Recreation

Working Americans 1880-2009 Volume X: Sports & Recreation focuses on the lighter side of life in America. Examining professional sports to amateur sports to leisure time and recreation, this interesting volume illustrates how Americans had fun from the Civil War to the present time. Intriguing profiles in each decade-long chapter are supplemented with information on current events, community issues, pricing of the times and news articles to give the reader a broader understanding of what was happening in that individual's world and how it shaped their life. To further explore the life and times of these individuals, each chapter includes several other helpful elements: Historical Snapshots, Timelines, News Features, Selected Prices, and Illustrations. Readers will be able to examine the growth of professional sports and how ticket prices changed over the years, look at what games were popular, find out how early Americans spent their leisure time and get and understanding of the importance of recreation in any time period.

Hardcover ISBN 978-1-59237-441-0, 600 pages, $145.00

The Encyclopedia of Warrior Peoples & Fighting Groups

Many military groups throughout the world have excelled in their craft either by fortuitous circumstances, outstanding leadership, or intense training. This new second edition of *The Encyclopedia of Warrior Peoples and Fighting Groups* explores the origins and leadership of these outstanding combat forces, chronicles their conquests and accomplishments, examines the circumstances surrounding their decline or disbanding, and assesses their influence on the groups and methods of warfare that followed. Readers will encounter ferocious tribes, charismatic leaders, and daring militias, from ancient times to the present, including Amazons, Buffalo Soldiers, Green Berets, Iron Brigade, Kamikazes, Peoples of the Sea, Polish Winged Hussars, Teutonic Knights, and Texas Rangers. With over 100 alphabetical entries, numerous cross-references and illustrations, a comprehensive bibliography, and index, the *Encyclopedia of Warrior Peoples and Fighting Groups* is a valuable resource for readers seeking insight into the bold history of distinguished fighting forces.

"Especially useful for high school students, undergraduates, and general readers with an interest in military history." –Library Journal

Hardcover ISBN 978-1-59237-116-7, 660 pages, $165.00 | Ebook ISBN 978-1-59237-172-3 www.greyhouse.com/ebooks.htm

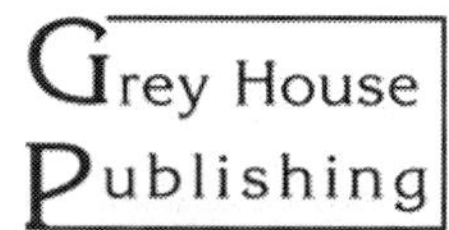

Speakers of the House of Representatives, 1789-2009

Beginning with Frederick Muhlenberg in 1789 and stretching to Nancy Pelosi, the first female Speaker of the House, this new reference work provides unique coverage of this important political position. Presiding over the House of Representatives and second the United States presidential line of succession, this position has particular influence over US politics. Features include: thoughtfully-written Biographies of each of the 52 Speakers of the House, all with photos; several full-length Essays, each covering an interesting and thought-provoking topic pertinent to the formation, history and current events surrounding the Speaker; Primary Documents, for added sources of research, include important articles, resignation letters, speeches and letters; several helpful Appendices: Years Served in Congress before Becoming Speaker, Speakers & Party Control of the Presidency, Dates of Election & States Represented, Speaker Firsts; a Chronology of Elections and Important Events, a comprehensive Bibliography and a cumulative Index. This new resource brings together a wealth of information on individual Speakers, the history of the position and its changing role in US politics. This resource will be a valuable addition to public libraries, high schools, university libraries along with history and political science collections.

Hardcover ISBN 978-1-59237-404-5, 500 pages, $135.00 | Ebook ISBN 978-1-59237-483-0 www.greyhouse.com/ebooks.htm

The Encyclopedia of Rural America: the Land & People

History, sociology, anthropology, and public policy are combined to deliver the encyclopedia destined to become the standard reference work in American rural studies. From irrigation and marriage to games and mental health, this encyclopedia is the first to explore the contemporary landscape of rural America, placed in historical perspective. With over 300 articles prepared by leading experts from across the nation, this timely encyclopedia documents and explains the major themes, concepts, industries, concerns, and everyday life of the people and land who make up rural America. Entries range from the industrial sector and government policy to arts and humanities and social and family concerns. Articles explore every aspect of life in rural America. *Encyclopedia of Rural America*, with its broad range of coverage, will appeal to high school and college students as well as graduate students, faculty, scholars, and people whose work pertains to rural areas.

"This exemplary encyclopedia is guaranteed to educate our highly urban society about the uniqueness of rural America. Recommended for public and academic libraries." -Library Journal

Two Volumes, Hardcover, ISBN 978-1-59237-115-0, 800 pages, $250.00

The Encyclopedia of Invasions & Conquests, From the Ancient Times to the Present

This second edition of the popular *Encyclopedia of Invasions & Conquests*, a comprehensive guide to over 150 invasions, conquests, battles and occupations from ancient times to the present, takes readers on a journey that includes the Roman conquest of Britain, the Portuguese colonization of Brazil, and the Iraqi invasion of Kuwait, to name a few. New articles will explore the late 20th and 21st centuries, with a specific focus on recent conflicts in Afghanistan, Kuwait, Iraq, Yugoslavia, Grenada and Chechnya. In addition to covering the military aspects of invasions and conquests, entries cover some of the political, economic, and cultural aspects, for example, the effects of a conquest on the invade country's political and monetary system and in its language and religion. The entries on leaders – among them Sargon, Alexander the Great, William the Conqueror, and Adolf Hitler – deal with the people who sought to gain control, expand power, or exert religious or political influence over others through military means. Revised and updated for this second edition, entries are arranged alphabetically within historical periods. Each chapter provides a map to help readers locate key areas and geographical features, and bibliographical references appear at the end of each entry. Other useful features include cross-references, a cumulative bibliography and a comprehensive subject index. This authoritative, well-organized, lucidly written volume will prove invaluable for a variety of readers, including high school students, military historians, members of the armed forces, history buffs and hobbyists.

"Engaging writing, sensible organization, nice illustrations, interesting and obscure facts, and useful maps make this book a pleasure to read." –ARBA

Hardcover ISBN 978-1-59237-114-3, 598 pages, $165.00 | Ebook ISBN 978-1-59237-171-6 www.greyhouse.com/ebooks.htm

Encyclopedia of Prisoners of War & Internment

This authoritative second edition provides a valuable overview of the history of prisoners of war and interned civilians, from earliest times to the present. Written by an international team of experts in the field of POW studies, this fascinating and thought-provoking volume includes entries on a wide range of subjects including the Crusades, Plains Indian Warfare, concentration camps, the two world wars, and famous POWs throughout history, as well as atrocities, escapes, and much more. Written in a clear and easily understandable style, this informative reference details over 350 entries, 30% larger than the first edition, that survey the history of prisoners of war and interned civilians from the earliest times to the present, with emphasis on the 19th and 20th centuries. Medical conditions, international law, exchanges of prisoners, organizations working on behalf of POWs, and trials associated with the treatment of captives are just some of the themes explored. Entries are arranged alphabetically, plus illustrations and maps are provided for easy reference. The text also includes an introduction, bibliography, appendix of selected documents, and end-of-entry reading suggestions. This one-of-a-kind reference will be a helpful addition to the reference collections of all public libraries, high schools, and university libraries and will prove invaluable to historians and military enthusiasts.

"Thorough and detailed yet accessible to the lay reader. Of special interest to subject specialists and historians; recommended for public and academic libraries." - Library Journal

Hardcover ISBN 978-1-59237-120-4, 676 pages, $165.00 | Ebook ISBN 978-1-59237-170-9 www.greyhouse.com/ebooks.htm

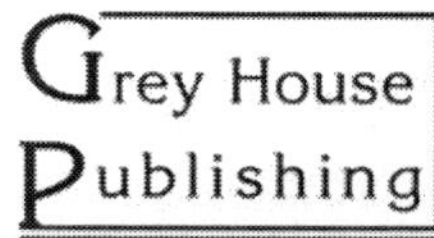

From Suffrage to the Senate, America's Political Women

From Suffrage to the Senate is a comprehensive and valuable compendium of biographies of leading women in U.S. politics, past and present, and an examination of the wide range of women's movements. This reference work explores American women's path to political power and social equality from the struggle for the right to vote and the abolition of slavery to the first African American woman in the U.S. Senate and beyond. The in-depth coverage also traces the political heritage of the abolition, labor, suffrage, temperance, and reproductive rights movements. The alphabetically arranged entries include biographies of every woman from across the political spectrum who has served in the U.S. House and Senate, along with women in the Judiciary and the U.S. Cabinet and, new to this edition, biographies of activists and political consultants. Bibliographical references follow each entry. For easy reference, a handy chronology is provided detailing 150 years of women's history. This up-to-date reference will be a must-purchase for women's studies departments, high schools and public libraries and will be a handy resource for those researching the key players in women's politics, past and present.

"An engaging tool that would be useful in high school, public, and academic libraries looking for an overview of the political history of women in the US." –Booklist

Two Volumes, Hardcover ISBN 978-1-59237-117-4, 1,160 pages, $199.00 | Ebook ISBN 978-1-59237-227-0 www.greyhouse.com/ebooks.htm

An African Biographical Dictionary

This landmark second edition is the only biographical dictionary to bring together, in one volume, cultural, social and political leaders – both historical and contemporary – of the sub-Saharan region. Over 800 biographical sketches of prominent Africans, as well as foreigners who have affected the continent's history, are featured, 150 more than the previous edition. The wide spectrum of leaders includes religious figures, writers, politicians, scientists, entertainers, sports personalities and more. Access to these fascinating individuals is provided in a user-friendly format. The biographies are arranged alphabetically, cross-referenced and indexed. Entries include the country or countries in which the person was significant and the commonly accepted dates of birth and death. Each biographical sketch is chronologically written; entries for cultural personalities add an evaluation of their work. This information is followed by a selection of references often found in university and public libraries, including autobiographies and principal biographical works. Appendixes list each individual by country and by field of accomplishment – rulers, musicians, explorers, missionaries, businessmen, physicists – nearly thirty categories in all. Another convenient appendix lists heads of state since independence by country. Up-to-date and representative of African societies as a whole, An African Biographical Dictionary provides a wealth of vital information for students of African culture and is an indispensable reference guide for anyone interested in African affairs.

"An unquestionable convenience to have these concise, informative biographies gathered into one source, indexed, and analyzed by appendixes listing entrants by nation and occupational field." –Wilson Library Bulletin

Hardcover ISBN 978-1-59237-112-9, 667 pages, $165.00 | Ebook ISBN 978-1-59237-229-4 www.greyhouse.com/ebooks.htm

African American Writers

A timely survey of an important sector of American letters, *African American Writers* covers the role and influence of African American cultural leaders, from all walks of life, from the 18th century to the present. Readers will explore what inspired various African-American writers to create poems, plays, short stories, novels, essays, opinion pieces and numerous other works, and how those writings contributed to culture in America today. With 200 new entries, over 35% larger than the previous edition, this edition features over 100 new Author biographies, for a total of 500, with illustrations, cover the important events in a writer's life, education, major works, honors and awards, and family and important associates; more Genre Tables, covering newspapers, journals, book publishers, online resources, illustrators and more, each with an introduction and listings of top authors in each genre, their pen names, key publications and awards; new Topical entries, including writing collaboratives, book clubs, celebrity authors and self-publishing; new Author Tables, covering additional authors in multiple genres, with author name, pen name, birth year, genre and more; an Appendix of Writers by Genre; a Chronology of Writers; a Chronology of Firsts, with interesting facts, from the first narrative written by an African-American slave, to the first African-American to receive the Nobel prize for literature; a list of Abbreviations and a Cumulative Index. More than a collection of biographies, this important work traces the evolution of African-American writers, their struggles, triumphs, and legacy, this volume is not to be missed. A comprehensive, easy to use source that will complement the reference collection of any public, high school or university library, and will prove useful to all university humanities and African American studies reference collections.

"No other single work seeks to include all past and present African American writers of significance in such an affordable format ... an appealing choice for all public and academic libraries." –Library Journal

Hardcover ISBN 978-1-59237-291-1, 667 pages, $165.00 | Ebook ISBN 978-1-59237-302-4 www.greyhouse.com/ebooks.htm

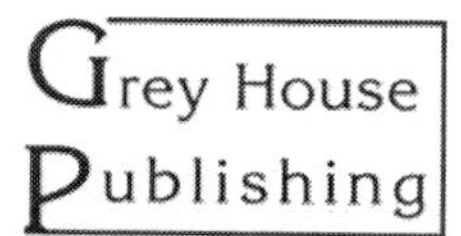

American Environmental Leaders, From Colonial Times to the Present

A comprehensive and diverse award winning collection of biographies of the most important figures in American environmentalism. Few subjects arouse the passions the way the environment does. How will we feed an ever-increasing population and how can that food be made safe for consumption? Who decides how land is developed? How can environmental policies be made fair for everyone, including multiethnic groups, women, children, and the poor? *American Environmental Leaders* presents more than 350 biographies of men and women who have devoted their lives to studying, debating, and organizing these and other controversial issues over the last 200 years. In addition to the scientists who have analyzed how human actions affect nature, we are introduced to poets, landscape architects, presidents, painters, activists, even sanitation engineers, and others who have forever altered how we think about the environment. The easy to use A–Z format provides instant access to these fascinating individuals, and frequent cross references indicate others with whom individuals worked (and sometimes clashed). End of entry references provide users with a starting point for further research.

"Highly recommended for high school, academic, and public libraries needing environmental biographical information." –Library Journal/Starred Review

Two Volumes, Hardcover ISBN 978-1-59237-119-8, 900 pages $195.00 | Ebook ISBN 978-1-59237-230-0
www.greyhouse.com/ebooks.htm

World Cultural Leaders of the Twentieth & Twenty-First Centuries

World Cultural Leaders of the Twentieth & Twenty-First Centuries is a window into the arts, performances, movements, and music that shaped the world's cultural development since 1900. A remarkable around-the-world look at one-hundred-plus years of cultural development through the eyes of those that set the stage and stayed to play. This second edition offers over 120 new biographies along with a complete update of existing biographies. To further aid the reader, a handy fold-out timeline traces important events in all six cultural categories from 1900 through the present time. Plus, a new section of detailed material and resources for 100 selected individuals is also new to this edition, with further data on museums, homesteads, websites, artwork and more. This remarkable compilation will answer a wide range of questions. Who was the originator of the term "documentary"? Which poet married the daughter of the famed novelist Thomas Mann in order to help her escape Nazi Germany? Which British writer served as an agent in Russia against the Bolsheviks before the 1917 revolution? A handy two-volume set that makes it easy to look up 450 worldwide cultural icons: novelists, poets, playwrights, painters, sculptors, architects, dancers, choreographers, actors, directors, filmmakers, singers, composers, and musicians. *World Cultural Leaders of the Twentieth & Twenty-First Centuries* provides entries (many of them illustrated) covering the person's works, achievements, and professional career in a thorough essay and offers interesting facts and statistics. Entries are fully cross-referenced so that readers can learn how various individuals influenced others. An index of leaders by occupation, a useful glossary and a thorough general index complete the coverage. This remarkable resource will be an important acquisition for the reference collections of public libraries, university libraries and high schools.

"Fills a need for handy, concise information on a wide array of international cultural figures."-ARBA

Two Volumes, Hardcover ISBN 978-1-59237-118-1, 900 pages, $199.00 | Ebook ISBN 978-1-59237-231-7
www.greyhouse.com/ebooks.htm

Political Corruption in America: An Encyclopedia of Scandals, Power, and Greed

The complete scandal-filled history of American political corruption, focusing on the infamous people and cases, as well as society's electoral and judicial reactions. Since colonial times, there has been no shortage of politicians willing to take a bribe, skirt campaign finance laws, or act in their own interests. Corruption like the Whiskey Ring, Watergate, and Whitewater cases dominate American life, making political scandal a leading U.S. industry. From judges to senators, presidents to mayors, *Political Corruption in America* discusses the infamous people throughout history who have been accused of and implicated in crooked behavior. In this new second edition, more than 250 A–Z entries explore the people, crimes, investigations, and court cases behind 200 years of American political scandals. This unbiased volume also delves into the issues surrounding Koreagate, the Chinese campaign scandal, and other ethical lapses. Relevant statutes and terms, including the Independent Counsel Statute and impeachment as a tool of political punishment, are examined as well. Students, scholars, and other readers interested in American history, political science, and ethics will appreciate this survey of a wide range of corrupting influences. This title focuses on how politicians from all parties have fallen because of their greed and hubris, and how society has used electoral and judicial means against those who tested the accepted standards of political conduct. A full range of illustrations including political cartoons, photos of key figures such as Abe Fortas and Archibald Cox, graphs of presidential pardons, and tables showing the number of expulsions and censures in both the House and Senate round out the text. In addition, a comprehensive chronology of major political scandals in U.S. history from colonial times until the present. For further reading, an extensive bibliography lists sources including archival letters, newspapers, and private manuscript collections from the United States and Great Britain. With its comprehensive coverage of this interesting topic, *Political Corruption in America: An Encyclopedia of Scandals, Power, and Greed* will prove to be a useful addition to the reference collections of all public libraries, university libraries, history collections, political science collections and high schools.

"...this encyclopedia is a useful contribution to the field. Highly recommended." - CHOICE
"Political Corruption should be useful in most academic, high school, and public libraries." Booklist

Two Volumes, Hardcover ISBN 978-1-59237-297-3, 500 pages, $195.00 | Ebook ISBN 978-1-59237-308-6
www.greyhouse.com/ebooks.htm

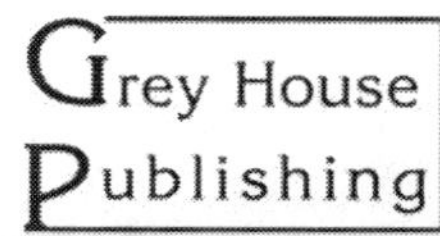

Encyclopedia of Religion & the Law in America

This informative, easy-to-use reference work covers a wide range of legal issues that affect the roles of religion and law in American society. Extensive A–Z entries provide coverage of key court decisions, case studies, concepts, individuals, religious groups, organizations, and agencies shaping religion and law in today's society. This *Encyclopedia* focuses on topics involved with the constitutional theory and interpretation of religion and the law; terms providing a historical explanation of the ways in which America's ever increasing ethnic and religious diversity contributed to our current understanding of the mandates of the First and Fourteenth Amendments; terms and concepts describing the development of religion clause jurisprudence; an analytical examination of the distinct vocabulary used in this area of the law; the means by which American courts have attempted to balance religious liberty against other important individual and social interests in a wide variety of physical and regulatory environments, including the classroom, the workplace, the courtroom, religious group organization and structure, taxation, the clash of "secular" and "religious" values, and the relationship of the generalized idea of individual autonomy of the specific concept of religious liberty. Important legislation and legal cases affecting religion and society are thoroughly covered in this timely volume, including a detailed Table of Cases and Table of Statutes for more detailed research. A guide to further reading and an index are also included. This useful resource will be an important acquisition for the reference collections of all public libraries, university libraries, religion reference collections and high schools.

Hardcover ISBN 978-1-59237-298-0, 500 pages, $135.00 | Ebook ISBN 978-1-59237-309-3 www.greyhouse.com/ebooks.htm

The Religious Right, A Reference Handbook

Timely and unbiased, this third edition updates and expands its examination of the religious right and its influence on our government, citizens, society, and politics. This text explores the influence of religion on legislation and society, while examining the alignment of the religious right with the political right. The coverage offers a critical historical survey of the religious right movement, focusing on its increased involvement in the political arena, attempts to forge coalitions, and notable successes and failures. The text offers complete coverage of biographies of the men and women who have advanced the cause and an up to date chronology illuminate the movement's goals, including their accomplishments and failures. Two new sections complement this third edition, a chapter on legal issues and court decisions and a chapter on demographic statistics and electoral patterns. To aid in further research, *The Religious Right*, offers an entire section of annotated listings of print and non-print resources, as well as of organizations affiliated with the religious right, and those opposing it. Comprehensive in its scope, this work offers easy-to-read, pertinent information for those seeking to understand the religious right and its evolving role in American society. A must for libraries of all sizes, university religion departments, activists, high schools and for those interested in the evolving role of the religious right.

" Recommended for all public and academic libraries." - Library Journal

Hardcover ISBN 978-1-59237-113-6, 600 pages, $165.00 | Ebook ISBN 978-1-59237-226-3 www.greyhouse.com/ebooks.htm

Human Rights in the United States: A Dictionary and Documents

This two volume set offers easy to grasp explanations of the basic concepts, laws, and case law in the field, with emphasis on human rights in the historical, political, and legal experience of the United States. Human rights is a term not fully understood by many Americans. Addressing this gap, the new second edition of *Human Rights in the United States: A Dictionary and Documents* offers a comprehensive introduction that places the history of human rights in the United States in an international context. It surveys the legal protection of human dignity in the United States, examines the sources of human rights norms, cites key legal cases, explains the role of international governmental and non-governmental organizations, and charts global, regional, and U.N. human rights measures. Over 240 dictionary entries of human rights terms are detailed—ranging from asylum and cultural relativism to hate crimes and torture. Each entry discusses the significance of the term, gives examples, and cites appropriate documents and court decisions. In addition, a Documents section is provided that contains 59 conventions, treaties, and protocols related to the most up to date international action on ethnic cleansing; freedom of expression and religion; violence against women; and much more. A bibliography, extensive glossary, and comprehensive index round out this indispensable volume. This comprehensive, timely volume is a must for large public libraries, university libraries and social science departments, along with high school libraries.

"...invaluable for anyone interested in human rights issues ... highly recommended for all reference collections."
- American Reference Books Annual

Two Volumes, Hardcover ISBN 978-1-59237-290-4, 750 pages, $225.00 | Ebook ISBN 978-1-59237-301-7
www.greyhouse.com/ebooks.htm

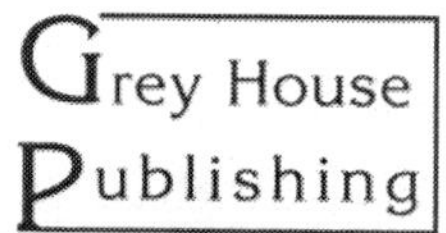

The Comparative Guide to American Elementary & Secondary Schools, 2009/10

The only guide of its kind, this award winning compilation offers a snapshot profile of every public school district in the United States serving 1,500 or more students – more than 5,900 districts are covered. Organized alphabetically by district within state, each chapter begins with a Statistical Overview of the state. Each district listing includes contact information (name, address, phone number and web site) plus Grades Served, the Numbers of Students and Teachers and the Number of Regular, Special Education, Alternative and Vocational Schools in the district along with statistics on Student/Classroom Teacher Ratios, Drop Out Rates, Ethnicity, the Numbers of Librarians and Guidance Counselors and District Expenditures per student. As an added bonus, *The Comparative Guide to American Elementary and Secondary Schools* provides important ranking tables, both by state and nationally, for each data element. For easy navigation through this wealth of information, this handbook contains a useful City Index that lists all districts that operate schools within a city. These important comparative statistics are necessary for anyone considering relocation or doing comparative research on their own district and would be a perfect acquisition for any public library or school district library.

"This straightforward guide is an easy way to find general information. Valuable for academic and large public library collections." –ARBA

Softcover ISBN 978-1-59237-436-6, 2,400 pages, $125.00 | Ebook ISBN 978-1-59237-238-6 www.greyhouse.com/ebooks.htm

The Complete Learning Disabilities Directory, 2009

The Complete Learning Disabilities Directory is the most comprehensive database of Programs, Services, Curriculum Materials, Professional Meetings & Resources, Camps, Newsletters and Support Groups for teachers, students and families concerned with learning disabilities. This information-packed directory includes information about Associations & Organizations, Schools, Colleges & Testing Materials, Government Agencies, Legal Resources and much more. For quick, easy access to information, this directory contains four indexes: Entry Name Index, Subject Index and Geographic Index. With every passing year, the field of learning disabilities attracts more attention and the network of caring, committed and knowledgeable professionals grows every day. This directory is an invaluable research tool for these parents, students and professionals.

"Due to its wealth and depth of coverage, parents, teachers and others... should find this an invaluable resource." -Booklist

Softcover ISBN 978-1-59237-368-0, 900 pages, $150.00 | Online Database: http://gold.greyhouse.com Call (800) 562-2139 for quote

Educators Resource Directory, 2009/10

Educators Resource Directory is a comprehensive resource that provides the educational professional with thousands of resources and statistical data for professional development. This directory saves hours of research time by providing immediate access to Associations & Organizations, Conferences & Trade Shows, Educational Research Centers, Employment Opportunities & Teaching Abroad, School Library Services, Scholarships, Financial Resources, Professional Consultants, Computer Software & Testing Resources and much more. Plus, this comprehensive directory also includes a section on Statistics and Rankings with over 100 tables, including statistics on Average Teacher Salaries, SAT/ACT scores, Revenues & Expenditures and more. These important statistics will allow the user to see how their school rates among others, make relocation decisions and so much more. For quick access to information, this directory contains four indexes: Entry & Publisher Index, Geographic Index, a Subject & Grade Index and Web Sites Index. *Educators Resource Directory* will be a well-used addition to the reference collection of any school district, education department or public library.

"Recommended for all collections that serve elementary and secondary school professionals." –Choice

Softcover ISBN 978-1-59237-397-0, 800 pages, $145.00 | Online Database: http://gold.greyhouse.com Call (800) 562-2139 for quote

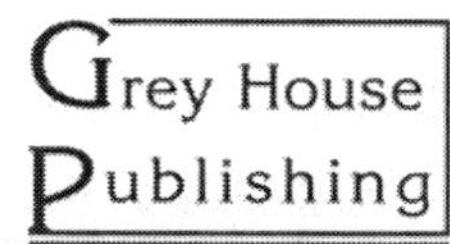

Profiles of New York | Profiles of Florida | Profiles of Texas | Profiles of Illinois | Profiles of Michigan | Profiles of Ohio | Profiles of New Jersey | Profiles of Massachusetts | Profiles of Pennsylvania | Profiles of Wisconsin | Profiles of Connecticut & Rhode Island | Profiles of Indiana | Profiles of North Carolina & South Carolina | Profiles of Virginia | Profiles of California

The careful layout gives the user an easy-to-read snapshot of every single place and county in the state, from the biggest metropolis to the smallest unincorporated hamlet. The richness of each place or county profile is astounding in its depth, from history to weather, all packed in an easy-to-navigate, compact format. Each profile contains data on History, Geography, Climate, Population, Vital Statistics, Economy, Income, Taxes, Education, Housing, Health & Environment, Public Safety, Newspapers, Transportation, Presidential Election Results, Information Contacts and Chambers of Commerce. As an added bonus, there is a section on Selected Statistics, where data from the 100 largest towns and cities is arranged into easy-to-use charts. Each of 22 different data points has its own two-page spread with the cities listed in alpha order so researchers can easily compare and rank cities. A remarkable compilation that offers overviews and insights into each corner of the state, each volume goes beyond Census statistics, beyond metro area coverage, beyond the 100 best places to live. Drawn from official census information, other government statistics and original research, you will have at your fingertips data that's available nowhere else in one single source.

"The publisher claims that this is the 'most comprehensive portrait of the state of Florida ever published,' and this reviewer is inclined to believe it...Recommended. All levels." –Choice on Profiles of Florida

Each Profiles of... title ranges from 400-800 pages, priced at $149.00 each

America's Top-Rated Cities, 2009

America's Top-Rated Cities provides current, comprehensive statistical information and other essential data in one easy-to-use source on the 100 "top" cities that have been cited as the best for business and living in the U.S. This handbook allows readers to see, at a glance, a concise social, business, economic, demographic and environmental profile of each city, including brief evaluative comments. In addition to detailed data on Cost of Living, Finances, Real Estate, Education, Major Employers, Media, Crime and Climate, city reports now include Housing Vacancies, Tax Audits, Bankruptcy, Presidential Election Results and more. This outstanding source of information will be widely used in any reference collection.

"The only source of its kind that brings together all of this information into one easy-to-use source. It will be beneficial to many business and public libraries." –ARBA

Four Volumes, Softcover ISBN 978-1-59237-410-6, 2,500 pages, $195.00 | Ebook ISBN 978-1-59237-233-1
www.greyhouse.com/ebooks.htm

America's Top-Rated Smaller Cities, 2008/09

A perfect companion to *America's Top-Rated Cities*, *America's Top-Rated Smaller Cities* provides current, comprehensive business and living profiles of smaller cities (population 25,000-99,999) that have been cited as the best for business and living in the United States. Sixty cities make up this 2004 edition of America's Top-Rated Smaller Cities, all are top-ranked by Population Growth, Median Income, Unemployment Rate and Crime Rate. City reports reflect the most current data available on a wide-range of statistics, including Employment & Earnings, Household Income, Unemployment Rate, Population Characteristics, Taxes, Cost of Living, Education, Health Care, Public Safety, Recreation, Media, Air & Water Quality and much more. Plus, each city report contains a Background of the City, and an Overview of the State Finances. *America's Top-Rated Smaller Cities* offers a reliable, one-stop source for statistical data that, before now, could only be found scattered in hundreds of sources. This volume is designed for a wide range of readers: individuals considering relocating a residence or business; professionals considering expanding their business or changing careers; general and market researchers; real estate consultants; human resource personnel; urban planners and investors.

"Provides current, comprehensive statistical information in one easy-to-use source... Recommended for public and academic libraries and specialized collections." –Library Journal

Two Volumes, Softcover ISBN 978-1-59237-284-3, 1,100 pages, $195.00 | Ebook ISBN 978-1-59237-234-8
www.greyhouse.com/ebooks.htm

Profiles of America: Facts, Figures & Statistics for Every Populated Place in the United States

Profiles of America is the only source that pulls together, in one place, statistical, historical and descriptive information about every place in the United States in an easy-to-use format. This award winning reference set, now in its second edition, compiles statistics and data from over 20 different sources – the latest census information has been included along with more than nine brand new statistical topics. This Four-Volume Set details over 40,000 places, from the biggest metropolis to the smallest unincorporated hamlet, and provides statistical details and information on over 50 different topics including Geography, Climate, Population, Vital Statistics, Economy, Income, Taxes, Education, Housing, Health & Environment, Public Safety, Newspapers, Transportation, Presidential Election Results and Information Contacts or Chambers of Commerce. Profiles are arranged, for ease-of-use, by state and then by county. Each county begins with a County-Wide Overview and is followed by information for each Community in that particular county. The Community Profiles within the county are arranged alphabetically. *Profiles of America* is a virtual snapshot of America at your fingertips and a unique compilation of information that will be widely used in any reference collection.

A Library Journal Best Reference Book "An outstanding compilation." –Library Journal

Four Volumes, Softcover ISBN 978-1-891482-80-9, 10,000 pages, $595.00

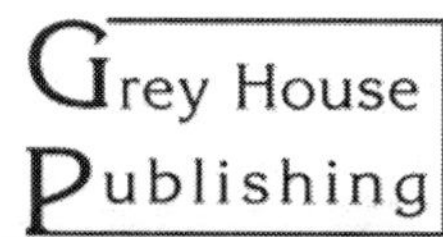

The Comparative Guide to American Suburbs, 2009/10

The Comparative Guide to American Suburbs is a one-stop source for Statistics on the 2,000+ suburban communities surrounding the 50 largest metropolitan areas – their population characteristics, income levels, economy, school system and important data on how they compare to one another. Organized into 50 Metropolitan Area chapters, each chapter contains an overview of the Metropolitan Area, a detailed Map followed by a comprehensive Statistical Profile of each Suburban Community, including Contact Information, Physical Characteristics, Population Characteristics, Income, Economy, Unemployment Rate, Cost of Living, Education, Chambers of Commerce and more. Next, statistical data is sorted into Ranking Tables that rank the suburbs by twenty different criteria, including Population, Per Capita Income, Unemployment Rate, Crime Rate, Cost of Living and more. *The Comparative Guide to American Suburbs* is the best source for locating data on suburbs. Those looking to relocate, as well as those doing preliminary market research, will find this an invaluable timesaving resource.

"Public and academic libraries will find this compilation useful...The work draws together figures from many sources and will be especially helpful for job relocation decisions." – Booklist

Softcover ISBN 978-1-59237-432-8 1,700 pages, $130.00 | Ebook ISBN 978-1-59237-235-5 www.greyhouse.com/ebooks.htm

The American Tally: Statistics & Comparative Rankings for U.S. Cities with Populations over 10,000

This important statistical handbook compiles, all in one place, comparative statistics on all U.S. cities and towns with a 10,000+ population. *The American Tally* provides statistical details on over 4,000 cities and towns and profiles how they compare with one another in Population Characteristics, Education, Language & Immigration, Income & Employment and Housing. Each section begins with an alphabetical listing of cities by state, allowing for quick access to both the statistics and relative rankings of any city. Next, the highest and lowest cities are listed in each statistic. These important, informative lists provide quick reference to which cities are at both extremes of the spectrum for each statistic. Unlike any other reference, *The American Tally* provides quick, easy access to comparative statistics – a must-have for any reference collection.

"A solid library reference." -Bookwatch

Softcover ISBN 978-1-930956-29-2, 500 pages, $125.00 | Ebook ISBN 978-1-59237-241-6 www.greyhouse.com/ebooks.htm

The Asian Databook: Statistics for all US Counties & Cities with Over 10,000 Population

This is the first-ever resource that compiles statistics and rankings on the US Asian population. *The Asian Databook* presents over 20 statistical data points for each city and county, arranged alphabetically by state, then alphabetically by place name. Data reported for each place includes Population, Languages Spoken at Home, Foreign-Born, Educational Attainment, Income Figures, Poverty Status, Homeownership, Home Values & Rent, and more. Next, in the Rankings Section, the top 75 places are listed for each data element. These easy-to-access ranking tables allow the user to quickly determine trends and population characteristics. This kind of comparative data can not be found elsewhere, in print or on the web, in a format that's as easy-to-use or more concise. A useful resource for those searching for demographics data, career search and relocation information and also for market research. With data ranging from Ancestry to Education, *The Asian Databook* presents a useful compilation of information that will be a much-needed resource in the reference collection of any public or academic library along with the marketing collection of any company whose primary focus in on the Asian population.

"This useful resource will help those searching for demographics data, and market research or relocation information... Accurate and clearly laid out, the publication is recommended for large public library and research collections." -Booklist

Softcover ISBN 978-1-59237-044-3, 1,000 pages, $150.00

The Hispanic Databook: Statistics for all US Counties & Cities with Over 10,000 Population

Previously published by Toucan Valley Publications, this second edition has been completely updated with figures from the latest census and has been broadly expanded to include dozens of new data elements and a brand new Rankings section. The Hispanic population in the United States has increased over 42% in the last 10 years and accounts for 12.5% of the total US population. For ease-of-use, *The Hispanic Databook* presents over 20 statistical data points for each city and county, arranged alphabetically by state, then alphabetically by place name. Data reported for each place includes Population, Languages Spoken at Home, Foreign-Born, Educational Attainment, Income Figures, Poverty Status, Homeownership, Home Values & Rent, and more. Next, in the Rankings Section, the top 75 places are listed for each data element. These easy-to-access ranking tables allow the user to quickly determine trends and population characteristics. This kind of comparative data can not be found elsewhere, in print or on the web, in a format that's as easy-to-use or more concise. A useful resource for those searching for demographics data, career search and relocation information and also for market research. With data ranging from Ancestry to Education, *The Hispanic Databook* presents a useful compilation of information that will be a much-needed resource in the reference collection of any public or academic library along with the marketing collection of any company whose primary focus in on the Hispanic population.

"This accurate, clearly presented volume of selected Hispanic demographics is recommended for large public libraries and research collections."-Library Journal

Softcover ISBN 978-1-59237-008-5, 1,000 pages, $150.00

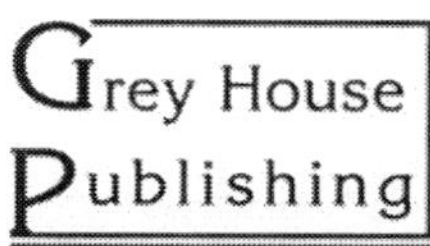

Ancestry in America: A Comparative Guide to Over 200 Ethnic Backgrounds

This brand new reference work pulls together thousands of comparative statistics on the Ethnic Backgrounds of all populated places in the United States with populations over 10,000. Never before has this kind of information been reported in a single volume. Section One, Statistics by Place, is made up of a list of over 200 ancestry and race categories arranged alphabetically by each of the 5,000 different places with populations over 10,000. The population number of the ancestry group in that city or town is provided along with the percent that group represents of the total population. This informative city-by-city section allows the user to quickly and easily explore the ethnic makeup of all major population bases in the United States. Section Two, Comparative Rankings, contains three tables for each ethnicity and race. In the first table, the top 150 populated places are ranked by population number for that particular ancestry group, regardless of population. In the second table, the top 150 populated places are ranked by the percent of the total population for that ancestry group. In the third table, those top 150 populated places with 10,000 population are ranked by population number for each ancestry group. These easy-to-navigate tables allow users to see ancestry population patterns and make city-by-city comparisons as well. This brand new, information-packed resource will serve a wide-range or research requests for demographics, population characteristics, relocation information and much more. *Ancestry in America: A Comparative Guide to Over 200 Ethnic Backgrounds* will be an important acquisition to all reference collections.

"This compilation will serve a wide range of research requests for population characteristics ... it offers much more detail than other sources." –Booklist

Softcover ISBN 978-1-59237-029-0, 1,500 pages, $225.00

Weather America, A Thirty-Year Summary of Statistical Weather Data and Rankings

This valuable resource provides extensive climatological data for over 4,000 National and Cooperative Weather Stations throughout the United States. Weather America begins with a new Major Storms section that details major storm events of the nation and a National Rankings section that details rankings for several data elements, such as Maximum Temperature and Precipitation. The main body of Weather America is organized into 50 state sections. Each section provides a Data Table on each Weather Station, organized alphabetically, that provides statistics on Maximum and Minimum Temperatures, Precipitation, Snowfall, Extreme Temperatures, Foggy Days, Humidity and more. State sections contain two brand new features in this edition – a City Index and a narrative Description of the climatic conditions of the state. Each section also includes a revised Map of the State that includes not only weather stations, but cities and towns.

"Best Reference Book of the Year." –Library Journal

Softcover ISBN 978-1-891482-29-8, 2,013 pages, $175.00 | Ebook ISBN 978-1-59237-237-9 www.greyhouse.com/ebooks.htm

Crime in America's Top-Rated Cities

This volume includes over 20 years of crime statistics in all major crime categories: violent crimes, property crimes and total crime. *Crime in America's Top-Rated Cities* is conveniently arranged by city and covers 76 top-rated cities. Crime in America's Top-Rated Cities offers details that compare the number of crimes and crime rates for the city, suburbs and metro area along with national crime trends for violent, property and total crimes. Also, this handbook contains important information and statistics on Anti-Crime Programs, Crime Risk, Hate Crimes, Illegal Drugs, Law Enforcement, Correctional Facilities, Death Penalty Laws and much more. A much-needed resource for people who are relocating, business professionals, general researchers, the press, law enforcement officials and students of criminal justice.

"Data is easy to access and will save hours of searching." –Global Enforcement Review

Softcover ISBN 978-1-891482-84-7, 832 pages, $155.00

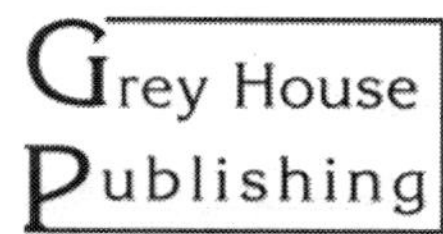

The Complete Directory for People with Disabilities, 2009

A wealth of information, now in one comprehensive sourcebook. Completely updated, this edition contains more information than ever before, including thousands of new entries and enhancements to existing entries and thousands of additional web sites and e-mail addresses. This up-to-date directory is the most comprehensive resource available for people with disabilities, detailing Independent Living Centers, Rehabilitation Facilities, State & Federal Agencies, Associations, Support Groups, Periodicals & Books, Assistive Devices, Employment & Education Programs, Camps and Travel Groups. Each year, more libraries, schools, colleges, hospitals, rehabilitation centers and individuals add *The Complete Directory for People with Disabilities* to their collections, making sure that this information is readily available to the families, individuals and professionals who can benefit most from the amazing wealth of resources cataloged here.

"No other reference tool exists to meet the special needs of the disabled in one convenient resource for information." –Library Journal

Softcover ISBN 978-1-59237-367-3, 1,200 pages, $165.00 | Online Database: http://gold.greyhouse.com Call (800) 562-2139 for quote

The Complete Learning Disabilities Directory, 2009

The Complete Learning Disabilities Directory is the most comprehensive database of Programs, Services, Curriculum Materials, Professional Meetings & Resources, Camps, Newsletters and Support Groups for teachers, students and families concerned with learning disabilities. This information-packed directory includes information about Associations & Organizations, Schools, Colleges & Testing Materials, Government Agencies, Legal Resources and much more. For quick, easy access to information, this directory contains four indexes: Entry Name Index, Subject Index and Geographic Index. With every passing year, the field of learning disabilities attracts more attention and the network of caring, committed and knowledgeable professionals grows every day. This directory is an invaluable research tool for these parents, students and professionals.

"Due to its wealth and depth of coverage, parents, teachers and others… should find this an invaluable resource." -Booklist

Softcover ISBN 978-1-59237-368-0, 900 pages, $150.00 | Online Database: http://gold.greyhouse.com Call (800) 562-2139 for quote

The Complete Directory for People with Chronic Illness, 2009/10

Thousands of hours of research have gone into this completely updated edition – several new chapters have been added along with thousands of new entries and enhancements to existing entries. Plus, each chronic illness chapter has been reviewed by a medical expert in the field. This widely-hailed directory is structured around the 90 most prevalent chronic illnesses – from Asthma to Cancer to Wilson's Disease – and provides a comprehensive overview of the support services and information resources available for people diagnosed with a chronic illness. Each chronic illness has its own chapter and contains a brief description in layman's language, followed by important resources for National & Local Organizations, State Agencies, Newsletters, Books & Periodicals, Libraries & Research Centers, Support Groups & Hotlines, Web Sites and much more. This directory is an important resource for health care professionals, the collections of hospital and health care libraries, as well as an invaluable tool for people with a chronic illness and their support network.

"A must purchase for all hospital and health care libraries and is strongly recommended for all public library reference departments." –ARBA

Softcover ISBN 978-1-59237-415-1, 1,200 pages, $165.00 | Online Database: http://gold.greyhouse.com Call (800) 562-2139 for quote

The Complete Mental Health Directory, 2008/09

This is the most comprehensive resource covering the field of behavioral health, with critical information for both the layman and the mental health professional. For the layman, this directory offers understandable descriptions of 25 Mental Health Disorders as well as detailed information on Associations, Media, Support Groups and Mental Health Facilities. For the professional, The Complete Mental Health Directory offers critical and comprehensive information on Managed Care Organizations, Information Systems, Government Agencies and Provider Organizations. This comprehensive volume of needed information will be widely used in any reference collection.

"… the strength of this directory is that it consolidates widely dispersed information into a single volume." –Booklist

Softcover ISBN 978-1-59237-285-0, 800 pages, $165.00 | Online Database: http://gold.greyhouse.com Call (800) 562-2139 for quote

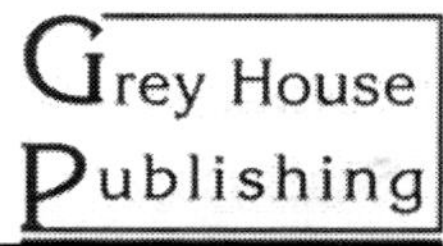

The Comparative Guide to American Hospitals, Second Edition

This new second edition compares all of the nation's hospitals by 24 measures of quality in the treatment of heart attack, heart failure, pneumonia, and, new to this edition, surgical procedures and pregnancy care. Plus, this second edition is now available in regional volumes, to make locating information about hospitals in your area quicker and easier than ever before. The Comparative Guide to American Hospitals provides a snapshot profile of each of the nations 4,200+ hospitals. These informative profiles illustrate how the hospital rates when providing 24 different treatments within four broad categories: Heart Attack Care, Heart Failure Care, Surgical Infection Prevention (NEW), and Pregnancy Care measures (NEW). Each profile includes the raw percentage for that hospital, the state average, the US average and data on the top hospital. For easy access to contact information, each profile includes the hospital's address, phone and fax numbers, email and web addresses, type and accreditation along with 5 top key administrations. These profiles will allow the user to quickly identify the quality of the hospital and have the necessary information at their fingertips to make contact with that hospital. Most importantly, *The Comparative Guide to American Hospitals* provides easy-to-use Regional State by State Statistical Summary Tables for each of the data elements to allow the user to quickly locate hospitals with the best level of service. Plus, a new 30-Day Mortality Chart, Glossary of Terms and Regional Hospital Profile Index make this a must-have source. This new, expanded edition will be a must for the reference collection at all public, medical and academic libraries.

"These data will help those with heart conditions and pneumonia make informed decisions about their healthcare and encourage hospitals to improve the quality of care they provide. Large medical, hospital, and public libraries are most likely to benefit from this weighty resource."-Library Journal

Four Volumes Softcover ISBN 978-1-59237-182-2, 3,500 pages, $325.00 | Regional Volumes $135.00 |
Ebook ISBN 978-1-59237-239-3 www.greyhouse.com/ebooks.htm

Older Americans Information Directory, 2008

Completely updated for 2008, this sixth edition has been completely revised and now contains 1,000 new listings, over 8,000 updates to existing listings and over 3,000 brand new e-mail addresses and web sites. You'll find important resources for Older Americans including National, Regional, State & Local Organizations, Government Agencies, Research Centers, Libraries & Information Centers, Legal Resources, Discount Travel Information, Continuing Education Programs, Disability Aids & Assistive Devices, Health, Print Media and Electronic Media. Three indexes: Entry Index, Subject Index and Geographic Index make it easy to find just the right source of information. This comprehensive guide to resources for Older Americans will be a welcome addition to any reference collection.

"Highly recommended for academic, public, health science and consumer libraries..." –Choice

1,200 pages; Softcover ISBN 978-1-59237-357-4, $165.00 | Online Database: http://gold.greyhouse.com Call (800) 562-2139 for quote

The Complete Directory for Pediatric Disorders, 2009/10

This important directory provides parents and caregivers with information about Pediatric Conditions, Disorders, Diseases and Disabilities, including Blood Disorders, Bone & Spinal Disorders, Brain Defects & Abnormalities, Chromosomal Disorders, Congenital Heart Defects, Movement Disorders, Neuromuscular Disorders and Pediatric Tumors & Cancers. This carefully written directory offers: understandable Descriptions of 15 major bodily systems; Descriptions of more than 200 Disorders and a Resources Section, detailing National Agencies & Associations, State Associations, Online Services, Libraries & Resource Centers, Research Centers, Support Groups & Hotlines, Camps, Books and Periodicals. This resource will provide immediate access to information crucial to families and caregivers when coping with children's illnesses.

"Recommended for public and consumer health libraries." –Library Journal

Softcover ISBN 978-1-59237-430-4, 1,200 pages, $165.00 | Online Database: http://gold.greyhouse.com Call (800) 562-2139 for quote

The Directory of Drug & Alcohol Residential Rehabilitation Facilities

This brand new directory is the first-ever resource to bring together, all in one place, data on the thousands of drug and alcohol residential rehabilitation facilities in the United States. The Directory of Drug & Alcohol Residential Rehabilitation Facilities covers over 1,000 facilities, with detailed contact information for each one, including mailing address, phone and fax numbers, email addresses and web sites, mission statement, type of treatment programs, cost, average length of stay, numbers of residents and counselors, accreditation, insurance plans accepted, type of environment, religious affiliation, education components and much more. It also contains a helpful chapter on General Resources that provides contact information for Associations, Print & Electronic Media, Support Groups and Conferences. Multiple indexes allow the user to pinpoint the facilities that meet very specific criteria. This time-saving tool is what so many counselors, parents and medical professionals have been asking for. *The Directory of Drug & Alcohol Residential Rehabilitation Facilities* will be a helpful tool in locating the right source for treatment for a wide range of individuals. This comprehensive directory will be an important acquisition for all reference collections: public and academic libraries, case managers, social workers, state agencies and many more.

"This is an excellent, much needed directory that fills an important gap..." –Booklist

Softcover ISBN 978-1-59237-031-3, 300 pages, $135.00

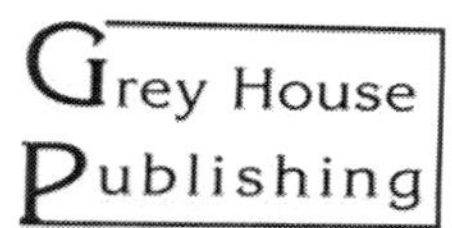

The Directory of Hospital Personnel, 2009

The Directory of Hospital Personnel is the best resource you can have at your fingertips when researching or marketing a product or service to the hospital market. A "Who's Who" of the hospital universe, this directory puts you in touch with over 150,000 key decision-makers. With 100% verification of data you can rest assured that you will reach the right person with just one call. Every hospital in the U.S. is profiled, listed alphabetically by city within state. Plus, three easy-to-use, cross-referenced indexes put the facts at your fingertips faster and more easily than any other directory: Hospital Name Index, Bed Size Index and Personnel Index. *The Directory of Hospital Personnel* is the only complete source for key hospital decision-makers by name. Whether you want to define or restructure sales territories... locate hospitals with the purchasing power to accept your proposals... keep track of important contacts or colleagues... or find information on which insurance plans are accepted, *The Directory of Hospital Personnel* gives you the information you need – easily, efficiently, effectively and accurately.

"Recommended for college, university and medical libraries." -ARBA

Softcover ISBN 978-1-59237-402-1, 2,500 pages, $325.00 | Online Database: http://gold.greyhouse.com Call (800) 562-2139 for quote

The HMO/PPO Directory, 2009

The HMO/PPO Directory is a comprehensive source that provides detailed information about Health Maintenance Organizations and Preferred Provider Organizations nationwide. This comprehensive directory details more information about more managed health care organizations than ever before. Over 1,100 HMOs, PPOs, Medicare Advantage Plans and affiliated companies are listed, arranged alphabetically by state. Detailed listings include Key Contact Information, Prescription Drug Benefits, Enrollment, Geographical Areas served, Affiliated Physicians & Hospitals, Federal Qualifications, Status, Year Founded, Managed Care Partners, Employer References, Fees & Payment Information and more. Plus, five years of historical information is included related to Revenues, Net Income, Medical Loss Ratios, Membership Enrollment and Number of Patient Complaints. Five easy-to-use, cross-referenced indexes will put this vast array of information at your fingertips immediately: HMO Index, PPO Index, Other Providers Index, Personnel Index and Enrollment Index. *The HMO/PPO Directory* provides the most comprehensive data on the most companies available on the market place today.

"Helpful to individuals requesting certain HMO/PPO issues such as co-payment costs, subscription costs and patient complaints. Individuals concerned (or those with questions) about their insurance may find this text to be of use to them." -ARBA

Softcover ISBN 978-1-59237-369-7, 600 pages, $325.00 | Online Database: http://gold.greyhouse.com Call (800) 562-2139 for quote

Medical Device Register, 2009

The only one-stop resource of every medical supplier licensed to sell products in the US. This award-winning directory offers immediate access to over 13,000 companies - and more than 65,000 products – in two information-packed volumes. This comprehensive resource saves hours of time and trouble when searching for medical equipment and supplies and the manufacturers who provide them. Volume I: The Product Directory, provides essential information for purchasing or specifying medical supplies for every medical device, supply, and diagnostic available in the US. Listings provide FDA codes & Federal Procurement Eligibility, Contact information for every manufacturer of the product along with Prices and Product Specifications. Volume 2 - Supplier Profiles, offers the most complete and important data about Suppliers, Manufacturers and Distributors. Company Profiles detail the number of employees, ownership, method of distribution, sales volume, net income, key executives detailed contact information medical products the company supplies, plus the medical specialties they cover. Four indexes provide immediate access to this wealth of information: Keyword Index, Trade Name Index, Supplier Geographical Index and OEM (Original Equipment Manufacturer) Index. *Medical Device Register* is the only one-stop source for locating suppliers and products; looking for new manufacturers or hard-to-find medical devices; comparing products and companies; know who's selling what and who to buy from cost effectively. This directory has become the standard in its field and will be a welcome addition to the reference collection of any medical library, large public library, university library along with the collections that serve the medical community.

"A wealth of information on medical devices, medical device companies... and key personnel in the industry is provide in this comprehensive reference work... A valuable reference work, one of the best hardcopy compilations available." -Doody Publishing

Two Volumes, Hardcover ISBN 978-1-59237-373-4, 3,000 pages, $325.00

The Directory of Health Care Group Purchasing Organizations, 2008

This comprehensive directory provides the important data you need to get in touch with over 800 Group Purchasing Organizations. By providing in-depth information on this growing market and its members, *The Directory of Health Care Group Purchasing Organizations* fills a major need for the most accurate and comprehensive information on over 800 GPOs – Mailing Address, Phone & Fax Numbers, E-mail Addresses, Key Contacts, Purchasing Agents, Group Descriptions, Membership Categorization, Standard Vendor Proposal Requirements, Membership Fees & Terms, Expanded Services, Total Member Beds & Outpatient Visits represented and more. Five Indexes provide a number of ways to locate the right GPO: Alphabetical Index, Expanded Services Index, Organization Type Index, Geographic Index and Member Institution Index. With its comprehensive and detailed information on each purchasing organization, *The Directory of Health Care Group Purchasing Organizations* is the go-to source for anyone looking to target this market.

"The information is clearly arranged and easy to access...recommended for those needing this very specialized information." –ARBA

1,000 pages; Softcover ISBN 978-1-59237-287-4, $325.00 | Online Database: http://gold.greyhouse.com Call (800) 562-2139 for quote

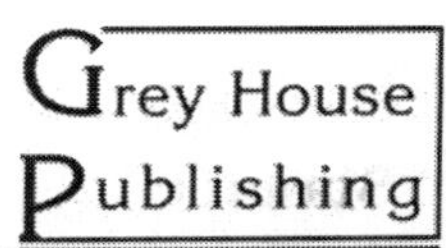

Canadian Almanac & Directory, 2009

The Canadian Almanac & Directory contains sixteen directories in one – giving you all the facts and figures you will ever need about Canada. No other single source provides users with the quality and depth of up-to-date information for all types of research. This national directory and guide gives you access to statistics, images and over 100,000 names and addresses for everything from Airlines to Zoos - updated every year. It's Ten Directories in One! Each section is a directory in itself, providing robust information on business and finance, communications, government, associations, arts and culture (museums, zoos, libraries, etc.), health, transportation, law, education, and more. Government information includes federal, provincial and territorial - and includes an easy-to-use quick index to find key information. A separate municipal government section includes every municipality in Canada, with full profiles of Canada's largest urban centers. A complete legal directory lists judges and judicial officials, court locations and law firms across the country. A wealth of general information, the *Canadian Almanac & Directory* also includes national statistics on population, employment, imports and exports, and more. National awards and honors are presented, along with forms of address, Commonwealth information and full color photos of Canadian symbols. Postal information, weights, measures, distances and other useful charts are also incorporated. Complete almanac information includes perpetual calendars, five-year holiday planners and astronomical information. Published continuously for 160 years, *The Canadian Almanac & Directory* is the best single reference source for business executives, managers and assistants; government and public affairs executives; lawyers; marketing, sales and advertising executives; researchers, editors and journalists.

Hardcover ISBN 978-1-59237-370-3, 1,600 pages, $325.00

Associations Canada, 2009

The Most Powerful Fact-Finder to Business, Trade, Professional and Consumer Organizations

Associations Canada covers Canadian organizations and international groups including industry, commercial and professional associations, registered charities, special interest and common interest organizations. This annually revised compendium provides detailed listings and abstracts for nearly 20,000 regional, national and international organizations. This popular volume provides the most comprehensive picture of Canada's non-profit sector. Detailed listings enable users to identify an organization's budget, founding date, scope of activity, licensing body, sources of funding, executive information, full address and complete contact information, just to name a few. Powerful indexes help researchers find information quickly and easily. The following indexes are included: subject, acronym, geographic, budget, executive name, conferences & conventions, mailing list, defunct and unreachable associations and registered charitable organizations. In addition to annual spending of over $1 billion on transportation and conventions alone, Canadian associations account for many millions more in pursuit of membership interests. *Associations Canada* provides complete access to this highly lucrative market. *Associations Canada* is a strong source of prospects for sales and marketing executives, tourism and convention officials, researchers, government officials - anyone who wants to locate non-profit interest groups and trade associations.

Hardcover ISBN 978-1-59237-401-4, 1,600 pages, $325.00

Financial Services Canada, 2009/10

Financial Services Canada is the only master file of current contacts and information that serves the needs of the entire financial services industry in Canada. With over 18,000 organizations and hard-to-find business information, Financial Services Canada is the most up-to-date source for names and contact numbers of industry professionals, senior executives, portfolio managers, financial advisors, agency bureaucrats and elected representatives. Financial Services Canada incorporates the latest changes in the industry to provide you with the most current details on each company, including: name, title, organization, telephone and fax numbers, e-mail and web addresses. *Financial Services Canada* also includes private company listings never before compiled, government agencies, association and consultant services - to ensure that you'll never miss a client or a contact. Current listings include: banks and branches, non-depository institutions, stock exchanges and brokers, investment management firms, insurance companies, major accounting and law firms, government agencies and financial associations. Powerful indexes assist researchers with locating the vital financial information they need. The following indexes are included: alphabetic, geographic, executive name, corporate web site/e-mail, government quick reference and subject. *Financial Services Canada* is a valuable resource for financial executives, bankers, financial planners, sales and marketing professionals, lawyers and chartered accountants, government officials, investment dealers, journalists, librarians and reference specialists.

Hardcover ISBN 978-1-59237-416-8, 900 pages, $325.00

Directory of Libraries in Canada, 2009/10

The Directory of Libraries in Canada brings together almost 7,000 listings including libraries and their branches, information resource centers, archives and library associations and learning centers. The directory offers complete and comprehensive information on Canadian libraries, resource centers, business information centers, professional associations, regional library systems, archives, library schools and library technical programs. *The Directory of Libraries in Canada* includes important features of each library and service, including library information; personnel details, including contact names and e-mail addresses; collection information; services available to users; acquisitions budgets; and computers and automated systems. Useful information on each library's electronic access is also included, such as Internet browser, connectivity and public Internet/CD-ROM/subscription database access. The directory also provides powerful indexes for subject, location, personal name and Web site/e-mail to assist researchers with locating the crucial information they need. *The Directory of Libraries in Canada* is a vital reference tool for publishers, advocacy groups, students, research institutions, computer hardware suppliers, and other diverse groups that provide products and services to this unique market.

Hardcover ISBN 978-1-59237-427-4, 850 pages, $325.00

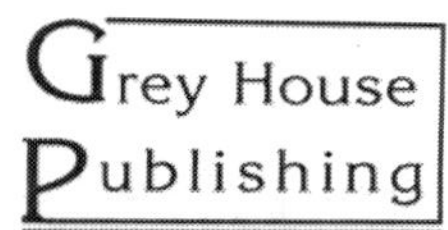

Canadian Environmental Directory, 2009

The Canadian Environmental Directory is Canada's most complete and only national listing of environmental associations and organizations, government regulators and purchasing groups, product and service companies, special libraries, and more! The extensive Products and Services section provides detailed listings enabling users to identify the company name, address, phone, fax, e-mail, Web address, firm type, contact names (and titles), product and service information, affiliations, trade information, branch and affiliate data. The Government section gives you all the contact information you need at every government level – federal, provincial and municipal. We also include descriptions of current environmental initiatives, programs and agreements, names of environment-related acts administered by each ministry or department PLUS information and tips on who to contact and how to sell to governments in Canada. The Associations section provides complete contact information and a brief description of activities. Included are Canadian environmental organizations and international groups including industry, commercial and professional associations, registered charities, special interest and common interest organizations. All the Information you need about the Canadian environmental industry: directory of products and services, special libraries and resource, conferences, seminars and tradeshows, chronology of environmental events, law firms and major Canadian companies, *The Canadian Environmental Directory* is ideal for business, government, engineers and anyone conducting research on the environment.

Softcover ISBN 978-1-59237-374-1, 900 pages, $325.00

Canadian Parliamentary Guide, 2009

An indispensable guide to government in Canada, the annual *Canadian Parliamentary Guide* provides information on both federal and provincial governments, courts, and their elected and appointed members. The Guide is completely bilingual, with each record appearing both in English and then in French. The Guide contains biographical sketches of members of the Governor General's Household, the Privy Council, members of Canadian legislatures (federal, including both the House of Commons and the Senate, provincial and territorial), members of the federal superior courts (Supreme, Federal, Federal Appeal, Court Martial Appeal and Tax Courts) and the senior staff for these institutions. Biographies cover personal data, political career, private career and contact information. In addition, the Guide provides descriptions of each of the institutions, including brief historical information in text and chart format and significant facts (i.e. number of members and their salaries). The Guide covers the results of all federal general elections and by-elections from Confederations to the present and the results of the most recent provincial elections. A complete name index rounds out the text, making information easy to find. No other resources presents a more up-to-date, more complete picture of Canadian government and her political leaders. A must-have resource for all Canadian reference collections.

Hardcover ISBN 978-1-59237-417-5, 800 pages, $184.00